AF335621

Advances in Experimental Medicine and Biology

Advances in Internal Medicine

Volume 956

More information about this series at http://www.springer.com/series/13780

Md. Shahidul Islam

Editor

Hypertension: from basic research to clinical practice

Volume 2

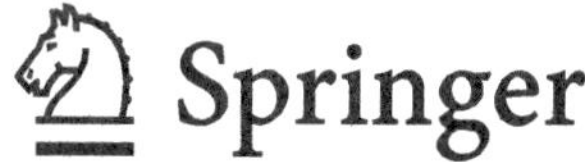 Springer

Editor
Md. Shahidul Islam
Karolinska Institutet
Department of Clinical Science and Education
  Södersjukhuset
Stockholm, Sweden

Department of Internal Medicine and Emergency Medicine
Uppsala University Hospital
Uppsala, Sweden

ISSN 0065-2598   ISSN 2214-8019   (electronic)
Advances in Experimental Medicine and Biology
ISSN 2367-0177   ISSN 2367-0185   (electronic)
Advances in Internal Medicine
ISBN 978-3-319-44250-1   ISBN 978-3-319-44251-8   (eBook)
DOI 10.1007/978-3-319-44251-8

Library of Congress Control Number: 2017940396

This Springer imprint is published by Springer Nature
The registered company is Springer International Publishing AG
The registered company address is: Gewerbestrasse 11, 6330 Cham, Switzerland

Contents

Adv Exp Med Biol - Advances in Internal Medicine (2017) 2: 1–2
DOI 10.1007/5584_2017_30
© Springer International Publishing AG 2016
Published online: 15 March 2017

Hypertension: From Basic Research to Clinical Practice

Md. Shahidul Islam

Keywords

Hypertension in high-income countries • Hypertension in middle-income countries • Hypertension in low-income countries • Hypertension in the world • Books on hypertension • Update on hypertension

Hypertension increases the risks of end-organ injury, maternal/fetal vulnerability, and total mortality. Throughout the world, it kills about 7.5 million people every year. During 1975–2015, the number of adults with hypertension increased from 594 million to more than 1.1 billion, mostly due to the increase in the low-income and middle-income countries (NCD Risk Factor Collaboration 2016, Lancet 15 Nov, 2016).

Blood pressure, even the so-called resting blood pressure, is inherently variable depending on innumerable factors. Doctors and nurses must follow the appropriate methods and procedures for measuring blood pressure. Blood pressure measured in the clinic, at home, or by ambulatory blood pressure monitoring yields different values that need careful interpretations.

At first sight, management of hypertension is fairly straightforward. In reality, this can sometimes be frustrating both for the doctors and for the patients. Many patients with hypertension remain undiagnosed for years; many others are wrongly diagnosed and unnecessarily treated for decades. Many people receiving tablets for hypertension are not adequately treated due to poor compliance, side effects of medicines, or inappropriate choice of medicines by the physicians. Compliance of patients must be assessed and improved by keeping treatment regimens simple, by involving the patients in the decision-making process, and above all without blaming the patients for poor compliance.

When it comes to target blood pressure, one size does not fit all. It seems the goals need to be personalized depending on many factors like the risks of cardiovascular diseases, albuminuria, age, sex, diabetes, orthostatism, and gestational age. For instance, blood pressure reduction in the elderly hypertensive patients reduces morbidity and mortality but needs to be done carefully taking into consideration the increased sensitivity of this group of patients to side effects.

M.S. Islam (✉)
Department of Clinical Science and Education, Södersjukhuset. Karolinska Institutet. Research Center, 3rd floor, S-118 83 Stockholm, Sweden

Department of Emergency Care and Internal Medicine, Uppsala University Hospital, Uppsala, Sweden
e-mail: Shahidul.Islam@ki.se

About 10% of hypertensive patients have resistant hypertension. About 20% of these patients have primary hyperaldosteronism. Others may have renal artery stenosis, obstructive sleep apnea syndrome, chronic kidney disease, Liddle syndrome, pheochromocytoma and paraganglioma, and glucocorticoid excess. Evaluate hypertension due to suspected primary mineralocorticoid excess states using some algorithm that includes functional, imaging, and genetic tests, in consultation with the endocrinologists. Treat the conditions depending on the diagnosis; for instance, treat Liddle syndrome with amiloride. Investigate for rare conditions like pheochromocytomas and paragangliomas, when clinically suspected. You need to be familiar with the perioperative, operative, and postoperative management of these patients. When you suspect an endocrine hypertension, do the preliminary tests, and then if your clinical suspicion is supported by the tests, refer the patient to an endocrinologist.

Management of hypertension in some patient groups merits special considerations. These include elderly patients with hypertension, hypertension in pregnancy, transplant patients with hypertension, and hypertension in patient on hemodialysis.

In pregnancy, you need to distinguish between chronic hypertension, chronic hypertension with superimposed preeclampsia, gestational hypertension, and preeclampsia/eclampsia. It is important to discontinue medicines with known fetal adverse effects, e.g., angiotensin-converting enzyme inhibitors, angiotensin receptor blockers, mineralocorticoid receptor blockers, and statins before conception. The exact blood pressure target for treatment of chronic hypertension in pregnancy is not known, but it has been shown that less tight control of chronic hypertension in pregnancy does not result in poorer maternal or fetal outcome. Use drugs like labetalol, nifedipine, thiazide diuretics, and clonidine that are safe in pregnancy.

Extensive basic researches are revealing fascinating pathophysiological mechanisms of hypertension and are identifying potential molecular targets for developing new drugs. These include the toll-like receptors and damage-associated molecular patterns (DAMPs), asymmetric dimethylarginine (ADMA), interleukin-17α, interleukin-6, interferon-γ, endothelin-1 receptors, and aminopeptidase A that converts angiotensin II to angiotensin III, to name only a few. Metabolomic, lipidomic, pharmacometabolomic, candidate gene polymorphism, and genome-wide association (GWAS) studies are being used to obtain insights into the pathophysiological processes leading to hypertension.

It is important to keep up to date, but it is becoming increasingly difficult, even for the experts. *Hypertension: From Basic Research to Clinical Practice* includes a wide range of articles on selected issues that are important for the beginners as well as the experts engaged in research and clinical practice in the field of hypertension.

Reference

NCD Risk Factor Collaboration (NCD-RisC). Worldwide trends in blood pressure from 1975 to 2015: a pooled analysis of 1479 population-based measurement studies with 19.1 million participants. Lancet 2017; 389:35–55

Adv Exp Med Biol - Advances in Internal Medicine (2017) 2: 3–19
DOI 10.1007/5584_2016_83
© Springer International Publishing AG 2016
Published online: 9 October 2016

Understanding Blood Pressure Variation and Variability: Biological Importance and Clinical Significance

Gary D. James

Abstract

Variability is a normative property of blood pressure necessary for survival which likely contributes to morbidity and mortality through allostatic load. Because of its allostatic and adaptive properties blood pressure responses to peculiar situations like the visit to the clinic can lead to the misdiagnosis of hypertension. Cuff methods of blood pressure measurement can also create blood pressure variation when there really is none. There are also physiological differences between populations related to their evolutionary history that likely further affect the extent of population differences in 24-h blood pressure variability. Quantifying the sources and extent of blood pressure variability can be done using natural experimental models and through the evaluation of ecological momentary data. It is very likely that the results of population studies of blood pressure variability and morbidity and mortality risk are inconclusive because the parameters used to assess blood pressure variability do not reflect the actual nature of blood pressure allostasis.

Keywords

Blood pressure variability • Allostasis • Allostatic load

1   Introduction

In 1988, Peter Sterling and Joseph Eyre (1988) introduced the physiological concept of allostasis, which literally means "stability through change" to describe the behavior of

G.D. James (✉)
Department of Anthropology, Binghamton University, 13902 Binghamton, NY, USA
e-mail: gdjames@binghamton.edu

dynamic physiological functions. The idea is that variation in physiological parameters occurs as a means of adaptation, so that there is a nexus between external conditions and the body's ability to meet the demands imposed by them which is all regulated by the brain. Thus, there is no "dynamic steady state" or setpoint in these functions meaning that they do not maintain homeostasis, but rather there is a multitude of stable states that occur as responses to continuously changing environmental demands. In introducing this concept, Sterling and Eyre used blood pressure as an exemplar, because of its inherent variability. In fact, variation is what gives blood pressure its adaptive value (James 1991, 2013), and is perhaps its single most important normative property, since without it human beings would not survive (James 2013).

The inherent variability in blood pressure was first recognized by Stephen Hales in his pioneering experiments in the horse that were reported in 1733, in which he endeavored to evaluate the nature of the arterial pulse using a cannula inserted into the crural artery (O'Rourke 1990; Pickering 1991). The oscillations he observed in the blood pulses where such that he concluded that any instantaneous measure of the blood pressure would never be exactly the same over the lifetime of the animal (Parati et al. 1992). Through the nineteenth century anecdotal evidence regarding blood pressure variation in humans accumulated, and in 1897 Riva-Rocci in his description of sphygmomanometry reported that the actual procedure of making a blood pressure measurement could induce an increase in pressure so large as to affect the process of obtaining valid data (Parati et al. 1992). Seen from the perspective of allostasis, what this observation meant is that the mere occluding of the artery is enough of a stressor to initiate a physiological response which will change blood pressure.

Nikolai Korotkoff, a field surgeon during the Russo-Japanese war discovered the auscultatory technique of blood pressure measurement using the sphygommanometric method of Riva-Rocci and a stethoscope, reporting on the sounds that bear his name to the Imperial Military Medical Academy in St. Petersburg, Russia in 1905 (Paskalev et al. 2005). Since the sounds could be coupled to the cuff pressure registered on the mercury column of the sphygmomanometer, numeric values could be assigned to both the blood pulse maxima and minima (systole and diastole) based upon the appearance and disappearance of sound. With this important insight, blood pressure level, as well as variation over time could be quantified.

Through the first half of the twentieth century, a variety of observations regarding blood pressure variation using auscultatory and intra-arterial techniques both outside and inside the clinic were made. First, numerous laboratory studies demonstrated that typically occurring variation in physiological habitus and the environment such as postural change, respiration, exercise, and external temperature all profoundly affected the variability of blood pressure (e.g. James 1991; Pickering 1991; Rowell 1986). There were also studies indicating that there was substantial variability in "resting blood pressure" by venue and over time. One of particular note was the report by Ayman and Goldshine (1940) who trained hypertensive patients or their family members in how to take blood pressures at home. They found that these measurements differed from clinic measurements by as much as 70/36 mmHg, a difference which persisted over 6 months. Other studies around that time suggested that the emotional or psychological state of the person could affect the reliability of resting ausculted blood pressure measurements (e.g. Levy et al. 1944; Rogers and Palmer 1944), and there were also data to suggest that variation in a person's pressure could be influenced by the familiarity between the patient and the person taking the pressure (Shapiro et al. 1954) as well as the gender of the person taking the pressure (Comstock 1957). During this time, the variation in resting blood pressure in and out of the office that was related to the patient's response to the procedure or circumstances (which from an allostatic perspective is an adaptive adjustment to the perceived stressfulness of the situation) was seen medically as something that confounded accurate clinical assessment and thus needed to be minimalized.

In the 1960s there was an increasing number of studies examining blood pressure variability outside the laboratory and clinic. These studies emerged with the technical development of the Remler® ambulatory blood pressure recorder which required that subjects manually inflate the cuff (see Hinman et al. 1962; Kain et al. 1964; Sokolow et al. 1966), and with the development of intra-arterial devices that measured pressure continuously (Richardson et al. 1964). A classic study by Bevan et al. (1969) employing an intra-arterial device provided data that showed just how variable blood pressure could be over the course of a typical day. This case study and others like it unambiguously showed that blood pressure levels were tied directly to what someone was feeling and doing as well as the circumstances. These data clearly indicated that blood pressure did not maintain a homeostatic "steady state" but rather allostatically changed to meet the demands of the circumstance.

As ambulatory blood pressure monitoring technology improved from the 1970' through the 2000s, the effects of various typical behaviors on blood pressures were evaluated, first using intra-arterial devices and later using automatic ambulatory blood pressure monitors that employed either auscultatory or oscillometric technology (James 2013; Pickering 1991). These studies, often undertaken by non-medical researchers, were designed to quantify the amount of intraindividual blood pressure variation over the course of a day associated with psychological, sociological, and environmental sources using data from larger scale population samples. Their purpose was to evaluate how the things that people do, think and experience as part of their lifestyle relate to the development of sustained high blood pressure and subsequent cardiovascular pathology (James 2013). The upshot of the results of these studies is that the extent of out of office blood pressure variation and its relation to pathology may not only be determined by both the mix and psychological appraisal of the activities and relationships that are experienced by a subject during the course of a day, but also by the duration and frequency of the experience of these factors over a lifetime (James 2007, 2013).

Over the past decade, there has been interest in evaluating the morbidity and mortality risk of circadian, diurnal or nocturnal blood pressure variation and the question has been raised as to whether variability should be treated (Asayama et al. 2015; Flores 2013; Palatini et al. 2014; Parati et al. 2015). The purpose of this brief overview is to critically examine blood pressure variability and variation both within and outside the office, separating its adaptive function from possible pathology using the perspective of the allostasis paradigm.

2 Are There Multiple Intrinsic Biological Rhythms That Contribute to Blood Pressure Variability?

From an allostatic perspective, all the measurable variation in blood pressure is related to beat-to-beat changes in the actions of the heart which in turn, are triggered by the actions of the brain (Sterling 2004). There are factors that acutely (very short time frame) influence the pulse wave of blood as it is ejected from the heart, such as respiration (Pickering 1991). Other than the acute metabolically interactive processes that are related to the maintenance of life (e.g. the need for tissue oxygen exchange and the release of carbon dioxide and other metabolic byproducts through exhaling), all other blood pressure variation occurs to adapt people to their circumstance, largely through the effects of numerous humoral and hormonal inputs that are regulated by the brain's response to external and internal stimuli (Sterling 2004).

Circadian blood pressure variation, most notably that related to the biobehavioral changes from waking to sleep reflect adaptive responses to habitual activity and postural variation associated with everyday life processes and sleep (James 2013; James et al. 2015). Other potential rhythms such as seasonal variation (Parati et al. 1992; Pickering 1991) likely arise from beat to beat adjustments to ambient temperature (transitions from heat to cold) and the various seasonal behavioral and social changes that are tied to culturally relevant seasonal traditions (James 1991, 2013; James and Baker 1995; James et al. 1990b).

Since blood pressure change is an adaptive process, changes in seated clinic auscultatory blood pressures over longer time frames such as monthly or yearly, must reflect either (1) changed social or psychological conditions experienced by the patient that are influencing the patients perceptions of the circumstance in the clinic; (2) changes in the underlying cardiovascular structure so that the system that is generating the pressure is itself changed or changing; or (3) perhaps both (Gerin and James 2010; Jhalani et al. 2005; Kleinert et al. 1984; Pickering 1991).

There is also a difference in evaluating blood pressure variability from invasive beat-to-beat assessments (based on continuous intraarterial or plethysmographic measurements) and non-invasive techniques, where a cuff occlusion method is employed and systolic and diastolic pressures are determined over a 20–30 s time frame using the appearance and disappearance of audible sound, high frequency signal components, or by examining a reflective waveform generated inside the blood pressure cuff (Pickering and Blank 1995) (see Fig. 1). In evaluating beat to beat pulse tracings, the diastolic (nadir) and systolic (zenith) pressures of the pulse are directly connected and influence one another whereas auscultatory or oscillometric systolic and diastolic pressures are estimates not tied to a particular pulse. Beat-to beat systolic and diastolic measurements will change in tandem with externally driven stimuli, however, the time it takes for the bladder-cuff assembly to deflate and re-establish blood flow is long enough to miss the effects of hormonal inputs as they happen, so that the factors affecting systolic pressure may be different than those affecting diastolic pressure (Blank et al. 1995). This difference will give a false impression of the amplitude of the blood pulse, possibly creating variation where there really is none. This variation is an artifact of the measurement technique.

In addition to the time frame issue that affects the variation of pulse pressure, added variability

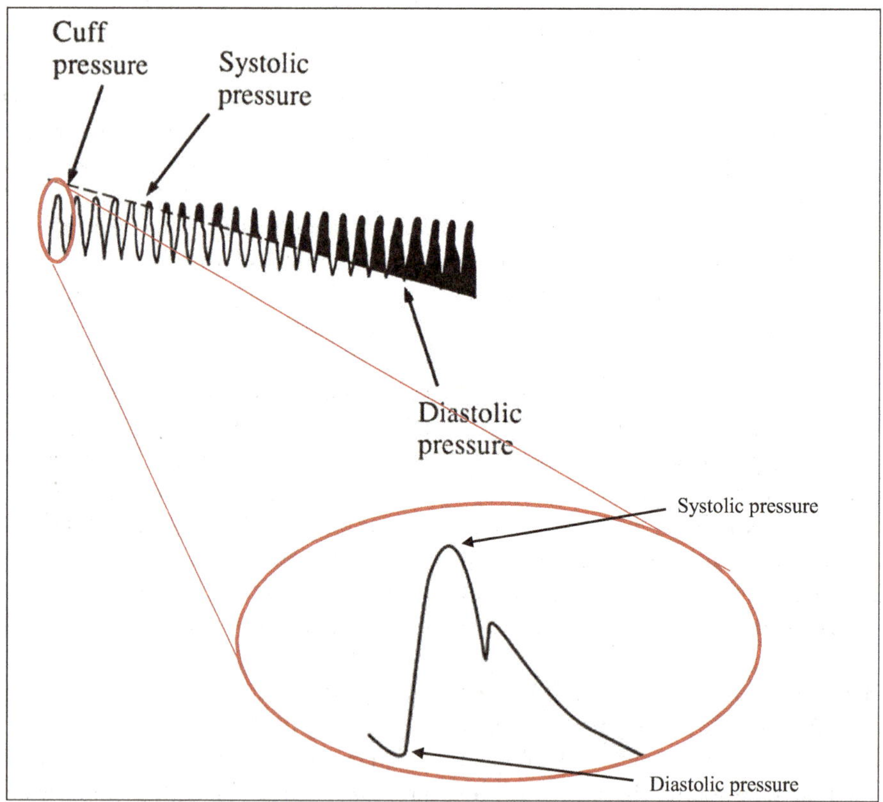

Fig. 1 Differences between the recorded systolic and diastolic pressures from intraarterial or plethysmographic measurements (depicted in the *circular insert*) and a cuff measured pressure where systolic and diastolic pressure are tied to the Korotkoff phase I and phase V sounds

can be created using cuff-based measurement methods by simply changing the position of the cuff relative to the heart when cuff deflation occurs (Pickering 1991; James et al. 2015). For example, blood pressure during sleep can appear to be quite variable, but that variation may be due to simple factors such as changes in sleep position, so that depending upon whether the pressure is taken while a subject is on their left or right side, or on their back or stomach, it can appear to change by 15 mmHg or more (James et al. 2015). Cuff position could also increase waking pressure variation during an ambulatory monitoring as well, also depending upon the position of the arm during cuff deflation (Pickering 1991).

So, are there different types of blood pressure variability that need to be considered clinically? It seems unlikely, because if blood pressure change is adaptive, meaning it changes to meet the circumstance, then all blood pressure variability must be beat-to-beat and what gives the impression of shorter and longer term variation patterns is the general patterning of life experiences, momentary reactions, and the intermittency of clinic or ambulatory measurements.

3 White Coat Hypertension, Masked Hypertension and the Life Experience of Visiting the Clinic

Seen from the perspective of the patient, going to the doctor is an event! The environment of the clinic, office, or hospital is uniquely different from every other place that the patient goes. Allostatically, a blood pressure taken during the event (being in the clinic) will reflect the patient's adaptive response to it. As Riva-Rocci noted (see above), arterial occlusion is enough of a stimulus to initiate an increase in blood pressure, but because the taking of a blood pressure is also an entirely unique social interaction involving a physician, nurse, or other medical professional and the patient, there will also be effects related to the perceptions of the patient connected to that interaction. Even if the pressure

is taken by an automatic device with no one present, that situation still requires an adaptive response from the patient. When the blood pressure response to this peculiar environment exceeds the average response to all other daily environments, the patient is said to exhibit a white coat effect, but if that effect leads to ausculted blood pressure measurements that exceed 140/90 (hypertension Rubicon) the patient is diagnosed with white coat hypertension. Whether blood pressure responds with an acute heightened response in the clinic may largely depend on prior patient experiences with the setting and prior relationships with the people within it.

That a blood pressure measurement can be profoundly influenced by the perceptions of the patient was dramatically demonstrated by Mancia and colleagues (1987) in their classic study in which blood pressure readings were continuously taken intra-arterially on one arm while a nurse or physician took an ausculted blood pressure from the other. The intra-arterial measurements showed that relative to the pressure prior to the ausculted measurement interaction with the physician, there was an increase of some 23/18 mmHg when the physician took the ausculted pressure. Further, the increase in pressure by the physician was about twice the effect seen when a nurse took the pressure.

What did the patient perceive that lead to the increase in pressure? A more recent study by Jhalani et al. (2005) provides some answers. They examined the acute effects of anxiety and expectancy on clinic measured pressures and found that when assessed as a specific office related effect, anxiety had a substantial influence on increasing pressure in the office. In their study, they measured anxiety before, during, and after blood pressure was measured. They also showed that there is an effect related to the patients' expectations about what their blood pressure measurement will be. Their findings suggest that prior experience can trigger anxiety regarding this peculiar environment and the relationships within it, so that the blood pressure response is elevated. These psychological factors will lead to a diagnosis of hypertension if the ausculted numbers exceed 140/90.

Masked hypertension is defined by the precise opposite effect seen with white coat hypertension. Specifically in these patients, adaptation to the peculiar clinical environment requires less of a response than an average of the responses to all other events outside the clinic. Rather than being made anxious, they may be calmed by the setting and interpersonal interactions. Interestingly, masked hypertension is seen not so much a relaxed adaptation as it is an absence of high risk behaviors which elevate pressure outside the clinic such as alcohol consumption, smoking, or contraceptive use (see Longo et al. 2005 for example).

Studies have been done which have evaluated the morbidity and mortality risk associated with the diagnosed conditions of white coat and masked hypertension which are defined from the average blood pressure in the clinic and the average blood pressure response to all other conditions during the day (e.g. everything not in the clinic). Pierdomenico and Cuccurullo (2011) did a metaanalysis comparing the risk for cardiac and cerebral events among patients who were diagnosed as normotensive, white coat hypertensive, masked hypertensive and essential hypertensive based on the out of clinic-inside clinic blood pressure difference and found that white coat and normotensive patients had similar risk as did the masked hypertensives and essential hypertensives. This kind of finding suggests that inside clinic-outside clinic variation may not be important to cardiovascular health, and that in fact, the determination of who really has hypertension should be made from average pressure experienced across many different situations and not from the peculiar setting of the clinic or office.

4 Ambulatory Blood Pressure Variability as a Risk Factor

Given that blood pressure is a response to ambient conditions, it would stand to reason that an evaluation of the relationship between its circadian variation and morbidity or mortality would necessarily involve assessing the appropriateness of the pressure responses to the various external

and internal conditions that drive the continuous changes (see Zanstra and Johnston 2011 for example). However, virtually every study that examines blood pressure variation as a risk factor for cardiac or cerebral events ignores the dynamic interplay between blood pressure and the specific environmental demands an individual confronts during daily life. Instead, studies of blood pressure variation and vascular risk focus on the event predictability of some measure of the statistical dispersion or cumulative differences of the sample of blood pressures taken with a non-invasive ambulatory blood pressure monitor over the course of one 24-h period (a day) or the average waking-sleep blood pressure transitions (either "dipping"-the difference between average waking pressure and average sleep pressure, or the "morning surge"-the difference between various pressures prior to and just after morning awakening), (see for example Asayama et al. 2015; Hansen et al. 2010; Palatini et al. 2014; Parati et al. 2015; Taylor et al. 2015). These measures are examined only with regard to a possible linear relationship; that is, the studies only address the question of whether risk is related to being too low or too high on the various parameter scales. The inconsistent results from these studies, where some suggest variability is an important risk factor and others find little or no effect has spurred a controversy as to whether blood pressure variation should be a target for treatment (e.g. Asayama et al. 2015). Before this type of issue can be addressed, it is useful to examine what each indicator of the variability, or variation in these risk related studies is measuring. Are the indexes and parameters that are employed in these studies suitable and meaningful indicators of blood pressure variability?

Standard deviations (SD) or coefficients of variation (CV) are measures of the dispersion around a mean of a variable that is normally distributed. These are calculated from presumably random samples of a population of measurements. However, if the distribution of the overall population is not normal and the sampling is unrepresentative and small, these measures will be biased, inaccurate, and uninformative (Cochran 1977). Given that 100,000 or more systolic and diastolic pressures are generated over a 24-h period, and non-invasive ambulatory monitors sample perhaps 50 of those (5/100ths of 1 % of all those generated) which vary with time and conditions in a systematic way (pressures change to adapt the person to continuously changing circumstances) what is the value of the SD or CV of that sample in predicting risk? Parati et al. (1992) some 25 years ago noted that these kinds of measures don't tell you anything about how single values, as collected, are distributed around the mean. Do the pressures spread out or is there perhaps a bimodal shape? Many odd distributions could provide the same calculated SD or CV. These measures do not provide any information about the pattern and extent of individual pressure responses, and because as noted above, what needs to be evaluated in an assessment of how variability affects pathology is the appropriateness of the variation, they really are unsuitable variability indicators for examining morbidity and mortality risk.

Furthermore, the SD and CV as indicators of 24-h blood pressure variation are poorly reproducible over 24-h (see for example, James et al. 1990a; and the review by Asayama et al. 2015). In our study, we compared 24-h variability in normotensive and hypertensive patients over 2 weeks. Figure 3 shows the timing and spacing of each measurement on each day for both groups of subjects. Note how different the days are. This disparity is actually typical when comparing daily non-invasive ambulatory monitoring data. What we found is that people did different things on different days, and while there were enough pressures to provide a reasonably stable average over time, the varying mix of conditions and times when pressures were taken, were poorly matched day to day. This mismatch profoundly affected the distribution of the pressures around the mean, rendering the distributionally tied measures of variation (SD, CV) irreproducible (James et al. 1990a).

The "average real variability" (ARV24) has also been used as an indicator of blood pressure variability and is defined as the mean of the absolute differences of consecutive non-invasive ambulatory measurements. The effects of this parameter on the predictability of events are small or inconclusive (e.g. Asayama et al. 2015; Hansen et al. 2010). Bearing in mind that each of the sequential blood pressures taken by non-invasive ambulatory monitors are a response to the ambient condition in which they are taken, the ARV24 can go up or down depending upon what the person confronts and is doing during the day. What this quantity really represents is a summary score of the differences between peak blood pressure responses to some indeterminate number of sequential unknown stressors. Ultimately, the magnitude of this parameter depends solely upon the variability of the environments experienced and the behavior/emotional responses of the patient (James 1991, 2013). Thus, a patient who is monitored on a day where they are inactive, remain at home and are emotionally stable will have low ARV24, whereas one that performs multiple varying tasks, transitions through many daily microenvironments (goes to work, out to dinner, etc.) and experiences an array of emotions will have a high ARV24. Since the blood pressure changes are adaptive and are a normative response to the tribulations of everyday life, it is not clear from the studies that have used this parameter why high (or low) values of ARV24 would be indicative of pathology or health.

The other variation measures used in risk studies are "dipping" and the "morning surge." These are measures of blood pressure change between the state of waking and the state of sleep. Conceptually, dipping refers to the blood pressure transition from waking to sleep, whereas the morning surge refers to the transition from sleep to waking. Operationally, there is no consistent definition for either measure across studies, although with dipping, a Rubicon of 10 % decline, particularly for systolic pressure seems to be the popular demarcation line for normalcy and pathology, although there is no definitive reason why this value is the clinically relevant cut-point (Asayama et al. 2015; Flores 2013; Taylor et al. 2015). Again, seeing blood pressure as an adaptive response, the waking average that is used to determine dipping is based on a mean of values that are tied to the conditions experienced on the day of study. So depending upon whether a person had a difficult day or an easy day, the waking average could be higher or lower. There are ample data showing that excessive psychological stress during the day can also carry over and increase sleep pressure (see James et al. 1989 for example), so non-dipping may occur on a given night simply because it was a stressful waking day. Another problem with the concept of dipping is that it assumes that all people experience just the two distinctive periods (waking and sleep) over the day, so that "waking" and "sleep" happen during the day and night. This presumption is demonstrably false as there are plentiful data showing that waking-sleep patterns can change with age and that this affects the circadian patterns of adaptive blood pressure responses in ways that confound the determination of dippers and non-dippers (see Ice et al. 2003). Likewise, whatever pressure(s) chosen to define the post- awakening point and the low pre-awakening point in defining the morning surge are also adaptive responses to the conditions when they are measured, so that its relative magnitude may be related to any number of factors affecting both sets of measurements. And, as previously noted, there are also other issues with "sleep" pressures taken by a cuff occlusion method that have to do with the position of the cuff relative to the heart that will influence the level and variability of "sleep" blood pressures (James et al. 2015).

It is not surprising that waking-sleep transition measures are often found to have poor reproducibility as well as differential effects in different populations (Asayama et al. 2015; Taylor et al. 2015). Patterns of behavior, stress, and sleep quality vary from day to day, and all these are factors that may be influenced by the cultural background and occupation of the patient (James 2007). While there may be theoretical reasons to believe that the variability in blood pressure associated with wakefulness and sleep ought to have health implications, the operationalization of the concepts using non-invasive ambulatory measurements are inadequate because they don't embrace the adaptive nature of blood pressure which makes it impossible to define what normative transitions ought to be. Without a clear definition of normalcy, there

is no way to coherently use these measures for treatment purposes (Flores 2013).

So, after evaluating the nature of the parameters that have been employed to assess the morbidity and mortality risk of blood pressure variability in large international and community based populations, it appears that none of them are meaningful indicators of what is or is not appropriate variability, and therefore can't really address the question of whether blood pressure variability ought to be treated.

5 Ambulatory Blood Pressure Variation: How Do You Measure It?

To understand why blood pressure varies during the day, you need to have information regarding the ambient conditions when measurements are made. If blood pressure is responding to these conditions during everyday life, you need to be able to show that as they change, so does blood pressure.

Several means have been used to classify the conditions of ambulatory blood pressure measurements. While direct observation of subjects wearing the monitor has been used (e.g. Ice et al. 2003), for most studies of blood pressure variation, subjects have self-reported the ambient conditions of each blood pressure measurement in a diary, which have taken on a variety of forms, from pencil and paper to hand held computers as has been discussed (see James 2007, 2013). Most behavioral studies of blood pressure variation have not been conducted with a focus toward allostasis, or even understanding cardiovascular adaptation. Rather, studies have simply defined the sources of diurnal blood pressure variation, or evaluated whether people with specific characteristics differ in their responses to similar lifestyle related stimuli (Gerin and James 2010; James 2013).

Studies designed to evaluate what affects blood pressure variation and by how much have generally taken two forms. As has been noted (James 2007, 2013), the first approach is one where each blood pressure measurement is assessed with regard to simultaneously recorded circumstances reported in a diary (often called ecological momentary data) using inferential statistical models (see for example Brondolo et al. 1999; Gump et al. 2001; James et al. 1986; Kamarck et al. 2002; Kamarck et al. 1998; Schwartz et al. 1994). In this analysis, the sources of blood pressure variation are separated based on the reported diary entries (such as the posture of the subject, the location of the subject, etc.). The proportion of variation associated with each is quantified, as is the number of mmHg the alternative levels of each (such as posture-standing, sitting, reclining) contribute to either increasing or decreasing the values of individual blood pressure measurements. In evaluating blood pressure variation this way, the choice of diary reporting alternatives is critical. The potential sources of variation chosen to have reported in the diary and how they get recorded will dictate how the variation in blood pressure gets analyzed (James 2007, 2013). Analysis of ecological momentary blood pressure data has been undertaken using raw (e.g. Brondolo et al. 1999; Kamarck et al. 2003; Schwartz et al. 1994) and standardized e.g. (Brown et al. 1998; Ice et al. 2003; James et al. 1986) data. The estimated effect sizes from different studies using these approaches vary considerably, due in part to the fact that there is no consensus as to what ought to be the standard value against which sources of variation should be measured, but also because of the demographic and cultural diversity of the groups studied (James 2007, 2013).

The second form employs what might be termed a "natural experiment" which has been discussed at length elsewhere (see James 1991, 2007, 2013). However in brief, natural experiments are studies in which there are a priori design elements that define predictable dynamically changing behaviors or situations that occur during a typical day (James 2013). This kind of study is done by anthropologists and human population biologists, and it is an approach that has its roots in psychological and psychophysiological paradigms in which blood pressure reactivity to various stressful tasks are evaluated in the laboratory, (see for example, Pickering and Gerin 1990; Linden et al. 2003;

Kamarck et al. 2003). In these laboratory experiments, a baseline condition is established and then the subject undertakes a series of predefined tasks that will elicit a response. The difference between the baseline measurements and those during the tasks define the magnitude of blood pressure reactivity (James 2013). Because they are conducted in a laboratory, there are controls in the experiment such that specific effects can be isolated, measurements can be taken in a systematic way, and all the participants experience the same protocol. Control groups can also be included in the experiment. Moving this experimental paradigm to a "natural" setting (e.g. into real life and outside the laboratory) requires modification because no true baseline can be established. But, a "natural experiment" can be designed where blood pressure changes can be evaluated as people move from situation to situation (such as their work and home situations) during the course of their everyday lives. For example, a person who lives in a suburb and commutes to an urban workplace every day likely has a structured, urban work environment where economic related activities occur, where social interactions take place with non-relative co-workers, and where a specific occupational hierarchy dictates the nature of social relationships (James 2013). The characteristics of this situation diverge sharply with that of the suburban home, where domestic tasks and leisure activity happen in a social context where interactions are with relatives and neighbors (James 2013). The variation in blood pressure required to adapt to these relatively predictable situations can be assessed by comparing the average blood pressure while in them with that during overnight sleep, or more specifically, while the person is quietly recumbent in a dark room acting as a pseudo-baseline.

In assessing blood pressure variability, it is important to realize that the blood pressure distributional parameters that come from an array of measurements will be related since they are determined from a single vascular system that has specific structural and functional properties. That is, the mean and variance of the population of pressures measured over the course of 24-h on the same person will be related. This is called heteroscadasticity and it is well known (Pickering 1991). Thus, people with lower 24 h average blood pressure will tend to have a narrower range of blood pressures diurnally than those with higher average pressures. Pickering (1991) has noted that this heteroscadasticity is probably related to underlying arterial structural differences such as stiffness and/or other functional factors such as differences in vasoactive hormone receptor density or sensitivity (see for example, van Berge-Landry and James (2008).

Over the past 30 years numerous studies have been conducted that have identified various psychological, social and behavioral parameters that are associated with increased ambulatory blood pressure variation. These effects have been summarized in a number of reviews (see for example, Gerin and James 2010; James 2007,

2013; Zanstra and Johnston 2011). In brief, mood variation, postural variation, situational variation, and activity variation all contribute significantly to diurnal blood pressure variation. These effects are further modified by seasonal (temperature) effects, dietary effects (e.g. sodium intake), alcohol consumption, smoking, specific social interactions (such as with spouses) and among employed people, the appraisal of job strain (Gerin and James 2010; James 2013; Zanstra and Johnston 2011). Any given effect can be small, but a blood pressure measurement is a response to all that are relevant when the measurement occurs, so that the impact of each of the factors is additive and can lead to substantial circadian blood pressure variation. An example of how this variation is additive is shown in Fig. 2.

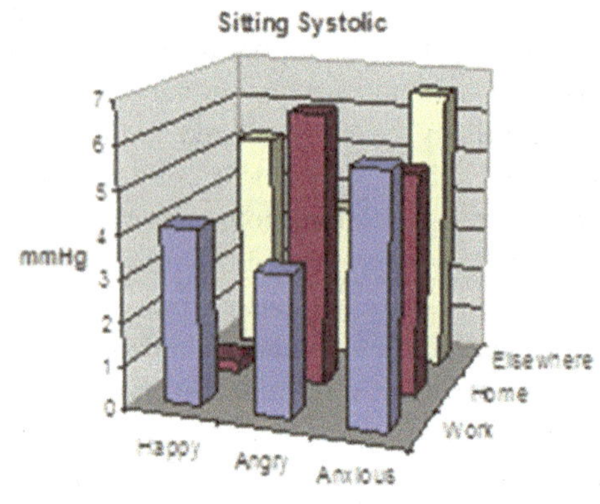

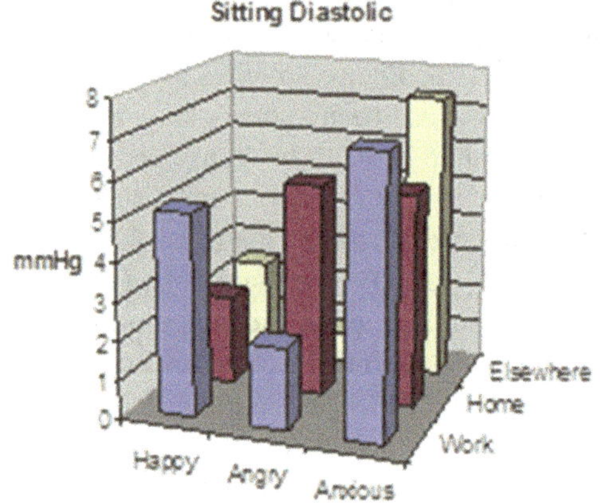

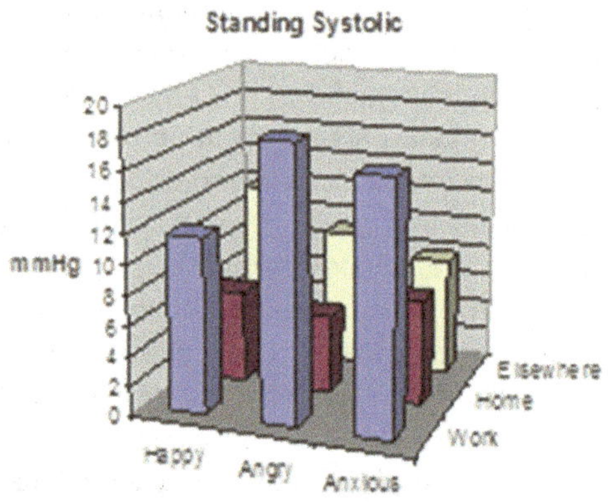

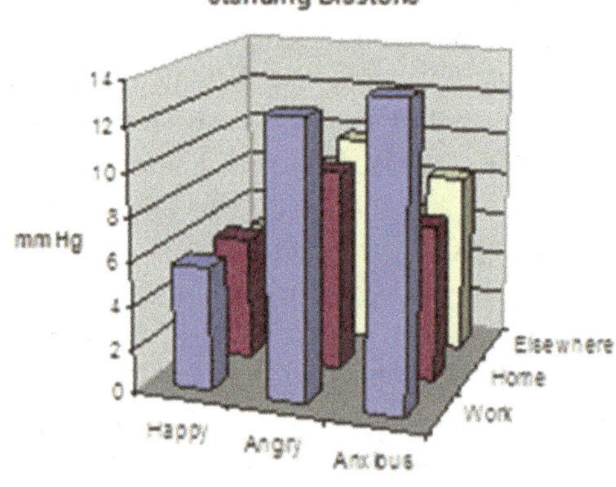

Fig. 2 The amount of diurnal blood pressure variation associated with variation in posture (sitting, standing), situation (work, home, and elsewhere) and reported emotional state (happy, angry, anxious) on daily blood pressure (Data from James et al. 1988). The variation is defined as mmHg from the 24-h mean, and is based on the assumption that the measure of dispersion around the 24-h mean (standard deviation) is 10 (Modified from James 2013)

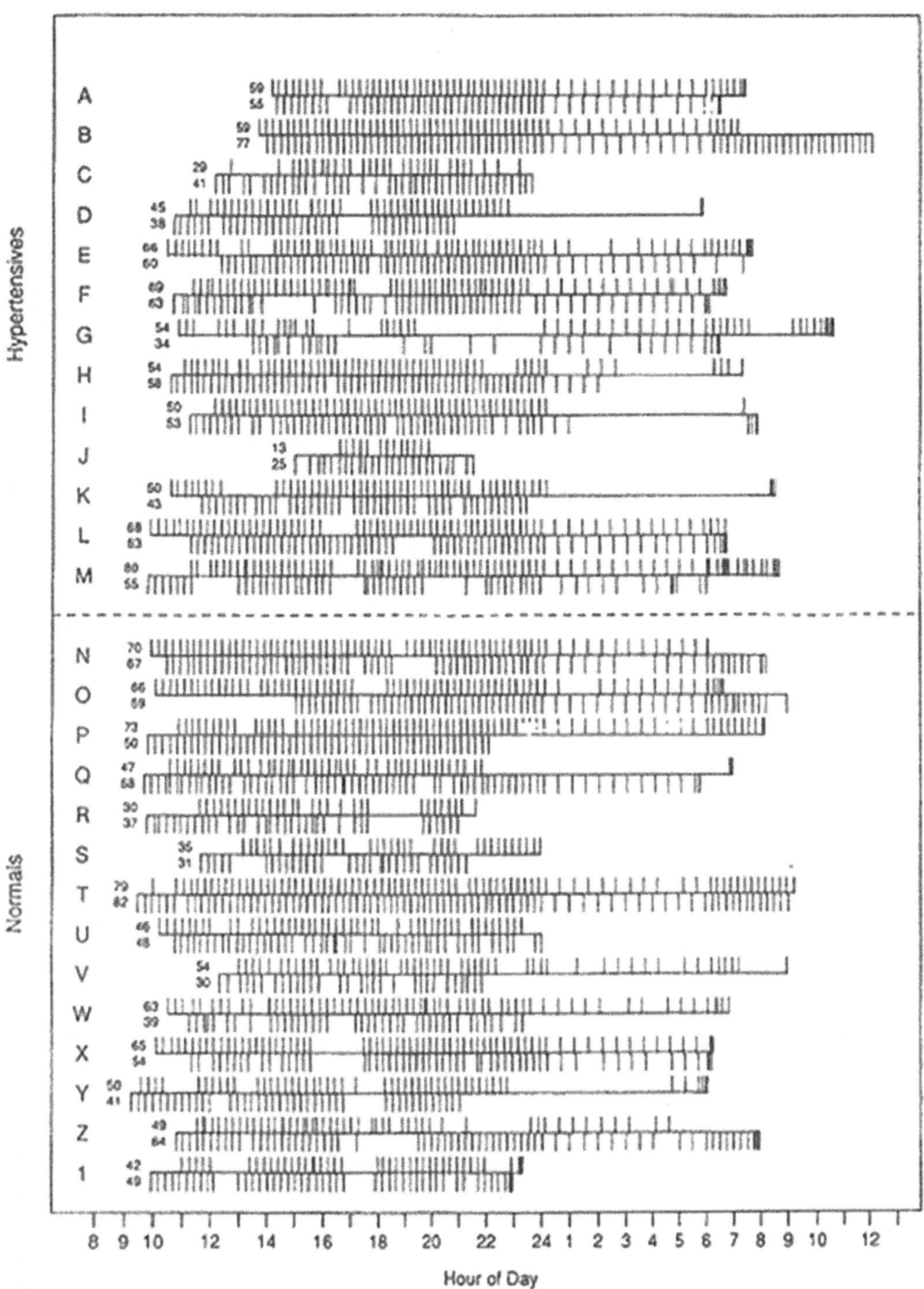

Fig. 3 The pattern of blood pressure measurements taken 2 weeks apart, in normotensive and hypertensive patients using a non-invasive ambulatory blood pressure monitor. Note the different numbers of pressures taken each time and the differences in the time spread between pressures. Test-retest correlations between the systolic/diastolic SDs were 0.18 and 0.22 respectively (Modified from James et al. 1990a)

In the example, note that the size of the estimated blood pressure adjustments associated with the mix of ecological momentary factors varies considerably. A closer examination of the effects shows that they are more or less additive with regard to blood pressure variation. Each set of factor alternatives defines a momentary state typically experienced by a person. From the figure it is easy to see that the allostatic change in blood pressure from one state to another can be substantial. Because a change in habitus from sitting to standing, or a mood change from happy to angry could happen almost instantly, it is clear that the process of allostasis, as reflected in blood pressure variation, is also instantaneous.

6 The Effects of Human Evolution on Blood Pressure Variation

As has been previously discussed (James 1991, 2010, 2013; James and Baker 1995), there has been physiological evolution in our species, some of which has been driven by climate and diet, so that there are various population or ethnic group physiological differences that can affect how an individual's blood pressure varies (James and Baker 1995; Young et al. 2005; James 2010, 2013). The influences of these genetic differences are the result of natural selection and are reflected in populational variation in blood pressure responses to environmental stressors such as prolonged cold temperature and dietary salt.

Current evolutionary evidence suggests that all modern human populations are descended from tropical "heat adapted" ancestors in Africa, somewhere between 100,000 and 200,000 years ago (Smith 2010), and it is also true that modern sub-Saharan African populations retain that heat adapted physiology, or more precisely a physiology adapted to a mostly hot, wet environment (Hanna and Brown 1979; James 2010, 2013; Young et al. 2005). However, many present day populations currently live in and have survived in temperate and freezing climates for millennia. When cold or freezing conditions are experienced in the unprotected human, there is a sympathetically driven constriction of peripheral arteries, particularly in the hands and feet that is designed to conserve body heat, which, if left unchecked, will lead to significant tissue damage in theses appendages (e.g. frostbite) (James and Baker 1995). To combat the tissue damage, ancestral human populations who migrated out of Africa over the past 100,000 years or so to ecosystems characterized by temperate and cold climates evolved a peripheral cold induced vasodilatory (CIVD) response through natural selection (Steegmann 1975). CIVD is a periodic release of the arterial constriction which suffuses the cold peripheral tissues with blood, rewarming them so that they are protected from frostbite for a time (James and Baker 1995). However, what this also means is that populations who did not migrate to these colder ecosystems (those remaining in Africa) did not develop this form of cold adaptation since such a response was unnecessary in tropical climates (James and Baker 1995). Numerous studies have found that African-American populations (whose migration to colder climate environments is very recent evolutionarily) show a generally more intense vasoconstrictive response to peripheral cold stress, with either inadequate or no CIVD (James and Baker 1995; Steegmann 1975). The increased cold pressor response among African-Americans is most often noted in studies of hand emersion in freezing water, however, research has also shown that cold to the face also elicits the accentuated pressor response among African-Americans (Anderson et al. 1988; Treiber et al. 1990) and that African-Americans may further exhibit heightened myocardial and vasoconstrictive reactivity during passive exposure to ambient temperatures from 8 to 10 °C (Kelsey et al. 2000). What these findings mean is that the typical outside exposure of the face during the cold of winter is probably sufficient to elicit the enhanced pressor and vasoconstrictive responses among African-Americans.

Why this is significant from the perspective of blood pressure variation is that the sympathetically driven peripheral vasoconstriction that is induced by cold stress increases blood pressure (Pickering and Gerin 1990). It is thus possible that African Americans living in the temperate and freezing climates of North America or Europe experience chronic cold stress through the winter months, potentially experiencing more chronic vasoconstriction due the their enhanced cold pressor response and inadequate CIVD which in turn will increase the overall variability of their circadian pressure relative to other population groups (James 2013; James and Baker 1995). This possibility is supported by studies which suggest that sympathetic hormone receptors among African-Americans may be more sensitive than those of European-Americans (Mills et al. 1995), and that the diurnal variation in blood pressure of African-Americans is more accentuated than that of European-Americans in relation to diurnal changes in catecholamines (Van Berge-Landry et al. 2008).

There are also two salient aspects of heat adapted physiology, or more precisely a physiology adapted to the mostly hot, wet environment in which *Homo sapiens* evolved: the ability to (1) profusely sweat and (2) retain salt (sodium). The latter is important because salt availability is limited in tropical ecosystems (James 2010; James and Baker 1995; Young et al. 2005). A geographic cline from the equator to the poles of "heat adapted" allelic variants from 5 functional genetic sites that affect salt retention and blood vessel tone has been reported by Young et al. (2005). Specifically, in their study, DNA samples from 53 geographically dispersed populations from the equator to the poles suggest that native populations living within 10° of the equator (hot, salt poor environments) have an average 74 % "heat adapted" allelic variants, while populations within 10° of the arctic (cold, salt rich environments) have only 43 % "heat adapted" variants. Based on this distribution, the authors hypothesized that the frequency of "heat adapted" alleles declined as our African ancestors colonized ecosystems that were cooler and salt rich and then rose again among groups that migrated from those areas back to more salt poor tropical climates (Young et al. 2005; James

2010, 2013). They further argued that since the "heat adapted" alleles facilitate salt retention and excessive dietary salt intake can contribute to the development of hypertension, populations with an increased numbers of "heat adapted" alleles are more susceptible to hypertension, particularly if they have migrated in more recent times to cooler salt rich ecosystems or who have had salt substantially increased in their diets (Young et al. 2005). It has been suggested that these genetic findings may partially explain the higher prevalence of hypertension and cardiovascular morbidity in African-American populations, at least as it may relate to variation of salt in the diet (James 2010, 2013). What this also means, however, is that blood pressure variation related to salt intake may be different depending upon the evolutionary history of the population being evaluated.

To summarize, evolutionarily developed differences in peripheral cold responses and salt and fluid retention likely affect allostatic blood pressure responses. However, in a broader context, what these studies suggest is that the extent to which blood pressure may vary, or move to presumptively adaptive states in response to challenges may depend upon how natural selection has shaped an individual's physiology. That is, the same set of conditions may lead to completely different blood pressure responses due to the fact that their physiologies differ as a consequence of natural selective processes that occurred in their ancestral populations. These underlying physiological differences should thus be considered when evaluating allostatic blood pressure variation in studies that examine ethnically diverse groups.

7 Rethinking Blood Pressure Variability and Morbidity and Mortality Risk

In a more recent discussion, Sterling (2004) contrasted the basis of allostasis with that of homeostasis, which defines physiological processes in terms of maintaining a stable internal environment. That is, in the homeostatic paradigm, the purpose of physiological regulation is to restrict internal parameters to specific "setpoints" so that substantial variation or deviation from that value is seen as pathology, indicating some mechanism is "broken" and needs correcting. In many ways, the current medical evaluation of blood pressure in this manner dramatically affects how blood pressure variability and morbidity/mortality risk studies are carried out. Essentially, studies are designed to assess the impact of too much or too little variability, so that if the amount is extreme, it must mean that that there is underlying pathology in the pressure maintenance feedback loops. I think it is not an unreasonable observation these studies have not provided the kind of results that would be clinically helpful. In fact, some researchers have concluded from the results that blood pressure variability is simply not an important clinical issue (see Asayama et al. 2015).

However, if blood pressure is treated as something that is normatively variable as would be the case in the allostasis paradigm, then the relationship between blood variability and pathology takes on a completely different dimension. In 1998, McEwen (1998) introduced the term "allostatic load" to describe the long term pathological effects of systems that undergo allostasis, or adaptation through change. "Allostatic load" can be defined as the wear and tear that the body experiences due to repeated cycles of allostasis as well as the inefficient turning on or shutting off of the regulatory responses. Morbidity and mortality can ensue from the effects of four types of allostatic load. The first type is the "repeated hits" to the system that result from long term normative continuous changes from minimal to maximal values. The second type is a lack of adaptation or habituation, where an accentuated initial response to acute stressors that should attenuate over time does not. The third type would emerge from prolonged accentuated responses where a maximal response is attained but then never attenuates after the stressor is removed and the fourth type would result from an inadequate response to stressors where substantial changes would be the appropriate adaptation, but instead there is minimal

response. While these types are described as separate possibilities, any or all types of allostatic load might contribute to physiological decline of an individual's cardiovascular system over time. Thus, following the principles of allostatic load, the variability of blood pressure that would contribute to morbidity and mortality is an intrinsic inevitable property of the cardiovascular system, but inappropriate variability in the form of lack of habituation, and prolonged excessive or prolonged inadequate responses to typical daily conditions and stressors could accelerate the pathological process. Thus, variability might not be something that you would treat, but it would be a marker indicating there is something else wrong. Appropriate variability to daily life events could be defined from studies of the sources of variability (see above). What one might then look for clinically is change in the extent of variability associated with events over time, and if there is change, find out what caused the change and if possible, treat it.

8 Conclusions

Variability is a normative property of blood pressure necessary for survival which likely contributes to morbidity and mortality through allostatic load. Because of its allostatic and adaptive properties blood pressure responses to peculiar situations like a visit to the clinic can lead to the misdiagnosis of hypertension. Cuff methods of blood pressure measurement can also create blood pressure variation when none exists. There are also physiological differences between populations related to their evolutionary history that likely further affect the extent of population differences in 24-h blood pressure variability. Quantifying the sources and extent of blood pressure variability can be done using natural experimental models and through the evaluation of ecological momentary data. Finally it is very likely that the results of population studies of blood pressure variability and morbidity and mortality risk are inconclusive because the parameters used to assess blood pressure variability do not reflect the actual nature of blood pressure allostasis.

References

Anderson NB, Lane LD, Muranaka M, Williams RB Jr, Houseworth SJ (1988) Racial differences in blood pressure and forearm vascular responses to the cold face stimulus. Psychosom Med 50:57–63

Asayama K, Fang-Fei W, Hara A, Hansen TW, Li Y, Staessen JA (2015) Prognosis in relation to blood pressure variability; con side of the argument. Hypertension 65:1170–1179. doi:10.1161/HYPERTENSIONAHA.115.04808

Ayman D, Goldshine AD (1940) Blood pressure determinations by patients with essential hypertension: the difference between clinic and home readings before treatment. Am J Med Sci 200:465–474

Bevan AT, Honor AJ, Stott FH (1969) Direct arterial pressure recording in unrestricted man. Clin Sci 36:329–344

Blank SG, Mann SJ, James GD, West JE, Pickering TG (1995) Isolated elevation of diastolic blood pressure: real or artifact? Hypertension 26:383–389

Brondolo E, Karlin W, Alexander K, Bubrow A, Schwartz J (1999) Workday communication and ambulatory blood pressure: implications for the reactivity hypothesis. Psychophysiology 36:86–94

Brown DE, James GD, Nordloh L (1998) Comparison of factors affecting daily variation of blood pressure in Filipino-American and Caucasian nurses in Hawaii. Am J Phys Anthropol 106:373–383

Cochran WG (1977) Sampling techniques. Wiley, New York

Comstock GW (1957) An epidemiological study of blood pressure levels in a biracial community in the southern United States. Am J Hyg 65:271–315

Flores JS (2013) Blood pressure variability: a novel and important risk factor. Can J Cardiol 29:557–563

Gerin W, James GD (2010) Psychosocial determinants of hypertension: laboratory and field models. Blood Press Monit 15:93–99

Gump BB, Polk DE, Kamarck TW, Shiffman S (2001) Partner interactions are associated with reduced blood pressure in the natural environment: ambulatory blood pressure monitoring evidence from a healthy, multi-ethnic adult sample. Psychosom Med 63:423–433

Hanna JM, Brown DA (1979) Human heat tolerance: biological and cultural adaptations. Yearb Phys Anthropol 22:163–186

Hansen TW, Thijs L, Li Y, Boggia J, Kikuya M, Björklund-Bodegård K et al (2010) Prognostic value of reading-to-reading blood pressure variability over 24 hours in 8938 subjects from 11 populations. Hypertension 55:1049–1057

Hinman AT, Engel BT, Bickford AF (1962) Portable blood pressure recorder: accuracy and preliminary use in evaluating intra-daily variation in pressure. Am Heart J 63:663–668

Ice GH, James GD, Crews DE (2003) Blood pressure variation in the institutionalized elderly. Coll Antropol 27:47–55

James GD (1991) Blood pressure response to the daily stressors of urban environments: methodology, basic concepts, and significance. Yearb Phys Anthropol 34:189–210

James GD (2007) Evaluation of journals, diaries, and indexes of worksite and environmental stress. In: White WH (ed) Clinical hypertension and vascular disease: blood pressure monitoring in cardiovascular medicine and therapeutics, 2nd edn. The Humana Press, Totowa, pp 39–58

James GD (2010) Climate-related morphological variation and physiological adaptations in Homo Sapiens. In: Larsen CS (ed) A companion to biological anthropology. Wiley-Blackwell, Malden, pp 153–166

James GD (2013) Ambulatory blood pressure variation: allostasis and adaptation. Auton Neurosci Basic Clin 177:87–94

James GD, Baker PT (1995) Human population biology and blood pressure: evolutionary and ecological considerations and interpretations of population studies. In: Laragh JH, Brenner BM (eds) Hypertension: pathophysiology, diagnosis and management. Raven Press, Ltd, New York, pp 115–126

James GD, Yee LS, Harshfield GA, Blank S, Pickering TG (1986) The influence of happiness, anger and anxiety on the blood pressure of borderline hypertensives. Psychosom Med 48:502–508

James GD, Yee LS, Harshfield GA, Pickering TG (1988) Sex differences in factors affecting the daily variation of blood pressure. Soc Sci Med 26:1019–1023

James GD, Cates EM, Pickering TG, Laragh JH (1989) Parity and perceived job stress elevate blood pressure in young normotensive working women. Am J Hypertens 2:637–639

James GD, Yee LS, Pickering TG (1990a) Winter-summer differences in the effects of emotion, posture, and place of measurement on blood pressure. Soc Sci Med 31:1213–1217

James GD, Pickering TG, Schlussel YR, Clark LA, Denby L, Pregibon D (1990b) Measures of reproducibility of blood pressure variability measured by non-invasive ambulatory blood pressure monitors. J Ambul Monit 3(2):139–147

James GD, Bovbjerg DH, Hill LA (2015) Daily environmental differences in blood pressure and heart rate variability in healthy premenopausal women. Am J Hum Biol 27:136–138. doi:10.1002/ajhb.22609

Jhalani J, Goyala T, Clemow L, Schwartz JE, Pickering TG, Gerin W (2005) Anxiety and outcome expectations predict the white-coat effect. Blood Press Monit 10:317–319

Kain HK, Hinman AT, Sokolow M (1964) Arterial blood pressure measurements with a portable recorder in hypertensive patients: variability and correlation with 'casual' pressure. Circulation 30:882–892

Kamarck TW, Schiffman SM, Smithline L, Goodie JL, Paty JA, Gnys M, Jong JY (1998) Effects of task strain, social conflict, on ambulatory cardiovascular activity: life consequences of recurring stress in a multiethnic adult sample. Health Psychol 17:17–29

Kamarck TW, Janicki DL, Shiffman S, Polk DE, Muldoon MF, Liebenauer LL, Schwartz JE (2002) Psychosocial demands and ambulatory blood pressure: a field assessment approach. Physiol Behav 77:699–704

Kamarck TW, Schwartz JE, Janiki DL, Schiffman S, Raynor DA (2003) Correspondence between laboratory and ambulatory measures of cardiovascular reactivity: a multilevel modeling approach. Psychophysiology 40:675–683

Kelsey RM, Alpert BS, Patterson SM, Barnard M (2000) Racial differences in hemodynamic responses to environmental thermal stress among adolescents. Circulation 101:2284–2289

Kleinert HD, Harshfield GA, Pickering TG, Devereux RB, Sullivan PA, Marion RM et al (1984) What is the value of home blood pressure measurement in patients with mild hypertension? Hypertension 6:574–578

Levy RL, Hillman CC, Stroud WD, White PD (1944) Transient hypertension: Its significance in terms of later development of sustained hypertension and cardiovascular-renal disease. J Am Med Assoc 126:829–833

Linden W, Gerin W, Davidson K (2003) Cardiovascular reactivity: status quo and a research agenda for the new millennium. Psychosom Med 65:5–8

Longo D, Dorigatti F, Palatini P (2005) Masked hypertension in adults. Blood Press Monit 10:307–310

Mancia G, Parati G, Pomidossi G, Grassi G, Casadei R, Zanchetti A (1987) Alerting reaction and rise in pressure during management by physician and nurse. Hypertension 9:209–215

McEwen BS (1998) Protective and damaging effects of stress mediators. N Engl J Med 338:171–179

Mills PJ, Dimsdale JE, Ziegler MG, Nelesen RA (1995) Racial differences in epinephrine and beta 2-adrenergic receptors. Hypertension 25:88–91

O'Rourke MF (1990) What is blood pressure? Am J Hypertens 3:803–810

Palatini P, Reboldi G, Beilin LJ, Casiglia E, Eguchi K, Imai Y et al (2014) Added predictive value of night-time blood pressure variability for cardiovascular events and mortality: the Ambulatory Blood Pressure International Study. Hypertension 64:487–493. doi:10.1161/HYPERTENSIONAHA.114.03694

Parati G, Mutti E, Omboni S, Mancia G (1992) How to deal with blood pressure variability. In: Brunner H, Waeber B (eds) Ambulatory blood pressure recording. Raven Press, Ltd, New York, pp 71–99

Parati G, Ochoa JE, Lombardi C, Bilo G (2015) Blood pressure variability: assessment, predictive value, and potential as a therapeutic target. Curr Hypertens Rep 17:23. doi:10.1007/s11906-015-0537-1

Paskalev D, Kircheva A, Krivoshiev S (2005) A centenary of auscultatory blood pressure measurement: a tribute to Nikolai Korotkoff. Kidney Blood Press Res 2:259–263. doi:10.1159/000090084

Pickering TG (1991) Ambulatory monitoring and blood pressure variability. Science Press, London

Pickering TG, Blank SG (1995) Blood pressure measurement and ambulatory pressure monitoring: evaluation of available equipment. In: Laragh JH, Brenner BM (eds) Hypertension: pathophysiology. diagnosis and management, 2nd edn. Raven Press, Ltd., New York, pp 1939–1952

Pickering TG, Gerin W (1990) Cardiovascular reactivity in the laboratory and the role of behavioral factors in hypertension: a critical review. Ann Behav Med 12:3–16

Pierdomenico SD, Cuccurullo F (2011) Prognostic value of white-coat and masked hypertension diagnosed by ambulatory monitoring in initially untreated subjects: an updated meta-analysis. Am J Hypertens 24:52–58

Richardson DW, Honour AJ, Fenton GW, Stott FH, Pickering GW (1964) Variation in pressure throughout the day and night. Clin Sci 26:445–460

Rogers WF, Palmer RS (1944) Transient hypertension as a military risk: its relation to essential hypertension. N Engl J Med 230:39–42

Rowell LB (1986) Human circulation: regulation during physical stress. Oxford University Press, New York

Schwartz JE, Warren K, Pickering TG (1994) Mood, location and physical position as predictors of ambulatory blood pressure and heart rate: application of a multilevel random effects model. Ann Behav Med 16:210–220

Shapiro A, Meyers T, Reier MF, Ferris EB (1954) Comparison of blood pressure response to Veriloid and to the doctor. Psychosom Med 16:478–488

Smith FH (2010) Species, populations, and assimilation in later human evolution. In: Larsen CS (ed) A companion to biological anthropology. Wiley-Blackwell, Malden, pp 357–378

Sokolow M, Werdegar D, Kain HK, Hinman AT (1966) Relationship between level of blood pressure measured casually and by portable recorders and severity of complications in essential hypertension. Circulation 34:279–298

Steegmann AG (1975) Human adaptation to cold. In: Damon A (ed) Physiological anthropology. Oxford University Press, New York, pp 130–166

Sterling P (2004) Principles of allostasis: optimal design, predictive regulation, pathophysiology, and rational therapeutics. In: Schulkin J (ed) Allostasis, homeostasis, and the costs of physiological adaptation. Cambridge University Press, Cambridge, pp 17–64

Sterling P, Eyer J (1988) Allostasis: a new paradigm to explain arousal pathology. In: Fisher S, Reason J (eds) Handbook of life stress. Wiley, New York, pp 629–649

Taylor KS, Heneghan CJ, Stevens RJ, Adams EC, Nunan D, Ward A (2015) Heterogeneity of prognostic studies of 24-hour blood pressure variability:

systematic review and meta-analysis. PLoS ONE 10 (5), e0126375. doi:10.1371/journal.pone.0126375

Treiber FA, Musante L, Braden D, Arensman F, Strong WB, Levy M, Leverett S (1990) Racial differences in hemodynamic responses to the cold face stimulus in children and adults. Psychosom Med 52:286–296

Van Berge-Landry HM, Bovbjerg DH, James GD (2008) The relationship between waking-sleep blood pressure and catecholamine changes in African American and European American women. Blood Press Monit 13:257–262

Young JH, Chang YC, Kim JD, Chretien J, Levine MA, Ruff CB, Wang N, Chakravarti A (2005) Differential susceptibility to hypertension is due to selection during the out-of-Africa expansion. PLoS Genet 1(6), e82

Zanstra YJ, Johnston DW (2011) Cardiovascular reactivity in real life settings: measurement, mechanisms and meaning. Biol Psychol 86:98–105

Adv Exp Med Biol - Advances in Internal Medicine (2017) 2: 21–35
DOI 10.1007/5584_2016_96
© Springer International Publishing AG 2016
Published online: 16 December 2016

Novel Pathophysiological Mechanisms in Hypertension

Rohan Samson, Andrew Lee, Sean Lawless, Robert Hsu, and Gary Sander

Abstract

Hypertension is the most common disease affecting humans and imparts a significant cardiovascular and renal risk to patients. Extensive research over the past few decades has enhanced our understanding of the underlying mechanisms in hypertension. However, in most instances, the cause of hypertension in a given patient continues to remain elusive. Nevertheless, achieving aggressive blood pressure goals significantly reduces cardiovascular morbidity and mortality, as demonstrated in the recently concluded SPRINT trial. Since a large proportion of patients still fail to achieve blood pressure goals, knowledge of novel pathophysiologic mechanisms and mechanism based treatment strategies is crucial. The following chapter will review the novel pathophysiological mechanisms in hypertension, with a focus on role of immunity, inflammation and vascular endothelial homeostasis. The therapeutic implications of these mechanisms will be discussed where applicable.

Keywords

Hypertension • Pathophysiology • Immune system • Neuro-inflammation • Bone marrow • RAAS • AT_2 receptor • Angiotensin- (1–7) • Mineralocorticoid receptor • VEGF • ADMA

1   Introduction

Hypertensive cardiovascular disease represents a complex spectrum of pathophysiological abnormalities associated with the biomarker of high blood pressure. Our understanding of the complex processes that lead to essential hypertension

R. Samson (✉), A. Lee, S. Lawless, R. Hsu, and G. Sander
Tulane University Heart and Vascular Institute, Tulane School of Medicine, 1430 Tulane Avenue, SL-48, New Orleans, LA 70112, USA
e-mail: rsamson@tulane.edu

has significantly increased over the past few decades. Established pathophysiological mechanisms in essential hypertension include: heightened sympathetic nervous system activity (SNS), alterations in the renin-angiotensin-aldosterone (RAAS) system, excess of sodium-retaining hormones and vasoconstrictors and lack of vasodilators (such as prostacyclin, nitric oxide (NO), and natriuretic peptides), disturbances in the kallikrein–kinin system, abnormalities of resistance vessels and renal microvasculature, and increased vascular growth factor activity (James et al. 2014; Takamura et al. 1999; Davies 2008).

Despite numerous advancements in our understanding of the pathophysiological mechanisms and in treatment strategies however, hypertension continues to remain the most common disease in humans. Novel pathophysiologic mechanisms and mechanism based treatment strategies need to be urgently explored to improve blood pressure control and cardiovascular outcomes in hypertensive patients. The following review summarizes some the key pathophysiological mechanisms in hypertension that have been recently described. Novel insights into the role of the immune system, neuroinflammation and bone marrow in hypertension will be first discussed. Next, recent evidence describing the vasculo-protective effect of the RAAS pathway and the vaso-deleterious effect of the mineralocorticoid receptor will be addressed. Alterations in vascular homeostasis and nitric oxide pathways through vascular endothelial growth factor (VEGF) inhibitors and asymmetric dimethylarginine (ADMA) will be considered last (Kandavar et al. 2011; Calhoun et al. 2000). "Finally, the effect of vascular endothelial growth factor (VEGF) inhibitors and asymmetric dimethylarginine (ADMA) on vascular homeostasis and nitric oxide pathways will be considered."

2 Immune System

Initial evidence for the contribution of the immune system (IS) to hypertension came from studies that demonstrated that immunosuppression lowered blood pressure in rats with partial renal infarction (White and Grollman 1964). In later studies, Olsen noted that mononuclear cells in rats adhered to and infiltrated damaged endothelium in response to angiotensin (Ang)-II infusion (Olsen 1970). Furthermore, athymic mice displayed blunted hypertensive responses and subsequent treatment with anti-thymocyte serum and cyclophosphamide reduced blood pressure (Olsen 1970; Bendich et al. 1981). Altered antibody production was also noted in the spontaneously hypertensive rat (Dzielak 1991; Takeichi et al. 1988; Takeichi and Boone 1976; Purcell et al. 1993). After these early studies in the 1980s, the link between the IS and hypertension remained unexplored for more than two decades. However, with the advent of new molecular tools and genetically engineered animal models, the field of immunology has grown tremendously, offering investigators greater insight into the role of the immune cells, cytokines and cell trafficking in hypertension.

2.1 T-Cell

Knock-out mice lacking recombinant activating genes (RAG) 1 or 2 develop a diminished response to Ang-II or DOCA salt challenge (Guzik et al. 2007). Hypertension was associated with perivascular adipose tissue and adventitial aggregation of effector type T-cells in RAG1$^{-/-}$ mice. Hypertensive response was restored with an adoptive T-cell transfer into RAG1$^{-/-}$ mice. Blunted hypertensive response to stress and recovery following T-cell transfer was further noted in RAG1$^{-/-}$ mice (Guzik et al. 2007).

Severe combined immunodeficiency in mice prevents development of hypertension (Crowley et al. 2010). Reduced hypertension was similarly observed in Dahl-sensitive rats with RAG1 gene knockout (Mattson et al. 2013). Adoptive transfer of regulatory T lymphocyte (Tregs) that suppress innate and adaptive immune responses prevented Ang II-induced blood pressure elevation, vascular stiffness and inflammation (Barhoumi et al. 2011; Muller et al. 2002). Vasculo-protective effects of Tregs have been further demonstrated in aldosterone-induced vascular dysfunction and hypertension (Kasal et al.

2012). Mycophenolate mofetil, a T cell suppressing agent improved blood pressure and renal inflammation in several animal models (Bravo et al. 2007; Franco et al. 2007; Herrera et al. 2006). In a small study of hypertensive patients with rheumatoid arthritis and psoriasis, Mycophenolate reduced blood pressure (Herrera et al. 2006).

2.2 Innate Immunity

Macrophage colony stimulating factor knockout mice, deficient in macrophages and monocytes, exhibit minimal response to Ang-II infusion and unaltered endothelium dependent vasodilation (De Ciuceis et al. 2005). This animal model, known as the osteoporosis spontaneous mutation mice, are further resistant to DOCA-salt hypertension (Ko et al. 2007). Increased aortic monocytes/macrophages and inflammation (as inferred by vascular cell adhesion molecule-1, cyclooxygenase 2, and inducible nitric oxide synthase mRNA) develops in response to Ang-II. Using lysozyme M–targeting of the diphtheria toxin receptor to delete monocytes, Wenzel et al. preempted the vascular alterations and hypertension caused by Ang-II (Wenzel et al. 2011). Transferring monocytes to these mice restored hypertension in these mice.

2.3 Cytokines

Hypertension causes infiltration of effector T cells and monocytes/macrophages in the perivascular regions of both large arteries and arterioles and the kidneys (Olsen 1970; Guzik et al. 2007; Wenzel et al. 2011). Potent cytokines locally released by these cells cause deleterious effects on the vasculature and renal function: this contributes to sustained hypertension and end organ damage. The role of important cytokines in hypertension, namely: interleukin-17A (IL-17A), interleukin 6 (IL-6), and Interferon-γ (IFN- γ) are discussed below:

Interleukin 17 Production of IL-17A is increased in hypertensive patients and mice exposed to Ang-II (Madhur et al. 2010). Minimal hypertensive response and endothelial dysfunction in response to Ang-II was reported in IL-17A deficient mice. Increase in vascular superoxide production and infiltration with T cells was significantly reduced in IL-17A deficient mice. Elevated blood pressure in mice given IL-17A infusion is attributed to conformational changes in endothelial nitric oxide synthase (eNOS) and the resultant decrease in nitric oxide (NO) (Fleming et al. 2001; Piazza et al. 2014). Recently, Amador et al. found that treatment with spironolactone reversed the increase in circulating T_H17 cells and normalized IL-17A mRNA in the heart and kidney of rats with DOCA-salt hypertension (Amador et al. 2014). Antibody against IL-17A reduced blood pressure and collagen-1 levels in the heart and kidney (Amador et al. 2014). Further, collagen deposits and aortic stiffening were absent in IL-17A−/− mice in contrast to the marked collagen deposits and aortic stiffening in Ang-II and DOCA-salt–induced hypertension (Wu et al. 2014).

Interleukin 6 IL-6 is produced by various cells of the IS and has been found to contribute to hypertension. Higher levels of IL-6 seen in hypertensive patients are reversed by Ang-II-receptor blockade (Vázquez-Oliva et al. 2005). Treatment with spironolactone blocks angiotensin II mediated increase in IL-6 levels (Luther et al. 2006). Mice deficient in IL-6 have minimal increase in blood pressure in response to a high salt diet and angiotensin-II (Lee et al. 2006). Activity of epithelial sodium channel is enhanced by IL6 in cultured collecting duct cells (Li et al. 2010). Apart from these direct effects, IL-6 transforms regulatory CD4+T cells to IL-17 producing phenotype, further contributing to hypertension.

Interferon-γ IFN- γ promotes angiotensinogen expression in both hepatocytes and renal proximal tubular cells (Jain et al. 2006; Satou et al. 2012). Angiotensinogen is further converted into Ang-I and Ang-II (Kobori et al. 2007). Locally produced Ang-II acts through various sodium ion transporters to increase sodium uptake and volume in the proximal and distal tubules. Kamat el al recently demonstrated perturbations in sodium transporters in IFN-γ deficient mice, thereby promoting natriuresis and sodium reabsorption (Kamat et al. 2015). Thus, in addition to modifying RAAS systems locally IFN-γ alters expression of renal sodium transporters thereby impacting the sodium and water balance.

2.4 Novel Mechanisms of T Cell Activation

Role of Isoketals Recent studies have revealed new mechanisms of T cell activation in hypertension, a phenomenon that was unexplained despite the large body of evidence supporting a role of the IS in hypertension (Kirabo et al. 2014). Upregulation of NADPH oxidase in dendritic cells promotes production of reactive oxygen species. Oxidation of arachidonic acid leads to formation of γ-ketoaldehydes or isoketals. Protein lysines and isoketals combine in dendritic cells to make immunogenic proteins that are then presented to T cells resulting in T cell activation and proliferation (Miyashita et al. 2014). Further, isoketals independently promote cytokine production in dendritic cells and T cells. Isoketal scavenger 2 hydroxybenzylamine halts dendritic cells from producing cytokines and T cell activation. Additionally, a blunted hypertensive response was noted in mice receiving dendritic cells from donors treated with 2 hydroxybenylamine (Kirabo et al. 2014; McMaster et al. 2015).

Toll-Like Receptors and Damage Associated Molecular Patterns Ubiquitously expressed in the immune cells and the cardiovascular system, toll-like receptors (TLRs) recognize and initiate inflammatory responses to dangerous molecules (Frantz et al. 2007; Matzinger 2002). Aside from pathogens, endogenous molecules produced following cellular injury or death (damage-associated molecular patterns (DAMPs)) also activate TLRs (Theodora Szasz 2013). Recent investigations have highlighted the inflammatory

properties of mitochondrial DNA as a result of TLR activation (Oka et al. 2012; Zhang et al. 2010). TLRs promote vascular dysfunction, low-grade inflammation and release of pro-inflammatory cytokines, all contributing to hypertension (Bomfim et al. 2012; Liang et al. 2013; De Batista et al. 2014; Singh and Abboud 2014). Initial innate IS TLRs response to DAMPs may thus be a necessary precursor of the adaptive IS activation observed in hypertension (McCarthy et al. 2014). Low complexity of TLR signaling pathway and availability of specific inhibitors may lead to the development of novel anti-hypertensive drugs.

3 Neuro-Inflammation

The association between hypertension and inflammation in the brain is evident from studies in animal models of hypertension demonstrating elevated levels of cytokines such leukotriene-B, nuclear factor-κb, TNF-α, IL-1β, and IL-6 in the brain (Waki et al. 2013; Santisteban et al. 2015; Cardinale et al. 2012; Song et al. 2014). Angiotensin converting enzyme (ACE) and Ang-II upregulate neuronal inflammatory pathways (Marc and Llorens-Cortes 2011; Agarwal et al. 2013; Shi et al. 2014). Exposure of cardioregulatory forebrain structures to TNF-α, IL-1β heightens SNS activity and blood pressure while anti-inflammatory drugs pentoxyphylline and minocycline attenuate the development of hypertension (Xue et al. 2016; Wei et al. 2015; Sriramula et al. 2013).

Innate IS activation through microglial cells also promotes SNS activity, peripheral inflammation and hypertension (Masson et al. 2015; Shi et al. 2010). Under normal conditions, microglial cells act to promote immune homeostasis within the brain environment. Upon activation of microglia through pathological insults or alterations in homeostasis, there is an induction of centrally produced proinflammatory cytokines, thereby contributing neuro-inflammation, and consequently, hypertension (Agarwal et al. 2013; de Kloet et al. 2015). Inhibition of microglial activation attenuates SNS activity, peripheral inflammation and hypertension (Santisteban et al. 2015; Shi et al. 2014).

4   Bone Marrow

The impact of peripheral and neuro-inflammation in hypertension has been described thus far. The relationship between the IS and the brain in hypertension was, however, poorly understood until recent investigations revealed a critical role of the bone marrow in regulating peripheral and neuro-inflammation in hypertension (Santisteban et al. 2015). As a site of inflammatory cell generation and convergence of CNS and IS, the BM was suggested as an ideal link between inflammatory system and hypertension. Indeed, the BM of spontaneously hypertensive rat had increased levels of inflammatory cells and cytokines, as well as migration of these cells into the hypothalamic paraventriuclar nucleus (Santisteban et al. 2015). Minocycline, through its anti-inflammatory effects, prevented both peripheral and neuro-inflammation, thereby attenuating hypertension (Santisteban et al. 2015).

SNS Effect on BM Hematopoietic stem and progenitor (HSPC) stem cell homeostasis is regulated by SNS via adrenergic nerve fibers that richly innervate the bone marrow. Central sympathetic outflow stimulates HSPC mobilization and release into circulation (Hanoun et al. 2015; Méndez-Ferrer et al. 2008). Multiple mechanisms contribute to this upregulation of HSPCs from the BM by sympathetic stimulation, including granulocyte-colony stimulating factor induced osteoblast suppression, modulation of the Wnt-B – catenin pathway, and substance P-mediated nociceptive signaling (Katayama et al. 2006; Spiegel et al. 2007; Amadesi et al. 2012). Ang-II increases HSPC proliferation in BM and inflammatory monocyte production in the spleen (Kim et al. 2016). Conversely, disruption of sympathetic tone impairs HSPC mobilization (Lucas et al. 2012).

SNS Effect on the Immune System Autonomic regulation of the IS seems to play an important role in hypertension (Scheiermann et al. 2013; Ganta 2005). Chronic Ang-induced hypertension animal models express inflammatory monocytes in BM, spleen and peripheral blood, contributing to hypertension (Santisteban et al. 2015; Swirski et al. 2009). Independent of the SNS effect on the BM, norepinephrine induces memory T cell production of cytokines in the vasculature and the kidneys (Marvar et al. 2010; Slota et al. 2015; Trott et al. 2014). Norepinephrine increases recruitment of immune cells from BM, while acetylcholine opposes this effect (Zubcevic et al. 2014). Lastly, renal denervation inhibits IS activation and preempts renal inflammation in Ang-II induced hypertension (Xiao et al. 2015).

Thus, a positive feedback loop is established, whereby neuro-inflammation contributes to sympathoexcitation, which then promotes activation of the IS and stem/progenitor cells in BM. In turn, this can exacerbate central inflammation generating a vicious proinflammatory cycle (Fig. 1) (Young and Davisson 2015). Extravasation of proinflammatory precursors from the BM to hypothalamic paraventricular nucleus causing neuro-inflammation in Ang-II–induced hypertension has been demonstrated (Santisteban et al. 2015; Spiegel et al. 2007). Mechanisms of extravasation of BM cells into the brain are currently unknown.

5   Vasculo-Protective RAAS Pathways

RAAS blockade generates alternate metabolites of Ang that can exert an anti-hypertensive effect. Vasculo-protective RAS pathways include Angiotensinase A-Ang III-Ang II type 2 (AT_2) receptor pathway and ACE 2-Ang-(1–7)-Mas receptor pathway (Te Riet et al. 2015).

5.1 AT_2 Receptor Pathway

Upregulation of AT_2 receptors counteracts the vaso-deleterious effects of angiotensin (AT_1) type 1 receptor. Mice deficient in AT_2 receptor exhibit increased blood pressure and baroreflex

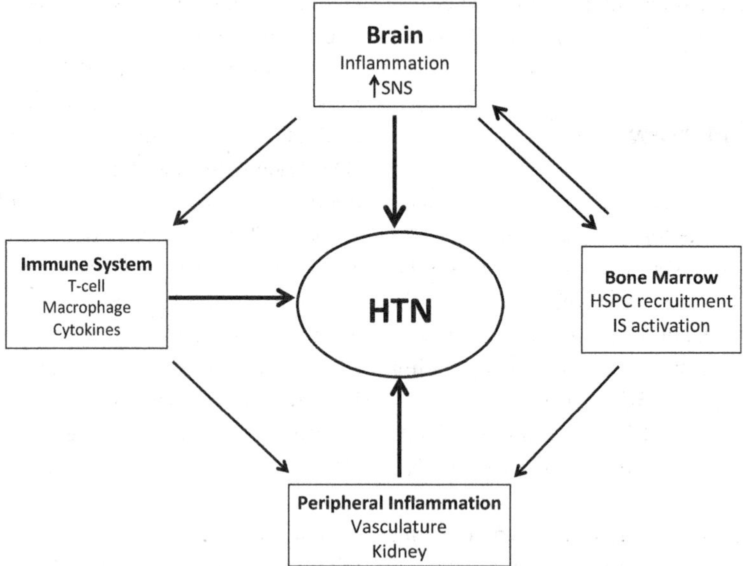

Fig. 1 Role of Immune system activation, brain and bone marrow in hypertension. Immune system activation via T cells, macrophages and various cytokines results in central and peripheral inflammation in the vasculature and kidney contributing to hypertension. Neuro-inflammation from hypertensive stimuli promotes sympathetic nervous system (SNS) activity causing hypertension. SNS activity in bone marrow increases recruitment and release of hematopoietic stem cell progenitors (HSPC) and cytokines, furthering the pro-inflammatory state

sensitivity, and decreased pressure-natriuresis and AT_1 receptor expression (Gross et al. 2004; Tanaka et al. 1999; Gembardt et al. 2008). Overexpression of AT_2 receptor reverses these effects (Tsutsumi et al. 1999). Four AT_2 agonist molecules are currently being developed for clinical use in hypertension namely: peptidergic agonists β-Tyr4-Ang II, β-Ile5-Ang II and LP2-3 and the non-peptide agonist Compound 21 (C21). AT_2 receptor mediated aortic vasodilation was reported in mice treated with peptidergic agonists (Jones et al. 2011; Wagenaar et al. 2013). Interestingly, vasodilatory effects of AT_2 receptor are appreciated most on a background of partial AT_1 receptor blockade (Esch et al. 2009; Sevá Pessôa et al. 2012). Indeed, simultaneous administration of β-Ile5-Ang II and candesartan lowered BP in spontaneously hypertensive rat (Jones et al. 2011).

5.2 ACE2-Ang-(1–7)-Mas Receptor Pathway

Angiotensin converting enzyme 2 (ACE 2) acts on angiotensin II to produce angiotensin (Ang)-(1–7) (Santos et al. 2003). Interaction of Ang-(1–7) and Mas receptor oppose AT_1 receptor functions. Further, Ang-(1–7) bind to AT_2 receptors and even AT_1 receptors at high doses. Several cardiovascular benefits have been attributed to Ang-(1–7), however its role in hypertension at present is unclear (Te Riet et al. 2015). Ang (1–7) has weak vasodilatory effects and has not uniformly exhibited anti-hypertensive effects in animal models (Sevá Pessôa et al. 2012; Durik et al. 2012).

Nevertheless, therapeutic options utilizing the vasoprotective effects of Ang-(1–7) have been explored. Cyclodextrin-encapsulated Ang-(1–7), non-peptide drug AVE0091 and peptide drug CGEN856S have shown BP-lowering effects in hypertensive animals (Sevá Pessôa et al. 2012; Ferreira et al. 2010).

Anti-hypertensive effects of ACE 2 have also been questioned. Overexpression of ACE 2 does lower blood pressure, however, its ability of degrade Ang-II could also account for anti-hypertensive effect (Gurley et al. 2006). Hypotension due to ACE 2 agonists Diminazine and XNT was recently shown to be independent of

ACE2-Ang-(1–7)-Mas pathway further weakening the evidence in support of its role in the pathogenesis of hypertension (Haber et al. 2014).

5.3 Alamandine

Alamandine, a recently discovered hormone of RAS, shares similar biological structure and activity to that of Ang-(1–7) including promotion of vasodilation and anti-hypertensive effects. ACE 2 hydrolyzation of Ang A and decarboxylation of Ang-(1–7) have both been shown to produce this endogenous peptide within the body (Villela et al. 2014). Lautner et al. demonstrated that alamandine interacts with its own specific MrgD receptor (Mas-related G-protein coupled receptor, member D) (Lautner et al. 2013). Oral administration of alamandine as a HP-B Cyclodextrin inclusion compound produced long term anti-hypertensive effect in spontaneously hypertensive rats (Lautner et al. 2013). Moreover, microinjections of almandine into the medullary brain demonstrated cardiovascular effects similar to that of Ang-(1–7), indicating a possible central role of BP control by alamandine (Villela et al. 2014; Mendoza-Torres et al. 2015). Further studies are required to delineate the role Alamandine plays in the RAAS, and as a anti-hypertensive agent.

5.4 Angiotensin III Inhibitors

Angiotensin III is a recognized AT_2 receptor agonist in the kidney and vasculature (Kemp et al. 2012). However, in the brain, it is believed to be the preferred AT_1 receptor agonist and therefore can cause hypertension (Wright et al. 2003). Aminopeptidase A inhibitors that act preferentially in the CNS to block Ang II conversion to Ang III are being developed. An orally administered prodrug (RB150), that converts to an aminopeptidase A inhibitor EC33 in the brain, exhibited antihypertensive effects in animal models. RB 150 is currently being evaluated in a phase Ib clinical study (Gao et al. 2014).

6 Aldosterone Mineralocorticoid Receptor Pathway

Aldosterone hormone activation of mineralocorticoid receptors (MR), a member of the steroid receptor family, is known to promote vascular cell oxidative stress, inflammation, proliferation, migration and extracellular matrix production (McCurley and Jaffe 2012; Lother and Hein 2016). Vaso-deleterious effects caused by MR activation include: vasoconstriction, atherosclerosis, and vascular remodeling and fibrosis (Lother and Hein 2016; Udelson et al. 2010). Nishiyama et al. demonstrated in animal models that mineralocorticoid-induced hypertension is associated with increased vascular oxidative stress and ROS production (McCurley and Jaffe 2012; Nishiyama and Abe 2004; Iglarz et al. 2004). Subsequently, MR antagonism showed a decrease in NADPH-oxidase activity, resulting in less ROS production, and thus lower BP (Keidar et al. 2003; Sanz-Rosa et al. 2005).

Activation of MR in the vascular bed is also associated with increased expression of proinflammatory factors including ICAM1, monocyte chemoattractant protein (MCP-1), cytokines, placental growth factor (PGF), COX-2 and transcription factor NF-κB (McCurley and Jaffe 2012; Rocha et al. 2002). Aortas from patients with atherosclerosis demonstrated a decrease in PGF and connective tissue growth factor when treated with spironolactone (a MR antagonist) (Jaffe et al. 2010; Newfell et al. 2011). Furthermore, the controlled Prevention and Treatment of Hypertension With Algorithm-Based Therapy (PATHWAY)-2-clinical trial showed a decrease in blood pressure by 8.7 mmHg with spironolactone treatment in patients with resistant hypertension (Lother and Hein 2016; MacDonald et al. 2015). Such findings support the role of MR-activation induced inflammation as a contributing factor to hypertension. However, further trials exploring the use of MR antagonists as anti-hypertensive agents are required to confirm these results.

7 VEGF Inhibitors

Anti-angiogenesis therapy targeting vascular endothelial growth factor (VEGF) and its receptors as treatment for anti-tumor growth has long been associated with adverse side effects of hypertension and renal toxicity manifesting as proteinuria and renal function impairment (Lankhorst et al. 2016; van den Meiracker and Danser 2016). Physiologically, VEGF mediates vasodilation through increased nitric oxide (NO) production by upregulating the NOS gene expression and increased endothelial NOS phosphorylation (Hood et al. 1998; Shen et al. 1999). The subsequent decrease in NO availability following VEGF inhibition contributes to the pathogenesis of hypertension during anti-angiogenesis therapy (van den Meiracker and Danser 2016; Facemire et al. 2009). Recent investigations of the role of the Endothelin (ET) system, specifically Endothelin-1, suggest this system as a more significant contributor to the rise in BP compared to NO deprivation. A rise in ET-1 is noted with administration of sunitinib, a receptor tyrosine kinase (RTK) inhibitor that targets VEGF receptors (Kappers et al. 2010). Endothelin-1 (ET-1) interacts with G-protein-coupled membrane bound ET_A and ET_B receptors on vascular smooth muscle to mediate vasoconstriction. Furthermore, ET_A receptor antagonism prevented anti-angiogenic induced hypertension in mice (Li et al. 2012). Currently, there is no established guideline for reversing hypertension induced by VEGF-targeted therapies (Hayman et al. 2012).

8 Asymmetric Dimethylarginine

Asymmetric dimethyarginine (ADMA) is a naturally occurring amino acid synthesized when arginine residues in proteins undergo methylation by arginine methyltransferases (PRMTs) (Vallance and Leiper 2004; Vallance et al. 1992). An additional by-product of this interaction is N^G-monomethyl- L-arginine (L-NMMA), a methylarginine similar to ADMA in its biological activity. Following hydrolysis of methylated proteins ADMA and L-NMMA are released in the cytosol. ADMA is found in various tissues, circulates in plasma and is excreted in urine (Vallance and Leiper 2004). In addition to renal clearance, ADMA is extensively metabolized by dimethylarginine dimethyl aminohydrolases (DDAHs) resulting in conversion to citrulline (Achan et al. 2003).

Both ADMA and L-NMMA competitively inhibit all three isoforms NOS, thereby causing vasoconstriction, impaired endothelium-mediated vasodilatation, increased endothelial adhesiveness, and hypertension (Vallance et al. 1992; Achan et al. 2003; Hasegawa et al. 2007; Kielstein et al. 2004; Barba et al. 2000; Böger et al. 2000). Targeted deletion of DDAH gene and use of specific inhibitors of DDAH lead to accumulation of ADMA, a reduction in NO signaling and subsequent vascular dysfunction, increased systemic vascular resistance and blood pressure (Leiper et al. 2007). Transgenic mice overexpressing DDAH demonstrated reduced ADMA levels and increased cardiac NO levels. However, transgenic mice showed no changes in systemic BP compared to wild type controls under normal conditions (Hasegawa et al. 2007). Two-week treatment with angiotensin II increased ADMA levels, cardiac oxidative stress and vascular injury while DDAH overexpression attenuated these changes (Hasegawa et al. 2007). Conversely, Jacobi et al. reported no increase in ADMA levels following 4-week Ang II infusion (Jacobi et al. 2008). Overexpression of DDAH however attenuated ang-II medicated end organ damage (Jacobi et al. 2008).

Small clinical studies have noted an association between hypertension and increased ADMA levels (Surdacki et al. 1999; Perticone et al. 2005). Larger scale clinical studies have however not corroborated these findings (Meinitzer et al. 2007; Schnabel et al. 2005). Trials evaluating the effect of antihypertensive agents on ADMA levels have yielded conflicting results. Some investigators reported significant reductions in ADMA levels following treatment with RAS, (Chen et al. 2002; Delles et al. 2002; Ito et al. 2002; Napoli et al. 2004; Aslam et al. 2006) while others have failed to confirm these findings (Fliser et al. 2005; Warnholtz et al. 2007). Differences in study design, treatment regimens, methods of determining ADMA levels may account for the discrepant findings of the aforementioned studies.

ADMA has been shown to have a negative correlation with endothelial-dependent vasodilation (EDV) and a positive correlation with carotid artery intima-media thickness (IMT) in hypertensive patients with administration of salbutamol and nitroglycerine (Serg et al. 2011). Cakar and colleagues evaluated arterial stiffness markers for endothelial dysfunction and found that ADMA levels significantly correlated with augmentation index (Aix) and CRP levels. However, there was no correlation between PWV and central aortic pressure (CAP) and ADMA (Cakar et al. 2015). Similarly, the PREVENCION study showed that ADMA and NMMA did not predict carotid-femoral PWV, blood pressure or hemodynamic abnormalities (Chirinos et al. 2008). Therefore, while it is very clear that ADMA plays a role in endothelial dysfunction and can cause significant changes in vascular flow, it still remains to be seen whether ADMA directly play a role in hypertension.

Therapeutic approaches specifically targeting ADMA pathways have been studied. Increased L-citrulline supplementation overcame ADMA inhibition, resulting in improved NO production in porcine hearts (Xuan et al. 2015). The effects of L-arginine on endothelial function, blood pressure, and ADMA levels in patients with hypertension (NCT02392767) and in patients with preeclampsia are currently being evaluated (NCT00275158).

9 Conclusion

The recently concluded SPRINT trial has suggested that achieving aggressive blood pressure targets reduces cardiovascular morbidity and mortality. This will require more aggressive and complex treatment regimens, in most cases with multi-drug protocols. In order to achieve better blood pressure control, it is imperative to understand the mechanisms that lead to increased blood pressure. Knowledge of the causative mechanisms will allow informed selection of agents and combinations that are additive and even synergistic. Such an approach will in turn allow the fashioning "personalized" treatment regimens that will maximally benefit each patient individually.

References

Achan V, Broadhead M, Malaki M, Whitley G, Leiper J, MacAllister R et al (2003) Asymmetric dimethylarginine causes hypertension and cardiac dysfunction in humans and is actively metabolized by dimethylarginine dimethylaminohydrolase. Arterioscler Thromb Vasc Biol 23(8):1455–1459

Agarwal D, Dange RB, Raizada MK, Francis J (2013) Angiotensin II causes imbalance between pro- and anti-inflammatory cytokines by modulating GSK-3β in neuronal culture. Br J Pharmacol 169(4):860–874

Amadesi S, Reni C, Katare R, Meloni M, Oikawa A, Beltrami AP et al (2012) Role for substance p-based nociceptive signaling in progenitor cell activation and angiogenesis during ischemia in mice and in human subjects. Circulation 125(14):1774, –86–S1–19

Amador CA, Barrientos V, Peña J, Herrada AA, González M, Valdés S et al (2014) Spironolactone decreases DOCA-salt-induced organ damage by blocking the activation of T helper 17 and the downregulation of regulatory T lymphocytes. Hypertension 63(4):797–803

Aslam S, Santha T, Leone A, Wilcox C (2006) Effects of amlodipine and valsartan on oxidative stress and plasma methylarginines in end-stage renal disease patients on hemodialysis. Kidney Int 70(12):2109–2115

Barba G, Vallance PJ, Strazzullo P, MacAllister RJ (2000) Effects of sodium intake on the pressor and renal responses to nitric oxide synthesis inhibition in normotensive individuals with different sodium sensitivity. J Hypertens 18(5):615–621

Barhoumi T, Kasal DA, Li MW, Shbat L, Laurant P, Neves MF et al (2011) T regulatory lymphocytes prevent angiotensin II-induced hypertension and vascular injury. Hypertension 57(3):469–476

Bendich A, Belisle EH, Strausser HR (1981) Immune system modulation and its effect on the blood pressure of the spontaneously hypertensive male and female rat. Biochem Biophys Res Commun 99 (2):600–607

Böger RH, Bode-Böger SM, Tsao PS, Lin PS, Chan JR, Cooke JP (2000) An endogenous inhibitor of nitric oxide synthase regulates endothelial adhesiveness for monocytes. J Am Coll Cardiol 36(7):2287–2295

Bomfim GF, Dos Santos RA, Oliveira MA, Giachini FR, Akamine EH, Tostes RC et al (2012) Toll-like receptor 4 contributes to blood pressure regulation and vascular contraction in spontaneously hypertensive rats. Clin Sci 122(11):535–543

Bravo Y, Quiroz Y, Ferrebuz A, Vaziri ND, Rodríguez-Iturbe B (2007) Mycophenolate mofetil administration reduces renal inflammation, oxidative stress, and arterial pressure in rats with lead-induced hypertension. Am J Physiol Renal Physiol 293(2):F616–F623

Cakar M, Bulucu F, Karaman M, Ay SA, Kurt Ö, Balta Ş et al (2015) Asymmetric dimethylarginine and augmentation index in newly diagnosed patients with hypertension. Angiology 66(1):43–48

Calhoun DA, Bakir SE, Oparil S, DiMarco J (2000) Etiology and pathogenesis of essential hypertension. In: Cardiology. Mosby International, London

Cardinale JP, Sriramula S, Mariappan N, Agarwal D, Francis J (2012) Angiotensin II-induced hypertension is modulated by nuclear factor-κBin the paraventricular nucleus. Hypertension 59(1):113–121

Chen J-W, Hsu N-W, Wu T-C, Lin S-J, Chang M-S (2002) Long-term angiotensin-converting enzyme inhibition reduces plasma asymmetric dimethylarginine and improves endothelial nitric oxide bioavailability and coronary microvascular function in patients with syndrome X. Am J Cardiol 90(9):974–982

Chirinos JA, David R, Bralley JA, Zea-Díaz H, Muñoz-Atahualpa E, Corrales-Medina F et al (2008) Endogenous nitric oxide synthase inhibitors, arterial hemodynamics, and subclinical vascular disease: the PREVENCION Study. Hypertension 52(6):1051–1059

Crowley SD, Song Y-S, Lin EE, Griffiths R, Kim H-S, Ruiz P (2010) Lymphocyte responses exacerbate angiotensin II-dependent hypertension. Am J Physiol Regul Integr Comp Physiol 298(4):R1089–R1097

Davies PF (2008) Hemodynamic shear stress and the endothelium in cardiovascular pathophysiology. Nat Clin Pract Cardiovasc Med 6(1):16–26

De Batista PR, Palacios R, Martín A, Hernanz R, Médici CT, Silva MASC, et al (2014) Toll-like receptor 4 upregulation by angiotensin II contributes to hypertension and vascular dysfunction through reactive oxygen species production. Huang Y, editor. PLoS ONE. 9(8):e104020

De Ciuceis C, Amiri F, Brassard P, Endemann DH, Touyz RM, Schiffrin EL (2005) Reduced vascular remodeling, endothelial dysfunction, and oxidative stress in resistance arteries of angiotensin II-infused macrophage colony-stimulating factor-deficient mice: evidence for a role in inflammation in angiotensin-induced vascular injury. Arterioscler Thromb Vasc Biol 25(10):2106–2113

de Kloet AD, Liu M, Rodríguez V, Krause EG, Sumners C (2015) Role of neurons and glia in the CNS actions of the renin-angiotensin system in cardiovascular control. Am J Physiol Regul Integr Comp Physiol 309(5):R444–R458

Delles C, Schneider MP, John S, Gekle M, Schmieder RE (2002) Angiotensin converting enzyme inhibition and angiotensin II AT1-receptor blockade reduce the levels of asymmetrical N(G), N(G)-dimethylarginine in human essential hypertension. Am J Hypertens 15 (7 Pt 1):590–593

Durik M, Sevá Pessôa B, Roks AJM (2012) The renin-angiotensin system, bone marrow and progenitor cells. Clin Sci 123(4):205–223

Dzielak DJ (1991) Immune mechanisms in experimental and essential hypertension. Am J Physiol 260(3 Pt 2): R459–R467

Esch JHM, Schuijt MP, Sayed J, Choudhry Y, Walther T, Jan Danser AH (2009) AT2 receptor-mediated vasodilation in the mouse heart depends on AT1A receptor activation. Br J Pharmacol 148(4):452–458

Facemire CS, Nixon AB, Griffiths R, Hurwitz H, Coffman TM (2009) Vascular endothelial growth factor receptor 2 controls blood pressure by regulating nitric oxide synthase expression. Hypertension 54 (3):652–658

Ferreira AJ, Santos RAS, Bradford CN, Mecca AP, Sumners C, Katovich MJ et al (2010) Therapeutic implications of the vasoprotective axis of the renin-angiotensin system in cardiovascular diseases. Hypertension 55(2):207–213

Fleming I, Fisslthaler B, Dimmeler S, Kemp BE, Busse R (2001) Phosphorylation of Thr(495) regulates Ca(2+)/calmodulin-dependent endothelial nitric oxide synthase activity. Circ Res 88(11):E68–E75

Fliser D, Wagner K-K, Loos A, Tsikas D, Haller H (2005) Chronic angiotensin II receptor blockade reduces (intra)renal vascular resistance in patients with type 2 diabetes. J Am Soc Nephrol 16(4):1135–1140

Franco M, Martínez F, Quiroz Y, Galicia O, Bautista R, Johnson RJ et al (2007) Renal angiotensin II concentration and interstitial infiltration of immune cells are correlated with blood pressure levels in salt-sensitive hypertension. Am J Physiol Regul Integr Comp Physiol 293(1):R251–R256

Frantz S, Ertl G, Bauersachs J (2007) Mechanisms of disease: Toll-like receptors in cardiovascular disease. Nat Clin Pract Cardiovasc Med 4(8):444–454

Ganta CK (2005) Central angiotensin II-enhanced splenic cytokine gene expression is mediated by the sympathetic nervous system. Am J Physiol Heart Circ Physiol 289(4):H1683–H1691

Gao J, Marc Y, Iturrioz X, Leroux V, Balavoine F, Llorens-Cortes C (2014) A new strategy for treating hypertension by blocking the activity of the brain renin-angiotensin system with aminopeptidase A inhibitors. Clin Sci. 2nd edn. Portland Press Limited 127(3):135–148

Gembardt F, Heringer-Walther S, van Esch JHM, Sterner-Kock A, van Veghel R, Le TH et al (2008) Cardiovascular phenotype of mice lacking all three subtypes of angiotensin II receptors. FASEB J 22(8):3068–3077

Gross V, Obst M, Luft FC (2004) Insights into angiotensin II receptor function through AT2 receptor knockout mice. Acta Physiol Scand 181(4):487–494

Gurley SB, Allred A, Le TH, Griffiths R, Mao L, Philip N et al (2006) Altered blood pressure responses and normal cardiac phenotype in ACE2-null mice. J Clin Invest 116(8):2218–2225

Guzik TJ, Hoch NE, Brown KA, McCann LA, Rahman A, Dikalov S et al (2007) Role of the T cell in the genesis of angiotensin II induced hypertension and vascular dysfunction. J Exp Med 204(10):2449–2460

Haber PK, Ye M, Wysocki J, Maier C, Haque SK, Batlle D (2014) Angiotensin-converting enzyme 2–independent action of presumed angiotensin-converting enzyme 2 activatorsNovelty and significance. Hypertension 63(4):774–782

Hanoun M, Maryanovich M, Arnal-Estapé A, Frenette PS (2015) Neural regulation of hematopoiesis, inflammation, and cancer. Neuron 86(2):360–373

Hasegawa K, Wakino S, Tatematsu S, Yoshioka K, Homma K, Sugano N et al (2007) Role of asymmetric dimethylarginine in vascular injury in transgenic mice overexpressing dimethylarginie dimethylamino-hydrolase 2. Circ Res 101(2):e2–e10

Hayman SR, Leung N, Grande JP, Garovic VD (2012) VEGF inhibition, hypertension, and renal toxicity. Curr Oncol Rep 14(4):285–294

Herrera J, Ferrebuz A, MacGregor EG, Rodríguez-Iturbe B (2006) Mycophenolate mofetil treatment improves hypertension in patients with psoriasis and rheumatoid arthritis. J Am Soc Nephrol 17(12 Suppl 3):S218–S225

Hood JD, Meininger CJ, Ziche M, Granger HJ (1998) VEGF upregulates ecNOS message, protein, and NO production in human endothelial cells. Am J Physiol 274(3 Pt 2):H1054–H1058

Iglarz M, Touyz R, Viel E, Amiri F, Schiffrin E (2004) Involvement of oxidative stress in the profibrotic action of aldosteroneInteraction with the renin-angiotensin system. Am J Hypertens 17(7):597–603

Ito A, Egashira K, Narishige T, Muramatsu K, Takeshita A (2002) Angiotensin-converting enzyme activity is involved in the mechanism of increased endogenous nitric oxide synthase inhibitor in patients with type 2 diabetes mellitus. Circ J 66(9):811–815

Jacobi J, Maas R, Cordasic N, Koch K, Schmieder RE, Böger RH et al (2008) Role of asymmetric dimethylarginine for angiotensin II-induced target organ damage in mice. Am J Physiol Heart Circ Physiol 294(2):H1058–H1066

Jaffe IZ, Newfell BG, Aronovitz M, Mohammad NN, McGraw AP, Perreault RE et al (2010) Placental growth factor mediates aldosterone-dependent vascular injury in mice. J Clin Invest 120(11):3891–3900

Jain S, Shah M, Li Y, Vinukonda G, Sehgal PB, Kumar A (2006) Upregulation of human angiotensinogen (AGT) gene transcription by interferon-gamma: involvement of the STAT1-binding motif in the AGT promoter. Biochim Biophys Acta 1759(7):340–347

James PA, Oparil S, Carter BL, Cushman WC, Dennison-Himmelfarb C, Handler J et al (2014) 2014 evidence-based guideline for the management of high blood pressure in adults: report from the panel members appointed to the Eighth Joint National Committee (JNC 8). JAMA 311:507–520

Jones ES, Del Borgo MP, Kirsch JF, Clayton D, Bosnyak S, Welungoda I et al (2011) A single beta-amino acid substitution to angiotensin II confers AT2 receptor selectivity and vascular function. Hypertension 57(3):570–576

Kamat NV, Thabet SR, Xiao L, Saleh MA, Kirabo A, Madhur MS et al (2015) Renal transporter activation during angiotensin-II hypertension is blunted in interferon-γ−/− and interleukin-17A−/− mice. Hypertension 65(3):569–576

Kandavar R, Higashi Y, Chen W, Blackstock C, Vaughn C, Sukhanov S et al (2011) The effect of nebivolol versus metoprolol succinate extended release on asymmetric dimethylarginine in hypertension. J Am Soc Hypertens 5(3):161–165

Kappers MHW, van Esch JHM, Sluiter W, Sleijfer S, Danser AHJ, van den Meiracker AH (2010) Hypertension induced by the tyrosine kinase inhibitor sunitinib is associated with increased circulating endothelin-1 levels. Hypertension 56(4):675–681

Kasal DA, Barhoumi T, Li MW, Yamamoto N, Zdanovich E, Rehman A et al (2012) T regulatory lymphocytes prevent aldosterone-induced vascular injury. Hypertension 59(2):324–330

Katayama Y, Battista M, Kao W-M, Hidalgo A, Peired AJ, Thomas SA et al (2006) Signals from the sympathetic nervous system regulate hematopoietic stem cell egress from bone marrow. Cell 124(2):407–421

Keidar S, Hayek T, Kaplan M, Pavlotzky E, Hamoud S, Coleman R et al (2003) Effect of eplerenone, a selective aldosterone blocker, on blood pressure, serum and macrophage oxidative stress, and atherosclerosis in apolipoprotein E–deficient mice. J Cardiovasc Pharmacol 41(6):955–963

Kemp BA, Bell JF, Rottkamp DM, Howell NL, Shao W, Navar LG et al (2012) Intrarenal angiotensin III is the predominant agonist for proximal tubule angiotensin type 2 receptors. Hypertension 60(2):387–395

Kielstein JT, Impraim B, Simmel S, Bode-Böger SM, Tsikas D, Frölich JC et al (2004) Cardiovascular effects of systemic nitric oxide synthase inhibition with asymmetrical dimethylarginine in humans. Circulation 109(2):172–177

Kim S, Zingler M, Harrison JK, Scott EW, Cogle CR, Luo D et al (2016) Angiotensin II regulation of proliferation, differentiation, and engraftment of hematopoietic stem cells. Hypertension 67(3):574–584

Kirabo A, Fontana V, de Faria APC, Loperena R, Galindo CL, Wu J et al (2014) DC isoketal-modified proteins activate T cells and promote hypertension. J Clin Invest 124(10):4642–4656

Ko EA, Amiri F, Pandey NR, Javeshghani D, Leibovitz E, Touyz RM et al (2007) Resistance artery remodeling in deoxycorticosterone acetate-salt hypertension is dependent on vascular inflammation: evidence from m-CSF-deficient mice. Am J Physiol Heart Circ Physiol 292(4):H1789–H1795

Kobori H, Nangaku M, Navar LG, Nishiyama A (2007) The intrarenal renin-angiotensin system: from physiology to the pathobiology of hypertension and kidney disease. Pharmacol Rev 59(3):251–287

Lankhorst S, Danser AHJ, van den Meiracker AH (2016) Endothelin-1 and antiangiogenesis. Am J Physiol Regul Integr Comp Physiol 310(3):R230–R234

Lautner RQ, Villela DC, Fraga-Silva RA, Silva N, Verano-Braga T, Costa-Fraga F et al (2013) Discovery and characterization of alamandine: a novel component of the renin-angiotensin system. Circ Res 112 (8):1104–1111

Lee DL, Sturgis LC, Labazi H, Osborne JB, Fleming C, Pollock JS et al (2006) Angiotensin II hypertension is attenuated in interleukin-6 knockout mice. Am J Physiol Heart Circ Physiol 290(3):H935–H940

Leiper J, Nandi M, Torondel B, Murray-Rust J, Malaki M, O'Hara B et al (2007) Disruption of methylarginine metabolism impairs vascular homeostasis. Nat Med 13 (2):198–203

Li K, Guo D, Zhu H, Hering-Smith KS, Hamm LL, Ouyang J et al (2010) Interleukin-6 stimulates epithelial sodium channels in mouse cortical collecting duct cells. Am J Physiol Regul Integr Comp Physiol 299 (2):R590–R595

Li F, Hagaman JR, Kim H-S, Maeda N, Jennette JC, Faber JE et al (2012) eNOS deficiency acts through endothelin to aggravate sFlt-1-induced pre-eclampsia-like phenotype. J Am Soc Nephrol 23(4):652–660

Liang C-F, Liu JT, Wang Y, Xu A, Vanhoutte PM (2013) Toll-like receptor 4 mutation protects obese mice against endothelial dysfunction by decreasing NADPH oxidase isoforms 1 and 4. Arterioscler Thromb Vasc Biol 33(4):777–784

Lother A, Hein L (2016) Vascular mineralocorticoid receptors: linking risk factors, hypertension, and heart disease. Hypertension 68(1):6–10

Lucas D, Bruns I, Battista M, Méndez-Ferrer S, Magnon C, Kunisaki Y et al (2012) Norepinephrine reuptake inhibition promotes mobilization in mice: potential impact to rescue low stem cell yields. Blood 119(17):3962–3965

Luther JM, Gainer JV, Murphey LJ, Yu C, Vaughan DE, Morrow JD et al (2006) Angiotensin II induces interleukin-6 in humans through a mineralocorticoid receptor-dependent mechanism. Hypertension 48 (6):1050–1057

MacDonald TM, Williams B, Caulfield M, Cruickshank JK, McInnes G, Sever P et al (2015) Monotherapy versus dual therapy for the initial treatment of hypertension (PATHWAY-1): a randomised double-blind controlled trial: Figure 1. BMJ Open 5(8): e007645

Madhur MS, Lob HE, McCann LA, Iwakura Y, Blinder Y, Guzik TJ et al (2010) Interleukin 17 promotes angiotensin II-induced hypertension and vascular dysfunction. Hypertension 55(2):500–507

Marc Y, Llorens-Cortes C (2011) The role of the brain renin–angiotensin system in hypertension: implications for new treatment. Prog Neurobiol 95(2):89–103

Marvar PJ, Thabet SR, Guzik TJ, Lob HE, McCann LA, Weyand C et al (2010) Central and peripheral mechanisms of T-lymphocyte activation and vascular inflammation produced by angiotensin II-induced hypertension. Circ Res 107(2):263–270

Masson GS, Nair AR, Silva Soares PP, Michelini LC, Francis J (2015) Aerobic training normalizes autonomic dysfunction, HMGB1 content, microglia activation and inflammation in hypothalamic paraventricular nucleus of SHR. Am J Physiol Heart Circ Physiol 309(7):H1115–H1122

Mattson DL, Lund H, Guo C, Rudemiller N, Geurts AM, Jacob H (2013) Genetic mutation of recombination activating gene 1 in Dahl salt-sensitive rats attenuates hypertension and renal damage. Am J Physiol Regul Integr Comp Physiol 304(6):R407–R414

Matzinger P (2002) The danger model: a renewed sense of self. Science 296(5566):301–305

McCarthy CG, Goulopoulou S, Wenceslau CF, Spitler K, Matsumoto T, Webb RC (2014) Toll-like receptors and damage-associated molecular patterns: novel links between inflammation and hypertension. Am J Physiol Heart Circ Physiol 306(2):H184–H196

McCurley A, Jaffe IZ (2012) Mineralocorticoid receptors in vascular function and disease. Mol Cell Endocrinol 350(2):256–265

McMaster WG, Kirabo A, Madhur MS, Harrison DG (2015) Inflammation, immunity, and hypertensive end-organ damage. Circ Res 116(6):1022–1033

Meinitzer A, Seelhorst U, Wellnitz B, Halwachs-Baumann G, Boehm BO, Winkelmann BR et al (2007) Asymmetrical dimethylarginine independently predicts total and cardiovascular mortality in individuals with angiographic coronary artery disease (the Ludwigshafen Risk and Cardiovascular Health study). Clin Chem 53(2):273–283

Méndez-Ferrer S, Lucas D, Battista M, Frenette PS (2008) Haematopoietic stem cell release is regulated by circadian oscillations. Nature 452(7186):442–447

Mendoza-Torres E, Oyarzún A, Mondaca-Ruff D, Azocar A, Castro PF, Jalil JE et al (2015) ACE2 and vasoactive peptides: novel players in cardiovascular/renal remodeling and hypertension. Ther Adv Cardiovasc Dis 9(4):217–237

Miyashita H, Chikazawa M, Otaki N, Hioki Y, Shimozu Y, Nakashima F et al (2014) Lysine pyrrolation is a naturally-occurring covalent modification involved in the production of DNA mimic proteins. Sci Rep 4:5343

Muller DN, Shagdarsuren E, Park J-K, Dechend R, Mervaala E, Hampich F et al (2002) Immunosuppressive treatment protects against angiotensin II-induced renal damage. Am J Pathol 161(5):1679–1693

Napoli C, Sica V, de Nigris F, Pignalosa O, Condorelli M, Ignarro LJ et al (2004) Sulfhydryl angiotensin-converting enzyme inhibition induces sustained reduction of systemic oxidative stress and improves the nitric oxide pathway in patients with essential hypertension. Am Heart J 148(1):172

Newfell BG, Iyer LK, Mohammad NN, McGraw AP, Ehsan A, Rosano G et al (2011) Aldosterone regulates vascular gene transcription via oxidative stress-dependent and -independent pathways. Arterioscler Thromb Vasc Biol 31(8):1871–1880

Nishiyama A, Abe Y (2004) Aldosterone and renal injury. Folia Pharmacol Jpn 124(2):101–109

Oka T, Hikoso S, Yamaguchi O, Taneike M, Takeda T, Tamai T et al (2012) Mitochondrial DNA that escapes from autophagy causes inflammation and heart failure. Nature 485(7397):251–255

Olsen F (1970) Type and course of the inflammatory cellular reaction in acute angiotensin-hypertensive vascular disease in rats. Acta Pathol Microbiol Scand A 78(2):143–150

Perticone F, Sciacqua A, Maio R, Perticone M, Maas R, Böger RH et al (2005) Asymmetric dimethylarginine, L-arginine, and endothelial dysfunction in essential hypertension. J Am Coll Cardiol 46(3):518–523

Piazza M, Taiakina V, Guillemette SR, Guillemette JG, Dieckmann T (2014) Solution structure of calmodulin bound to the target peptide of endothelial nitric oxide synthase phosphorylated at Thr495. Biochemistry 53 (8):1241–1249

Purcell ES, Wood GW, Gattone VH (1993) Immune system of the spontaneously hypertensive rat: II. Morphology and function. Anat Rec 237(2):236–242

Rocha R, Martin-Berger CL, Yang P, Scherrer R, Delyani J, McMahon E (2002) Selective aldosterone blockade prevents angiotensin II/salt-induced vascular inflammation in the rat heart. Endocrinology 143 (12):4828–4836

Santisteban MM, Ahmari N, Carvajal JM, Zingler MB, Qi Y, Kim S et al (2015) Involvement of bone marrow cells and neuroinflammation in hypertension. Circ Res 117(2):178–191

Santos RAS, Silva ACS, Maric C, Silva DMR, Machado RP, de Buhr I et al (2003) Angiotensin-(1–7) is an endogenous ligand for the G protein-coupled receptor Mas. Proc Natl Acad Sci 100(14):8258–8263

Sanz-Rosa D, Oubiña MP, Cediel E, Heras N de L, Aragoncillo P, Balfagón G, et al (2005) Eplerenone reduces oxidative stress and enhances eNOS in SHR: vascular functional and structural consequences. Antioxidants & Redox Signaling. Mary Ann Liebert, Inc. 2 Madison Avenue Larchmont, NY 10538 USA 7 (9–10):1294–1301

Satou R, Miyata K, Gonzalez-Villalobos RA, Ingelfinger JR, Navar LG, Kobori H (2012) Interferon-γ biphasically regulates angiotensinogen expression via a JAK-STAT pathway and suppressor of cytokine signaling 1 (SOCS1) in renal proximal tubular cells. FASEB J 26(5):1821–1830

Scheiermann C, Kunisaki Y, Frenette PS (2013) Circadian control of the immune system. Nat Rev Immunol 13(3):190–198

Schnabel R, Blankenberg S, Lubos E, Lackner KJ, Rupprecht HJ, Espinola-Klein C et al (2005) Asymmetric dimethylarginine and the risk of cardiovascular events and death in patients with coronary artery disease: results from the AtheroGene Study. Circ Res 97 (5):e53–e59

Serg M, Kampus P, Kals J, Zagura M, Muda P, Tuomainen T-P et al (2011) Association between asymmetric dimethylarginine and indices of vascular function in patients with essential hypertension. Blood Press 20(2):111–116

Sevá Pessôa B, van der Lubbe N, Verdonk K, Roks AJM, Hoorn EJ, Danser AHJ (2012) Key developments in renin–angiotensin–aldosterone system inhibition. Nat Rev Nephrol 9(1):26–36

Shen BQ, Lee DY, Zioncheck TF (1999) Vascular endothelial growth factor governs endothelial nitric-oxide synthase expression via a KDR/Flk-1 receptor and a protein kinase C signaling pathway. J Biol Chem 274 (46):33057–33063

Shi P, Diez-Freire C, Jun JY, Qi Y, Katovich MJ, Li Q et al (2010) Brain microglial cytokines in neurogenic hypertension. Hypertension 56(2):297–303

Shi P, Grobe JL, Desland FA, Zhou G, Shen XZ, Shan Z et al (2014) Direct pro-inflammatory effects of prorenin on microglia. Block ML, editor. PLoS ONE 9(10):e92937

Singh MV, Abboud FM (2014) Toll-like receptors and hypertension. Am J Physiol Regul Integr Comp Physiol 307(5):R501–R504

Slota C, Shi A, Chen G, Bevans M, Weng N-P (2015) Norepinephrine preferentially modulates memory CD8 T cell function inducing inflammatory cytokine production and reducing proliferation in response to activation. Brain Behav Immun 46:168–179

Song X-A, Jia L-L, Cui W, Zhang M, Chen W, Yuan Z-Y et al (2014) Inhibition of TNF-α in hypothalamic paraventricular nucleus attenuates hypertension and cardiac hypertrophy by inhibiting neurohormonal excitation in spontaneously hypertensive rats. Toxicol Appl Pharmacol 281(1):101–108

Spiegel A, Shivtiel S, Kalinkovich A, Ludin A, Netzer N, Goichberg P et al (2007) Catecholaminergic neurotransmitters regulate migration and repopulation of immature human CD34+ cells through Wnt signaling. Nat Immunol 8(10):1123–1131

Sriramula S, Cardinale JP, Francis J (2013) Inhibition of TNF in the brain reverses alterations in RAS components and attenuates angiotensin II-induced hypertension. Bonini MG, editor. PLoS ONE. Public Library of Science 8(5):e63847

Surdacki A, Nowicki M, Sandmann J, Tsikas D, Boeger RH, Bode-Boeger SM et al (1999) Reduced urinary excretion of nitric oxide metabolites and increased plasma levels of asymmetric dimethylarginine in men with essential hypertension. J Cardiovasc Pharmacol 33 (4):652–658

Swirski FK, Nahrendorf M, Etzrodt M, Wildgruber M, Cortez-Retamozo V, Panizzi P et al (2009) Identification of splenic reservoir monocytes and their deployment to inflammatory sites. Science 325 (5940):612–616

Takamura Y, Shimokawa H, Zhao H, Igarashi H, Egashira K, Takeshita A (1999) Important role of endothelium-derived hyperpolarizing factor in shear stress-induced endothelium-dependent relaxations in the rat mesenteric artery. J Cardiovasc Pharmacol 34 (3):381–387

Takeichi N, Boone CW (1976) Spontaneous rosette formation of rat thymus cells with guinea pig erythrocytes. Cell Immunol 27(1):52–59

Takeichi N, Hamada J, Takimoto M, Fujiwara K, Kobayashi H (1988) Depression of T cell-mediated immunity and enhancement of autoantibody production by natural infection with microorganisms in spontaneously hypertensive rats (SHR). Microbiol Immunol 32(12):1235–1244

Tanaka M, Tsuchida S, Imai T, Fujii N, Miyazaki H, Ichiki T et al (1999) Vascular response to angiotensin II is exaggerated through an upregulation of AT1 receptor in AT2 knockout mice. Biochem Biophys Res Commun 258(1):194–198

Te Riet L, van Esch JHM, Roks AJM, van den Meiracker AH, Danser AHJ (2015) Hypertension: renin-angiotensin-aldosterone system alterations. Circ Res 116(6):960–975

Theodora Szasz GFB (2013) The Toll way to hypertension: role of the innate immune response. Endocrinol Metab Synd 02(02)

Trott DW, Thabet SR, Kirabo A, Saleh MA, Itani H, Norlander AE et al (2014) Oligoclonal CD8+ T cells play a critical role in the development of hypertension. Hypertension 64(5):1108–1115

Tsutsumi Y, Matsubara H, Masaki H, Kurihara H, Murasawa S, Takai S et al (1999) Angiotensin II type 2 receptor overexpression activates the vascular kinin system and causes vasodilation. J Clin Invest 104(7):925–935

Udelson JE, Feldman AM, Greenberg B, Pitt B, Mukherjee R, Solomon HA et al (2010) Randomized, double-blind, multicenter, placebo-controlled study evaluating the effect of aldosterone antagonism with eplerenone on ventricular remodeling in patients with mild-to-moderate heart failure and left ventricular systolic dysfunction. Circ Heart Fail 3 (3):347–353

Vallance P, Leiper J (2004) Cardiovascular biology of the asymmetric dimethylarginine:dimethylarginine dimethylaminohydrolase pathway. Arterioscler Thromb Vasc Biol 24(6):1023–1030

Vallance P, Leone A, Calver A, Collier J, Moncada S (1992) Accumulation of an endogenous inhibitor of nitric oxide synthesis in chronic renal failure. Lancet 339(8793):572–575

van den Meiracker AH, Danser AHJ (2016) Mechanisms of hypertension and renal injury during vascular endothelial growth factor signaling inhibition. Hypertension 68(1):17–23

Vázquez-Oliva G, Fernández-Real JM, Zamora A, Vilaseca M, Badimón L (2005) Lowering of blood pressure leads to decreased circulating interleukin-6 in hypertensive subjects. J Hum Hypertens 19 (6):457–462

Villela DC, Passos-Silva DG, Santos RAS (2014) Alamandine: a new member of the angiotensin family. Curr Opin Nephrol Hypertens 23(2):130–134

Wagenaar GTM, Laghmani EH, Fidder M, Sengers RMA, de Visser YP, de Vries L et al (2013) Agonists of MAS oncogene and angiotensin II type 2 receptors attenuate cardiopulmonary disease in rats with neonatal hyperoxia-induced lung injury. Am J Physiol Lung Cell Mol Physiol 305(5):L341–L351

Waki H, Hendy EB, Hindmarch CCT, Gouraud S, Toward M, Kasparov S et al (2013) Excessive leukotriene B4 in nucleus tractus solitarii is prohypertensive in spontaneously hypertensive rats. Hypertension 61 (1):194–201

Warnholtz A, Ostad MA, Heitzer T, Thuneke F, Fröhlich M, Tschentscher P et al (2007) AT1-receptor blockade with irbesartan improves peripheral but not coronary endothelial dysfunction in patients with stable coronary artery disease. Atherosclerosis 194 (2):439–445

Wei S-G, Yu Y, Zhang Z-H, Felder RB (2015) Proinflammatory cytokines upregulate sympathoexcitatory mechanisms in the subfornical organ of the rat. Hypertension 65(5):1126–1133

Wenzel P, Knorr M, Kossmann S, Stratmann J, Hausding M, Schuhmacher S et al (2011) Lysozyme M-positive monocytes mediate angiotensin II-induced arterial hypertension and vascular dysfunction. Circulation 124(12):1370–1381

White FN, Grollman A (1964) Autoimmune factors associated with infarction of the kidney. Nephron 1:93–102

Wright JW, Tamura-Myers E, Wilson WL, Roques BP, Llorens-Cortes C, Speth RC et al (2003) Conversion of brain angiotensin II to angiotensin III is critical for pressor response in rats. Am J Physiol Regul Integr Comp Physiol 284(3):R725–R733

Wu J, Thabet SR, Kirabo A, Trott DW, Saleh MA, Xiao L et al (2014) Inflammation and mechanical stretch promote aortic stiffening in hypertension through activation of p38 mitogen-activated protein kinase. Circ Res 114(4):616–625

Xiao L, Kirabo A, Wu J, Saleh MA, Zhu L, Wang F et al (2015) Renal denervation prevents immune cell activation and renal inflammation in angiotensin II-induced hypertension. Circ Res 117(6):547–557

Xuan C, Lun L-M, Zhao J-X, Wang H-W, Wang J, Ning C-P et al (2015) L-citrulline for protection of endothelial function from ADMA–induced injury in porcine coronary artery. Sci Rep 5:10987

Xue B, Thunhorst RL, Yu Y, Guo F, Beltz TG, Felder RB et al (2016) Central renin-angiotensin system activation and inflammation induced by high-fat diet sensitize angiotensin II-elicited hypertension. Hypertension 67(1):163–170

Young CN, Davisson RL (2015) Angiotensin-II, the brain, and hypertension. Hypertension 66 (5):920–926

Zhang Q, Raoof M, Chen Y, Sumi Y, Sursal T, Junger W et al (2010) Circulating mitochondrial DAMPs cause inflammatory responses to injury. Nature 464 (7285):104–107

Zubcevic J, Jun JY, Kim S, Perez PD, Afzal A, Shan Z et al (2014) Altered inflammatory response is associated with an impaired autonomic input to the bone marrow in the spontaneously hypertensive rat. Hypertension 63(3):542–550

Adv Exp Med Biol - Advances in Internal Medicine (2017) 2: 37–59
DOI 10.1007/5584_2016_169
© Springer International Publishing AG 2016
Published online: 19 November 2016

Pathophysiological Mechanisms and Correlates of Therapeutic Pharmacological Interventions in Essential Arterial Hypertension

Francesco Maranta, Roberto Spoladore, and Gabriele Fragasso

Abstract

Treating arterial hypertension (HT) remains a hard task. The hypertensive patient is often a subject with several comorbidities and metabolic abnormalities. Clinicians everyday have to choose the right drug for the single patient among the different classes of antihypertensives. Apart from lowering blood pressure, a main therapeutic target should be that of counteracting all the possible pathophysiological mechanisms involved in HT itself and in existing/potential comorbidities. All the ancillary positive and negative effects of the administered drugs should be considered: in particular, since hypertensive patients are often glucose intolerant/diabetic, carrier of serum lipids disorder, have already developed atherosclerotic diseases and endothelial dysfunction, they should not be treated with drugs negatively interfering with these conditions but with molecules that, if possible, improve them. The main pathophysiological mechanisms and correlates of therapeutic pharmacological interventions in essential HT are reviewed here.

Keywords

Hypertension • Therapy • Pathophysiology • ACE-inhibition • RAAS inhibition • Beta-blockers • Thiazides diuretics • Metabolic syndrome • Side effects • Hyperglycemia

1   Introduction

Arterial hypertension (HT) is one of the most frequent cardiovascular diseases that physicians have to face during their routine clinical activity.

F. Maranta, R. Spoladore, and G. Fragasso (✉)
Clinical Cardiology, Heart Failure Unit, IRCCS San Raffaele Scientific Institute, Milan, Italy
e-mail: fragasso.gabriele@hsr.it

Even if official guidelines are regularly issued by several societies and organizations, treating HT remains a hard task. Clinicians have to choose the right drug for the individual patient trying to stay within the guidelines and considering at the same time the comorbidities and the pathophysiological mechanisms at the base of HT in that specific case (Fragasso et al. 2012). Recently the situation has become more complex owing to the fact that, after a long period, multiple guidelines, scientific statements and consensus documents have been published: although they are endorsed by highly regarded organizations, they follow different processes for development, transparency, objectives and several central recommendations (Ripley and Baumert 2016). The discordance among different guidelines and documents has led to more uncertainty than clarity, being source of intense debate. There are, among the others, differences in the drugs recommended for initial treatment strategies: in particular, some guidelines (e.g. those by the European Society of Cardiology, ESC (Mancia et al. 2013)), differently from the others, consider all the pharmacological classes suitable for the initiation of antihypertensive treatment and indicate that preference should be given to some agents only in specific conditions (e.g. concomitant heart failure -HF-, coronary artery disease -CAD-). It should be considered that significant ancillary effects of different drug classes may be important from a pathophysiological point of view but these additional effects are usually not taken into account by institutional guidelines, since these are mostly focused on the demonstration of hard endpoints reduction. Moreover, it should be noted that the hypertensive patient is often a subject with concomitant cardiovascular conditions (e.g. dyslipidemia, diabetes…) and comorbidities that require special attention to define the best therapy.

In this chapter, the main antihypertensive pharmacological interventions will be described in the light of the common pathophysiological mechanisms at the base of HT; additional positive and negative effects of the administered drugs will also be addressed to provide an overview of the elements that should be considered trying to define the proper therapy in each individual patient.

2 Brief Review of the Mechanisms of Arterial Hypertension

A more detailed description of the pathophysiological alterations at the base of HT is far from the aim of this chapter; here we review the principal elements necessary to initiate pharmacological interventions. Blood pressure is the product of cardiac output and peripheral vascular resistance: despite this simple physiological definition, its level is determined by many physiological systems that are connected by complex interactions.

HT is generally classified as primary (essential) or secondary. HT is defined secondary when a clear cause (such as a renal or endocrine disorder) can be identified. On the contrary, essential HT, that represents the majority of cases, can be described as multifactorial in origin: basically there are multiple interactions between genetic and environmental factors that influence blood pressure through several mechanisms, that are known only in part. The main pathophysiological elements described are an increased adrenergic tone, an over-activation of the renin/angiotensin/aldosterone system (RAAS) and renal-adrenal mechanisms (with differences in patients with low and high renin HT) with sodium retention (Laragh and Sealey 1991; Brunner et al. 1973). Fundamentally, essential HT can be described as a primitive defect in renal excretion of sodium and/or an excessive rise of vascular tone that cannot be ascribed to single mechanisms but that has to be considered as the result of many factors affecting catecholamine and sodium homeostasis (Mendlowitz et al. 1964). The different factors involved can influence each other: in particular, the overactive sympathetic nervous system further activates the RAAS system and influences the ability of the kidneys to excrete sodium (favoring also water retention and blood volume elevation) (Mancia et al. 2006). Similarly, the peripheral vascular resistances are increased because of altered autonomic regulation, increased RAAS activity level, as well as structural alterations of arterial vessels. Resistance arteries might have an important role in the development of HT and its complications (Bohlen 1986): recent studies have shown that the media-lumen ratio of small arteries has a prognostic value for cardiovascular events in hypertensive patients (Park and Schiffrin 2001). Moreover, altered vascular integrity determines endothelial dysfunction: impaired endothelium-dependent vasorelaxation has been observed in patients with essential HT (Panza et al. 1993) and in several animal models. It is clearly established that endothelial dysfunction is an important prognostic factor for the development of atherosclerosis and cardiovascular events (Modena et al. 2002). Antihypertensive drugs trying to favorably affect outcomes in HT should be able to counteract the multiple known mechanisms that sustain increased blood pressure, to possibly induce vascular structural reverse remodeling and to exert a positive effect on impaired endothelial dysfunction.

Several other derived and/or correlated factors can also be present and contribute to the pathogenesis and morbidity associated with essential HT: among them, insulin resistance, lipid metabolism abnormalities and, in general, metabolic syndrome. These also represent part of the basic factors involved in the risk for the development of CAD and, in general, have a great prognostic weight; therefore, when treating the hypertensive patient, their control is a major target. Moreover, it should never be forgotten that, usually, clinical practice has to face subjects with a complex health status due to many different comorbidities (not only cardiovascular or metabolic).

3 Diuretics

The increase in blood volume is an important pathophysiological element present in many forms of HT, which in turn increases cardiac output by the Frank-Starling relationship. For this reason, diuretics, which enhance the removal of sodium and water by the kidneys and thereby decrease blood volume, can exert a clear antihypertensive effect, as shown in many studies. It should be noted, on the other hand, that the exact mechanism for reduction of blood pressure by diuretics is not yet completely understood: extracellular volume reduction is first observed, followed by decrease of vascular resistance (Bennett et al. 1977; Freis 1983). To explain this latter mechanism it has been hypothesized that diuretics may have an independent direct effect on vascular smooth muscle, but this has not been confirmed by substantial data. It has also been proposed that the persistent small reduction in body sodium might decrease the interstitial fluid volume and that a reduced smooth muscle cell sodium concentration could secondarily reduce intracellular calcium concentration, modifying cells reactivity to contractile stimuli (Insel and Motulsky 1984). On the other side, it should be considered that diuretics cause a reactive increase in sympathetic and RAAS activity, following their initial effect, resulting in opposed vasoconstriction and reduced sodium loss and enhancing side metabolic effects of these agents (Grassi et al. 2003; Burnier and Brunner 1992).

Among diuretics, thiazides are the most commonly used agents for HT treatment. Thiazides act inhibiting the sodium-chloride transporter in the distal part of the nephron and they are particularly different from the loop diuretics not only because of the site of action but also for their longer duration of action: a prolonged natriuretic effect better counteracts sodium retention and this is a crucial aspect to achieve some persistent volume depletion.

Thiazide diuretics have been the mainstay of antihypertensive treatment for almost 40 years, since the first Joint National Committee (JNC) report in the late seventies; in JNC 7 (2003) they were still suggested as the initial therapy in most patients with HT (Chobanian et al. 2003). Diuretics have also been confirmed as a first-line choice in the last European Society of Cardiology (ESC) HT guidelines (Mancia et al. 2013), JNC 8 (James et al. 2014) and in the statement by the American Society of Hypertension and the International Society of

Hypertension (ASH/ISH) (Weber et al. 2014), where they are particularly recommended in older adults and in black patients. Recently, some molecules have been distinguished from hydrochlorothiazide (HCTZ) and standard thiazides: among these thiazide-like agents, chlorthalidone and indapamide, in particular, are preferred to conventional diuretics by NICE guidelines (National Institute for Health and Clinical Excellence, http://www.nice.org.uk/guidance/cg127). This point has been a matter of great debate: even if the evidence about clinical outcomes benefits seems stronger for the thiazide-like diuretics, the latest ESC guidelines underlined that a real recommendation can not be given in favor of a specific drug from the available data, especially when considering the lack of randomized head-to-head comparisons (Mancia et al. 2013).

The main data supporting the use of diuretics in HT come from the ALLHAT (Antihypertensive and Lipid-Lowering Treatment to Prevent Heart Attack Trial) (Davis et al. 1996), the SHEP (Systolic Hypertension in the Elderly Program) (Kostis et al. 2005) and the HYVET (Hypertension in the Very Elderly Trial) studies (Beckett et al. 2008). The ALLHAT, in particular, was a randomized, double-blind trial designed to determine whether treatment with amlodipine (a calcium channel blocker, CCB), lisinopril (an ACE-inhibitor, ACE-I) or an alpha-adrenergic blocker (doxazosin) reduced the incidence of fatal CAD and nonfatal myocardial infarction more than chlorthalidone in high-risk hypertensive patients; secondary end-points were all-cause mortality and major cardiovascular events, including congestive heart failure (HF). Results showed no significant differences in primary outcome between the drugs; however, there were differences in secondary outcomes (not in mortality): compared with chlorthalidone, new-onset HF occurred more frequently in patients randomized to the other pharmacological strategies (ALLHAT Collaborative Research Group 2000; ALLHAT Officers and Coordinators for the ALLHAT Collaborative Research Group 2002). Certainly, these results and the real value of the ALLHAT study have

been widely debated, receiving several criticisms (Messerli 2001; Weber 2003). Among the others, it should be noted that diuretic therapy was withdrawn in several patients at the time of enrollment (>90 % of patients were on antihypertensive therapy before entering the study): many of them had a history of previous myocardial infarction or hypertensive cardiomyopathy and withdrawal of diuretics in such patients could have increased the risk of developing HF. Moreover, even if data from the initial major outcome trials showed that thiazides globally improved prognosis in hypertensive patients, subsequent studies showed that their association with an ACE-I was less effective in reducing cardiovascular events than the association of the same ACE-I with a CCB (Jamerson et al. 2008): these data should be taken into account, even though coming from one isolated trial that needs further replication.

Apart from all the possible considerations about outcomes data, a main point to take into account is that thiazides may potentially cause several vascular and metabolic abnormalities that negatively influence the global cardiovascular risk. Since thiazides inhibit the reabsorption of sodium in the early distal tubule, more sodium reaches the most distal part of the nephron and stimulates the exchange with potassium by aldosterone-sensitive transporters (that are particularly active in the presence of an activated RAAS): for this reason, hypokalemia can be precipitated (Zillich et al. 2006; Shafi et al. 2008), enhancing the risk of arrhythmias. The incidence of hypokalemia can be reduced by the use of low doses of diuretic and by the combination with potassium-retaining agents (e.g. ACE-I). Similar observations have been done also for hypomagnesemia, even if usual doses of diuretics rarely cause magnesium deficiency (Wilcox 1999). Studies have shown that thiazides decrease urate excretion, with the risk of increasing blood uric acid, possibly causing gout in predisposed subjects (for which only low doses should be used) (Reungjui et al. 2008; Franse et al. 2000). Calcium retention might also happen and produce hypercalcemia: this can have a positive effect in older adults, reducing the risk of fractures due to osteoporosis (LaCroix et al. 1990), but can be harmful in hyper-parathyroid patients.

Additional important side effects of diuretics involve lipid and glucose metabolism. Data coming from several trials show that thiazides cause changes in blood lipids: total and low-density lipoprotein (LDL) cholesterol and triglycerides seem to increase in relation to diuretic dose (Kasiske et al. 1995); moreover, even if total cholesterol level does not change, the ratio of apolipoprotein B to A might rise and high-density lipoprotein (HDL) cholesterol could be reduced (Lindholm et al. 2003). From a practical point of view, it is advisable to monitor blood lipids during diuretic therapy and to recommend a low-fat diet. Among the others, indapamide seems to have no/small effects on lipid profile (Ames 1996).

Impaired insulin-sensitivity and the risk of new onset diabetes are other recognized critical points of thiazides (Ferrari et al. 1991; Eriksson et al. 2008; Gupta et al. 2008). In the ALLHAT trial the thiazide-treated group compared with the other treatment groups showed a significant increase in incidence of diabetes; this increment apparently was not associated to increased mortality (Whelton et al. 2005). Similar results were found in the SHEP trial, comparing chlorthalidone with placebo (Kostis et al. 2005). For this reason, some Authors have suggested that thiazides as initial therapy for hypertension might achieve superior cardiovascular disease outcomes in older hypertensive patients even with the metabolic syndrome, as compared with treatment with CCBs and ACE-Is (ALLHAT Officers and Coordinators for the ALLHAT Collaborative Research Group 2002), and that the effects on glucose homeostasis may depend only from the use of higher doses (ALLHAT Collaborative Research Group 2000). It should be considered, however, that the follow-up of these trials was conducted for a limited period of time while HT is usually diagnosed in middle-aged patients and, therefore, the course of the disease (and therapy) may last for 25–30 years: it can be surmised that a relatively short study period might not be enough to determine with adequate predictive value the outcomes for a disease of longer duration, when the secondary effects of therapies on cardiovascular risk factors could become manifest. The issue of long-term consequences of thiazides appears even more important when considering that HT and metabolic syndrome are rampant and increasing numbers of adolescents are developing obesity and HT. Hyperuricemia and hypokalemia may also contribute to the exacerbation of the metabolic syndrome in response to thiazides, creating a vicious circle (Burnier and Brunner 1992). In any case, the potential diabetogenic effect of diuretics is still a matter of great debate and further research is needed (Carter et al. 2008). In addition to these problematic aspects, it has been observed that thiazides do not reduce vascular oxidative stress and do not improve endothelial dysfunction (Zhou et al. 2008).

In the light of all the facts presented, it seems that diuretics have no pleiotropic vasoprotective effects beyond lowering blood pressure. Furthermore, when administered in animal model in combination with an ACE-I, thiazides were shown to abolish the anti-atherosclerotic effect of the latter; it is unknown whether this also applies to humans (Fonseca et al. 2003). It should be noted that many side and metabolic effects are dose dependent: in fact, since it has been shown that lower doses of diuretics achieve a blood pressure reduction similar to the higher ones, the use of low-dose thiazide is an important point to reduce potential metabolic problems associated to this therapy.

It can be reasonably affirmed that, even if thiazides are still indicated as a possible first-line choice by most HT guidelines, several reservations and concerns exist in prescribing them as a first-line antihypertensive drug over the other agents, particularly in high-risk patients. Furthermore, quality of life (QOL) is an important issue when choosing drug therapies, especially considering that many hypertensive patients are asymptomatic and it would be unpleasant to create symptoms due to drug prescription: from this point of view diuretics have been consistently associated with low QOL, making their systematic prescription less

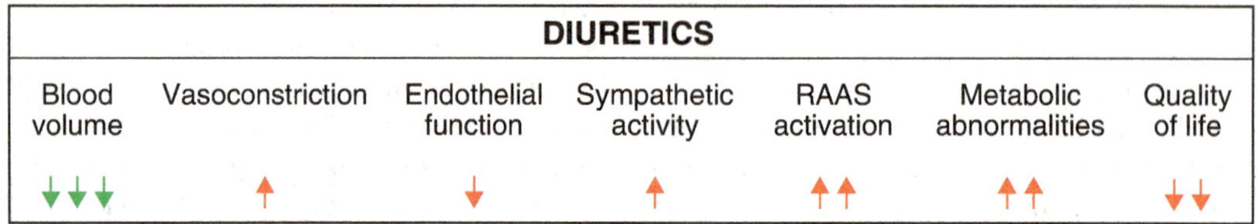

Fig. 1 Main pharmacological effects of diuretics on the single pathophysiological factors (*RAAS* Renin Angiotensin Aldosterone System, *Red/green arrow* negative/ positive effect, *Bidirectional flat arrow* neutral effect, Quantity of *upward/downward arrows*: *1* mild, *2* moderate, *3* great effect)

attractive than other approaches. Some data suggest that erectile dysfunction might be observed more commonly with thiazides than with other antihypertensive; this can be an important factor negatively influencing the QOL (Wassertheil-Smoller et al. 1992). Figure 1 summarizes the effects of diuretics on the principal mechanisms and correlates of HT.

Loop diuretics have less space in HT, unless they are administered for other indications (e.g. HF) in combination with other drugs. Thiazides become ineffective when renal function is severely impaired: even if this point has been recently questioned by a pilot study (Dussol et al. 2012), in this case thiazides could be replaced by loop diuretics.

Potassium-sparing diuretics have to be combined with another diuretic (e.g. amiloride with HCTZ) to exert an effective antihypertensive effect and this combination could be useful also to prevent diuretic-induced hypokalemia. Although they have never been tested in large studies (promising results come from small randomized trials, apart from HF trials) (Roush et al. 2016; Pitt et al. 1999), aldosterone receptor antagonists can be used as third/fourth line drugs in treating patients with resistant hypertension (Mancia et al. 2013; Dahal et al. 2015): this may be because aldosterone excess can contribute to resistant hypertension and some cases of primary aldosteronism might be undetected.

4　Beta-Blocking Agents

Present HT guidelines are not concordant on the role of beta-blockers (BBs). JNC 8 no longer recommends BBs for initial antihypertensive therapy (James et al. 2014); this confirms the previous JNC 7, that at the same time listed some compelling indications for the use of BBs in hypertensive patients with other cardiovascular diseases (e.g. HF or previous myocardial infarction) (Chobanian et al. 2003). Similarly, the NICE guidelines state that BBs are not a preferred initial treatment; exceptions are considered for patients intolerant to ACE-Is and angiotensin II receptors (ARBs), women of childbearing potential and people with evidence of increased sympathetic drive: apart from these conditions, BBs are relegated to fourth- or even fifth-line choices (National Institute for Health and Clinical Excellence, http://www.nice.org.uk/guidance/cg127). On the contrary, ESC guidelines do not exclude BBs as one of the options for fist-line antihypertensive pharmacological strategy (Mancia et al. 2013); similarly to JNC 7, European guidelines reported some suggested indications for the use of BBs and the other antihypertensive agents in specific conditions (see Table 1).

The beta-adrenergic signaling system acts through different receptors (Brodde et al. 2006). In brief, it should be taken into account that beta$_1$-adrenoreceptors are situated on the cardiac sarcolemma and their stimulation increases heart rate, the rate and force of myocardial contraction, the reuptake of cytosolic calcium (lusitropic effect) and the rate of conduction. Beta$_2$-receptors, on the other hand, are mainly located on bronchial and vascular smooth muscle cells, where they mediate the dilating effect of epinephrine; there is a significant proportion of beta$_2$-receptors also in the myocardium that might have additional inhibitory action modulating the level of adrenergic activation.

Table 1 Drugs to be preferred in specific conditions

Condition	Drug
Asymptomatic organ damage	
Renal dysfunction	ACE inhibitor, ARB
Clinical CV event	
Previous myocardial infarction	BB, ACE inhibitor, ARB
Angina pectoris	BB, CCB
Heart failure	Diuretic, BB, ACE inhibitor, ARB, mineralocorticoid receptor antagonist
Atrial fibrillation, ventricular rate control	BB, non-dihydropyridine CCB
Peripheral artery disease	ACE inhibitor, CCB
Other	
Metabolic syndrome	ACE inhibitor, ARB, CCB
Diabetes mellitus	ACE inhibitor, ARB

Adapted from ESC guidelines
ACE angiotensin-converting enzyme, *ARB* angiotensin receptor blocker, *BB* beta-blocker, *CCB* calcium channel blocker, *CV* cardiovascular

Beta$_3$-receptors are a more recently recognized type of beta-receptor that have been found in many tissues: even if their specific role remains to be fully elucidated, they appear to be involved, among the others, in the control of thermogenesis and urinary bladder relaxation (Balligand 2013). A main cardiovascular effect of beta$_3$-receptors seems to be the endothelium-dependent vasorelaxation by production of nitric oxide. Moreover, even if further research is needed, there are some evidences that these receptors may have a cardioprotective role in myocardial hypertrophy and HF, counteracting the known adverse effects of beta$_1$ and beta$_2$ overactivation and modulating left ventricular relaxation and inotropism (Balligand 2013).

BBs have several antihypertensive mechanisms: along with their chronotropic and inotropic negative effects that reduce cardiac output, they exert central adrenergic inhibition and decrease the renal release of renin (negatively influencing also the activity of RAAS). At the beginning, these mechanisms do not lead to a significant fall in blood pressure, since there is a reflex increase in peripheral vascular resistance with tendency to normotension: alfa-adrenergic vasoconstriction, in particular, is not properly counteracted by the vasodilator component of epinephrine because of the vascular beta$_2$ blockade (Vatner and Hintze 1983). A later action of BBs on prejunctional receptors of the sympathetic terminal neurons inhibits the release of norepinephrine, possibly explaining the subsequent reduction of peripheral resistance and late antihypertensive effect. BBs retaining a vasodilatory property (see ensuing paragraph) determine an early decrease in vascular resistance and blood pressure. Additionally, like most other antihypertensive agents, beta-blockers probably also lower blood pressure through interference with a not yet identified vasoconstrictor mechanism (Man in't Veld et al. 1988). Apparently, no significant effect on circulating blood volume is exerted (Weidmann et al. 1976). In relation to RAAS activation, BBs have been shown to yield either a neutral (Balansard et al. 1977; Fagard et al. 1976) or a mildly inhibitory effect (Ishizaki et al. 1983; Pitkäjärvi et al. 1979), with apparently no relation with blood pressure fall.

According to their pharmacological characteristics, different subclasses of BBs can be distinguished. The first-generation molecules (e.g. propranolol) are non-selective agents, blocking beta$_1$ and beta$_2$ receptors. They have been superseded by cardioselective blockers (such as atenolol, metoprolol, bisoprolol): the greater β1 than β2 affinity is dose dependent and is less with higher doses. A third generation class of BBs is represented by agents with vasodilatory activity that depends by two main mechanisms: direct vasodilation mediated by the release of nitric oxide (as for nebivolol and carvedilol) (Chen et al. 2013) and additional alfa-blockade (as for labetalol and carvedilol). Some BBs (pindolol and acebutolol) have an intrinsic sympathomimetic activity, stimulating smooth muscle cells to relax. As described further in the text, vasodilating agents carry a better metabolic profile that might represent an added value in treating hypertensive patients.

As stated above, even if BBs have been commonly used as first-line treatment for HT, at present they have been downgraded in most guidelines since several evidences have questioned their efficacy in preventing death and cardiovascular outcomes. A first meta-analysis by Messerli et al. found that BBs were ineffective in preventing CAD, cardiovascular and all-cause mortality in comparison with diuretics in patients older than 60 years (Messerli et al. 1998). Another systematic review by Calberg et al., including 9 randomized clinical trials, showed that atenolol had a blood pressure-lowering effect similar to that of other antihypertensive drugs, but cardiovascular mortality and stroke were higher with atenolol (Messerli et al. 1998): these results were confirmed also by two subsequent larger meta-analysis evidencing that BBs are no better than any other antihypertensive at preventing heart attacks and are less effective at preventing strokes (Lindholm et al. 2005; Bradley et al. 2006). A more recent Cochrane meta-analysis, updating a previous one, was performed on 13 randomized controlled trials and reported that patients treated with BBs showed higher total mortality and more cardiovascular events than CCBs (not diuretics and RAAS blockers) and higher incidence of stroke than CCBs and RAAS inhibitors; the different classes of agents were found similar for CAD (Wiysonge et al. 2007). It should be underlined that in the majority of the studies included in the meta-analysis atenolol was the most used BB, therefore any extrapolation to other BBs should be done with caution: in particular, as addressed in the ensuing text, some limitations of the old BBs seem not to be shared by third-generation molecules (Ram 2010). Moreover, the Authors acknowledged the low quality of the available evidence. The main arguments supporting the fact that ESC guidelines did not exclude BBs from the first-line pharmacological options are similar to these observations: in general, it has been recognized that evidence against their use appeared to be mixed and globally not strong enough (Mancia et al. 2013). In fact, differently from the analysis presented above, another large meta-analysis on 147 trials showed that all classes of antihypertensive drugs had a similar effect in reducing myocardial infarction and stroke for a given reduction in blood pressure and, in particular, BBs were highly effective in preventing cardiovascular events in patients with recent myocardial infarction and HF (Law et al. 2009). Moreover, incidence of cardiovascular outcomes was found to be similar for BBs and other drugs in the revision of trials realized by the Blood Pressure Lowering Treatment Trialists' Collaboration, giving the message that reducing blood pressure is what apparently really counts (Czernichow et al. 2011). Nevertheless, as a consequence of all observations, several authorities consider that at present even if it would be incorrect to affirm that BBs have no effect in patients with primary HT, probably their effect should be considered suboptimal (Lindholm et al. 2005). BBs appear to be less effective than RAAS blockers and CCBs also in delaying or reverting hypertensive organ damage (e.g. left ventricular hypertrophy, arterial remodeling..). In any case, the importance of sympathetic nervous system activation in the pathogenesis of HT and the utility of BBs in certain compelling indications for cardiovascular diseases indicate that these drugs still have an important role for many hypertensive patients.

Several reasons have been considered to explain the relative lower efficacy of BBs found in some studies. One possible mechanism has been suggested by the Conduit Artery Function Evaluation (CAFE) study (a substudy of the Anglo-Scandinavian Cardiac Outcomes -ASCOT- Trial): treatment with BBs resulted in reduced brachial blood pressure with a lesser reduction of central (aortic) and pulse pressure in comparison to the other agents (Williams et al. 2006). Indeed, it has been shown that distinct antihypertensive drugs produce different blood pressure effects peripherally vs centrally (Morgan et al. 2004) and that changes in peripheral artery pressure do not accurately reflect changes in central pressure following different drug interventions. In particular, it seems that the effect of BBs on central aortic pressure is overestimated by brachially-measured blood pressure whereas the effects of ACE-i and

CCBs are underestimated. Moreover, from a hemodynamic point of view, it was shown that BBs increased blood pressure variability and this correlated with trends in stroke risk (Rothwell et al. 2010).

Additional observations suggest that most traditional BBs produce several deleterious metabolic and vascular effects, which could negatively affect the prognosis of hypertensive patients (Ram 2010; Fragasso et al. 2009). As stated above, BBs may induce peripheral vasoconstriction that not only can be particularly detrimental in the context of atherosclerosis but is also one of the determinants of insulin resistance, a pathologic condition directly correlated with the severity of HT (Taddei et al. 2001; Ferrannini et al. 1987; Schiffrin and Deng 1996). The loss of insulin sensitivity is also associated with endothelial dysfunction, a pathophysiological factor present in many patients with HT that has a relevant prognostic weight. BBs have been shown to impair vasodilation, to induce endothelial dysfunction (that can contribute to vasoconstriction) and to deteriorate glucose homeostasis in hypertensive patients (Lithell 1991): atenolol has been found to increase the risk of new-onset diabetes in predisposed patients (Gupta et al. 2008), particularly when used in combination with diuretics. Additionally, old generations BBs have also been consistently shown to favor the increase of body weight, because of the inhibition of lipolysis in adipose tissue, and to adversely affect lipid metabolism, with tendency to an increase in plasma triglyceride and lowering of HDL cholesterol (Eliasson et al. 1981). In general, it could be stated that old generation BBs yield a metabolic profile not dissimilar from diuretics. Attention should be paid to diabetic patients not only for the possible metabolic side effects but also for the risk of masking the symptoms of hypoglycemia. Along with all these issues, BBs may affect QOL also by causing insomnia, depression (due to low arousal of central nervous system), erectile dysfunction and easy fatigability (which can limit significantly the ability to perform exercise).

As previously outlined, BBs may yield differential metabolic and vascular effects among different molecules. In particular, in more recent years, the development of the third-generation vasodilatory BBs has determined a reassessment of the ancillary metabolic effects of this class of drugs and some of the past reservations may apply less or not at all to the new agents (Kalinowski et al. 2003). ESC guidelines have also underlined the potential ameliorating effects of new generations BBs and this fact was another valid reason to keep BBs among first-line treatment options (Mancia et al. 2013).

Carvedilol, compared to metoprolol, was shown not to negatively affect glycemic control and to improve some components of the metabolic syndrome in hypertensive patients with diabetes (Bakris et al. 2004a). Similar results were obtained with nebivolol, that was superior in terms of insulin sensitivity and fibrynolitic balance (reducing plasminogen activator inhibitor-1 antigen concentrations) (Ayers et al. 2012); a reduction of oxidative stress was also observed (Kaiser et al. 2006; Celik et al. 2006; Rizos et al. 2003). The glucose-neutral effect of nebivolol has been observed even when added to diuretics. Accordingly, new BBs have been seen to reduce vasoconstriction and endothelial dysfunction (Mason et al. 2005; Pasini et al. 2008). It has also been proven that nebivolol reduces central aortic pressure and induces regression of left ventricular hypertrophy to a greater extent than metoprolol (Kampus et al. 2011). Vasodilation may be important not only for blood pressure reduction, but also for better tolerability; nebivolol has been shown to improve QOL (Van Bortel et al. 2008; Kendall 1989). In any case, apart from these pathophysiological observations, it should be noted that at present there are no strong outcome data to support the use of third-generation BBs as antihypertensives, even if both carvedilol and nebivolol have shown good results in HF (Mancia et al. 2013). General main contraindications to BBs are bronchospasm (in particular BBs are not safe in patients with asthma), sinus/atrio-ventricular node dysfunction, active peripheral vascular disease (also considering the Raynaud phenomenon) and coronary

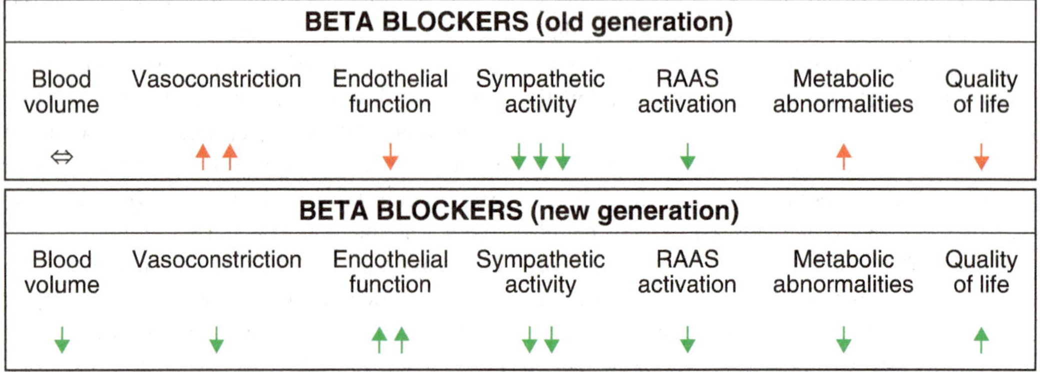

Fig. 2 Main pharmacological effects of beta-blockers on the single pathophysiological factors (*RAAS* Renin Angiotensin Aldosterone System, *Red/green arrow* negative/ positive effect, *Bidirectional flat arrow* neutral effect, Quantity of *upward/downward arrows*: *1* mild, *2* moderate, *3* great effect)

vasospasm. Figure 2 synthesizes the effects of traditional and new generation BBs on principal factors involved in the pathogenesis, maintenance and induction of complications in essential HT.

5   Calcium Channel Blockers

CCBs have gained a great role among the treatments for HT and are recommended as a first-line option by all the guidelines, in particular for older and black patients (Mancia et al. 2013; National Institute for Health and Clinical Excellence, http://www.nice.org.uk/guidance/ cg127). This class of agents comprises two main subclasses, dihydropyridines (DHPs, e.g. nifedipine and amlodipine) and nondihydropyridines (Non-DHPs, verapamil and diltiazem), extensively studied in hypertensive patients (Nathan et al. 2005). The pharmacological property shared by all the CCBs is the selective inhibition of L-type calcium channel, whose main role is to allow the entrance of calcium ions required for initiation of contraction via calcium-induced calcium release from the sarcoplasmic reticulum. This channel is present in vascular smooth muscle cells and in the myocardium: distinction between DHPs and Non-DHPs depends on the different molecular binding site (Opie 1996). DHPs show a greater vascular selectivity (with modest direct cardiac effects),

while Non-DHPs act also on the atrioventricular and sinoatrial node (with negative chronotropic effect and conduction delay) and have significant negative inotropic effect, more evident in patients with already altered myocardial function. The main anti-hypertensive mechanism of CCBs is arteriolar dilation due to blockade of vascular calcium channels (Braunwald 1982). A certain diuretic effect is also observed (particularly with short-acting DHPs as nifedipine): DHPs may increase glomerular filtration rate and renal plasma flow by antagonizing the intrarenal effects of angiotensin II and/or norepinephrine with vasodilatation of renal afferent arterioles, thereby resulting in increased natriuresis and diuresis (Loutzenhiser and Epstein 1985; Chellingsworth et al. 1990; Madeddu et al. 1987). The initial diuretic and natriuretic effects of most calcium channel blockers probably persist with long-term usage (Kaplan 1989; Epstein and De Micheli 1992) but the natriuresis resulting from nifedipine may be transient (Ene et al. 1985). In any case, CCBs acts independently of sodium intake.

The reduction in blood pressure achieved by CCBs stimulates a reflex activation of counter-regulatory mechanisms, with increased sympathetic activity and stimulation of RAAS: these systems determine tachycardia, increased myocardial contractility and tendency to increased systemic vascular resistance. The reflex release of norepinephrine is particularly stimulated by DHPs (Hamada et al. 1998), whereas verapamil tends to decrease plasma catecholamines levels (Bonadue et al. 1997; Kailasam et al. 1995; Vaage-Nilsen and Rasmussen 1998), yielding a sympatholytic effect. Moreover, verapamil and diltiazem control reflex tachycardia through their action on sinoatrial node and by reducing the influence of sinoaortic baroreceptors on heart rate, facilitating the reflex vagal control on the cardiac pacemaker by the afferent cardiopulmonary vagal receptors (Staszewska-Woolley 1987) and attenuating the sympathetic and parasympathetic components of the baroreceptor reflex (Giudicelli et al. 1984).

CCBs of both subclasses appear to be effective antihypertensive agents and most clinical trial data showed that they compare well with other drugs (Nathan et al. 2005); moreover, some meta-analysis have suggested that CCBs determine a better protection against stroke (Law et al. 2009; Blood Pressure Lowering Treatment Trialists' Collaboration 2005; Verdecchia et al. 2005), although the reason is not fully understood. Potential harmful effects of CCBs have been previously reported (Psaty et al. 1997; Furberg et al. 1995). Observational studies and systematic overviews led to the suspect of an increased risk for cardiovascular events with some agents of this therapeutic class. In particular, short-acting nifedipine may precipitate myocardial ischemia as a consequence of the acute adrenergic reflex stimulation and sudden blood pressure fall: this pathophysiological mechanism might be enhanced in presence of CAD, with special hazard in high-risk patients in the immediate post-myocardial infarction period or in those with unstable angina (Marwick 1996; Turnbull 2003; Opie et al. 1995). The possibility of a "coronary steal" phenomenon has been considered too. Initial data suggested also pro-arrhythmic and pro-hemorrhagic effects.

At present, only long-acting CCBs are recommended for HT and several long-term studies have shown their safety and efficacy. Data from the ASCOT-Blood Pressure Lowering Arm (ASCOT-BPLA) trial showed that amlodipine (with possible addition of ACE-I as required) reduced major cardiovascular events and diabetes development compared to atenolol-based strategy (Dalhöf et al. 2005). Moreover, the more recent Avoiding Cardiovascular Events in Combination Therapy in Patients Living with Systolic Hypertension (ACCOMPLISH) trial, a large morbidity and mortality study comparing the effects of two different antihypertensive combination strategies on major fatal and nonfatal cardiovascular events, was stopped earlier because treatment with the ACE-I benazepril plus amlodipine was more effective than treatment with the ACE-I and diuretic (Jamerson et al. 2008). The trend to increased HF in patients treated with CCBs compared to ACE-I and BBs remains an important debated issue. This observation has been found in several trials and confirmed in a recent systematic review (Shibata et al. 2010): certainly, these findings should be considered in accordance with the important role of BBs and ACE-i in established HF treatment and with the superior results of CCBs-ACE-i combination in hypertensive patients. It should be also considered that, as reported as a criticism for the ALLHAT trial, the results against CCBs might be due to the design of the trials, with withdrawal of previous therapies in compensated patients (Mancia et al. 2013; Zanchetti 2012). Nevertheless, the reflex sympathetic activation stimulated by DHPs might indeed yield a negative role in HF patients (Muiesan et al. 1986).

As already recognized when interpreting the results of the ASCOT-BPLA trial, the effects of CCBs might not be entirely explained only by the better control of blood pressure. A first point to underline is that CCBs have also been shown to interact with endothelial function. The lack of functional calcium channels on endothelial cells suggests that CCBs might modify the function of mediators specifically released by the endothelium: it has been observed that some CCBs promote the release of nitric oxide (Salomone et al. 1995; 1996). Furthermore, nitric oxide and endothelin, initially identified as specific products of endothelium, are also produced by other cells: this production may be altered by some CCBs and not necessarily related to calcium channel blockade (Godfraind and Salomone 1996). Some experimental data suggest data CCBs might modify the expression of the endothelin gene (Huang et al. 1993). Moreover, it has been shown that amlodipine, nifedipine and lacidipine (two DHPs) determined a lower progression of carotid atherosclerosis than BBs. (Zanchetti et al. 2002) In the end, CCBs have no effects on potassium, glucose, uric acid and lipid metabolism: this metabolic-neutral profile and the beneficial effects on endothelial function could explain, at least in part, the lower incidence of new metabolic syndrome and diabetes observed in patients treated with CCBs in comparison to other agents (particularly BBs and diuretics). CCBs have shown also a greater effectiveness in reducing left ventricular hypertrophy (Fagard et al. 2009).

A final important point to consider is the role of CCBs in relation to progression of renal dysfunction and their use in patients with chronic kidney disease. CCBs determine no impairment of renal function. Moreover, the ALLHAT trial showed that renal function was better preserved in patients treated with amlodipine (ALLHAT Officers and Coordinators for the ALLHAT Collaborative Research Group 2002). On the other hand, the value of CCBs in patients with proteinuria and elevated creatinine is uncertain (Kloke et al. 1998), with a differential renoprotective effect between DHPs and Non-DHPs. In people with proteinuric renal disease, progressive increases in proteinuria and a more rapid decline in kidney function were noted in patients treated with DHPs in comparison to those treated with ACE-I or ARB (Lewis et al. 2001; Wright et al. 2002). In contrast, several small long-term clinical studies using Non-DHPs have demonstrated reductions in proteinuria and slower declines in glomerular filtration rate but not reduced progression towards end-stage renal disease (Bakris et al. 1996; 1998; 2004b; Smith et al. 1998). In agreement with these observations, the Kidney Disease Outcomes Quality Initiative Blood Pressure guidelines recognized that Non-DHPs alone or in combination with an ACE-I or an ARB are preferable in hypertensive patients with proteinuria of >300 mg/dl, as well as in those with impaired kidney function (Kidney Disease Outcomes Quality Initiative (K/DOQI) 2004). In general, if DHPs are used in hypertensive patients with chronic kidney disease, it is considered prudent to add CCBs after ACE-I or ARB, to achieve a balanced dilation of the afferent and efferent renal arterioles avoiding excessive glomerular pressure and flow.

In terms of main side effects, DHPs are more problematic, since peripheral edema (especially ankle edema) and flushing may be a problem for some patients (Papavassiliou et al. 2001; Weir 2003). Conversely, Non-DHPs appear better tolerated, at least when compared to old generation BBs (Fletcher et al. 1989), even though constipation may represent a relevant problem in a significant proportion of patients treated with verapamil, particularly in the elderly. Major contraindications to DHPs are represented by severe aortic stenosis or obstructive hypertrophic cardiomyopathy (to avoid excess pressure gradient). Left ventricular systolic dysfunction is a contraindication to CCBs. Non-DHPs should not be used in known sinoatrial or atrioventricular nodal disease, in almost all cases of ventricular tachycardia and in patients with pre-excitation. The use of Non-DHPs with concomitant BBs therapy is discouraged, since cardiac effects might be harmfully enhanced. On the contrary, CCBs may be useful in patients with stable and vasospastic angina, Raynaud phenomenon (to obtain peripheral vasodilation) or supraventricular tachy-arrhythmias (to control heart rate with Non-DHPs). Figure 3 synthesizes the effects of DHPs and Non-DHPs on principal factors involved in the pathogenesis, maintenance and induction of complications in essential hypertension.

6 RAAS Blockers: ACE-Inhibitors and Angiotensin Receptor Blockers

RAAS plays a central role in the control of blood pressure as well as global cardiovascular and renal function and certainly its deregulation is a major pathophysiological factor involved in HT

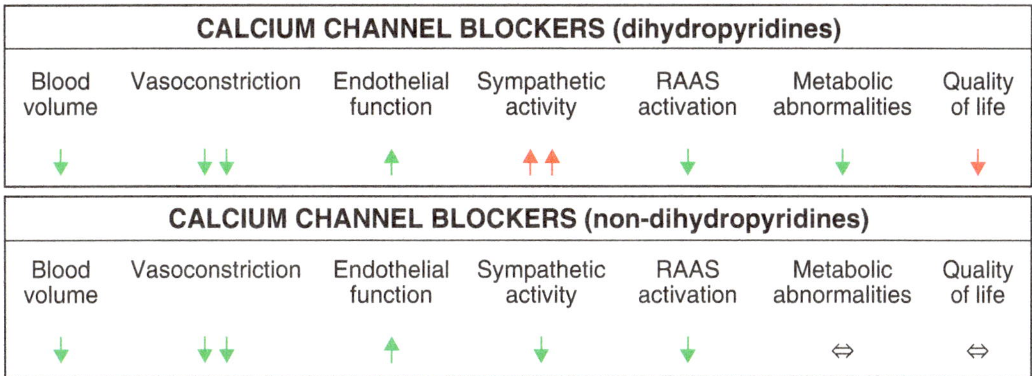

Fig. 3 Main pharmacological effects of calcium channel blockers on the single pathophysiological factors (*RAAS* Renin Angiotensin Aldosterone System, *Red/green arrow* negative/positive effect, *Bidirectional flat arrow* neutral effect, Quantity of *upward/downward arrows*: *1* mild, *2* moderate, *3* great effect)

and in the pathogenesis of many other cardiovascular and renal diseases: it is clear that RAAS should be a main pharmacological target (Castro-Chaves et al. 2010). Renin controls the first and rate-limiting step of the RAAS, determining the conversion of angiotensinogen to angiotensin-I and representing an interesting point to reduce the activity of the whole system. A direct renin blocker (aliskiren) has been recently introduced (Azizi et al. 2006): despite several theoretical attractive features and initial enthusiasm, its development for clinical use has been limited and some clinical trials have been stopped for adverse events (see ensuing paragraph), underlining the need for further research. On the contrary, over the years, important results have been obtained with ACE-Is and ARBs. The angiotensin-converting enzyme (ACE) realizes the central conversion of angiotensin-I to angiotensin-II, the metabolite that activates angiotensin receptors. ACE-Is, therefore, reduce the complex and diffuse effects of angiotensin-II and RAAS, lowering arteriolar resistance and increasing venous capacity, finally increasing cardiac output. Moreover, renal vascular resistance is lowered (with specific relaxation of the efferent arterioles) and aldosterone release decreased, enhancing diuresis and natriuresis with concomitant reduction of blood volume (Sánchez et al. 1985; Atlas et al. 1979). ACE is found mainly in the vascular endothelium of the lungs, even if present in all vascular beds,

and is a relatively nonspecific enzyme. Bradykinin and other tachykinins are further substrates of ACE and thus the inhibition of conversion results in accumulation of these molecules: even if they cause some of the most frequent side effects of this class of drugs, it has been suggested that decreased degradation of bradykinin might also play a role in ACE-Is induced vasodilation (Remme 1997; Su et al. 2000). In the long term competitive inhibition of ACE could result in a reactive increase in renin and angiotensin I levels, possibly reducing the effect of ACE-Is. Moreover, it should be noted that angiotensin-II is partially generated through non-ACE pathways, that are unaffected by ACE-Is (Dzau 1989). For these reasons, to overcome some problems of ACE-Is and to achieve a more intense RAAS blockade, ARBs have been developed: these molecules act selectively blocking the major angiotensin-II receptor subtype (AT-1) (Burnier and Brunner 2000). The main antihypertensive mechanisms are similar to those of ACE-Is.

Consistently with the central pathogenic role of RAAS, ACE-Is have been found to be beneficial for treating HF (The SOLVD Investigators 1991), achieving effective secondary prevention in CAD and slowing the progression toward end-stage renal disease (Hannedouche et al. 1994). ACE-Is are a main first-line option for HT treatment, particularly for younger patients, those with high-renin HT (more than a third of all hypertensive patients) and chronic kidney disease patients. ACE-I should also be preferentially used in hypertensive patients with diabetes, HF or CAD (particularly post-infarction) (Mancia et al. 2013). Meta-analysis of outcome trials in hypertensive patients have shown that ACE-Is are effective in reducing events (particularly HF and heart attacks) and mortality (Blood Pressure Lowering Treatment Trialists' Collaboration 2007), even if apparently less protective against stroke in comparison with diuretics with or without BBs and with CCBs. The HOPE (Heart Outcomes Prevention Evaluation) trial found that the use of ramipril provided substantial additional cardiovascular protection in high-risk patients (HOPE (Heart Outcomes Prevention Evaluation) Study Investigators 2000). This result was reproduced by the EUROPA (Efficacy of perindopril in reduction of cardiovascular events among patients with stable coronary artery disease) trial in patients with known CAD, where a significant reduction in myocardial infarction was observed compared to placebo (Fox and EURopean trial On reduction of cardiac events with Perindopril in stable coronary Artery disease Investigators 2003). On the other hand, the perindopril protection against recurrent stroke study (PROGRESS), enrolling patients with a previous stroke or transient ische-mic attack, found that only the subgroup receiv-ing both perindopril and indapamide had reduced stroke recurrence: it has therefore been suggested that in that context the association of ACE-i and diuretic may be more effective in reducing blood pressure and, therefore, events (PROGRESS Collaborative Group 2001). However, the most recent ACCOMPLISH trial, as state above, showed that ACE-I plus amlodipine was more effective than treatment with the ACE-I and diuretic in reducing morbidity and mortality (Jamerson et al. 2008). It has been suggested by the results of several studies that ACE-Is have beneficial effects that are at least partially inde-pendent from the blood pressure-lowering action. They yield no effects on total cholesterol, LDL cholesterol and triglycerides, while some evidences suggest that HDL fraction is increased (Sasaki and Arakawa 1989). Moreover, improved insulin sensitivity (Paolisso et al. 1992) and reduced diabetes incidence have also been observed after ACE-I therapy (Andraws and Brown 2007). This better metabolic profile might be associated also to endothelial function improvement (De Gennaro et al. 2005) and reduced sympathetic activity induced by ACE-Is (Imai et al. 1982). Last but not least, they have been found to inhibit cardiac and vas-cular remodeling associated with chronic cardio-vascular diseases (Abdulla et al. 2007). Figure 4 summarizes the effects of ACE-Is on the princi-pal mechanisms and correlates of HT.

ACE-Is are generally well tolerated and improve QOL (Croog et al. 1986), provided that their administration does not cause cough, the most frequent side effect (due to bradykinin metabolites accumulation). Angioedema is the most severe, but rare, side effect (Israeli and Hall 1992). Additionally they may induce hyperkalemia and contribute to renal function deterioration, especially in patients with an already impaired renal function. Nevertheless, since early mild worsening of renal function in the setting of ACE-Is initiation appears to repre-sent a benign event that is not associated with a loss of benefit from continued therapy, ACE-Is administration should not be discontinued and is

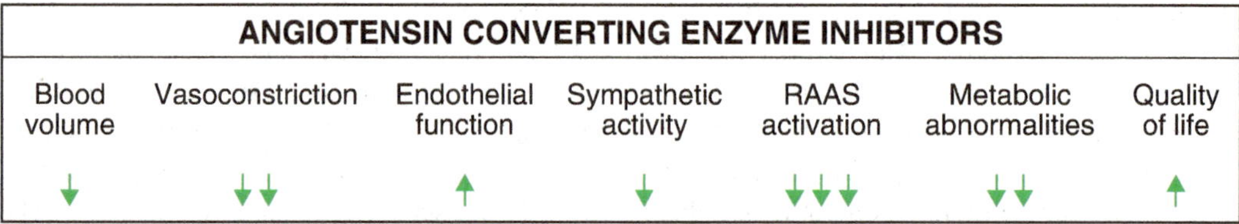

Fig. 4 Main pharmacological effects of angiotensin converting enzyme inhibitors on the single pathophysio-logical factors (*RAAS* Renin Angiotensin Aldosterone System, *Red/green arrow* negative/positive effect, *Bidi-rectional flat arrow* neutral effect, Quantity of *upward/downward arrows*: *1* mild, *2* moderate, *3* great effect)

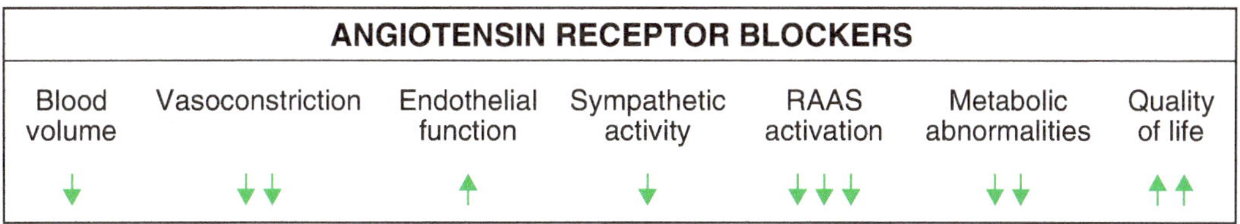

Fig. 5 Main pharmacological effects of angiotensin receptor blockers on the single pathophysiological factors (*RAAS* Renin Angiotensin Aldosterone System, *Red/green arrow* negative/positive effect, *Bidirectional flat arrow* neutral effect, Quantity of *upward/downward arrows*: *1* mild, *2* moderate, *3* great effect)

advised also in these conditions (Testani et al. 2011). ACE-Is are contraindicated in patients with bilateral renal artery stenosis and during pregnancy.

ARBs have been tested in large outcome trials, proving their role as antihypertensive agents. A major systematic review comparing ACE-Is and ARBs reported similar blood pressure control and outcomes (Matchar et al. 2008a): even if there is evidence for better tolerability, at present no superiority of ARBs have been proven concerning hard endpoints. ACE-Is remain a preferred choice for many physicians because of the lower cost and long-term experience with their use, reserving ARBs for ACE-Is intolerant patients. ARBs are also approved for chronic kidney disease (particularly diabetic nephropathy) (Kidney Disease Outcomes Quality Initiative (K/DOQI) 2004) and as an alternative to ACE-Is in HF (McMurray et al. 2012). Moreover, the two classes of drugs share similar contraindications. Similarly to ACE-Is, ARBs have a beneficial effect on endothelial function, probably because of their antioxidant effect (Huang et al. 2007; Flammer et al. 2007), and a good metabolic profile (Kintscher et al. 2007; Vitale et al. 2005; Aksnes et al. 2007). In general, ARBs are well tolerated (Weber et al. 2003): in particular, the occurrence of cough is significantly lower (Matchar et al. 2008b). It should be noted that some data have suggested a possible association between ARBs and cancer (Sipahi et al. 2010): a subsequent large meta-analysis found no evidence of increased cancer incidence (Pfeffer 2013). Another controversy regarded the possible increase of myocardial infarction (Strauss et al. 2006), but also in this case a more comprehensive analysis of available

data dismissed initial doubts (Bangalore et al. 2011). Figure 5 summarizes the effects of ARBs on the principal mechanisms and correlates of HT.

The combination of an ACE-I and an ARB has been proposed in the hope that more complete blockade of the RAAS would lead to better blood-pressure control and potentially major nephron-protective and cardio-protective effects. However, data from the ONTARGET study shattered the idea of dual RAAS blockade not only for hypertension but also for nephron-protection, since the combination produced similar cardiovascular outcomes but increased hypotension and renal dysfunction (Yusuf et al. 2008). Figure 5 synthesizes the effects of ARBs on principal factors involved in the pathogenesis, maintenance and induction of complications in essential hypertension.

7 Other Drugs

In this chapter, the most used antihypertensive drugs have been discussed extensively. Some additional classes are represented by alpha1-blockers, direct vasodilators, centrally active agents and the direct renin inhibitor (aliskiren).

Regarding alpha1-blockers (e.g. prazosin, doxazosin), ESC and NICE guidelines are non-committal: there is neither indication nor refusal but they are mentioned as a possible add-on option for resistant HT. Certainly the disappointing results of the ALLHAT trial had an important role in limiting the use of alpha1-blockers, since the group treated with doxazosin showed a higher incidence of HF. However, as discussed above in detail, several limitations of that study should be considered when interpreting its findings: in particular, the confounding effect of prior treatment drugs should be taken into account, since the replacement of diuretic with the study drug might have precipitated HF in previously compensated, but predisposed, patients. At the same time, positive evidences came from other trials: among the others, the Treatment of Mild Hypertension (TOMH) study showed that doxazosin reduced blood pressure as much as the other first-line agents with good QOL (Study et al. 1993) and the ASCOT trial reported an impressive reduction of blood pressure with the addition of doxazosin as a third line drug in patients who had not responded to their initial treatments (amlodipine plus perindopril or atenolol plus thiazide) (Chang et al. 2006). Alpha1-blockers have an interesting metabolic profile: it has been observed a decrease in total and LDL cholesterol with HDL increase and a reduced or neutral effect on plasma glucose with improved insulin sensitivity (Kabra 2014). Moreover, the amelioration of endothelial function and the reduction in arterial stiffness have been described. Overall, according to their pharmacological profile, alpha1-blockers may be an option in particular for those patients with metabolic syndrome or in males with benign prostatic hyperplasia (in whom symptomatic relief is provided) (McConnell et al. 2003); the positive effect on impotence described might be desirable for younger patients (Grimm et al. 1997). Drowsiness and postural hypotension, with the risk of syncope, are possible main side effects, which can rise some concerns of safety, even if their incidence have been reduced by new controlled release formulations (or with multiple-step dose titration of normal preparations) (Nerurkar and Ved 2014). In general, QOL is good and these drugs combine well with other antihypertensives. Combined alpha1 and alpha2-blockers (e.g. phentolamine) are used only for pheocromocytoma. As said above, some BBs (e.g. carvedilol and labetalol) have limited alpha-blocking activity; labetalol maintain a place for acute intravenous use in hypertensive crises.

Direct vasodilators (hydralazine and minoxidil) and central adrenergic inhibitors (e.g. reserpine, methyldopa and clonidine) have a limited role at present; methyldopa is the best validated antihypertensive for pregnancy HT.

Aliskiren, the first direct renin inhibitor, appeared as a very promising new approach to block the RAAS at its activation step but some initial disappointing results heavily compromised its introduction as antihypertensive agent. The ALiskiren Trial in Type 2 Diabetes Using Cardio-renal End-points (ALTITUDE) showed no real benefit on top of other RAAS blockers in these patients at high risk of cardiovascular and renal events and was stopped because of the higher incidence of adverse events, renal complications, hyperkalemia and hypotension in the treatment arm (Parving et al. 2012). Other evidences, in any case, suggest that when used as monotherapy, aliskiren could lower blood pressure with an efficacy comparable with other RAS blockers (Jordan et al. 2007), providing dose-dependent and sustained 24-h efficacy, which is enhanced by concomitant diuretic (Oh et al. 2007). The ACCELERATE was a small study assessing in hypertensive patients the effects of treatment with aliskiren compared to amlodipine and their combination; similar blood pressure reduction was found with single agents and a larger fall when drugs were combined (Brown et al. 2011). A larger trial, A Randomized Controlled Trial of Aliskiren in the Prevention of Major Cardiovascular Events in Elderly People (APOLLO), evaluating aliskiren alone or in combination with a thiazide or a CCB, has been prematurely interrupted by the sponsor in agreement with Health Authorities for feasibility reasons, despite no evidence of harm in the aliskiren-treated group (Teo et al. 2014).

8 Conclusions

Current guidelines do not recommend treatment strategies on the basis of the mechanisms of elevated blood pressure in individual patients because clinical trial data supporting such an approach are limited. However, we think that better approaches to individualizing antihypertensive therapy to achieve optimal clinical outcomes and optimal patient adherence are needed. Anti-hypertensive therapy should take into account those factors most likely involved in the single patient and all possible pathogenic components should be considered. Since the main goal of any anti-hypertensive therapy is the correction of blood pressure levels that, in the majority of cases, requires multiple therapies, combinations of drugs differently regulating specific pathophysiological mechanisms should be preferred. This approach should also be applied in the present fashionable trend of single pill associated drugs. In fact, apart from lowering blood pressure, the main therapeutic target in treating arterial hypertension should be that of counteracting all the possible pathophysiological mechanisms involved in hypertension itself and in existing/potential co-morbidities. All the ancillary positive and negative effects of the administered drugs should not be dismissed. Hypertensive patients are often glucose intolerant/diabetic, carrier of serum lipids disorder, have already developed atherosclerotic diseases and therefore should be treated with drugs not interfering with these conditions and, if possible, rather improving them. A simple scheme which comprises the following factors commonly considered at work in hypertension, alone or in combination, should be: increased blood volume, increased RAAS activity, increased sympathetic activity, endothelial dysfunction, glucose and lipid metabolism abnormalities. These parameters are not always evaluated directly, but can be evinced by taking into account simple factors such as body mass index, heart rate, presence of arrhythmias, presence of atherosclerosis in specific vascular districts, routine blood testing, somatic symptoms of hyperarousal. Last but not least, quality of life is also of great importance in the choice of treatment. As summarized in the present chapter, from a pathophysiological point of view, ACE-Is and ARBs should at present be considered as the most appropriate drugs for the treatment of arterial hypertension and its correlates, especially in the high-risk patient.

References

Abdulla J, Barlera S, Latini R et al (2007) A systematic review: effect of angiotensin converting enzyme-inhibition on left ventricular volumes and ejection fraction in patients with a myocardial infarction and in patients with left ventricular dysfunction. Eur J Heart Fail 9:129–135

Aksnes TA, Seljeflot I, Torjesen PA et al (2007) Improved insulin sensitivity by the angiotensin II-receptor blocker losartan is not explained by adipokines, inflammatory markers, or whole blood viscosity. Metabolism 56:1470–1477

ALLHAT Officers and Coordinators for the ALLHAT Collaborative Research Group (2000) Major cardiovascular events in hypertensive patients randomized to doxazosin vs chlorthalidone: the Antihypertensive and Lipid-Lowering Treatment to Prevent Heart Attack Trial (ALLHAT). JAMA 283:1967–1975

ALLHAT Officers and Coordinators for the ALLHAT Collaborative Research Group (2002) Major outcomes in high-risk hypertensive patients randomized to angiotensin-converting enzyme inhibitor or calcium channel blocker vs diuretic: the Antihypertensive and Lipid-Lowering Treatment to Prevent Heart Attack Trial (ALLHAT). JAMA 288:2981–2997

Ames RP (1996) A comparison of blood lipid and blood pressure responses during the treatment of systemic hypertension with indapamide and with thiazides. Am J Cardiol 77:12b–16b

Andraws R, Brown DL (2007) Effect of inhibition of the renin-angiotensin system on development of type 2 diabetes mellitus (meta-analysis of randomized trials). Am J Cardiol 99:1006–1012

Atlas SA, Case DB, Sealey JE et al (1979) Interruption of the renin-angiotensin system in hypertensive patients by captopril induces sustained reduction in aldosterone secretion, potassium retention and natriuresis. Hypertension 1:274–280

Ayers K et al (2012) Differential effects of nebivolol and metoprolol on insulin sensitivity and plasminogen activator inhibitor in the metabolic syndrome. Hypertension 59:893–898

Azizi M et al (2006) Renin inhibition with aliskiren. where are we now, and where are we going. J Hypertens 24:243–256

Bakris GL, Copley JB, Vicknair N et al (1996) Calcium channel blockers versus other antihypertensive therapies on progression of NIDDM associated nephropathy. Kidney Int 50:1641–1650

Bakris GL, Weir MR, DeQuattro V et al (1998) Effects of an ACE inhibitor/calcium antagonist combination on proteinuria in diabetic nephropathy. Kidney Int 54:1283–1289

Bakris GL, Fonseca V, Katholi RE et al (2004a) Metabolic effects of carvedilol vs metoprolol in patients with type 2 diabetes mellitus and hypertension: a randomized controlled trial. JAMA 292:2227–2236

Bakris GL, Weir MR, Secic M et al (2004b) Differential effects of calcium antagonist subclasses on markers of nephropathy progression. Kidney Int 65:1991–2002

Balansard P, Chabrillat Y, Paulin R et al (1977) Effect of atenolol, a new cardioselective beta- blocker, on plasma renin activity in treatment of hypertension. Acta Cardiol 32:229–243

Balligand JL (2013) Beta3-adrenoreceptors in cardiovasular diseases: new roles for an "old" receptor. Curr Drug Deliv 10:64–66

Bangalore S et al (2011) Angiotensin receptor blockers and risk of myocardial infarction. Meta-analyses and trial sequential analyses of 147,020 patients from randomised trials. BMJ 342:d22–d34

Beckett N, et al.: for the HYVET Study Group (2008) Treatment of hypertension in patients 80 years of age or older. N Engl J Med 358:1887–1898

Bennett WM, McDonald WJ, Kuehnel E et al (1977) Do diuretics have antihypertensive properties independent of natriuresis? Clin Pharmacol Ther 22:499–504

Blood Pressure Lowering Treatment Trialists' Collaboration (2005) Effects of different blood pressure-lowering regimens on major cardiovascular events in individuals with and without diabetes mellitus: results of prospectively designed overviews of randomized trials. Arch Intern Med 165:1410–1419

Blood Pressure Lowering Treatment Trialists' Collaboration (2007) Blood pressure-dependent and independent effects of agents that inhibit the renin angiotensin system. J Hypertens 25:951–958

Bohlen HG (1986) Localization of vascular resistance changes during hypertension. Hypertension 8:181–183

Bonadue D, Petretta M, Ianniciello A et al (1997) Comparison of verapamil versus felodipine on heart rate variability after acute myocardial infarction. Am J Cardiol 79:564–569

Bradley HA, Wiysonge CS, Volmink JA et al (2006) How strong is the evidence for use of beta- blockers as first-line therapy for hypertension? Systematic review and meta-analysis. J Hypertens 24:2131–2141

Braunwald E (1982) Mechanism of action of calcium-channel-blocking agents. N Engl J Med 307:1618–1627

Brodde OE et al (2006) Cardiac adrenoceptors. physiological and pathophysiological relevance. J Pharmacol Sci 100:323–337

Brown MJ et al (2011) Aliskiren and the calcium channel blocker amlodipine combination as an initial treatment strategy for hypertension control (ACCELERATE): a randomised, parallel-group trial. Lancet 377:312–320

Brunner HR, Sealey JE, Laragh JH (1973) Renin subgroups in essential hypertension. Further analysis of their pathophysiological and epidemiological characteristics. Circ Res 32:99–105

Burnier M, Brunner HR (1992) Neurohormonal consequences of diuretics in different cardiovascular syndromes. Eur Heart J 13:G28–G33

Burnier M, Brunner HR (2000) Angiotensin II receptor antagonists. Lancet 355:637–645

Carter BL, Einhorn PT, Brands M, et al.; Working Group from the National Heart, Lung, and Blood Institute (2008) Thiazide-induced dysglycemia: call for research from a working group from the national heart, lung, and blood institute. Hypertension 52:30–36

Castro-Chaves P, Cerqueira R, Pintalhao M et al (2010) New pathways of the renin–angiotensin system: the role of ACE2 in cardiovascular pathophysiology and therapy. Export Opin Ther Targets 14:485–496

Celik T, Iyisoy A, Kursaklioglu H et al (2006) Comparative effects of nebivolol and metoprolol on oxidative stress, insulin resistance, plasma adiponectin and soluble P-selectin levels in hypertensive patients. J Hypertens 24:591–596

Chang C et al (2006) The effect on blood pressure and lipid profiles of doxazosin GITS as a third-line antihypertensive agent in the Anglo-Scandinavian Cardiac Outcomes Trial (ASCOT). J Hypertens 24:S3

Chellingsworth MC, Kendall MJ, Lote CJ et al (1990) Diuresis and natriuresis after dihydropyridines: role of prostaglandin E. J Hum Hypertens 4:241–245

Chen J et al (2013) The effects of carvedilol on cardiac structural remodeling: the role of endogenous nitric oxide in the activity of carvedilol. Mol Med Rep 7 (4):1155–1158

Chobanian AV, Bakris GL, Black HR et al (2003) Seventh report of the Joint National Committee on prevention, detection evaluation, and treatment of high blood pressure. Hypertension 42:1206–1252

Croog SH, Levine S, Testa MA et al (1986) The effects of antihypertensive therapy on the quality of life. N Engl J Med 314:1657–1664

Czernichow S, Blood Pressure Lowering Treatment Trialists' Collaboration et al (2011) The effects of blood pressure reduction and different blood pressure-lowering regimens on major cardiovascular events according to baseline blood pressuremeta-analysis of randomized trials. J Hypertens 29:4–16

Dahal K, Kunwar S, Rijal J, Alqatahni F, Panta R, Ishak N, Russell RP (2015) The effects of aldosterone antagonists in patients with resistant hypertension: a meta-analysis of randomized and nonrandomized studies. Am J Hypertens 28:1376–1385

Dalhöf B et al (2005) Prevention of cardiovascular events with an antihypertensive regimen of amlodipine adding perindopril as required versus atenolol adding bendroflumethiazide as required, in the Anglo-Scandinavian Cardiac Outcomes Trial-Blood Pressure Lowering Arm (ASCOT-BPLA). A multicentre randomised controlled trial. Lancet 366:895–906

Davis BR, Cutler JA, Gordon DJ et al (1996) Rationale and design for the Antihypertensive and Lipid Lowering Treatment to Prevent Heart Attack Trial (ALLHAT): ALLHAT Research Group. Am J Hypertens 9:342–360

De Gennaro CV, Rigamonti A et al (2005) Angiotensin-converting enzyme inhibition and angiotensin AT1-receptor antagonism equally improve endothelial vasodilator function in L- NAME-induced hypertensive rats. Eur J Pharmacol 516:253–259

Dussol B et al (2012) A pilot study comparing furosemide and hydrochlorothiazide in patients with hypertension and stage 4 or 5 chronic kidney disease. J Clin Hypertens 14:32–37

Dzau VJ (1989) Multiple pathways of angiotensin production in the blood vessel wall: evidence, possibilities and hypotheses. J Hypertens 7:933–936

Eliasson K, Lins LE, Rössner S (1981) Serum lipoprotein changes during atenolol treatment of essential hypertension. Eur J Clin Pharmacol 20:335–338

Ene MD, Williamson PJ, Roberts CJC et al (1985) The natriuresis following oral administration of the calcium antagonists-nifedipine and nitrendipine. Br J Clin Pharmacol 19:423–427

Epstein M, De Micheli AG (1992) Natriuretic effects of calcium antagonists. In: Epstein M (ed) Calcium antagonists in clinical medicine. Hanley and Belfus, Philadelphia, pp 349–366

Eriksson JW, Jansson PA, Carlberg B et al (2008) Hydrochlorothiazide, but not Candesartan, aggravates insulin resistance and causes visceral and hepatic fat accumulation: the mechanisms for the diabetes preventing effect of Candesartan (MEDICA) Study. Hypertension 52:1030–1037

Fagard R, Amery A, Deplaen JF et al (1976) Plasma renin concentration and the hypotensive effect of bendrofluazide and of atenolol. Clin Sci Mol Med Suppl 3:215s–217s

Fagard RH, Celis H, Thijs L, Wouters S (2009) Regression of left ventricular mass by anti-hypertensive treatment: a meta-analysis of randomized comparative studies. Hypertension 54:1084–1091

Ferrannini E, Buzzigoli G, Bonadonna R et al (1987) Insulin resistance in essential hypertension. N Engl J Med 317:350–357

Ferrari P, Rosman J, Weidmann P (1991) Antihypertensive agents, serum lipoproteins and glucose metabolism. Am J Cardiol 67:26B–35B

Flammer AJ, Hermann F, Wiesli P et al (2007) Effect of losartan, compared with atenolol, on endothelial function and oxidative stress in patients with type 2 diabetes and hypertension. J Hypertens 25:785–791

Fletcher AE, Chester PC, Hawkins CM et al (1989) The effects of verapamil and propranolol on quality of life in hypertension. J Hum Hypertens 3:125–130

Fonseca FA, Ihara SS, Izar MC et al (2003) Hydrochlorothiazide abolishes the anti-atherosclerotic effect of quinapril. Clin Exp Pharmacol Physiol 30:779–785

Fox KM, EURopean trial On reduction of cardiac events with Perindopril in stable coronary Artery disease Investigators (2003) Efficacy of perindopril in reduction of cardiovascular events among patients with stable coronary artery disease: randomised, double-blind, placebo-controlled, multicentre trial (the EUROPA study). Lancet 362:782–788

Fragasso G, Cera M, Margonato A (2009) Different metabolic effects of selective and non- selective beta-blockers rather than mere heart rate reduction may be the mechanism by which beta- blockade prevents cardiovascular events. J Am Coll Cardiol 53:2105

Fragasso G, Maranta F, Montanaro C, Salerno A, Torlasco C, Margonato A (2012) Pathophysiologic therapeutic targets in hypertension: a cardiological point of view. Expert Opin Ther Targets 16:179–193

Franse LV, Pahor M, Di Bari M et al (2000) Serum uric acid, diuretic treatment and risk of cardiovascular events in the Systolic Hypertension in the Elderly Program. J Hypertens 18:1149–1154

Freis ED (1983) How diuretics lower blood pressure. Am Heart J 106:185–187

Furberg CD, Psaty BM, Meyer JV (1995) Nifedipine. Dose-related increase in mortality in patients with coronary heart disease. Circulation 92:1326–1331

Giudicelli JF, Berdeaux A, Edouard A et al (1984) Attenuation by diltiazem of arterial baroreflex sensitivity in man. Eur J Clin Pharmacol 26:675–679

Godfraind D, Salomone S (1996) Calcium antagonists and endothelial function: focus on nitric oxide and endothelin. Cardiovasc Drugs Ther 10:439–446

Grassi G, Seravalle G, Dell'Oro R et al (2003) Comparative effects of candesartan and hydrochlorothiazide on blood pressure, insulin sensitivity, and sympathetic drive in obese hypertensive individuals: results of the CROSS study. J Hypertens 21:1761–1769

Grimm RH et al (1997) Long-term effects on sexual function of five antihypertensive drugs and nutritional hygienic treatment in hypertensive men and women. Treatment of Mild Hypertension Study (TOMHS). Hypertension 29:8–14

Gupta AK, Dahlof B, Dobson J et al (2008) Determinants of new-onset diabetes among 19,257 hypertensive patients randomized in the Anglo-Scandinavian Cardiac Outcomes Trial--Blood Pressure Lowering Arm and the relative influence of antihypertensive medication. Diabetes Care 31:982–988

Hamada T, Watanabe M, Kaneda T et al (1998) Evaluation of changes in sympathetic nerve activity and heart rate in essential hypertensive patients induced by amlodipine and nifedipine. J Hypertens 16:111–118

Hannedouche T, Landais P, Goldfarb B et al (1994) Randomised controlled trial of enalapril and β blockers in non-diabetic chronic renal failure. BMJ 309:833–837

HOPE (Heart Outcomes Prevention Evaluation) Study Investigators (2000) Effects of an angiotensin-converting-enzyme inhibitor, ramipril, on cardiovascular events in high-risk patients. N Engl J Med 342:145–153

Huang S, Simonson MS, Dunn MJ (1993) Manidipine inhibits endothelin-1-induced [Ca2+]i signaling but potentiates endothelin's effect on c-fos and c-jun induction in vascular smooth muscle and glomerular mesangial cells. Am Heart J 125:589–597

Huang BS, Ahmad M, Tan J et al (2007) Sympathetic hyperactivity and cardiac dysfunction post- MI: different impact of specific CNS versus general AT1 receptor blockade. J Mol Cell Cardiol 43:479–486

Imai Y, Abe K, Seino M et al (1982) Captopril attenuates pressor responses to norepinephrine and vasopressin through depletion of endogenous angiotensin II. Am J Cardiol 49:1537–1539

Insel PA, Motulsky HJ (1984) A hypothesis linking intracellular sodium, membrane receptors, and hypertension. Life Sci 34:1009–1013

Ishizaki T, Oyama Y, Suganuma T et al (1983) A dose ranging study of atenolol in hypertension: fall in blood pressure and plasma renin activity, beta-blockade and steady-state pharmacokinetics. Br J Clin Pharmacol 16:17–25

Israeli ZH, Hall WD (1992) Cough and angioneurotic edema associated with angiotensin- converting enzyme inhibitor therapy; a review of the literature and pathophysiology. Ann Intern Med 117:234–242

Jamerson K, Weber MA, Bakris GL et al (2008) Benazepril plus amlodipine or hydrochlorothiazide for hypertension in high-risk patients. N Engl J Med 359:2417–2428

James PA, Oparil S, Carter BL et al (2014) Evidence-based guideline for the management of high BP in adults. JAMA 311:507–520

Jordan J et al (2007) Direct renin inhibition with aliskiren in obese patients with arterial hypertension. Hypertension 49:1047–1055

Kabra NK (2014) Alpha blockers and metabolic syndrome. J Assoc Physicians India 62:13–16

Kailasam MT, Parmer RJ, Cervenka JH et al (1995) Divergent effects of dihydropyridine and phenylalkylamine calcium channel antagonist classes on autonomic function in human hypertension. Hypertension 26:143–149

Kaiser T, Heise T, Nosek L et al (2006) Influence of nebivolol and enalapril on metabolic parameters and arterial stiffness in hypertensive type 2 diabetic patients. J Hypertens 24:1397–1403

Kalinowski L, Dobrucki LW, Szczepanska-Konkel M et al (2003) Third-generation beta-blockers stimulate nitric oxide release from endothelial cells through ATP efflux: a novel mechanism for antihypertensive action. Circulation 107:2747–2752

Kampus P et al (2011) Differential effects of nebivolol and metoprolol on central aortic pressure and left ventricular wall thickness. Hypertension 57:1122–1128

Kaplan NM (1989) Calcium entry blockers in the treatment of hypertension: current status and future prospects. JAMA 262:817–823

Kasiske BL et al (1995) Effects of antihypertensive therapy on serum lipids. Ann Intern Med 122:133–141

Kendall MJ (1989) Pharmacology of third generation beta blockers: greater benefits, fewer risks. J Cardiovasc Pharmacol 14:S4–S8

Kidney Disease Outcomes Quality Initiative (K/DOQI) (2004) K/DOQI clinical practice guidelines on hypertension and antihypertensive agents in chronic kidney disease. Am J Kidney Dis 43:1–290

Kintscher U, Bramlage P, Paar WD et al (2007) Irbesartan for the treatment of hypertension in patients with the metabolic syndrome: a subanalysis of the Treat to Target post authorization survey. Prospective observational, two armed study in 14,200 patients. Cardiovasc Diabetol 6:12

Kloke HJ, Branten AJ, Huysmans FT et al (1998) Antihypertensive treatment of patients with proteinuric renal diseases: risks or benefits of calcium channel blockers? Kidney Int 53:1559–1573

Kostis JB, Wilson AC, Freudenberger RS, SHEP Collaborative Research Group et al (2005) Long-term effect of diuretic-based therapy on fatal outcomes in subjects with isolated systolic hypertension with and without diabetes. Am J Cardiol 95:29–35

LaCroix AZ et al (1990) Thiazide diuretic agents and the incidence of hip fracture. New Engl J Med 322:286–290

Laragh JH, Sealey JE (1991) Renin angiotensin aldosterone system and the renal regulation of sodium, potassium, and blood pressure homeostasis. In: Windhager EE (ed) Handblock of physiology. Renal physiology Oxford University Press, New York, pp 1409–1541

Law MR, Morris JK, Wald NJ (2009) Use of blood pressure lowering drugs in the prevention of cardiovascular disease: meta-analysis of 147 randomised trials in the context of expectations from prospective epidemiological studies. BMJ 338:b1665

Lewis EJ, Hunsicker LG, Clarke WR et al (2001) Renoprotective effect of the angiotensin receptor antagonist irbesartan in patients with nephropathy due to type 2 diabetes. N Engl J Med 345:851–860

Lindholm LH et al (2003) Metabolic outcome during 1 year in newly detected hypertensives. results of the Antihypertensive Treatment and Lipid Profile in a North of Sweden Efficacy Evaluation (ALPINE study). J Hypertens 21:1563–1574

Lindholm LH, Carlberg B, Samuelsson O (2005) Should beta blockers remain first choice in the treatment of primary hypertension? A meta-analysis. Lancet 366:1545–1553

Lithell HO (1991) Effect of antihypertensive drugs on insulin, glucose, and lipid metabolism. Diabetes Care 14:203–209

Loutzenhiser R, Epstein M (1985) Effects of calcium antagonists on renal hemodynamics. Am J Physiol 249:F619–F629

Madeddu P, Oppes M, Soro A et al (1987) Natriuretic effect of acute nifedipine administration is not mediated by the renal kallikrein-kinin system. J Cardiovasc Pharmacol 9:536–540

Man in't Veld AJ, Van den Meiracker AH, Schalekamp MA (1988) Do beta-blockers really increase peripheral vascular resistance? Review of the literature and new observations under basal conditions. Am J Hypertens 1:91–96

Mancia G, Dell'Oro R, Quarti-Trevano F et al (2006) Angiotensin-sympathetic system interactions in cardiovascular and metabolic disease. J Hypertens Suppl 24:S51–S56

Mancia G, Fagard R, Narkiewica K et al (2013) 2013 ESH/ESC guidelines for the management of arterial hypertension: the Task Force for the Management of Arterial Hypertension of the European Society of Hypertension (ESH) and of the European Society of Cardiology (ESC). Eur Heart J 34:2159–2219

Marwick C (1996) FDA gives calcium channel blockers clean bill of health but warns of short- acting nifedipine hazards. JAMA 275:423–424

Mason RP, Kalinowski L, Jacob RF et al (2005) Nebivolol reduces nitroxidative stress and restores nitric oxide bioavailability in endothelium of black Americans. Circulation 112:3795–3801

Matchar DB et al (2008a) Systematic review. Comparative effectiveness of angiotensin-converting enzyme inhibitors and angiotensin II receptor blockers for treating essential hypertension. Ann Intern Med 148:16–29

Matchar DB, McCrory DC, Orlando LA et al (2008b) Systematic review: comparative effectiveness of angiotensin-converting enzyme inhibitors and angiotensin II receptor blockers for treating essential hypertension. Ann Intern Med 148:16–29

McConnell JD et al (2003) The long-term effect of doxazosin, finasteride, and combination therapy on the clinical progression of benign prostatic hyperplasia. N Engl J Med 349:2387–2398

McMurray JJ et al (2012) ESC guidelines for the diagnosis and treatment of acute and chronic heart failure 2012. Eur J Heart 33:1787–1847

Mendlowitz M, Gitlow SE, Wolf RL et al (1964) Mechanisms in essential hypertension. Dis Chest 45:360–364

Messerli FH (2001) Doxazosin and congestive heart failure. J Am Coll Cardiol 38:1295–1296

Messerli FH et al (1998) Are beta-blockers efficacious as first-line therapy for hypertension in the elderly? A systematic review. JAMA 279:1903–1907

Modena MG, Bonetti L, Coppi F et al (2002) Prognostic role of reversible endothelial dysfunction in hypertensive postmenopausal women. J Am Coll Cardiol 40:505–510

Morgan T, Lauri J, Bertram D et al (2004) Effect of different antihypertensive drug classes on central aortic pressure. Am J Hypertens 17:118–123

Muiesan G, Agabiti-Rosei E, Romanelli G et al (1986) Adrenergic activity and left ventricular function during treatment of essential hypertension with calcium antagonists. Am J Cardiol 57:44D–49D

Nathan S, Pepine CJ, Bakris GL (2005) Calcium antagonists: effects on cardio-renal risk in hypertensive patients. Hypertension 46:637–642

National Institute for Health and Clinical Excellence. Hypertension (CG127). Web site http://www.nice.org.uk/guidance/cg127. Accessed 2 Oct 2014.

Nerurkar RP, Ved JK (2014) Clinical pharmacology of alpha-1 blockers improving drug-profile through novel formulations. J Assoc Physicians India 62:9–12

Oh BH et al (2007) Aliskiren, an oral renin inhibitor, provides dose-dependent efficacy and sustained 24-hour blood pressure control in patients with hypertension. J Am Coll Cardiol 49:1157–1163

Opie LH (1996) Calcium channel antagonists in the treatment of coronary artery disease. fundamental pharmacological properties relevant to clinical use. Prog Cardiovasc Dis 38:273–290

Opie LH et al (1995) Nifedipine and mortality. grave defects in the dossier. Circulation 92:1068–1073

Panza JA, Casino PR, Kilcoyne CM, Quyumi AA (1993) Role of nitric oxide in the abnormal endothelium-dependent vascular relaxation of patients with essential hypertension. Circulation 87:1468–1474

Paolisso G, Gambardella A, Verza M et al (1992) ACE inhibition improves insulin-sensitivity in aged insulin-resistant hypertensive patients. J Hum Hypertens 6:175–179

Papavassiliou MV, Vyssoulis GP, Karpanou EA et al (2001) Side effects of antihypertensive treatment with calcium channel antagonists. Am J Hypertens 14:114A

Park JB, Schiffrin EL (2001) Small artery remodeling is the most prevalent (earliest?) form of target organ damage in mild essential hypertension. J Hypertens 19:921–930

Parving HH, Brenner BM, McMurray JJ, de Zeeuw D, Haffner SM, Solomon SD, Chaturvedi N, Persson F, Desai AS, Nicolaides M, Richard A, Xiang Z, Brunel P, Pfeffer MA; ALTITUDE Investigators (2012) Cardiorenal end points in a trial of aliskiren for type 2 diabetes. N Engl J Med 367:2204–2213

Pasini AF, Garbin U, Stranieri C et al (2008) Nebivolol treatment reduces serum levels of asymmetric dimethylarginine and improves endothelial dysfunction in essential hypertensive patients. Am J Hypertens 21:1251–1257

Pfeffer MA (2013) Cancer in cardiovascular drug trials and vice versa. A personal perspective. Eur Heart J 34:1089–1094

Pitkäjärvi T, Ylitalo P, Metsä-Ketelä T et al (1979) The effects of a beta 1-blocking agent, atenolol, on blood pressure, plasma renin activity and prostaglandin F2 alpha excretion in patients with essential hypertension. Acta Med Scand 206:107–113

Pitt B, Zannad F, Remme WJ, Cody R, Castaigne A, Perez A, Palensky J, Wittes J (1999) The effect of spironolactone on morbidity and mortality in patients with severe heart failure. Randomized Aldactone Evaluation Study Investigators. N Engl J Med 341:709–717

PROGRESS Collaborative Group (2001) Randomised trial of a perindopril-based blood pressure lowering regimen among 6,105 individuals with previous stroke or transient ischaemic attack. Lancet 358:1033–1041

Psaty BM, Smith NL, Siscovick DS et al (1997) Health outcomes associated with antihypertensive therapies used as first-line agents. A systematic review and meta-analysis. JAMA 277:739–745

Ram CV (2010) Beta-blockers in hypertension. Am J Cardiol 106:1819–1825

Remme WJ (1997) Bradykinin-mediated cardiovascular protective actions of ACE inhibitors. A new dimension in anti-ischaemic therapy? Drugs 54(Suppl 5):59–70

Reungjui S, Pratipanawatr T, Johnson RJ et al (2008) Do thiazides worsen metabolic syndrome and renal disease? The pivotal roles for hyperuricemia and hypokalemia. Curr Opin Nephrol Hypertens 17:470–476

Ripley TL, Baumert M (2016) Controversies among the hypertension guidelines. J Pharm Pract 29:5–14

Rizos E, Bairaktari E, Kostoula A et al (2003) The combination of nebivolol plus pravastatin is associated with a more beneficial metabolic profile compared to that of atenolol plus pravastatin in hypertensive patients with dyslipidemia: a pilot study. J Cardiovasc Pharmacol Ther 8:127–134

Rothwell PM et al (2010) Effects of beta blockers and calcium-channel blockers on within-individual variability in blood pressure and risk of stroke. Lancet Neurol 9:469–480

Roush GC, Ernst ME, Kostis JB, Yeasmin S, Sica DA (2016) Dose doubling, relative potency, and dose equivalence of potassium-sparing diuretics affecting blood pressure and serum potassium: systematic review and meta-analyses. J Hypertens 34:11–19

Salomone S, Morel N, Godfraind T (1995) Effects of 8-bromocyclic GMP and verapamil on depolarization-evoked Ca 2+ signal and contraction in rat aorta. Br J Pharmacol 114:1731–1737

Salomone S, Silva LM, Morel N et al (1996) Facilitation of the vasorelaxant action of calcium antagonists by basal nitric oxide in depolarized artery. Naunyn Schmiedebergs Arch Pharmacol 354:505–512

Sánchez RA, Marcó E, Gilbert HB et al (1985) Natriuretic effect and changes in renal haemodynamics induced by enalapril in essential hypertension. Drugs 30(Suppl 1):49–58

Sasaki J, Arakawa K (1989) Effect of captopril on high-density lipoprotein subfractions in patients with mild to moderate essential hypertension. Clin Ther 11:129–134

Schiffrin LE, Deng LY (1996) Structure and function of resistance arteries of hypertensive patients treated with a ß-blocker or a calcium channel antagonist. J Hypertens 14:1247–1255

Shafi T, Appel LJ, Miller ER 3rd et al (2008) Changes in serum potassium mediate thiazide- induced diabetes. Hypertension 52:1022–1029

Shibata MC, León H, Chatterley T et al (2010) Do calcium channel blockers increase the diagnosis of heart failure in patients with hypertension? Am J Cardiol 106:228–235

Sipahi I, Debanne SM, Rowland DY et al (2010) Angiotensin-receptor blockade and risk of cancer: meta-analysis of randomised controlled trials. Lancet Oncol 11:627–636

Smith AC, Toto R, Bakris GL (1998) Differential effects of calcium channel blockers on size selectivity of proteinuria in diabetic glomerulopathy. Kidney Int 54:889–896

Staszewska-Woolley J (1987) Modification by diltiazem, a calcium antagonist, of the pulmonary vagal and cardiac sympathetic chemoreflexes in the dog. Clin Exp Pharmacol Physiol 14:455–464

Strauss MH et al (2006) Angiotensin receptor blockers may increase risk of myocardial infarction. Unraling the ARB-MI paradox. Circulation 114:838–854

Su JB, Hoüel R, Héloire F (2000) Stimulation of bradykinin B(1) receptors induces vasodilation in conductance and resistance coronary vessels in conscious dogs: comparison with B(2) receptor stimulation. Circulation 101:1848–1853

Taddei S, Virdis A, Ghiadoni L et al (2001) Effect of calcium antagonist or beta blockade treatment on nitric oxide-dependent vasodilation and oxidative stress in essential hypertensive patients. J Hypertens 19:1379–1386

Teo KK et al (2014) Aliskiren alone or with other antihypertensives in the elderly with borderline and stage 1 hypertension: the APOLLO trial. Eur Heart J 35(26):1743–1751

Testani JM, Kimmel SE, Dries DL et al (2011) Prognostic importance of early worsening renal function after initiation of Angiotensin-converting enzyme inhibitor therapy in patients with cardiac dysfunction. Circ Heart Fail 4:685–691

The SOLVD Investigators (1991) Effect of enalapril on survival in patients with reduced left ventricular ejection fractions and congestive heart failure. N Engl J Med 325:293–302

TOMH Study, Neaton JD, et al. Treatment of Mild Hypertension study (TOMH) (1993) Final results. JAMA 270:713–724

Turnbull F (2003) Effects of different blood-pressure-lowering regimens on major cardiovascular events: results of prospectively-designed overviews of randomised trials. Lancet 362:1527–1535

Vaage-Nilsen M, Rasmussen V (1998) Effect of Verapamil on heart rate variability after an acute myocardial infarction. Cardiovasc Drugs Ther 12:285–290

Van Bortel LM, Fici F, Mascagni F (2008) Efficacy and tolerability of nebivolol compared with other antihypertensive drugs: a meta-analysis. Am J Cardiovasc Drugs 8:35–44

Vatner SF, Hintze TH (1983) Mechanism of constriction of large coronary arteries by β- adrenergic receptor blockade. Circ Res 53:389–400

Verdecchia P, Reboldi G, Angeli F, Gattobigio R, Bentivoglio M, Thijs L, Staessen JA, Porcellati C (2005) Angiotensin-converting enzyme inhibitors and calcium channel blockers for coronary heart disease and stroke prevention. Hypertension 46:386–392

Vitale C, Mercuro G, Castiglioni C et al (2005) Metabolic effect of telmisartan and losartan in hypertensive patients with metabolic syndrome. Cardiovasc Diabetol 4:6

Wassertheil-Smoller S, Oberman A, Blaufox MD et al (1992) The Trial of Antihypertensive Interventions and Management (TAIM) Study. Final results with regard to blood pressure, cardiovascular risk, and quality of life. Am J Hypertens 5:37–44

Weber MA (2003) The ALLHAT report: a case of information and misinformation. J Clin Hypertens 5:9–13

Weber MA, Bakris GL, Neutel JM et al (2003) Quality of life measured in a practice-based hypertension trial of an angiotensin receptor blocker. J Clin Hypertens 5:322–329

Weber MA, Schiffrin EL, White WB et al (2014) Clinical practice guidelines for the management of hypertension in the community. A statement by the American Society of Hypertension and the International Society of Hypertension. J Hypertens 32:3–15

Weidmann P, Beretta-Piccoli C, Ziegler W et al (1976) Interrelations between blood pressure, blood volume, plasma renin and urinary catecholamines during beta-blockade in essential hypertension. Klin Wochenschr 54:765–773

Weir MR (2003) Incidence of pedal edema formation with dihydropyridine calcium channel blockers: issues and practical significance. J Clin Hypertens 5:330–335

Whelton P, Barzilay J, Cushman WC et al (2005) Clinical outcomes in antihypertensive treatment of type 2 diabetes, impaired fasting glucose concentration, and normoglycemia: Antihypertensive and Lipid-Lowering Treatment to Prevent Heart Attack Trial (ALLHAT). Archives Intern Med 165:1401–1409

Wilcox CS (1999) Metabolic and adverse effects of diuretics. Semin Nephrol 19:557–568

Williams B, Lacy PS, Thom SM et al (2006) Differential impact of blood pressure-lowering drugs on central aortic pressure and clinical outcomes: principal results of the Conduit Artery Function Evaluation (CAFE) study. Circulation 113:1213–1225

Wiysonge CS, Bradley H, Mayosi BM et al (2007) Beta-blockers for hypertension. Cochrane Database Syst Rev 1:CD002003

Wright JT Jr, Bakris G, Greene T et al (2002) Effect of blood pressure lowering and antihypertensive drug class on progression of hypertensive kidney disease: results from the AASK trial. JAMA 288:2421–2431

Yusuf S, Teo KK, Pogue J, et al for the ONTARGET investigators (2008) Telmisartan, ramipril, or both in patients at high risk for vascular events. N Engl J Med 358:1547–1559

Zanchetti A (2012) Calcium channel blockers in hypertension. In: Black HR, Elliott WJ (eds) Hypertension, a companion to Braunwald heart disease. Elsevier, Philadelphia, pp 204–218

Zanchetti A et al (2002) On behalf of the ELSA Investigators. Calcium antagonist lacidipine slows down progression of asymptomatic carotid atherosclerosis. Principal results of the European Lacidipine Study on Atherosclerosis (ELSA), a randomized, double-blind, long-term trial. Circulation 106:2422–2427

Zhou MS, Schulman IH, Jaimes EA et al (2008) Thiazide diuretics, endothelial function, and vascular oxidative stress. J Hypertens 26:494–500

Zillich AJ, Garg J, Basu S et al (2006) Thiazide diuretics, potassium, and the development of diabetes: a quantitative review. Hypertension 48:219–224

Adv Exp Med Biol - Advances in Internal Medicine (2017) 2: 61–84
DOI 10.1007/5584_2016_147
© Springer International Publishing AG 2016
Published online: 19 October 2016

Impact of Salt Intake on the Pathogenesis and Treatment of Hypertension

Petra Rust and Cem Ekmekcioglu

Abstract

Excessive dietary salt (sodium chloride) intake is associated with an increased risk for hypertension, which in turn is especially a major risk factor for stroke and other cardiovascular pathologies, but also kidney diseases. Besides, high salt intake or preference for salty food is discussed to be positive associated with stomach cancer, and according to recent studies probably also obesity risk. On the other hand a reduction of dietary salt intake leads to a considerable reduction in blood pressure, especially in hypertensive patients but to a lesser extent also in normotensives as several meta-analyses of interventional studies have shown. Various mechanisms for salt-dependent hypertension have been put forward including volume expansion, modified renal functions and disorders in sodium balance, impaired reaction of the renin-angiotensin-aldosterone-system and the associated receptors, central stimulation of the activity of the sympathetic nervous system, and possibly also inflammatory processes.

Not every person reacts to changes in dietary salt intake with alterations in blood pressure, dividing people in salt sensitive and insensitive groups. It is estimated that about 50–60 % of hypertensives are salt sensitive. In addition to genetic polymorphisms, salt sensitivity is increased in aging, in black people, and in persons with metabolic syndrome or obesity. However, although mechanisms of salt-dependent hypertensive effects are increasingly known, more research on measurement, storage and kinetics of sodium, on physiological properties, and genetic determinants of salt sensitivity are necessary to harden the basis for salt reduction recommendations.

P. Rust
Institute of Nutritional Sciences, University of Vienna,
Althanstrasse 14, 1090 Vienna, Austria

C. Ekmekcioglu (✉)
Institute of Environmental Health, Centre for Public
Health, Medical University of Vienna,
Kinderspitalgasse 15, 1090 Vienna, Austria
e-mail: cem.ekmekcioglu@meduniwien.ac.at

Currently estimated dietary intake of salt is about 9–12 g per day in most countries of the world. These amounts are significantly above the WHO recommended level of less than 5 g salt per day. According to recent research results a moderate reduction of daily salt intake from current intakes to 5–6 g can reduce morbidity rates. Potential risks of salt reduction, like suboptimal iodine supply, are limited and manageable. Concomitant to salt reduction, potassium intake by higher intake of fruits and vegetables should be optimised, since several studies have provided evidence that potassium rich diets or interventions with potassium can lower blood pressure, especially in hypertensives.

In addition to dietary assessment the gold standard for measuring salt intake is the analysis of sodium excretion in the 24 h urine. Spot urine samples are appropriate alternatives for monitoring sodium intake. A weakness of dietary evaluations is that the salt content of many foods is not precisely known and information in nutrient databases are limited. A certain limitation of the urine assessment is that dietary sources contributing to salt intake cannot be identified.

Salt reduction strategies include nutritional education, improving environmental conditions (by product reformulation and optimization of communal catering) up to mandatory nutrition labeling and regulated nutrition/ health claims, as well as legislated changes in the form of taxation.

Regarding dietary interventions for the reduction of blood pressure the Dietary Approaches to Stop Hypertension (DASH) diet can be recommended. In addition, body weight should be normalized in overweight and obese people (BMI less than 25 kg/m^2), salt intake should not exceed 5 g/day according to WHO recommendations (<2 g sodium/day), no more than 1.5 g sodium/d in blacks, middle- and older-aged persons, and individuals with hypertension, diabetes, or chronic kidney disease, intake of potassium (~4.7 g/day) should be increased and alcohol consumption limited. In addition, regular physical activity (endurance, dynamic resistance, and isometric resistance training) is very important.

Keywords

Physiology of sodium chloride • Renin-angiotensin-aldosterone system • Hypertension • Cardiovascular diseases • Salt sensitivity • Mechanisms of salt induced hypertension • Salt intake • Assessment of salt intake • Salt intake recommendations • Salt reduction strategies

Debates on whether current salt intake is too high for health reasons are ongoing for years. To take on the worldwide non-communicable disease challenge the recommendation for dietary salt reduction is one of the top priority actions of the WHO and member nations are stimulated to take action too (WHO and FAO Expert Consultation 2003; WHO 2012, 2014). Convincing scientific and medical evidence which associates excessive sodium intake to high blood pressure and secondary consequences such as cardiovascular disease (CVD), stroke, and cardiac-related mortality supports these efforts (Aburto et al. 2013a). Nevertheless, concerns have been raised that a low sodium intake may adversely affect health by influencing blood lipids and insulin resistance (Nakandakare et al. 2008). This is in conflict with numerous recommendations and strategies of scientific institutions and professional health associations which have faced sodium reduction in the population to reduce these hazards.

This critical review summarizes the nutritional physiology of sodium chloride and the effect of salt intake on hypertension and other diseases. Putative mechanisms, determinants of salt sensitivity and the role of potassium in hypertension will be discussed separately. Furthermore potential dangers of a low salt diet and strategies for a reduction of salt intake will also be addressed in separate chapters.

1 Physiology of Sodium Chloride

Sodium chloride (NaCl, or common salt) is an ionic compound required to perform a variety of essential functions. Sodium is the major cation and chloride the major anion in the extracellular fluid. The concentration of Na^+ in the extracellular fluid is regulated at about 135–145 mmol/L; the distribution of Cl^- follows this of Na^+ with an extracellular concentration of about 110 mmol/L. Therefore, Na^+ and Cl^- are mainly responsible for the osmolarity of the extracellular fluid and constitute the most important electrolytes in the regulation of body fluids (Elmadfa and Leitzmann 2015; Gibney et al. 2009).

The intestinal tract absorbs nearly all dietary sodium, and the kidneys retain more than 90 % of the filtered Na^+. As a consequence of excessive excretion of sodium by extreme vomiting, diarrhea, or sweating blood sodium concentrations can drop and cause hyponatremia (serum sodium concentrations less than 135 mmol/l). Without treatment hyponatremia can lead to osmosis with the central nervous being especially vulnerable. Headache, confusion, or in the worst coma could

be the consequence. Many diseases such as those of the kidneys, cancer, and heart disease can be associated with low blood sodium levels. On the contrary, especially dehydration and also more seldom rapid intake of large quantities of sodium can result in hypernatremia leading to neurological symptoms (Stipanuk and Caudill 2006).

Besides its importance with respect to the regulation of the water and fluid balance, sodium is vital for the excitation of muscle and nerve cells and is also partly involved in the control of the acid-base balance. Moreover, sodium helps to release digestive secretions and controls the absorption of some nutrients, such as amino acids, glucose, galactose, and water.

The renin-angiotensin-aldosterone system (RAAS), plays a key role in the regulation of sodium balance and blood pressure. Under normal physiological conditions a low salt diet stimulates RAAS by an increased release of renin from the juxtaglomerular cells of the kidneys which leads to an increase of angiotensin I stimulating angiotensin converting enzyme (ACE) in the lungs and release of angiotensin II. Angiotensin II is a potent vasoconstrictor and it stimulates aldosterone secretion from the adrenal cortex resulting in especially late tubular Na^+ and water reabsorption with increases in blood volume and blood pressure. In response to a high salt diet the RAAS is suppressed to some extent (Majid et al. 2015; Rassler 2010).

2 Dietary Requirements of Sodium Chloride

In terms of "how much" it should be noted that the human body contains about 0.15 % by weight sodium and chloride, respectively. This means that total body sodium as well as chloride have been considered at 60 mmol (1.38 g)/kg body weight or about 100 g for a 70 kg human.

For balance in the body the amount consumed must be equal to the amount lost. By estimation of obligatory losses in urine and faeces (1 mmol/day), and sweat (2–4 mmol/day) a minimum requirement of 1 mmol (23 mg) per 100 kcal or 24 mmol (550 mg) sodium per day was calculated for healthy adults. When sweating heavily sodium loss is more than 0.5 g and required intake increases. Accordingly, under normal living conditions and physical activity an intake of 5 g salt per day is considered to be sufficient. Highest sodium retention of 1.2 mmol/day was shown in newborn due to their rapid growth during the first 4 month of life. During pregnancy and lactation there is an additional need of sodium of 3 and 6 mmol/day, respectively. People with large losses, like patients with cystic fibrosis, require substitution (Deutsche Gesellschaft für Ernährung (DGE), Österreichische Gesellschaft für Ernährung, Schweizerische Gesellschaft für Ernährung (SGE) (Hrsg.) 2015).

The human body tolerates a large range of sodium intake being considerably different between cultures (0.2 g/day in Yanomami Indians (Brazil) up to 10.3 g/day in northern parts of Japan). Maximum adaptation of sodium urine excretion permits an intake of 0.18 g (about 8 mmol) per day with a minimum loss of sweat. However it is uncertain that a diet with such low sodium content can meet the need of other nutrients (Institute of Medicine 2005).

3 Assessment of Salt Intake

The most common methods used to measure sodium intake are 24-h dietary recall, food frequency questionnaire (FFQ), or food record with their advantages and limitations. Although dietary sodium intake is very complex, useful informations can be obtained by these methods when measurement errors like underreporting or underestimation of amounts during a 24 h dietary recall or limited food selection of a FFQ are considered.

However, in a previous study Kersting et al. for example showed that urinary sodium excretion was 1.4–1.7 times higher than the sodium intake estimated by dietary records (3-day food diary). This implies that sodium intake assessed by dietary reports may be underreported by an average of 29–41 % (Kersting et al. 2006).

A major challenge of dietary assessment is that sodium intake is highly correlated with total energy intake whereby underreporting of food intake leads to underestimation of sodium intake. In addition, sodium content in recipes is highly variable as well as salt used in home cooking and at the table. A FFQ is a less reliable estimate of intake but provides good information of sources of sodium intake which is essential for public health interventions. Nevertheless, dietary assessment also enables recognition of relationships between sodium intake and supply with other nutrients or dietary pattern associated with specific diseases (McLean 2014).

In addition to dietary assessment, urine sodium excretion is measured as an indicator of salt intake. As more than 90 % of consumed sodium is absorbed and excreted in the urine (Holbrook et al. 1984), 24-h urine sodium excretion has been considered as the gold standard to assess dietary sodium intake. In hot climates and among highly physically active people the losses through sweat and faeces can be higher than 10 % which have been estimated under normal conditions. A correlation of 0.75 between sodium intake measured by a nutrition survey and 24-h urine sodium excretion over a 9-day collection were calculated by Luft and colleagues (Luft et al. 1982). To minimize errors caused by under-/overcollection of urine samples 24-h urine creatinine excretion can be assessed. Under physiological conditions, 24-h urine creatinine excretion is influenced only to a minor extent by kidney function itself, but correlates mainly with muscle mass and dietary meat ingestion. To assess completeness of urine collection para-aminobenzoic acid tables can be used. However there are limitations like decreased excretion with increasing age or interaction with other medications (McLean 2014).

Alternatively spot urine samples can be collected and evaluated. This requires correction for urine tonicity, which is accomplished by referring to urine creatinine (Kawasaki et al. 1993; Tanaka et al. 2002; Toft et al. 2014). Because creatinine excretion depends on proportion of muscle mass, which is lower in women, older people, and individuals with lower body weight formula to correct creatinine excretion were developed. By adjusting for estimated creatinine excretion the correlation of spot urine sodium-to-creatinine ratio with 24-h urine sodium can be improved (Rhee et al. 2014). Actually several formulae have been developed but no single formula has been accepted for international use. This is challenging because validity of estimates is different between women and men as well as in different ethnic groups (McLean 2014).

Spot urine samples have greater intra-individual variability of sodium concentrations than 24 h samples and therefore are a poor predictor of individual sodium intake but an appropriate tool for monitoring. Huang et al. (2016) confirm in their systematic review and meta-analysis that estimates of mean population salt intake determined from spot urine samples were comparable to estimates based upon 24-h urine collection with a sensitivity of 97 % and specificity of 100 % for the 5 g/day WHO threshold (Huang et al. 2016). These results support that estimates of NaCl intake evaluated by spot urine samples can be used to make decisions on salt reduction programmes and evaluation of strategies. Nonetheless, the authors recognised an overestimation of intake by the equations at lower levels of intake and an underestimation at higher salt intake levels. Therefore, the collection of 24-h urine in a subsample is recommended.

Measuring sodium excretion in urine underestimates dietary salt intake due to unrecognised loss in sweat which is approximately 400 mg/day (equivalent to ~ 1 g NaCl) (Maughan and Leiper 1995). This amount of sodium is almost equal to the intake of sodium from natural food sources (400–500 mg/day) and therefore compensates losses by sweat whereby urine sodium excretion reflects actual salt intake quite well (Mattes 1990).

While a limitation of the urine assessment is that dietary sources contributing to salt intake cannot be identified, a weakness of the dietary evaluations is that the salt content of many foods is not precisely known and information in nutrient databases are limited.

4 Recommendations for Salt Intake

Dietary sodium is consumed mainly as salt: NaCl = Na (g) × 2.54

> 1 mmol sodium corresponds to 23.0 mg,
>   1 mmol chloride to 35.5 mg;
> 1 g NaCl consists of ~ 17 mmol sodium and chloride each.

The Word Health Organization (WHO) recommends a maximum salt intake of 5 g/day, equivalent of one teaspoon (WHO 2012). Due to the suggested potential to prevent and control non-communicable diseases the WHO has recommended reduction of salt intake in the extent of 30 % by 2025 (WHO 2013a). For children younger than 9 month no salt should be added to food. For children aged 18 months to 3 years, salt intake should be no more than 2 g per day (WHO 2012; WHO 2016). Based on the WHO recommendation the European Society of Hypertension/European Society of Cardiology (ESH/ESC) guidelines also propose to reduce dietary salt intake to 5 g/day for the management of hypertension (Mancia et al. 2013).

The Dietary Reference Intake (DRI) recommendation for sodium intake is less than 2.3 g/day (~6 g NaCl/day; UL = maximum level of daily nutrient intake) for healthy adults. The Adequate Intake (AI) is defined as an amount to obtain a nutritionally adequate diet and to meet the needs for sweat losses which result from recommended levels of physical activity (Institute of Medicine 2013). As most people consume far too much sodium this recommendation is set at an upper limit. Special population groups including hypertension patients should limit sodium consumption to 1.5 g/day. Thus, the American Heart Association advice to eat no more than 1.5 g of sodium per day for optimal heart health (American Heart Association 2016).

Table 1 Sodium intake recommendations

Life stage	AI (g/day) (DRI 2004)	UL (g/day) (DRI 2004)	Estimate value for min. intake (g/day) (DGE et al. 2015)
Infants:			**Infants:**
0–6 month	0.12	Not determinable	0– < 4 month: 0.1
7–12 month	0.37		4– < 12 month: 0.18
Children:			**Children:**
1–3 year	1.0	1.5	1– < 4 year: 0.3
4–8 year	1.2	1.9	4– < 7 year: 0.41
			7– < 10 year: 0.46
			10– < 13 year: 0.51
			13– < 15 year: 0.55
Adults:			**Adolescents/Adults:**
9– > 70 year	1.5	2.3	0.55
Pregnancy	1.5	2.3	
Lactation	1.5	2.3	

Deutsche Gesellschaft für Ernährung (DGE) et al. (2015), Institute of Medicine (2005)

The estimate value for minimum intake according to DACH reference values is about 550 mg/day for adolescents and adults (Deutsche Gesellschaft für Ernährung (DGE) et al. 2015) (Table 1).

Similar to the recommendations in USA, the Scientific Committee on Food established as acceptable range of sodium intakes for adults 25–150 mmol/day (0.6–3.5 g/day) (SCF 1993). The Reference Nutrient Intake in UK is 70 mmol/day (1.6 g/day) (Dietary reference values for food energy and nutrients for the United Kingdom 1991). The current sodium intake across Europe is much higher than the amounts required for normal function. For the reason that increased sodium intake is associated with high blood pressure, which in turn could result in cardiovascular and renal diseases, salt reduction is highly recommended.

5 Salt Intake and Hypertension

According to the WHO hypertension is the number one risk factor for mortality worldwide (WHO 2009). Furthermore hypertension is the primary contributor to DALYS (Disability-Adjusted Life Years) in the world (Lim et al. 2012) and a major risk factor for cardiovascular diseases, heart failure, kidney disease including nephrosclerosis, and retinopathy. Several factors are associated with a high blood pressure, such as especially genetic predispositions, but also age, overweight and obesity, low physical activity, and chronic stress (Dorner et al. 2013). In addition, there is convincing evidence that the diet, in front salt (sodium chloride) intake, has significant effects on the blood pressure (Dorner et al. 2013; Appel et al. 2006). The fact that sodium plays a prominent role in managing blood pressure has been well established for long now (Ekmekcioglu et al. 2013). Many trials have been published, showing that a reduction of sodium intake is associated with a reduction in systolic and diastolic blood pressure, especially in hypertensive but also in normotensive persons (He and MacGregor 2002).

Already in 1904 Ambard und Beaujard published a study showing the blood pressure rising effects of salt (Ambard and Beaujard 1904). More than 40 years later Dr. Walter Kempner impressively presented that an extreme salt deficient rice diet could lower the blood pressure of patients with severe hypertension for an average of 47 mmHg systolic and 21 mmHg diastolic (Kempner 1948). These remarkable effects are comparable with an intensive, modern antihypertensive drug therapy. However only approx. 60 % of Dr. Kempners hypertensive patients reacted on salt reduction with noteable lowering of blood pressure. These patients are known as salt sensitive. This is described below (Dorner et al. 2013; Luft et al. 1979).

In the last decades the effects of salt on human blood pressure was investigated in several epidemiological and interventional studies. In one of the most famous and global, the Intersalt study, which included 32 countries and 52 different populations, it was shown that a 100 mmol higher urinary sodium excretion was associated with an average 6 or 3 mmHg higher systolic blood pressure (with or without adjustment for body mass index) (Elliott et al. 1996). Furthermore in a high British sample of more than 23 000 persons in the age of 45–79 years those with the lowest salt intake showed an average 7.2/3.0 mmHg (systolic/diastolic) lower blood pressure compared to the group with the highest intake. (Khaw et al. 2004).

Several interventional studies looked at the effect of salt reduction on blood pressure in hypertensive and normotensive individuals. Most of the studies lasted 2–8 weeks and the daily salt reduction was in the range of 4.3–9.3 g/day. This resulted in a reduction of blood pressure in the range of 3.9–5.9/ 1.9–3.8 mmHg (systolic/diastolic) in hypertensives and 1.2–2.4/0.3–1.1 mmHg (systolic/diastolic) in normotensives as a half a dozen meta-analyses have calculated (Fig. 1) (Aburto et al. 2013a; He and MacGregor 2002; Kotchen et al. 2013; Midgley et al. 1996; Cutler et al. 1997; Graudal et al. 1998; He et al. 2013).

In a recent meta-analysis, by including 103 studies, Mozaffarian and coworkers found a strong evidence for a linear dose-response effect with each reduction of sodium intake by 2.3 g/day (equivalent to approx. 5.8 g salt) being associated with a reduction of 3.82 mmHg systolic blood pressure (Mozaffarian et al. 2014).

Also the blood pressure of children is beneficially affected by salt reduction. In a large study in 650 children, a reduction in salt intake of 15–20 % through changes in food purchasing and in preparation practices in the schools' kitchens resulted in a significant fall in blood pressure after 6 months (Ellison et al. 1989), and in a meta-analysis by He and MacGregor of controlled trials it was concluded that an average reduction in salt intake by 42 % in children is associated with immediate decreases in blood pressure and, if continued, may prevent the subsequent rise in blood pressure with age (He and MacGregor 2006).

In addition to adverse effects on blood pressure a high salt consumption also may lead to other adverse outcomes on the cardiovascular system, such as endothelial dysfunction, and ventricular hypertrophy (Baldo et al. 2015; Du Cailar et al. 1992; Todd et al. 2010; Oberleithner et al. 2007). For example the acute intake of salt impairs the flow-mediated dilation of the brachial artery in healthy individuals (Dickinson et al. 2011). Importantly, excess salt intake also impairs endothelium-dependent dilation in salt resistant humans (DuPont et al. 2013).

Regarding cardiovascular risk recent meta-analyses calculated a reduced risk in cardiovascular events of approximately 10–20 % for a lower vs. higher salt intake (He and MacGregor 2011; Strazzullo et al. 2009).

5.1 Mechanisms of Salt-Dependent Hypertension

Arterial blood pressure is dependent on the cardiac output (heart rate × stroke volume) and total peripheral vascular resistance. Short and long term mechanisms are involved in the regulation of blood pressure by influencing these two variables (Porth 2009). In the short-term arterial and cardiopulmonary baroreflexes regulate mean arterial blood pressure by mainly modulating the activity of the autonomic nervous system. On the longer term especially endocrine mechanisms, in front the RAAS and vasopressin are involved in the regulation of blood pressure with the kidneys playing an important role.

Studies from Guyton from the early 60s showed that sodium loading lead to extracellular volume expansion and volume loaded hypertension in the context of induced renal dysfunction in dogs (Farquhar et al. 2015). This was in

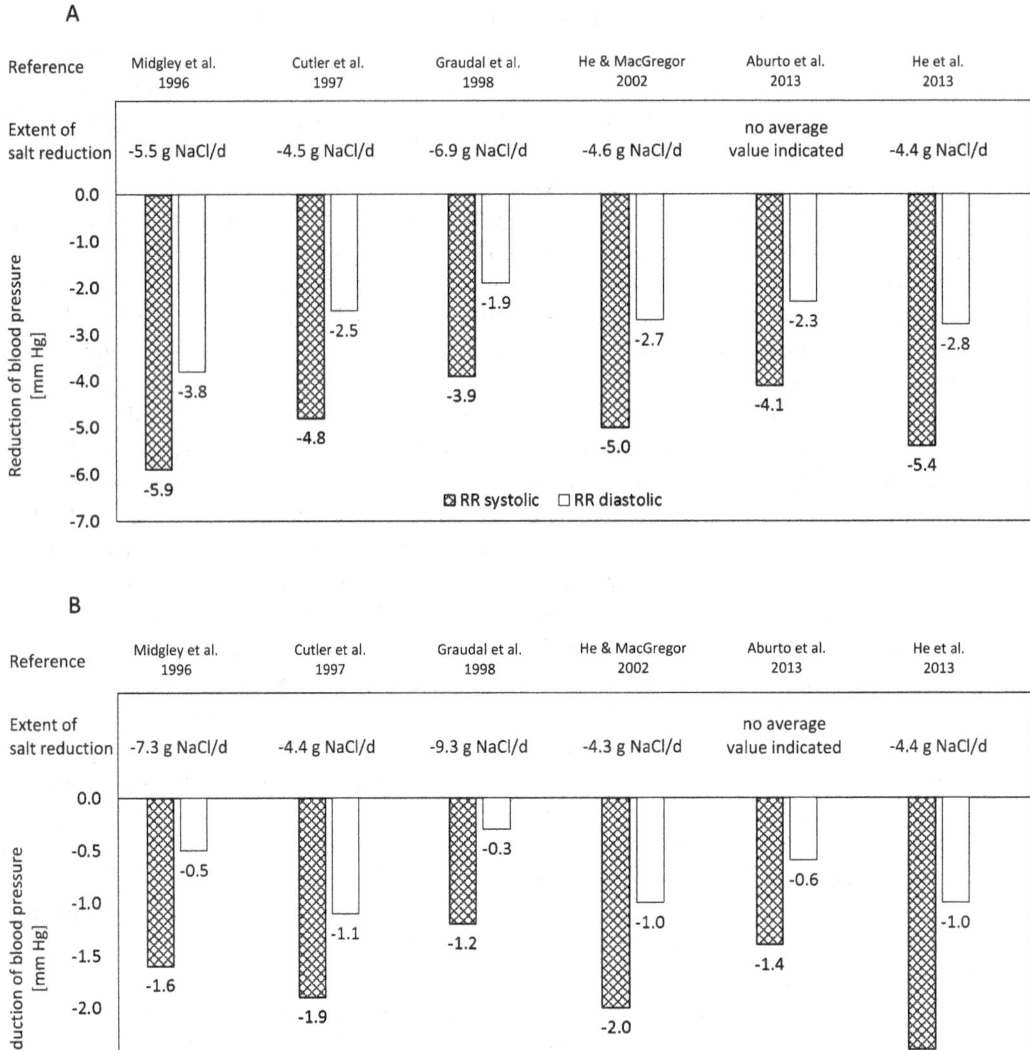

Fig. 1 (**a**) Effect of a salt reduction on the blood pressure of hypertensive patients. (**b**) Effect of a salt reduction on the blood pressure of normotensive persons. Average values are given for salt and blood pressure reduction

accordance with clinical studies in patients with chronic kidney disease (Koomans et al. 1982). Also according to Guyton, a rise in blood pressure above the pressure natriuresis equilibrium point, leads to an increase in sodium and water excretion, in turn lowering the blood pressure towards the previous levels (Guyton 1990; Luzardo et al. 2015). In salt sensitive individuals, the pressure natriuresis relationship is shifted to the right, meaning that higher blood pressure levels are necessary to increase renal sodium excretion and to maintain sodium balance (Guyton et al. 1972).

As mentioned before mean blood pressure is primarily dependent on (stroke) volume and peripheral vascular resistance. So salt induced increases in extracellular volume, and related to this stroke volume, would especially exert blood pressure raising effects if peripheral resistance does not decline compensatory (Schmidlin et al. 2007). Therefore, an unchanged or increased peripheral resistance, in association with a salt-induced increase in cardiac output, would result in a salt-dependent blood pressure response, as shown in African Americans (Schmidlin et al. 2007).

Also an impaired reaction of the RAAS during a sodium manipulation may be linked to a salt sensitive blood pressure response. In this regard it is assumed that angiotensin II type 1 receptors may be involved in sodium-induced increases in blood pressure (Crowley et al. 2005). These are found in systemic as well as renal vasculature, and also in the central nervous system, where they are important for blood pressure and/or fluid volume regulation. In this regard high salt intake increases several components of the central RAAS, such as angiotensin II and aldosterone, in addition to the AT1 receptor, renin and ACE expression (Baldo et al. 2015; Huang et al. 2006). For example mice lacking renal angiotensin II type 1 receptors become salt sensitive (Mangrum et al. 2002). Furthermore the ChineseGenSalt studies identified angiotensin II type 1 gene variants as predictive of salt sensitivity (Gu et al. 2010).

In addition to the RAAS also modulation of the autonomic nervous system may be involved in salt sensitive hypertension. For example it is suggested that in rodents a salt induced central stimulation of the activity of the sympathetic nervous system leads to a rise in blood pressure (Farquhar et al. 2015; Brooks et al. 2005; Stocker et al. 2010). In humans for example, salt-sensitive individuals react with a higher increase in heart rate to mental stress compared to salt-resistant controls (Buchholz et al. 2003). A stimulatory effect of sodium on angiotensin II may also increase sympathetic outflow (Guild et al. 2012). Furthermore sodium induced temporary increases in osmolality may also affect sympathetic outflow (Farquhar et al. 2006). On the other hand also an acute, drastic lowering of sodium intake may activate the sympathetic nervous system in humans (Anderson et al. 1989). This can be explained as a stress reaction to acute salt (and volume) depletion.

The kidneys have a prominent role in salt dependent hypertension. Several experimental findings in genetically hypertensive rat strains provided evidence that renal mechanisms and disorders in sodium balance are involved in salt sensitive hypertension (Majid et al. 2015). Further evidence to the critical role of the kidneys in the development of hypertension stems from monogenic forms of human hypertension with abnormalities in tubular sodium transport leading to increased sodium reabsorption (Lifton et al. 2001; Shimkets et al. 1994).

Furthermore relating to animal studies it is suggested that serum- and glucocorticoid-inducible kinase (SGK), a downstream mediator of mineralocorticoid receptors (MRs) that activates the epithelial sodium channel in renal tubules, may be involved in the adaptation to salt and the pathogenesis of hypertension (Luzardo et al. 2015; Farjah et al. 2003). In Dahl salt-sensitive hypertensive rats for example, sodium intake upregulates the expression of SGK1, suggesting that MRs are activated in an aldosterone-independent manner (Farjah et al. 2003). Furthermore, an impairment of renal sodium excretion could be also due to renal inflammation, as suggested in experimental models (Rodriguez-Iturbe et al. 2012).

5.2 Salt Sensitivity

The blood pressure response to changes in sodium intake varies considerably among individuals. Whereas some persons can eat high amounts of salt without any or marginal effects on their blood pressure, others would react with a significant rise in blood pressure as a consequence of a sodium-rich diet indicating that the response to changes in blood pressure by dietary sodium is variable dividing the people in salt-sensitive and insensitive groups (Kawasaki et al. 1978; Luft et al. 1991). Weinberger et al. defined salt sensitivity if at least a 10 % increase in mean arterial pressure is found after a high salt vs. low salt challenge. Persons having smaller increases were defined as salt-resistant (Weinberger 1996). However, in general there is no clear consensus on the definition of salt sensitivity in clinical practice (Luzardo et al. 2015; Rodriguez-Iturbe and Vaziri 2007).

In the literature approx. 50 % of hypertensives are estimated to be salt sensitive (Felder et al. 2013). In particular genetic polymorphisms have been linked to salt sensitivity, hypertension and cardiovascular disease (Trudu et al. 2013). Possible candidate genes include especially those that increase or decrease the expression of proteins which are involved in renal sodium transport (Armando et al. 2015). In addition to hypertensives and genetic polymorphisms salt sensitivity is especially also increased in aging (Weinberger and Fineberg 1991), in black people (Jenni and Suter 2011), and in persons with metabolic syndrome or obesity (Chen et al. 2009; Fujita 2014).

What is also important is that salt sensitivity in normotensive adults predicts future hypertension (Weinberger and Fineberg 1991; Sullivan 1991). Furthermore salt sensitivity has been associated with increased mortality in normal and hypertensive persons (Weinberger 2002).

6   High Salt Intake and Other Diseases

In addition to cardiovascular diseases a high dietary salt intake was also shown to be associated with an increased risk for gastric cancer and kidney disease. Furthermore in the last years there is accumulating evidence for a link between high dietary salt intake and risk for overweight and obesity.

6.1   Stomach Cancer

A recent meta-analysis of prospective cohort studies showed that dietary salt intake is directly associated with risk of gastric cancer, with progressively increasing risk across consumption levels (D'Elia et al. 2012). Furthermore 24 % of stomach cancer cases in the UK in 2010 were suggested to be attributed to high salt consumption (Parkin 2011). Various mechanisms, including an increased gastric *H. pylori* colonization, mutations, or exposure to carcinogens such as N-nitroso compounds from certain salty foods,

are hypothesized to be involved in a higher gastric cancer risk by high dietary salt intake (Ge et al. 2012). According to the International Systematic Literature Review (2015) of the World Cancer Research Fund there were not enough data to conduct dose-response meta-analysis. The review did not observe a significant association comparing the highest versus lowest salt intake (measured by food frequency questionnaire) as well as comparing the highest versus lowest added salt intake. Nonetheless a significant positive association was observed for stomach cancer and with salted food intake and comparing preference for salty food versus no preference (Norat et al. 2015).

6.2   Renal Disease

Epidemiological studies reported an association between dietary salt intake and urinary albumin excretion, independent of blood pressure (du Cailar et al. 2002). In this regard it is known that urinary albumin levels are a risk factor for the development and progression of kidney disease and are also strong predictors for cardiovascular risk (Cerasola et al. 2010). In an interventional study in three ethnic groups, a reduction in salt intake of about 3.2 g per day over 6 weeks lead to significant reductions in blood pressure and urinary albumin excretion (He et al. 2009). Furthermore it was demonstrated that reduced salt intake may lower the risk of estimated glomerular filtration rate decline (Lin et al. 2010).

6.3   Obesity

Dietary salt induces hyperosmolar thirst in the hypothalamus leading to higher water intake and renal water excretion (Cowley et al. 1983). Many people, especially children and adolescents, prefer caloric, sugar-sweetened beverages (SSBs) instead of tap water or low energy drinks (Duffey et al. 2012). In a cross-sectional study in young British children and adolescents it was demonstrated that 31 % of total fluid intake were by SSBs (He et al. 2008) and a difference of 1 g/day in salt intake was associated with a difference of 100 and 27 g/day in total fluid and

SSBs consumption, respectively. Other studies also found a positive association between urinary sodium excretion/dietary salt intake and beverage consumption (Alexy et al. 2012; Grimes et al. 2013).

In a recent paper by Ma et al. in a collective of 458 British children and 785 adults it was demonstrated that salt intake was higher in overweight and obese individuals (Ma et al. 2015). A 1-g/day increase in salt intake was associated with an increase in the risk of obesity by 28 % (CI 95 %:1.12–1.45) in children and 26 % (CI 95 %: 1.16–1.37) in adults after adjusting for various factors. The results were independent from energy intake suggesting that other mechanisms such as higher consumption of sugar-sweetened soft drinks might have played a role. An experimental study for example showed that high dietary sodium intake in rats leads to higher plasma leptin concentrations and excessive accumulation of white adipose fat compared with the rats with lower salt intake (Fonseca-Alaniz et al. 2007).

Also human studies in healthy adolescents suggest a positive association between dietary salt intake and subcutaneous abdominal adipose tissue, independent of energy intake (Zhu et al. 2014). Future studies will gain more insight into the mechanisms between dietary salt intake and obesity.

In summary, the negative effects of a high sodium/salt intake are not only restricted to the cardiovascular and renal systems, but may also adversely affect our metabolism and energy intake. However, it should also be mentioned that regarding nutrition not only a low dietary intake of salt, but also a higher consumption of potassium-rich fruit and vegetables, as important components of a healthy diet, has preventive effects on chronic diseases including hypertension (Boeing et al. 2012). For example, several publications in the last years provided a high degree of evidence that a Dietary Approaches to Stop Hypertension (DASH)-style diet, which is based on fruits and vegetables with low-fat dairy products and low in saturated and total fat, exerts blood pressure lowering and cardioprotective effects (Dorner et al. 2013; Appel et al. 1997; Salehi-Abargouei et al. 2013).

7 Potassium and Hypertension

The association between potassium and blood pressure was already put forward for the first time in 1928 by W.L. Addison (Bulpitt 1981). Ever since then, many trials suggested or showed the blood pressure lowering effects of potassium. These were summarized and analysed in a handful of meta-analyses (Cappuccio and MacGregor 1991; Whelton et al. 1997; Dickinson et al. 2006; Aburto et al. 2013b; Geleijnse et al. 2003). All of these provided evidence that potassium rich diets or interventions with potassium can lower blood pressure, especially in hypertensives. In the most recent meta-analysis by Aburto et al. (Aburto et al. 2013b) it was for example shown that a higher potassium intake in the range of 90–120 mmol/day reduced blood pressure and was associated with a lower risk of stroke incidence. However, dietary amounts above 120 mmol/day seem to be not associated with additional beneficial effects. In addition, in combination with a recommended sodium intake of less than 2 g/day (about 5 g/day salt), sodium/potassium ratios with positive health effects can be obtained according to the authors. Furthermore, it was concluded that potassium may be more effective in reducing blood pressure at higher levels of sodium intake, consistent with previous findings (Whelton et al. 1997). The largest benefit was analysed when sodium intake was more than 4 g/day. However, potassium is also beneficial at lower intake values of sodium (Aburto et al. 2013b). In this regard, a recent meta-analysis found that potassium has relevant blood pressure reducing effects in hypertensive patients with salt-rich diets (van Bommel and Cleophas 2012). The effects were in the magnitude of −9.5 mmHg (95 % CI: −10.8 to −8.1) for systolic and −6.4 mmHg for diastolic blood pressure values (95 % CI: −7.3 to −5.6). Patients with reduced salt intake showed little effects from potassium treatment. Concomitantly to these results in the recent PURE study, a prospective cohort study of 102 216 participants from 18 countries with average cardiovascular risk, it was shown that a high salt intake was more strongly associated with increased blood pressure in individuals with lower potassium excretion (Mente et al. 2014).

Finally, the advantages of dietary potassium on blood pressure may be strongest in salt-sensitive individuals (Dietary Guidelines Advisory Committee 2010). Therefore it is reasonable and important to not only recommend salt reduction but also to increase potassium intake (Aaron and Sanders 2013).

Potassium might exert blood pressure lowering effects through many pathways (reviewed in (Ekmekcioglu et al. 2016)). These include (1) stimulation of natriuresis, (2) improvement of endothelial function and NO release, (3) stimulation of the sodium/potassium pump and plasma membrane potassium channels leading to endothelial hyperpolarization and decrease in cytosolic smooth muscle calcium, and (4) decrease in the activity of the sympathetic nervous system with vascular smooth muscle relaxation.

Some authors also suggest an antioxidant effect of dietary potassium (Ishimitsu et al. 1996). Carotid artery rings from rabbits fed a low potassium diet for example showed an approximately 100 % higher formation of superoxide anions, enhanced norepinephrine contraction, and suppressed acetylcholine relaxation (Yang et al. 1998). In addition, dietary potassium supplementation suppressed ROS overproduction in injured arteries of salt-loaded Dahl S rats (Kido et al. 2008).

8 Potential Dangers of a Low-Salt Diet

A considerable restriction of sodium in the diet may bear some potential dangers (Burnier et al. 2015). One of these is iodine insufficiency, which is common in Alpine countries such as Austria (Burnier et al. 2015). The iodization of salt is an important and cost efficient strategy to combat iodine deficiency and related to this hypothyroidism in the general population. Reducing salt intake in the population may worsen the iodine status of especially people with suboptimal or marginal iodine intake.

Different scenarios could estimate the dietary supply of iodine in case of salt reduction. For the Netherlands for example it was estimated that up to 10 % of the population would have an insufficient iodine supply when the dietary salt intake would be reduced by 50 % (Vandevijvere 2012; Verkaik-Kloosterman et al. 2010). A strategy to overcome this problem could be to increase the iodine content of salt.

Furthermore a low salt diet could increase the risk of volume depletion and hypotension in patients with acute dehydration or diarrhoea. Also, in elderly people, reducing salt in the diet could lead to altered food taste, which in turn my increase the risk of low energy intake and malnutrition (Zeanandin et al. 2012).

Although the benefits of salt reduction on blood pressure and human health is overwhelming there are also few studies showing an inverse or J-shaped association meaning that not only a high but also a low dietary salt intake might be associated with adverse health outcomes, especially on the cardiovascular system (Van Horn 2015).

For example the results of the ONTARGET and TRANSCEND trials in 28,880 people at high cardiovascular risk showed a J-shaped association with an increased risk for cardiovascular mortality in those consuming <3 g or >7 g sodium (approximately < 7.5 salt or 17.5 g salt) per day (O'Donnell et al. 2011). A similar association was shown in the PURE study with low (<3 g/day) or high (≥ 7 g/day) sodium intakes being associated with higher risk of death or major vascular events (O'Donnell et al. 2014). A J-shaped relationship for all-cause or cardiovascular mortality was also shown in patients with type 1 and 2 diabetes mellitus, respectively (Thomas et al. 2011; Saulnier et al. 2014). An inverse association was reported in the Flemish Study on Genes, Environment and Health Outcomes and the European Project on Genes in Hypertension with an increased risk for cardiovascular disease (CVD) mortality in the lowest tertile of sodium intake (Stolarz-Skrzypek et al. 2011).

Since there are few indications that a low salt diet seems to be also, at least in part, associated with an increased incidence of cardiovascular events and mortality, the important 2 questions are: what are the reasons for these negative outcomes and what are the suggested mechanisms? Is this due to the low sodium/salt intake per se or to one or more additional factors that might affect patients' survival? Another question might be whether the low salt intake in the patients is a consequence or a cause of their disease. This limiting issue is defined as reverse causality meaning that compromised patients may consume less sodium, because of medical advice or an illness-related reduction in food consumption (Cobb et al. 2014). It may also be relevant that some of the studies showing J-shaped or inverse associations included sick persons or were based on secondary analyses of studies not primarily intended to test these relationships.

One further major drawback in these studies are suboptimal methods in the assessment of sodium intake including food frequency questionnaires, or spot or overnight urine collection (Cobb et al. 2014).

9 Strategies for Reduction of Salt Intake

For millions of years, dietary salt intake was very low (0.1–1 g/day). Main source of NaCl was meat containing about 1.2 g/kg (Ha 2014; MacGregor and de Wardener 1998). Until the invention of the refrigerator great amounts of salt were used for cooking and preserving foods whereby around the nineteenth century salt intake reached a peak comparable to amounts of about 9–12 g/day, significantly above recommended levels (Brown et al. 2009). A comparison of world salt consumption observed highest consumption in Asian people, followed by Europeans, people in Middle East and North Africa, USA/Canada, Australia/New Zealand, Latin America and the Caribbean, Oceania, and Sub Saharan Africa (Powles et al. 2013).

Within the "WHO Global Strategy on Diet, Physical Activity and Health" an action plan to control and prevent non-communicable diseases has been established. A primary goal is the reduction of salt (WHO 2013a). Since now most Europeans consume salt above the recommended level of less than 5 g/day (<2 g sodium/day).

Studies found that in industrial countries only 5–10 % of sodium intake comes from food naturally rich in sodium bicarbonate, sodium glutamate, and sodium citrate like smoked meat, processed foods, and canned vegetables. 75–80 % of daily sodium consumption comes from processed food like bread, cereals and bakery products, meat and meat products, cheese and dairy products, fish products, ready-to-eat meals, and salty snacks, 10–15 % from table salt added during cooking or at the table (European Commission 2012), while in developing countries salt used for seasoning is much more important. For example in China and Japan soy sauce contributes significantly to salt intake. Worldwide, the sodium content of processed foods plays a more important role compared to that of natural foods.

Many studies detected a wide range of sodium content within various food categories. Also salt content of products of global brands varied in different countries. This may be due to traditional diet habits and taste preferences of different population groups. Certain individuals such as men, adolescents, and people with lower socioeconomic status consume greater amounts of salt, supposing that these population groups consume more meat, high-sodium processed and packaged foods than other consumer groups.

Opportunities for supporting the reduction of salt intake to moderate levels are manifold and varied. They reach from nutritional education, improving environmental conditions (make the healthier choices the easier choices) up to mandatory nutrition labeling and regulated nutrition/health claims, as well as legislated changes in the form of taxation. Current knowledge makes the importance of combining reformulation approaches, improvement of the quality of communal catering, and education to raise awareness evident.

Ekmekcioglu et al. established a simple model of how salt intake can be reduced in the population. This model emphasises the need for a holistic approach in the improvement of optimal salt intake (Fig. 2) (Ekmekcioglu et al. 2013).

9.1 Association Between Knowledge on Salt and Salt-Related Dietary Practices

Gathering and exploiting knowledge about the awareness of the people on the relationship between salt consumption and health or disease risk, about levels of uptake, and drivers of salt intake, provide the basis for improving the current situation.

Therefore, Newson et al. evaluated self-rated and calculated salt intake, sources of salt consumption, concern in salt reduction, knowledge about salt intake recommendations, and importance of salt reduction in health issues in eight countries (Germany, Austria, United States of America, Hungary, India, China, Brazil, and South Africa) by a comprehensive web-based questionnaire. Mean salt intake calculated from data of the FFQ was 9.5 g per day, ranging from 7 to 13 g/day. On average 83 % of salt intake was derived from In-Home-Foods and 17 % came from Out-of the House-Consumption. While people perceive that salt added during cooking is the main source of intake, calculated data recognised processed food as a primary source. There was also a misperception of personal intake. One third of participants were not interested in salt reduction and only 13 % of all participants could correctly identify the salt intake recommendations (Newson et al. 2013). Although, numerous studies showed that consumers were able to identify the health risks associated with high salt intake, their knowledge of recommendations, and of foods that contribute most salt to their diet is poor. Therefore, findings support the importance of information, of increasing awareness, and motivation, as well as reformulation of food stuff (Newson et al. 2013).

Most important for behavioural changes according to the health belief model (Janz and Becker 1984) is motivation which can be achieved by increasing awareness, information, and therefore self-efficacy (Ekmekcioglu et al. 2013).

Individuals affected by diseases like hypertension become aware of the importance of behavioural changes and are more motivated to change dietary habits compared to healthy people. Nakano and colleagues for example showed that regular 20-min educational sessions with nutritionists can be effective in lowering urinary sodium excretion, ambulatory BP monitoring (ABPM), and clinic BP in hypertensive patients (Nakano et al. 2016). This study is probably the first that demonstrates the effectiveness of patient education for hypertension management. Participants who didn't reach the goal of 6 g/day tended to have higher BMI and therefore had a higher salt intake because of their higher food consumption. The effect of potassium can be excluded because urinary excretions were the same in the intervention and control groups. Due to the short duration of the study (12 weeks) patients didn't lose weight, which might have an impact on blood pressure. Limitations might be the small sample size of 51 participants in the education group and 44 in the control group, the Hawthorne effect and different medications (Nakano et al. 2016).

9.2 Reduction of Salt Intake by Reformulation

Part of the strategies to reduce salt consumption is cooperating with food companies to reduce the amount of salt in processed foods and improving consumers' awareness of the impact of salt on human health.

This can be achieved through limiting salt by food reformulation. Since the WHO launched the "Global Strategy on Diet, Physical Activity and Health" to limit the levels of salt in foods, many companies have reformulated their products and reduced salt content by 10–40 % in many food categories including bread, breakfast cereals, processed meat, cheese, soups and sauces, ready-to-eat meals as well as snacks.

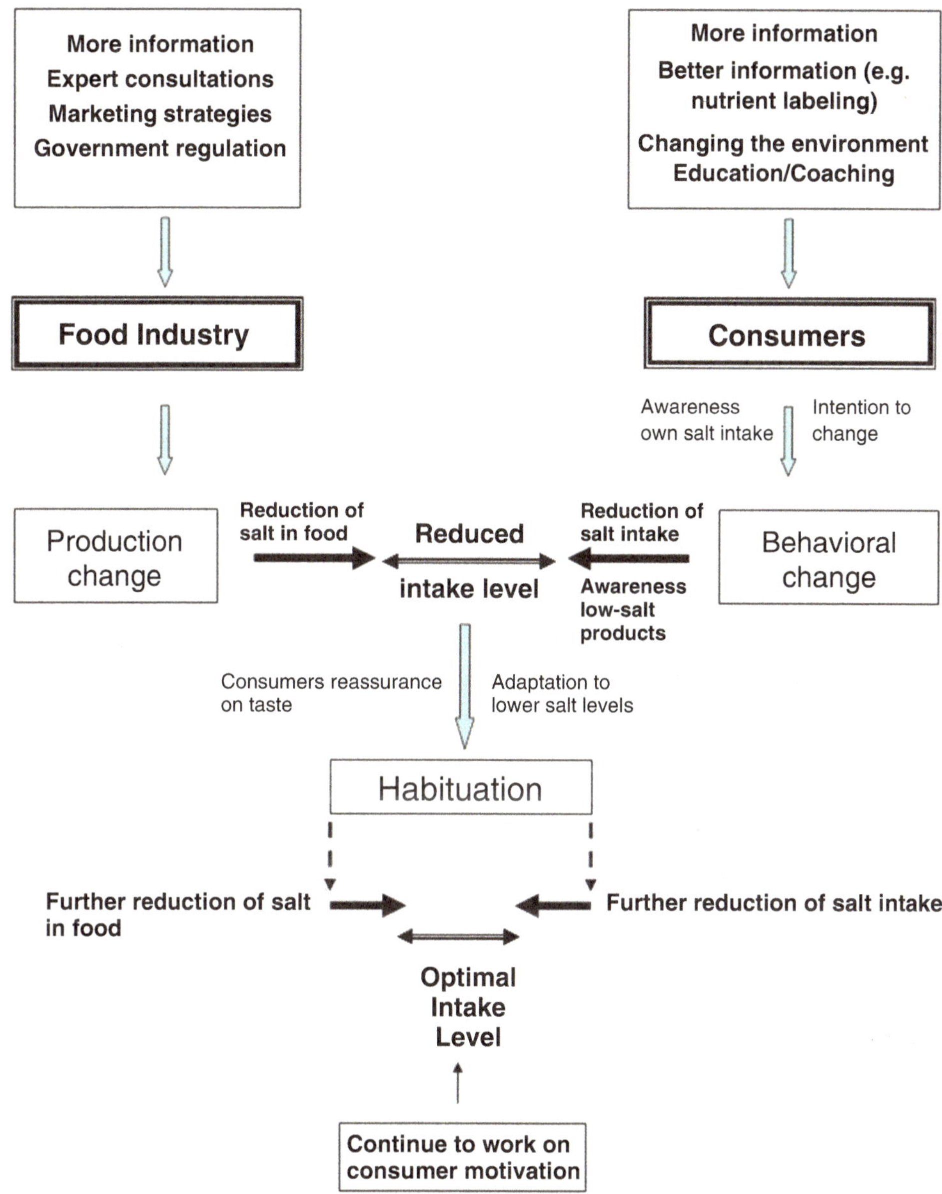

Fig. 2 A simple model of how dietary salt intake can be reduced in population (The figure is taken from Ekmekcioglu et al. (Ekmekcioglu et al. 2013). With kind permission from S. Karger AG, Medical and Scientific Publishers, 4009 Basel, Switzerland)

Sodium is responsible for the taste of a food by enhancing other aromatic ingredients and suppressing bitterness (Dötsch et al. 2009). Therefore, salt content in food stuff increases acceptance. But the human salt taste receptors can adapt to low salt concentrations (Blais et al. 1986) which makes a small, stepwise reduction of sodium content without reduced product acceptance possible, which in turn means that a cooperation of all manufacturers is required.

Beside the stepwise approach, salt reduction strategies include an increased use of spices and taste enhancers (Wilson and Incles 2012).

To ensure food safety and preservation in some cases addition of antimicrobial agents is necessary. Replacement of NaCl by KCl by 30–40 % has been made in meat and dairy products without any adverse effects on microorganism growth (Harper and Getty 2012). Even though, potassium chloride has similar antimicrobial effects and technological function, its application is limited because of its metallic and bitter off-taste (Buttriss 2013).

Salt reduction in bread and bakery products can be achieved by a stepwise sodium reduction of 5 % per week until 25 %, substitution of sodium chloride by potassium chloride (up to 10 %), and use of organic acids such as acetic and lactic acid. Replacement of NaCl up to 50 % by other salts/salt mixtures (potassium or magnesium chloride, potassium lactate, sodium diacetate), use of phosphates to promote water binding capacity of the proteins, and use of flake salt in dry-cured meat products are strategies used in reformulation of meat and meat products. Salt reduction in cheese is more difficult to manage than in bread and most meat products because salt controls the ripening process. Despite 30–40 % sodium reduction, taste and acceptance of ready-to-eat meals can be improved by the use of salt substitutes like potassium chloride and natural flavour enhancers (e.g. yeast extract or natural aroma sources such as garlic and herbs like oregano, rosemary). The composition of snacks can be optimised by the use of smaller salt particles which induce an increased initial perception of saltiness, as well as the use of spices (Kloss et al. 2015).

As protected designation of origin (PDO) products such as Parmesan, Prosciutto di Parma, Feta, and Camembert de Normandie must be produced according to traditional methods reducing salt content by reformulation is limited within these food stuffs (Wilson and Incles 2012).

In the meantime, impressive success stories can be reported on collaborations with food companies to reduce salt content followed by a decrease in blood pressure and in mortality rate related to heart disease and stroke (Ekmekcioglu et al. 2013). Thus, reformulation has along with

Table 2 Nutrition claims to salt/sodium content

Nutrition claim	Sodium content	Equivalent salt content
	(per 100 g or 100 ml)	(per 100 g or 100 ml)
No added sodium/salt	0.12 g	0.30 g
Sodium-free/ salt-free	0.005 g	0.01 g
Very low sodium/salt	0.04 g	0.10 g
Low sodium/salt	0.12 g	0.30 g

Commission Regulation (EU) No 1047 (2012)

other approaches such as healthier food choice editing, portion size control, as well as clear and comprehensible information provision, potential to increase the opportunities of healthier choices to improve public health. However, reformulation alone doesn't have the impact to provide a complete solution to the challenge of improving eating patterns and nutrient supply.

9.3 Reduction of Salt Intake by Legal Provision

Taxation of "unhealthy" high sodium food is discussed controversy. By introducing a tax for salty snacks (salt content of more than 1 g/100 g; for condiments >5 g/100 g) in Hungary in 2011 (0.8 €/kg salt) sales of salty snacks decreased by 26 %. Food prices influence food consumption on the one hand (Duffey et al. 2010), and changes consumer behaviour on the other hand by increased awareness of negative health effects.

Referring to salt/sodium content there are four nutrition claims (Table 2).

"A claim stating that sodium/salt has not been added to a food and any claim likely to have the same meaning for the consumer may only be made where the product does not contain any added sodium/salt or any other ingredient containing added sodium/salt and the product contains no more than 0.12 g sodium, or the equivalent value for salt, per 100 g or 100 ml.

A claim that a food is sodium-free or salt-free, and any claim likely to have the same meaning for the consumer, may only be made where the product contains no more than 0.005 g of sodium, or the equivalent value for salt, per 100 g or per 100 ml.

A claim that a food is very low in sodium/salt, and any claim likely to have the same meaning for the consumer, may only be made where the product contains no more than 0.04 g of sodium, or the equivalent value for salt, per 100 g or per 100 ml. This claim shall not be used for natural mineral waters and other waters.

A claim that a food is low in sodium/salt, and any claim likely to have the same meaning for the consumer, may only be made where the product contains no more than 0.12 g of sodium, or the equivalent value for salt, per 100 g or per 100 ml. For waters, other than natural mineral waters falling within the scope of Directive 80/777/EEC, this value should not exceed 2 mg of sodium per 100 ml." (Commission Regulation (EU) No 1047 (2012)).

There is one authorized health claim for foods with low or reduced sodium: "Reducing consumption of sodium contributes to the maintenance of normal blood pressure" in the European Union (EFSA 2011).

Different labeling confuses consumers because most of them are not aware that salt content is 2.54 times higher than sodium concentration. Therefore, the European Parliament and the Council determined in 2011 by The Regulation (EU) No 1169/2011 on the provision of food information to consumers that the term salt instead of sodium must be used on food labels (Regulation (EU) No 1169/2011 (2011)). In Finland warning labels must be used for products with high salt content, in the United Kingdom, there is a voluntary traffic light label and as front-of-package labeling the guideline daily amount (GDA) system is used (WHO 2013b). Food labeling is most effective in promoting buyers awareness and can help consumer make the healthier choice. Additionally this motivates food companies to reduce salt in their products.

Webster et al. evaluated global salt reduction initiatives and recognized that 59 countries from 83 cooperate with food industry to reduce salt. Most of the countries established voluntary targets while South Africa and Argentina had mandatory targets for many food products, and six European countries (Belgium, Bulgaria, Greece, Hungary, the Netherlands and Portugal) had mandatory targets for bread amongst others. Salt reductions in bread ranged from 6 % in Belgium to 38 % in Chile. For other products, reductions between 5 % (cornflakes, USA) and 81 % (frozen peas, USA) have been observed (Webster et al. 2014). Because consumer's knowledge on salt content in food is limited these partnerships are very important for public health concern.

The EATWELL research project (www. eatwellproject.eu) (Interventions to Promote Healthy Eating Habits: Evaluation and Recommendations) conducted between 2009 and 2013 evaluated the effectiveness of healthy eating interventions in EU Member States. Main topics were policies supporting informed choice (nutrition education, labelling), and changing the market environment (taxes, food reformulation, regulation of school and workplace meals). A common recommendation is to gather more and better evidence (Traill et al. 2013).

10 Practical Recommendations for Moderate Salt Intake

Well known dietary patterns for treatment of elevated blood pressure are the Dietary Approaches to Stop Hypertension (DASH) diet and the OmniHeart diet. The DASH diet is rich in fruits, vegetables, low-fat dairy products, contains poultry, fish, and nuts, whereas only small amounts of red meat, sweets, and sugar-containing beverages are consumed. Macronutrient composition is about 58 % carbohydrate, 15 % protein, and 27 % fat; sodium intake less than 2.3 g/day. Compared to a typical American diet DASH is reduced in saturated fat and total fat, modestly increased in protein (Sacks et al. 2001).

Because the types of macronutrients (carbohydrate, protein, or unsaturated fat) replacing saturated fat has been discussed controversial, slight variations of DASH have been evaluated within the Optimal Macronutrient Intake Trial to

Prevent Heart Disease (OmniHeart). The OmniHeart diet is a carbohydrate-rich diet which allows partially substituting carbohydrate with protein or unsaturated fat, similar to a Mediterranean-style diet. This offers more flexibility and makes it easier to eat a heart-healthy diet (Swain et al. 2008).

Generally, a DASH eating plan consists of 7–8 servings grains and grain products; 4–5 servings vegetables and fruits, each; 2–3 servings low-fat dairy products; 2 or less servings lean meats, poultry, and fish; 2–3 servings fats and oils per day, and 4–5 servings of nuts, seeds, dry beans, and peas; 5 or less servings sweets per week (U.S. Department of Health and Human Services 2003).

Along with the recommendations of the DASH diet, body weight should be reduced in overweight and obese people (BMI less than 25 kg/m^2), salt intake not exceed 5 g/day (<2.3 g sodium/day, no more than 1.5 g/day in blacks, middle- and older-aged persons, and individuals with hypertension, diabetes, or chronic kidney disease), intake of potassium (~4.7 g/day) should be increased and alcohol consumption limited to max. 10 g/day for female and 20 g/day for male (Appel, on Behalf of the American Society of Hypertension Writing Group 2009).

Yokoyama et al. described an association between vegetarian diets and lower blood pressure in their meta-analysis including 7 controlled trials and 32 observational studies. It remains to be clarified which type of vegetarian diet is most effective (Yokoyama et al. 2014).

Additionally, regular physical activity can lower blood pressure. There is evidence that 150 min physical activity per week may support antihypertensive medication. The American College of Sports Medicine recommends primarily endurance physical activity supplemented by resistance exercise in moderate-intensity (40–< 60 % of VO$_2$R) for at least 30 min daily (Pescatello et al. 2004). A Systematic Review and Meta-analysis done by Cornelissen and Smart concluded that endurance, dynamic resistance, and isometric resistance training lower SBP and DBP, whereas combined training lowers only DBP. Isometric resistance training is suggested for the largest SBP reductions (Cornelissen and Smart 2013).

The burden of hypertension raises with increasing prevalence of obesity. Therefore, weight reduction and control is very important in prevention and therapy of hypertension. A meta-analysis of 25 RCTs showed blood pressure reduction of ~1 mm Hg for each kilogram of body weight loss (Neter et al. 2003).

Salt reduction is difficult to achieve because in industrialised countries ~80 % of salt intake comes from industrial produced foods.

Average amount of salt consumed per daily food intake is about:

- 1 g from basic unprocessed foods (vegetables, potatoes, grain, milk, meat)
- 2–3 g from bread and bakery products
- 3–5 g from sausages, ham, cured meat products, cheese, fish sauce
- 4–5 g from industrially processed products like preserves/fish products and home-made dishes
- 1–2 g from salt added at the table

Therefore avoid adding salt at the table, and season with herbs and spices. Always read the food label and reduce consumption of ready-to-eat meals with high amounts of salt.

11 Conclusion

The positive relationship between salt and blood pressure is known since more than 100 years. Accumulating evidence especially began in the 1940s where severe arterial hypertension has been cured by drastic lowering of salt intake by the Kempner rice and fruit diet. In the 1950s Lewis K. Dahl observed a blood pressure lowering effect by a low-salt diet in rats with salt-sensitive hypertension. Most of the subsequent studies showed beneficial effects of a low salt diet on blood pressure. However, also some negative papers were published, which failed to find a relationship between salt and blood pressure. While selection of study participants (more salt sensitive people like elderly or people with hypertension) can increase likelihood of the positive association between salt intake and blood pressure, dietary and other lifestyle factors like intake of potassium (from fruit and vegetable sources), physical activity level, as well as alcohol consumption have also to be considered (Drueke 2016).

A few studies also suggested that a low salt diet may have detrimental health outcomes, especially regarding cardiovascular diseases and mortality. (O'Donnell et al. 2014; Graudal et al. 2014). A recent study by Mente at al. for example observed an association between low sodium intake and increased risk of cardiovascular events and mortality in both hypertensive and normotensive individuals (Mente et al. 2016).

More reliable randomised controlled trials, as well as research on measurement, storage and kinetics of sodium, on physiological properties, and genetic determinants of salt sensitivity are necessary to explain these negative outcomes of a low salt diet. However, according to the current overwhelming state of knowledge people with hypertension and high sodium intake should be advised to lower their salt intake.

Dislcosure Statement The authors declare to have no conflict of interest.

References

Aaron KJ, Sanders PW (2013) Role of dietary salt and potassium intake in cardiovascular health and disease: a review of the evidence. Mayo Clin Proc 88 (9):987–995

Aburto NJ, Ziolkovska A, Hooper L, Elliott P, Cappuccio FP, Meerpohl JJ (2013a) Effect of lower sodium intake on health: systematic review and meta-analyses. BMJ 346:f1326

Aburto NJ, Hanson S, Gutierrez H, Hooper L, Elliott P, Cappuccio FP (2013b) Effect of increased potassium intake on cardiovascular risk factors and disease: systematic review and meta-analyses. BMJ 346:f1378

Alexy U, Cheng G, Libuda L, Hilbig A, Kersting M (2012) 24 h-Sodium excretion and hydration status in children and adolescents--results of the DONALD Study. Clin Nutr 31(1):78–84

Ambard L, Beaujard E (1904) Causes de l'hypertension artérielle. Arch Gén Méd 81:520–533

American Heart Association. Sodium and salt. Available from: http://www.heart.org/HEARTORG/Healthy Living/HealthyEating/HealthyDietGoals/Sodium-Salt -or-Sodium-Chloride_UCM_303290_Article.jsp#.V5 IbrTVUjbl: accessed October 2016

Anderson EA, Sinkey CA, Lawton WJ, Mark AL (1989) Elevated sympathetic nerve activity in borderline hypertensive humans. Evidence from direct intraneural recordings. Hypertension 14(2):177–183

Appel LJ, on Behalf of the American Society of Hypertension Writing Group (2009) ASH position paper: dietary approaches to lower blood pressure. J Clin Hypertens 11(7):358–368

Appel LJ, Moore TJ, Obarzanek E, Vollmer WM, Svetkey LP, Sacks FM et al (1997) A clinical trial of the effects of dietary patterns on blood pressure. DASH Collaborative Research Group. N Engl J Med 336(16):1117–1124

Appel LJ, Brands MW, Daniels SR, Karanja N, Elmer PJ, Sacks FM (2006) Dietary approaches to prevent and treat hypertension: a scientific statement from the American Heart Association. Hypertension 47 (2):296–308

Armando I, Villar VA, Jose PA (2015) Genomics and pharmacogenomics of salt-sensitive hypertension. Curr Hypertens Rev 11(1):49–56

Baldo MP, Rodrigues SL, Mill JG (2015) High salt intake as a multifaceted cardiovascular disease: new support from cellular and molecular evidence. Heart Fail Rev 20(4):461–474

Blais CA, Pangborn RM, Borhani NO, Ferrell MF, Prineas RJ, Laing B (1986) Effect of dietary sodium restriction on taste responses to sodium chloride: a longitudinal study. Am J Clin Nutr 44(2):232–243

Boeing H, Bechthold A, Bub A, Ellinger S, Haller D, Kroke A et al (2012) Critical review: vegetables and fruit in the prevention of chronic diseases. Eur J Nutr 51(6):637–663

Brooks VL, Haywood JR, Johnson AK (2005) Translation of salt retention to central activation of the sympathetic nervous system in hypertension. Clin Exp Pharmacol Physiol 32(5–6):426–432

Brown IJ, Tzoulaki I, Candeias V, Elliott P (2009) Salt intakes around the world: implications for public health. Int J Epidemiol 38(3):791–813

Buchholz K, Schachinger H, Wagner M, Sharma AM, Deter HC (2003) Reduced vagal activity in salt-sensitive subjects during mental challenge. Am J Hypertens 16(7):531–536

Bulpitt CJ (1981) Sodium excess or potassium lack as a cause of hypertension: a discussion paper. J R Soc Med 74(12):896–900

Burnier M, Wuerzner G, Bochud M (2015) Salt, blood pressure and cardiovascular risk: what is the most adequate preventive strategy? A Swiss perspective. Front Physiol 6:227

Buttriss JL (2013) Food reformulation: the challenges to the food industry. Proc Nutr Soc 72(01):61–69

Cappuccio FP, MacGregor GA (1991) Does potassium supplementation lower blood pressure? A meta-analysis of published trials. J Hypertens 9(5):465–473

Cerasola G, Cottone S, Mule G (2010) The progressive pathway of microalbuminuria: from early marker of renal damage to strong cardiovascular risk predictor. J Hypertens 28(12):2357–2369

Chen J, Gu D, Huang J, Rao DC, Jaquish CE, Hixson JE et al (2009) Metabolic syndrome and salt sensitivity of blood pressure in non-diabetic people in China: a dietary intervention study. Lancet 373(9666):829–835

Cobb LK, Anderson CA, Elliott P, Hu FB, Liu K, Neaton JD et al (2014) Methodological issues in cohort studies that relate sodium intake to cardiovascular disease outcomes: a science advisory from the American Heart Association. Circulation 129(10):1173–1186

Commission Regulation (EU) No 1047/2012 of 8 November 2012 amending Regulation (EC) No 1924/2006 with regard to the list of nutrition claims Text with EEA relevance (2012)

Cornelissen VA, Smart NA (2013) Exercise training for blood pressure: a systematic review and meta-analysis. J Am Heart Assoc 2(1)

Cowley AW Jr, Skelton MM, Merrill DC, Quillen EW Jr, Switzer SJ (1983) Influence of daily sodium intake on vasopressin secretion and drinking in dogs. Am J Physiol 245(6):R860–R872

Crowley SD, Gurley SB, Oliverio MI, Pazmino AK, Griffiths R, Flannery PJ et al (2005) Distinct roles for the kidney and systemic tissues in blood pressure regulation by the renin-angiotensin system. J Clin Invest 115(4):1092–1099

Cutler JA, Follmann D, Allender PS (1997) Randomized trials of sodium reduction: an overview. Am J Clin Nutr 65(2 Suppl):643S–651S

D'Elia L, Rossi G, Ippolito R, Cappuccio FP, Strazzullo P (2012) Habitual salt intake and risk of gastric cancer: A meta-analysis of prospective studies. Clin Nutr 31(4):489–498

Deutsche Gesellschaft für Ernährung (DGE), Österreichische Gesellschaft für Ernährung, Schweizerische Gesellschaft für Ernährung (SGE) (Hrsg.) (2015) Die Referenzwerte für die Nährstoffzufuhr. Neustadt an der Weinstraße: Umschau Buchverlag

Dickinson HO, Nicolson DJ, Campbell F, Beyer FR, Mason J (2006) Potassium supplementation for the management of primary hypertension in adults. The Cochrane database of systematic reviews (3): CD004641

Dickinson KM, Clifton PM, Keogh JB (2011) Endothelial function is impaired after a high-salt meal in healthy subjects. Am J Clin Nutr 93(3):500–505

Dietary Guidelines Advisory Committee (2010) Report of the dietary guidelines advisory committee on the dietary guidelines for Americans, 2010, to the Secretary of Agriculture and the Secretary of Health and Human Services. Agricultural Research Service

Dietary reference values for food energy and nutrients for the United Kingdom (1991) Report of the Panel on Dietary Reference Values of the Committee on Medical Aspects of Food Policy. Rep Health Soc Subj (Lond) 41:1–210

Dorner TE, Genser D, Krejs G, Slany J, Watschinger B, Ekmekcioglu C et al (2013) [Hypertension and nutrition. Position paper of the Austrian Nutrition Society]. Herz 38(2):153–162

Dötsch M, Busch J, Batenburg M, Liem G, Tareilus E, Mueller R et al (2009) Strategies to reduce sodium consumption: a food industry perspective. Crit Rev Food Sci Nutr 49(10):841–851

Drueke TB (2016) Salt and health: time to revisit the recommendations. Kidney Int 89(2):259–260

Du Cailar G, Ribstein J, Daures JP, Mimran A (1992) Sodium and left ventricular mass in untreated hypertensive and normotensive subjects. Am J Physiol 263 (1 Pt 2):H177–H181

du Cailar G, Ribstein J, Mimran A (2002) Dietary sodium and target organ damage in essential hypertension. Am J Hypertens 15(3):222–229

Duffey KJ, Gordon-Larsen P, Shikany JM, Guilkey D, Jacobs DR Jr et al (2010) Food price and diet and health outcomes: 20 years of the cardia study. Arch Intern Med 170(5):420–426

Duffey KJ, Huybrechts I, Mouratidou T, Libuda L, Kersting M, De Vriendt T et al (2012) Beverage consumption among European adolescents in the HELENA study. Eur J Clin Nutr 66(2):244–252

DuPont JJ, Greaney JL, Wenner MM, Lennon-Edwards SL, Sanders PW, Farquhar WB et al (2013) High dietary sodium intake impairs endothelium-dependent dilation in healthy salt-resistant humans. J Hypertens 31(3):530–536

EFSA Panel on Dietetic Products, Nutrition and Allergies (2011) Scientific opinion on the substantiation of health claims related to foods with reduced amounts of sodium and maintenance of normal blood pressure (ID 336, 705, 1148, 1178, 1185, 1420) pursuant to Article 13(1) of Regulation (EC) No 1924/2006. EFSA J 9(6):2237

Ekmekcioglu C, Blasche G, Dorner TE (2013) Too much salt and how we can get rid of it. Forschende Komplementarmedizin 20(6):454–460

Ekmekcioglu C, Elmadfa I, Meyer AL, Moeslinger T (2016) The role of dietary potassium in hypertension and diabetes. J Physiol Biochem 72(1):93–106

Elliott P, Stamler J, Nichols R, Dyer AR, Stamler R, Kesteloot H et al (1996) Intersalt revisited: further analyses of 24 hour sodium excretion and blood pressure within and across populations. Intersalt Cooperative Research Group. BMJ 312(7041):1249–1253

Ellison RC, Capper AL, Stephenson WP, Goldberg RJ, Hosmer DW Jr, Humphrey KF et al (1989) Effects on blood pressure of a decrease in sodium use in institutional food preparation: the Exeter-Andover Project. J Clin Epidemiol 42(3):201–208

Elmadfa I, Leitzmann C (2015) Ernährung des Menschen. Verlag Eugen Ulmer, Stuttgart

European Commission (2012) Survey on Members States' – Implementation of the EU salt reduction framework

Farjah M, Roxas BP, Geenen DL, Danziger RS (2003) Dietary salt regulates renal SGK1 abundance: relevance to salt sensitivity in the Dahl rat. Hypertension 41(4):874–878

Farquhar WB, Wenner MM, Delaney EP, Prettyman AV, Stillabower ME (2006) Sympathetic neural responses to increased osmolality in humans. Am J Physiol Heart Circ Physiol 291(5):H2181–H2186

Farquhar WB, Edwards DG, Jurkovitz CT, Weintraub WS (2015) Dietary sodium and health: more than just blood pressure. J Am Coll Cardiol 65(10):1042–1050

Felder RA, White MJ, Williams SM, Jose PA (2013) Diagnostic tools for hypertension and salt sensitivity testing. Curr Opin Nephrol Hypertens 22(1):65–76

Fonseca-Alaniz MH, Brito LC, Borges-Silva CN, Takada J, Andreotti S, Lima FB (2007) High dietary sodium intake increases white adipose tissue mass and plasma leptin in rats. Obesity 15(9):2200–2208

Fujita T (2014) Mechanism of salt-sensitive hypertension: focus on adrenal and sympathetic nervous systems. J Am Soc Nephrol 25(6):1148–1155

Ge S, Feng X, Shen L, Wei Z, Zhu Q, Sun J (2012) Association between habitual dietary salt intake and risk of gastric cancer: a systematic review of observational studies. Gastroenterol Res Pract 2012:808120

Geleijnse JM, Kok FJ, Grobbee DE (2003) Blood pressure response to changes in sodium and potassium intake: a metaregression analysis of randomised trials. J Hum Hypertens 17(7):471–480

Gibney MJ, Vorster HH, Kok FJ (2009) Introduction to human nutrition. Wiley-Blackwell, West Sussex

Graudal NA, Galloe AM, Garred P (1998) Effects of sodium restriction on blood pressure, renin, aldosterone, catecholamines, cholesterols, and triglyceride: a meta-analysis. JAMA 279(17):1383–1391

Graudal N, Jurgens G, Baslund B, Alderman MH (2014) Compared with usual sodium intake, low- and excessive-sodium diets are associated with increased mortality: a meta-analysis. Am J Hypertens 27(9):1129–1137

Grimes CA, Riddell LJ, Campbell KJ, Nowson CA (2013) Dietary salt intake, sugar-sweetened beverage consumption, and obesity risk. Pediatrics 131(1):14–21

Gu D, Kelly TN, Hixson JE, Chen J, Liu D, Chen JC et al (2010) Genetic variants in the renin-angiotensin-aldosterone system and salt sensitivity of blood pressure. J Hypertens 28(6):1210–1220

Guild SJ, McBryde FD, Malpas SC, Barrett CJ (2012) High dietary salt and angiotensin II chronically increase renal sympathetic nerve activity: a direct telemetric study. Hypertension 59(3):614–620

Guyton AC (1990) The surprising kidney-fluid mechanism for pressure control--its infinite gain! Hypertension 16(6):725–730

Guyton AC, Coleman TG, Cowley AV Jr, Scheel KW, Manning RD Jr, Norman RA Jr (1972) Arterial pressure regulation. Overriding dominance of the kidneys in long-term regulation and in hypertension. Am J Med 52(5):584–594

Ha SK (2014) Dietary salt intake and hypertension. Electrolyte Blood Press 12(1):7–18

Harper NM, Getty KJ (2012) Effect of salt reduction on growth of Listeria monocytogenes in meat and poultry systems. J Food Sci 77(12):M669–M674

He FJ, MacGregor GA (2002) Effect of modest salt reduction on blood pressure: a meta-analysis of randomized trials. Implications for public health. J Hum Hypertens 16(11):761–770

He FJ, MacGregor GA (2006) Importance of salt in determining blood pressure in children: meta-analysis of controlled trials. Hypertension 48(5):861–869

He FJ, MacGregor GA (2011) Salt reduction lowers cardiovascular risk: meta-analysis of outcome trials. Lancet 378(9789):380–382

He FJ, Marrero NM, MacGregor GA (2008) Salt intake is related to soft drink consumption in children and adolescents: a link to obesity? Hypertension 51(3):629–634

He FJ, Marciniak M, Visagie E, Markandu ND, Anand V, Dalton RN et al (2009) Effect of modest salt reduction on blood pressure, urinary albumin, and pulse wave velocity in white, black, and Asian mild hypertensives. Hypertension 54(3):482–488

He FJ, Li J, MacGregor GA (2013) Effect of longer term modest salt reduction on blood pressure: Cochrane systematic review and meta-analysis of randomised trials. BMJ 346:f1325

Holbrook J, Patterson K, Bodner J, Douglas L, Veillon C, Kelsay J et al (1984) Sodium and potassium intake and balance in adults consuming self-selected diets. Am J Clin Nutr 40(4):786–793

Huang BS, Amin MS, Leenen FH (2006) The central role of the brain in salt-sensitive hypertension. Curr Opin Cardiol 21(4):295–304

Huang L, Crino M, Wu JH, Woodward M, Barzi F, Land MA et al (2016) Mean population salt intake estimated from 24-h urine samples and spot urine samples: a systematic review and meta-analysis. Int J Epidemiol 45:239–250

Institute of Medicine (2005) Panel on dietary reference intakes for electrolytes and water. DRI, dietary reference intakes for water, potassium, sodium, chloride, and sulfate. National Academy Press

Institute of Medicine (2013) Sodium intake in populations: assessment of evidence. In: Strom BL, Yaktine AL, Oria M (eds) The National Academies Press, Washington, DC

Ishimitsu T, Tobian L, Sugimoto K, Everson T (1996) High potassium diets reduce vascular and plasma lipid peroxides in stroke-prone spontaneously hypertensive rats. Clin Exp Hypertens 18(5):659–673

Janz NK, Becker MH (1984) The health belief model: a decade later. Health Educ Behav 11(1):1–47

Jenni B, Suter PM (2011) Help – doctor must I avoid salt? Praxis 100(21):1271–1280

Kawasaki T, Delea CS, Bartter FC, Smith H (1978) The effect of high-sodium and low-sodium intakes on blood pressure and other related variables in human subjects with idiopathic hypertension. Am J Med 64(2):193–198

Kawasaki T, Itoh K, Uezono K, Sasaki H (1993) A simple method for estimating 24 h urinary sodium and potassium excretion from second morning voiding urine specimen in adults. Clin Exp Pharmacol Physiol 20(1):7–14

Kempner W (1948) Treatment of hypertensive vascular disease with rice diet. Am J Med 4(4):545–577

Kersting M, Rehmer T, Hilbig A (2006) Ermittlung des Kochsalzkonsums in Verzehrserhebungen anhand der Kochsalzausscheidung im Urin: eine Sonderauswertung der DONALD Studie. Abschlussbericht Forschungsprojekt (05HS048).

Khaw KT, Bingham S, Welch A, Luben R, O'Brien E, Wareham N et al (2004) Blood pressure and urinary sodium in men and women: the Norfolk Cohort of the European Prospective Investigation into Cancer (EPIC-Norfolk). Am J Clin Nutr 80(5):1397–1403

Kido M, Ando K, Onozato ML, Tojo A, Yoshikawa M, Ogita T et al (2008) Protective effect of dietary potassium against vascular injury in salt-sensitive hypertension. Hypertension 51(2):225–231

Kloss L, Meyer JD, Graeve L, Vetter W (2015) Sodium intake and its reduction by food reformulation in the European Union — a review. NFS J 1:9–19

Koomans HA, Roos JC, Boer P, Geyskes GG, Mees EJ (1982) Salt sensitivity of blood pressure in chronic renal failure. Evidence for renal control of body fluid distribution in man. Hypertension 4(2):190–197

Kotchen TA, Cowley AW Jr, Frohlich ED (2013) Salt in health and disease--a delicate balance. N Engl J Med 368(26):2531–2532

Lifton RP, Gharavi AG, Geller DS (2001) Molecular mechanisms of human hypertension. Cell 104(4):545–556

Lim SS, Vos T, Flaxman AD, Danaei G, Shibuya K, Adair-Rohani H et al (2012) A comparative risk assessment of burden of disease and injury attributable to 67 risk factors and risk factor clusters in 21 regions, 1990–2010: a systematic analysis for the Global Burden of Disease Study 2010. Lancet 380 (9859):2224–2260

Lin J, Hu FB, Curhan GC (2010) Associations of diet with albuminuria and kidney function decline. Clin J Am Soc Nephrol 5(5):836–843

Luft FC, Rankin LI, Bloch R, Weyman AE, Willis LR, Murray RH et al (1979) Cardiovascular and humoral responses to extremes of sodium intake in normal black and white men. Circulation 60(3):697–706

Luft FC, Fineberg NS, Sloan RS (1982) Overnight urine collections to estimate sodium intake. Hypertension 4:494–498

Luft FC, Miller JZ, Grim CE, Fineberg NS, Christian JC, Daugherty SA et al (1991) Salt sensitivity and resistance of blood pressure. Age and race as factors in physiological responses. Hypertension 17(1 Suppl): I102–I108

Luzardo L, Noboa O, Boggia J (2015) Mechanisms of salt-sensitive hypertension. Curr Hypertens Rev 11(1):14–21

Ma Y, He FJ, MacGregor GA (2015) High salt intake: independent risk factor for obesity? Hypertension 66 (4):843–849

MacGregor GA, de Wardener HE (1998) Salt, diet and health: Neptune's poisoned Chalice; The origin of high blood pressure. Cambridge University Press, Cambridge, p 233

Majid DSA, Prieto MC, Navar LG (2015) Salt-sensitive hypertension: perspectives on intrarenal mechanisms. Curr Hypertens Rev 11(1):38–48

Mancia G, Fagard R, Narkiewicz K, Redon J, Zanchetti A, Böhm M et al (2013) ESH/ESC Guidelines for the management of arterial hypertension. The Task Force for the management of arterial hypertension of the European Society of Hypertension (ESH) and of the European Society of Cardiology (ESC) 34(28):2159–2219

Mangrum AJ, Gomez RA, Norwood VF (2002) Effects of AT(1A) receptor deletion on blood pressure and sodium excretion during altered dietary salt intake. Am J Physio Renal Physiol 283(3):F447–F453

Mattes RD (1990) Discretionary salt and compliance with reduced sodium diet. Nutr Res 10(12):1337–1352

Maughan RJ, Leiper JB (1995) Sodium intake and post-exercise rehydration in man. Eur J Appl Physiol Occup Physiol 71(4):311–319

McLean RM (2014) Measuring population sodium intake: a review of methods. Nutrients 6(11):4651–4662

Mente A, O'Donnell MJ, Rangarajan S, McQueen MJ, Poirier P, Wielgosz A et al (2014) Association of urinary sodium and potassium excretion with blood pressure. N Engl J Med 371(7):601–611

Mente A, O'Donnell M, Rangarajan S, Dagenais G, Lear S, McQueen M et al (2016) Associations of urinary sodium excretion with cardiovascular events in individuals with and without hypertension: a pooled analysis of data from four studies. Lancet 388:465–475

Midgley JP, Matthew AG, Greenwood CM, Logan AG (1996) Effect of reduced dietary sodium on blood pressure: a meta-analysis of randomized controlled trials. JAMA 275(20):1590–1597

Mozaffarian D, Fahimi S, Singh GM, Micha R, Khatibzadeh S, Engell RE et al (2014) Global sodium consumption and death from cardiovascular causes. N Engl J Med 371(7):624–634

Nakandakare ER, Charf AM, Santos FC, Nunes VS, Ortega K, Lottenberg AMP et al (2008) Dietary salt restriction increases plasma lipoprotein and inflammatory marker concentrations in hypertensive patients. Atherosclerosis 200(2):410–416

Nakano M, Eguchi K, Sato T, Onoguchi A, Hoshide S, Kario K (2016) Effect of intensive salt-restriction education on clinic, home, and ambulatory blood pressure levels in treated hypertensive patients during a 3-month education period. J Clin Hypertens 18(5):385–392

Neter JE, Stam BE, Kok FJ, Grobbee DE, Geleijnse JM (2003) Influence of weight reduction on blood pressure: a meta-analysis of randomized controlled trials. Hypertension 42(5):878–884

Newson RS, Elmadfa I, Biro G, Cheng Y, Prakash V, Rust P et al (2013) Barriers for progress in salt reduction in the general population. An international study. Appetite 71:22–31

Norat T, Chan D, Vingeliene S, Aune D, Abar L, Vieira AR, Navarro D (2015) World Cancer Research Fund International Systematic Literature Review. The associations between food, nutrition and physical activity and the risk of stomach cancer London: World Cancer Research Fund. 2015.

O'Donnell MJ, Yusuf S, Mente A, Gao P, Mann JF, Teo K et al (2011) Urinary sodium and potassium excretion and risk of cardiovascular events. JAMA 306(20):2229–2238

O'Donnell M, Mente A, Rangarajan S, McQueen MJ, Wang X, Liu L et al (2014) Urinary sodium and potassium excretion, mortality, and cardiovascular events. N Engl J Med 371(7):612–623

Oberleithner H, Riethmuller C, Schillers H, MacGregor GA, de Wardener HE, Hausberg M (2007) Plasma sodium stiffens vascular endothelium and reduces nitric oxide release. Proc Natl Acad Sci U S A 104 (41):16281–16286

Parkin DM (2011) 7. Cancers attributable to dietary factors in the UK in 2010. IV. Salt. Br J Cancer 105 (Suppl 2):S31–S33

Pescatello LSFB, Fagard R, Farquhar WB, Kelley GA, Ray CA, American College of Sports Medicine (2004) American College of Sports Medicine position stand. Exercise and hypertension. Med Sci Sports Exerc 36(3):533–553

Porth CM (2009) Disorders of blood pressure regulation. In: Hannon RA, Pooler C, Porth CM, (eds). Porth's pathophysiology: Lippincott

Powles J, Fahimi S, Micha R, Khatibzadeh S, Shi P, Ezzati M et al (2013) Global, regional and national sodium intakes in 1990 and 2010: a systematic analysis of 24 h urinary sodium excretion and dietary surveys worldwide. BMJ Open 3(12):e003733

Rassler B (2010) The renin-angiotensin system in the development of salt-sensitive hypertension in animal models and humans. Pharmaceuticals 3(4):940–960

Regulation (EU) (2011) No 1169/2011 of the European Parliament and of the Council of 25 October 2011 on the provision of food information to consumers, amending Regulations (EC) No 1924/2006 and (EC) No 1925/2006 of the European Parliament and of the Council, and repealing Commission Directive 87/250/EEC, Council Directive 90/496/EEC,

Commission Directive 1999/10/EC, Directive 2000/13/EC of the European Parliament and of the Council, Commission Directives 2002/67/EC and 2008/5/EC and Commission Regulation (EC) No 608/2004 Text with EEA relevance

Rhee M-Y, Kim J-H, Shin S-J, Gu N, Nah D-Y, Hong K-S et al (2014) Estimation of 24-hour urinary sodium excretion using spot urine samples. Nutrients 6 (6):2360–2375

Rodriguez-Iturbe B, Vaziri ND (2007) Salt-sensitive hypertension--update on novel findings. Nephrol Dial Transplant 22(4):992–995

Rodriguez-Iturbe B, Franco M, Tapia E, Quiroz Y, Johnson RJ (2012) Renal inflammation, autoimmunity and salt-sensitive hypertension. Clin Exp Pharmacol Physiol 39(1):96–103

Sacks FM, Svetkey LP, Vollmer WM, Appel LJ, Bray GA, Harsha D et al (2001) Effects on blood pressure of reduced dietary sodium and the Dietary Approaches to Stop Hypertension (DASH) diet. N Engl J Med 344 (1):3–10

Salehi-Abargouei A, Maghsoudi Z, Shirani F, Azadbakht L (2013) Effects of Dietary Approaches to Stop Hypertension (DASH)-style diet on fatal or nonfatal cardiovascular diseases--incidence: a systematic review and meta-analysis on observational prospective studies. Nutrition 29(4):611–618

Saulnier PJ, Gand E, Hadjadj S (2014) Sodium and cardiovascular disease. N Engl J Med 371 (22):2135–2136

SCF (1993) Reports of the Scientific Committee on Food (31st series). Commission of the European Community, Luxembourg

Schmidlin O, Sebastian AF, Morris RC Jr (2007) What initiates the pressor effect of salt in salt-sensitive humans? Observations in normotensive blacks. Hypertension 49(5):1032–1039

Shimkets RA, Warnock DG, Bositis CM, Nelson-Williams C, Hansson JH, Schambelan M et al (1994) Liddle's syndrome: heritable human hypertension caused by mutations in the beta subunit of the epithelial sodium channel. Cell 79(3):407–414

Stipanuk MH, Caudill MA (2006) Biochemical, physiological, and molecular aspects of human nutrition. Elsevier Inc., St Louis

Stocker SD, Madden CJ, Sved AF (2010) Excess dietary salt intake alters the excitability of central sympathetic networks. Physiol Behav 100(5):519–524

Stolarz-Skrzypek K, Kuznetsova T, Thijs L, Tikhonoff V, Seidlerova J, Richart T et al (2011) Fatal and nonfatal outcomes, incidence of hypertension, and blood pressure changes in relation to urinary sodium excretion. JAMA 305(17):1777–1785

Strazzullo P, D'Elia L, Kandala NB, Cappuccio FP (2009) Salt intake, stroke, and cardiovascular disease: meta-analysis of prospective studies. BMJ 339:b4567

Sullivan JM (1991) Salt sensitivity. Definition, conception, methodology, and long-term issues. Hypertension 17(1 Suppl):I61–I68

Swain JF, McCarron PB, Hamilton EF, Sacks FM, Appel LJ (2008) Characteristics of the diet patterns tested in the optimal macronutrient intake trial to prevent heart disease (OmniHeart): options for a heart-healthy diet. J Am Diet Assoc 108(2):257–265

Tanaka T, Okamura T, Miura K, Kadowaki T, Ueshima H, Nakagawa H et al (2002) A simple method to estimate populational 24-h urinary sodium and potassium excretion using a casual urine specimen. J Hum Hypertens 16(2):97–103

Thomas MC, Moran J, Forsblom C, Harjutsalo V, Thorn L, Ahola A et al (2011) The association between dietary sodium intake, ESRD, and all-cause mortality in patients with type 1 diabetes. Diabetes Care 34(4):861–866

Todd AS, Macginley RJ, Schollum JB, Johnson RJ, Williams SM, Sutherland WH et al (2010) Dietary salt loading impairs arterial vascular reactivity. Am J Clin Nutr 91(3):557–564

Toft U, Cerqueira C, Andreasen AH, Thuesen BH, Laurberg P, Ovesen L et al (2014) Estimating salt intake in a Caucasian population: can spot urine substitute 24-hour urine samples? Eur J Prev Cardiol 21 (10):1300–1307

Traill WB, Mazzocchi M, Niedźwiedzka B, Shankar B, Wills J (2013) The EATWELL project: recommendations for healthy eating policy interventions across Europe. Nutr Bull 38(3):352–357

Trudu M, Janas S, Lanzani C, Debaix H, Schaeffer C, Ikehata M et al (2013) Common noncoding UMOD gene variants induce salt-sensitive hypertension and kidney damage by increasing uromodulin expression. Nat Med 19(12):1655–1660

U.S. Department of Health and Human Services (2003) Your guide to lowering blood pressure: NIH Publication No. 03–5232; 2003. Available from: https://www. nhlbi.nih.gov/files/docs/public/heart/hbp_low.pdf

van Bommel E, Cleophas T (2012) Potassium treatment for hypertension in patients with high salt intake: a meta-analysis. Int J Clin Pharmacol Ther 50 (7):478–482

Van Horn L (2015) Dietary sodium and blood pressure: how low should we go? Prog Cardiovasc Dis 58 (1):61–68

Vandevijvere S (2012) Sodium reduction and the correction of iodine intake in Belgium: Policy options. Arch Public Health 70(1):10

Verkaik-Kloosterman J, Van't Veer P, Ocke MC (2010) Reduction of salt: will iodine intake remain adequate in The Netherlands? Br J Nutr 104(11):1712–1718

Webster J, Trieu K, Dunford E, Hawkes C (2014) Target Salt 2025: a global overview of national programs to encourage the food industry to reduce salt in foods. Nutrients 6(8):3274

Weinberger MH (1996) Salt sensitivity of blood pressure in humans. Hypertension 27(3 Pt 2):481–490

Weinberger MH (2002) Salt sensitivity is associated with an increased mortality in both normal and hypertensive humans. J Clin Hypertens 4(4):274–276

Weinberger MH, Fineberg NS (1991) Sodium and volume sensitivity of blood pressure. Age and pressure change over time. Hypertension 18(1):67–71

Whelton PK, He J, Cutler JA, Brancati FL, Appel LJ, Follmann D et al (1997) Effects of oral potassium on blood pressure. Meta-analysis of randomized controlled clinical trials. JAMA 277(20):1624–1632

WHO (2009) Global health risks: mortality and burden of disease attributable to selected major risks, vol vi. World Health Organization, Geneva, 62 pp

WHO (2012) Guideline sodium intake for adults and children. WHO Press, Geneva

WHO (2013a) Global action plan for the prevention and control of noncommunicable diseases 2013–2020. World Health Organization, Geneva

WHO (2013b) Mapping salt reduction initiatives in the WHO European Region

WHO (2014) Global strategy on diet, physical activity and health. World Health Organization, Geneva

WHO (2016) What is the maximum acceptable daily salt intake for children? World Public Health Organisation. Available from: http://www.euro.who. int/en/health-topics/disease-prevention/nutrition/ news/news/2011/10/reducing-salt-intake/frequently-asked-questions-about-salt-in-the-who-european-region

WHO, FAO Expert Consultation (2003) Diet, nutrition and the prevention of chronic diseases. World Health Organ Tech Rep Ser 916(i–viii)

Wilson RKE, Incles M (2012) Evaluation of technological approaches to salt reduction. Leatherhead Food Research

Yang BC, Li DY, Weng YF, Lynch J, Wingo CS, Mehta JL (1998) Increased superoxide anion generation and altered vasoreactivity in rabbits on low-potassium diet. Am J Physiol 274(6 Pt 2):H1955–H1961

Yokoyama Y, Nishimura K, Barnard ND, Takegami M, Watanabe M, Sekikawa A et al (2014) Vegetarian diets and blood pressure: a meta-analysis. JAMA Intern Med 174(4):577–587

Zeanandin G, Molato O, Le Duff F, Guerin O, Hebuterne X, Schneider SM (2012) Impact of restrictive diets on the risk of undernutrition in a free-living elderly population. Clin Nutr 31(1):69–73

Zhu H, Pollock NK, Kotak I, Gutin B, Wang X, Bhagatwala J et al (2014) Dietary sodium, adiposity, and inflammation in healthy adolescents. Pediatrics 133(3):e635–e642

Adv Exp Med Biol - Advances in Internal Medicine (2017) 2: 85–96
DOI 10.1007/5584_2016_49
© Springer International Publishing AG 2016
Published online: 15 July 2016

Principles of Blood Pressure Measurement – Current Techniques, Office vs Ambulatory Blood Pressure Measurement.

Annina S. Vischer and Thilo Burkard

Abstract

Blood pressure measurement has a long history and a crucial role in clinical medicine. Manual measurement using a mercury sphygmomanometer and a stethoscope remains the Gold Standard. However, this technique is technically demanding and commonly leads to faulty values. Automatic devices have helped to improve and simplify the technical aspects, but a standardised procedure of obtaining comparable measurements remains problematic and may therefore limit their validity in clinical practice. This underlines the importance of less error-prone measurement methods such as ambulatory or home blood pressure measurements and automated office blood pressure measurements. These techniques may help to uncover patients with otherwise unrecognised or overestimated arterial hypertension. Additionally these techniques may yield a better prognostic value.

Keywords

Blood pressure measurement • Office blood pressure • Home blood pressure • Ambulatory blood pressure measurement • Arterial pressure waveform • Pulse-transit time measurement • Blood pressure devices • Arterial hypertension

A.S. Vischer (✉) and T. Burkard
Medical Outpatient and Hypertension Clinic, ESH Hypertension Centre of Excellence, University Hospital Basel, Basel, Switzerland

Department of Cardiology, University Hospital Basel, Basel, Switzerland
e-mail: Annina.Vischer@usb.ch

1   The History of Blood Pressure Measurement

The history of blood pressure (BP) measurement was reviewed in detail by Eoin O'Brien and Desmond Fitzgerald [1]. The following summarises the main points:

1.1 Direct Measurement of Systolic Blood Pressure

As long as 4000 years ago, Chinese Emperor Huang-Ti was aware of the changing characteristics of the pulse and realised, that people who eat too much salt had hard pulses and tended to suffer strokes. However, it took until the first half of the eighteenth century for Stephen Hales to undertake his famous experiment demonstrating that blood rose to a height of 8 ft and 3 in. in a glass tube positioned in the carotid artery of a horse [1].

1.2 Indirect Measurement of Blood Pressure

Indirect measurement of BP was made possible by sphygmographs, which were first invented by Karl Vierordt in 1855. Sphygmographs applied pressure to the radial artery, while an oscillating metal tip recorded the pulse wave on a strip of smoked paper driven by a clockwork motor [1].

In 1880 Samuel Siegfried Ritter von Basch developed a device he called the sphygmomanometer, which consisted of a rubber pelotte or bulb filled with water with a thin membrane on one side, which was pressed to the radial artery while the pulse was palpated. Water was pressed out into the closed arm of the manometer. The point of disappearance of the pulse was taken as systolic pressure [1].

Later, water-filled cuffs were applied instead of the pelotte, which applied pressure to the entire arm. Kymographs and oscillometers were added, and the size of the devices was reduced, bringing these devices into clinical medicine. Harvey Cushing was the first to advocate putting BP in the bedside chart [1].

Nicolai Sergeivich Korotkoff described what is today called Korotkoff sounds in 1905. The next advancement was an occluding arm cuff developed by Scipione Riva Rocci. The pressure was recorded by a mercury manometer [1].

As early as 1918, focus was set on parameters like patient anxiety, posture of the patient, arm level and the number of measurements needed to be recorded for an accurate diagnosis – factors, which did not lose importance over time [1].

1.3 Ambulatory Measurement of Blood Pressure

In 1904 the basic idea for ambulatory blood pressure measurement (ABPM) was born as Theodore Janeway drew attention to the variability of BP and its response to stressors such as surgery, tobacco and anxiety [1]. 60 years later, Sir George Pickering was the first to show the constant fall of BP during sleep and the fluctuation of BP over 24 h [2]. The first intra-arterial ABPM was performed in 1966 [3]. The first truly portable non-invasive ABPM device was described by Hinman et al. in 1962 [4]. The device weighed 5.5 lbs (2.5 kg) and had to be manually inflated. To overcome the pitfalls of intermittent measurements, the first servo-plethysmomanometer based on the vascular unloading principle using a light source and photocell in a finger cuff was developed in the 1970s [1].

2 Definition and Classification of Hypertension

There is a continuous relationship between BP and vascular mortality above 115 mmHg systolic blood pressure (sBP), obscuring a clear distinction between normotension and hypertension solely based on sBP and diastolic BP (dBP) values [5]. Additionally, sBP and dBP are normally distributed in the general population [6]. However, cut-off BP values are necessary to simplify the diagnostic approach and to facilitate the decision about treatment. The widely accepted office BP measurement (OBPM) cut-off values and the corresponding World Health Organization (WHO) classification of hypertension are depicted in Table 1 [7]. These cut-off values are based on the evidence of a meta-analysis from 1994 showing that above these BP values patients benefit from antihypertensive therapy [8].

Data on a classification of hypertension based on ABPM and home blood pressure measurements (HBPM) are scarce and there is no widely accepted classification beyond the cut-off values for the diagnosis of hypertension, which are provided in Table 2. The National Institute for Health Care Excellence (NICE) guidelines for the management of hypertension advocate a classification based on mean daytime ABPM or HBPM values, derived from a study which directly compared directly OBPM and ABPM measurements in 8529 patients [9, 10]. This may have the limitation that the corresponding stages of the measurement types may not reflect the same cardiovascular risk because of different blood pressure patterns (e.g. white coat hypertension) and different prognostic values of the measurement techniques. Both will later be discussed in detail.

By NICE, stage 1 hypertension is suggested as OBPM $\geq$140/90 mmHg and daytime ABPM/HBPM $\geq$135/85 mmHg and stage 2 as OBPM $\geq$ 160/100 mmHg and daytime ABPM/HBPM $\geq$ 150/95 mmHg [9, 10]. There is no equivalent for stage 3 hypertension proposed [10].

Table 1 Classification of hypertension according to office blood pressure values (mmHg) [7]

Category	Systolic BP		Diastolic BP
Optimal	<120	and	<80
Normal	120–129	and/or	80–84
High normal	130–139	and/or	85–89
Grade 1 hypertension	140–159	and/or	90–99
Grade 2 hypertension	160–179	and/or	100–109
Grade 3 hypertension	$\geq$180	and/or	$\geq$110
Isolated systolic hypertension	$\geq$140	and	<90

Table 2 Cut-off values for office, ambulatory and home blood pressure measurements (mmHg)

Modality	Systolic BP	Diastolic BP
OBPM	140	90
ABPM: 24 h-mean	130	80
ABPM: Awake	135	85
ABPM: Sleep	120	70
HBPM	135	85

Modified after [7]

2.1 White Coat Hypertension

White coat hypertension (WCH) is defined as a BP pattern where OBP values are elevated at repeated visits, but within normal limits out of the office, either on ABPM or HBPM (Table 3 and Fig. 1) [7]. The prevalence of WCH has been described in about 5–65 % of patients with newly diagnosed hypertension [11, 12]. There is an ongoing debate on whether patients with WCH have the same long-term cardiovascular risk as truly normotensive subjects, underlining the importance of its detection [7].

2.2 Masked Hypertension

Masked hypertension is defined as normal BP in the office, with elevated BP values out of the medical environment, shown by ABPM or HBPM (Table 3 and Fig. 1). The phenomenon

Table 3 Definition of white-coat hypertension and masked hypertension

White-coat hypertension	Masked hypertension
Treated or untreated patients with office BP $\geq$ 140/90 mmHg AND	Treated or untreated patients with office BP < 140/90 mmHg AND
24-h ABPM < 130/80 mmHg AND	24-h ABPM $\geq$ 130/80 mmHg AND/OR
Awake ABPM < 135/85 mmHg AND	Awake ABPM $\geq$ 135/85 mmHg AND/OR
Sleep measurement < 120/70 mmHg OR	Sleep measurement $\geq$ 120/70 mmHg OR
Home BP < 135/85 mmHg	Home BP $\geq$ 135/85 mmHg

Modified after [37]

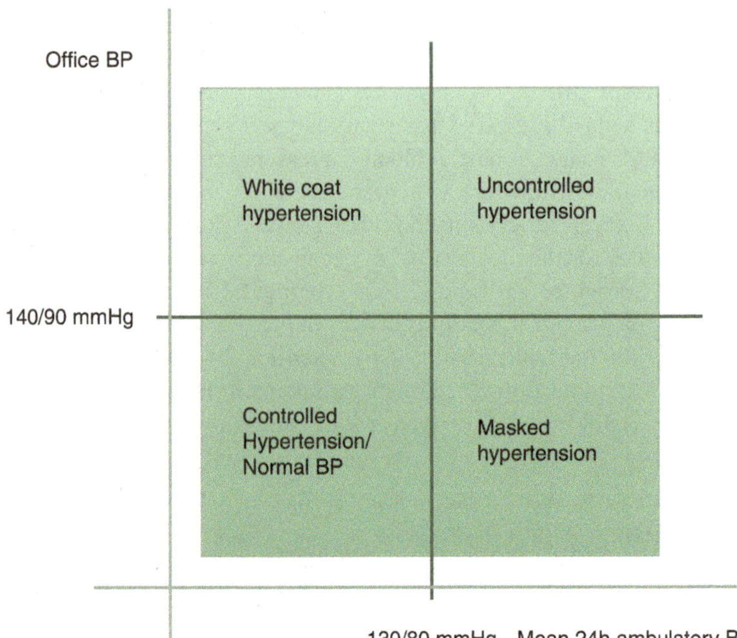

Fig. 1 Definition of different blood pressure (BP) patters when combining in-office and out-of-office BP measurements (Modified after [13])

of masked hypertension has been described in up to 37 % of patients with arterial hypertension under an intensified therapy [13]. Masked hypertension is frequently associated with other risk factors such as asymptomatic organ damage and increased risk of diabetes and sustained hypertension [7]. The cardiovascular risk seems to be as high as in patients with sustained hypertension [14].

3 Office Blood Pressure Measurement

As common practice over decades and until today, OBPM is measured using a brachial pressure cuff and auscultation of the brachial artery to identify the appearance and disappearance of Korotkoff sounds. Over the last years, automated BP measurement devices have reached the market and are now widely accepted in guidelines and used in outpatient clinics, hospitals and by people at home [7, 10].

3.1 Manual Blood Pressure Measurement Technique

In order to receive comparable results, the environment should be standardised as much as possible [10]. The technique is accurately described in the National Institute for Health Care Excellence (NICE) and European Society of Hypertension (ESH) guidelines [10] and summarised in the following:

The patient should be rested and relaxed in a seated position for at least 3–5 min and rested before beginning BP measurements [7, 10]. The arm is out-stretched, in line with the mid-sternum and supported [10]. Further requirements for the environment are shown in Table 4. An appropriately sized cuff (as indicated by markings, see also the paragraph on Cuffs) is wrapped around the upper arm and connected to a manometer [10]. While palpating the brachial pulse, the cuff is rapidly inflated to 20 mmHg above the point where the brachial pulse disappears [10]. This pressure should be noted, as it is the approximate systolic pressure [10]. The cuff should then be re-inflated to 20 mmHg above

Table 4 Principles of office and home blood pressure measurement

Conditions for blood pressure measurements
5 min rest, 30 min without smoking/caffeine
Seated, back supported, arm outstretched, resting on the table
Correct cuff bladder placement
Immobile, legs uncrossed, not talking, relaxing
Repeated readings at 1–2 min intervals
Results written down (if device without memory)

Modified after [10, 32]

Table 5 Recommended cuff sizes [20]

Arm circumference	Cuff size	Cuff measurement
22–26 cm	Small adult	12 × 22 cm
27–34 cm	Adult	16 × 30 cm
35–44 cm	Large adult	16 × 36 cm
45–52 cm	Adult thigh	16 × 42 cm

this point [10]. The stethoscope should be placed over the brachial artery ensuring complete skin contact without clothing in between [10]. Then, the cuff is slowly deflated at 2–3 mmHg per second listening for the Korotkoff sounds [10]. The first sound appearing with the brachial pulse (phase I Korotkoff sound) is the systolic pressure [10]. At this point, the pulse pressure wave overcomes the obstruction caused by the cuff with its maximal pressure [10]. Intermediate sounds follow as the cuff pressure drops, with muffling and then complete disappearance of sounds (phase V Korotkoff sounds) indicating the diastolic pressure [10]. At this point the residual diastolic arterial pressure is sufficient to overcome the pressure caused by the cuff, leading to a normal arterial diameter without systolic blood flow murmurs [10]. The cuff is then quickly deflated completely [7, 10]. At least two BP measurements should be taken in the sitting position, spaced 1–2 min apart, adding more measurements if the first two are quite different (in daily practice more than 2–5 mmHg difference) and the average of the measurements should be used [7]. More measurements are recommended in patients with arrhythmia (i.e. atrial fibrillation) [7]. In case of elevated OBPM, the diagnosis of hypertension should be confirmed in a second visit, usually 1–4 weeks after the initial investigation or preferably with the use of ABPM [10, 15, 16].

In case of a significant (>10 mmHg) and consistent systolic BP difference between the arms, the arm with the higher BP values should be used [7]. A BP difference of >10 mmHg may help to identify patients in need of further vascular assessment, whereas a BP difference of $\geq$ 15 mmHg may be an indicator of peripheral vascular disease, pre-existing cerebrovascular disease, increased cardiovascular mortality and increased all-cause mortality [17].

3.2 Conditions and Environment

BP is maintained through a combination of mechanical, neuronal and endocrine self-regulating systems in the body [10]. There is a considerable variability of BP due to respiration, emotion, exercise, meals, tobacco, alcohol, temperature, bladder distension, etc. [18]. Additionally, BP is influenced by age, race, and circadian variation [18]. Therefore attention should be paid to these circumstances.

3.3 Cuffs

A cuff is an inelastic cloth that encircles the arm and encloses an inflatable rubber bladder [18]. Present-day cuffs consist of an inflatable cloth-enclosed bladder which encircles the arm and is secured by Velcro or by tucking in the tapering end [10]. The width of the bladder is recommended to be about 40 %, and its length 80 % of the arm circumference [10]. Both cuffs that are too narrow and cuffs that are too short will lead to falsely high BP measurements [19]. A bladder which is too large will lead to an underestimation of BP [18]. Recommended cuff sizes are stated in Table 5 [20]. Arm cuffs are preferred, as cuffs fitting on the finger or wrist are often inaccurate and should therefore not be recommended [15].

3.4 Devices

There is a range of manual and automatic BP measurement devices available. For clinical decision making devices need to be validated according to standardised protocols and their accuracy should be checked on a regular basis through calibration in a technical laboratory [7, 21]. A list of currently recommended devices can be found online [22].

3.4.1 Mercury Sphygmomanometers

Mercury sphygmomanometers have traditionally been used to measure BP [10]. They are reliable and provide the reference standard for indirect BP measurement [10]. However, there are significant safety and economic concerns about the toxic effects of mercury [10]. Therefore, in most European countries, mercury sphygmomanometers are no longer available – but still are used as reference devices for the validation of automated measurement devices e.g. in the international protocol for the validation of BP measuring devices by the ESH [7, 23, 24].

Non-mercury devices working with a similar system are available and provide a suitable alternative to mercury devices when manual measurement is required [10].

3.4.2 Aneroid Sphygmomanometers

Aneroid sphygmomanometers measure pressure through a lever and bellows system [10]. In general, they are less accurate than mercury sphygmomanometers and their alternatives, especially over time [10].

3.4.3 Automated Blood Pressure Measurement Devices

Auscultatory or oscillometric automated devices are now commonly used in hospitals and primary care [7, 10]. Certified devices are listed on the webpage of the Dabl Educational Trust [22].

3.4.4 Comparison of Auscultatory and Oscillometric Techniques

Automated devices are easy to use and less error-prone. Techniques using manual devices are more complex and time consuming. Failure to accurately identify the Korotkoff sounds, tendency of physicians to round readings up or down and observer prejudice are common mistakes with manual readings [10].

Mercury manometer technique tend to result in higher BP values than oscillometric devices [25]. This may be due to the fact that oscillometric devices calculate BP from oscillations based on "maximum buckling" of the brachial artery under the cuff, which is nearly equal to the mean arterial pressure. Systolic and diastolic BP values are thus calculated from this mean by device-specific algorithms, rather than directly measured [26]. Therefore it is crucial for clinical decision making to use automated devices which are validated according to a standardised protocol [24]. With thus validated devices the abovementioned effects are clinically not significant.

3.5 Advantages

OBPM has been the cornerstone of hypertension diagnosis and management for over 100 years and is the basis for most studies on hypertension [27]. Even the most recent BP outcome studies like the SPRINT trial and the HOPE-3 trial rely on OBPM with specific measurement procedures in each study [28, 29]. Elevated OBPM predicts cardiovascular events (Fig. 2) [30]. Automated OBPM means to take the mean of multiple BP readings recorded with a fully automated device with the patient resting quietly, alone, in the office or clinic, which was reported to deliver results closer to ABPM [31].

3.6 Disadvantages

A single office BP reading does not represent a patient's true BP [32]. Errors may be due to patients' alerting reaction to the measurement procedure and setting (i.e. white coat effect). With OBPM there is a lack of relevant information on BP during usual daytime activities and during sleep [32].

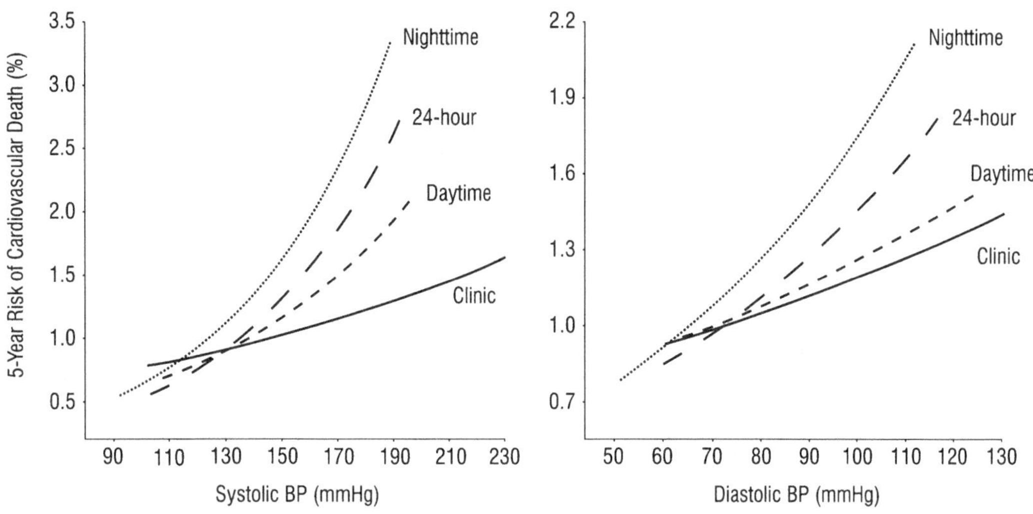

Fig. 2 Adjusted 5-year risk of cardiovascular death in the study cohort of 5292 patients for OBPM and ABPM. Multiple Cox regression was used to calculate the relative risk with adjustment for baseline characteristics including gender, age, presence of diabetes mellitus, history of cardiovascular events, and smoking status (Reprinted with permission from [42])

Table 6 Common mistakes during routine in-hospital BP measurements and their possible influence

Error	Frequency %	Variation in mmHg
Single measurement	96	Mean + 8 mmHg
Arm not at heart level	69	Ca 1.6 mmHg/cm difference
Conversation during measurement	41	Up 20 % increase sBP/dBP
Simultaneous ear temperature measurement	58	Unknown
Simultaneous pulse-oximetry	82	Unknown
Supine, semi-recumbent	39	Ca 8 mmHg sBP
Wrong cuff size	36	Overestimated BP (10–50 mmHg)
Legs crossed	15	Mean + 2–8 mmHg sBP

Modified after [20, 34]

3.7   Caveats

There is a high variability with a mean difference of approximately +20 mmHg sBP between OBPM measurements of primary care physicians and specifically trained research assistants, even after short training [33]. Possible pitfalls in daily practice may be faulty position such as legs crossed, back or arm unsupported, talking during the measurement or insufficient number of readings [33]. The influence of different pitfalls is summarised in Table 6.

In routine in-patient BP measurements, e.g. during nurse-rounds, a variety of procedural errors occur in a very high percentage, affecting the accuracy of BP measurements [34]. These mistakes include utilising non-validated devices, obtaining only a single BP reading, lack of rest prior to the reading, inadequate patient position (arm not at heart level, back not supported, legs crossed, semi-recumbent or supine patient position), misplacement of the cuff or use of an inadequate cuff and finally, conversations with the patient during the reading (see also Table 6) [34].

4   Home Blood Pressure Measurement

4.1   Technique

To guide clinical decisions by HBPM measurements should be taken in a standarised manner as defined by the European Society of Hypertension guidelines for blood pressure monitoring at home [32]. Principles of correct HBPM are summarised in Table 4 and are largely similar to the previously described OBPM procedure.

Frequent measurements produce average values which are more reproducible and reliable than OBPM [10]. Usually, the average of BP measurements over several days, e.g. morning and evening values of 5–7 days, can be helpful in the guidance of treatment decisions [15]. Recommendations on the number and frequency of measurements are collected in Table 7.

4.2   Devices

For HPBM, oscillometric devices which measure the BP on the upper arm are most commonly used; there are – in theory – devices for measurement on the wrist or the finger [10]. However, finger and wrist cuff devices are generally not recommended [32]. Electronic devices are most commonly used, as they are simpler to use and probably more reliable than a sphygmomanometer [15]. An updated list of validated devices is provided by the Dabl Educational Trust website [22].

Table 7 Number of measurements in home blood pressure monitoring

Number and frequency of blood pressure measurements
Mean of 5–7 days of measurements
Two measurements for each session,
Morning and evening sessions per day (before drug intake and before eating)
First day of each monitoring period may be discarded
Long-term follow-up: one to two measurements per week may be considered

Modified after [10, 32]

4.3   Advantages

The presence of a doctor can increase intra-arterially measured BP by 25 mmHg [35], therefore methods which do not include another person are of interest. With HBPM, a large number of measurements during the day and also over several days, weeks or months are possible [32]. The effect of treatment can be assessed at different times of the day and over extended periods [32]. Values attained from HBPM have a good reproducibility [32]. Elevated home BP values have been shown to predict cardiovascular morbidity and cardiovascular, non-cardiovascular and all-cause mortality [30]. The predictive value is thereby stronger compared to OBPM [36]. The costs remain relatively low [32]. Patients get involved in their hypertension management, which may improve both the patients' compliance to treatment and hence their hypertension control [32]. Today, most devices store BP values digitally, which can be printed or directly transmitted in order to prevent reporting bias [32].

4.4   Disadvantages

HBPM has many advantages, but also some disadvantages, such as the need of patient training, the possibility of inaccurate devices used by the patients, measurement errors (e.g. due to arrhythmias), limited reliability of BP values reported by patients (i.e. reporting bias), and induction of anxiety, resulting in excessive monitoring [32]. Occasionally, patients may change their treatment on the basis of causal home measurements without a doctor's guidance [32]. There is still an uncertainty about normality thresholds and therapeutic targets [32]. However, the main disadvantage is that night recordings are not possible and hence a lack of prognostic information through night-time values and dipping pattern [32].

5 Ambulatory Blood Pressure Measurement

5.1 Technique

For ABPM, patients are provided with an ABPM device, which measures BP during 24–72 h at predefined time intervals. Detailed guidelines for the use of ABPM were published by the European Society of Hypertension and the National Institute for Health and Care Excellence [11, 31, 37, 38]. Patients should be instructed about manual deflation, missed readings, and machine location [10]. They should also gain a basic understanding of how the device works [10]. An appropriately sized cuff is obligatory (see Cuffs) [10]. If one arm gives a higher reading at baseline, then this arm should be used subsequently [10], however in general the non-dominant arm will lead to as little interference with daily activities as possible [37]. Patients should be asked to write diary records of activities and sleeping times [10]. Sleeping times can also be estimated by using fixed-narrow time intervals in which the retiring and rising periods are eliminated and only a daytime period from 0900 to 2100 h and night-time period from 0100 to 0600 h is recorded [37]. By this definition, variations of time spent in bed depending on age or culture can be reduced, however information on the white-coat window, the early phase of night sleep, when dipping can be most evident, as well as the morning surge of BP, which may be associated with cardiovascular events, are reduced as well [37]. Therefore, this definition is usually reserved for research purposes [37]. In countries, where a daytime siesta is common practice, a record of sleeping times both during day and night is important and ABPM software should be able to adjust for this, as otherwise nocturnal BP dipping may be underestimated [37].

Blood pressure is measured automatically at repeated intervals (usually every 20 min at day-time and every 30 min at night) over 24 h, while patients continue their daily routines [10]. Patients should engage in normal activities, but should refrain from strenuous exercise and, at the time of cuff inflation, stop moving and talking and keep the arm still at heart level [7].

5.2 Devices

ABPM monitors include a cuff and bladder connected to electronic sensors which detect changes in cuff pressure and allow BP to be measured oscillometrically [10]. Systolic and diastolic pressure readings are deduced from the shape of these oscillometric pressure changes using a specific algorithm [10]. The cuff is inflated by a battery powered compressor [10].

Devices differing in size, weight, noise level, data manipulation and costs are available [10]. They should be validated and internationally recommended [10, 22].

5.3 Advantages

In order to overcome the previously mentioned problems of OBPM, techniques for obtaining automated ambulatory BP profiles over 24 h or more have been developed [37]. In comparison to OBPM, a larger number of readings can be collected during an ABPM [37]. Through this, a profile of BP behaviour during the patient's daily activities can be provided [37]. BP can not only be influenced by the presence of a doctor [35], but also by emotion, exercise, temperature [39] and even by certain actions like car driving [40], or sexual activity [41]. ABPM have been shown to be prognostically superior to office BP readings (Fig. 2) [30, 42]. Especially night-time BP appears to be the best predictor of adverse outcome, independently of either clinic or ambulatory awake measurements [42, 43]. Also, ABPM may uncover a masked hypertension, with the need for more aggressive therapy (Table 3 and Fig. 1) [13]. ABPM has a great potential to reduce misdiagnosis of arterial hypertension, as it may detect white coat hypertension and should therefore be recommended before the start of antihypertensive drugs

[10, 16]. The use of ABPM for diagnosing arterial hypertension in patients with elevated OBPM is time- and cost-effective and is implemented in current guidelines [10, 16, 44].

5.4 Disadvantages

The main disadvantage of ABPM is its limited availability [37, 38]. Also, it may cause discomfort to the patient, particularly at night [37, 38]. Patients may therefore be reluctant to use it, specifically for repeat measurements [37, 38].

There may be a limited reproducibility, particularly when the procedure is not standardised [37]. However changes in ABPM appear to depend mostly on changes in body weight and reaction to medical environment [45].

Generally oscillometric devices are used, which may lead to erroneous readings in some individuals, especially in those with cardiac arrhythmias [37, 38].

6 The Future: Newer Techniques

New devices are placed on the marked on a regular basis. Validated and hence recommended devices can be found online [22]. A selection of recently studied devices is subsequently described.

6.1 Arterial Pressure Waveform

Measurement of the arterial pressure waveform was made possible with a device called Finapres (FINger Arterial PRESsure) and was introduced in the 1980s [46]. The Finapres, which reconstructs a brachial BP waveform from a finger BP waveform, was initially found to correlate with intra-atrial measurements after one supine return to flow calibration, correcting the waveform-estimated finger pressure with a calibration through an upper-arm oscillometric cuff [47]. However, later it was suggested that although the Finapres fulfilled the accuracy requirements for the mean BP and diastolic BP, the Finapres systolic BP measurements did not fulfil the criteria of the Association for the Advancement of Medical Instrumentation [48]. The improved apparatus, the Finometer, compensates for the distortion of the pressure waveform along the arm artery [49]. As a calibration, it measures the brachial BP in a traditional way and then corrects the finger pressure accordingly [49]. Additionally, the Finometer corrects for the hydrostatic height of the finger in respect to the heart level and has upgraded filtering software [49]. Dabl Educational Trust, however, does currently not recommend its used due to incomplete validation [22].

6.2 Pulse-Transit Time Measurement

An alternative technique to estimate beat-to-beat BP is the so-called pulse-transit time measurement (PTT) technique. With this technique, a beat-to-beat determination of the PTT on the basis of a finger photo-plethysmography and a three-channel electrocardiogram is done. PTT is the time-interval between the R-wave on the ECG and the arrival of the corresponding pulse-wave at the finger-plethysmograph. When a specific PTT is calibrated to the systolic and diastolic values of a single standard BP measurement, changes of PTT can be translated into changes of BP values by the application of a stretch strain model and specific algorithms [50]. One commercially available device is the Somnotouch-NIBP (Somnomedics GmbH, Randersacker, Germany), which implements the technique in a watch, which is connected to the finger-plethysmograph and the three channel ECG leads. With the appropriate software an ABPM can be combined with a 24-h-ECG and a nocturnal pulse oximetry. The Somnotouch-NIBP was validated for clinical use according to the European Society of Hypertension protocol and the signal was stable under short-term conditions [51]. The validity of the 24-h BP values derived by the PTT device compared to conventional ABPM values needs to be determined.

References

1. O'Brien E, Fitzgerald D (1994) The history of blood pressure measurement. J Hum Hypertens 8(2):73–84
2. Richardson DW, Honour AJ, Fenton GW, Stott FH, Pickering GW (1964) Variation in arterial pressure throughout the day and night. Clin Sci 26:445–460
3. Bevan AT, Honour AJ, Stott FH (1969) Direct arterial pressure recording in unrestricted man. Br Heart J 31 (3):387–388
4. Hinman AT, Engel BT, Bickford AF (1962) Portable blood pressure recorder. Accuracy and preliminary use in evaluating intradaily variations in pressure. Am Heart J 63:663–668
5. Lewington S, Clarke R, Qizilbash N, Peto R, Collins R, Prospective Studies Collaboration (2002) Age-specific relevance of usual blood pressure to vascular mortality: a meta-analysis of individual data for one million adults in 61 prospective studies. Lancet Lond Engl 360(9349):1903–1913
6. Pickering G (1972) Hypertension. Definitions, natural histories and consequences. Am J Med 52(5):570–583
7. Mancia G, Fagard R, Narkiewicz K, Redón J, Zanchetti A, Böhm M et al (2013) 2013 ESH/ESC Guidelines for the management of arterial hypertension: the Task Force for the management of arterial hypertension of the European Society of Hypertension (ESH) and of the European Society of Cardiology (ESC). J Hypertens 31(7):1281–1357
8. Collins R, MacMahon S (1994) Blood pressure, antihypertensive drug treatment and the risks of stroke and of coronary heart disease. Br Med Bull 50 (2):272–298
9. Head GA, Mihailidou AS, Duggan KA, Beilin LJ, Berry N, Brown MA et al (2010) Definition of ambulatory blood pressure targets for diagnosis and treatment of hypertension in relation to clinic blood pressure: prospective cohort study. BMJ 340:c1104
10. National Clinical Guideline Centre (UK) (2011) Hypertension: the clinical management of primary hypertension in adults: update of clinical guidelines 18 and 34 [Internet]. London: Royal College of Physicians (UK); [cited 2016 Feb 21]. (National Institute for Health and Clinical Excellence: Guidance). Available from: http://www.ncbi.nlm.nih.gov/books/NBK83274/
11. Zeller A, Sigle J-P, Battegay E, Martina B (2005) Value of a standard urinary dipstick test for detecting microalbuminuria in patients with newly diagnosed hypertension. Swiss Med Wkly 135(3–4):57–61
12. Piper MA, Evans CV, Burda BU, Margolis KL, O'Connor E, Whitlock EP (2015) Diagnostic and predictive accuracy of blood pressure screening methods with consideration of rescreening intervals: a systematic review for the U.S. Preventive Services Task Force. Ann Intern Med 162(3):192–204
13. Lehmann MV, Zeymer U, Dechend R, Kaiser E, Hagedorn I, Deeg E et al (2013) Ambulatory blood pressure monitoring: is it mandatory for blood pressure control in treated hypertensive patients?: prospective observational study. Int J Cardiol 168 (3):2255–2263
14. Hänninen M-RA, Niiranen TJ, Puukka PJ, Kesäniemi YA, Kähönen M, Jula AM (2013) Target organ damage and masked hypertension in the general population: the Finn-Home study. J Hypertens 31(6):1136–1143
15. Weber MA, Schiffrin EL, White WB, Mann S, Lindholm LH, Kenerson JG et al (2014) Clinical practice guidelines for the management of hypertension in the community: a statement by the American Society of Hypertension and the International Society of Hypertension. J Clin Hypertens Greenwich Conn 16(1):14–26
16. Siu AL, U.S. Preventive Services Task Force (2015) Screening for high blood pressure in adults: U.S. Preventive Services Task Force recommendation statement. Ann Intern Med 163(10):778–786
17. Clark CE, Taylor RS, Shore AC, Ukoumunne OC, Campbell JL (2012) Association of a difference in systolic blood pressure between arms with vascular disease and mortality: a systematic review and meta-analysis. Lancet Lond Engl 379(9819):905–914
18. Beevers G, Lip GY, O'Brien E (2001) ABC of hypertension. Blood pressure measurement. Part I-sphygmomanometry: factors common to all techniques. BMJ 322(7292):981–985
19. Thulin T, Andersson G, Scherstén B (1975) Measurement of blood pressure--a routine test in need of standardization. Postgrad Med J 51(596):390–395
20. Pickering TG, Hall JE, Appel LJ, Falkner BE, Graves J, Hill MN et al (2005) Recommendations for blood pressure measurement in humans and experimental animals: part 1: blood pressure measurement in humans: a statement for professionals from the Subcommittee of Professional and Public Education of the American Heart Association Council on High Blood Pressure Research. Circulation 111(5):697–716
21. O'Brien E, Waeber B, Parati G, Staessen J, Myers MG (2001) Blood pressure measuring devices: recommendations of the European Society of Hypertension. BMJ 322(7285):531–536
22. dabl Educational Trust – Table of recommended devices by category [Internet]. [cited 2016 Mar 26]. Available from: http://www.dableducational.org/sphygmomanometers/recommended_cat.html
23. O'Brien E, Pickering T, Asmar R, Myers M, Parati G, Staessen J et al (2002) Working Group on Blood Pressure Monitoring of the European Society of Hypertension International Protocol for validation of blood pressure measuring devices in adults. Blood Press Monit 7(1):3–17
24. O'Brien E, Atkins N, Stergiou G, Karpettas N, Parati G, Asmar R et al (2010) European Society of Hypertension International Protocol revision 2010 for the validation of blood pressure measuring devices in adults. Blood Press Monit 15(1):23–38
25. Landgraf J, Wishner SH, Kloner RA (2010) Comparison of automated oscillometric versus auscultatory blood pressure measurement. Am J Cardiol 106 (3):386–388

26. Kiers HD, Hofstra JM, Wetzels JFM (2008) Oscillometric blood pressure measurements: differences between measured and calculated mean arterial pressure. Neth J Med 66(11):474–479

27. Parati G, Bilo G, Mancia G (2004) Blood pressure measurement in research and in clinical practice: recent evidence. Curr Opin Nephrol Hypertens 13 (3):343–357

28. SPRINT Research Group, Wright JT, Williamson JD, Whelton PK, Snyder JK, Sink KM et al (2015) A Randomized Trial of Intensive versus Standard Blood-Pressure Control. N Engl J Med 373 (22):2103–2116

29. Lonn EM, Bosch J, López-Jaramillo P, Zhu J, Liu L, Pais P et al (2016) Blood-Pressure Lowering in Intermediate-Risk Persons without Cardiovascular Disease. N Engl J Med 2

30. Niiranen TJ, Mäki J, Puukka P, Karanko H, Jula AM (2014) Office, home, and ambulatory blood pressures as predictors of cardiovascular risk. Hypertension 64 (2):281–286

31. Myers MG, Godwin M, Dawes M, Kiss A, Tobe SW, Kaczorowski J (2012) Conventional versus automated measurement of blood pressure in the office (CAMBO) trial. Fam Pract 29(4):376–382

32. Parati G, Stergiou GS, Asmar R, Bilo G, de Leeuw P, Imai Y et al (2008) European Society of Hypertension guidelines for blood pressure monitoring at home: a summary report of the Second International Consensus Conference on Home Blood Pressure Monitoring. J Hypertens 26(8):1505–1526

33. Sebo P, Pechère-Bertschi A, Herrmann FR, Haller DM, Bovier P (2014) Blood pressure measurements are unreliable to diagnose hypertension in primary care. J Hypertens 32(3):509–517

34. Holland M, Lewis PS (2014) An audit and suggested guidelines for in-patient blood pressure measurement. J Hypertens 32(11):2166–2170; discussion 2170

35. Mancia G, Bertinieri G, Grassi G, Parati G, Pomidossi G, Ferrari A et al (1983) Effects of blood-pressure measurement by the doctor on patient's blood pressure and heart rate. Lancet Lond Engl 2 (8352):695–698

36. Ward AM, Takahashi O, Stevens R, Heneghan C (2012) Home measurement of blood pressure and cardiovascular disease: systematic review and meta-analysis of prospective studies. J Hypertens 30 (3):449–456

37. O'Brien E, Parati G, Stergiou G, Asmar R, Beilin L, Bilo G et al (2013) European Society of Hypertension position paper on ambulatory blood pressure monitoring. J Hypertens 31(9):1731–1768

38. Parati G, Stergiou G, O'Brien E, Asmar R, Beilin L, Bilo G et al (2014) European Society of Hypertension practice guidelines for ambulatory blood pressure monitoring. J Hypertens 32(7):1359–1366

39. Watson RD, Stallard TJ, Flinn RM, Littler WA (1980) Factors determining direct arterial pressure and its variability in hypertensive man. Hypertension 2 (3):333–341

40. Littler WA, Honour AJ, Sleight P (1973) Direct arterial pressure and electrocardiogram during motor car driving. Br Med J 2(5861):273–277

41. Littler WA, Honour AJ, Sleight P (1974) Direct arterial pressure, heart rate and electrocardiogram during human coitus. J Reprod Fertil 40(2):321–331

42. Dolan E, Stanton A, Thijs L, Hinedi K, Atkins N, McClory S et al (2005) Superiority of ambulatory over clinic blood pressure measurement in predicting mortality: the Dublin outcome study. Hypertension 46 (1):156–161

43. Hermida RC, Ayala DE, Mojón A, Fernández JR (2012) Sleep-time blood pressure and the prognostic value of isolated-office and masked hypertension. Am J Hypertens 25(3):297–305

44. Lovibond K, Jowett S, Barton P, Caulfield M, Heneghan C, Hobbs FDR et al (2011) Cost-effectiveness of options for the diagnosis of high blood pressure in primary care: a modelling study. Lancet Lond Engl 378(9798):1219–1230

45. Palatini P, Mormino P, Canali C, Santonastaso M, De Venuto G, Zanata G et al (1994) Factors affecting ambulatory blood pressure reproducibility. Results of the HARVEST Trial. Hypertension and Ambulatory Recording Venetia Study. Hypertension 23 (2):211–216

46. Sleight P (1985) Ambulatory blood pressure monitoring. Hypertension 7(2):163–164

47. Guelen I, Westerhof BE, van der Sar GL, van Montfrans GA, Kiemeneij F, Wesseling KH et al (2008) Validation of brachial artery pressure reconstruction from finger arterial pressure. J Hypertens 26(7):1321–1327

48. Silke B, McAuley D (1998) Accuracy and precision of blood pressure determination with the Finapres: an overview using re-sampling statistics. J Hum Hypertens 12(6):403–409

49. Schutte AE, Huisman HW, van Rooyen JM, Malan NT, Schutte R (2004) Validation of the Finometer device for measurement of blood pressure in black women. J Hum Hypertens 18(2):79–84

50. Gesche H, Grosskurth D, Küchler G, Patzak A (2012) Continuous blood pressure measurement by using the pulse transit time: comparison to a cuff-based method. Eur J Appl Physiol 112(1):309–315

51. Bilo G, Zorzi C, Ochoa Munera JE, Torlasco C, Giuli V, Parati G (2015) Validation of the Somnotouch-NIBP noninvasive continuous blood pressure monitor according to the European Society of Hypertension International Protocol revision 2010. Blood Press Monit 20(5):291–294

Adv Exp Med Biol - Advances in Internal Medicine (2017) 2: 97–107
DOI 10.1007/5584_2016_151
© Springer International Publishing AG 2016
Published online: 19 October 2016

Blood Pressure Self-Measurement

Stefan Wagner

Abstract

Blood pressure self-measurement has been used extensively as part of several clinical processes including in the home monitoring setting for mitigating white coat effect and gaining more detailed insights into the blood pressure variability of patients over time. Self-measurement of BP is also being used as part of telemonitoring and telemedicine processes, as well as in the waiting rooms and self-measurement rooms of general practice clinics, specialized hospital department's outpatient clinics, and in other types of care facilitates and institutions.

The aim of this review is to provide an overview of where, when, and how blood pressure self-measurement is being used, which official clinical guidelines and procedures are available for its implementation, as well as the opportunities and challenges that are related to its use.

Keywords

Blood pressure • Self-measurement • Hypertension • Home blood pressure monitoring • Office blood pressure measurement • Automated office blood pressure measurement • Ambulatory blood pressure measurement • Guidelines • Recommendations

1 Significance of Blood Pressure Measurements

Blood pressure measurements are important in the diagnosis and monitoring of patients suffering from hypertension or receiving BP lowering medication, as well as for patients in high risk groups, including diabetics, kidney disease patients, and pregnant women suffering from pre-eclampsia (Campbell and McKay 1999; Pickering 1991; Pierdomenico et al. 2009). Hypertension is estimated to be affecting a quarter of the world's adult population with a prevalence as high as 50 % for senior citizens (Wagner et al. 2012a; Santamore et al. 2008).

S. Wagner (✉)
Aarhus University, Finlandsgade 22, 8200 Aarhus, Denmark
e-mail: sw@eng.au.dk

BP measurements are primarily performed in the clinical or in the home setting. In the clinical setting the BP measurements performed by healthcare staff, including medical doctors and trained nurses is called Office BP measurement (OBPM).

OBPM is considered to be the cornerstone of hypertension diagnosis with most evidence on the clinical importance of hypertension and benefits of treatment coming from studies using this technique (Parati et al. 2008). However, OBPM has important limitations, including the inability of OBPM to collect information on BP during usual daytime activities and during sleep, also known as the true blood pressure of the patient (Pickering 1996). Other limitations of OBPM include measurement bias originating from the clinical measurement context and conditions under which the measurement is performed, including the anxiety some patients feel during this process, also known as the white coat effect, which we shall discuss in more detail later (Parati et al. 2008).

Another alternative method for clinical use is called automated office blood pressure (AOBP). It is based on an automated BP device, where the cuff is mounted by a healthcare professional, after which a series of measurements automatically is taken by the device with 1–2 min interval (Leung et al. 2016).

As an alternative to OBPM, measurements in the home setting have proven successful for obtaining valid measurements (Pickering et al. 2008; AbuDagga et al. 2010). Measurements in the home setting may be done using either ambulatory blood pressure devices (ABPM) which are typically worn by the patient for a single 24-h diagnostic period and provides a long range of samples typically at 15–30 min intervals, or automatic home blood pressure devices used for obtaining point measurements typically spanning several days, mornings and afternoons. Both ambulatory and home devices have proven their ability to provide reliable measurements, while home BP devices are more cost effective, less obtrusive and easier to use for the patient than ambulatory BP devices (Pickering et al. 2005a).

Blood pressure self-measurement can also be performed by patients in outpatient clinics and other clinical settings, e.g. in waiting rooms or special self-measurement rooms, as an alternative or supplement to home measurements, using the same BP device types and following the same techniques as in the home setting (Wagner et al. 2012a). In recent years, a range of additional BP devices targeting the clinical self-measurement context has been validated for clinical use.

In the clinic, measurements are either performed by healthcare professionals or as part of a self-measurement procedure handled by the patient themselves. The main motivation for introducing self-measurements relates to a phenomenon known as the white coat effect. Here patients are showing higher blood pressure readings at the clinic than at home, possibly due to the anxiety some people experience during a visit to the clinic or due to the presence of healthcare staff. This is estimated to affect as many as 20 % of all patients (Pickering et al. 2008; AbuDagga et al. 2010). White coat effect is also frequently used as one of the main arguments for home BP monitoring (Parati et al. 2010). Other incentives for increased use of self-measurement in the clinic include a higher number of samples, e.g. several blood pressures readings as opposed to a single point measurement, as well as reduced strain on healthcare personnel.

2 Home Blood Pressure Monitoring

Self-monitoring of blood pressure by patients at home, also known as self-measured blood pressure (SMBP) monitoring, or home blood pressure monitoring (HBPM), is being increasingly used in many countries. SMBP and HBPM have been well received by hypertensive patients and other patient groups that require monitoring of their BP, such as kidney disease patients, diabetics, and pregnant women with BP related complications (Abdoh et al. 2003). HBPM has been shown to predict health outcomes better than office BP measurements (Bobrie et al. 2004; Asayama et al. 2004), and has been found to lower BP compared with usual care (Uhlig et al. 2013).

HBPM is usually performed using a validated blood pressure measurement device using either manual log book entries (paper and pen) or by utilizing the automatic memory of most modern BP devices (Parati et al. 2008). As an alternative, HBPM may also be done as part of a telemedicine or telemonitoring system setup (Parati et al. 2010). Here, the blood pressure device is usually part of a connected system that is able to automatically record data and relay these to the healthcare professionals, e.g. through the use of a secure web based system (Santamore et al. 2008).

Hypertension guidelines provided by the European Society of Hypertension (ESH) and the American Heart Association (AHA) have endorsed the use of HBPM in clinical practice as a useful supplement or alternative to conventional office measurements, especially in patients suspected of possible white coat effect (Parati et al. 2010; Pickering et al. 2005b).

The use of HBPM holds several advantages over conventional office blood pressure (BP) measurement: (1) it provides multiple measurements of BP over time allowing health professionals better insights into the causes and progression of elevated BP (Parati et al. 2010); (2) HPBM measurements are made in the usual environment of each individual, usually the home settings, away from the clinical setting, a setting known to cause white coat effect (Pickering 1996); (3) HBPM is more closely related to hypertension-induced target organ damage and predicts the risk of cardiovascular events better than conventional OBPM office measurements (Bobrie et al. 2004; Asayama et al. 2004; O'Brien et al. 2003); (4) HBPM can detect the white-coat and masked hypertension phenomena, and it shares most of the above features with 24-h ambulatory BP monitoring (ABPM) (Parati et al. 2010).

Compared with ABPM, HBPM provides measurements over a much longer period, is more cost efficient, more widely available, more convenient for patients particularly for repeated measurements, and has been shown to improve patients' adherence to treatment and hypertension control rates (Pickering et al. 2008, 2010; Parati et al. 2010;). Furthermore, HBPM can in theory be continued indefinitely, allowing the patient to self-monitor BP progression over time. However, unlike ABPM, HBPM does not allow for the monitoring of BP during sleep, leisure activities or at work, and does not support the quantification of short-term BP variability, e.g. in 15–30 min intervals.

One of the major shortcomings of HBSM is the design of the BP devices, most of which are based on designs targeting healthcare professionals (Wagner et al. 2012b). Thus, most HBSM devices validated for clinical use does not ensure that patients are adhering to the measurement regiment they have been provided with by their healthcare professional (Parati et al. 2010). This includes not being able to verify the time of day to take their measurements and the number of measurements to take, usually 2–3 measurements each morning and 2–3 each afternoon/evening depending on the provider guidelines, as well as a lack of meeting the guidelines for use of self-measurement in general (Pickering et al. 2005b).

HBPM may be perceived by healthcare professionals and patients to be more time consuming than OBPM, requiring the patient to be instructed in proper use, registering the equipment for lending, and testing and calibrating the equipment after use (Pickering et al. 2008). Furthermore, in case of manual paper based BP schemas or logbooks, the individual measurements needs to be checked for consistency, average values must be calculated and entered into the patient record, or alternatively, data needs to be entered into a decision support system (e.g. an electronic patient record system), for automatic calculations (Santamore et al. 2008). All of these mandatory activities are also error-prone and may result in low quality data sets (Wagner et al. 2012b).

3 Self-Monitoring vs. Self-Measurements

We need to distinguish between self-monitoring of BP in the home setting and time limited self-measurement of BP (BPSM). Self-monitoring is usually used to describe a series of self-measurements over time, usually in the home setting where it is called HBPM, whereas BPSM self-measurement often is constituted as a single point of measurement, or a series of single point measurements, e.g. performed in the clinic's waiting room (Wagner et al. 2012b). As such, BPSM can be viewed as being situated somewhere between the OBPM and HBPM methods with characteristics from both, and should thus be treated and studied in its own right. Thus, some of the challenges associated with OBPM could still apply to BPSM, including bias stemming from the anxiety of attending a clinical setting, something usually associated with the white coat effect phenomenon. However, as with HBPM, the reliability of BPSM measurements depends on the ability and willingness of the individual patient to comply with the provided guidelines (Wagner et al. 2012b). As we shall discus later in further detail, this is one of the major shortcomings of HBPM and BPSM when using state of the art equipment and methods.

4 Blood Pressure Self-Measurement in the Clinic

As an alternative to both OBPM and HBPM, some clinics provide the possibility of letting their patients self-measure their BP before consultation relying on patients performing BPSM in the clinic waiting room or similar. It has not yet been investigated whether this mitigates the white coat effect to the same extent as HBPM and ABPM. While the patient is still in the clinic, the patient is no longer in the same room as the healthcare professional, which could possibly help mitigate the white coat effect of some patients. This has not yet been studied in sufficient detail, and the mere presence of the patient in a clinical setting could cause similar symptoms of anxiety as with white coat hypertension, resulting in increased BP measurements. However, like with HBPM the BPSM process in the clinic requires the patient to follow the same range of recommendations as in HBPM in order to be valid and even though careful instructions and training are provided, BPSM may still be associated with problems.

Current state-of-the-art BP devices used in the HBPM and BPSM setups are not capable of sensing incorrect usage (Wagner et al. 2012a). Therefore, the ability of the patients to adhere to the instructions and related BPSM recommendations is very important. Only measurements following the recommendations are considered reliable (Campbell and McKay 1999; Pickering 1991; Pierdomenico et al. 2009). Thus, non-adherent patient behavior could lead to potential misdiagnoses and possibly result in inappropriate medication (Pickering et al. 2008; AbuDagga et al. 2010).

5 HBPM and BPSM in Clinical Practice

There are important prerequisites for the optimal application of HBPM and BPSM in clinical practice. HBPM and BPSM should be performed by patients who have been trained under medical supervision, and trained nurses and/or pharmacists can have an important part in the implementation of HBPM and BPSM in daily practice and in the diffusion of correct recommendations. Training should include information regarding hypertension, natural occurring and context induced BP variability, proper conditions and procedures to follow for self-monitoring, advice on equipment choice based on validation status (clinical or home use), technical features, price and individual experience, and its proper use and interpretation of results (Parati et al. 2010).

The HBPM and BPSM techniques, when applied using automated electronic devices, is not particularly complex and can easily be explained to most patient groups during a single training session. This could be combined with subsequent periodic verification of correct monitoring performance during office visits or visits by home nurses. Recent studies indicate that even well-trained patients are not following the recommended procedure over time, indicating the need for continuous control measures (Wagner et al. 2013a).

Also, in some patients, in particular elderly with motor or cognitive impairment as well as in young children, the support of a trained nurse, a friend or a relative, may be needed (Parati et al. 2010). Telephonic or video link assistance for patients having doubts or problems with correct HBPM performance could also prove to be useful. A standardized BP logbook structured according to the required monitoring schedule is useful for ensuring the accuracy of data reporting and for improving adherence to measurements schedule (Parati et al. 2010). Manufacturers can facilitate reliable HBPM and BPSM by providing devices with a range of cuffs for varying arm sizes and capable of automatically calculating average BP, and even for the detection of incorrect behavior during measurements. The provision of telemedicine or telemonitoring facilities may be of further advantage to some groups, particularly chronic patient groups.

6 Guidelines on Self-Measurement

A range of guidelines on the self-measurement procedure to follow for HBPM and BPSM, as well as the conditions under which they should be performed exist. Care should be taken to follow these recommendations, as the level of compliance can greatly affect the measured BP levels. These set of recommendations differs between organizations such as the AHA and the ESH (see Table 1).

Healthcare professionals should also be aware of any national or local guidelines to follow, as well, as even the smallest deviations in protocol could result in differences in the resulting measurement levels.

Table 1 Comparison of ESH and AHA guidelines on HBPM procedure and schedule

ESH guidelines	AHA guidelines
Measurement procedure and schedule:	Measurement procedure and schedule:
Seven-day home measurements (minimum of 3 days). At initial assessment, when assessing treatment effects, and in the long-term follow-up before each clinic/office visit. Take two readings morning (before drug intake if treated) and two readings evening (before eating). Readings should be 1–2 min apart. Long-term follow-up: less frequent measurements (for example, once or twice per week) could be regularly performed aimed at reinforcing compliance, although isolated readings should never be used for diagnostic purposes. Overuse of the method and self-modification of treatment should be avoided.	Take multiple readings. Each time you measure, take two or three readings one minute apart and record all the results. Measure at the same time daily. It is important to take the readings at the same time each day, such as morning and evening, or as your healthcare professional recommends. Accurately record all your results. Keep a record of all of your readings, including the date and time taken. Share your blood pressure records with your healthcare team. Some monitors have built-in memory to store your readings; if yours does, take it with you to your appointments. Some monitors may also allow you to upload your readings to a secure web site.

6.1 Monitoring Schedule

Most guidelines suggest that for the initial evaluation of blood pressure levels, including for the diagnosis of hypertension, as well as for the assessment of the effects of antihypertensive treatment including changes in drug or dose, HBPM should be performed daily during at least 3 days before the appointment at the clinic (Parati et al. 2010; Pickering et al. 2005b). Duplicate measurements should be obtained in the morning before drug intake, and in the evening before eating. Measurements of the first monitoring day are usually higher and unstable and are excluded. Well-treated hypertensive patients may also perform regular home BP measurements as a long-term follow-up, e.g. once per week, with the additional aim to reinforce their treatment compliance levels, but the diagnostic value of such long-term measurements is not well-established (Parati et al. 2010).

6.2 Measurement Recommendations

Common to all guidelines, it is recommended that the cuff should be wrapped around the arm with its inflatable bladder centered on the arm with the lower edge of the cuff approximately 2–3 cm above the bend of the elbow. The bladder should always be positioned at the heart level. Also, the measurement should be performed in a quiet room and the patient should remain seated comfortably, not moving during measurements, with the arm resting on a table or other support. Also, the patient should not talk during measurements, and refrain from talking in the minutes before the measurement is taken if feasible.

Please note the subtle differences between ESH and AHA guidelines, where AHA requires the upper arm to be supported at heart level, while ESH only requires the cuff to be placed at heart level. In a recent study by O'brien et al. from 2003, it was found that the forearm also should be at the level of the heart as denoted by the mid-sternal level. Dependency of the arm below heart level leads to an overestimation of systolic and diastolic pressures and raising the arm above heart level leads to underestimation. According to O'brien et al. the magnitude of this error can be as great as 10 mmHg for systolic and diastolic readings, underlining that the source of arm position errors are especially important for the sitting and standing positions. Furthermore, there is evidence that even with a patient in the supine position, an error of up to 5 mmHg for diastolic pressure may occur if the arm is not supported at heart level (O'Brien et al. 2003).

BP measurement results should be reported in a paper schema or logbook format immediately after each measurement according to both ESH and AHA guidelines (Parati et al. 2010; Pickering et al. 2005b). Alternatively, memory equipped devices can store the readings with time and date for each measurement. BP devices designed for telemedicine and telemonitoring purposes are also capable of sending data to a

Table 2 Comparison of ESH and AHA guidelines on HBPM recommendations

ESH guidelines	AHA guidelines
Measurement recommendations:	Measurement recommendations:
At least 5-min rest, 30 min without smoking, meal, caffeine intake or physical exercise. Seated position in a quiet room, back supported, arm supported (for example, resting on the table). Subject immobile, legs uncrossed, not talking and relaxed. Correct cuff bladder placement at heart level. Results immediately reported in a specific logbook or stored in device memory.	Make sure the cuff fits. Measure around your upper arm and choose a monitor that comes with the correct size cuff. Be still, do not smoke, drink caffeinated beverages or exercise within the 30 min before measuring your blood pressure. Sit correctly. Sit with your back straight and supported (on a dining chair, for example, rather than a sofa). Your feet should be flat on the floor; do not cross your legs. Your arm should be supported on a flat surface (such as a table) with the upper arm at heart level. Make sure the middle of the cuff is placed directly above the eye of the elbow. Check your monitor's instructions for an illustration or have your healthcare provider show you how.

computer or tablet device, and even to an online record system, such as the OpenTele telemedicine system (Wagner 2015). Such systems can distinguish data originating from different device users, removing such bias. Sometimes devices are used to measure BP in other family members and it is important to ensure that these are not erroneously included into a patient BP measurement data set (Parati et al. 2010). Finally, in the rare case of a significant and consistent BP difference between arms, defined as more than 10 mmHg, the physician should advise the patient to use the arm with the highest BP values for HBPM and BPSM purposes (Pickering et al. 2005b).

As may be seen in the comparison of ESH vs AHA guidelines in Tables 1 and 2, there are several differences in measurement procedure and schedule as well as measurement recommendations. For instance, the ESH highlight the need to take the measurements before drug intake (in the morning) and before eating (in the evening). Guidelines from other organizations differ even more, including guidelines from the British Hypertension Society that recommends two measurements be taken in the seated position with 1 min apart in the morning and evening for 4–7 days, ensuring a relaxed, temperate setting, with the patient quiet and seated, and their arm outstretched and supported. No other indications are provided, e.g. on rest time before the first measurement (NICE 2011).

6.3 Interpretation of HBPM

The average of a series of measurements taken following the chosen set of guidelines should be used for the clinical decisions based on HBPM and BPSM readings. Casual, isolated home

Table 3 Comparison of ESH and AHA guidelines on interpretation of measurements

ESH guidelines	AHA guidelines
Interpretation of measurements:	Interpretation of measurements:
Average BP from several monitoring days should be considered. BP values measured on the first monitoring day should be discarded.. Mean home systolic BP greater than or equal to 135 mmHg and/or diastolic BP greater than or equal to 85 mmHg should be considered as elevated. Systolic and diastolic home BP less than 130 and less than 80 mmHg, respectively, should be considered normal in most subjects. In high-risk subjects home BP targets should probably be lower.	Optimal blood pressure is less than 120/80 mmHg (systolic pressure should be less than 120 mmHg and diastolic pressure should be less than 80 mmHg). Consult your healthcare professional if you get several high readings. A single high reading of blood pressure is not an immediate cause for alarm. However, if you get a high reading, take your blood pressure several more times and consult your healthcare professional to make sure you (or your monitor) do not have a problem. When blood pressure reaches a systolic (top number) of 180 or higher OR diastolic (bottom number) of 110 or higher, emergency medical treatment is required.

measurements can be very misleading and should not by themselves constitute the basis for clinical decisions. The users should be informed that BP may vary between measurements and be instructed not to be alarmed by lone standing high or low BP measurements. Optimal blood pressure is defined as systolic pressure less than 120 mmHg and diastolic pressure less than 80 mmHg. Average systolic home BP greater than or equaling 135 mm Hg and/or diastolic greater than or equaling 85 mm Hg indicates elevated BP. The levels of 'normal' and 'optimal' home BP are still under investigation, provisionally suggested values being below 130 mmHg systolic and below 80 mmHg diastolic for normal home BP (Parati et al. 2010) (Table 3).

7 Challenges of HBPM and BPSM

7.1 Patients Ability to Report Self-Measured BP Data

There are several well-known challenges associated with both BPSM in general and HBPSM in particular, including failure to correctly report self-measured data, as well as failure to comply with one or more recommendations as described in the guidelines provided by the healthcare professional. A recent study by Wagner et. al. of 113 chronic kidney disease patients self-measuring in the outpatient clinic, in a special purpose self-measurement room, found that over a third of the participants failed to self-report accurately, either omitting, doubling, rounding, or even fabricating one or more parameters in one or more of their measurements. This represents a challenge to the validity of the data being self-reported by patients (Wagner et al. 2013a). These findings are in line with previous work in the area studying HBPM (Johnson et al. 1999; Mengden et al. 1998; Myers 1998). In these studies patients were equipped with home BP devices, but where not informed that the devices were capable of storing the measurements automatically in device memory. This was done in order to investigate the participant's ability to correctly self-report measurements. After a period of self-monitoring and filling out of the paper records, these records were compared with BP device memory values. In total, more than half the patients had either omitted or fabricated readings indicating unacceptable levels of reporting bias, in line with previous work (Wagner et al. 2013a). In a later study on HBPM using a telemedicine web-based system and a home BP device, 161 patients' ability to accurately report self-measured BP data was investigated (Santamore et al. 2008). The study compared the self-reported data from the web, being manually input by the patients after each measurement, with the data stored in the memory of the devices. The authors found that around 16 % of the reported data deviated from the actual data stored in the device memory, which is significantly less reporting error compared with previous work (Johnson et al. 1999; Mengden et al. 1998; Myers 1998). Also, the study found the average reporting error to be below 4 mmHg, and thus not of major importance to the prognostic value for diagnostic or monitoring purposes (Santamore et al. 2008). The lower error rate reported in this study could be due to participants entering data into a web solution rather than keeping a paper logbook. This implies that the participants were aware of technology being involved and thus presumably less likely to be tempted to misreport. Also, as we cannot expect all patient types to be able to utilize a web solution for self-reporting of data, it could indicate that the Santamore study included a population with higher competencies than was the case in the four related studies. Of the five presented studies, only the first investigated adherence to the recommendations, such as rest time before measurement, talking, and noise levels, the other four focusing solely on the patients' ability to correctly and accurately self-report BPSM data. These findings provides us with an indication of the challenges related to relying on HBPM and BPSM obtained in the unsupervised setting with regard to patients' ability to accurately report self-measured data, but not on their ability to self-measure reliably.

In conclusion, self-reported data should not be trusted to be accurate with currently available technology. Either the use of device memory or telemonitoring and telemedicine solutions should be used to overcome reporting-bias.

7.2 Patient Adherence to the Recommendations

A recent study of kidney disease patients who were trained to self-measure their BP at regular intervals at special purpose self-measurement room at an outpatient clinic found that only 8 % of patients adhered to the required rest time before taking the first measurement (Wagner et al. 2013a). Rest time is considered one of the most central requirements for patients to comply with in order to provide a valid rested BP reading, and failing to rest at least 5 min could cause unacceptable bias to the measurement if not properly adhered to (Pickering 1991; Pickering et al. 2008). The study found that less than half of all measurements, including the second and third measurement, where performed after the required 5 min rest time. Furthermore, when analysing the overall ability of participants to adhere to the recommendations: "no talking", "legs not crossed", "back supported", and being in a "quiet setting", the study found that none of the participants followed all of the five recommendations, while most participants did avoid talking during measurements (Wagner et al. 2013a). Not complying with just a single of these HBPM recommendations has been shown to potentially create significant bias to the measurement, in effect rendering the data unusable or even harmful (Campbell and McKay 1999; Pickering 1991; Campbell et al. 1990). As no single participant were able to follow all of the five measured recommendations, and only a minority adhered to four out of five, and less than half adhered to two out of five, this indicates a serious challenge associated with the BPSM method.

In a related study, 81 pregnant diabetic women were observed self-measuring BP while preparing for their weekly or bi-weekly medical consultation in the waiting room of the outpatient clinic. The study found that the pregnant diabetics predominantly did not adhere to given instructions when performing BPSM in the waiting room (Wagner et al. 2013b).

In conclusion, these two chronic patient groups, both of which being well trained in BPSM guidelines and techniques, failed to follow their training.

Likewise, in a recent study of healthy pregnant women's ability to perform BPSM as part of a screening process for pre-eclampsia, where an interactive system provided partial guidance, including on rest time, time between measurements, and number of measurements (a total of three measurements), the authors found that most participants (85 %) performed exactly the three required BP measurements when guided throughout the process by an interactive video screen (Sandager et al. 2013). The remaining performed either four (12 %) or five measurements (3 %) respectively, the system allowing for additional measurements (Sandager et al. 2013). There were also three incidents of "premature measurements" typically taken within 15–60 s after the patient was first seated. However, these three patients eventually managed to wait a further 5 min before taking the next measurement, achieving three valid measurements in the end. The ability to recover from the erroneous process is likely due to the context-aware adherence aid which would subsequently inform the patient of the insufficient rest time and instruct her to redo the measurement when a premature measurement was detected. Also, one patient had actually rested sufficiently before starting the measurement process, but continued to take an additional two measurements after the system had indicated the successful receipt of the required three measurements. The authors also observed adequate patient adherence to the recommendations with regard to rest time in general where 96 % complied (Pickering et al. 2010). Compared with the non-guided results of 8 % compliance reported by the authors in (Wagner et al. 2013a), this indicates the relevance for proper interactive guidance. Also, refraining

from talking during measurements was adhered to by 98 % of patients, without interactive guidance, which is in line with previous results. However, the recommendation on keeping legs not crossed was only adhered to in 85 % of measurements, while back supported was only adhered to by 44 % of the patients. Common to the recommendations "legs not crossed" and "back supported", was that no interactive feedback was provided during the BPSM process. Inadequate patient adherence to these recommendations could cause critical bias and erroneously increased BP levels (Pickering et al. 2010).

These results indicate that patients primarily comply to recommendations when they are actively guided. Using instructions and passive adherence aids did not seem to be sufficient for ensuring reliable measurements. Thus, it should be considered whether interactive aware adherence aids should be introduced to verify and aid during the BPSM and HBPM processes (Wagner et al. 2013c).

Within the field of telemedicine, several state-of-the-art platforms exists that features BP measurement and automatic data collection in order to avoid reporting errors. This includes the Intel Health Guide (IHG), which has been used in several telemedicine studies (Intel 2011; Takahashi et al. 2012). The IHG allows the patient to take the recommended three successive measurements, after which it automatically calculates the average values and reports the data to the healthcare provider, thus enforcing correct reporting procedure eliminating the risk of reporting bias. The IHG also features the capability of enforcing a one minute wait between the three measurements as recommended in most guidelines. However, the system does not have any context-aware sensors, and cannot check whether the patient has remained silent and still during measurements, or observed the proper rest time. It does feature a range of interactive questionnaires, allowing the user to self-report whether he or she has rested sufficiently, been drinking coffee, or smoking cigarettes. Similar systems include the Tunstall Mymedic (Tunstall 2011), and the Bosch Health

Buddy (Koff et al. 2009), which both features automatic collection of BP data and interactive questionnaires, thus avoiding reporting errors, but still relying on self-reporting for relevant context. However, none of these three systems supports the detection of patients not following the recommendations during BPSM and HBPM.

8 Conclusion

HBPM and BPSM are valuable tools in the daily management of hypertension. However, due to the lack of medical supervision during the measurement process, care should be taken to carefully instruct patients of the risks associated with it.

Conflict of Interest No conflict of interests exists.

References

Abdoh AA, Krousel-Wood MA, Re RN (2003) Accuracy of telemedicine in detecting uncontrolled hypertension and its impact on patient management. Telemed J E Health 9(4):315–323

AbuDagga A, Resnick HE, Alwan M (2010) Impact of blood pressure telemonitoring on hypertension outcomes: a literature review. Telemed J E Health 16 (7):830–838

Asayama K, Ohkubo T, Kikuya M, Metoki H, Hoshi H, Hashimoto J et al (2004) Prediction of stroke by self-measurement of blood pressure at home versus casual screening blood pressure measurement in relation to the Joint National Committee 7 classification: the Ohasama study. Stroke 35(10):2356–2361

Bobrie G, Chatellier G, Genes N, Clerson P, Vaur L, Vaisse B et al (2004) Cardiovascular prognosis of masked hypertension detected by blood pressure self-measurement in elderly treated hypertensive patients. JAMA 291(11):1342–1349

Campbell NRC, McKay DW (1999) Accurate blood pressure measurement: why does it matter? Can Med Assoc J 161(3):277–278

Campbell NR, Chockalingam A, Fodor JG, McKay DW (1990) Accurate, reproducible measurement of blood pressure. CMAJ 143(1):19–24

Intel Corporation (2011) Intel health guide PHS6000. Available at: http://www.intel.com/corporate/ healthcare/emea/eng/healthguide/pdfs/Health_Guide_ Product_Brief.pdf. Accessed 1 Jan 2011

Johnson KA, Partsch DJ, Rippole LL, McVey DM (1999) Reliability of self-reported blood pressure measurements. Arch Intern Med 159(22):2689–2693

Koff P, Jones RH, Cashman JM, Voelkel NF, Vandivier R (2009) Proactive integrated care improves quality of life in patients with COPD. Eur Respir J 33 (5):1031–1038

Leung AA, Nerenberg K, Daskalopoulou SS, McBrien K, Zarnke KB, Dasgupta K et al (2016) Hypertension Canada's 2016 Canadian Hypertension Education Program Guidelines for blood pressure measurement, diagnosis, assessment of risk, prevention, and treatment of hypertension. Can J Cardiol 32(5):569–588

Mengden T, Hernandez Medina RM, Beltran B, Alvarez E, Kraft K, Vetter H (1998) Reliability of reporting self-measured blood pressure values by hypertensive patients. Am J Hypertens 11 (12):1413–1417

Myers MG (1998) Self-measurement of blood pressure at home: the potential for reporting bias. Blood Press Monit 3(Suppl 1):S19–S22

NICE (2011) Hypertension in adults: diagnosis and management. NICE guidelines [CG127]

O'Brien E, Asmar R, Beilin L, Imai Y, Mallion JM, Mancia G et al (2003) European Society of Hypertension recommendations for conventional, ambulatory and home blood pressure measurement. J Hypertens 21(5):821–848

Parati G, Stergiou GS, Asmar R, Bilo G, de Leeuw P, Imai Y et al (2008) European Society of Hypertension guidelines for blood pressure monitoring at home: a summary report of the second international consensus conference on home blood pressure monitoring. J Hypertens 26(8):1505–1526

Parati G, Stergiou GS, Asmar R, Bilo G, De Leeuw P, Imai Y et al (2010) European Society of Hypertension practice guidelines for home blood pressure monitoring. J Hum Hypertens 24(12):779–785

Pickering TG (1991) Ambulatory monitoring and blood pressure variability. Science Press, London

Pickering T (1996) Recommendations for the use of home (self) and ambulatory blood pressure monitoring. Am J Hypertens 9(1):1–11

Pickering TG, Hall JE, Appel LJ, Falkner BE, Graves J, Hill MN et al (2005a) Recommendations for blood pressure measurement in humans and experimental animals: Part 1: blood pressure measurement in humans: a statement for professionals from the Subcommittee of Professional and Public Education of the American Heart Association Council on High Blood Pressure Research. Hypertension 45(1):142–161

Pickering TG, Hall JE, Appel LJ, Falkner BE, Graves J, Hill MN et al (2005b) Recommendations for blood pressure measurement in humans and experimental animals: part 1: blood pressure measurement in humans: a statement for professionals from the Subcommittee of Professional and Public Education of the American Heart Association Council on High Blood Pressure Research. Circulation 111(5):697–716

Pickering TG, Miller NH, Ogedegbe G, Krakoff LR, Artinian NT, Goff D et al (2008) Call to action on use and reimbursement for home blood pressure monitoring: executive summary: a joint scientific statement from the American Heart Association, American Society Of Hypertension, and Preventive Cardiovascular Nurses Association. Hypertension 52 (1):1–9

Pickering TG, White WB, Giles TD, Black HR, Izzo JL, Materson BJ et al (2010) When and how to use self (home) and ambulatory blood pressure monitoring. J Am Soc Hypertens 4(2):56–61

Pierdomenico SD, Di Nicola M, Esposito AL, Di Mascio R, Ballone E, Lapenna D et al (2009) Prognostic value of different indices of blood pressure variability in hypertensive patients. Am J Hypertens 22(8):842–847

Sandager P, Lindahl C, Schlütter JM et al (2013) Context-aware patient guidance during blood pressure self-measurement. In: Proceedings of the Iadis International Conference E-health 2013, Eh 2013: University of Twente

Santamore WP, Homko CJ, Kashem A, McConnell TR, Menapace FJ, Bove AA (2008) Accuracy of blood pressure measurements transmitted through a telemedicine system in underserved populations. Telemed J E Health 14(4):333–338

Takahashi PY, Pecina JL, Upatising B, Chaudhry R, Shah ND, Van Houten H, et al (2012) A randomized controlled trial of telemonitoring in older adults with multiple health issues to prevent hospitalizations and emergency department visits. Arch Intern Med 256(1)

Tunstall Limited (2011) Telehealth solutions. Available at: Online: http://www.tunstall.co.uk/Our-products/Telehealth-solutions. Accessed 1 Jan 2011.

Uhlig K, Patel K, Ip S, Kitsios GD, Balk EM (2013) Self-measured blood pressure monitoring in the management of hypertension: a systematic review and meta-analysis. Ann Intern Med 159(3):185–194

Wagner S (2015) Telemedicine systems engineering, First edn. Medivate Publishing

Wagner S, Toftegaard TS, Bertelsen OW (2012a) Challenges in blood pressure self-measurement. Int J Telemed Appl

Wagner S, Toftegaard TS, Bertelsen OW (2012b) Challenges in blood pressure self-measurement. Int J Telemed Appl:2

Wagner S, Buus NH, Jespersen B, Toftegaard TS, Bertelsen OW (2013a) Measurement adherence in the blood pressure self-measurement room. Telemed J E Health (in press)

Wagner S, Kamper, Christina. H., Toftegaard, Thomas S., Bertelsen OW (2013b) Blood pressure self-measurement in the obstetric waiting room. J Telemed e-Health

Wagner S, Toftegaard TS, Bertelsen OW (2013c) Introducing the Adherence Strategy Engineering Framework (ASEF). Methods Inf Med 52(3):220–230

Adv Exp Med Biol - Advances in Internal Medicine (2017) 2: 109–116
DOI 10.1007/5584_2016_177
© Springer International Publishing AG 2016
Published online: 16 December 2016

Ambulatory Blood Pressure Monitoring in the Diagnosis and Treatment of Hypertension

Md. Shahidul Islam

Abstract

Clinicians should take initiatives to establish ambulatory blood pressure monitoring (ABPM) services in their own practice, or to ensure that they have access to such services elsewhere. Whenever possible, ABPM should be performed in suitable cases, where it is likely to deliver clinically useful information for making a correct diagnosis, or for tailoring the anti-hypertensive treatment regimen for each individual patient. ABPM is clinically useful, among others, for identifying people with "masked normotension", "masked hypertension", "sleep-time hypertension", and "reduced decline of sleep-time blood pressure". This review briefly outlines the rationales for the use of ABPM, interpretations of the ABPM-derived parameters, and the advantages of ABPM in decision making in the management of hypertension.

Keywords

White-coat hypertension • White-coat effect • Isolated office hypertension • Hypertension in pregnancy • Obstructive sleep apnea syndrome • Resistant hypertension • Non-dipper • Dipping pattern • Normal values for blood pressure

M.S. Islam (✉)
Department of Clinical Science and Education, Karolinska Institutet, Research Center, 3rd Floor, 118 83 Stockholm, Sweden

Department of Emergency Medicine and Internal Medicine, Uppsala University Hospital, Uppsala, Sweden
e-mail: shahidul.islam@ki.se

1 Introduction

A fundamental property of blood pressure (BP) is its variability, which is essential for adaptation to numerous changes in the prevailing circumstances. Thus, blood pressures measured at the doctors' offices or clinics are the results of the adaptive responses to, for example, the anxieties and expectations of the patients in those special situations and environments.

These BPs do not represent the BPs measured outside the clinic at various time points during the days and the nights. In this respect, ambulatory blood pressure monitoring (ABPM) over a 24-h or 48-h period provides more representative information than BP measurements in the office. However, ABPM is expensive, technically more difficult, not available in many of the developing countries, and not widely available even in many centers in the developed countries.

If available, clinicians should use ABPM generously for the diagnosis of, and the follow up of the treatment of hypertension (O'Brien 2016). The technique should be made available more widely both in the primary care centers as well as in the hospital clinics. If the ABPM services do not exist, then the clinicians should take initiatives, and influence the decision makers to make the technique available to the patients at affordable costs.

In this review, I shall address some selected issues for a better understanding of the rationale, and the utility of ABPM, in an attempt to persuade clinicians to use the technique more liberally in their practices. I shall also touch upon some practical issues, which may help clinicians feel comfortable in using the technique, interpreting the results, and making treatment decisions more correctly. For more comprehensive information on ABPM, clinicians may read some recent reviews and guidelines (O'Brien et al. 2013; Parati et al. 2014; Hermida et al. 2013a).

2 When Should Clinicians Use ABPM?

Even when freely available, use of ABPM for all patients will not be cost effective. Physicians need to make decisions about the use of ABPM in individual cases based on sound clinical judgment and experience, even in the absence of convincing evidence, or clear guidelines. In principle, it should be used to identify eventual discrepancies between the office blood pressure measurement (OBPM) and the ABPM. ABPM should be performed, in selected cases, preferably for two consecutive 24 h periods, for confirming the diagnosis of different forms of hypertension, for evaluating the severity of the condition during a 24-h period, for diagnosing sleep-time hypertension, for identifying the dipping patterns, episodes of hypertension or hypotension, and for identifying the patients with autonomic failures (O'Brien et al. 2013). In the following paragraphs, I shall briefly describe some of these conditions.

1. "Masked normotension" (more often called "isolated office-hypertension" or "white-coat hypertension"):

Some patients, who are not on any antihypertensive medicines, have high blood pressure (BP) on repeated measurements (usually day time awake BP) at the doctors' office (OBPM). If ABPM is not available, most doctors will label these patients as hypertensive patients, and they will do so rightly in about 80 % of the cases. However, they will be wrong in about 20 % of the cases, who actually have normal BP (as evidenced from ABPM), but are wrongly diagnosed as hypertensive patients and treated unnecessarily by antihypertensive medicines, often for the rest of their lives. This is a serious problem for the patients and is expensive for the society, and it must be avoided.

Men who have high office BP ($>140/90$) but whose mean 24-h BP is normal (i.e. $\leq 130/80$ mmHg), do not have hypertension, and should not be treated with antihypertensive drugs (O'Brien et al. 2013). These people have "masked normotension" (also called "white-coat hypertension", or "isolated office- hypertension"), and identification of these people by ABPM is important. They cannot be identified by home blood pressure monitoring (HBPM), which cannot measure sleep-time BP, an important marker of cardiovascular disease (CVD) risk. These people should be followed up by ABPM within two years, if they do not have an increased risk for CVD (e.g. diabetes, chronic kidney disease, or past CVD), or within one year, if they have an increased CVD risk.

In the USA, the Centers for Medicare and Medicaid Services approves reimbursement for the use of ABPM for identification of people with "masked normotension". Early use of ABPM for the diagnosis of "masked normotension" is recommended, among others, by the Canadian Hypertension Education Program (CHEF), UK National Institute for Health and Clinical Excellence (NICE), the European Society of Hypertension, and the International Society for Chronobiology (O'Brien et al. 2013; Hermida et al. 2013a; Gelfer et al. 2015; Krause et al. 2011). U.S. Preventive Services Task Force (USPSTF) concludes that ABPM is the reference standard for confirming elevated office BP results to avoid misdiagnosis and overtreatment of persons with isolated office-hypertension (Piper et al. 2015). ABPM before starting treatment of hypertension is cost-effective (Lovibond et al. 2011).

It should be noted that if office BP is $\geq 180/110$, doctors need to start treatment without waiting for ABPM. First-time ABPM should not be done for patients who are on ≤ 2 antihypertensive medicines. If they are on ≥ 3 antihypertensive medicines then they should be tested by ABPM to confirm if they have true resistant hypertension (see below).

2. "Masked hypertension":

Many people, who are not on any antihypertensive medicines, have normal office BP measured on repeated occasions. It is important for clinicians to keep in mind that about 10 % of these people may have hypertension, despite normal office BP ("masked hypertension"). In some cases "masked hypertension" is due to sleep-time hypertension. "Masked hypertension" is common and is associated with increased risk for CVD events (Hermida et al. 2012; Booth et al. 2016). If the diagnosis of hypertension is missed in people with "masked hypertension", they will remain untreated with increased risk for CVD. For the diagnosis of "masked hypertension", clinicians should use ABPM whenever they suspect the condition.

3. "Sleep-time hypertension" and "dipping" or "rising" patterns of BP:

Sleep-time hypertension and the "dipping" or "rising" patterns of BP during sleep-time can be identified only by using 24-h ABPM (preferably on two consecutive days). It should be noted that for defining the wake-time BP and the sleep time BP, it is common and convenient to use arbitrary fixed clock hours, for example, wake-time BP defined as BP measured during 09:00–21:00, and sleep-time BP defined as those during 01:00–06:00. However, presentation of ABPM results in terms of clock hours can be misleading. For accurately measuring the average wake-time and sleep-time BPs, people undergoing ABPM must note down in a diary the times of retiring to the bed at night, and the times of awakening in the morning, and the ABPM results must be presented in terms of "hours from bedtime" (Hermida et al. 2013a).

Some people have normal office BP, and normal ABPM-derived mean wake-time BP, but high ABPM-derived mean sleep-time BP. The latter is an independent, and a better predictor of CVD morbidity and mortality compared to the office BP or ABPM-derived mean wake-time BP, or mean 24 h BP (Hermida et al. 2016). Sleep-time relative systolic BP (SBP) decline has additional prognostic value. Sleep time relative SBP decline or "dipping" is calculated as $100\times$ (mean wake-time SBP − mean sleep-time SBP)/mean wake-time SBP. Sleep-time relative SBP decline is a continuous variable but it is conventional to divide people into four groups based on the decline: people who have >10 % decline in sleep-time SBP compared to the wake-time SBP are called "dippers"; those who have <10 % decline are called "non-dippers"; those who have >20 % decline are called "extreme dippers"; and those who have <0 % decline are called "risers". It should be noted that in shift-workers, the circadian rhythm of BP is reversed. They have peak BP at about 10:00–11:00 (Sternberg et al. 1995).

The frequency of sleep-time hypertension, "non-dipping", "reduced-dipping" or "riser" patterns of BP is high (as high as 65–81 %) in the elderly people, type 2 diabetes, chronic kidney disease, obstructive sleep apnea and other sleep disorders, resistant hypertension, obesity and pregnancy (Hermida et al. 2016; Mojon et al. 2013; Ayala et al. 2013). Moreover, about 20 % "normotensive" people are "non-dippers", and thus have increased CVD risk. ABPM should be performed when sleep-time hypertension, "reduced dipping", "non-dipping" or "rising" patterns of sleep-time BP are suspected. Identification of sleep-time hypertension and the "non-dippers" is clinically useful, since some of these patients can be treated by administering some of the antihypertensive medicines, in full dose, at the bed-time (not traditional BID regimen) (Hermida et al. 2016).

4. Resistant hypertension:

Hypertension that is not controlled by lifestyle changes and therapeutic doses of ≥ 3 antihypertensive medicines (including a diuretic, unless contraindicated) is called resistant hypertension. Thus, all patients who need ≥ 4 medicines for control of BP have resistant hypertension. Diagnosis of resistant hypertension based on OBPM can often be wrong because of the well-known "white-coat effect". In one large study, 37.5 % of the "resistant hypertension" patients diagnosed by OBPM had "white-coat resistant hypertension", and 62.5 % had true resistant hypertension, as verified by ABPM (de la Sierra et al. 2011). ABPM is essential for a correct diagnosis of resistant hypertension (Lazaridis et al. 2015). It is also useful for guiding the treatment of hypertension in these patients. When any treatment of these patients is modified in any way, the results of such modifications should be evaluated by repeating ABPM within the ensuing three months.

5. Evaluation of the treatment of hypertension:

ABPM is useful for choosing the optimal treatment regimen for any individual hypertensive patient, and to monitor if the treatment has resulted in the desired BP goals. Follow up of patients by repeated ABPM can allow changes of treatments, reduction of multidrug treatment or even total withdrawal of anti-hypertensive medicines and improved BP control (Grin et al. 1993; Staessen et al. 1997).

Some patients who are on the treatment by antihypertensive medicines have high BP measured at the office, but have normal or lower BP measured by ABPM. Some patients have normal wake-time BP, but high sleep-time BP. Some patients have reduced decline of sleep-time BP. Some patients develop symptoms suggestive of hypotension during the treatment with anti-hypertensive medicines. Ideally, antihypertensive medicines should reduce BP in a homogeneous and smooth manner throughout the day and the night. In reality, many long-acting BP-lowering medicines do not reduce BP homogeneously over an entire 24-h period. Thus, long-acting BP-lowering medicines taken once only in the morning may not reduce sleep-time BP or may not induce adequate decline of the sleep-time BP. If some BP lowering medicines are taken at the bed-time, it can reduce the sleep-time hypertension, and restore the normal dipping pattern in some patients (Hermida et al. 2013b).

6. ABPM in pregnancy

For ABPM in pregnancy, doctors should use only those ABPM devices that have been validated for use in pregnancy. ABPM is clinically useful in early pregnancy to distinguish the women who have true hypertension from those who have "masked normotension" or "white-coat hypertension". In one study about 50 % of the women, who were diagnosed for the first time by OBPM to have hypertension, had actually "masked normotension" or "white-coat hypertension" as confirmed by ABPM (Brown et al. 2005). There is no conclusive evidence that ABPM can predict pre-eclampsia. In gestational hypertension and pre-eclampsia, the frequency of sleep-time hypertension is high, but these patients also have wake-time hypertension (Brown et al. 2001).

Normally, BP in pregnant women is lower than that in non-pregnant women. In normal pregnancy BP successively decreases up to the middle of pregnancy and then successively increases up to the delivery. BP ranges and the upper normal values for 24 h BP and sleep-time BP (defined as mean + 2 standard deviation), in different weeks of pregnancy have been reported by several groups and one such set of values are given below (O'Brien et al. 2013; Higgins 2001):

9–17 weeks: 24 h BP: 101/60-118/71. Upper normal value for 24 h BP: 121/73. Sleep-time BP: 93/50-109/64. Upper normal value for Sleep-time BP: 110/64.

18–22 weeks: 24 h BP: 96/56-127/78. Upper normal value for 24 h BP: 126/76. Sleep-time BP: 88/46-120/68. Upper normal value for sleep-time BP: 114/66.

26–30 weeks: 24 h BP: 97/56-133/84. Upper normal value for 24 h BP: 128/78. Sleep-time BP: 87/46-125/76. Upper normal value of Sleep-time BP: 117/68.

31–40 weeks: 24 h BP: 103/57-136/85. Upper normal value for 24 h BP: 131/82. Sleep-time BP: 85/46-131/77. Upper normal value for sleep-time BP: 123/72.

ABPM is also useful than OBPM for diagnosing sustained hypertension during late post-partum period in women who had gestational hypertension or pre-eclampsia during pregnancy (Mangos et al. 2012).

3 Reference Values for ABPM

Reference values for ambulatory BPs are lower than those for office BP. Based on the CVD outcome, the following diagnostic threshold values have been recommended for ambulatory BPs (Hermida et al. 2013a). For adult men, mean wake-time BP: 135/85 mmHg, and mean sleep-time BP: 120/70 mmHg (Kikuya et al. 2007). For adult women, mean wake-time BP: 125/80 mmHg, mean sleep-time BP: 110/65 mmHg (Hermida et al. 2013c). For high risk patients (e.g. those with diabetes, chronic kidney disease, previous CVD events) of both sexes, mean wake-time BP: 120/75 mmHg, and mean sleep-time BP: 105/60 mmHg (Hermida et al. 2013a).

4 Performing ABPM and Interpreting the Results

Doctors working in the primary care centers or in hospital clinics should take initiatives to establish their own ABPM services, if those do not already exist. Price of ABPM device with software in 2016 is around 2500 USD. Alternatively, doctors should know where to refer their patients to for ABPM. Doctors and nurses responsible for ABPM services and analysis of the results must receive appropriate training, and keep themselves updated.

Many automated ABPM devices that measure blood pressure by oscillometric method are available. These devices do not measure the SBP and the DBP directly; rather they measure the mean arterial BP and then deduce the SBP and DBP from the oscillometric pressure changes by using algorithms that are often kept secret and are specific to the respective devices. For this reason, it is important to use devices that have been independently validated by internationally accepted protocols, for their accuracy, for use in different patient groups (e.g. in the elderly, in pregnancy). For a list of recommended ABPM devices check this website: http://www.dableducational.org/sphygmomanometers/devices_3_abpm.html. The devices should be recalibrated yearly by companies that meet the ISO 9001 standards. The batteries should be checked regularly. The software must be able to generate a standardized report, including the raw BP and heart-rate data, blood pressure plots, software generated mean wake-time and sleep-time BP, and sleep-time BP decline (dipping in %) (Omboni et al. 2015).

At the outset, it is necessary to assess whether the patient is able to understand and follow the instructions, and cooperate during the ABPM process. Patients must receive a number of clear verbal and written instructions. On the day of the monitoring, they will carry on their normal activities as much as possible, but they must avoid physical exercise and activities that may interfere with the recording of representative BP values (e.g. driving and day-time sleeping). The ABPM devices give a beep sound a few seconds before starting the inflation of the cuff. At the time of the inflation, the person will stand still or sit down, without talking, with the arm relaxed at the heart level. At night, the beep sound must be shut off, but the monitor must stay on, and it can be placed on the patient´s side. If the device is removed for short periods, for example, for a shower, it should be switched off. They must maintain a diary where they note down the times of retirement to the bed at night, waking in the morning, meals, taking medicines, and other events. They must know how to switch off the device, when needed, and exactly when and where they should return the device.

Measure the arm circumference, and BP in both arms, and apply a blood pressure cuff of appropriate size to the dominant arm. If there is >10 mmHg difference in BP between the arms then use the arm with higher BP for ABPM. The patient should not be able to see the BP values displayed on the device during the monitoring. Program the ABPM device to measure BP at 15–60 min intervals (often at 20–30 min intervals during the wake-time, and at 60 min interval during the sleep-time). It should be noted that, the reproducibility of the BP patterns depends more on the duration of monitoring (preferably for 24 h on two consecutive days) than on the sampling rate (Hermida et al. 2013d).

At the time of interpreting the ABPM results, it is first of all essential to check if the monitoring has been done satisfactorily (Omboni et al. 2015). If ABPM records ≥70 % of the scheduled measurements, ≥20 valid measurements during the wake-time and ≥7 measurements during the sleep-time, than it can be accepted as a satisfactory monitoring (Parati et al. 2014). The monitoring cannot be accepted as entirely satisfactory if data are lacking for more than two, consecutive hourly intervals, if the patient sleeps during the night for less than 6 h or more than 12 h, or if the measurements were done during exercise, driving, excessive movement, or during unusual emotional stress (Hermida et al. 2013a). Look at the BP traces for episodes of high or low BPs. A report of analysis of the ABPM should include the dates of the performance of the monitoring, comments on the quality of the recording, mean 24 h BP, mean wake-time BP, mean sleep-time BP, and degree of "dipping" in percent.

5   Difficulties of ABPM

The main problem with ABPM is that it is either not widely available or not used by doctors even when it is readily available. OBPM is faster, cheaper and more convenient to most doctors. Some patients may find ABPM inconvenient especially during the sleep-time and especially if ABPM has to be done repeatedly. Some people do not tolerate ABPM at all and others fail to follow the instructions despite clear instructions, making good quality monitoring difficult. It may be difficult to perform ABPM in some very obese people and results can be wrong if cuffs of appropriate size are not used. In atrial fibrillation ABPM is less accurate in measuring the diastolic BP but ABPM is not contraindicated in this condition.

6   Concluding Remarks

Numerous researches over past three decades have established ABPM as an evidence-based and cost-effective gold-standard for the diagnosis and treatment of hypertension. Use of ABPM can reduce misdiagnosis, and unnecessary treatment, and lead to better control of BP. Clinicians should use ABPM whenever possible and take initiatives to establish ABPM services where those do not exist.

Acknowledgement Financial support was obtained from Karolinska Institutet, Stockholm, Uppsala County Council, and Uppsala University Hospital.

Conflict of Interest None

References

Ayala DE, Moya A, Crespo JJ, Castineira C, Dominguez-Sardina M, Gomara S et al (2013) Circadian pattern of ambulatory blood pressure in hypertensive patients with and without type 2 diabetes. Chronobiol Int 30 (1–2):99–115

Booth JN III, Diaz KM, Seals SR, Sims M, Ravenell J, Muntner P et al (2016) Masked hypertension and cardiovascular disease events in a prospective cohort of blacks: the Jackson heart study. Hypertension 68 (2):501–510

Brown MA, Davis GK, McHugh L (2001) The prevalence and clinical significance of nocturnal hypertension in pregnancy. J Hypertens 19(8):1437–1444

Brown MA, Mangos G, Davis G, Homer C (2005) The natural history of white coat hypertension during pregnancy. BJOG 112(5):601–606

de la Sierra A, Segura J, Banegas JR, Gorostidi M, de la Cruz JJ, Armario P et al (2011) Clinical features of 8295 patients with resistant hypertension classified on the basis of ambulatory blood pressure monitoring. Hypertension 57(5):898–902

Gelfer M, Dawes M, Kaczorowski J, Padwal R, Cloutier L (2015) Diagnosing hypertension: evidence supporting the 2015 recommendations of the Canadian Hypertension Education Program. Can Fam Physician 61 (11):957–961

Grin JM, McCabe EJ, White WB (1993) Management of hypertension after ambulatory blood pressure monitoring. Ann Intern Med 118(11):833–837

Hermida RC, Ayala DE, Mojon A, Fernandez JR (2012) Sleep-time blood pressure and the prognostic value of isolated-office and masked hypertension. Am J Hypertens 25(3):297–305

Hermida RC, Smolensky MH, Ayala DE, Portaluppi F (2013a) 2013 ambulatory blood pressure monitoring recommendations for the diagnosis of adult hypertension, assessment of cardiovascular and other hypertension-associated risk, and attainment of therapeutic goals. Chronobiol Int 30(3):355–410

Hermida RC, Rios MT, Crespo JJ, Moya A, Dominguez-Sardina M, Otero A et al (2013b) Treatment-time regimen of hypertension medications significantly affects ambulatory blood pressure and clinical characteristics of patients with resistant hypertension. Chronobiol Int 30(1–2):192–206

Hermida RC, Ayala DE, Mojon A, Fontao MJ, Chayan L, Fernandez JR (2013c) Differences between men and women in ambulatory blood pressure thresholds for diagnosis of hypertension based on cardiovascular outcomes. Chronobiol Int 30(1–2):221–232

Hermida RC, Ayala DE, Fontao MJ, Mojon A, Fernandez JR (2013d) Ambulatory blood pressure monitoring: importance of sampling rate and duration–48 versus 24 hours–on the accurate assessment of cardiovascular risk. Chronobiol Int 30(1–2):55–67

Hermida RC, Ayala DE, Smolensky MH, Fernandez JR, Mojon A, Portaluppi F (2016) Sleep-time blood pressure: unique sensitive prognostic marker of vascular risk and therapeutic target for prevention. Sleep Med Rev 14

Higgins JR, de Swiet M (2001) Blood-pressure measurement and classification in pregnancy. Lancet 357 (9250):131–135

Kikuya M, Hansen TW, Thijs L, Bjorklund-Bodegard K, Kuznetsova T, Ohkubo T et al (2007) Diagnostic thresholds for ambulatory blood pressure monitoring based on 10-year cardiovascular risk. Blood Press Monit 12(6):393–395

Krause T, Lovibond K, Caulfield M, McCormack T, Williams B (2011) Management of hypertension: summary of NICE guidance. BMJ 343:d4891

Lazaridis AA, Sarafidis PA, Ruilope LM (2015) Ambulatory blood pressure monitoring in the diagnosis, prognosis, and management of resistant hypertension: still a matter of our resistance? Curr Hypertens Rep 17 (10):78

Lovibond K, Jowett S, Barton P, Caulfield M, Heneghan C, Hobbs FD et al (2011) Cost-effectiveness of options for the diagnosis of high blood pressure in primary care: a modelling study. Lancet 378(9798):1219–1230

Mangos GJ, Spaan JJ, Pirabhahar S, Brown MA (2012) Markers of cardiovascular disease risk after hypertension in pregnancy. J Hypertens 30(2):351–358

Mojon A, Ayala DE, Pineiro L, Otero A, Crespo JJ, Moya A et al (2013) Comparison of ambulatory blood pressure parameters of hypertensive patients with and without chronic kidney disease. Chronobiol Int 30 (1–2):145–158

O'Brien E (2016) Why is it that we continue to deny patients ambulatory blood pressure monitoring? Hypertension 67(3):484–487

O'Brien E, Parati G, Stergiou G, Asmar R, Beilin L, Bilo G et al (2013) European society of hypertension position paper on ambulatory blood pressure monitoring. J Hypertens 31(9):1731–1768

Omboni S, Palatini P, Parati G (2015) Standards for ambulatory blood pressure monitoring clinical reporting in daily practice: recommendations from the Italian Society of Hypertension. Blood Press Monit 5

Parati G, Stergiou G, O'Brien E, Asmar R, Beilin L, Bilo G et al (2014) European Society of Hypertension practice guidelines for ambulatory blood pressure monitoring. J Hypertens 32(7):1359–1366

Piper MA, Evans CV, Burda BU, Margolis KL, O'Connor E, Whitlock EP (2015) Diagnostic and predictive accuracy of blood pressure screening methods with consideration of rescreening intervals: a systematic review for the U.S. Preventive Services Task Force. Ann Intern Med 162(3):192–204

Staessen JA, Byttebier G, Buntinx F, Celis H, O'Brien ET, Fagard R (1997) Antihypertensive treatment based on conventional or ambulatory blood pressure measurement. A randomized controlled trial. Ambulatory Blood Pressure Monitoring and Treatment of Hypertension Investigators. JAMA 278(13):1065–1072

Sternberg H, Rosenthal T, Shamiss A, Green M (1995) Altered circadian rhythm of blood pressure in shift workers. J Hum Hypertens 9(5):349–353

Adv Exp Med Biol - Advances in Internal Medicine (2017) 2: 117–127
DOI 10.1007/5584_2016_97
© Springer International Publishing AG 2016
Published online: 9 October 2016

Treatment of Hypertension: Which Goal for Which Patient?

Faiçal Jarraya

Abstract

Hypertension remains the most important risk factor for cardiovascular disease. If antihypertensive drugs choice is well guided today, blood pressure (BP) target still a subject of controversies. Residual risk is matter of debate and the lower- the better dogma is come back again regarding to data reported from recent trials. The J curve, reason for European Society of Hypertension Guidelines reappraisal in 2009, is criticized by recent data. The one goal (<140/90 mmHg) fit 90 mmg 90 mmHg) fit all should be adapted as a personalized goal guided by evidence generated by randomized controlled trials. Target controversy is back because of the results of ACCORD and SPRINT trials challenging the common systolic BP target less 140 mmHg to less than 120 mmHg. The first was performed in diabetic patients and the second in patients at high cardiovascular risk; elderly aged of 75 years and above, or patients with chronic kidney disease, or with pre-existing subclinical or clinical cardiovascular disease or a Framingham 10-year cardiovascular disease risk score of 15 % or above, however non diabetic. If the first trial was negative, SPRINT reports a huge reduction of the composite primary outcome, which included myocardial infarction, other acute coronary syndromes, stroke, heart failure or death from cardiovascular causes by 25 %, and the risk of death from all causes by 27 %, when target systolic BP is lower than 120 mmHg compared to lower than 140 mmHg. However, BP was measured by automated office BP technique which correlates more with home BP measurement than auscultatory office BP measurement. Also, only significant less heart failure in the intensive arm was driving the difference in mortality favoring the intensive arm in SPRINT. The greater use of diuretics may have

F. Jarraya (✉)
Research Unit 12ES14, Faculty of Medicine, Sfax
University, Sfax, Tunisia

Nephrology Department, H. Chaker University Hospital,
Sfax 3029, Tunisia
e-mail: Jarraya_faical@yahoo.fr

demasked latent heart failure in hypertensive patients with rather high cardiovascular risk.

More convincing data suggest that BP should be diagnosed early and treatment should be started at BP level of 140 mmHg and above, based on an office BP measurement, confirmed by an out-of-office BP measurement. Target systolic BP should be less than 140 mmHg if BP is measured by classic auscultatory method, less than 120 mmHg in high risk patients if BP is measured by automated office BP measurement. These targets are relevant in elderly patients if no orthostatic hypotension occurred, patients with non proteinuric chronic kidney disease (eGFR $<$ 60 ml/mn/1.73 m^2) and patients with cardiovascular disease or a Framingham score more than 15 %. However attention should be taken on diastolic BP if lower than 70 mmHg because of an increasing risk of ischemic heart event and on renal function since acute renal failure is more frequently reported at these low targets.

In diabetic patients, SBP target should be less than 140 mmHg according to ACCORD trial. However, for patients with protein-creatinine ratio >500 mg/g (albumin-creatinine ratio $>$ 300 mg/g), with or without diabetes, lower SBP target should be proposed for renal protection aiming SBP $<$ 130 mmHg as recommended by KDIGO guidelines.

In patients at low or intermediate risk, without cardiovascular disease, SBP should start to be treated when SBP is above 140 mmHg, and when treated, target BP should be less than 140 mmHg as reported by HOPE-3 trial.

Keywords

Hypertension in the diabetics • Hypertension in the elderly • Blood pressure goals • Hypertension and cardiovascular prevention • Hypertension and microvascular complications • SPRINT trial • ACCORD trial • Ambulatory blood pressure measurement

1   Introduction

Cardiovascular diseases are a worldwide leading cause of mortality and morbidity, even in most developing countries, as Tunisia, where cardiovascular mortality is the leader, accounting for about 29 % causes of deaths (Hajem and Hsairi 2013). Hypertension remains the most important risk factor. According to the recently published global, regional and national comparative risk assessment of 79 behavioral, environmental and occupational, and metabolic risks or clusters of risks in 188 countries, (GBD 2013 Risk Factors Collaborators 2015), high systolic blood pressure (BP) accounted for 6.9 million deaths in 1990 and 10.4 million deaths in 2013 with a 49.1 % progression and 208.1 million DALYs (disability-adjusted life-years) in 2013. This data contrast with the emergence of many treatment choices for hypertension in the last three decades, reflecting the magnitude of this clinical problem and highlighting that the treatment of hypertension remains difficult.

If BP was measured since eighteenth century by Stephen Hales (Lewis 1994), we have to wait for the contribution of the Framingham Heart Study to recognize that high BP is an eminent cardiovascular risk factor (Kannel et al. 1961). The Veterans Administration Cooperative Study on Antihypertensive Agents was the first study demonstrating in 1967 the benefit of BP reduction ([no authors listed] 1967). It included men with diastolic BP (DBP) of 115–129 mmHg. The treatment, including hydrochlorothiazide, reserpine and hydralazine hydrochloride, caused a remarkable average BP reduction of systolic/diastolic (SBP/DBP) by 43/30 mmHg in the active treatment arm. This reduction resulted in a reduction of cardiovascular events after only 11 months follow-up, with 21 fatal or morbid events in placebo arm as opposed to one event in the active treatment arm. The study was therefore stopped prematurely. The second larger Veterans Administration Cooperative Study conducted in patients with milder hypertension (HTN) confirmed the effect of BP control on stroke and congestive heart failure occurrence ([no authors listed] 1970). From then on, several questions were raised: what is the definition of HTN? at which level of BP should one start to treat? and down to which level should BP be reduced to obtain the highest protective effect?

2 Definition of Hypertension

The best definition of HTN at a personnel point of view was given by G. Rose (1980); indeed, hypertension is the level of arterial BP at which the benefits of intervention exceed those of inaction. However, it is difficult to translate this definition to the daily practice, there is a need for a numerical definition. Earlier in 1980s and early 1990s the definition of HTN was BP > 160/ 95 mmHg, up to 1993 where the definition of HTN was reduced to a level equal or above 140/90 mmHg. This definition still adopted nowadays by all guidelines.

The definition of HTN relates an attributable risk to a BP level. In most populations and age groups, there is a linearly relationship between systolic blood pressure (SBP) and risk of cardiovascular mortality, cardiovascular events and strokes. Among patients younger than 65 years, there is a progressive increase in the risk of stroke and coronary artery disease with a parallel increase in SBP. Increasing risk is, however, not equivalent for DBP. For the population of

65 years old and above, the risk continues to increase with the increase of SBP, however, a reversal occurs with the DBP where the risk of cardiovascular events increases with the rise of DBP but also with the fall of it, showing a J curve (Neaton and Wentworth 1992).

The Multiple Risk Factor Intervention Trial (MRFIT) assessed the combined influence of BP, serum cholesterol level, and cigarette smoking on death from coronary heart disease (CHD) for 316,099 men screened in whom 6327 deaths from CHD have been identified after an average follow-up of 12 years. Strong graded relationships between SBP above 110 mmHg, and DBP above 70 mmHg and mortality due to CHD were evident. SBP was a stronger predictor than DBP; however, the greater risk was attributed to the highest SBP ($\geq$160 mmHg) and the lowest DBP (<70 mmHg) highlighting the pulse pressure as a powerful actor in this coronary artery disease related death risk (Neaton and Wentworth 1992). The definition of HTN based on DBP in the 1960s was therefore not justified. However all current guidelines define HTN without focusing on the non linearity of the risk attributed to DBP with a fixed SBP level.

In Joint National Committee 7 guidelines (Chobanian et al. 2003) and ESH 2007 guidelines (ESH-ESC Task Force on the Management of Arterial Hypertension 2007) was introduced the terms of Pre-Hypertension (BP 120–139/ 80–89 mmHg) and High-normal BP (BP 130–139/85–90 mmHg) respectively. In fact, a stepwise increase in cardiovascular event rates was noted in persons with higher baseline blood-pressure categories.

The Framingham Heart Study investigated 6859 subjects, 35–64 years of age, free from cardiovascular disease and HTN (Vasan et al. 2001). As compared with optimal BP (<120/80 mmHg), high-normal BP (130–139/ 85–89 mmHg) was associated with a risk-factor–adjusted hazard ratio for cardiovascular disease of 2.5 (95 % CI, 1.6–4.1) in women and 1.6 (95 % CI, 1.1–2.2) in men. However, the 10-year cumulative incidence of cardiovascular disease was lower in younger individuals; 4 %

for women and 8 % for men; than in older subjects (those from 65 to 90 years old), the incidence was 18 % for women and 25 % for men.

These data should make HTN definition change to 130/85 mmHg or even lower, however; there is a need for data showing that reduction of BP from 130 to less than 120 mmHg for SBP will induce a reduction of cardiovascular events. Also, the definition of HTN takes in account the economic challenge of BP reduction from 140/90 to 130/85 mmHg; even if controlling BP with medication is unquestionably one of the most cost-effective methods of reducing premature cardiovascular morbidity and mortality (Elliott 2003). This evidence has many limits since BP reduction by treatment should reduce the risk of development of renal, cerebral and cardiovascular diseases to validate starting treatment at the level of which risk is increased.

3 Impact of Blood Pressure Control

An increasing number of trials have provided evidence that antihypertensive therapy to attain BP control provides a relative cardiovascular protection. The best evidence was shown by trials reporting BP reduction with antihypertensive treatment compared to placebo or no antihypertensive treatment. The last on date was HYVET trial including 3845 patients aged 80 or older who were randomized to active treatments or placebo without antihypertensive medications (Beckett et al. 2008).

According to the intention-to-treat analysis and as compared to the baseline value 173.0/90.8 mmHg, SBP/DBP values obtained while the patient was seated had fallen by a mean of 14.5 $\pm$ 18.5/6.8 $\pm$ 10.5 mmHg in the placebo group and by 29.5 $\pm$ 15.4/12.9 $\pm$ 9.5 mmHg in the active-treatment group at 2 years. This reduction of SBP/DBP by active treatment was associated with a 30 % reduction in the rate of fatal or nonfatal stroke (p: 0.06), a 39 % reduction in the rate of death from stroke (p: 0.05), a 21 % reduction in the rate of death from any cause (p: 0.02), a 23 % reduction in the rate of death from cardiovascular causes (p: 0.06), and a 64 % reduction in the rate of heart failure (p < 0.001).

A meta-analysis including 11 randomized controlled trials and 67,475 individuals compared antihypertensive therapy with placebo and aimed to investigate whether the benefits of BP-lowering drugs are proportional to baseline cardiovascular risk. Patients were risk stratified according to their estimated 5-year risk of having a major cardiovascular event. Lowering BP provides similar relative protection at all levels of baseline cardiovascular risk, but progressively greater absolute risk reductions were obtained when baseline risk increases, yielding to a possible benefit for more intense BP reduction in high risk patients (Blood Pressure Lowering Treatment Trialists' Collaboration 2014).

More recently, Thomopoulos et al. (2014) reported a meta-analysis on the effects at different baseline and achieved blood pressure levels on cardiovascular disease. Results of this meta-analysis favor BP-lowering treatment even in grade 1 hypertension at low-to-moderate risk, and lowering SBP/DBP to less than 140/90 mmHg. Achieving less than 130/80 mmHg appears safe, but only adds further significant reduction in stroke and all-cause death. Is it important to achieve earlier BP target on the occurrence of cardiovascular outcomes?. A response strand was generated by the VALUE Trial. This study (Julius et al. 2004) compared the effect on cardiovascular morbidity and mortality of a calcium channel blocker based strategy versus an angiotensin II receptor blocker based strategy in a high cardiovascular risk population. An unexpected equivalence between the two strategies was reported. The result was explained, in part, by a significantly better earlier BP control achieved in the amlodipine group. In fact, after the first month of treatment, SBP is on average 4 mmHg lower, DBP by 2.1 mmHg lower (p <0.0001). A respective difference of 2 and 1.6 mmHg persists after the sixth month until the end of the study (p <0.001).

It is so clearly proved that control of BP results in saving lives and reducing cardiovascular death and events. The debate becomes down to which level BP should be dropped?

4 Is the Lower the Better? – The Dogma of J Curve

Observational studies show a direct linear relationship between SBP/DBP values as low as 115–110 and 75–70 mmH respectively, and cardiovascular events, without evidence within this range of a J curve phenomenon. The Prospective Studies Collaboration (Lewington et al. 2002) performed a meta-analysis including one million adults from 61 prospective trials. Authors reported that within each decade of age at death, the proportional difference in the risk of vascular death associated with a given absolute difference in usual BP is about the same down to at least 115 mmHg usual SBP and 75 mmHg usual DBP, below which there is little evidence.

At ages 40–69 years, each difference of 20 mm Hg usual SBP is associated with more than a twofold difference in the stroke death rate, and with twofold differences in the death rates from ischemic heart disease and from other vascular causes.

So, evidence that achieving lower BP targets by treatment may enhance protection in hypertensive patients at higher risk, yielded ESH/ESC task force (for the management of arterial hypertension- 2007guidelines) to suggest that target BP should be at least <130/80 mmHg in diabetics and in high or very high risk patients, such as those with associated clinical conditions (stroke, myocardial infarction, renal dysfunction, proteinuria) (ESH-ESC Task Force on the Management of Arterial Hypertension 2007).

The evidence available on the BP targets of antihypertensive treatment has been reviewed by Zanchetti et al. (2009). In uncomplicated hypertensive patients, SBP reduced to less than 140 mmHg with active treatment was associated with a difference in outcome. This evidence supports the recommendation of guidelines to reduce SBP to less than 140 mmHg in the general population of patients with grade 1 or 2 hypertension and low or moderate total cardiovascular risk. However, for the elderly hypertensive patients, these authors reported no trial evidence in support of the guidelines recommendation to adopt the less than 140 mmHg SBP target in this population suggesting a target SBP of less than 150 mmHg.

When considering diabetic patients, lower BP goal less than 130/80 mmHg is also not supported by incontrovertible trial evidence. Even if HOT (Hansson et al. 1998) and Syst-Eur (Tuomilehto et al. 1999) trials, reported a greater absolute reduction of cardiovascular outcomes for a small BP difference in diabetic but not in nondiabetic hypertensive patients, these data were not confirmed by ACCORD trial (ACCORD Study Group 2010). This landmark trial in diabetic population tested a strict BP control (SBP less than 120 mmHg) compared to a standard target (SBP less than 140 mmHg) on the primary composite outcome (nonfatal myocardial infarction, nonfatal stroke, or death from cardiovascular causes). The only benefit reported was significant fewer strokes, but counterbalanced by a significant high level of serious adverse events as hypotension and fall of eGFR to less than 30 ml/mn/1.73 m^2.

STENO-2 trial showed a significant reduction of microvascular complications 8 years and all cardiovascular events 13 years after study start with an intense treatment strategy including a BP < 130/80 mmHg versus less strict strategy with a standard BP goal of 130–139 mmHg in type 2 diabetic patients with microalbuminuria (Gaede et al. 2003, 2008). However, the positive results attributed to the intense strategy cannot be directly attributed to a strict BP target, since the two groups were not comparable elsewhere. This study however, highlights the importance of a combined optimal strategy to reduce cardiovascular and microvascular events in type 2 diabetes.

Out of cardiovascular prevention, there are solid data regarding the benefits of a SBP target less than 130 mmHg when considering diabetic patients with proteinuria aiming to reduce renal events (end stage renal disease). The meta analysis of Bakris et al. (2000) considering type 2 diabetic patients with proteinuria reported less estimated glomerular filtration rate loss (eGFR) when BP is under 130/85 than at 140/90 mmHg. In type 2 diabetic patients without proteinuria, however, no evidence was reported by ACCORD trial (ACCORD study Group 2010).

The Kidney Disease Improving Global Outcome KDIGO clinical practice guideline for the management of BP in chronic kidney disease outlined the strict target of BP < 130/80 mmHg only in patients with abnormal albumin excretion rate, meaning those with microalbuminuria or A2 category as defined by urine albumin-creatinine ratio more than 30 mg/g or A3 category (severely increased) as defined by urine albumin-creatinine ratio above 300 mg/g or Protein-creatinine ratio above 500 mg/g, with or without diabetes (Kidney Disease: Improving GlobalOutcomes (KDIGO) Blood Pressure Work Group 2012). However, since microalbuminuria is also a marker of vascular damage, defining target BP based on the presence of microalbuminuria should consider the presence of subclinical coronary heart disease (Jarraya et al. 2013).

In diabetic patients with coronary heart disease, as for those without diabetes, no evidence have been reported for a better cardiovascular outcome with a tight control of BP (<130 mmHg) versus usual control (130–139 mmHg). However, patients with uncontrolled HTN develop more cardiovascular events. In the 6400 type 2 diabetes patients with coronary artery disease of the INVEST trial, patients who achieved SBP of 130–140 mmHg had better outcome than those with value >140 mmHg. However, there is no additional benefit observed in the group achieving target SBP <130 mmHg (Cooper-DeHoff et al. 2010).

Moreover, this INVEST trial reported evidence of J curve, not for stroke, but for coronary events with a nadir DBP of 70 mmHg, compromising coronary blood flow at diastolic phase, in patients with already narrowing coronary arteries by atheroma reducing blood flow (Messerli et al. 2006).

The irbesartan Diabetic Nephropathy Trial (IDNT) included diabetic patients with proteinuric diabetic nephroipathy. The primary end point included doubling of serum creatinine, development of end stage renal disease or death. It was significantly reduced by an ARB, irbesartan than a calcium channel blocker, amlodipine, although BP was similarly reduced (Lewis et al. 2001). Investigating independent and additive impact of BP control on renal outcomes in the IDNT trial, Pohl et al reported a linear relationship between SBP and development of renal endpoint (end stage renal disease or doubling of serum creatinine), without a nadir down to less than 121 mmHg. However, for the same patients, reduction of SBP was associated with an increase in the relative risk of death when SBP <121 mmHg, showing a J curve (Pohl et al. 2005).

In general, the benefits of increasingly intensive therapy must be weighed against the potentially increased incidence of serious side effects associated with such a regimen, as the acute reduction of eGFR reported in ACCORD trial with a significantly more hypotension in the intensive BP lowering arm. (ACCORD Study Group et al. 2010).

As far as goals of treatment are concerned, the 2009 ESH guidelines update document recommends that SBP pressure should be lowered below 140 mmHg (and DBP below 90 mmHg) in all hypertensive patients, irrespective of their grade of risk (Mancia et al. 2009). On the basis of the results of clinical studies, it is advisable to lower BP to values within the range 130–139 mmHg for systolic and 80–85 mmHg for diastolic as recommended by the French Society of Hypertention (SFHTA) in their 2013 guidelines on hypertension (Blacher et al. 2013). Thus, it appears by this reappraisal, that the concept of lower BP goals, to be pursued in diabetics or very high risk patients, is no longer recommended because there is no evidence from trials of a greater benefit, nor can the procedure be regarded as easily achievable in current clinical practice.

The update document of guideline underlines the so-called "J-curve phenomenon" related to an increase rather than a reduction in the incidence of coronary events when BP values are below

120–125 for systolic and 70–75 for diastolic. It suggests not to lower blood pressure values too much, particularly in patients with a history of a previous coronary event. This recommendation was confirmed and adopted in the 2013 ESH/ESC guidelines (Task Force for the Management of Arterial Hypertension of the European Society of Hypertension and the European Society of Cardiology 2013).

5 SPRINT Guided Goal of BP on Treatment: The Lower the Better Finally Approved?

After the failing of ACCORD (ACCORD Study Group 2010) to validate low BP target for diabetic patients, the Systolic Blood Pressure Intervention Trial (SPRINT) aimed to challenge the SBP target less than 120 mmHg versus usual SBP target less than 140 mmHg in patients with a high cardiovascular risk (SPRINT Research Group et al. 2015). This study excludes diabetic patients already tested in ACCORD trial, patients with polycystic kidney disease investigated in the HALT Progression of Polycystic Kidney Disease Study (Schrier et al. 2014), patients with excessive proteinuria >1 g/24 h already investigated in MDRD trial and REIN trial (Peterson et al. 1995; Ruggenenti et al. 2005) and patients who already developed a stroke investigated in the Secondary Prevention of Small Sub-cortical Strokes 5PS3 trial (The SPS3 Study Group 2013) and also tested in the ESH-CHL-SHOT trial (Zanchetti et al. 2016).

SPRINT (SPRINT Research Group et al. 2015) is the largest study that tested how maintaining SBP at a lower level than currently recommended will impact mortality, cardiovascular and kidney diseases. It enrolled 9361 participants aged 50 years and older in about 100 medical centers and clinical practices throughout the USA and Puerto Rico from 2009 to 2013.

The study population included 2636 elderly aged of 75 years and above, 2646 patients with chronic kidney disease as defined by an eGFR rate $<$ 60 ml/min/1.73 m^2 and 1877 patients with pre-existing subclinical or clinical cardiovascular disease or a Framingham 10-year cardiovascular disease risk score of 15 % or above. This study included also about 35 % female 29.9 % black and 10.5 % Hispanic.

The study participants were randomly allocated into two groups. The standard treatment group received an average of 1.8 BP medications to achieve a target of less than 140 mmHg; the intensive treatment group received an average of 2.8 BP medications to achieve a target of less than 120 mmHg.

SPRINT results were awaited for 2018, but the significant preliminary results were announced on September 11, 2015 (National Heart, Lung, and Blood Institute 2015). The intensive intervention, that achieves a target SBP of 120 mmHg, reduced the rate of the composite primary outcome, which included myocardial infarction, other acute coronary syndromes, stroke, heart failure or death from cardiovascular causes by 25 %, and the risk of death from all causes by 27 %, compared to the target SBP of less than 140 mmHg.

Results were largely mediated and commented by medical journals (Kjeldsen et al. 2016a; Taler 2016; Cohen and Townsend 2016; Nilsson 2016) but also media such as *New York Times* (2015) that headed "lower blood pressure guidelines could be lifesaving".

These results were supported by the conclusions of two meta-analyses. The first pooled data from SPRINT and ACCORD trials and showed that the primary endpoint still in favor of BP reduction <120/80 mmHg (Perkovic and Rodgers 2015). The meta-analysis by Xie et al. (2016) included randomized controlled trials with at least 6 months' follow-up that randomly assigned participants to more intensive versus less intensive BP-lowering treatment, with different BP targets or different BP changes from baseline. It showed that after randomization, patients in the more intensive BP-lowering treatment group had mean BP levels of 133/76 mm Hg, compared with 140/81 mm Hg in the less intensive treatment group. Intensive BP lowering treatment achieved relative risk reductions for major cardiovascular events (14 % [95 % CI 4–22]), myocardial infarction (13 % [0–24]), stroke (22 % [10–32]), albuminuria (10 % [3–16]), and retinopathy progression (19 % [0–34]), but without effects on heart failure (15 % [−11 to 34]), cardiovascular death (9 % [−11 to 26]), total mortality (9 % [−3 to 19]), or end-stage kidney disease (10 % [−6 to 23]). Severe hypotension was more frequent in the more intensive treatment regimen (RR 2.68 [1.21–5.89], p = 0.015), but the absolute excess was small (0.3 % *vs* 0.1 % per person-year for the duration of follow-up).

Furthermore, recent analyses of BP targets in two large outcome trials, VALUE (Kjeldsen et al. 2016b) and ONTARGET (Verdecchia et al. 2015), have refuted the concept of increase of cardiovascular events when BP is lower than we usually accept during treatment of HTN. However, the major benefit is achieved with BP control less than 140/90 mmHg, while there is only some limited additional stroke protection with consistent BP control less than 130/80 mmHg (Mancia et al. 2016).

The SPRINT trial failed to show significant reduction in stroke, acute coronary syndrome or myocardial infarction that composed the primary outcome, unlike heart failure which was significantly reduced by 43 % (p 0.002). Less heart failure in the intensive arm was driving the difference in mortality favoring the intensive arm in SPRINT. Patients included in intensive arm were up-titrated in BP medication and received one more antihypertensive drug frequently a diuretic. A thiazide-type diuretic was prescribed for 54.9 versus 33.3 % and aldosterone antagonists for 8.7 versus 4 % patients, respectively in the intense and the usual arm. The greater use of diuretics may have demasked latent heart failure in hypertensive patients with rather high cardiovascular risk (Thoma et al. 2016).

The earlier stop of SPRINT trial than originally planned by the director of the National Heart, Lung and Blood Institute (NHLBI) based on the recommendation of the Data Safety Monitoring Board, makes interpretation of secondary outcomes results difficult since underpowered for that.

However, the way of BP measurement should be considered when interpreting SPRINT results. In fact, BPs in SPRINT were measured with patients seated in a quiet room without talking and taken as an average of three measurements with an automated device that was preset to wait 5 min before measurements without the observer being present. This technique called automated office BP measurement is known to reduce the "white coat" effect. It correlates tightly with the average daytime BP measured by ambulatory blood pressure monitoring, and up to 20 mmHg lower than conventional auscultatory SBP measured at the office (Myers et al. 2012).

Positive results reported by SPRINT should also be balanced by the harmful of this strategy. The number needed to harm in the trial is important, 100 for hypotension, 167 for syncope, 125 for electrolyte abnormalities and 62 for acute kidney injury (respectively +1 %, +0.6, +0.8 % and +1.6 absolute risk increase). Just a reminder of the number needed to treat to reach the primary outcome is 61 and the absolute risk reduction is −1.6 % (Thoma et al. 2016).

SPRINT included patients with SBP starting from 130 mmHg. That seems to validate crucial definition of high BP since the normal high BP or pre-hypertension are terms introduced in guidelines but does not already justify starting antihypertensive treatment. As reported at the baseline characteristics of the study participants, only 9.2 and 9.6 % respectively from intensive and standard treatment groups were not using antihypertensive agents. That means others patients are currently using antihypertensive treatments and their BP are controlled at 130 mmHg and above. So we can't validate to start treating patients at high risk from the latter cut off. In the same rationale, the Heart Outcomes Prevention Evaluation (HOPE)-3 Trial randomly assigned 12,705 participants at intermediate risk who did not have cardiovascular disease to receive either candesartan at a dose of 16 mg per day plus hydrochlorothiazide at a dose of 12.5 mg per day or placebo (Lonn et al. 2016). The mean BP of the participants at baseline was 138.1/81.9 mmHg; the decrease in BP was 6.0/3.0 mmHg greater in the active-treatment group than in the placebo group. This study doesn't report any benefice on composite primary (death from cardiovascular causes, nonfatal myocardial infarction, or nonfatal stroke) nor secondary outcomes (resuscitated cardiac arrest, heart failure, and revascularization) after a median follow-up of 5.6 years. However, with the sub-group analysis, patients with upper third of SBP > 143.5 mmHg who were in the active-treatment group had significantly lower rates of the first and second primary outcomes than those in the placebo group. The pre-hypertension should not be treated, even if the cardiovascular risk is higher than at normal BP.

6   In Summary, Which BP Goal for Which Patient?

BP should be diagnosed early and treatment should be started at BP level of 140 mmHg and above, based on an office BP measurement, confirmed by an out-of-office BP measurement. Target SBP should be less than 140 mmHg if BP is measured by classic auscultatory method, less than 120 mmHg in high risk patients if BP is measured by automated office BP measurement. These targets are relevant in elderly patients if no orthostatic hypotension occurred, patients with non proteinuric chronic kidney disease (eGFR < 60 ml/mn/1.73 m^2) and patients with cardiovascular disease or a Framingham score more than 15 %. However attention should be taken on DBP if lower than 70 mmHg because of an increasing risk of ischemic heart event and on renal function since acute renal failure is more frequently reported at these low targets.

In diabetic patients, SBP target should be less than 140 mmHg according to ACCORD trial. However, for patients with albumin-creatinine ratio > 300mg/g or Protein-creatinine ratio > 500mg/g, with or without diabetes, lower SBP target should be proposed for renal protection aiming SBP < 130 mmHg as recommended by KDIGO guidelines.

In patients at low or intermediate risk, without cardiovascular disease, SBP should start to be treated when SBP is above 140 mmHg, and when treated, target BP should be less than 140 mmHg as reported by HOPE-3 trial.

Finally, superiority of ambulatory over office BP measurement in predicting mortality and cardiovascular events should be promoted when treating hypertension (Dolan et al. 2005; Sega et al. 2005). Validated target BP are SBP less than 135 mmHg for home BP measurement and 130, 135 and 120 mmHg for respectively 24 h, daytime and nighttime period (Task Force for the Management of Arterial Hypertension of the European Society of Hypertension and the European Society of Cardiology 2013).

References

[no authors listed] (1967) Effects of treatment on morbidity in hypertension. Results in patients with diastolic blood pressure averaging 115 through 129mmhg. JAMA 202:1028–1034

[no authors listed] (1970) Effects of treatment on morbidity in hypertension. II. Results in patients with diastolic blood pressure averaging 90 through 114mmhg. JAMA 213:1143–1052

ACCORD Study Group, Cushman WC, Evans GW, Byington RP et al (2010) Effects of intensive blood-pressure control in type 2 diabetes mellitus. N Engl J Med 362:1575–1585

Bakris GL, Williams M, Dworkin L et al (2000) Preserving renal function in adults with hypertension and diabetes: a consensus approach. National Kidney Foundation Hypertension and Diabetes Executive Committees Working Group. Am J Kidney Dis 36:646–661

Beckett NS, Peters R, Fletcher AE, et al. for the HYVET Study Group (2008) Treatment of hypertension in patients 80 years of age or older. N Engl J Med 358:1887–1898

Blacher J, Halimi JM, Hanon O et al (2013) Prise en charge de l'hypertension artérielle de l'adulte. Recommandations 2013 de la Société française d'hypertension artérielle. Presse Med 42:819–825

Blood Pressure Lowering Treatment Trialists' Collaboration (2014) Blood pressure-lowering treatment based on cardiovascular risk: a meta-analysis of individual patient data. Lancet 384:591–598

Chobanian AV, Bakris GL, Black HR, National Heart, Lung, and Blood Institute Joint National Committee on Prevention, Detection, Evaluation, and Treatment of High Blood Pressure, National High Blood Pressure Education Program Coordinating Committee et al (2003) The seventh report of the Joint National Committee on Prevention, Detection, Evaluation, and Treatment of High Blood Pressure: the JNC 7 report. JAMA 289:2560–2572

Cohen DL, Townsend RR (2016) Which patients does the SPRINT study not apply to and what are the appropriate blood pressure goals in these populations? J Clin Hypertens (Greenwich) 18:477–478

Cooper-DeHoff RM, Gong Y, Handberg EM et al (2010) Tight blood pressure control and cardiovascular outcomes among hypertensive patients with diabetes and coronary artery disease. JAMA 304:61–68

Dolan E, Stanton A, Thijs L et al (2005) Superiority of ambulatory over clinic blood pressure measurement in predicting mortality: the Dublin outcome study. Hypertension 46:156–161

Elliott WJ (2003) The economic impact of hypertension. J Clin Hypertens (Greenwich) 5(3 Suppl 2):3–13

ESH-ESC Task Force on the Management of Arterial Hypertension (2007) Guidelines 2007 ESH-ESC practice guidelines for the management of arterial hypertension. J Hypertens 25:1751–1762

Gaede P, Vedel P, Larsen N et al (2003) Multifactorial intervention and cardiovascular disease in patients with type 2 diabetes. N Engl J Med 348:383–393

Gaede P, Lund-Andersen H, Parving HH et al (2008) Effect of a multifactorial intervention on mortality in type 2 diabetes. N Engl J Med 358:580–591

GBD 2013 Risk Factors Collaborators (2015) Global, regional, and national comparative risk assessment of 79 behavioural, environmental and occupational, and metabolic risks or clusters of risks in 188 countries, 1990–2013: a systematic analysis for the Global Burden of Disease Study 2013. Lancet 386:2287–2323

Hajem S, Hsairi M (2013) Le système national d'information sur les causes de décès: Diagnostic de situation et principaux résultats. National Institute of Public Health, Ministry of Heath, Tunisia

Hansson L, Zanchetti A, Carruthers SG et al (1998) Effects of intensive bloodpressure lowering and low-dose aspirin in patients with hypertension: principal results of the Hypertension Optimal Treatment (HOT) randomised trial. HOT Study Group. Lancet 351:1755–1762

Jarraya F, Lakhdar R, Kammoun K et al (2013) Microalbuminuria: a useful marker of cardiovascular disease. Iran J Kidney Dis 7:178–86

Julius S, Kjeldsen SE, Weber M et al (2004) Outcomes in hypertensive patients at high cardiovascular risk treated with regimens based on valsartan or amlodipine: the VALUE randomized trial. Lancet 363:2022–2031

Kannel WB, Dawber TR, Kagan A et al (1961) Factors of risk in the development of coronary heart disease–six year follow-up experience. The Framingham Study. Ann Intern Med 55:33–50

Kidney Disease: Improving Global Outcomes (KDIGO) Blood Pressure Work Group (2012) KDIGO clinical practice guideline for the management of blood pressure in chronic kidney disease. Kidney Int (Suppl.) 2:337–414

Kjeldsen SE, Narkiewicz K, Hedner T et al (2016a) The SPRINT study: outcome may be driven by difference in diuretic treatment demasking heart failure and study design may support systolic blood pressure target below 140 mmHg rather than below 120 mmHg. Blood Press 25:63–66

Kjeldsen SE, Berge E, Bangalore S et al (2016b) No evidence for J-shaped curve in treated hypertensive patients with increased cardiovascular risk: the VALUE trial. Blood Press 25:83–92

Lewington S, Clarke R, Qizilbash N, Prospective Studies Collaboration et al (2002) Age-specific relevance of usual blood pressure to vascular mortality: a meta-analysis of individual data for one million adults in 61 prospective studies. Lancet 360:1903–1913

Lewis O (1994) Stephen Hales and the measurement of blood pressure. J Hum Hypertens 8:865–871

Lewis EJ, Hunsicker LG, Clarke WR et al (2001) Renoprotective effect of the angiotensin-receptor antagonist irbesartan in patient with nephropathy due to type 2 diabetes. N Engl J Med 345:851–860

Lonn EM, Bosch J, Lopez-Jaramillo P, et al. for the HOPE-3 Investigators (2016) Blood-pressure lowering in intermediate-risk persons without cardiovascular disease. N Engl J Med. doi:10.1056/NEJMoa1600175. [Epub ahead of print]

Mancia G, Laurent S, Agabiti-Rosei E et al (2009) Reappraisal of European guidelines on hypertension management: a European Society of Hypertension Task Force document. J Hypertens 27:2121–2158

Mancia G, Kjeldsen SE, Zappe DH et al (2016) Cardiovascular outcomes at different on-treatment blood pressures in the hypertensive patients of the VALUE trial. Eur Heart J 37:955–964

Messerli F, Mancia G, Conti R et al (2006) Dogma disputed: can aggressively lowering blood pressure in hypertensive patients with coronary artery disease be dangerous? Ann Intern Med 144:884–893

Myers MG, Godwin M, Dawes M et al (2012) Conventional versus automated measurement of blood pressure in the office (CAMBO) trial. Fam Pract 29:376–382

National Heart, Lung, and Blood Institute (2015) Landmark NIH study shows intensive blood pressure management may save lives. Available from http://www.nhlbi.nih.gov/news/pressreleases/2015/landmark-nih-study-showsintensive-blood-pressure-management-may-save-lives.webpage. Accessed 11 Sept 2015

Neaton JD, Wentworth D (1992) Serum cholesterol, blood pressure, cigarette smoking, and death from coronary heart disease. Overall findings and differences by age for 316 099 white men. Multiple Risk Factor Intervention Trial Research Group. Arch Intern Med 152:56–64

New York Times (2015) Lower blood pressure guidelines could be "lifesaving", federal study says. Available from http://www.nytimes.com/2015/09/12/health/bloodpressure-study.html. Webpage accessed 8 Oct 2015

Nilsson PM (2016) Blood pressure strategies and goals in elderly patients with hypertension. Exp Gerontol.

doi:10.1016/j.exger.2016.04.018 [Epub ahead of print]

Perkovic V, Rodgers A (2015) Redefining blood-pressure targets — SPRINT starts the marathon. N Engl J Med 373:2175–2178

Peterson JC, Adler S, Burkart JM et al (1995) Blood pressure control, proteinuria and the progression of renal disease. Ann Intern Med 123:754–762

Pohl MA, Blumenthal S, Cordonnier DJ, et al. for the Collaborative Study Group (2005) Independent and additive impact of blood pressure control and angiotensin II receptor blockade on renal outcomes in the Irbesartan diabetic nephropathy trial: clinical implications and limitations. J Am Soc Nephrol 16:3027–3037

Rose G (1980) Epidemiology. In: Marshall AJ, Barrett DW (eds) The hypertensive patient. Pitman Medical, Kent, pp 1–21

Ruggenenti P, Perna A, Loriga G et al (2005) Blood-pressure control for renoprotection in patients with non-diabetic chronic renal disease (REIN-2): multicentre randomized controlled trial. Lancet 365:939–946

Schrier RW, Abebe KZ, Perron RD, et al. for the HALT-PKD Trial Investigators (2014) Blood pressure in early autosomal dominant polycystic kidney disease. N Engl J Med 371:2255–2266

Sega R, Facchetti R, Bombelli M et al (2005) Prognostic value of ambulatory and home blood pressures compared with office blood pressure in the general population: follow-up results from the Pressioni Arteriose Monitorate e Loro Associazioni (PAMELA) study. Circulation 111:1777–1783

SPRINT Research Group, Wright JT Jr, Williamson JD, Whelton PK et al (2015) A randomized trial of intensive versus standard blood-pressure control. N Engl J Med 373:2103–2116

Taler SJ (2016) How does SPRINT (Systolic Blood Pressure Intervention Trial) direct hypertension treatment targets for CKD? Am J Kidney Dis. doi:10.1053/j.ajkd.2016.02.045. [Epub ahead of print]

Task Force for the Management of Arterial Hypertension of the European Society of Hypertension and the European Society of Cardiology (2013) **2013 ESH/ESC practice Guidelines** for the management of arterial hypertension. J Hypertens 31:1281–1357

The SPS3 Study Group (2013) Effects of blood pressure targets in patients with recent lacunar strokes. Lancet 382:507–515

Thoma G, Nally JV, Pohl MA (2016) Interpreting SPRINT: how low should you go? Cleve Clin J Med 83:187–195

Thomopoulosa C, Parati G, Zanchetti A (2014) Effects of blood pressure lowering on outcome incidence in hypertension: 2. Effects at different baseline and achieved blood pressure levels – overview and meta-analyses of randomized trials. J Hypertens 32:2296–2304

Tuomilehto J, Rastenyte D, Birkenhager WH et al (1999) Effects of calcium-channel blockade in older patients with diabetes and systolic hypertension. Systolic hypertension in Europe Trial Investigators. N Engl J Med 340:677–684

Vasan RS, Larson MG, Leip EP et al (2001) Impact of high-normal blood pressure on the risk of cardiovascular disease. N Engl J Med 345:1291–1297

Verdecchia P, Reboldi G, Angeli F et al (2015) Systolic and diastolic blood pressure changes in relation with myocardial infarction and stroke in patients with coronary heart disease. Hypertension 65:108–114

Xie X, Atkins E, Lv J et al (2016) Effects of intensive blood pressure lowering on cardiovascular and renal outcomes: updated systematic review and meta-analysis. Lancet 387:435–443

Zanchetti A, Grassi G, Mancia G (2009) When should antihypertensive drug treatment be initiated and to what levels should systolic blood pressure be lowered? A critical reappraisal. J Hypertens 27:923–934

Zanchetti A, Liu L, Mancia G, ESH-CHL-SHOT trialinvestigators et al (2016) Continuation of the ESH-CHL-SHOT trial after publication of the SPRINT: rationale for further study on blood pressure targets of antihypertensive treatment after stroke. J Hypertens 34:393–6

Adv Exp Med Biol - Advances in Internal Medicine (2017) 2: 129–147
DOI 10.1007/5584_2016_77
© Springer International Publishing AG 2016
Published online: 19 October 2016

Adherence to Treatment in Hypertension

Carlos Menéndez Villalva, Xosé Luís López Alvarez-Muiño,
Trinidad Gamarra Mondelo, Alfonso Alonso Fachado,
and Joaquín Cubiella Fernández

Abstract

The lack of adherence to treatment in hypertension affects approximately 30 % of patients. The elderly, those with several co-morbidities, social isolation, low incomes or depressive symptoms are the most vulnerable to this problem. There is no ideal method to quantify the adherence to the treatment. Indirect methods are recommended in clinical practice. Any intervention strategy should not blame the patient and try a collaborative approach. It is recommended to involve the patient in decision-making. The clinical interview style must be patient-centered including motivational techniques. The improvement strategies that showed greater effectiveness in the compliance of hypertension treatment were: treatment simplification, appointment reminders systems, blood pressure self-monitoring, organizational improvements and nurse and pharmacists care. The combination of different interventions are recommended against isolated interventions.

Keywords

Hypertension • Patient compliance • Medication adherence

C.M. Villalva (✉) and X.L.L. Alvarez-Muiño
Mariñamansa-A Cuña Health Center, Galician Health Service, Centro de Saúde Marinamansa – A Cuña, Dr. Peña Rey 2b, SERGAS (Servicio Galego de Saúde), CP 32005 Ourense, Spain
e-mail: carlos.menendez.villalva@sergas.es; joseluis.lopez.alvarez@sergas.es

T.G. Mondelo
Pontedeva Health Center, Galician Health Service, Ourense, Spain
e-mail: maria.trinidad.gamarra.Mondelo@sergas.es

A.A. Fachado
Carballo Health Center, Galician Health Service, Corunna, Spain
e-mail: alfonso.alonso.fachado@sergas.es

J.C. Fernández
University Hospital Center of Ourense, Ourense, Spain
e-mail: joaquin.cubiella.fernandez@sergas.es

1 Introduction

High blood pressure (hypertension) is a chronic disease. Several measures, such as habits of life, diet and medication, are required for its control. It is widely known that the greater efficacy of nowadays available treatments does not correspond with an increase in the number of controlled patients. So, it is important to measure compliance and study which factors might influence it. Approximately 50 % of patients with a hypertension prescription will stop it during the first year and only 50–66 % of the remaining patients will keep with the treatment prescribed. As a result, only 25–34 % of patients with hypertension will have a good control of their blood pressure (BP) figures (Morris et al. 2006). The lack of adherence to treatment is a common phenomenon, especially in chronic conditions. According to data from the World Health Organization (WHO), adherence to long-term treatment of chronic diseases in developed countries is around 50 %, with rates even lower in developing countries. Therefore, non-compliance of the chronic treatments and their clinical and economic consequences is considered a priority public health issue (WHO 2004).

There is no personality profile associated with the low-adherent patient to medical treatments. On the other hand, non-adherence is difficult to predict and the point of view expressed by the health-professionals does not correlate with the actual compliance. In fact, it is no more accurate than throwing a coin in the air (Medding et al. 2012). Patients with hypertension have characteristics that favors poor compliance (Table 1). It is often difficult to follow the health professional recommendations in chronic and asymptomatic problems. It is hard to become aware of the need of a long-term treatment. Hypertension diagnosis at the age of forty, can mean a loss of vigor and vitality for the patient. Sometimes it can cause a denial reaction and an economic and social burden that hinders acceptance of treatment (Kaplan et al. 2016). Curiously, the adherence of the prescription is unrelated to the implementation of lifestyle

Table 1 Major predictors of non-adherence to treatments

Dependent on the Patient
Chronic process
Asymptomatic disease
Lack of knowledge of the disease by the patient
Lack of confidence in the benefit of the treatment by the patient
Missing scheduled appointments
Presence of psychological problems
Cognitive impairment
Social isolation
Dependent on the Treatment
Complexity or long duration of treatment
Adverse effects of medication
Inadequate patient-physician relationship
Fragmented attention: lack of coordination
Absence of scheduled periodic appointments
Cost of medication

changes. So, the decision to quit smoking or doing exercise is not associated with greater adherence to the medication. Patients want to know why should they take medication, which benefits and side effects can be expected, the cost and what would happen if they do not follow the therapeutic guidelines. Health professionals, in general, communicate poorly with their patients and provide little information about medical prescriptions (Fuster 2012).

2 Consequences of Non-compliance

Several results from adherence studies are available. Thus in a study involving more than 18,000 patients followed during 4.6 years, good adherence to antihypertensive treatment involves a lesser degree of morbidity and mortality (HR 0.62 (0.40–0)) (Mazzaglia et al. 2009). Deficiency in compliance has an impact in most of cases in an increase in costs. These are generated due to an increase in hospitalizations and visits to the outpatient centers and emergency departments as well as changes in doses and prescriptions and more invasive diagnostic tests required (Hughes et al. 2001). Only in the United States, approximately 125,000 deaths per year and 33–69 % of the hospital admissions are related to the lack of adherence to treatment, with an estimated total cost of 100 billion dollars annually: 25 billion corresponded to admissions and 70 billion to loss of productivity and premature death (Osterberg and Blaschke 2005; Ho et al. 2006; Dezii 2000; McCarthy 1998; Berg et al. 1993).

Patients with cardiovascular disease that fail to comply with their treatment regimen, have an 80 % increase in the risk of death in the first 120 days after an acute myocardial infarction (Newby et al. 2006). Non adherence to medication increases the risk of death from stroke in patients with hypertension (OR 3.81 (2.35; 3.20)) (Mayor 2013). Another study has shown that patients with diabetes, hypertension, high cholesterol, and heart failure, had higher hospitalization rates if they were low adherent (13 % vs 30 % for diabetics; 19 % vs. 28 % in hypertension) (New England Healthcare 2009). On the other side, there is a study pointing out a possible overestimation of the effect of poor compliance on the final outcomes (LaFleur et al. 2011).

3 Concept of Compliance

We can define *compliance* as the degree to which the behavior of the patient, in terms of medication, a diet or lifestyle changes, meets up clinical prescription or medical advice. Since compliance implies somehow blaming the patient, other terms have been used. As an example, *adherence* is defined as the capacity and willingness to comply with a prescribed therapeutic regimen (Sackett and Haynes 1976; Inkster et al. 2006). It is important to distinguish, as Haynes highlights (Haynes et al. 2008) between adherence and concordance in treatments. **Adherence** is the degree in which a patient meets the prescription ordered by his doctor, but sometimes this can have a guilty connotation. The **concordance** would be the degree of agreement on the treatment achieved by the patient and the physician. Three prerequisites are required in order that the patient has a good

adhesion to treatment: it must be acceptable, understandable and personally manageable (James et al. 2016).

The Spanish Society of Hypertension Working Group on Compliance defines compliance as the extent that the patient assumes the rules or advices given by the physician or health professional, both from the point of view of lifestyle or the pharmacological treatment recommended. It shows the degree of overlap between the guidance given by the professional and the fulfillment by the patient after a fully reasoned decision (Márquez Contreras et al. 1998).

4 Types of Non-compliance

Non-compliance is a dynamic concept that may affect all phases of the clinical process from the first contact with the doctor until the end of the treatment. There is consensus in the literature that patients taking at least 80 % of the tablets are considered compliant.

On the basis of the Medication Event Monitoring System (MEMS) several patterns of non-compliance have been described (Márquez 2008; Márquez et al. 2012):

Compliers

- Absolute complier: person who takes quite the 100 % of medication
- Masked complier: person who takes more than 80 % of medication
- Sporadic failure: Non compliance with the treatment one to six times a month
- Over complier: person who takes more than 100 % of medication.

Non Complier

- Absolute breach: person who takes less than 50 % of medication.
- Partial non-compliance: individuals taking between 50 and 80 %.

- <u>Medication abandonment</u>: patients definitely stop taking their medication.

Others Patterns

- <u>Drug holidays</u>: individuals who do not take their medication for three days.
- <u>Predicted non-compliance</u>: repetitive non adherence at certain times.
- <u>White coat effect</u>: non compliers individuals that take their medications the days before an appointment.
- <u>Time table non-compliance</u>: do not take the medication at the scheduled hours medication hours.
- <u>Mixed non-compliers</u>: coexistence of two or more associated patterns.

With the advent of integrated electronic prescribing and dispensing data they can be classified in (Tamblyn et al. 2014; Fischer et al. 2010):

<u>Primary non adherence</u>: it was defined as failing to fill a new incident prescription.

<u>Persistence or secondary non adherence</u>: the patient stop taking medications soon after filling the first prescription

5 Factors Involved

The general factors involved in adherence of the treatments can be classified in (Rosenson et al. 2016):

- <u>Cognitive losses</u> cause forgetfulness of dose or loss of ability to understand the impact of treatments
- <u>Psychopathology</u>: the depression, anxiety or high levels of hostility may affect compliance
- <u>Functional illiteracy</u> affects to the compression of the treatments.
- The <u>interaction with the professionals</u> of health may improve compliance using non-technical words and involving the patients in the decisions.
- The <u>lost in the clinical follow-up</u> of patients with chronic diseases affects the adhesion and the final objectives of the treatment

The most frequent barriers are related to the characteristics **of the patient and disease** (simple forgetfulness, ignorance of the chronic disease condition, retirement (Kivimäki et al. 2013), poor social, health or family support and personal decision of the patient to give up treatment). Some are also dependent on the **characteristics of the treatment** (side effects, long-term therapies, difficult to understand or to take, inadequate communication, price) (Baroletti and Dell'Orfano 2010). Although age is not a risk factor per se, there are several studies that suggest that non-adherence, intentional or not, is a problem in aged patients. This is due, in part, to the lack of understanding of the schemes available and the forgetfulness, favored by the high proportion of elderly people who live alone, the impairment of cognitive function, the prevalence of co-morbidities and the polimedication (Horne et al. 2005; Wang et al. 2014)

An interesting systematic review with qualitative research methodology concludes that patients with hypertension link together stress and the presence of symptoms (Marshall et al. 2012). This perception justifies treatment abandonment when they perceive less stress or less symptoms. Sometimes they stop treatment if they are afraid of side effects or a possible addiction to treatment. No ethnic or countries differences were detected. A factor who influence in the adherence to treatment is the **patient-physician relationship.** It is important to know the beliefs and expectations of the patient, as well as the socio-familial support. It is the family in many cases that acts as a reminder of the treatment and can promote a change of conduct. The success of treatment depends on both: therapist and patient. For a solid grip, the doctor requires technics and tools in communication skills (Sanson-Fisher and Clover 1995).

6 Prevalence of Treatment Adherence

According to a systematic reviews, the prevalence of non-compliance with HTA treatment in the world is, at average, 30 % and probably this is one of the main causes of the lack of control of hypertension (Tamblyn et al. 2014; Cramer et al. 2008). The therapeutic compliance prevalence ranges between 40 and 90 % according to the method used to measure, the disease and the population studied. In this sense, Choo and collaborators (Choo et al. 1999) they assessed the validity of self-reported compliance, pharmacy records and counting tablets as measures of antihypertensive drugs compliance against the MEMS standard. Hansen (Hansen et al. 2009) and Horne (Horne et al. 2010) also compared different methods of measurement of compliance, with figures between 80 and 90 %. Other authors that also used MEMS system as control, found a compliance rate around 80 % (Zeller et al. 2007; Santschi et al. 2008). In a series that evaluated the compliance evolution in 3553 patients during 20 years, an increase in compliance was detected, although the final rate was 67.47 % (Márquez et al. 2006). This contrasts with a study performed in non-industrialized countries where the average compliance was 40 % even after using the same method (Qureshi et al. 2007). Besides, Schoenthaler found a compliance rate of 56 % in African Americans (Schoenthaler and Ogedegbe 2008).

The different studies available show conflicting results. It is difficult to obtain significant relations with the compliance variable, as long as this variables depends largely on individual factors that are difficult to assess. Some works highlight that the presence of other chronic diseases associated to high blood pressure adversely affect taking medication: multiple drugs are required for the control of the diseases. So, patients with high cardiovascular risk sometimes use 4 or more drugs to control several diseases that can cause undesired side effects and trigger low adhesion (Morris et al. 2006; Chapman et al. 2005; Gregorie et al. 2006; Sicras et al. 2006). DiMateo and collaborators published a meta-analysis of studies published over nearly six decades. They concluded that patients with severe disease and a poor state of health should be identified as of great risk of being non-compliant with treatment (DiMatteo et al. 2007).

To achieve the therapeutic objectives in hypertension, health professional must consider that each patient has priorities in health and that each person has an **"acceptable therapeutic load"**; i.e. the maximum number of medications that are considered reasonable to take every day. This number varies from person to person and the physician needs to know it in order to plan treatment (van Duijn et al. 2011). Some authors suggest that non adherence to treatment is induced by the health system. They propose a **"minimally disruptive medicine"** (May et al. 2009; Dabrh et al. 2015) with 4 principles: determine the load weight which is acceptable for each patient, enhance coordination in clinical practice with an holistic vision, increase the knowledge of the co-morbidity in clinical practice, and prioritize the patient autonomy and its perspective.

7 Methods to Measure Adherence

It is necessary to know the degree of adherence both to make decisions on the follow-up of the patient as to assess the outcome of clinical trials. There are several methods to measure compliance and are classified into direct and indirect (Márquez 2008; MacFadyen and Struthers 1997). In general, the former tend to be more sensitive and specific, but less acceptable to the more invasive.

Direct methods measure the amount of drug, metabolites, or markers found in some body fluids. Methods are more objective and specific but expensive and inaccessible in primary care. They are also inefficient for short half-life drugs. The use of liquid chromatography-mass spectrometry analysis for antihypertensive drugs in urine analysis can detect low compliance in patients with

Table 2 Indirect methods for evaluating compliance of hypertension

Method		Advantages	Disadvantages	Validation[a]			
				S	S	PPV	NPV
Based on the table count	Simple count of tablets	Objective, quantifiable	It takes time. It does not detect the drug intake. High price	Gold standard in research studies			
	Medication Event Monitoring System (MEMS)						
Based on the clinical interview	Haynes-Sackett test	Simple, quick. Useful in clinical practice	It overestimates the adhesion	0.33	0.93	0.73	0.69
	Test of Morysky			0.49	0.68	0.48	0.68
Other methods	Professional judgment	Simple, fast	Vague	0.28	0.78	0.44	0.64
	Assistance to appointments	Simple	It also depends on the health care organization	0.71	0.83	0.43	0.65
	Improvement of disease	Simple, easy to apply	Interference from other factors such as co-morbidities	0.53	0.62	0.46	0.68
	Knowledge of disease	Simple	Dependent on the level of culture of the patient	0.82	0.41	0.46	0.79

[a]From Márquez (2008)

S sensitivity, *S* specificity, *PPV* positive predictive value, *NPV* negative predictive value

refractory hypertension (Jung et al. 2013; Tomaszewski et al. 2014).

Indirect methods are simple and economic, useful in the clinic, but their disadvantage is that they are not objective and tend to overestimate the adherence to the treatment. They are based on the quantification of the number of tablets or on clinical interviews. These are the most widely used (Table 2).

7.1 Clinical Interview-Based Methods Most Commonly Used Are

7.1.1 Haynes-Sackett or Self-Reported Compliance Test (Sackett et al. 1975)

It consists of two parts. The first part avoids a direct question, and in a friendly environment, the following sentence is inserted:

> "the majority of patients have difficulty taking their tablets, do you have difficulty in taking all your own?".

This approach eases the identification of poor adhesion. If the answer is Yes, the patient is non-compliant, and he will be questioned on the tablets taken in the last month. The authors considered complier a patient whose percentage of self-reported compliance is between 80 and 110 % (Stephenson et al. 1993).

7.1.2 Morinsky-Green Test (Morisky Medication Adherence Scale-4 Items, MMAS-4) (Morisky et al. 1986)

It is a questionnaire that can help the professional to identify the poor adherence to antihypertensive treatment. This method has been validated for several chronic diseases, although it was initially developed by Morinsky, Green and Levine to assess compliance with medication in patients with arterial hypertension. A patient is considered a good complier if answers correctly to 4 questions conducted, interspersed in a cordial way, during a conversation about her illness:

1. Do you ever forget to take the drugs for your illness?;
2. Do you take your medication at the indicated hours?;
3. Do you stop taking your medication when you feel well?

4. If you ever feel ill, do you quit your treatment?

There is a **version of the questionnaire with 8 items (MMAS-8)** (Morisky et al. 2008; Gallagher et al. 2015) It also includes questions on the reasons for non-adherence. It is useful to propose improvement strategies with the patient. The authors determinate low adhesion if the patient has less than 6 correct answers, average adhesion between 6 and 8 and high adhesion if 8 questions are correct.

1. Do you sometimes forget your high blood pressure pills?
2. Over the last two weeks, were there any days that you did not take your high blood pressure medicine?
3. Have you ever cut back or stopped taking your medication without telling your doctor because you felt worse when you took it?
4. Do you sometimes forget to bring along your medication when you travel or leave home?
5. Did you take your hight blood pressure medicine yesterday?
6. Do you sometimes stop taking your medicine when you feel your blood pressure is under control?
7. Taking medication everyday is a real inconvenience for some people. Do you ever feel hassled about sticking to your blood pressure treatment plan?
8. How often do you have difficulty remenbering to take all your blood pressure medication?

7.2 Methods Based on Tablet Quantification

7.2.1 Medication Event Monitoring System (MEMS)

They use the **Medication Event Monitoring System (MEMS).** These are monitoring systems based on a computerized registration. A microchip placed on the top of the container records the date and the time in which the container is opened. This method is often regarded as the gold standard to measure the adhesion. However, it only detects the opening, not the drug intake, it is not useful in routine clinical practice and it is expensive (Choo et al. 1999; Rosen et al. 2004).

7.2.2 Simple Tablets Count

It is a simple and objective method that compares the number of pills remaining in the container, taking into account the prescribed and the time elapsed between the prescription and the moment when they are measured. A patient is considered good compliant when has consumed 80–100 % of the prescribed tablets. This method tends to overestimate compliance when the patient assumes that it is controlled or if the drug is consumed by another member of the family (Bond and Hussar 1991).

7.3 Additional Compliance Estimations (Márquez et al. 2006)

- There are other practical measures, although less used as the *Batalla test*. This test analyze the degree of *knowledge that the patient has of his illness,* assuming that the greater patient awareness, the more compliant he will be.
- *The health professional judgement*: based on the opinion of the doctor or the nurse on the patient. The compliance is considered according to the health professional criteria.
- The *assistance to scheduled appointments:* if the patient does not attend the appointments, he is considered a bad compliant.
- *Method based on the improvement of the treated disease*: If hypertension is controlled that would indicate us that the patient is a good complier.
- *Method based on the medication collection*: It is based on the quantification of the medication withdrawn from the pharmacy. The computer records (e-prescribing) report if the patient goes to renew prescriptions on time.

Usually, patients tend to overestimate their adherence to medication, and unless a patient fails to respond to therapy, it is difficult detect a low compliance. If the patient affirms he is a good complier in the clinical interview and we are suspecting non-compliance, we will have to check medication collection in the chemist records and count the tablets used either in the clinic or at home. The count can be masked indicating the patient that we are simultaneously evaluation the expiration. This is the method of choice for general research, but if you want to know the pattern of non-compliance the count will be used through MEMS.

8 Improvement Strategies

8.1 Doctor-Patient Relationship and Treatment Compliance

The style of communication preferred to improve the performance of treatments is a patient-centered style. Thus, it is useful to ask how the patient understands his illness ("what do you known about hypertension?, Which organs can be affected? Do you think that you can control it?). In this way we explore their attitudes and expectations. Patients who understand the personal consequences of their risk factors can manage better the information. In a structured way and to advance in the knowledge of the beliefs of the patient on the arterial hypertension we can use questionnaires based on the Self-Regulatory Model (Ross et al. 2004).

Patients often express their fears to take several drugs or become dependent on them (eg: "When I have to take so many medications, I feel old" "When my labs are normal, I can quit treatment"). Therefore we should ask about the compliance in a non-punitive manner and in the context of the particular values of the patients (eg: "it's hard to take so many pills, How many times does it happen to you?"). Clinicians must have a long-term perspective and see failures as a learning tool.

The communication strategy to improve adherence should include: the use of non-technical language adapted to the cultural level of each person, personal experience in other drug use, discuss with the patient expectations of benefit and adverse effects, modify ideas and misconceptions, incorporate the preferences of the patient in the treatment plan, give written instructions in a clear and simple way, recommend pill boxes to organize the medication, involve family members, discuss the need to keep the medication despite feeling well. Try to improve the adhesion with a confrontational style with the patient is rarely useful (James et al. 2016).

8.1.1 Shared Decision Making (SDM)

Involving the patient in decision-making and a collaborative integration is beneficial in the management of chronic diseases. We have studies in hypertensive patients where shared decision-making strategy improves therapeutic adherence and control of hypertension. There are studies with SDM in several health care professionals such as physicians, pharmacists, nurses and dieticians. This strategy also showed benefit in poorly controlled hypertension patients with computer-based decision-making tools (van Duijn et al. 2011; Houle et al. 2014; Buhse et al. 2015; Tinsel et al. 2013; Buchholz et al. 2012; Abel and Barksdale 2012; Paasche-Orlow 2011; Roshanov et al. 2011).

8.1.2 Motivational Interview

The motivational interview technics based on the stages of change model of Prochaska and Di Clemente demonstrated some benefit in lifestyle and adherence to treatments (Miller and Rollnick 2013). There are three systematic reviews of clinical trials performed with this technique that presents a statistically significant improvement over conventional interventions with an estimated OR 1.55 (1.40; 1.71). The benefit is particularly promising in weight loss, alcohol and tobacco consumption, sedentary life style self-monitoring and treatment adherence (Lundahl et al. 2013). O'Halloran meta-analysis was performed with studies on people with chronic diseases (O'Halloran et al. 2014). VanBuskirk published another systematic review on primary care population with good results for weight loss and blood pressure. The motivational interview seems to be useful in clinical settings and one single session can improve the willingness to change and an action for health goals for behavior changes (VanBuskirk and Wetherell 2014).

The benefit of the motivational interview has been validated in different healthcare professionals: physicians, nurses and pharmaceuticals (Stewart et al. 2014; Klamerus et al. 2014; Ma et al. 2014; Drevenhorn et al. 2012). The health professional must know in which stage of change is the patient for lifestyles or taking medication changes, as long as the management strategy is different in each stage. The stage of the change of the patient can be classified as shown below:

- Not thinking about it at all (pre-contemplation stage)
- Thinking about it (contemplation stage)
- Ready to start planning (preparation stage)
- Ready to implement it (Action stage)
- Already making the change (Maintenance stage)

8.2 Factors Associated with Disease and Treatment

We have three Cochrane reviews on different intervention studies to improve compliance and control of hypertension. The different interventions can be classified as:

8.2.1 Health Education to Patients and Professionals

Trials of educational interventions to patients or professionals in general are not related to significant reductions in blood pressure. Clinical studies show that the effects of reducing the BP with changes in lifestyle can be equivalent to monotherapy with drug but the main drawback is the low level of adhesion as time passes (Elmer et al. 2006). There is a consensus that when patients get the information material available in press, pharmacies, medical clinics or other public places offices, it can have a favorable effect on information and motivation of the persons concerned (Guthrie et al. 2007).

A Cochrane review (Glynn et al. 2010) including 20 randomized clinical trials (RCTs) educational interventions directed to the patient was performed. The combination of the results of all RCTs produced mixed results. The mean difference in systolic blood pressure (SBP) and diastolic (DBP) was not statistically significant. With respect on the blood pressure control, there was a trend towards an improvement in the control (Odds Ratio 0.83; 95 % CI: 0.75–0.91). In the same systematic review, ten RCT with educational interventions directed to the health professional were analyzed. These interventions were not associated with a significant decrease in SBP and DBP, nor with a significant increase in the blood pressure control.

The tendency to minimize the high figures of the BP by the physician is denominated therapeutic inertia. Medical training programs significantly reduce therapeutic inertia therapeutic although with fewer benefits than expected (Redon et al. 2010; Luders et al. 2010).

8.2.2 Reminder Systems

Glynn reviewed eight RCTs with interventions aimed at reminding the patient appointments and encourage self-monitoring of the efficacy of the treatment. The systems were diverse: from postcards, phone reminder notices by text messages to computer feedbacks. Pooled results were associated with an improvement during follow-up (Odds Ratio of losses to follow up 0.4; 95 % CI: 0.3–0.5). However, we have the study could not determine which reminder system was the most effective (Glynn et al. 2010).

The impact of information and communication technologies in general, and particularly the computerized decision support systems, is discussed in detail in the health security report published by the European Commission in 2007. The report argues that these systems can prevent medical errors and adverse events, promote the participation of the patient with an advantage due to cooperation and adherence (OECD www.oecd.org; Russell et al. 2009).

New technologies, allow that more patients can be controlled, the contacts may be more frequent, with a greater chance to address their concerns, adapt treatment and ultimately improve the adhesion. However, it is important to note that these new care delivery models do not represent a substitute for visits to the physician's office. Rather, they offer support for the strategy of establishing a good relationship between the patient and the health care professionals. Studies using communication technologies have demonstrated that there are many ways to communicate with patients, with the theoretical advantage of appropriate adjustment and effective care plans.

8.2.3 Treatment Simplification

Adherence to treatment can also be improved through treatment simplification (Claxton et al. 2001) A Cochrane review reviewed nine RCTs on treatment simplification (Schroeder et al. 2004). The simplified dosing regimens improved compliance in seven of the nine studies, with an improvement in the fulfillment that varied from 8 to 19.6 %. Studies that were made using MEMS showed improvement in compliance when one dose a day was used instead of two. The type of antihypertensive drug is related with compliance. Thus, in the meta-analysis published by Kronish et al., the highest adhesion was found with angiotensin II-receptor blokers and angiotensine-converting enzyme inhibitors, the lowest with beta blockers and diuretics (Kronish et al. 2011).

It is more likely to achieve the goals of blood pressure control in patients with higher blood pressure values with combination therapy. We have recent studies that have shown that patients receiving fixed-dose combination therapy have a lower abandonment rate (Corrao et al. 2010). The use of polypills (fixed-dose drug combinations) greatly simplifies the number and doses of drugs and is an interesting field to improve adhesion. Polypills lowers cost of production and distribution, improve accessibility to treatment especially in middle and low income countries (Muntner et al. 2011).

8.2.4 Pharmacists and Nurses Care

Several studies show a greater reduction of the BP in groups with multidisciplinary care teams, when compared with the conventional approach. Nurses and pharmacists either within a clinic or in the community are beneficial in reducing the BP. The participation of nurses and pharmacists in the management of hypertension has obtained benefit when they are involved in the patient education, advice and evaluation of adherence to the treatment. The contribution of nurses may be particularly important for the implementation of the changes of life style (Carter et al. 2009; Walsh et al. 2006). A recent study confirms the positive effect of pharmacists interventions on compliance (Hedegaard et al. 2015).

The systematic review conducted by Glynn in 2010 brought together 12 RCTs with pharmacists or nurses care. Pooled results show that the mean for the SBP difference was from − 13 to 0 mmHg. And the DBP was from − 8 to 0 mmHg. With respect to the degree of blood pressure control, the results were not significant (odds ratio ranged from 0.1 to 0.9). The authors of the review conclude that these health professionals care can be an excellent way to provide assistance, since the majority of RCTs are associated with better control of blood pressure (Glynn et al. 2010).

8.2.5 Self-Monitoring

There are 18 RCTs evaluating the effect of self-monitoring of the AP by the patient that wer analyzed in a systematic review (Glynn et al. 2010). The pooled data showed that self-monitoring was associated with a significant reduction in the mean SBP: − 2.5 mmHg (95 % CI: − 3.7 to − 1.3 mmHg). The mean DBP showed a more modest decline of − 1.8 mmHg (95 % CI: − 2.4 to − 1.2 mmHg). With regard to the control of blood pressure, there was no significant improvement (Odds Ratio 0.97; 95 % CI: 0.81–1.16). In this line, Uhlig concluded that self-monitoring of blood pressure drops blood pressure compared to usual care, but the effect beyond the 12 months is uncertain in a meta-analysis published in 2013 (Uhlig et al. 2013). Tele-monitoring at home proved to be useful in patients with hypertension. Several studies have confirmed that the electronic transmission of the self-BP monitoring favors better adhesion to the regime of treatment and is a more effective control of hypertension (McManus et al. 2010; Morak et al. 2012; Shea and Chamoff 2012; Parati et al. 2009).

8.2.6 Interventions to Improve the Provision of Care Services

The systematic review published by Glynn et al. in 2010 (Glynn et al. 2010) analyzed 9 RCTs with organizational interventions to improve care for hypertensive patients. Pooling of results from the individual RCTs produced mixed results. The largest clinical trial, the Hypertension Detection and follow-up Program (HDFP) (The effect of treatment on mortality in mild hypertension results of the Hypertension Detection and Follow up Program 1982) that included around 10.940 people, obtained appreciable reductions both in sBP and dBP. After a five year follow-up period, these reductions in blood pressure were associated with a 28.6 % significant reduction in mortality from all causes. The organizational measures of this study consisted of a free of charge care, active follow-up visits on a regular basis and a steps use of antihypertensive drug therapy.

8.3 Factors Related to the Health System

8.3.1 Costs

Recently, an increase in compliance was found in those patients taking generic drugs when compared with those taking registered trademark drugs. Besides, a reduction in the vascular events was also founds (Gragne et al. 2014). These data were obtained in populations with low incomes, so it cannot be extrapolated to other populations where the drug cost may be less important for adhesion. Other studies confirm that the price of prescription drugs influences the therapeutic non-compliance. An example is a study that showed that patients who had had a cardiac event and subsequently did not have to pay a high price for their medication, presented a better performance and were less likely to have recurrences of the heart disease (Susan 2015; Chourdhy et al. 2011).

Sometimes, when the price of drugs is high, some patients skipped doses or do not continue with the prescription when it finishes. This makes the physicians that the prescribed medication was not enough with a subsequent unnecessary dose increase. Health care co-payment policies can lead to the patient to use fewer medicines or to choose the cheapest. Although this can avoid using unnecessary medicines, they can also cause harm when treatments for the control of chronic diseases are abandoned (Baroletti and Dell'Orfano 2010; Luiza et al. 2015) The minimum dose required should be prescribed using generics, and informing the patient about the most cheap available drugs. The use of cheaper medication tries to reduce costs and prevent barriers in the access to medication (Kaplan et al. 2016). Today, we have generic drugs and cheap options in all classes of antihypertensive medication (Choudhry et al. 2016).

8.3.2 Social Support and Self-Help Groups

There are interesting studies of community-based intervention on cardiovascular problems among adult assistance programs similar to other self-help organizations. They do not require the active presence of doctors or nurses and focuses on the empowerment of the patient and the formation of "expert patients" and community agents. Their results indicate an improvement in adhesion and achievement of the objectives of cardiovascular health in chronic diseases (Fuster et al. 2011; Vedanthan et al. 2014).

Interventions have also been developed in order to organize a network of social support in relation to physical activity, sodium intake, weight control or reduction of alcohol consumption. As an example, the project "walking with a friend to health" intends to include the community in the prevention measures and hypertension control. In this way, it obtains support for early intervention, prevention, and treatment of high blood pressure through the organizations of patients and relatives. So, the relatives of the patients and their support network become supporters of the treatment plan (Fishman 1995).

The incorporation of the family, the community, and organizations is a key factor for success in the improvement of adhesion. Living alone is a major cause of non-compliance. Accordingly, a poor perception of social support received by the patient is linked to reduced physical activity and poor adherence to the diet. Several research studies have concluded that social support improves adherence to treatment in hypertensive patients. In this way, patients who have wide social support networks or those who are married or in couple indeed, have better adherence. Social support is also essential when long-term treatment are planned that require continuous actions by the patient (DiMatteo 2004; Oegdegbe et al. 2004; Bosworth 2010). It is not only necessary an increase in family support. Research has shown that participation in patient groups is an effective strategy of motivation (Sherbourne et al. 1992; Coull et al. 2004). There is substantial evidence that support between pairs of patients can improve adherence to therapy and, at the same time, reduces the amount of time spent by the health care professionals to care for chronic diseases (WHO 2004).

8.4   Multiple Interventions

As the therapeutic non-compliance is complex issue that is influenced by variety of factors it seems logical to design interventions with multiple strategies to try to improve it. In this sense, there are studies with multiple interventions such as: reminders, pill containers, self-monitoring of blood pressure, treatment simplification, pharmacists or nurses support, family interventions, or the provision of educational material to the patient; that achieved improvements in compliance (Marquez et al. 2006). In this sense, the COM99 study (Pladevall et al. 2010) confirmed that combination of strategies is always more effective than a single one.

In another systematic review on adherence Haynes (Haynes et al. 2008) and his collaborators analyzed 70 RCTs and found 83 types of different interventions. They conclude that multifactorial interventions are most effective in modifying the adherence to long-term therapies. These studies included combinations of information, reminders, self-monitoring, reinforcement, counseling, family therapy, psychological therapy, crisis intervention, telephone follow-up and support care. Due to the heterogeneity of the studies they could not evaluate the individual effect of each strategy on the control of hypertension, or which combination was the most effective. With respect to the quantification of the effect of interventions the authors are cautious and conclude that even the most effective interventions did not result in great improvements in adherence and treatment outcomes. Marquez and colleagues refer that these interventions can control BP in two out of three patients with high cardiovascular risk and a poor BP control and the number needed to treat to prevent one patient with poor hypertension control is five (Márquez et al. 2012). In Table 3 we present a summary of the practical strategies to improve adherence.

9   Recommendations of the Clinical Practice Guidelines

9.1   European Society of Hypertension (ESH/ESC) Guideline

European society of hypertension (ESH/ESC) guideline (ESH/ESC 2013) give great relevance to the low level of compliance observed, especially in elderly and poor patients, due to its influence in prognosis and healthcare costs. They emphasize that low adherence to treatment is the most important reason for poor control of the BP and that this fact has been fully documented (Lee et al. 2006; Gale et al. 2011;

Table 3 Interventions to improve adherence: practical strategies

Type of intervention	
Physician related	Before you increase the medication think about compliance. Enter medication in a step ahead fashion. Use the minimum effective dose to avoid side effects. Avoid therapeutic inertia
Relationship doctor – patient	Explain the indication of each pill and its side effects. Report of the blood pressure values. Ask for adherence with a non-confrontational style. Use the motivational interview techniques: in the event of poor compliance, identify in which stage of change the patient is
	Involve the patient in decision-making
	Note the mood of the patient and its cognitive function
Treatment simplification	Use the minimum number of drugs and minimum number of possible dose
	Use fixed-dose combinations
	Recommend the use of pill boxes and organizers for medication
	Associate taking medication with a routine of the patient. Provide written information
Reminders	Keep the contact with the patient. Schedule an annual review and share with him the clinical situation. Use reminders: telephone, computer or postal. Contact patients that are not attending the clinic. Check the collection of medication in the pharmacy records
Self-monitoring of BP	Recommend self-monitoring blood pressure
Cost of drugs	Use cheap and generic drugs
Collaboration with other professionals	Promote the control of hypertension by pharmacists and nurses.
	Incorporate organizational improvements in the care of hypertensive patients
Social support	Involve family members in the treatment
	Recommend self-help groups and patient forums.
Multiple interventions	Use at least three strategies together

Shanti and Maribel 2003; Krousel-Wood et al. 2011; Corrao et al. 2011; Mazzaglia et al. 2009).

With regard to **the identification of low adherence to treatment** in clinical practice they point out that there are difficulties because the information provided by the patient can be misleading and methods for objectively measuring the adherence to treatment have little application in daily medicine.

The guidelines make a series of recommendations to promote adherence to medication, with **the simplification of the drug regimen** as the isolated more effective recommendation. As in the previous guidelines, the 2013 ESH/ESC guidelines favor the use of combinations of two antihypertensive doses fixed in a single pill, since reducing the number of pills taken daily improves adhesion.

The guideline stresses the relevance of **reporting BP values**, even in visits that are not related to hypertension. They also recommended the use of **self- monitoring blood pressure** at home (Parati et al. 2010).

The European guidelines insist in avoiding the **therapeutic physician inertia** (Banegas et al. 2004), attitude that tends to minimize the relevance of high blood pressure levels. They point out that if high AP is detected, the reason must be searched. The most common causes are poor adherence to the prescribed regimen, the persistence of a white coat effect and the occasional or regular consumption of substances that increase BP.

On the other hand, they recommend **multifactorial interventions** and to enhance **the role of nurses** as a possible strategy to improve adherence to treatment (Berra et al. 2011). The guideline points out that multidisciplinary cardiovascular prevention programs co-ordinated by a professional nursing improve the control of risk factors, susceptibility to physical activity and adherence to treatment compared with usual care. Besides, it also improves the perception of the patient's health, especially in secondary prevention.

The **multidisciplinary team** -based care (Machado et al. 2007) with the participation of pharmacists and nurses can improve adhesion and reduce the BP and, thus, it is also recommended by the European guideline.

The ESH/ECH published its recommendations on how to organize the work team for the management of hypertension in centers of excellence (Stergiou et al. 2010). It recommends a close contact with the patient and the use of telemedicine to improve compliance with treatments, as well as the incorporation of other models for care continuity.

9.2 The NICE Guidelines

The NICE guidelines (2011) in his chapter on education and adherence in hypertension recommends

- Provide appropriate guidance and materials about the benefits of drugs and the unwanted side effects sometimes experienced in order to help people make informed choices
- People vary in their attitudes to their hypertension and their experience of treatment. It may be helpful to provide details of patient organizations that provide useful forums to share views and information
- Provide an annual review of care to monitor blood pressure, provide people with support and discuss their lifestyle, symptoms and medication
- Because evidence supporting interventions to increase adherence is inconclusive, only use interventions to overcome practical problems associated with non-adherence if a specific need is identified. Target the intervention to the need. Interventions might include:
  - suggesting that patients record their medicine-taking
  - encouraging patients to monitor their condition
  - simplifying the dosing regimen

- using alternative packaging for the medicine
- using a multi-compartment medicines system

9.3 The Recommendations of the Panel Members Appointed to the Eighth Joint National Committee (JNC 8)

The recommendations of the Panel Members Appointed to the Eighth Joint National Committee (JNC 8) (James et al. 2014) choose an individualized treatment strategy. This strategy should be adapted on the basis of the particular circumstances of the doctor, the preferences of the patient and the tolerance to the drug. Within each strategy, physicians should regularly assess BP, foster evidence-based interventions in lifestyle and adhesion. The Panel recognizes the importance of treatment adherence and medication costs but experts think that these issues are beyond the scope of their recommendations

9.4 Report of the American College of Cardiology Foundation Task Force on Clinical Expert Consensus Documents Developed in Collaboration with the American Academy of Neurology, American Geriatrics Society, American Society for Preventive Cardiology, American Society of Hypertension, American Society of Nephrology, Association of Black Cardiologists, and European Society of Hypertension

An important set of scientific societies (Aronow 2011) have made specific recommendations for elderly hypertensive patients. They conclude that "elderly patients who are taking more than

6 medications present a lower adherence to treatment. So clinicians must take account of polypharmacy and potential pharmacological interactions, as causes of low adherence to treatment".

10   Conclusions

1. The lack of adherence is very prevalent in hypertension with a multifactorial etiology.

2. Elderly patients, those with several co-morbidities, social isolation, low incomes or with depression are the most vulnerable to this problem.
3. There is no an ideal method to quantify the adherence to the treatment. Indirect methods are recommended in clinical practice.
4. Any intervention strategy should be based in not blaming the patient and a collaborative approach. It is recommended to involve the patient in decision-making. The clinical interview style must be patient-centered including motivational techniques.
5. The strategies that demonstrated greater effectiveness in hypertension treatment compliance were: treatment simplification, systems appointment reminders, self-monitoring of blood pressure, organizational improvements and nurse and pharmacists care.
6. Combined interventions are recommended instead of isolated interventions.

References

Abel WM, Barksdale DJ (2012) Freedom of choice and adherence to the health regimen for African Americans with hypertension. Adv Nurs Sci 35(4): E1–E8. doi:10.1097/ANS.0b013e31826b842f

Aronow WS (2011) ACCF/AHA 2011 expert consensus document on hypertension in the elderly. J Am Coll Cardiol 57(20):2037–2114

Banegas JR, Segura J, Ruilope LM, Luque M, Garcia-Robles R, Campo C et al (2004) Blood pressure control and physician management of hypertension in hospital hypertension units in Spain. Hypertension 43:1338–1344

Baroletti S, Dell'Orfano H (2010) Medication adherence in cardiovascular disease. Circulation 121:1455

Berg JS, Dischler J, Wagner DJ, Raia JJ, Palmer-Shevlin N (1993) Medication compliance: a healthcare problem. Ann Pharmacother 27(9 suppl):S1–S24

Berra K, Fletcher BJ, Hayman LL, Miller NH (2011) Global cardiovascular disease prevention: a call to action for nursing: the global burden of cardiovascular disease. J Cardiovasc Nurs 26:S1–S2

Bond WS, Hussar DA (1991) Detection methods and strategies for improving medication compliance. Am J Hosp Pharm 48:1987–1988

Bosworth H (2010) Improving patient treatment adherence. A clinician's guide. Springer, New York. ISBN 978-1-4419-5865-5

Buchholz A, Vach W, Siegel A, Dürk T, Loh A, Buchholz A et al (2012) Implementation of shared decision making by physician training to optimise hypertension treatment. Study protocol of a cluster-RCT. Cardiovasc Disord 12:73. doi:10.1186/1471-2261-12-73

Buhse S, Mühlhauser I, Kuniss N, Müller UA, Lehmann T, Liethmann K (2015) An informed shared decision making programme on the prevention of myocardial infarction for patients with type 2 diabetes in primary care: protocol of a cluster randomised, controlled trial. BMC Fam Pract 16:43. doi:10.1186/s12875-015-0257-2

Carter BL, Rogers M, Daly J, Zheng S, James PA (2009) The potency of team-based care interventions for hypertension: a meta-analysis. Arch Intern Med 169:1748–1755

Chapman RH, Benner JS, Petrilla AS, Tierce JS, Collins SR, Battleman DS et al (2005) Predictors of adherence with antihypertensive and lipid-lowering therapy. Arch Intern Med 165:1147–1152

Choo PW, Rand CS, Inui TS, Lee ML, Cain E (1999) Cordeiro – Breault et M to the validation of patient reports, automated adherence to antihypertensive therapy. Med Care 37(9):846–857

Choudhry NK, Denberg TD, Qaseem A, Clinical Guidelines Committee of the American College of Physicians (2016) Improving adherence to therapy and clinical outcomes while containing costs: opportunities from the greater use of generic medications: best practice advice from the Clinical Guidelines Committee of the American College of Physicians. Ann Intern Med 164:41

Chourdhy NK, Avon J, Glynn RJ et al (2011) Full coverage for preventive medication after myocardial infarction. N Engl J Med 365:2088

Claxton AJ, Cramer J, Pierce C (2001) A systematic review of the associations between dose regimens and medication compliance. Clin Ther 23:1296–1310

Corrao G, Parodi A, Zambon A, Heiman F, Filippi A, Cricelli C et al (2010) Reduced discontinuation of antihypertensive treatment by two-drug combination as first step. Evidence from daily life practice. J Hypertens 28:1584–1590

Corrao G, Parodi A, Nicotra F, Zambon A, Merlino L, Cesana G et al (2011) Better compliance to antihypertensive medications reduces cardiovascular risk. J Hypertens 29:610–618

Coull AJ, Taylor VH, Elton R, Murdoch PS, Hargreaves AD (2004) A randomised controlled trial of senior Lay Health Mentoring in older people with ischaemic heart disease: The Braveheart Project. Age Ageing 33:348–354

Cramer JA, Benedict A, Muszbek N, Keskinalsan A, Khan ZM (2008) The significance of compliance and persistence in the treatment of diabetes, hypertension and dyslipidaemia: a review. Int J Clin Pract 62:76–87

Dabrh A, Gallacher K, Boehmer KR, Hargraves IG, Mair FS (2015) Minimally disruptive medicine: the evidence and conceptual progress supporting a new era of healthcare. J R Coll Physicians Edinb 45:114–117

Dezii CM (2000) Medication noncompliance: what is the problem? Manag Care 9:7–12

DiMatteo MR (2004) Social support and patient adherence to medical treatment: a meta-analysis. Health Psychol 23(2):207–218

DiMatteo MR, Haskard KB, Williams SL (2007) Health beliefs, disease severity, and patient adherence. A meta-analysis. Med Care 45:521–528

Drevenhorn E, Bengtson A, Nilsson PM, Nyberg P, Kjellgren KI (2012) Consultation training of nurses for cardiovascular prevention – a randomized study of 2 years duration. Blood Press 21(5):293–299

Elmer PJ, Obarzanek E, Vollmer WM, Simons-Morton D, Stevens VJ, Young DR et al (2006) Effects of comprehensive lifestyle modification on diet, weight, physical fitness and blood pressure control: 18-month results of a randomized trial. Ann Intern Med 144:485–495

ESH/ESC (2013) ESH/ESC Guidelines for the management of arterial hypertension. http://eurheartj. oxfordjournals.org/content/34/28/2159

Fischer M, Stedman M, Lii J, Vogeli C, Shrank W, Brookhart A, Weissman J (2010) Primary medication non-adherence: analysis of 195930 electronic prescriptions. J Gen Intern Med 24(4):284–290

Fishman T (1995) The 90-Second Intervention: a patient compliance mediated technique to improve and control hypertension. Public Health Rep 110(2):173–178

Fuster V (2012) An alarming threat to secondary prevention: low compliance (lifestyle) and poor adherence (drugs). Rev Esp Cardiol 65(Supl 2):10–16

Fuster V, Kelly BB, Vedanthan R (2011) Promoting global cardiovascular health: moving forward. Circulation 123:1671–1678

Gale NK, Greenfield S, Gill P, Gutridge K, Marshall T (2011) Patient and general practitioner attitudes to taking medication to prevent cardiovascular disease after receiving detailed information on risks and benefits of treatment: a qualitative study. BMC Fam Pract 12:59

Gallagher BD, Muntner P, Moise N et al (2015) Are two commonly used self-report questionnaires useful for identifying antihypertensive medication nonadherence? J Hypertens 33:1108

Glynn LG, Murphy AW, Smith SM, Schroeder K, Fahey T (2010) Interventions used to improve control of blood pressure in patients with hypertension. Cochrane Database Syst Rev

Gragne JJ, Choudry NK, Kesselheim AS et al (2014) Comparative effectiveness of generic and brand-name statins on patient outcomes: a cohort study. Ann Intern Med 161:400

Gregorie JP, Moisan J, Gilbert R, Ciampi A, Milot A (2006) Predictors of self-reported compliance with antihypertensive drug treatment: a prospective study. Can J Cardiol 22:323–329

Guthrie B, Inkster M, Fahey T (2007) Tackling therapeutic inertia: role of treatment data in quality indicators. BMJ 335:542–544

Hansen RA, Kim MM, Song L, Tu W, Wu J, Murray MD (2009) Comparison of methods to asses medication adherence and classify non adherence. Ann Pharmacotner 43:413–422

Haynes RB, Ackloo E, Sahota N, McDonald HP, Yao X (2008) Interventions for enhancing medication adherence. Cochrane Database Syst Rev, Issue 2. Art. No.: CD000011. doi:10.1002/14651858.CD000011.pub3

Hedegaard U, Kjeldsen LJ, Pottegård A, Henriksen JE, Lambrechtsen J, Hangaard J, Hallas J (2015) Improving medication adherence in patients with hypertension: a randomized trial. Am J Med 128 (12):1351–1361, PMID: 26302142

Ho PM, Rumsfeld JS, Masoudi FA, McClure DL, Plomondon ME, Steiner JF et al (2006) Effect of medication nonadherence on hospitalization and mortality among patients with diabetes mellitus. Arch Intern Med 166(17):1836–1841

Horne R, Weinman J, Barber N, Elliott R, Myfanwy M (2005) Concordance, adherence and compliance in medicine taking. Report for the National Co-ordinating Centre for NHS Service Delivery and Organisation R & D (NCCSDO). http://www.sdo.nihr. ac.uk/files/project/76-final-report.pdf

Horne R, Clatworthy J, Hankins M (2010) High adherence and concordance within a clinical trial of antihypertensives. Chronic Illn 6:243–251

Houle SK, Chatterley T, Tsuyuki RT (2014) Multidisciplinary approaches to the management of high blood pressure. Curr Opin Cardiol 29(4):344–353. doi:10. 1097/HCO.0000000000000071

Hughes DA, Bagust A, Haycox A, Walley T (2001) Accounting for noncompliance in pharmacoeconomic evaluations. Pharmacoeconomics 19:1185–1197

Hypertension in adults: diagnosis and management NICE guidelines [CG127] Published date: August 2011 https://www.nice.org.uk/guidance/cg127/chapter/1-recommendations#patient-education-and-adherence-to-treatment

Inkster ME, Donnan PT, MacDonald TM (2006) Adherence to antihypertensive medication and association with patient and practice factors. J Hum Hypertens 20:295–297

James P, Oparil S, Pharm B, Cushman W (2014) 2014 Evidence-based guideline for the management of high blood pressure in adults. Report from the panel members appointed to the Eighth Joint National Committee (JNC 8). JAMA 311(5):507–520. doi:10.1001/jama.2013.284427

James LL, Dimsdale J, Solomon D (2016) Psychological factors affecting other medical conditions: management. www.uptodate.com. UpToDate

Jung O, Gechter JL, Wunder C, Paulke A, Bartel C, Geiger H et al (2013) Resistant hypertension? Assessment of adherence by toxicological urine analysis. J Hypertens 31:766–774

Kaplan N, Bakris G, Forman J (2016) Patient adherence and the treatment of hypertension. www.uptodate.com.UpToDate

Kivimäki M, Batty GD, Hamer M, Nabi H, Korhonen M, Huupponen R, Pentti J, Oksanen T, Kawachi I, Virtanen M, Westerlund H, Vahtera J (2013) Retirement seems to be a major risk factor: influence of retirement on nonadherence to medication for hypertension and diabetes. CMAJ 185(17):E784–E790, PMID: 24082018

Klamerus ML, Kerr EA, Bosworth HB, Schmittdiel JA, Heisler M (2014) Characteristics of diabetic patients associated with achieving and maintaining blood pressure targets in the Adherence and Intensification of Medications program. Chronic Illn 10(1):60–73. doi:10.1177/1742395313496590

Kronish IM, Woodward M, Sergie Z, Ogedegbe G, Falzon L, Mann DM (2011) Meta-analysis: impact of drug class on adherence to antihypertensives. Circulation 123(15):1611–1621, PMID: 21464050

Krousel-Wood M, Joyce C, Holt E, Muntner P, Webber LS, Morisky DE, Frohlich ED (2011) Predictors of decline in medication adherence: results from the cohort study of medication adherence among older adults. Hypertension 58:804–810

LaFleur J, Nelson RE, Sauer BC, Nebeker JR (2011) Overestimation of the effects of adherence on outcomes: a case study in healthy user bias and hypertension. Heart 97(22):1862–1869, PMID: 21586421

Lee JK, Grace KA, Taylor AJ (2006) Effect of a pharmacy care program on medication adherence and persistence, blood pressure and low-density lipoprotein cholesterol: a randomized controlled trial. JAMA 296:2563–2571

Luders S, Schrader J, Schmieder RE, Smolka W, Wegscheider K, Bestehorn K (2010) Improvement of hypertension management by structured physician education and feedback system: cluster randomized trial. Eur J Cardiovasc Prev Rehabil 17:271–279

Luiza VL, Chaves LA, Silva RM et al (2015) Pharmaceutical policies: effects of cap and copayment on rational use of medicines. Cochrane Database Syst Rev 5: CD007017

Lundahl BW, Moleni T, Burke BL, Butters R, Tollefson D, Butler C et al (2013) Motivational interviewing in medical care settings: a systematic review and meta-analysis of randomized controlled trials. Patient Educ Couns 93(2):157–168. doi:10.1016/j.pec.2013.07.012

Ma C, Zhou Y, Zhou W, Huang C (2014) Evaluation of the effect of motivational interviewing counselling on hypertension care. Patient Educ Couns 95 (2):231–237. doi:10.1016/j.pec.2014.01.011

MacFadyen RJ, Struthers AD (1997) The practical assessment of compliance with ACE-Inhibitor therapy-a novel approach. J Cardiovasc Pharmacol 29:119–124

Machado M, Bajcar J, Guzzo GC, Einarson TR (2007) Sensitivity of patient outcomes to pharmacist interventions. Part II: Systematic review and meta-analysis in hypertension management. Ann Pharmacother 41:1770–1781

Márquez E (2008) Evaluation of non-compliance in clinical practice. Hipertension 25:205–213

Márquez Contreras E, Casado Martínez JJ, Ramos Gómez J, Sáenz Soubrier S, Moreno García JP, Celotti Gómez B et al (1998) Influence of medical adherence in blood pressure levels in the treatment of hypertension. Hipertension 5:133–139

Márquez E, Gil V, Casado J, Martel N, de la Figuera M, Martín JL et al (2006a) Analysis of studies published on therapy non-compliance with hypertension treatment in spain between 1984 and 2005. Aten Primaria 38(6):325–332

Márquez E, Martell N, Gil VF, De la Figuera M, Casado JJ, Martín de Pablos JL et al (2006b) Efficacy of a home blood pressure monitoring programme on therapeutic compliance in hypertensión. The EAPACUM-HTA Study. J Hypertens 24:169–175

Márquez E, De la Figuera M, Franch J, Llisterri JL, Gil V, Martín de Pablos JL et al (2012) Do patients with high vascular risk take antihypertensive medication correctly? cumple-MEMS study. Rev Esp Cardiol 65:544–550

Marshall IJ, Wolfe CD, McKevitt C (2012) Lay perspectives on hypertension and drug adherence: systematic review of qualitative research. BMJ 345: e3953, PMID: 22777025

May C, Montori VM, Mair FS (2009) We need minimally disruptive medicine. BMJ 339:b2803, doi: http://dx.doi.org/10.1136/bmj.b2803

Mayor S (2013) Non-adherence to medication increases stroke risk in patients with high blood pressure. BMJ 347:f4586, PMID: 23863964

Mazzaglia G, Ambrosioni E, Alacqua M, Filippi A, Sessa E, Immordino V et al (2009) Adherence to antihypertensive medications and cardiovascular morbidity among newly diagnosed hypertensive patients. Circulation 120(16):1598–1605. doi:10.1161/circulationaha.108.830299

McCarthy R (1998) The price you pay for the drug not taken. Bus Health 16:27–33

McManus RJ, Mant J, Bray EP, Holder R, Jones MI, Greenfield S et al (2010) Telemonitoring and self-management in the control of hypertension (TASMINH2): a randomised controlled trial. Lancet 376:163–172

Medding J, Kerr E, Heisler M, Hofer T (2012) Physician assessments of medication adherence and decisions to intensify medications for patients with uncontrolled blood pressure: still no better than acoin toss. BMC Health Serv Res 12:270. doi:10.1186/1472-6963-12-270

Miller W, Rollnick S (2013) Motivational interviewing, 3rd edn. The Guilford Press, New York

Morak J, Kumpusch H, Hayn D, Modre-Osprian R, Schreier G (2012) Design and evaluation of a telemonitoring concept based on NFC-enabled mobile phones and sensor devices. IEEE Trans Inf Technol Biomed Publ IEEE Eng Med Biol Soc 16:17–23

Morisky DE, Green LW, Levine DM (1986) Concurrent and predictive validity of a self-reported measure of medication adherence. Med Care 24:67–74

Morisky DE, Ang A, Krousel-Wood M, Ward H (2008) Predictive validity of a medication adherence measure for hypertension control. J Clin Hypertens 10:348–354

Morris AB, Pharm D, Jingjin L, Kroenke K, Bruner-England TE, Young JM, Murray MD (2006) Factors associated with drug adherence and blood pressure control in patients with hypertension. Pharmacotherapy 26:483–492

Muntner P, Mann D, Wildman RP, Shimbo D, Fuster V, Woodward M (2011) Projected impact of polypill use among US adults: medication use, cardiovascular risk reduction, and side effects. Am Heart J 161:719–725

New England Healthcare Institute (2009) Thinking outside the pillbox. A system-wide approach to improving patient medication adherence for chronic disease. http://wwwnehi.net/uploads/full_report/pa_issue_brief__final.pdf

Newby LK, LaPointe NM, Chen AY, Kramer JM, Hammill BG, DeLong ER, Muhlbaier LH et al (2006) Long-term adherence to evidence-based secondary prevention therapies in coronary artery disease. Circulation 113:203–212

O'Halloran PD, Blackstock F, Shields N, Holland A, Iles R, Kingsley M et al (2014) Motivational interviewing to increase physical activity in people with chronic health conditions: a systematic review and meta-analysis. Clin Rehabil 28(12):1159–1171. doi:10.1177/0269215514536210

OECD Health Policy Studies. Improving health sector. Efficiency the role of information and communication technologies. Online at www.oecd.org/publishing/corrigenda

Oegdegbe G, Harrison M, Robbins L et al (2004) Barriers and facilitators of medicationa adherence in hypertensive African Americans: a qualitative study. Ethn Dis 14(1):3–12

Osterberg L, Blaschke T (2005) Adherence to medication. N Engl J Med 353(5):487–497

Paasche-Orlow M (2011) Caring for patients with limited health literacy: a 76-year-old man with multiple medical problems. JAMA 306(10):1122–1129. doi:10.1001/jama.2011.1203

Parati G, Omboni S, Albini F, Piantoni L, Giuliano A, Revera M et al (2009) Home blood pressure telemonitoring improves hypertension control in general practice. The TeleBPCare study. J Hypertens 27:198–203

Parati G, Stergiou GS, Asmar R, Bilo G, de Leeuw P, Imai Y et al (2010) European Society of Hypertension practice guidelines for home blood pressure monitoring. J Hum Hypertens 24:779–785

Pladevall M, Brotons C, Gabriel R, Arnau A, Suárez C, De la Figuera M et al (2010) Multicenter cluster-randomized trial of a mukltifactorial intervention to improve antihypertensive medication adherence and blood pressure control among patients at high cardiovascular risk (the COM99 study). Circulation 122:1183–1191

Qureshi NN, Hatcher J, Chaturvedi N, Jafar TH (2007) Effect of general practitioner education on adherence to antihypertensive drugs: cluster randomised controlled trial. BMJ 335:1030

Redon J, Coca A, Lazaro P, Aguilar MD, Cabanas M, Gil N et al (2010) Factors associated with therapeutic inertia in hypertension: validation of a predictive model. J Hypertens 28:1770–1777

Rosen MI, Rigsby MO, Salahi JT, Ryan CE, Cramer JA (2004) Electronic monitoring and counseling to improve medication adherence. Behav Res Ther 42 (4):409–422

Rosenson RS, Braun LT, Freeman MW, Gersh BJ, Rind DM (2016) Compliance with lipid altering medications and recommended lifestyle changes. www.uptodate.com. UpToDate.

Roshanov PS, Misra S, Gerstein HC, Garg AX, Sebaldt RJ, Mackay JA et al (2011) Computerized clinical decision support systems for chronic disease management: a decision-maker-researcher partnership systematic review. Implement Sci 6:92. doi:10.1186/1748-5908-6-92

Ross S, Walker A, MacLeod MJ (2004) Patient compliance in hypertension: role of illness perceptions and treatment beliefs. J Hum Hypertens 18(9):607–613

Russell M, Roe B, Beech R, Russell W (2009) Service developments for managing people with long-term conditions using case management approaches, an example from the UK. Int J Integr Care 9:e02

Sackett DL, Haynes RB (1976) Compliance with therapeutic regimens. The Johns Hopkins University Press, Baltimore

Sackett DL, Haynes RB, Gibson ES (1975) Randomized clinical trial of stategies for improving medication compliance in primary hypertension. Lancet 1:1205–1217

Sanson-Fisher R, Clover K (1995) Compliance in the treatment of hypertension. A need of action. Am J Hypertens 8:82S–88S

Santschi V, Rodonti N, Bugnon O, Burnier M (2008) Impact of electronic monitoring of drug adherence on blood pressure control in primary care: a cluster 12-month randomised controlled study. Eur J Intern Med 19:427–434

Schoenthaler A, Ogedegbe G (2008) Patients' perceptions of electronic monitoring devices affect medication adherence in hypertensive African Americans. Ann Pharmacotherar 42:647–652

Schroeder K, Fahey T, EbrahimS (2004) Interventions for improving adherence to treatment in patients with high blood pressure in ambulatory settings. Cochrane Database Syst Rev Issue 3. Art. No.: CD004804. doi:10.1002/14651858.CD004804

Shanti M, Maribel S (2003) Hypertension. World Health Organization. p 98–104

Shea K, Chamoff B (2012) Telehomecare communication and self-care in chronic conditions: moving toward a shared understanding. Worldviews Evid Based Nurs/ Sigma Theta Tau Int Honor Soc Nurs 9:109–116

Sherbourne C, Hays RD, Ordway L, DiMattteo HR (1992) Antecedents of adherence to medical recommendations: results from the Medical Outcomes Study. J Behav Med 1:447–468

Sicras A, Fernández J, Rejas J, García M (2006) Antihypertensive and/or lipid-lowering treatments pattern of compliance in hypertense and/or dyslipemic patients in Primary Care. An Med Interna 23:361–368

Stephenson BJ, Rowe BH, Haynes RB, Macharia WM, Leon G (1993) The rational clinical examination. Is this patient taking the treatment as prescribed? JAMA 269(21):2779–2781

Stergiou G, Myers MG, Reid JL, Burnier M, Narkiewicz K, Viigimaa M et al (2010) Setting-up a blood pressure and vascular protection clinic: requirements of the European Society of Hypertension. J Hypertens 28:1780–1781

Stewart K, George J, Mc Namara KP, Jackson SL, Peterson GM, Bereznicki LR et al (2014) Multifaceted pharmacist intervention to improve antihypertensive adherence: a cluster-randomized, controlled trial (HAPPy trial). J Clin Pharm Ther 39(5):527–534. doi:10.1111/jcpt.12185

Susan J (2015) USA grapples with high drug costs. Lancet 386:2127

Tamblyn R, Eguale T, Huang A, Winslade N, Doran P (2014) The incidence and determinants of primary non adherence with prescribed medication in primary care: a cohort study. Ann Intern Med 160:441–450

The effect of treatment on mortality in "mild" hypertension: results of the Hypertension Detection and Follow-up Program (1982) N Engl J Med 307:976–980

Tinsel I, Buchholz A, Vach W, Siegel A, Dürk T, Buchholz A et al (2013) Decision-making in antihypertensive therapy: a cluster randomised controlled trial. BMC Fam Pract 14:135. doi:10.1186/1471-2296-14-135

Tomaszewski M, White C, Patel P, Masca N, Damani R, Hepworth J et al (2014) High rates of non-adherence to antihypertensive treatment revealed by high-performance liquid chromatography-tandem mass spectrometry (HP LC-MS/MS) urine analysis. Heart 100:855–861

Uhlig K, Patel K, Ip S, Kitsios GD, Balk EM (2013) Self-measured blood pressure monitoring in the management of hypertension: a systematic review and meta-analysis. Ann Intern Med 159:185–194

van Duijn HJ, Belo JN, Blom JW, Velberg ID, Assendelft WJ (2011) Revised guidelines for cardiovascular risk management – time to stop medication? A practice-based intervention study. Br J Gen Pract 61(587): e347–e352. doi:10.3399/bjgp11X578025

VanBuskirk KA, Wetherell JL (2014) Motivational interviewing with primary care populations: a systematic review and meta-analysis. J Behav Med 37 (4):768–780. doi:10.1007/s10865-013-9527-4

Vedanthan R, Kamano JH, Naanyu V, Delong AK, Were MC, Finkelstein EA et al (2014) Optimizing linkage and retention to hypertension care in rural Kenya (LARK hypertension study): study protocol for a randomized controlled trial. Trials 15:143. doi:10. 1186/1745-6215-15-143

Walsh JM, McDonald KM, Shojania KG, Sundaram V, Nayak S, Lewis R et al (2006) Quality improvement strategies for hypertension management: a systematic review. Med Care 44:646–657

Wang W, Lau Y, Loo A, Chow A, Thompson DR (2014) Medication adherence and its associated factors among Chinese community-dwelling older adults with hypertension. Heart Lung 43(4):278–283, PMID: 24856232

WHO (2004) Adherence to long-therm therapics. Evidence for action. Geneva: World Health Organization. http://apps.who.int/iris/bitstream/10665/42682/1/9241545992.pdf

Zeller A, Schoroeder K, Peters T (2007) Electronic pillboxes (MEMS) to asses the relatioshep between medication adherence and and blood pressure control in primary care. Scand J Prim Health Care 25:202–207

Adv Exp Med Biol - Advances in Internal Medicine (2017) 2: 149–166
DOI 10.1007/5584_2016_36
© Springer International Publishing AG 2016
Published online: 13 December 2016

The Role of Beta-Blockers in the Treatment of Hypertension

John M. Cruickshank

Abstract

Importance

Two major guide-line committees (JNC-8 and NICE UK) have dropped beta-blockers as first-line therapy in the treatment of hypertension. Also, recent meta-analyses (that do not take age into account) have concluded that beta-blockers are inappropriate first-line agents in the treatment of hypertension. This review seeks to shed some light on the "rights and wrongs" of such actions and conclusions.

Objectives

Because the pathophysiology of primary/essential hypertension differs in elderly and younger subjects, the latter being closely linked to obesity and increased sympathetic nerve activity, the author sought to clarify the efficacy of beta-blockers in the younger/middle-aged group in reducing the risk of death, and cardiovascular end-points.

Evidence acquisition

Four searches were undertaken, utilising PubMed up to 31st Dec 2015. One search was under the terms "hypertension AND obesity AND sympathetic nerve activity". A second was "hypertension AND plasma nor-adrenaline/norepinephrine AND survival". A third was "beta-blockers or adrenergic beta-antagonists AND hypertension AND age AND stroke or myocardial infarction or death". A fourth was "meta-analysis of beta-blockers AND hypertension AND age AND death, stroke, myocardial infarction"

J.M. Cruickshank (✉)
Oxonian Cardiovascular Consultancy, 42 Harefield,
Long Melford, Suffolk CO10 9DE, UK
e-mail: johndtl@aol.com

Results

Diastolic (with or without systolic) hypertension, in contrast to isolated systolic hypertension, occurs primarily in younger subjects, and is linked to overweight/obesity and increased sympathetic nerve activity. In younger/middle-aged hypertensive subjects, high plasma norepinephrine levels are linked (independent of blood pressure) to an increased risk of future cardiovascular events and death. High resting heart rates (a surrogate for high sympathetic nerve activity) likewise predict premature all-cause death, coronary heart disease and cardiovascular events in younger hypertensive subjects. In this younger/middle-aged hypertensive group, antihypertensive agents that increase sympathetic nerve activity (diuretics, dihydropyridine calcium blockers, and angiotensin receptor blockers (ARBs)) do not decrease (and may increase) the risk of myocardial infarction, and are therefore inappropriate first-line agents in this age-group. By contrast, in younger/middle-aged hypertensive subjects (less than 60 years old), meta-analysis has shown that beta-blockers are significantly superior to randomised placebo, and at least as effective as randomised comparator agents, in reducing death/stroke/myocardial infarction. In this younger/middle-aged hypertensive group beta-blockers have been shown (vs randomised placebo or diuretics) to reduce the risk of myocardial infarction by 35–50 %, and stroke by 50–55 % (vs placebo), in non-smoker men. Atenolol was at least as effective as ACE-inhibition (captopril) in reducing all 7 cardiovascular endpoints (including stroke which was reduced by 50 %), vs less tight control of blood pressure, in obese hypertensive subjects with type-2 diabetes (UKPDS study); and after 20 years follow-up, atenolol was significantly (23 %) superior to the ACE-inhibitor in reducing the risk of all-cause death (beta-blockers have anti-cancer properties, which maybe relevant).

Conclusions and Relevance

Primary/essential hypertension in younger/middle-age is underpinned by high sympathetic nerve activity. In this age-group high resting heart rates and high plasma norepinephrine levels (independent of blood pressure) are linked to premature cardiovascular events and death. Thus, anti-hypertensive agents that increase sympathetic nerve activity ie diuretics, dihydropyridine calcium blockers, and ARBs, are inappropriate first-line choices in this younger age-group. Beta-blockers perform well vs randomised placebo and other antihypertensive agents regarding reduced risk of death/stroke/myocardial infarction in younger (<60 years) hypertensive subjects, and are a reasonable first-line choice of therapy (certainly in men). These facts should be reflected in the recommendations of guideline committees around the world.

Keywords

Hypertension • Age • Beta-blocker • Epinephrine • Norepinephrine • Stroke • Myocardial infarction • Smoking status

Abbreviations

BP   blood pressure
BB   beta-blocker

1   Introduction

There is much confusion regarding the role of beta-blockers (BB) in primary (or essential) hypertension, stemming from two main sources. Firstly there are differences among Guideline committees from the USA (James et al. 2014), Europe (Mancia et al. 2007) and UK (Krause et al. 2011), concerning the role of BBs; BBs are no longer recommended as first-line therapy for hypertension in the USA (James et al. 2014) and UK (Krause et al. 2011). Secondly, the results of 7 recent meta-analyses (Wu et al. 2013; Prospective Studies Collaboration 2002; Wiysonge and Opie 2013; Lindholm et al. 2005; Xue et al. 2015; Thomopoulos et al. 2015a, b) regarding appropriate first-line therapy for the treatment of hypertension, were not favourable to BBs (age was not taken into account).

Importantly, neither the USA-JNC-8 guidelines (James et al. 2014), nor the European guidelines (Mancia et al. 2007), take age into account (hypertension in the young/middle-aged is often associated with obesity and is underpinned by high sympathetic nerve activity, and this is a situation favourable to beta-blockade, or ACE-inhibitors which reduce sympathetic nerve activity – see later). Nevertheless, Europe views first-line beta-blockade to be similar to other classes of anti-hypertensive agents, the reduction in blood pressure (BP) being the important factor. In contrast JNC-8 no longer recommends first-line beta-blockade, primarily due to the poor results of atenolol (vs losartan) in the LIFE Study (Dahlof et al. 2002) involving elderly hypertensives. The UK NICE Committee (Krause et al. 2011) does take age into account, but gives the reason for omitting BBs as a first-line treatment of younger hypertensive patients, as 1. impaired efficacy in reducing stroke-risk. 2. a tendency to precipitate diabetes, and is

therefore the least cost effective option (vs - ACE-Is and ARBs) (Williams 2007). Unlike the USA, its near neighbour Canada does (like the UK NICE Committee) take age into account and (unlike the UK NICE Committee) recommends first-line beta-blockade for hypertensive subjects less than 60 years old (Khan et al. 2009 May).

This review seeks to shed a little light upon a confused situation regarding the role of BBs in the treatment of hypertension, based on views already expressed by the author (Cruickshank 2013).

2   Methods

Involved utilisation of the PubMed Search up to December 31st, 2015, under the search terms

1. "hypertension AND obesity AND sympathetic nerve activity", where 191 studies were identified, from which 3 (Grassi et al. 2004; Lambert et al. 2007; Huggett et al. 2003) relevant, illustrative, recent (from year 2000) publications were selected by mutual agreement between the author and a medical colleague.
2. "hypertension AND plasma noradrenaline/ norepinephrine AND survival", where 3 studies were identified, and one was selected (Peng et al. 2006). There was also reference to two recent reviews conducted by the author (Coats and Cruickshank 2014; Cruickshank 2014), relating to diuretics, dihydropyridine calcium channel blockers, and angiotensin receptor blockers (ARBs), and their effects on sympathetic nerve activity and the risk of myocardial infarction; this approach provided 11 references (Menon et al. 2009; No author listed 1980; Medical Research Working Party 1985; Leren and Heigeland 1986; Fogari et al. 2000; Estacio et al. 1998; Heuser et al. 2003; Moltzer et al. 2010; Strauss and Hall 2006, 2007).
3. A search was conducted under the terms "meta-analyses of beta-blockers AND hypertension AND age AND death, stroke, myocardial infarction". This search identified

5 studies, from which two were selected, being specific to BBs (Khan and McAlister 2006; Kuyper and Kahn 2014).

## 3	Results

1. Essential hypertension, obesity, sympathetic nervous activity, and prognostic/treatment implications.

The classic Framingham Heart Study began in 1948 with enrolment of 5209 men and women aged 28–62 years, and was enlarged in 1971 to include a further 5124 men and women who were the offspring (or their spouses) of the original participants; follow-up of subjects occurred every 2–4 years. Two of Framingham's conclusions (Franklin et al. 2005) were 1. The development of diastolic ($\pm$ systolic) hypertension was closely related to a younger age and an increased body mass index (BMI), and 2. The development of isolated systolic hypertension occurred in an older age-group, reflecting a stiffening/ageing of the arteries – Table 1. Certainly from a haemodynamic view-point, primary hypertension in the young and elderly differ markedly, with the former being linked primarily to a high cardiac output (Druktenis et al. 2007); in the elderly there is a fall in cardiac output (Palatini and Julius 2009; Sowers and Lester 2000), so that high blood pressure is dependent on an increased peripheral resistance.

Obese (defined as a BMI greater than 30 kg/m2) adolescents with hypertension experience a marked fall in BP after weight-loss following bariatric surgery, with 74 % becoming normotensive (Inge et al. 2016). In younger subjects, obesity (particularly central) is linked to a significant increase in sympathetic nerve activity (Grassi et al. 2004). The obesity-related high sympathetic nerve activity may be confined to men (Kostis et al. 2015), and be apparent mainly in muscle and kidney (Brooks et al. 2015). Obesity-related increases in sympathetic nerve activity are particularly apparent in the presence of hypertension (Lambert et al. 2007)- Fig. 1, or type-2 diabetes (Huggett et al. 2003). Even high-normal blood pressure is linked to increased muscle sympathetic nerve activity (Seravalle et al. 2015). The raised sympathetic nerve activity is associated with the release of leptin (so-called "thin hormone") from adipose tissue; leptin acts upon the hypothalamic region of the mid-brain, resulting in increased sympathetic nerve activity (Barnes and McDougal 2014). High insulin levels, associated with obesity-related insulin resistance, also act upon the hypothalamic region, resulting in heightened sympathetic nerve activity (Coats and Cruickshank 2014; Cruickshank 2014). This has important prognostic implications, as high norepinephrine (noradrenaline) levels are associated with the atherosclerotic process (Helin et al. 1970) and

Table 1 Different Predictors of Diastolic Hypertension (DH) ($\pm$ raised systolic – SDH) and Isolated Systolic Hypertension (ISH) – FRAMINGHAM Study

Predictors of Diastolic Hypertension ($\pm$ Systolic Hypertension) = DBP $\geq$ 90 mmHg ($\pm$ SBP $\geq$ 140 mmHg)	Predictors of Isolated Systolic Hypertension = SBP $\geq$ 140 mmHg + DBP $<$ 90 mmHg (wide P-P)
1. Young age	1. Older age
2. Male sex	2. Female Sex
3. High BMI at baseline	3. Increased BMI during follow-up (weak)
4. Increased BMI during follow-u	4. ISH arises more commonly from normal and high normal BP, than "burned out" diastolic hypertension
5. Main mechanism of DH and SDH is raised peripheral resistance	5. Only 18 % with new – onset ISH had a previous DBP $\geq$ 95 mmHg
	6. Main mechanism of ISH is increased arterial stiffness = aging of arteries

Franklin et al Circulat (2005)

(via an increased heart rate) coronary plaque rupture (Heidland and Strauer 2001a). It thus comes as no surprise that high plasma norepinephrine levels, independent of smoking and blood pressure levels, are powerful predictors of cardiovascular death and survival in 601 (354 men and 247 women) young/middle-aged hypertensive subjects (over a 6–7 year follow-up period (Peng et al. 2006) – Fig. 2. Importantly, high intra-lymphocyte beta-receptor density (Bmax) and cyclic adenosine monophosphate (AMP) levels predict (independent of BP) future myocardial infarctions, but not stroke (which relates to blood pressure) (Peng et al. 2006) – Fig. 3. In the Framingham Heart Study (Gillman et al. 1993), high resting heart rates, particularly over 85 bpm (a surrogate for increased sympathetic nerve activity), in young/middle-aged hypertensive subjects, have been shown to predict all-cause death and cardiovascular and coronary heart disease events for both hypertensive men – Fig. 4, and women over a 36 year follow-up period.

Though sympathetic nerve activity is increased in elderly hypertension (Yamada et al. 1989; Hart and Charkoudian 2014), this is not so within the kidney (Esler et al. 1984). There is also a marked reduction in beta-receptor

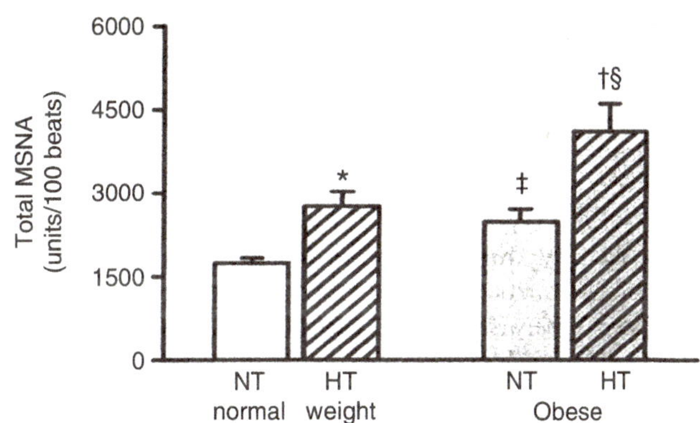

Fig. 1 Muscle sympathetic nerve activity (MSNA) in normal weight and obese, young/middle-aged normotensives (NT) and hypertensives (HT) (Lambert et al. 2007)

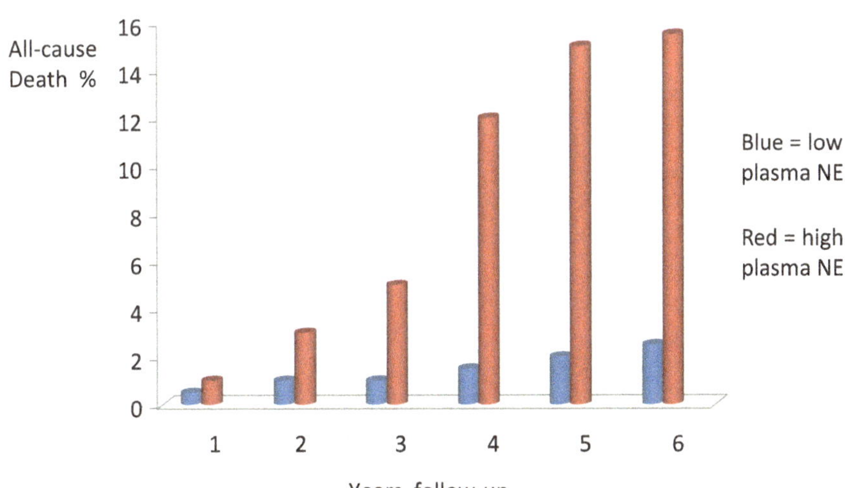

Fig. 2 601 middle-aged hypertensive subjects followed-up for 6–7 years; high plasma norepinephrine concentrations (NE) (>4.0 nmol/L = *red*) vs low (>4.0 nmol/L = *blue*) were associated with high levels of all-cause death (independent of blood pressure) (Peng et al. 2006)

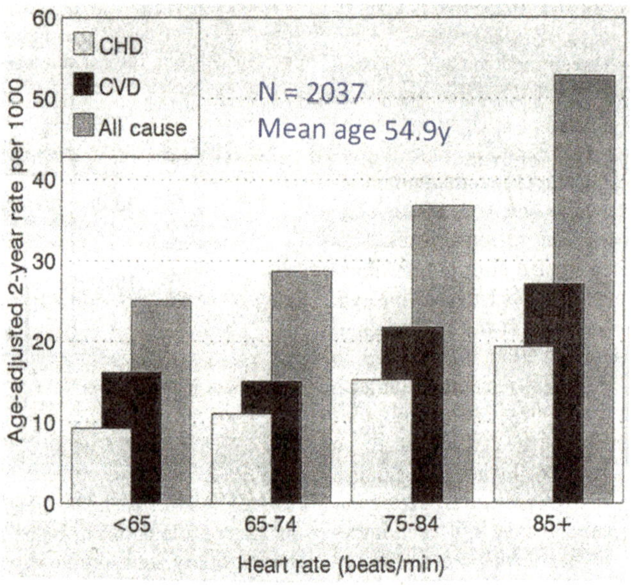

Fig. 3 Beta-receptor density (Bmax) and cAMP levels (in lymphocytes) as predictors of myocardial infarction(MI)and stroke in middle-aged hypertensives followed for 7 years (Peng et al. 2006)

Fig. 4 Framingham: Effect of resting heart rate on all-cause death, CHD and CVD events in untreated male hypertensives, followed-up for 36 years (Gillman et al. 1993)

affinity/sensitivity in this older age-group (Feldman et al. 1984; Tenero et al. 1990), which may explain the relative lack of efficacy of beta-blockers in the elderly – (see later).

In the above context, it is notable that antihypertensive agents that increase sympathetic nerve activity in young/middle-age, perform poorly in terms of reducing cardiovascular events in this age-group. Thus, thiazide-type diuretics increase sympathetic nerve activity (Menon et al. 2009), and in 3 studies involving diuretic therapy in young/middle-aged hypertensive subjects (No author listed 1980; Medical Research Working Party 1985; Leren and Heigeland 1986) there was no reduction in the risk of myocardial infarction (No author listed 1980; Medical Research Working Party 1985), and even a significant increase (Leren and Heigeland 1986), versus randomised placebo/non-treatment. Dihydropridine calcium blockers (felodipine, amlodipine, manidipine, and lacidipine) increase heart rate and plasma norepinephrine levels (Fogari et al. 2000), and in the ABCD study (Estacio et al. 1998) the investigation was terminated prematurely due to a significant excess of myocardial infarctions in the nisoldipine, vs the enalapril, group. Likewise, angiotensin receptor blockers (ARBs) increase sympathetic nerve activity in younger subjects (Heuser et al. 2003; Moltzer et al. 2010). Meta-analyses indicates that, in contrast to ACE-inhibitors, ARBs increase the risk of myocardial infarction (Strauss and Hall 2006; Straus and Hall 2007) Fig. 5, and in two subsequent placebo-controlled studies involving hypertension (Imai et al. 2011) and pre-hypertension plus diabetes (Haller et al. 2011), there was a significant excess if cardiovascular events in those receiving the ARB. Thus, prevention of myocardial infarction and cardiovascular events is not just about good control of BP. In contrast to ARBs, ACE-inhibition results in a reduction in sympathetic nerve activity (Noll et al. 1997) – see later.

2. The role of beta-blockers in the treatment of hypertension; the importance of age

2a. Beta-blockers and the atheromataous process

As myocardial infarction is the most common cardiovascular event in young/middle-aged essential hypertension (Medical Research Working Party 1985), it is important to note that beta-blockade is able to reverse the coronary atherosclerotic process. In a pooled analysis of four intravascular ultrasonography randomised, controlled trials in patients with coronary heart disease, over an 18–24 month time-interval, BBs (mainly atenolol and metoprolol) effected a significant (p < 0.001) regression of coronary artery atherosclerotic plaque (Sipahi et al. 2007). BBs also stabilise vulnerable coronary plaque. A study of 106 middle-aged patients who underwent coronary angiography twice within a 6 month period, revealed that high heart rates (>80 bpm) significantly increased, and BBs significantly decreased, the risk of atheromataous plaque disruption and rupture (a precursor to myocardial infarction) (Heidland and Strauer 2001b).

2b. Beta-blockers and control of blood pressure in the younger subject

Beta-2 blockade results in a rise in BP of about 7/5 mm Hg (Robb et al. 1985). Thus a moderately beta-1 selective agent like atenolol is more effective in lowering BP than a non-selective BB like propranolol (Zacharias and Cowen 1977). Atenolol, in turn, is less effective in lowering BP than highly beta-1 selective bisoprolol (Neutel et al. 1993). Indeed, in younger/middle-aged hypertensive subjects, bisoprolol is a more effective anti-hypertensive agent than the calcium blocker amlodipine, the alpha-blocker doxazosine, the ACE-inhibitor lisinopril, and the diuretic bendrofluozide (Deary et al. 2002), and angiotensin receptor

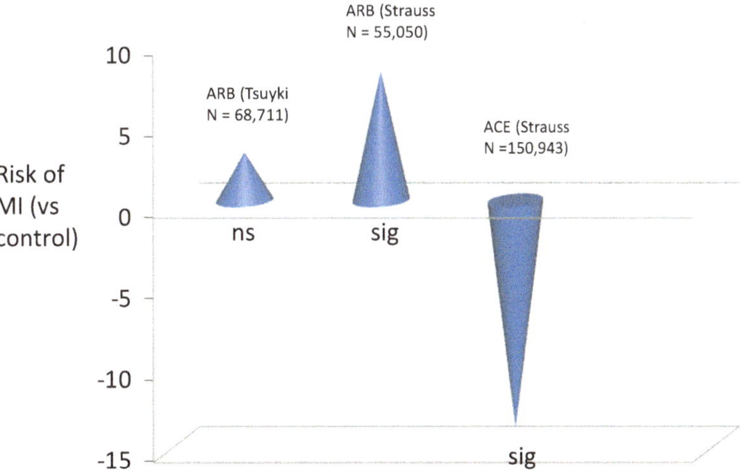

Fig. 5 Relative risk of myocardial infarction (MI) in meta-analyses of ARB and ACE-inhibitors: ARBs increase risk of MI. Strauss and Hall, Circulation 2006

blockers (ARBs) (Hiltunen et al. 2007), being at least as reno-protective as the latter (Parrinello et al. 2009).

2c. Beta-blockers and reduction of hard endpoints.

As already noted, recent meta-analyses that do not take age into account, are less than complimentary to BBs (Wu et al. 2013; Prospective Studies Collaboration 2002; Wiysonge and Opie 2013; Lindholm et al. 2005; Xue et al. 2015; Thomopoulos et al. 2015a, b; Dahlof et al. 2002). One (Wu et al. 2013) suggested that BBs increase all-cause mortality; another (Lindholm et al. 2005) indicated that first-line beta-blockade did not reduce all-cause mortality and was associated with only modest reductions in cardiovascular events (vs randomised placebo or non-treatment); another (Xue et al. 2015) suggested that BBs increase the risk of stroke; another (Thomopoulos et al. 2015a) indicated that BBs were inferior to renin-angiotensin system (RAS) inhibitors in preventing cardiovascular events and stroke; and finally 2 meta-analyses (Thomopoulos et al. 2015b; Dahlof et al. 2002) concluded that BBs were less effective than other agents in preventing stroke, and that reduction in coronary heart disease and all-cause death did not achieve statistical significance.

Two meta-analyses that do take age into account (Khan and McAlister 2006; Kuyper and Kahn 2014) arrive at very different conclusions to meta-analyses that do not. One meta-analysis (Khan and McAlister 2006) included 8 randomised placebo-controlled studies, and 9 randomised studies involving active agents (Williams 2007; Medical Research Working Party 1985; The IPPPSH Collaborative Group 1985; Coope and Warrender 1986; Dahlof et al. 1991; MRC Working Party 1992; Trial of secondary prevention with atenolol after transient ischemic attack or nondisabling stroke. The Dutch TIA Trial Study Group. Stroke 24:543–548 1993; Eriksson et al. 1995; Wilhelmsen et al. 1987; UK Prospective Diabetes Study Group 1998; Hansson et al. 1999a, b, 2000; Zanchetti et al. 2002; Pepine et al. 2003; Black et al. 2003; Dahlof et al. 2005). Compared to randomised placebo, in the younger/middle-aged hypertensive subject, with a mean age less than 60 years old, (admittedly and arbitrary cut-off point re definition of young/middle-aged) BBs were significantly superior to placebo in reducing the risk of death/stroke/MI – Fig. 6; with only a positive trend in the elderly – Fig. 7. When compared to randomised comparator anti-hypertensive drugs, there was a trend favouring BBs in younger hypertensive subjects Fig. 8, in contrast to those older than 60 years old, where BBs were significantly less effective in reducing the risk of death/stroke/myocardial infarction – Fig. 9. The other meta-analysis (Kuyper and Kahn 2014) involved 21 studies, comprising the same 17 studies as the first meta-analysis (Khan and McAlister 2006), plus an extra 4 studies in

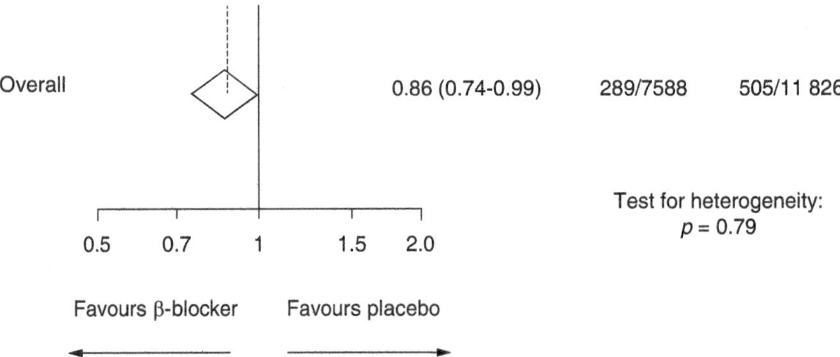

Fig. 6 A meta-analysis of 2 studies in the younger (<60y) hypertensive subject; beta-blockers significantly superior to randomised placebo in preventing all cause death/stroke/MI (Khan and McAlister 2006)

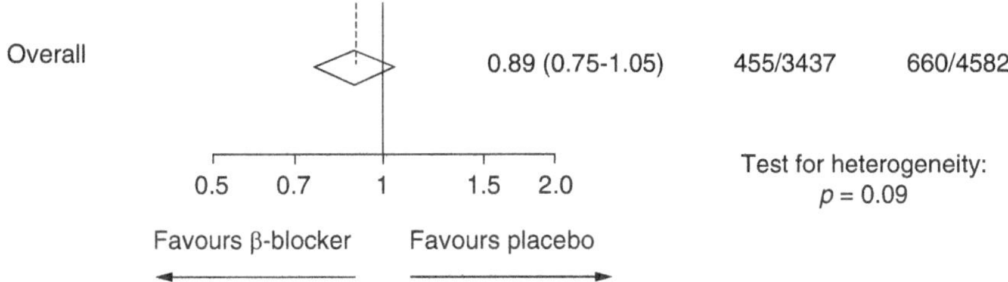

Fig. 7 Meta-analysis of 5 studies in the elderly hypertensive subject (>60y) – a strong trend favouring beta-blockers vs randomised placebo in the prevention of the composite death/stroke/MI (Khan and McAlister 2006)

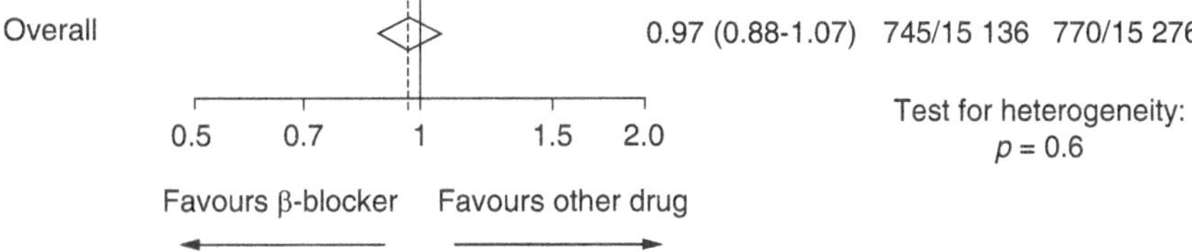

Fig. 8 A meta-analysis of 5 studies in the younger (<60y) hypertensive subject; a trend favouring beta-blockers vs. drug in preventing all cause death/stroke/MI (Khan and McAlister 2006)

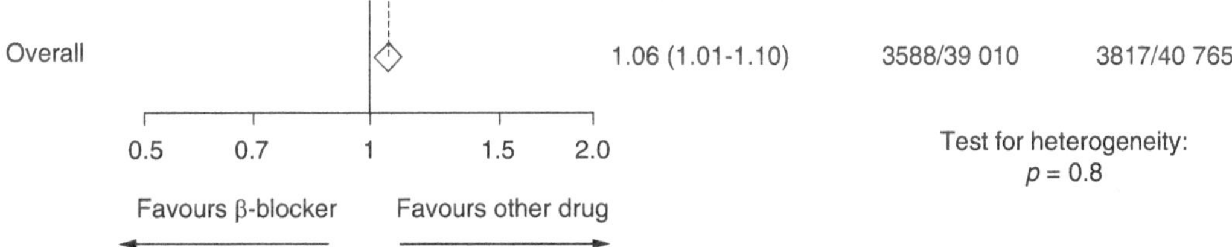

Fig. 9 A meta-analysis of 7 studies in the elderly (>60y) hypertensive subject; beta-blockers were significantly inferior to other drugs in preventing all-cause death/stroke/MI. Khan and McAlister

the younger group (3 studies compared propranolol with diuretic therapy (Veterans Administration Cooperative Study Group on Antihypertensive Agents 1982; Berglund et al. 1986; Yurenev et al. 1992), and the fourth – AASK study (Wright et al. 2002), compared metoprolol with amlodipine and ramipril in Black American hypertensive patients with renal disease). The conclusion was that in the young/middle-aged (less than 60 years old) both atenolol and non-atenolol beta-blockers were similarly effective in reducing cardiovascular endpoints, while in the elderly, atenolol (no other BBs have been studied) was associated with an increased risk of stroke. The second meta-analysis did not include the most recent results of the AASK study (Norris et al. 2006) in younger/middle-age subjects, which showed that metoprolol, amlodipine, and ramipril were similarly effective in reducing cardiovascular outcomes after 4 years of follow-up.

BBs thus have no role to play as first-line agents in the elderly hypertensive subject, unless myocardial ischemia is also present (Pepine et al. 2003), where atenolol was equivalent to the calcium blocker verapamil. The role of BBs in the elderly is as second-line therapy to either diuretics or calcium blockers, as evidenced in the MRC-elderly study (MRC Working Party 1992) and the large ALLHAT (The ALLHAT Officers and Coordinators for the ALLHAT Collaborative Research Group 2002) and SHEP (SHEP Cooperative Research Group 1991) studies, especially in the presence of the metabolic syndrome (SHEP Cooperative Research Group 1991).

3. Beta-blockers and prevention of stroke and all-cause death in younger/middle-aged hypertensive subjects; dispelling some myths

There is a perception that BBs do not reduce all-cause mortality (Wu et al. 2013; Prospective Studies Collaboration 2002; Wiysonge and Opie 2013; Lindholm et al. 2005), and are relatively ineffective in reducing the risk of stroke (Krause et al. 2011; Xue et al. 2015; Thomopoulos et al. 2015a, b; Dahlof et al. 2002; Williams 2007; Khan et al. 2009 May), in younger/middle-aged hypertensive subjects. The UKPDS-39 (UK Prospective Diabetes Study Group 1998) and MRC-1 (Medical Research Working Party 1985) studies give no credence to these perceptions. Concerning stroke-risk reduction in MRC-1 (Medical Research Working Party 1985) in non-smoking men, both non-selective propranolol and the diuretic bendrofluazide, vs randomised placebo, reduced the risk of stroke by 54 %. In UKPDS-38 (U.K. Prospective Diabetes Study Group 1998), where smoking was not taken into account, tight control (either atenolol or captopril) of blood pressure, vs less tight control (difference 10/5 mm hg), resulted in a significant 44 % reduction in the risk of stroke. UKPDS-39 (UK Prospective Diabetes Study Group 1998) examined the effect of atenolol and captopril in reducing macrovascular and microvascular complications over a 9 year follow-up period. Figure 10 shows the effect of the 2 agents in reducing the 7 primary endpoints (plus heart failure- a secondary end point) vs less-tight control of blood pressure. It is apparent that all 8 trends favoured the BB (over the ACE-I) which reduced stroke-risk by about 50 %, peripheral arterial disease-related endpoints by about 60 %, microvascular (kidney and eye) endpoints by about 45 %, and heart failure by about 65 %. Thus, the UKPDS-39 (UK Prospective Diabetes Study Group 1998) results, like MRC-1 (Medical Research Working Party 1985), deny totally the claim that BBs are relatively ineffective in preventing stroke in young/middle-aged hypertensive subjects.

The UKPDS patients were monitored for a further 10 years, with a median total follow-up time of 14.5 years (Holman et al. 2008). The trends favouring the beta-blocker over the ACE-inhibitor tended to persist, but now, in the case of all-cause death, there was a significant 23 % reduction in favour of atenolol – Fig. 11. There is thus no truth in the claim that BBs do not reduce all cause death (Wu et al. 2013; Prospective Studies Collaboration 2002; Wiysonge and Opie 2013; Lindholm et al. 2005).

In middle-aged patients with pre/mild hypertension plus stable myocardial ischemia (von Armin and for the TIBBS Investigators 1996), randomised to either highly beta-1 selective (cardioselective) bisoprolol or nifedipine SR, at

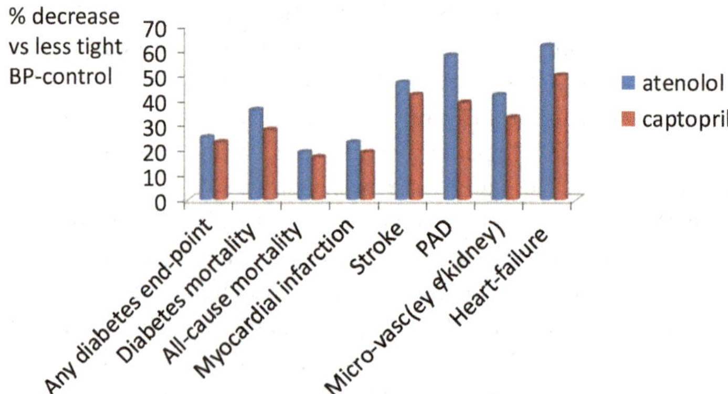

Fig. 10 UKPDS 39 – all primary end-point trends favour atenolol vs captopril when compared with less-tight BP control (BP diff 10/5 mm Hg)

1 year follow-up, event-free survival was significantly superior in those randomised to bisoprolol.

4. The possible mechanism of the reduction in all-cause death by long-term beta-blockade (in middle-age)

In UKPDS-39, apart from all-cause death, all other benefits of atenolol (relative to ACE-I) noted after the initial study (UK Prospective Diabetes Study Group 1998), tended to diminish with time (mean follow-up time 14.5 years) (Holman et al. 2008). So what other factors might be in evidence?

BBs have been observed by several authors, to modify the initiation and spread of various cancers. Certainly stress has been noted to hasten cancer-progression, probably via activation of tumour-associated beta-receptors by epinephrine and norepinephrine (Cole and Sood 2012; Fitzgerald 2012). Thus, beta-blockade has been noted to benefit 1. Breast cancer and prevent metastases (Cakir et al. 2002; Barron et al. 2011; Melhem-Bertrandt et al. 2011) 2. Colon cancer (Takezaki et al. 2001; Perrone et al. 2008) 3. Pancreatic cancer (Weddle et al. 2001; Zhang et al. 2010) 4. Melanoma (De Giorgi et al. 2012) 5. Lung cancer (Al-Wadei et al. 2012) 6. Neuroblastoma (Pasquier et al. 2013) 7. Prostate cancer (Perron et al. 2004; Grytli et al. 2013) –Table 2. This likely anti-cancer property of BBs is particularly important in the context of the increased risk of cancer in middle-aged hypertensive subjects (Harding et al. 2016).

5. The important beta-blocker/smoking interaction in younger/middle-aged hypertensive subjects

In three major prospective, randomised, hard-endpoint studies in middle-aged hypertensive subjects, cigarette smoking played a vital role in modifying the potential of the BB to reduce the risk of a cardiovascular event. The MRC-1 study (Medical Research Working Party 1985) compared non-selective propranolol with a

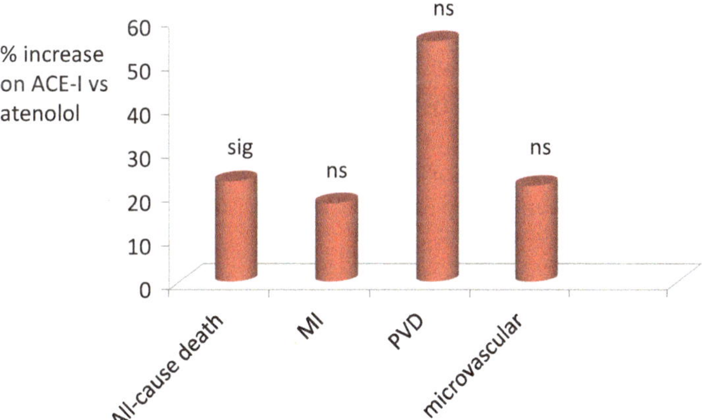

Fig. 11 UKPDS study 20 year follow-up (mean 14.5 years); significant (p < 0.05) 23 % increase in all-cause death on ACE-I (vs atenolol) (Holman et al. 2008)

Table 2 Cancers that may benefit from beta-blockade

Breast (Cakir et al. (2002); Barron et al. (2011); Melhem-Bertrandt et al. (2011))
Colon (Takezaki et al. (2001); Perrone et al. (2008))
Pancreas (Weddle et al. (2001); Zhang et al. (2010))
Melanoma (De Giorgi et al. (2012))
Lung (Al-Wadei et al. (2012))
Neuroblastoma (Pasquier et al. (2013))
Prostate (Perron et al. (2004); Grytli et al. (2013))

thiazide diuretic and placebo, in 17,354 subjects, of whom 30 % of men and 25 % of women were smokers, over a 5 year follow-up period. The IPPPSH study (The IPPPSH Collaborative Group 1985) compared non-selective oxprenolol with placebo, in 6357 subjects, of whom 29 % were smokers, over a 3–5 year follow-up period. The MAPPY study (Wikstrand et al. 1991) (an extension of the HAPPHY study (Wilhelmsen et al. 1987)) compared moderately selective metoprolol with a thiazide diuretic, in 3156 subjects, of whom 34 % were smokers, followed-up for 4 years.

In the case of myocardial infarction (about 3 times more common than stroke in the young/middle-aged hypertensive subject (Medical Research Working Party 1985)), the ability of the BB to reduce the risk of an event by 33–49 % (vs randomised placebo or diuretic therapy) in non-smokers, was not observed in smokers (Medical Research Working Party 1985; The IPPPSH Collaborative Group 1985; Wikstrand et al. 1991). Indeed, in the case of non-selective propranolol and oxprenolol, the risk of myocardial infarction was actually increased by 13–35 % in smokers – Fig. 12. A similar result relating to stroke was also noted in MRC-I (Medical Research Working Party 1985). In the MRC-elderly study (MRC Working Party 1992), atenolol (vs randomised placebo) increased the rate of cardiovascular events by 38 % in smokers, compared to a modest 16 % reduction in non-smokers.

How can these events relating to smokers be explained and avoided? Cigarette smoking is linked to a two-to threefold increase in plasma epinephrine (adrenaline) levels (Cryer et al. 1976). Epinephine stimulates beta-1, beta-2, and alpha receptors, and in the presence of non-selective beta-blockers (and to a lesser extent with only moderately beta-selective agents like metoprolol and atenolol) there is unopposed (total or partial) alpha-vasoconstriction, resulting in an increase in blood pressure (Tarnow and Muller 1991). This increase in blood pressure is about 30 mm Hg for non-selective BBs, and about 9–10 mm Hg for a moderately selective agent like metoprolol, compared to no change in blood pressure (vs control) with a highly beta-1 selective beta-blocker like bisoprolol (which permits full beta-2-stimulation-induced vasodilatation) (Wellstein et al. 1986; Smith and Teitler 1999). Thus, the adverse BB/hypertensive/smoking interaction can be avoided by high beta-1 selectivity (cardioselectivity).

6. The gender debate

The proven benefit of beta-blockade in younger/middle-aged hypertensive subjects has been confined to men. In the MRC-1 trial (Medical Research Working Party 1985), the reduction in all-cause death (vs placebo) was confined to active treatment (both diuretic and beta-blocker therapy) in men only (there was an increase in women). Also in the MRC-1 trial, the 33 %

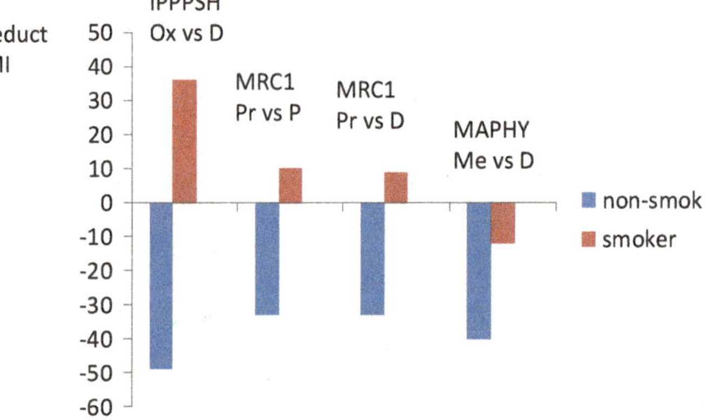

Fig. 12 BB/Smoking interaction, re reduction of myocardial infarction (MI) risk in young/mid-age hypertensives; P = placebo, D = diuretic, Ox = oxprenolol, Pr = propranolol, Me = metoprolol

reduction in coronary events in non-smoking men was confined to propranolol. Likewise in the IPPPSH study (The IPPPSH Collaborative Group 1985) involving young/middle-age hypertensive subjects, oxprenolol (vs placebo) significantly reduced cardiac events only in men, the opposite being the case for women. In the MAPHY study in male younger/middle-aged hypertensive subjects, metoprolol significantly reduced the risk of coronary events only in non-smokers. In the UKPDS-39 study (UK Prospective Diabetes Study Group 1998), 45 % were women, but the significant effects of atenolol (vs less-tight control of BP) were not analysed in terms of sexual gender.

7. Beta-blockers and Black hypertensive subjects

Black hypertensive patients usually have low plasma renin levels (Cruickshank and Prichard 1994), which were thought to account for the poor antihypertensive effect of propranolol, vs diuretics, in middle-aged Black subjects (Hammond et al. 1978). In contrast, highly beta-1 selective bisoprolol lowered BP equally in White and Black middle-aged hypertensive patients (Frishman et al. 1995; Prisant and Mensah 1996).

In the AASK Study (Norris et al. 2006), involving 1094 middle-aged African American patients with hypertension and renal dysfunction, after 4 years follow-up metoprolol, ramipril, and amlodipine all had similar effects in reducing the cumulative incidence of composite cardiovascular outcomes.

8. The importance of first-line therapy

The outcome of a drug trial is dependent on which therapy is given first-line. A classic example is the MRC-elderly study (MRC Working Party 1992). In that randomised placebo-controlled trial, there were 2 active, randomised therapy groups, namely 1. first-line diuretic, followed by (if necessary) add-on beta-blocker (atenolol), and 2. first-line beta-blocker, followed by (if necessary) add-on diuretic. Only first-line diuretic/second-line beta-blocker therapy was associated with significant risk-reduction regarding stroke, coronary events, and all cardiovascular events.

4 Summary and Recommendations

There is disagreement amongst leading Guideline Committees around the world on the role of beta-blockers in the treatment of hypertension. Unless age is taken into account, wrong conclusions will arise. Meta-analyses that do not consider age as a factor have been unfavourable to beta-blockers. By contrast, meta-analyses that include age as a factor, show that beta-blockers perform well in the younger/middle-age group (less than 60 years) in terms of preventing death/stroke/myocardial infarction (vs randomised placebo and other antihypertensive drugs).

Diastolic hypertension in younger/middle-aged subjects is closely associated with overweight/obesity and high sympathetic nerve activity. High sympathetic drive (independent of blood pressure) and high resting heart rates are linked to premature cardiovascular events and death in young/middle-aged hypertension. Antihypertensive drugs that increase sympathetic nerve activity (diuretics, dihydropyridine calcium blockers, and ARBs) are thus inappropriate first-line agents in younger/middle-aged hypertensive subjects. In this younger group, first-line beta-blockade was superior to placebo and diuretics in preventing myocardial infarction (certainly in non-smoker males). Beta-blockade was also at least as good as ACE-inhibition in reducing the risk of all 7 hard end-points (vs less-tight control of BP), including a 50 % reduction in stroke-risk, and was significantly superior in preventing all-cause death after long-term follow-up (beta-blockers have anti-cancer properties).

Thus, beta-blockade is a highly reasonable first-line choice in the treatment of the younger/ middle-aged hypertensive subject (certainly in non-smoker men). There is an urgent need for leading Guide-line Committees to be aware of the importance of obesity and the sympathetic nervous system in hypertension in the young/ middle-aged (and treatment implications), and for there to be a general consensus on the role of beta-blockers in the treatment of hypertension.

Conflicts of Interest The author has no conflicts of interest.

References

Al-Wadei HA, Al-wadei MH, Schuller HM (2012) Cooperative regulation of non-small cell lung carcinoma by nicotinic and beta-adrenergic receptors: a novel target for intervention. PLoS One 7:e29915. Epub 2012

Barnes MJ, McDougal DH (2014) Leptin into the rostral ventral lateral medulla (RVLM) augments renal sympathetic nerve activity and blood pressure. Front Neurosci 8:232

Barron TL, Conolly RM, Sharp L, Bennett K, Visvanathan K (2011) Beta-blockers and breast cancer mortality: a population-based study. J Clin Oncol 29:2635–2644

Berglund G, Andersin O, Widgren B (1986) Low-dose antihypertensive treatment with a thiazide diuretic is not diabetogenic. Acta Med Scand 220:419–424

Black HR, Elliot WJ, Grandits G, Grambcsh P, Lucente T, White WB et al (2003) Principal results of the Controlled Onset Verapamil Investigation Of Cardiovascular End Points (CONVINCE) Trial. JAMA 289:2073–2082

Brooks VL, Shi Z, Holwerda SW, Fadel PJ (2015) Obesity-induced increases in sympathetic nerve activity: sex matters. Auton Neurosci 187:18–26. doi:10. 1016/j.Autoneu.2014.11.006, Epub 2014 Nov 20

Cakir Y, Plummer HK, Tithof PK, Schuller HM (2002) Beta-adrenergic and arachidonic acid-mediated growth regulation of human breast cancer cell lines. Int J Oncol 21:153–157

Coats AJS, Cruickshank JM (2014) Hypertensive subjects with type-2 diabetes, the sympathetic nervous system, and treatment implications. Int J Cardiol 174:702–709

Cole SW, Sood AK (2012) Molecular pathways: beta-adrenergic signaling in cancer. Clin Cancer Res 18:1201–1206

Coope J, Warrender TS (1986) Randomised trial of treatment of hypertension in elderly patients in primary care. BMJ 293:1145–1151

Cruickshank JM (2013) Essential hypertension. People's Publishing House, Shelton

Cruickshank JM (2014) The unholy alliance between obesity, type-2 diabetes, the sympathetic nervous system, and hypertension in young/middle-aged subjects. J Mol Genet Med S1. http://dd.org/10.4172/1747-0862.S1-016

Cruickshank JM, Prichard BNC (1994) Beta-blockers in clinical practice (2nd edn). Churchill Livingstone, Edinburgh, pp 1–351

Cryer PE, Haymond MW, Satiago JV, Shar SP (1976) Norepinephrine and epinephrine release and adrenergic mediation of smoking-associated hemodynamic and metabolic events. N Engl J Med 295:573–577

Dahlof B, Lindholm LH, Hansson L, Schersten B, Ekbom T, Wester PO (1991) Morbidity and mortality in the Swedish Trial in Old Patients with hypertension (STOP-Hypertension). Lancet 338:1281–1285

Dahlof B, Devereux RB, Kjeldsen SE, Julius S, Beevers G, Faire U et al (2002) LIFE Study Group. Cardiovascular morbidity and mortality in the Losartan Intervention for Endpoint reduction in hypertension study (LIFE): a randomised trial against atenolol. Lancet 359:995–1003

Dahlof B, Sever PS, Poulter NR et al (2005) Prevention of cardiovascular events with an antihypertensive regimen of amlodipine adding perindopril as required versus atenolol adding bendroflumethiazide as required, in the Anglo-Scandanavian Cardiac Outcomes Trial-Blood Pressure Lowering Arm (ASCOT-BPLA): a multicentre randomised controlled trial. Lancet 366:895–906

De Giorgi V, Gandini S, Grazzini M, Benemai S, Marchionni N, Geppetti P (2012) Beta-blockers: a new and emerging treatment for melanoma. Recenti Prog Med 103:11–16

Deary AJ, Schumann AL, Murfeet H, Haydock SF, Foo RS, Brown MJ (2002) Double-blind, placebo controlled crossover comparison of 5 classes of drugs. J Hypertens 20:771–777

Druktenis JS, Roman MJ, Fabsitz RR, Lee ET, Best LG, Russel M et al (2007) Cardiac and systemic hemodynamic characteristics of hypertension and prehypertension in adolescents and young adults. The Strong Heart Study. Circulation 115:221–227

Eriksson S, Olofsson B-O, Wester P-O, for the TEST Study Group (1995) Atenolol in secondary prevention after stroke. Cerebrovasc Dis 5:21–25

Esler MO, Jennings GL, Johns J, Burke F, Little PJ, Leonard P (1984) Estimation of "total" renal, cardiac and splanchnic sympathetic nervous tone in essential hypertension from measurements of noradrenaline release. J Hypertens Suppl 2(3):S123–S125

Estacio RO, Jeffers BW, Hiatt W, Biggerstaff SL, Gifford N, Schrier RW (1998) The effect of nisoldipine as compared with enalapril on cardiovascular outcomes in patients with non-insulin-dependent diabetes and hypertension. N Engl J Med 338:645–652

Feldman RD, Limbird LE, Nadeau J, Robertson D, Wood AJ (1984) Alteration in leukocyte beta-receptor affinity with aging. A potential explanation for altered beta-adrenergic sensitivity in the elderly. N Engl J Med 310:815–819

Fitzgerald PJ (2012) Beta-blockers, norepinephrine, and cancer: an epidemiological viewpoint. Clin Epidemiol 4:151–156

Fogari R, Zoppi A, Coradi L, Preti P, Malalamani GD, Muellini A (2000) Effects of different dihydropyridine calcium antagonists on plasma norepinephrine in essential hypertension. J Hypertens 18:1871–1875

Franklin SS, Pio JR, Wong ND, Larson MG, Leip EP, Vasan RS et al (2005) Predictors of new-onset diastolic and systolic hypertension. The Framingham Heart Study. Circulation 111:1121–1127

Frishman WH, Burris JF, Mroczek WJ, Weir MR, Alemayehu D, Simon JS et al (1995) First-line therapy option with low-dose bisoprolol fumarate and low-dose hydrochlorthiazide in patients with stage 1 and stage 11 systemic hypertension. J Clin Pharmacol 35:182–188

Gillman MW, Kannel WB, Belanger A (1993) Influence of heart rate on mortality among persons with hypertension: the Framingham Study. Am Heart J 125:1148–1154

Grassi G, Dell Oro R, Facchini A, Quarti Trevano F, Bolla GB, Mancia G (2004) Effect of central and peripheral body fat distribution on sympathetic and baroreflex functionin obese normotensives. J Hypertens 22:236–239

Grytli HH, Fagerland MW, Fossa SD, Tasken KA, Hanheim LL (2013) Use of beta-blockers is associated with prostate cancer-specific survival in prostate cancer patients on androgen deprivation therapy. Prostate 73:250–260

Haller H, Ito S, Izzo JL, Januszewicz A, Katayama S, Menne J et al (2011) Olmesartan for the delay or prevention of microalbuminuria in type-2 diabetes. N Engl J Med 364;907–917

Hammond JJ, Kirkendall WM, Zama A, Thomas JC, Overturf ML (1978) Pindolol, propranolol and chlorthalidone in moderate hypertension. Pharmacologist 20:189

Hansson L, Linholm LH, Niskanen L, Lanke J, Hedner T, Niklason A et al (1999a) Effect of angiotensin-converting-enzyme inhibition compared with conventional therapy on cardiovascular morbidity and mortality in hypertension: the Captopril Prevention Project(CAPP)randomised trial. Lancet 353:611–616

Hansson L, Lindholm LH, Ekbom T, Dahlof B, Lanke J, Schersten B et al (1999b) Randomised trial of old and new antihypertensive drugs in elderly patients: cardiovascular mortality and morbidity in the Swedish Trial in Old Patients with Hypertension-2 study. Lancet 354:1751–1756

Hansson L, Hedner T, Lund-Johansen P, Kjeldsen SE, Lindholm LH, Syvertsen JO et al (2000) Randomised of effects of calcium antagonists compared with diuretics and beta-blockers on cardiovascular morbidity and mortality: the Nordic Diltiazem (NORDIL) study. Lancet 356:359–365

Harding JL, Sooriyakumaran M, Anstey KJ, Adam R, Balkau B, Brennan-Olsen S et al (2016) Hypertension, antihypertensive treatment and cancer incidence and mortality: a pooled collaborative analysis of 12 - Australian and New Zealand cohorts. J Hypertens 34:149–155

Hart EC, Charkoudian N (2014) Sympathetic neural regulation of blood pressure: influence of sex and age. Physiology (Bethesda) 29:8–15

Heidland UE, Strauer BE (2001) Left ventricular muscle mass and elevated heart rate are associated with coronary plaque disruption. Circulation 104:1477–1482

Helin P, Lorenzen I, Garbash C, Matthiessen ME (1970) Atherosclerosis in rabbit aorta induced by noradrenaline. The importance of the duration of noradrenaline action. Atherosclerosis 12:125–132

Heuser K, Vitkovsky J, Raasch W, Schmieder R, Schobel HP (2003) Elevation of sympathetic activity by eprosartan in young male subjects. Am J Hypertens 16:658–664

Hiltunen TP, Suonsyrja T, Hanilla-Handelberg T, Paarvonen KJ, Miettinen HE, Strandberg T et al (2007) Predictors of antihypertensive drug responses: initial data from a placebo-controlled, randomesed, cross-over study with foue antihypertensive drugs (The GENRES Study). Am J Hypertens 20 (3):311–318

Holman RR, Paul SK, Bethel MA, Neil HA, Matthews DR (2008) Long-term follow-up after tight control of blood pressure in type-2 diabetes. N Engl J Med 359:1565–1576

Huggett RJ, Scott EM, Gilbey SG, Stoker JB, Macintosh AF, Mary DA (2003) Impact of type-2 diabetes on sympathetic neural mechanisms in hypertension. Circulation 108:3097–4101

Imai E, Chan JC, Ito S, Yamasaki T, Kobayashi F, Hanada M et al (2011) Effects of olmesartan on renal and cardiovascular outcomes in type-2 diabetes with overt nephropathy: a multicentre, randomised, placebo-controlled study. Diabetologia 54:2978–2986

Inge TH, Courcoulas AP, Jenkins TM, Michalski MP, Helmrath MA, Brandt MD et al (2016) Weight loss and health status 3 years after bariatric surgery in adolescents. N Engl J Med 374:113–123

James PA, Oparil S, Carter BL, Cushman WC, Dennison-Himmelfarb C, Handler J et al (2014) 2014 evidence-based guideline for the management of high blood pressure in adults. Report from the panel members appointed to the Eighth Joint National Committee (JNC 8). JAMA 311:507–520

Khan N, McAlister FA (2006) Re-examining the efficacy of beta-blockers for the treatment of hypertension: a meta-analysis. CMAJ 174:1737–1742

Khan NA, Hemmelgarn B, Herman RJ, Bell CM, Mahon JL, Leiter LA et al (2009) The 2009 Canadian Hypertension Education Program recommendations for the management of hypertension: Part 2 – therapy. Can J Cardiol 25(5):287–298

Kostis V, Nilsson P, Grassi G, Mancia G, Redon J, Luft F et al (2015) New developments in the pathogenesis of obesity-induced hypertension. J Hypertens 33:1499–1508

Krause T, Lovibond K, Caufield M, McCormak T, Williams B (2011) Management of hypertension: summary of NICE guidelines. BMJ 343:d4891. doi:10.1136/bmj:d4891

Kuyper LM, Kahn NA (2014) Atenolol vs non-atenolol beta-blockers for the treatment of hypertension: a meta-analysis. Can J Cardiol 30(suppl 5):S47–S53

Lambert E, Straznicky N, Schlaich M, Esler MP, Haikerwal D, Brencley D et al (2007) Differing pattern of sympathoexcitation in normal- weight and obesity-related hypertension. Hypertension 50:862–868

Leren P, Heigeland A (1986) Coronary heart disease and treatment of hypertension. The Oslo Study. Am J Med 80:3–6

Lindholm LH, Carlberg B, Samuelsson O (2005) Should beta-blockers remain the first choice in the treatment of primary hypertension? A meta-analysis. Lancet 366:1545–1553

Mancia G, De Backer G, Dominiczak A, Cifcova R, Fagard R, Gernano G et al (2007) 2007 Guidelines forthe management of arterial hypertension. The task force for the management of arterial hypertension of the European Society of Hypertension (ESH) and of the European Society of Cardiology (ESC). Eur Heart J 28:1462–1536

Medical Research Working Party (1985) MRC trial of treatment of mild hypertension: principle results. BMJ 291:97–104

Melhem-Bertrandt A, Chavez-Macgreggor LX, Brown EN, Lee RT, Meric-Bernstam F et al (2011) Beta-blocker use is associated with improved relapse-free survival in patients with triple-negative breast cancer. J Clin Oncol 29:2645–2652

Menon DV, Arbique D, Wang Z, Adam-Huet B, Auchus RJ, Vongpatanasin W (2009) Differential effects of chlorthalidone versus spironolactone on muscle sympathetic nerve activity in hypertensive patients. J Clin Endocrinol Metab 94:1361–1366

Moltzer E, Mattace Raso FU, Karamermer Y, Boersma E, Webb GD, Simoons ML et al (2010) Comparison of candesartan versus metoprolol for treatment of systemic hypertension after repaired aortic coarctation. Am J Cardiol 105:217–222

MRC Working Party (1992) Medical Research Council trial of treatment of hypertension in older adults.: principal results. BMJ 304:405–412

Neutel JM, Smith DH, Ram CV, Kaplan NM, Papademetriou V, Fagan TC et al (1993) Application of ambulatory blood pressure monitoring in differentiating between antihypertensive agents. Am J Med 94:181–187

No author listed (1980) The Australian therapeutic trial in hypertension. Report by the Management Committee. Lancet 1:1261–1267

Noll G, Wenzel RR, de Marchi S, Shaw S, Luscher TF (1997) Differential effects of captopril and nitrates on muscle sympathetic nerve activity in volunteers. Circulation 95:2286–2292

Norris K, Bourgoigne J, Gassman J, Hibert L, Middleton J, Phillips RA et al (2006) Cardiovascular outcomes in the African American Study of Kidney Disease and Hypertension (AASK) Trial. Am J Kidney Dis 48:739–751

Palatini P, Julius S (2009) The role of cardiac autonomic function in hypertension and cardiovascular disease. Curr Hypertens Rep 11:199–205

Parrinello G, Paterna S, Torres D, Di Pasquale P, Mezzero M, La Rocca G et al (2009) One year renal and cardiac effect of bisoprolol versus losartan in recently diagnosed hypertensive patients. Clin Drug Investig 29:591–600

Pasquier E, Street J, Pouchy C, Carre M, Gifford AJ, Murray J et al (2013) Beta-blockers increase response to chemotherapy via direct anti-tumor and anti-angiogenic mechanisms in neuroblastoma. Br J Cancer 108:2485–2494

Peng Y-X, Shan J, Qi XY, Qi XY, Zhang SJ, Mu SP, Wang N et al (2006) The catecholamine-beta-adrenoceptor-cAMP system and prediction of cardiovascular events in hypertension. Clin Exp Pharmacol Physiol 33:27–231

Pepine CJ, Handberg EM, Cooper-DeHoff RM, Marks RG, Kowey P, Messerli FH et al (2003) A calcium antagonist vs a non-calcium antagonist hypertension treatment strategy for patients with coronary artery disease. The International Verapamil-Trandolapril Study (INVEST): a randomised controlled trial. JAMA 290:2805–2816

Perron L, Bairati L, Harel F, Meyer F (2004) Antihypertensive drug use and the risk of prostate cancer (Canada). Cancer Causes Control 15:535–541

Perrone MG, Notanicola M, Caruso MG, Tutino V, Scilimati A (2008) Upregulation of beta-3adrenergic receptor mRNA in human colon cancer: a preliminary study. Oncology 75:224–229

Prisant LM, Mensah GA (1996) Use of beta-adrenergic receptor blockers in blacks. J Clin Pharmacol 36:867–873

Prospective Studies Collaboration (2002) Age-specific relevance of usual blood pressure to vascular mortality: a meta-analysis of individual data for one million adults in 61 prospective studies. Lancet 360:1903–1913

Robb OJ, Petrie JC, Webster J, Harry J (1985) ICI 118,551 does not reduce blood pressure in hypertensive patients responsive to atenolol and propranolol. Br J Clin Pharmacol 19:541–542

Seravalle G, Lonati L, Buzzi S, Cairo M, Quarti Trevano F, Dell'Oro R et al (2015) Sympathetic nerve traffic and baroreflex function in optimal, normal, and high-normal blood pressure states. J Hypertens 33(7):1411–1417. doi:10.1097/HJH.000000000000567

SHEP Cooperative Research Group (1991) Prevention of stroke by antihypertensive drug treatment in older persons with isolated systolic hypertension. JAMA 265:3255–3264

Sipahi I, Tuzcu M, Wolski KE, Nicholls SJ, Schoenhagen P, Hu B et al (2007) Beta-blockers and progression of coronary atherosclerosis: pooled analysis of 4 intravascular ultrasonography trials. Am Int Med 147:10–18

Smith C, Teitler M (1999) Beta-blocker selectivity at cloned human beta-1 and beta-2 adrenergic receptors. Carsiovasc Drugs Ther 13:126–127

Sowers JR, Lester M (2000) Hypertension, hormones and aging. J Lab Clin Med 135:379–386

Straus MH, Hall AS (2007) Renin-angiotensin system and cardiovascular talk. Lancet 370:23–24

Strauss MH, Hall AS (2006) Angiotensin receptor blockers may increase the risk of myocardial infarction. Circulation 114:838–854

Takezaki T, Hamajima N, Maisuo K, Tanaka R, Hirai T, Kato T et al (2001) Association of polymorphisms in the beta-2 and beta-3 adrenoceptor genes with risk of colorectal cancer in Japanese. Int J Clin Oncol 6:117–122

Tarnow J, Muller RK (1991) Cardiovascular effects of low-dose epinephrine infusions in relation to the extent of pre-operative beta-blockade. Anaesthesiology 74:1035–1043

Tenero DM, Bottorf MB, Burlew BS, Williams JB, Lalande RL (1990) Altered beta-adrenergic sensitivity and protein binding to I-propranolol in the elderly. Cardiovasc Pharmacol 16:702–707

The ALLHAT Officers and Coordinators for the ALLHAT Collaborative Research Group (2002) Major outcomes in high-risk hypertensive patients randomised to ACE-inhibitor or calcium channel blocker vs diuretic. JAMA 288:2981–2997

The IPPPSH Collaborative Group (1985) Cardiovascular risk and risk factors in a randomised trial of treatment based on the beta-blocker oxprenolol: the International prospective primary prevention study in hypertension (IPPPSH). J Hypertens 3:379–392

Thomopoulos C, Parati G, Zanchetti A (2015a) Effects of blood pressure-lowering on outcome incidence in hypertension: 4. Effects of various classes of antihypertensive drugs –Overview and meta-analysis. J Hypertens 33:195–211

Thomopoulos C, Parati G, Zanchetti A (2015b) Effects of blood pressure-lowering on outcome incidence in hypertension: head-to-head comparisons of various classes of antihypertensive drugs – overview and meta-analyses. J Hypertens 33:1321–1341

Trial of secondary prevention with atenolol after transient ischemic attack or nondisabling stroke. The Dutch TIA Trial Study Group. Stroke 24:543–548 (1993)

U.K. Prospective Diabetes Study Group (1998) Tight blood pressure control and risk of macrovascular and microvascular complications in type-2 diabetes. UKPDS 38. BMJ 317:703–713

UK Prospective Diabetes Study Group (1998) Efficacy of atenolol and captopril reducing risk of macrovascular and microvascular complications of type-2 diabetes: UKPDS 39. BMJ 317:713–720

Veterans Administration Cooperative Study Group on Antihypertensive Agents (1982) Comparison of propranolol and hydrochlorthiazide for the initial treatment of hypertension. Results of long-term therapy. JAMA 248:2004–2011

von Armin T, for the TIBBS Investigators (1996) Prognostic significance of transient ischemic episodes: response to treatment shows improve prognosis. J Am Coll Cardiol 28:20–24

Weddle D, Tiihoff P, Williams M, Schuller HM (2001) Beta-adrenergic growth regulation of human cancer cell lines derived from pancreatic ductal carcinomas. Carcinogenesis 22:473–479

Wellstein A, Palm D, Belz GG (1986) Affinity and selectivity of beta-adrenoceptor antagonists in vitro. J Cardiovasc Pharmacol 8(Suppl):S36–S40

Wikstrand J, Warnold T, Tuomilehto J, Olsson G, Barber HJ, Eliasson K et al (1991) Metoprolol versus diuretics in hypertension. Morbidity results from MAPHY study. Hypertension 17:579–588

Wilhelmsen L, Bergland G, Elmfeldt D, Fitzsimons T, Holzgreve H, Hosie J et al (1987) Beta-blockers versus diuretics in hypertensive men: main results from the HAPPHY trial. J Hypertens 5:561–572

Williams B (2007) The obese hypertensive. The weight of evidence against beta-blockers. Circulation 115:1973–1974

Wiysonge CS, Opie LH (2013) Beta-blockers as initial therapy for hypertension. JAMA 310:1851–1852

Wright JT, Bakris GL, Green T (2002) Effect of blood pressure lowering and antihypertensive drug class on progression of hypertensive kidney disease. Results from the AASK trial. JAMA 288:2421–2431

Wu H-Y, Huang J-W, Lin H-J, Liao WC, Peng YS, Hung KY et al (2013) Comparative effectiveness of renin-angiotensin system blockers and of other antihypertensive drugs in patients with diabetes: systematic review and bayesian network meta-analysis. BMJ 347:f6008. doi:10.1136/bmj.f6008

Xue H, Lu Z, Tang, WL, Pang LW, Wang GM, Wong GW et al (2015). First-line drugs inhibiting the renin angiotensin system versus other first-line antihypertensive drug classes for hypertension. Cochrane Database Syst Rev 1:CD008170. doi:10.1002/14651858. CD008170.pub2

Yamada Y, Miyajima E, Tochicubo O, Matsukawa T, Isshi M (1989) Age related changes in muscle sympathetic nerve activity in essential hypertension. Hypertension 13:870–877

Yurenev AP, Dyakonova HG, Novikov ID (1992) Management of essential hypertension in patients with different degrees of left ventricular hyperterophy. Multicentre trial. Am J Hypertens 6(S):182S–189S

Zacharias FJ, Cowen KJ (1977) Comparison of propranolol and atenolol in hypertension. Postgrad Med J 53:111–113

Zanchetti A, Bond MG, Henning M, Neiss A, Mancia G, Dal Palu C et al (2002) Calcium antagonist lacidipine slows down progression asymptomatic carotid atherosclerosis. Principal results of the European lacidipine study on atherosclerosis (ELSA), a randonised, double-blind, long-term trial. Circulation 106:2422–2427

Zhang D, Ma QY, Hu HT, Zhang M (2010) Beta2-adrenergic antagonists suppress pancreatic cancer cell invasion by inhibiting CREB, NFkB and AP-1. Cancer Biol Ther 10:19–29

Adv Exp Med Biol - Advances in Internal Medicine (2017) 2: 167–180
DOI 10.1007/5584_2016_149
© Springer International Publishing AG 2016
Published online: 5 November 2016

Challenges in the Management of Hypertension in Older Populations

Lisa Pont and Tariq Alhawassi

Abstract

The prevalence of hypertension increases with age making it a significant health concern for older persons. Aging involves a range of physiological changes such as increases in arterial stiffness, widening pulse pressure, changes in renin and aldosterone levels, decreases in renal salt excretion, declining in renal function, changes in the autonomic nervous system sensitivity and function and changes to endothelial function all of which may not only affect blood pressure but may also affect individual response to pharmacotherapy used to manage hypertension and prevent end organ damage and other complications associated with poor blood pressure control.

Unlike many chronic conditions where there is limited evidence for management in older populations, there is good evidence regarding the management of hypertension in the elderly. The findings from multiple large, robust trials have provided a solid evidence-base regarding the management of hypertension in older adults, showing that reduction of blood pressure in older hypertensive populations is associated with reduced mortality and morbidity. Diuretics, agents action on the renin angiotensin system, beta blockers and calcium channel blockers have all been well studied in older populations both in view of the benefits associated with blood pressure lowering and the risks associated with associated adverse events. While all antihypertensive agents will lower blood pressure, when managing hypertension in older persons the choice of agent is dependent not only on the ability to lower blood pressure but also on the potential for harm with older persons. Understanding such potential harms in older populations is essential with older persons experiencing increased sensitivity to many of the adverse effects such as dizziness associated with the use of antihypertensive agents.

L. Pont (✉)
Centre for Health System and Safety Research, Australian Institute of Health Innovation, Macquarie University, North Ryde, Australia
e-mail: lisa.pont@mq.edu.au

T. Alhawassi
College of Pharmacy, King Saud University, Riyadh, Saudi Arabia

Despite the wealth of evidence regarding the benefits of managing hypertension in the old and very old, a significant proportion of older individuals with hypertension have suboptimal BP control. While there is good evidence supporting blood pressure lowering in older antihypertensive agents, these have not yet been optimally translated fully into clinical guidelines and clinical practice. There appear to be considerable differences between guidelines in terms of the guidance given to clinicians. Differences in interpretation of the evidence, as well as differences in study design and populations all contribute to differences in the guideline recommendations with respect to older populations, despite the strength of the underlying scientific evidence. Differences around who is considered "old" and what BP targets and management are considered appropriate may lead to confusion among clinicians and further contribute to the evidence-practice lag.

Keywords

Hypertension • Pharmacotherapy • Guidelines • Antihypertensive • Aged • Older • Drug therapy

Hypertension is the leading modifiable cause of mortality worldwide. The prevalence of hypertension increases with age making it a significant health concern for older persons. Unlike many chronic conditions, there is good evidence regarding the management of hypertension in the elderly exists and pharmacotherapy is the mainstay of treatment for most patients. Given predicted international increases in the elderly population and the wealth of evidence regarding management of hypertension in the elderly, understanding how the risks associated with hypertension increase with age as well as how physicians currently manage older patients with increased blood pressure is important. Furthermore, insight into current barriers to the provision of optimal management is essential if we are to meet the health needs of the growing older population.

1   Who Is Old?

Internationally the proportion of the population that is considered older is increasing. In 1950, 8 % of the population was aged over 65 years, this increased to 10 % in 2000 and is predicted to exceed 20 % by 2050.(Department of Economic and Social Affairs United Nations 2002) It has been estimated that life expectancy for those aged 65 years has increased by 19 years for men and 17 years for women over the past century.(Rai and Mulley 2007) Projections indicate that by 2050 there will be over 2 billion older persons worldwide.(Halter 2009) However while there is international agreement that the population is aging there is less agreement regarding who should be considered "old". (Gambert 1994) Aging encompasses a number of domains and different definitions focus on different aspects of the aging process. Chronological age is the simplest and most commonly used parameter to define age and refers simply to the number of years since birth. Yet aging is multidimensional and not just related to the duration of time in an individual's life. Physiologically, aging refers to the general and gradual changes that human body experiences over time. Physiological aging is characterized by declining functional capacity, decreasing fertility and increased mortality all of which may vary from individual to individual. (Kirkwood and Austad 2000; Masoro and Austad 2006) Such variation among older populations and how it affects their response to pharmacotherapy is one of the challenges facing clinicians in the management of hypertension among older populations.

2 Hypertension and Aging

Population aging presents a number of healthcare challenges. There are implications in terms of resources and funding, as well as in the type of care that is delivered. Non-communicable chronic diseases such as cardiovascular disease currently account for almost two-thirds of deaths worldwide. (Mathers and Loncar 2006; Daar et al. 2007) Cardiovascular disease contributes significantly to the disease burden, disability and death in both developed and developing countries (Beaglehole et al. 2008; Murray and Lopez 1997; Yang et al. 2008) with an increasing burden among the elderly..(Daar et al. 2007; Murray and Lopez 1997) Despite predicted increases in population aging, The World Health Organization (WHO) has predicted that ischemic heart disease and stroke will remain among the leading causes of death worldwide. (Mathers and Loncar 2006) Hypertension is a major risk factor for cardiovascular disease (Menotti et al. 2004; Lim et al. 2013), affecting up to one billion individuals internationally (Chobanian et al. 2003) (Kumar 2013). It is one of the leading cause of death worldwide (The World Health Organisation 2016). The prevalence of hypertension increases with age (Fagard 2002), with approximately 30 % of the population aged under 60 years being considered hypertensive. Once we start looking at older populations, the prevalence of hypertension doubles to over 60 % for those aged over 60 years, with even higher prevalence with further aging as demonstrated by data from both the UK Framingham study (Kannel and Gordan 1978; Vasan et al. 2002; Beckett et al. 2012) and the US National Health and Nutrition Survey (NHANES) (Lloyd-Jones et al. 2005). The NHANES data demonstrates that increases in hypertension prevalence begin in adulthood, with the prevalence doubling between the ages of 20 and 40 years, and doubling again between 40 and 60 years (Kannel and

Gordan 1978), while the Framingham study showed that this pattern continues with ongoing aging, with the prevalence of hypertension increasing from 27.3 % in those aged $\geq$ 60 years to 74.0 % in those aged over 80 years (Vasan et al. 2002).

Gender differences in the prevalence of hypertension have been noted in both younger and older populations. A number of studies have shown found that while the prevalence of hypertension is higher in younger males, this reverse after the age of 60, when the prevalence in females is greater than that in males (Halter 2009; Franklin et al. 1997; Mann 1992; Hajjar and Kotchen 2003; Primatesta and Poulter 2004; Trenkwalder et al. 1994; Gambassi et al. 1998).

Differences in the hypertension phenotype with respect to increases in systolic (SBP) compared with diastolic blood pressure (DBP) have also been reported in older hypertensive populations. Both systolic (SBP) and diastolic blood pressure (DBP) increase with age, (Franklin et al. 1997) however it has been proposed that DBP may plateau or even decrease from the age of 60 years, leaving the SBP to increase (Franklin et al. 2001). Such differences may account for the increase in isolated systolic hypertension that is noted among older populations. Increases in hypertension among older persons may be due to pathophysiological changes associated with aging such as increased peripheral vascular resistance due to arterial stiffening (Franklin et al. 1997; Mitchell et al. 2004). This increase in arterial stiffness with ageing is proposed to alter the normal hemodynamic patterns causing an increase in pulse wave velocity which is an index of arterial stiffness and a widening pulse pressure may account for age related decreases in DBP and increases in SBP (Mann 1992; Mitchell et al. 2004; Pinto 2007; Mackey et al. 2002). Other age related factors such as the changes in renin and aldosterone levels, decreases in renal salt excretion, declining in renal function, changes in the autonomic nervous system sensitivity and function and changes to endothelial function may further contribute to the increases in hypertension seen with aging (Halter 2009; Weinberger 1996; Fliser and Ritz 1998; Wallace et al. 2007). Age related life style changes such as decreased physical activity, changes in body fat composition, high sodium intake and obesity may further contribute to the development of hypertension among older persons. Moreover a synergistic effect on the risk of hypertension has been observed when multiple factors exist together (Halter 2009; Carretero and Oparil 2000; MacMahon et al. 1984; Barreto et al. 2001).

3 Pseudohypertension

Pseudohypertension is occasionally observed in older persons. In pseudohypertension, measurement of blood pressure using a sphygmomanometer results in a falsely elevated reading.(Kleman et al. 2013) This phenomenon is more common in older persons due to increased arterial stiffness, which results in falsely high reading upon blood pressure measurement due to the inability of the arteries to compress. Pseudohypertension is estimated to affect up to 7 % of patients with resistant hypertension (Kleman et al. 2013) and should be considered when older patients presenting with consistently elevated blood pressure over time but who show no signed of end organ damage or in those who treatment with antihypertensive agents result in ongoing symptoms of hypotension. In patients for whom pseudohypertension is suspected an intra-arterial blood pressure measurement is required.

3.1 Pharmacological Management of Hypertension in Older Populations

Unlike many conditions where limited evidence exists for management of those aged over 65 years due to the exclusion of older populations from clinical trials,(White 2010; Devlin 2010) the findings of multiple large, robust trials have provided a solid evidence-base regarding the management of hypertension in older adults. Adverse outcomes associated with poor blood pressure (BP) control in older persons have

been well documented. A Cochrane review of 12 clinical trials showed that the management of hypertension in people aged 60 years and over was associated with a reduction in mortality (Relative Risk (RR)) = 0.9, 95 % confidence interval ((CI) 0.84–0.97).(Musini et al. 2009) The same review reported pharmacological management of hypertension in older adults was associated with significant reductions in both cardiovascular (RR = 0.77, 95 % CI 0.68–0.86) and cerebrovascular mortality (RR = 0.66, 95 % CI 0.53–0.82). (Musini et al. 2009) While life-style interventions are generally considered first-line for the management of all persons with hypertension, the majority of hypertensive patients, including older persons, will require pharmacotherapy to adequately control their blood pressure (Wallace et al. 2007). There have been a number of large well-conducted clinical trials exploring pharmacological management of hypertension in older populations and there is good evidence for the use of a variety of different antihypertensive agents in the management of hypertension in older persons (Pimenta and Oparil 2012).

3.1.1 Thiazide and Thiazide – Like Diuretics

Thiazides diuretics are one of the oldest drug classes used in the treatment of hypertension. (Huebschmann et al. 2006) Evidence of their effectiveness in lowering BP and preventing the cardiovascular and cerebrovascular adverse outcomes associated with hypertension in older people has been provided by several clinical trials, including the Hypertension in the very elderly trial (HyVET) (Beckett et al. 2012), the Swedish Trial in Old Patients with Hypertension (STOP) (Dahlöf et al. 1991; Hansson et al. 1999) and the Antihypertensive and Lipid-Lowering Treatment to prevent Heart Attack Trial; (ALLHAT) (Officers et al. 2002) studies While not all of these studies specifically recruited older participants, the mean participant age for all 3 was over 65 years, making their findings particularly pertinent to older populations.

Use of thiazide and thiazide like diuretics for the management of hypertension in older persons has declined over the past decade (Primatesta and Poulter 2004; Trenkwalder et al. 1994; Triantafyllou et al. 2010; Prencipe et al. 2000; Psaty et al. 2002). There are a number of factors that may have contributed to this decline including increased use of other non-thiazide diuretics, particularly by older persons with complicated hypertension (Van Kraaij et al. 1998) the advent of newer antihypertensives such as Calcium channel blockers (CCBs) and agents acting on the Renin Angiotensin System (RAS) and caution by prescribers due to increased risk of potential adverse drug reactions associated with the use of thiazide diuretics in frail, older persons (Onder et al. 2001; Moser 1998). Despite this general decline, the use of thiazide diuretics for the management of hypertension in the older individual remains high (Bromfield et al. 2014; Rodriguez-Roca et al. 2013; Tu et al. 2006), especially in fixed-dose combination products where they are among the most commonly used antihypertensive agents (Primatesta and Poulter 2004; Trenkwalder et al. 1994; Triantafyllou et al. 2010; Prencipe et al. 2000; Rodriguez-Roca et al. 2013; Svetkey et al. 1996).

3.1.2 Agents Acting on the Renin-Angiotensin System (RAS)

There are three main three antihypertensive classes that act on the RAS. These are the angiotensin blocking agents (ARBs), the Angiotensin converting enzyme inhibitors (ACEI) and the direct renin inhibitors (DRI). The use of both ARBs (Triantafyllou et al. 2010; Bromfield et al. 2014; Rodriguez-Roca et al. 2013) and ACEIs (Primatesta and Poulter 2004; Trenkwalder et al. 1994; Triantafyllou et al. 2010; Psaty et al. 2002; Bromfield et al. 2014; Rodriguez-Roca et al. 2013; Svetkey et al. 1996; Barker et al. 1998; Prince et al. 2012) in older populations has increased over recent years and now surpasses the use of many other antihypertensive classes. The increase in use of these agents for the management of hypertension in older populations has been supported by clinical trials such as the Second Australian National Blood Pressure (ANBP2) (Wing et al. 2003). ANBP2 demonstrated that ACEI were superior

to thiazide diuretics in terms of cardiovascular outcomes in a population comprising 6083 older persons aged between 65 and 84 years. Despite benefits in cardiovascular outcomes no difference between ACEI and diuretics in terms of all cause mortality was observed. (Wing et al. 2003) In addition to increased use as monotherapy for the management of hypertension among older individuals, the use of ACEIs and ARBs in combination with other antihypertensive medications has also increased over recent years (Primatesta and Poulter 2004; Trenkwalder et al. 1994; Triantafyllou et al. 2010; Rodriguez-Roca et al. 2013; Svetkey et al. 1996). In contrast the uptake of aliskiren, a direct renin inhibitor has been slow. Aliskiren has been approved for use in older populations with hypertension since 2007 yet use of daily practice is limited in comparison to other antihypertensive agents (Bromfield et al. 2014; Rodriguez-Roca et al. 2013). The slow uptake of aliskiren for use among older persons may be in part due to concerns around limited efficacy and a poor safety profile (Parving et al. 2012; Gheorghiade et al. 2013).

3.1.3 Calcium Channel Blockers (CCBs)

Since the introduction of CCBs, the prescribing pattern of this antihypertensive medication class in older populations has increased both as monotherapy and combination therapy (Trenkwalder et al. 1994; Prencipe et al. 2000; Bromfield et al. 2014; Svetkey et al. 1996; Barker et al. 1998) and use remained steady until the mid 1990s (Psaty et al. 2002). Despite publication of the findings from the Systolic Hypertension in the Europe Trial (Syst-Eur) in 1997, which showed that treating 1000 patients for 5 years with a CCB prevented 29 strokes or 53 myocardial infarctions (MI), a decline in the use of CCB has generally been noticed in older and the very old patients since the mid-1990s. (Primatesta and Poulter 2004; Triantafyllou et al. 2010; Rodriguez-Roca et al. 2013) This decline may in part be due safety concerns with the use of CCBs older populations, including increased risk of cancer, MI and gastrointestinal haemorrhage with long-term use (Pahor et al. 1996a, b; Maclure et al. 1998).

3.1.4 Beta Blockers (BBs)

Beta blockers have been among the most commonly prescribed antihypertensive agents since their introduction into hypertension treatment (Psaty et al. 2002; Svetkey et al. 1996; Barker et al. 1998) However in recent years, use in older persons has declined following publication of a meta-analysis questioning the efficacy of the BB for hypertension and highlighting safety concerns, with an increased risk of stroke reported with use as monotherapy. (Larochelle et al. 2014) Consequently use of BBs for the management of hypertension in older populations has declined particularly as monotherapy for uncomplicated hypertension management. (Primatesta and Poulter 2004; Trenkwalder et al. 1994; Triantafyllou et al. 2010; Prencipe et al. 2000; Onder et al. 2001).

3.1.5 Alpha Blockers

While several studies have shown a slight increase in the use of alpha blockers in the management of hypertension in the old and very old (Psaty et al. 2002; Bromfield et al. 2014) in general, there has been a downward trend in the use of these agents (Trenkwalder et al. 1994; Rodriguez-Roca et al. 2013; Svetkey et al. 1996; Barker et al. 1998). This decline in use may be due to the poorer adverse effect profile of the alpha-blockers for older persons in comparison to newer agents such as the ACEI and ARBs, as well as to a lack of mortality evidence when compared with other antihypertensive agents.

3.1.6 Nitrates

While nitrates have an important role in the management of coronary artery disease, the lack of studies in older populations using nitrates for the management of hypertension have resulted in these drugs no longer having a major role in the management of hypertension. There has been some discussion around the potential benefit of nitrates for the management of hypertension in older populations, however to date they are not currently recommended in the main hypertension guidelines (Weber et al. 2014; Mancia et al. 2013a).

3.1.7 Choice of Antihypertensive Agent in Older Populations

While all antihypertensive agents will lower blood pressure, when managing hypertension in older persons the choice of agent is dependent not only on the ability to lower blood pressure but also on the potential for harm with older persons showing an increased sensitivity to many adverse effects. In general low dose thiazides, calcium channel blockers or agents acting on the renin angiotensin system appear to present the lowest risks for older populations.

3.2 Barriers to the Optimal Management of Hypertension in Older Persons

Despite the wealth of evidence regarding the benefits of managing hypertension in the old and very old, a significant proportion of older individuals with hypertension have suboptimal BP control (Falaschetti et al. 2014). A number of barriers to optimal blood pressure control in older persons have been identified. These barriers can be considered as system, prescriber or patient related (Alhawassi et al. 2015).

System–related barriers affecting blood pressure control in older populations include the variability in treatment recommendations for this population. (Schäfer et al. 2012; Psaty et al. 1995). While a number of clinical trials have been conducted in older populations, the extent to which this evidence has been incorporated into treatment guidelines and translated into practice remains unknown.

While older persons are often excluded from clinical trials for many conditions (Gross et al. 2002; Heiat et al. 2002), multiple large, well-designed trials exploring hypertension in older persons have been conducted (Dahlöf et al. 1991; Bulpitt et al. 2011). A Cochrane review published in 2009 reported 15 studies (n = 24,055 subjects) exploring the management of hypertension in those aged over 60 years (Musini et al. 2009). These findings demonstrated the considerable benefits of actively managing hypertension in older populations, as well as providing evidence regarding appropriate blood pressure (BP) targets and pharmacotherapy for this population.

Physician related barriers include differences in physician attitudes towards the risks and benefits of managing hypertension in older persons as well as differences in interpretation of the evidence. (Trenkwalder et al. 1994; Rodriguez-Roca et al. 2013).

Establishing the evidence is the first step in ensuring optimal care, yet it is well documented that there is a considerable lag in the translation of scientific evidence into current clinical practice. Moreover, incorporating the latest evidence into daily practice is something many physicians often find problematic (Spranger et al. 2004). One strategy aimed at minimizing the evidence-practice gap is the development and implementation of evidence based guidelines. Guidelines have the potential to improve care and improve patient outcomes (Grimshaw and Russell 1993) and multiple international guidelines for the management of hypertension exist.

Management of hypertension in older persons is one area where there appear to be considerable differences between guidelines in terms of the guidance given to clinicians. Differences in interpretation of the evidence, as well as differences in study design and populations all contribute to differences in the guideline recommendations with respect to older populations, despite the strength of the underlying scientific evidence. Differences around who is considered "old" and what BP targets and management are considered appropriate may lead to confusion among clinicians and further contribute to the evidence-practice lag and a recent systematic review of international hypertension guidelines found considerable variation in recommendations regarding the management of hypertension (Alhawassi et al. 2014).

4   Who Is Considered "Older" in International Guidelines?

In the 13 international guidelines for the management of hypertension included in the systematic review, three different age ranges were used to define older populations. Approximately half of the guidelines defined older populations as those aged 80 years or older, while other guidelines defined older populations as those above 65 years and one guideline included individuals aged over 60 years as older. To further add to the discussion, In the American Society of Hypertension/International Society of Hypertension (ASH/ISH) guideline (Weber et al. 2014), recommendations were given for the "middle aged to elderly population" which was defined as 55–80 years. The European Society of Cardiology (ESC) (Mancia et al. 2013a) and National Institute of Clinical excellence (NICE) (Jaques et al. 2013) guidelines referred explicitly to differing needs among older persons and provide recommendations for older populations aged below 80 years and those aged above 80.

5   BP Targets for Older Persons in the International Guidelines

In most international guidelines the same BP targets were used for younger and older populations. (Alhawassi et al. 2014) For the guidelines that did define hypertension, there was consensus that a higher BP reading was more acceptable in older persons with hypertension and that tighter blood pressure control could be considered for older populations. The majority of guidelines that provided specific BP targets for older populations defined a BP of 140/90 mmHg to be consistent with hypertension. The only guideline to provide a different BP target was the ASH/ISH guideline which specifying a slightly higher target BP of 150/90mmHG (Weber et al. 2014).

Despite the plentiful evidence supporting active management of hypertension in older persons, no guidelines specifically dedicated to the management of hypertension in the older populations were identified in the review. Specific information regarding the diagnosis and management of hypertension in older populations was included in all of the international hypertension guidelines included in the review, however there was considerable variation in the depth and scope of the recommendations. Such variation may reflect differences in the populations included in the landmark hypertension in older population studies. The HYVET (Hypertension in the very Elderly) (Bulpitt et al. 2011) recruited participants aged over 80, while the SHEP (Systolic Hypertension in the Elderly) (Perry et al. 1989) recruited those 60 years and over, and the STOP study (Swedish Trial in Old patients with Hypertension) those aged between 70 and 84 years (Dahlöf et al. 1991).

In general, there is consistency across all guidelines regarding recommendations that treatment be commenced in older individuals when systolic BP readings were above 140–150 mmHg and treatment titrated to achieve a target BP at the same level. However, despite the guideline recommendations debate continues regarding the optimal BP targets in older populations. Two Japanese studies, the JATOS (Japanese trial to assess optimal systolic BP in older hypertensive patients) (Group 2008) and VALISH (Valsartan in Elderly Isolated Systolic Hypertension) (Ogihara et al. 2010) studies failed to show an additional benefit in treating older individuals to a target of 140 mmHg systolic compared to a target of 160 mmHg, highlighting the clinical uncertainty in this area.

The major international hypertension treatment guidelines (Weber et al. 2014; Jaques et al. 2013; National Heart Foundation of Australia (National Blood Pressure and Vascular Disease Advisory Committee) 2010; James et al. 2014; Mancia et al. 2013b; Dasgupta et al. 2014; Luehr et al. 2012; Shimamoto et al. 2014) all support the use of pharmacotherapy for the management of hypertension in the elderly reflecting the findings of a 2008 meta-analysis that concluded that the benefits of pharmacotherapy for managing hypertension in older individuals is comparable to that in younger persons (Turnbull et al. 2008).

While most guidelines mentioned that tolerability of pharmacotherapy may be an issue for older persons, only two guidelines in this review discussed specific adverse effects in the elderly

such as orthostatic hypotension or falls. Antihypertensive medications have been linked with adverse outcomes in a number of studies (Tinetti et al. 1995; Rejnmark 2013; Sato and Akazawa 2013)

Given global increases in life expectancy, there is a need to re-consider how we define "older" populations as well as a need to ensure they are represented in clinical trials and included in evidence based clinical treatment guidelines.

6 Adverse Reactions and Antihypertensive Medications in the Elderly

One potential age related barrier associated with antihypertensive pharmacotherapy is an increased risk of adverse reactions (Monane et al. 1997). Adverse drug reactions (ADRs) are a significant health care problem, associated with significant morbidity and mortality worldwide. The World Health Organization (WHO) define an ADR as "the response to a drug that is noxious and unintended and occurs at doses normally used in man for the prophylaxis, diagnosis or therapy of disease, or for modification of physiological function". (National Heart Foundation of Australia (National Blood Pressure and Vascular Disease Advisory Committee) 2010) ADRs have a significant impact on heath, with between 5 and 7 % of all hospitalisations being due to an ADR and with a further 10–20 % of all hospitalized patient experiencing an ADR during their hospital admission (Davies et al. 2007, 2009; Pirmohamed et al. 2004). The burden associated with ADRs is considerable. Up to 6 % of all ADRs are fatal or have serious consequences (Moore et al. 1998; Wester et al. 2008; Lazarou et al. 1998; White et al. 1999).

Older persons have been shown to be at a high risk of ADRs. (Alhawassi et al. 2014) A systematic review estimated that at least one in ten older persons admitted to hospital will experience an ADRs, either leading to hospitalization or during hospitalization (Alhawassi et al. 2014). The very old, those aged over

80 years of age, are at an even higher risk of experiencing an ADR with up to 40 % of older adults medicine users experiencing an ADR. (Edwards and Aronson 2000; Talbot and Waller 2004) The increased risk of ADRs associated with aging is multifactorial. Physiological changes affecting pharmacokinetics and pharmacodynamics as well as increased clinical complexity, multimorbidity and polypharmacy have all been associated with an increased risk of an ADR in the elderly (Alhawassi et al. 2014).

Cardiovascular medicines, including antihypertensive medications have been associated with an increased risk of ADRs in the general adult population (Pirmohamed et al. 2004; Bond and Raehl 2006; Onder et al. 2002; Grossman and Messerli 2006; Stas et al. 2006; Bates et al. 1999; Field et al. 2004; Gribbin et al. 2010; Tinetti et al. 2014; Rende et al. 2013). One study found that over two thirds of adults using antihypertensive therapy has experienced an adverse reaction to their medication (National Heart Foundation of Australia (National Blood Pressure and Vascular Disease Advisory Committee) 2010; Olsen et al. 1999). Side effects associated with antihypertensive agents are well documented in the product information for each medication and it is well known that older persons are more sensitive to a number of antihypertensive side effects, such as hypotension. The Hypertension Detection and Follow-up Program study, although not mainly designed to study ADR, found that about 33 % patients had experienced at least one drug side effect and required antihypertensive medications discontinuation (Curb et al. 1985).

There have been a number of concerns regarding both the role of poorly controlled blood pressure and the use of antihypertensive agents with a number of common conditions in the elderly such as dementia and falls (Dharmarajan and Dharmarajan 2015). The use of centrally acting ACEI has been associated with reduced rates of cognitive decline (Gao et al. 2013). A systematic review of 18 observation studies comprising 1.3 million older individuals reported similar findings, suggesting that the benefits in terms of cognitive function appeared associated with both

CCBs and those medicines affecting the renin angiotensin system (Rouch et al. 2015). Given that these findings are based upon observational data it remains uncertain if the observed benefit in terms of cognitive decline is directly due to the use of the individual antihypertensive agents or if it is a benefit of optimising blood pressure control in older individuals.

Falls are a common adverse occurrence that increases in prevalence with age. While multiple factors such as cognitive function, comorbid conditions, functional status and environment may play a role in falls (Dharmarajan and Dharmarajan 2015), antihypertensive medications have long been recognised as contributing factors (Butt et al. 2013; Callisaya et al. 2014; Gribbin et al. 2011; Lee and Goeres 2015). However the evidence around the role of antihypertensive medications in falls is conflicting. A large meta-analysis exploring if any of the commonly used antihypertensive agents (thiazide diuretics, ACEI, ARBs, CCBs and BB) were associated with an increased risk of falls failed to confirm the association. Despite these findings there has been multiple studies demonstrating a dose dependent significant increase in the risk of falls with the use of antihypertensive medications across multiple antihypertensive agents (Butt et al. 2013; Callisaya et al. 2014; Gribbin et al. 2011; Lee and Goeres 2015). Given that all antihypertensive medications may cause hypotension, and that older persons appear to have an increased sensitivity to such effects, balancing the benefits of optimal blood pressure control with minimization and avoidance of adverse effects remains a challenge in clinical practice.

7 Conclusions

Antihypertensive medications are widely used by older persons and have critical role in decreasing hypertension related mortality and morbidity for older persons. However, achieving optimal blood pressure control may be challenging among older populations. Despite considerable high quality evidence regarding the benefits of blood pressure management in older persons, translation of this evidence into treatment recommendations in clinical guidelines remains problematic internationally. Furthermore increased medication related harm and adverse reactions associated with the aging further add to complexity to the optimal management of hypertension in older populations.

References

Alhawassi TM, Krass I, Bajorek BV, Pont LG (2014) A systematic review of the prevalence and risk factors for adverse drug reactions in the elderly in the acute care setting. Clin Interv Aging 9:2079–2086

Alhawassi TM, Krass I, Pont LG (2015) Prevalence, prescribing and barriers to effective management of hypertension in older populations: a narrative review. J Pharm Policy Pract 8:24

Barker WH, Mullooly JP, Linton KL (1998) Trends in hypertension prevalence, treatment, and control in a well-defined older population. Hypertension 31(1):552–559

Barreto SM, Passos VMA, Firmo JOA, Guerra HL, Vidigal PG, Lima-Costa MFF (2001) Hypertension and clustering of cardiovascular risk factors in a community in Southeast Brazil: the Bambuí Health and Ageing Study. Arq Bras Cardiol 77(6):576–581

Bates DW, Miller EB, Cullen DJ, Burdick L, Williams L, Laird N et al (1999) Patient risk factors for adverse drug events in hospitalized patients. Arch Intern Med 159(21):2553–2560

Beaglehole R, Ebrahim S, Reddy S, Voûte J, Leeder S (2008) Prevention of chronic diseases: a call to action. Lancet 370(9605):2152–2157

Beckett N, Peters R, Tuomilehto J, Swift C, Sever P, Potter J et al (2012) Immediate and late benefits of treating very elderly people with hypertension: results from active treatment extension to Hypertension in the Very Elderly randomised controlled trial. BMJ 344

Bond C, Raehl CL (2006) Adverse drug reactions in United States hospitals. Pharmacotherapy 26(5):601–608

Bromfield SG, Bowling CB, Tanner RM, Peralta CA, Odden MC, Oparil S et al (2014) Trends in hypertension prevalence, awareness, treatment, and control among US adults 80 years and Older, 1988–2010. J Clin Hypertens 16(4):270–276

Bulpitt C, Beckett N, Peters R, Leonetti G, Gergova V, Fagard R et al (2011) Blood pressure control in the Hypertension in the Very Elderly Trial (HYVET). J Hum Hypertens 26(3):157–163

Butt DA, Mamdani M, Austin PC, Tu K, Gomes T, Glazier RH (2013) The risk of falls on initiation of antihypertensive drugs in the elderly. Osteoporos Int 24(10):2649–2657

Callisaya ML, Sharman JE, Close J, Lord SR, Srikanth VK (2014) Greater daily defined dose of antihypertensive medication increases the risk of falls in older people--a population-based study. J Am Geriatr Soc 62(8):1527–1533

Carretero OA, Oparil S (2000) Essential hypertension part I: definition and etiology. Circulation 101(3):329–335

Chobanian AV, Bakris GL, Black HR, Cushman WC, Green LA, Izzo JL Jr et al (2003) The seventh report of the joint national committee on prevention, detection, evaluation, and treatment of high blood pressure: the JNC 7 report. JAMA 289(19):2560–2571

Curb JD, Borhani NO, Blaszkowski TP, Zimbaldi N, Fotiu S, Williams W (1985) Long-term surveillance for adverse effects of antihypertensive drugs. JAMA 253(22):3263–3268

Daar AS, Singer PA, Persad DL, Pramming SK, Matthews DR, Beaglehole R et al (2007) Grand challenges in chronic non-communicable diseases. Nature 450(7169):494–496

Dahlöf BHL, Lindholm L, Schersten B, Ekbom T, Wester P (1991) Morbidity and mortality in the Swedish trial in old patients with hypertension (STOP-Hypertension). Lancet 338(8778):1281–1285

Dasgupta K, Quinn RR, Zarnke KB, Rabi DM, Ravani P, Daskalopoulou SS et al (2014) The 2014 Canadian Hypertension Education Program recommendations for blood pressure measurement, diagnosis, assessment of risk, prevention, and treatment of hypertension. Canadian J Cardiol 30(5):485–501

Davies EC, Green CF, Mottram DR, Pirmohamed M (2007) Adverse drug reactions in hospitals: a narrative review. Curr Drug Saf 2(1):79–87

Davies EC, Green CF, Taylor S, Williamson PR, Mottram DR, Pirmohamed M (2009) Adverse drug reactions in hospital in-patients: a prospective analysis of 3695 patient-episodes. PLoS One 4(2):e4439

Department of Economic and Social Affairs United Nations (2002) World population ageing: 1950–2050. UN

Devlin G (2010) Women and elderly: subgroups underrepresented in clinical trials. Curr Opin Cardiol 25(4):335–339

Dharmarajan TS, Dharmarajan L (2015) Tolerability of antihypertensive medications in older adults. Drugs Aging 32(10):773–796

Edwards IR, Aronson JK (2000) Adverse drug reactions: definitions, diagnosis, and management. Lancet 356(9237):1255–1259

Fagard RH (2002) Epidemiology of hypertension in the elderly. Am J Geriatr Cardiol 11(1):23–28

Falaschetti E, Mindell J, Knott C, Poulter N (2014) Hypertension management in England: a serial cross-sectional study from 1994 to 2011. Lancet 383(9932):1912–1919

Field TS, Gurwitz JH, Harrold LR, Rothschild J, DeBellis KR, Seger AC et al (2004) Risk factors for adverse drug events among older adults in the ambulatory setting. J Am Geriatr Soc 52(8):1349–1354

Fliser D, Ritz E (1998) Relationship between hypertension and renal function and its therapeutic implications in the elderly. Gerontology 44(3):123–131

Franklin SS, Gustin W, Wong ND, Larson MG, Weber MA, Kannel WB et al (1997) Hemodynamic patterns of age-related changes in blood pressure The Framingham Heart Study. Circulation 96(1):308–315

Franklin SS, Jacobs MJ, Wong ND, Gilbert J, Lapuerta P (2001) Predominance of isolated systolic hypertension among middle-aged and elderly US hypertensives analysis based on National Health and Nutrition Examination Survey (NHANES) III. Hypertension 37(3):869–874

Gambassi G, Lapane K, Sgadari A, Landi F, Carbonin P, Hume A et al (1998) Prevalence, clinical correlates, and treatment of hypertension in elderly nursing home residents. Arch Intern Med 158(21):2377–2385

Gambert SR (1994) Who are the "elderly"? Geriatr Nephrol Urol 4(1):3–4

Gao Y, O'Caoimh R, Healy L, Kerins DM, Eustace J, Guyatt G et al (2013) Effects of centrally acting ACE inhibitors on the rate of cognitive decline in dementia. BMJ Open 3(7)

Gheorghiade M, Böhm M, Greene SJ, Fonarow GC, Lewis EF, Zannad F et al (2013) Effect of aliskiren on postdischarge mortality and heart failure readmissions among patients hospitalized for heart failure: the ASTRONAUT randomized trial. JAMA 309(11):1125–1135

Gribbin J, Hubbard R, Gladman JR, Smith C, Lewis S (2010) Risk of falls associated with antihypertensive medication: population-based case–control study. Age Ageing:afq092

Gribbin J, Hubbard R, Gladman J, Smith C, Lewis S (2011) Risk of falls associated with antihypertensive medication: self-controlled case series. Pharmacoepidemiol Drug Saf 20(8):879–884

Grimshaw JM, Russell IT (1993) Effect of clinical guidelines on medical practice: a systematic review of rigorous evaluations. Lancet 342(8883):1317–1322

Gross CP, Mallory R, Heiat A, Krumholz HM (2002) Reporting the recruitment process in clinical trials: who are these patients and how did they get there? Ann Intern Med 137(1):10–16

Grossman E, Messerli FH (2006) Long-term safety of antihypertensive therapy. Prog Cardiovasc Dis 49(1):16–25

Group JS (2008) Principal results of the Japanese trial to assess optimal systolic blood pressure in elderly hypertensive patients (JATOS). Hypertens Res 31(12):2115–2127

Hajjar I, Kotchen TA (2003) Trends in prevalence, awareness, treatment, and control of hypertension in the United States, 1988–2000. JAMA 290(2):199–206

Halter JB (2009) Hazzard's geriatric medicine and gerontology. McGraw-Hill Companies

Hansson LLL, Ekbom T, Dahlöf B, Lanke J, Scherstén B et al (1999) Randomised trial of old and new antihypertensive drugs in elderly patients: cardiovascular mortality and morbidity the Swedish Trial in Old Patients with Hypertension-2 study. Lancet 354(9192):1751–1756

Heiat A, Gross CP, Krumholz HM (2002) Representation of the elderly, women, and minorities in heart failure clinical trials. Arch Intern Med 162(15):1682–1688

Huebschmann AD, Bublitz C, Anderson RJ (2006) Are hypertensive elderly patients treated differently? Clin Interven Aging 1(3):289

James PA, Oparil S, Carter BL, Cushman WC, Dennison-Himmelfarb C, Handler J et al (2014) 2014 evidence-based guideline for the management of high blood pressure in adults: report from the panel members appointed to the Eighth Joint National Committee (JNC 8). JAMA 311(5):507–520

Jaques H, National Institute for H, Clinical E (2013) NICE guideline on hypertension. Eur Heart J 34(6):406–408

Kannel WB, Gordan T (1978) Evaluation of cardiovascular risk in the elderly: the Framingham study. Bull N Y Acad Med 54(6):573–591

Kirkwood TB, Austad SN (2000) Why do we age? Nature 408(6809):233–238

Kleman M, Dhanyamraju S, DiFilippo W (2013) Prevalence and characteristics of pseudohypertension in patients with "resistant hypertension". J Am Soc Hypertens 7(6):467–470

Kumar J (2013) Epidemiology of hypertension. Clinical Queries. Nephrology 2(2):56–61

Larochelle P, Tobe SW, Lacourcière Y (2014) β-blockers in hypertension: studies and meta-analyses over the years. Can J Cardiol 30(5):S16–S22

Lazarou J, Pomeranz BH, Corey PN (1998) Incidence of adverse drug reactions in hospitalized patients: a meta-analysis of prospective studies. JAMA 279(15):1200–1205

Lee DS, Goeres LM (2015) Higher antihypertensive dose increases risk of falls in older people. Evid Based Nurs 18(3):96

Lim SS, Vos T, Flaxman AD, Danaei G, Shibuya K, Adair-Rohani H et al (2013) A comparative risk assessment of burden of disease and injury attributable to 67 risk factors and risk factor clusters in 21 regions, 1990–2010: a systematic analysis for the Global Burden of Disease Study 2010. Lancet 380(9859):2224–2260

Lloyd-Jones DM, Evans JC, Levy D (2005) Hypertension in adults across the age spectrum: current outcomes and control in the community. JAMA 294(4):466–472

Luehr DWT, Burke R, Dohmen F, Hayes R, Johnson M, Kerandi H, Margolis K, Marshall M, O'Connor P, Pereira C, Reddy G, Schlichte A, Schoenleber M (2012) Hypertension diagnosis and treatment. Institute for Clinical Systems Improvement [Internet]. Updated November 2012. Available from: http://bit.ly/Hypertension1112

Mackey RH, Sutton-Tyrrell K, Vaitkevicius PV, Sakkinen PA, Lyles MF, Spurgeon HA et al (2002)

Correlates of aortic stiffness in elderly individuals: a subgroup of the Cardiovascular Health Study. Am J Hypertens 15(1):16–23

Maclure M, Dormuth C, Naumann T, McCormack J, Rangno R, Whiteside C et al (1998) Influences of educational interventions and adverse news about calcium-channel blockers on first-line prescribing of antihypertensive drugs to elderly people in British Columbia. Lancet 352(9132):943–948

MacMahon SW, Blacket RB, Macdonald GJ, Hall W (1984) Obesity, alcohol consumption and blood pressure in Australian men and women the National Heart Foundation of Australia Risk Factor Prevalence Study. J Hypertens 2(1):85–91

Mancia G, Fagard R, Narkiewicz K, Redon J, Zanchetti A, Böhm M et al (2013) 2013 ESH/ESC Guidelines for the management of arterial hypertension The Task Force for the management of arterial hypertension of the European Society of Hypertension (ESH) and of the European Society of Cardiology (ESC). Eur Heart J 34(28):2159–2219

Mann SJ (1992) Systolic hypertension in the elderly: pathophysiology and management. Arch Intern Med 152(10):1977–1984

Masoro EJ, Austad SN (2006) Handbook of the biology of aging. Academic press

Mathers CD, Loncar D (2006) Projections of global mortality and burden of disease from 2002 to 2030. PLoS Med 3(11):e442

Menotti A, Lanti M, Kafatos A, Nissinen A, Dontas A, Nedeljkovic S et al (2004) The role of a baseline casual blood pressure measurement and of blood pressure changes in middle age in prediction of cardiovascular and all-cause mortality occurring late in life: a cross-cultural comparison among the European cohorts of the Seven Countries Study. J Hypertens 22 (9):1683–1690

Mitchell GF, Parise H, Benjamin EJ, Larson MG, Keyes MJ, Vita JA et al (2004) Changes in arterial stiffness and wave reflection with advancing age in healthy men and women the Framingham Heart Study. Hypertension 43(6):1239–1245

Monane M, Bohn RL, Gurwitz JH, Glynn RJ, Levin R, Avorn J (1997) The effects of initial drug choice and comorbidity on antihypertensive therapy compliance* results from a population-based study in the elderly. Am J Hypertens 10(7):697–704

Moore N, Lecointre D, Noblet C, Mabille M (1998) Frequency and cost of serious adverse drug reactions in a department of general medicine. Br J Clin Pharmacol 45(3):301–308

Moser M (1998) Why are physicians not prescribing diuretics more frequently in the management of hypertension? JAMA 279(22):1813–1816

Murray CJ, Lopez AD (1997) Alternative projections of mortality and disability by cause 1990–2020: Global Burden of Disease Study. Lancet 349 (9064):1498–1504

Musini VM, Tejani AM, Bassett K, Wright JM (2009) Pharmacotherapy for hypertension in the elderly. Cochrane Database Syst Rev 2009(4):CD000028

National Heart Foundation of Australia (National Blood Pressure and Vascular Disease Advisory Committee) (2010) Guide to management of hypertension 2008. Updated December 2010. Accessed via https://heartfoundation.org.au/images/uploads/publications/HypertensionGuidelines2008to2010Update.pdf on April 15, 2016

Officers A, Coordinators for the ACRGTA, Lipid-Lowering Treatment to Prevent Heart Attack T (2002) Major outcomes in high-risk hypertensive patients randomized to angiotensin-converting enzyme inhibitor or calcium channel blocker vs diuretic: The Antihypertensive and Lipid-Lowering Treatment to Prevent Heart Attack Trial (ALLHAT). JAMA 288(23):2981–2997

Ogihara T, Saruta T, Rakugi H, Matsuoka H, Shimamoto K, Shimada K et al (2010) Target blood pressure for treatment of isolated systolic hypertension in the elderly: valsartan in elderly isolated systolic hypertension study. Hypertension 56(2):196–202

Olsen H, Klemetsrud T, Stokke HP, Tretli S, Westheim A (1999) Adverse drug reactions in current antihypertensive therapy: a general practice survey of 2586 patients in Norway. Blood Press 8(2):94–101

Onder G, Gambassi G, Landi F, Pedone C, Cesari M, Carbonin P et al (2001) Trends in antihypertensive drugs in the elderly: the decline of thiazides. J Hum Hypertens 15(5):291–297

Onder G, Pedone C, Landi F, Cesari M, Della Vedova C, Bernabei R et al (2002) Adverse drug reactions as cause of hospital admissions: results from the Italian Group of Pharmacoepidemiology in the Elderly (GIFA). J Am Geriatr Soc 50(12):1962–1968

Pahor M, Carbonin P, Guralnik J, Havlik R, Furberg C (1996a) Risk of gastrointestinal haemorrhage with calcium antagonists in hypertensive persons over 67 years old. Lancet 347(9008):1061–1065

Pahor M, Guralnik JM, Ferrucci L, Corti M-C, Salive ME, Cerhan JR et al (1996b) Calcium-channel blockade and incidence of cancer in aged populations. Lancet 348(9026):493–497

Parving H-H, Brenner BM, McMurray JJ, de Zeeuw D, Haffner SM, Solomon SD et al (2012) Cardiorenal end points in a trial of aliskiren for type 2 diabetes. N Engl J Med 367(23):2204–2213

Perry HM Jr, Smith WM, McDonald RH, Black D, Cutler JA, Furberg CD et al (1989) Morbidity and mortality in the Systolic Hypertension in the Elderly Program (SHEP) pilot study. Stroke 20(1):4–13

Pimenta E, Oparil S (2012) Management of hypertension in the elderly. Nat Rev Cardiol 9(5):286–296

Pinto E (2007) Blood pressure and ageing. Postgrad Med J 83(976):109–114

Pirmohamed M, James S, Meakin S, Green C, Scott AK, Walley TJ et al (2004) Adverse drug reactions as cause of admission to hospital: prospective analysis of 18 820 patients. BMJ 329(7456):15–19

Prencipe M, Casini A, Santini M, Ferretti C, Scaldaferri N, Culasso F (2000) Prevalence, awareness, treatment and control of hypertension in the elderly: results from a population survey. J Hum Hypertens 14(12):825–830

Primatesta P, Poulter NR (2004) Hypertension management and control among English adults aged 65 years and older in 2000 and 2001. J Hypertens 22 (6):1093–1098

Prince MJ, Ebrahim S, Acosta D, Ferri CP, Guerra M, Huang Y et al (2012) Hypertension prevalence, awareness, treatment and control among older people in Latin America, India and China: a 10/66 cross-sectional population-based survey. J Hypertens 30 (1):177–187

Psaty BM, Koepsell TD, Yanez ND, Smith NL, Manolio TA, Heckbert SR et al (1995) Temporal patterns of antihypertensive medication use among older adults, 1989 through 1992: an effect of the major clinical trials on clinical practice? JAMA 273(18):1436–1438

Psaty BM, Manolio TA, Smith NL, Heckbert SR, Gottdiener JS, Burke GL et al (2002) Time trends in high blood pressure control and the use of antihypertensive medications in older adults: the Cardiovascular Health Study. Arch Intern Med 162 (20):2325–2332

Rai GS, Mulley GP (2007) Elderly medicine: a training guide. Elsevier Health Sciences

Rejnmark L (2013) The ageing endocrine system: fracture risk after initiation of antihypertensive therapy. Nat Rev Endocrinol 9(4):189–190

Rende P, Paletta L, Gallelli G, Raffaele G, Natale V, Brissa N et al (2013) Retrospective evaluation of adverse drug reactions induced by antihypertensive treatment. J Pharmacol Pharmacotherap 4(Suppl1): S47

Rodriguez-Roca GC, Llisterri JL, Prieto-Diaz MA, Alonso-Moreno FJ, Escobar-Cervantes C, Pallares-Carratala V et al (2013) Blood pressure control and management of very elderly patients with hypertension in primary care settings in Spain. Hypertens Res 37(2):166–171

Rouch L, Cestac P, Hanon O, Cool C, Helmer C, Bouhanick B et al (2015) Antihypertensive drugs, prevention of cognitive decline and dementia: a systematic review of observational studies, randomized controlled trials and meta-analyses, with discussion of potential mechanisms. CNS Drugs 29(2):113–130

Sato I, Akazawa M (2013) Polypharmacy and adverse drug reactions in Japanese elderly taking antihypertensives: a retrospective database study. Drug Healthcare Patient Saf 5:143–150

Schäfer H-H, De Villiers JN, Sudano I, Dischinger S, Theus G-R, Zilla P et al (2012) Recommendations for the treatment of hypertension in the elderly and very elderly–a scotoma within international guidelines. Swiss Med Wkly Epub

Shimamoto K, Ando K, Fujita T, Hasebe N, Higaki J, Horiuchi M et al (2014) The Japanese Society of Hypertension Guidelines for the Management of Hypertension (JSH 2014). Hypertens Res 37 (4):253–387

Spranger CB, Ries AJ, Berge CA, Radford NB, Victor RG (2004) Identifying gaps between guidelines and clinical practice in the evaluation and treatment of patients with hypertension. Am J Med 117 (1):14–18

Stas S, Appesh L, Sowers J (2006) Metabolic safety of antihypertensive drugs: myth versus reality. Current Hypertens Rep 8(5):403–408

Svetkey LP, George LK, Tyroler HA, Timmons PZ, Burchett BM, Blazer DG (1996) Effects of gender and ethnic group on blood pressure control in the elderly. Am J Hypertens 9(6):529–535

Talbot J, Waller P (2004) Stephens' detection of new adverse drug reactions. Wiley, New York

The World Health Organisation (2016) Projections of mortality and causes of death, 2015 and 2030. Accessed via http://www.who.int/healthinfo/global_burden_disease/projections/en/on 15 April 2016

Tinetti ME, Inouye SK, Gill TM, Doucette JT (1995) Shared risk factors for falls, incontinence, and functional dependence. Unifying the approach to geriatric syndromes. JAMA 273(17):1348–1353

Tinetti ME, Han L, Lee DS, McAvay GJ, Peduzzi P, Gross CP et al (2014) Antihypertensive medications and serious fall injuries in a nationally representative sample of older adults. JAMA Intern Med 174 (4):588–595

Trenkwalder P, Ruland D, Stender M, Gebhard J, Trenkwalder C, Lydtin H et al (1994) Prevalence, awareness, treatment and control of hypertension in a population over the age of 65 years: results from the Starnberg Study on Epidemiology of Parkinsonism and Hypertension in the Elderly (STEPHY). J Hypertens 12(6):709

Triantafyllou A, Douma S, Petidis K, Doumas M, Panagopoulou E, Pyrpasopoulou A et al (2010) Prevalence, awareness, treatment and control of hypertension in an elderly population in Greece. Rural Remote Health 10(2):1225

Tu K, Campbell NR, Chen Z, McAlister FA (2006) Thiazide diuretics for hypertension: prescribing practices and predictors of use in 194,761 elderly patients with hypertension. Am J Geriatr Pharmacother 4(2):161–167

Turnbull F, Neal B, Ninomiya T, Algert C, Arima H, Barzi F et al (2008) Effects of different regimens to lower blood pressure on major cardiovascular events in older and younger adults: meta-analysis of randomised trials. BMJ 336(7653):1121–1123

Van Kraaij D, Jansen R, Gribnau F, Hoefnagels W (1998) Loop diuretics in patients aged 75 years or older: general practitioners' assessment of indications and possibilities for withdrawal. Eur J Clin Pharmacol 54 (4):323–327

Vasan RS, Beiser A, Seshadri S, Larson MG, Kannel WB, D'Agostino RB et al (2002) Residual lifetime risk for developing hypertension in middle-aged women and men: The Framingham Heart Study. JAMA 287(8):1003–1010

Wallace SM, McEniery CM, Mäki-Petäjä KM, Booth AD, Cockcroft JR, Wilkinson IB (2007) Isolated systolic hypertension is characterized by increased aortic stiffness and endothelial dysfunction. Hypertension 50 (1):228–233

Weber MA, Schiffrin EL, White WB, Mann S, Lindholm LH, Kenerson JG et al (2014) Clinical practice guidelines for the management of hypertension in the community a statement by the American Society of Hypertension and the International Society of Hypertension. J Hypertens 32(1):3–15

Weinberger MH (1996) Salt sensitivity of blood pressure in humans. Hypertension 27(3):481–490

Wester K, Jonsson AK, Spigset O, Druid H, Hagg S (2008) Incidence of fatal adverse drug reactions: a population based study. Br J Clin Pharmacol 65(4):573–579

White SM (2010) Including the very elderly in clinical trials. Anaesthesia 65(8):778–780

White TJ, Arakelian A, Rho JP (1999) Counting the costs of drug-related adverse events. Pharmacoeconomics 15(5):445–458

Wing LM, Reid CM, Ryan P, Beilin LJ, Brown MA, Jennings GL et al (2003) A comparison of outcomes with angiotensin-converting--enzyme inhibitors and diuretics for hypertension in the elderly. N Engl J Med 348(7):583–592

Yang G, Kong L, Zhao W, Wan X, Zhai Y, Chen LC et al (2008) Emergence of chronic non-communicable diseases in China. Lancet 372(9650):1697–1705

Adv Exp Med Biol - Advances in Internal Medicine (2017) 2: 181–189
DOI 10.1007/5584_2016_38
© Springer International Publishing AG 2016
Published online: 19 November 2016

Resistant Hypertension

Debbie Valsan, Umber Burhan, and Geoffrey Teehan

Abstract

Conservatively, ten million people in the USA alone may suffer from RH and may be similarly prevalent elsewhere. Given the strong linear correlation between hypertension and cardiovascular outcomes, better control is paramount. We favor a multi-pronged approach. It may not suffice to address this by pharmacologic means only. Careful attention to modifiable risk factors, particularly sodium intake, adhering to a proper diet (i.e. DASH), and avoiding agents, i.e. non-steroidals, that can elevate the blood pressure, is key. Frequent follow up to establish the right treatment regimen and home blood pressuring monitoring can have a strong impact on control. Finally, consideration of device therapy may be a more viable option in the future.

Keywords

Resistant hypertension • Hyperaldosteronism • Renovascular hypertension • Obstructive sleep apnea • Cushing syndrome • Chronic kidney disease • Liddle syndrome • Coarctation of aorta • Pheochromocytoma • Sympathectomy • Carotid sinus baroreceptor electrical stimulation

1   Introduction

Hypertension is the most common chronic disease in the developed world. Between 2005 and 2008, the National Health and Nutrition Examination Survey (NHANES) estimated that nearly one quarter of U.S. adults were hypertensive, and of those only one half were considered controlled. Therefore, adequate control is of utmost public health importance given the linear relationship between blood pressure and cardiovascular risk.

While essential hypertension (EH) usually results from a complex interaction between genetic traits and lifestyle factors such as weight, stress, and sodium intake, several other defined

D. Valsan, U. Burhan, and G. Teehan (✉)
Lankenau Medical Center, Lancaster Avenue, Suite 130, Wynnewood, PA, USA19096,
e-mail: gteehan1@gmail.com

forms of hypertension exist. Among these are white coat hypertension, masked hypertension, resistant hypertension (RH), refractory hypertension and pseudohypertension. This chapter will focus on RH which is defined as a blood pressure of >140/90 despite appropriate adherence to a regimen of three antihypertensive agents including a diuretic. Its actual prevalence unknown, estimates in several recent studies show it to be an increasingly common finding.

Therapy in RH, as in EH, requires not only pharmacologic intervention, but also lifestyle modification, careful scrutiny of pharmacologic and herbal remedies, supplements, and over the counter agents. Device therapy may offer promise in the future. Certain epidemiologic factors appear more prevalent in the RH population than in other hypertensive cohorts. Recognition of these patients is a challenge to clinicians but several clues may identify patients for targeted therapies.

In this chapter, we will describe the epidemiology, prognosis, disease states, diagnostic evaluation, non-pharmacologic and pharmacologic treatment of RH.

2 Establishing the Diagnosis

Distinguishing RH from other forms of hypertension is critical. The *sine qua non* of RH is a blood pressure > 140/90 on three maximally dosed/tolerated drugs including a well-dosed diuretic, preferably a thiazide or mineralocorticoid antagonist rather than a loop diuretic which tends to be less effective in blood pressure control (Sarafidis 2011). Correct blood pressure measuring is also critical and is described elsewhere (Kaplan and et al. 2010). Table 1 lists the forms of hypertension and associated diagnostic criteria.

3 Epidemiology

The actual prevalence of RH is unknown but estimates range from 8 to 15 % of all hypertensive subjects. An ethnically diverse cross-sectional study done in the Kaiser-Permanente system in Southern California between 2006 and 2007 revealed 12.8 % of all hypertensive individuals met criteria for RH. This was particularly common among males, those of black race, obese, and older subjects. Diabetes mellitus, ischemic heart disease, congestive heart failure, and chronic kidney disease (CKD) also associated with RH (Pimenta et al. 2012).

In the most recent National Health and Nutrition Examination Survey (NHANES) between 2005 and 2008, among 6000 adults with hypertension, 11.8 % had RH. Between 1988–1994 and 1999–2004 the prevalence was estimated to 5.5 and 8.5 % respectively. In today's terms,

Table 1 Lists the forms of hypertension and associated diagnostic criteria

Cause	Criteria
Essential hypertension	Lacks specific known/causative condition; genetics, diet, environmental factors play role
White coat hypertension	Office BP > 140/90 with reliable out of office readings < 140/90; Can confirm with ABPM[a]
Masked hypertension	Office BP < 140/90; home readings > 140/90
Pseudohypertension	Radial pulse remains palpable despite occlusion of brachial artery, the Osler Maneuver
Resistant hypertension	BP > 140/90 on 3 antihypertensives including a diuretic
Refractory hypertension	Like resistant hypertension but on 4 antihypertensives and less likely to respond to MRA[b] (Kaplan et al. 2010)

[a]Ambulatory blood pressure monitoring
[b]Mineralocorticoid antagonists

based on the latest NHANES data some 76 million Americans are hypertensive, of which 12 % or nine million individuals may be resistant (Pimenta et al. 2012; Persell 2011).

In the Antihypertensive and Lipid-Lowering Treatment To Prevent Heart Attack trial (ALLHAT), International Verapamil-Trandolapril Study (INVEST), and Avoiding Cardiovascular Events through Combination Therapy in Patients Living with Systolic Hypertension (ACCOMPLISH) trials RH was estimated at 8–15 % of these hypertensive cohorts (The ALLHAT Officers and Coordinators for the ALLHAT Collaborative Research Group 2002; Pepine et al. 1998; Jamerson et al. 2008).

4 Prognosis

Patients with RH are at greater risk for end organ damage such as left ventricular hypertrophy (LVH), CKD, and albuminuria than those patients who have controlled blood pressure (Sarafidis 2011).

Retrospectively, Daugherty et al. found that RH was significantly associated with a 47 % increased risk of adverse cardiovascular outcomes (Daugherty 2012). Armario studied 513 patients in a Spanish cohort with RH finding LVH by echocardiography in 57 %; 46 % had albuminuria (Armario 2011).

Successfully lowering blood pressure in RH may reduce cardiovascular events. Pisoni et al showed a 96 % reduction in cardiovascular events over 18 months with the use of 3 antihypertensive agents versus placebo in patients with severe diastolic hypertension (Pisoni 2009).

Sales et al demonstrated the additional clinical benefits of ambulatory blood pressure monitoring (ABPM) in RH and found that elevated systolic and diastolic blood pressures predicted cardiovascular and overall mortality (Salles et al. 2008).

5 RH: Associated Medical Conditions: Secondary Causes of Hypertension and Workup

Table 2 lists the most common causes of RH.

Table 2 Lists the most common causes of RH

Diagnosis	Etiology	Clues to its diagnosis
Primary aldosteronism	Bilateral hyperplasia, solitary adrenal adenoma	Hypokalemia, metabolic alkalosis, mild hypernatremia (Acelajado 2011).
Renovascular hypertension	Renal artery stenosis, fibromuscular dysplasia	Flash pulmonary edema with preserved systolic function, atherosclerotic disease, abdominal or femoral bruit, absent pedal pulses, assymetric kidneys on imaging (Cooper et al. 2014).
OSA	Partial or complete collapse of the airway during sleep	Fatigue, day time somnolence, poor sleep (Drager 2010)
CKD	Acute glomerulonephritis, APCKD, renal cell carcinoma, renin-producing tumors, vasculitis and chronic pyelonephritis	Elevated creatinine, abnormal urine studies (Thomas 2015)
Cushing syndrome	Excess endogenous or exogenous glucocorticoids	Moon facies, abdominal striae, truncal obesity, hirsuitism and kyphoscoliosis (Moneva 2002)
Coarctation of the aorta	Discrete narrowing in the region of the ligamentum arteriosum	Hypertension in the upper extremities with hypotension in the lower extremities, a systolic-diastolic murmur audible on the chest or back and a time delay between brachial and femoral pulses or pulse diminishment (Prisant 2004)
Liddle syndrome	Causal mutation of the beta subunit of the amiloride sensitive sodium channel	Hypokalemia, mild hypernatremia and metabolic alkalosis (Rose 2001)
Pheochromocytoma	Catecholamine-secreting tumors of the adrenal medulla and the sympathetic ganglia	Episodic headache, sweating, and tachycardia (Stein 1981)

5.1 Primary Hyperaldosteronism

Among patients with RH, primary hyperaldosteronism (PHA) is likely the most common identifiable cause. In an analysis of 88 patients with RH, 20 % had PHA (Calhoun et al. 2002). Acelajado et al. found a 17 % prevalence of RH due to PHA (Acelajado 2011).

Screening should occur in hypertensive subjects with unexplained or unprovoked hypokalemia, or if induced by diuretics, resisting correction. Those with a strong family history of hypertension, especially early-onset (<40 years), drug resistant hypertension, hypertensive with an adrenal "incidentaloma," should also be screened. Morning samples for plasma aldosterone concentration (PAC), plasma renin activity (PRA) and an aldosterone to renin ratio (ARR) are obtained. We suggest holding MRAs and continuing all other drugs to avoid accelerating hypertension.

An ARR above 20 is consistent with PHA. Additionally, a PAC of greater than 15 ng/dl yields a positive screening result. Twenty-four urinary aldosterone measurements confirm the diagnosis. Salt sensitivity is diagnosed when the Aldosterone levels are relatively high but fail to reach threshold values for PHA. These patients are highly responsive to MRAs but also to simple sodium restriction.

Computed tomography (CT) represents the best test for this for confirming an adrenal tumor. Incidental adrenal adenomas are found in 4 % of the general population on CT, and are particularly common after the age of 40. Proceeding to adrenal vein sampling is reasonable in the hypertensive patient over 40 with an adenoma. This can help lateralize the hormonal excess and direct surgical excision. In bilateral adrenal hyperplasia medical therapy with MRAs is best (Mantero 2000).

5.2 Renovascular Hypertension

Renovascular hypertension is common among hypertensive patients with multiple risk factors for atherosclerotic disease, particularly those with RH.

An abdominal bruit and known history of athereosclerosis and tobacco use are commonly seen. Patients challenged with ACE inhibitors (ACE I) or Angiotensin Receptor Blockers (ARB may get ischemic nephropathy due to the effects on Angiotensin II and the efferent renal arteriole. Bloodwork usually shows an elevated PRA and PAC. Once suspected, imaging modalities, particularly duplex ultrasonography, magnetic resonance angiography (MRA) and computed tomography angiography (CTA) are performed.

In duplex ultrasonography, reliable detection of RAS is operator dependent and sensitivity and specificity do not compare favorably with MRA or CTA. MRA confers the risk of gadolinium induced nephrogenic systemic fibrosis, a syndrome linked to individuals with a GFR <30 ml/min. CTA requires a significant volume of contrast and may be contraindicated in those with advancing CKD. Conventional intraarterial angiography can confirm diagnosis. Unfortunately, three separate trials have shown no benefit to interventional approaches relative to medical management and this often leads to a diagnostic quandary as to whether to pursue this diagnosis at all (Cooper et al. 2014; The Astral Trial Investigators 2009; Bax et al. 2009).

Therapy usually includes dual anti-platelet therapy, antihyperlipidemic drugs, and blood pressure control. Use of ACE I or ARB is generally discouraged due to the risk of ischemic nephropathy (Cooper et al. 2014).

5.3 Obstructive Sleep Apnea

Obstructive sleep apnea (OSA) occurs when there is a partial or complete collapse of the airway during sleep. Affecting nearly 2.4 % of adults, it is associated with mortality and cardiovascular risks (Drager 2010). The Ohasama study showed each 5 % deficiency in the normal decline in nocturnal blood pressure was associated with an approximate 20 % increase in risk of cardiovascular mortality (Ohkubo et al. 2000). The prevalence of OSA in hypertensive patients may be as high as 56 % and in resistant hypertensive patients, nearly 80 %.

Polysomnography confirms the diagnosis when the apnea hypopnea index (AHI) is greater than 5. Alajmi et al identified ten randomized controlled trials that found that the effects of CPAP on reduction of blood pressure were modest and not significant. Reductions in BP tended to be larger in patients with severe OSA (AHI > 30), and a trend for systolic BP reduction was associated with higher CPAP adherence (Alajmi 2007; Hyun 2015).

5.4 Chronic Kidney Disease

Broadly this diagnosis captures glomerular and vascular disorders, hypertension, diabetic kidney disease and other forms. The Chronic Renal Insufficiency Cohort (CRIC) investigators looked at nondialysis CKD patients. Fully 40 % of the cohort had RH and among these there was a higher risk of congestive heart failure and CKD progression versus those without RH (Thomas 2015).

Increased fluid and sodium retention and subsequent intravascular expansion leads to treatment resistance. Khosla et al found that MRAs are effective and safe to reach goal blood pressure amongst patients with diabetic nepheropathy when added to a triple antihypertensive regimen of diuretic, ACE I and Calcium Channel Blocker (CCB). Aside from the reduction of blood pressure, they are modestly antiproteinuric (Khosla 2009; Williams et al. 2015). Treating the underlying renal disorder may also be of some benefit.

5.5 Cushing Syndrome

Hypertension is present in 70–90 % of patients with Cushing's syndrome (Moneva 2002).

Screening consists of an early morning Cortisol reading which can be verified either by a low dose dexamethasone suppression test (DST) or measurement of a 24-h urinary free cortisol level.

Following DST a morning plasma cortisol level is drawn. Levels greater than 5 mg/dL are consistent with Cushing's Syndrome. Alternatively, a 24 h urine cortisol level over 55 mcg confirms the diagnosis. Further testing/imaging should follow to determine if there is an ectopic, pituitary or adrenal source. CT or MRI of the pituitary and adrenals should secure the diagnosis.

The therapy used in Cushing Syndrome to treat patients with hypertension is the same treatment of EH. The use of MRA may be particularly effective in patients with very high cortisol levels. In a study by Ulick et al, cortisol was the major mineralocorticoid in ectopic ACTH syndrome (Moneva 2002; Ulick et al. 1992).

5.6 Coarctation of the Aorta

Coarctation of the aorta accounts for approximately 6–8 % of congenital heart disease in infants and children. Although rare compared with other causes of secondary hypertension, accounting for only 0.2 % of the adult population, clinicians should be aware of the elements of physical exam abnormalities that can point to the diagnosis (Prisant 2004). Aortic imaging confirms the diagnosis. Early correction is advised (Prisant 2004; Yetman 1997).

5.7 Liddle Syndrome

Liddle Syndrome is a rare form of autosomal dominant hypertension. Clinically, hypertension usually begins in childhood. Genetic testing is available but costly. Diagnosis is often clinical. Despite a clinical presentation typical of primary aldosteronism, PRA and PAC are low. Potassium-sparing diuretics are the therapy of choice in Liddle syndrome (Rose 2001).

5.8 Pheochromocytoma

Pheochromocytomas account for fewer than 0.2 % cases of hypertension. Almost one half of these patients have RH whereas most of the rest have apparent EH (Stein 1981).

Once suspected, interfering medications, such as tricyclics and other psychoactive agents, in the screening and confirmation of the diagnosis should be discontinued 2 weeks prior to the assessment. Screening includes 24 h urinary and plasma catecholamine levels and may include MIBG scintigraphy. Although 10 % of pheochromocytomas are extra-adrenal, 95 % are intra-abdominal. CT or MRI of the abdomen are highly sensitive (98–100 %) but only 70 % specific due to the high prevalence of adrenal "incidentalomas." (Guerrero 2009)

Surgical resection is the definitive treatment. Preoperatively, therapy is aimed at controlling blood pressure and prevent intraoperative HTN. Phenoxybenzamine is the preferred drug of choice as well as propanolol which is initiated thereafter. This order of treatment is important to avoid stimulating unopposed alpha adrenergic receptors (Tauzin-Fin 2004).

6 RH: Lifestyle Factors/ Modifications

While establishing a secondary cause can allow the practitioner to address a specific issue, i.e. treating PHA with an MRA, often a secondary cause is elusive. In the **a** section below drug options will be discussed. As medical costs continue to climb, efforts to find inexpensive solutions to expensive problems is paramount. If the prevalence estimates of RH are correct at 8–15 % of the hypertensive population, the economic implications are astounding. This assumes that lowering blood pressure will lead to fewer cardiovascular, cerebrovascular and renal outcomes. Correcting modifiable risk factors may offer a very cost-sensitive way to approach this problem. The upcoming Triumph trial will look at an RH population and assess the value of exercise training, low sodium diet, DASH diet, and weight management (Blumenthal et al. 2015). Our current practice is to address these factors as we would in other hypertensive populations in the hopes the results will be similar. Table 3 lists many of the modifiable risk factors and the magnitude of their effects.

6.1 Sodium Consumption

The majority of patients with RH may consume more than 10 g of sodium per day. In a resistant population on a mean off 3–4 antihypertensive agents, Calhoun et al demonstrated that lower sodium intake (50 mmol/day vs 250 mmol) decreased blood pressures by 23/10 mmHg (office readings and ABPM) (Calhoun 2009). In current guidelines for hypertensive individuals, dietary sodium should be less than 100 mmol/day or 2.4 g of sodium chloride (Calhoun 2009). For salt sensitive patients, even lower amounts of sodium may be necessary. Two pivotal trials highlight the effect of sodium restriction and how it is magnified by Thiazide diuretic usage. Fothersby et al studied 17 untreated subjects with a mean systolic BP of 176 +/− 11 mmHg and simply applied an 80–100 mmol/day sodium restriction without any antihypertensive agents. The BP fell a disappointing 5/2 mmHg. Gavras et al however showed that by adding a thiazide diuretic to an austere sodium diet (10 mmol/day) BP fell 21/7 mmHg (Gavras 1981; Fothersby 1993).

Table 3 Lists many of the modifiable risk factors and the magnitude of their effects (James et al. 2014)

Factor	Goal	Estimated systolic BP effect
Sodium consumption	<5–6 g/day	8–14 mmHg
Ethanol intake	20–30 g/day for men	2–4 mmHg
	10–20 g/day for women	
Weight loss	BMI < 25 kg/m (2)	5–10 mmHg per 10 kg wt loss
Exercise	30 min daily aerobic exercise	4–9 mmHg
Diet	DASH diet	11 mmHg

6.2 Weight Loss

The Dietary Approaches to Stopping Hypertension (DASH) trial utilized a Mediterranean diet with low fat, high fiber, rich in calcium and potassium, and lowered systolic BP by 11 mmHg in just 2 weeks' time. When sodium restriction was added the BP fell a bit further but was less well-tolerated (Sacks et al. 2001). We target a BMI goal of < 25 kg/m^2. The German Hydra Trial demonstrated that for a BMI > 40 kg/m(2) vs < 25 kg/m(2), there was 5.3 fold increased risk of RH and a 3.2 fold risk of refractory hypertension (Sharma et al. 2004). The additive effect of exercise and alcohol moderation can be a useful adjunct.

6.3 Over the Counter Agents, Supplements, and Medications That Can Raise Blood Pressure

A growing trend toward alternative therapies exists and patients often seek "non-traditional" therapies to treat various maladies. Additionally, certain over the counter agents can raise the blood pressure and should be avoided, particularly in those with RH. Other agents are medically necessary, e.g. immunosuppressants in a transplant recipient and little can be done. Table 4 lists these and recommendations/comments.

6.4 Pharmacologic Therapy

While certain forms of RH mandate specific therapy, i.e. CPAP for OSA or adrenalectomy for an aldosterone secreting tumor, when there is no such directed therapy, there is little available data to guide treatment options. To satisfy the definition of RH, diuretic therapy is mandatory, and we prefer thiazides and mineralocorticoid antagonists to loop diuretics. Further, lacking much guidance in the literature we advocate using the first line agents from the Joint National Committee VIII recommendations which would include treating with an ACE I or ARB and a dihydropyridine CCB such as Amlodipine (James et al. 2014). The Pathways II trial showed that among those with RH, Aldactone was superior to Bisoprolol or Doxazosin for blood pressure control. The Resistant Hypertension Optimal Treatment Trial is a Brazilian study will compare spironolactone to clonidine as the best fourth agent to a standard regimen that includes diuretics, ace inhibitors/angiotensin receptor blockers and a calcium channel blocker (Williams et al. 2015; Krieger et al. 2014).

We further recommend those with RH purchase a blood pressure cuff, be instructed on proper use, and keep a diary of readings. Calibrating the cuff with an office cuff can be helpful. Ambulatory blood pressure monitoring

Table 4 Lists these and recommendations/comments (James et al. 2014)

Supplement/Drug/Herb	Comment
Nonsteroidal anti-inflammatory drugs	Salt-retention
Nasal decongestants	Vasoconstricting
Diet pills	Multiple mechanisms
Sympathomimetic agents	Tachycardia, vasoconstriction
Oral contraceptives	Multiple hormonal mechanisms
Steroids	Anabolic/Catabolic
Calcineurin inhibitors	Cyclosporine, Tacrolimus
Street drugs	Cocaine, Amphetamines, etc
Antidepressants	Venlafaxine, Monoamine oxidase inhibitors, Tricyclic Antidepressants, Fluoxetine
Herbal remedies	Arnica, Bitter Orange, Ephedra, Ginkgo, Ginseng, Guarana, Licorice, Senna, St. John's Wort

intuitively makes sense but is not reimbursed, is expensive and not widely available. Patients are counseled that controlling blood pressure may take weeks to months or longer and requires frequent follow up.

6.5   Device Therapy

In light of the prevalence of RH and hypertension in general, the inherent difficulties in effectively treating the disease(s), and potential impact of a successful non-pharmacological therapy, several different devices have been trialed. Unfortunately, the results have thus far been disappointing.

Surgical sympathectomy in the 1920s "cured" hypertension but at the expense of causing syncope and a host of other neurologic findings (Grimson et al. 1949). Catheter-based renal denervation resulted whereby an electrical pulse within the renal arterial lumen severs sympathetic fibers from the brain to the kidney. Initial results from the european Symplicity II investigators were promising (office blood pressure fell systolically by 32 mmHg versus placebo) but failed in a larger trial (Esler et al. 2010; Bhatt et al. 2014).

Carotid Sinus Baroreceptor Electrical Stimulators send an impulse to the brain that BP is actually higher reflexively causing reduction in sympathetic output, and lower BP. Of the 265 subjects with RH in the trial nearly 80 % of those treated experienced a 44 mmHg decline in systolic blood pressure. As the trial failed to meet 2 of its 5 pre-specified endpoints (short-term efficacy and procedure-related adverse events) it remains unapproved in the U.S. by the Food and Drug Administration (Bisognano 2011).

Central Arteriovenous Anastomosis creates a conduit anastomosis between large vessels, shunting substantial blood volume into high-capacity, low-resistance venous system, thereby decreasing total systemic vascular resistance and therefore BP. Lobo et al studied 88 patients with RH and found mean office systolic blood pressure and mean ambulatory blood pressure fell by 26.9 and 13.5 mmHg among those treated versus 3.7 and 0.5 mmHg not treated (Lobo 2015). Median and vagus nerve stimulators may offer promise as well but remain poorly studied.

Works Cited

Acelajado MC, Calhoun DA (2011) Aldosteronism and resistant hypertension. Int J Hypertens 2011:837817. doi:10.4061/2011/837817

Alajmi M (2007) Impact of continuous positive airway pressure therapy on blood pressure in patients with obstructive sleep apnea hypopnea: a meta analysis of randomized control trials. LUNG 185(2):67–72

Armario P (2011) Prevalence of target organ damage and metabolic abnormalities in resistant hypertension. Med Clin (Barc) 137(10):435–439

Bax L et al (2009) Stent placement in patients with atherosclerotic renal artery stenosis and impaired renal function: a randomized trial. Ann Intern Med 150:840–848

Bhatt D et al (2014) A controlled trial of renal denervation for resistant hypertension. N Engl J Med 370:1393–1401

Bisognano JD (2011) Baroflex activation lowers blood pressure in patients with resistant hypertension: results from the double-blind, randomized, placebo-controlled rheos pivotal trial. J Am Coll Cardiol 58 (7):765–73

Blumenthal JA et al (2015) Lifestyle modification for resistant hypertension: the TRIUMPH randomized clinical trial. Am Heart J 170(5):986–994

Calhoun D (2009) Effects of dietary sodium reduction on blood pressure in subjects with resistant hypertension: results from a randomized trial. Hypertension 54:475–481

Calhoun D (2010) Sleep and hypertension. CHEST 138 (2):434–443

Calhoun DA et al (2002) Hyperaldosteronism among black and white subjects with resistant hypertension. Hypertension 40:892–896

Cooper C et al (2014) Stenting and medical therapy for atherosclerotic renal- artery stenosis. N Engl J Med 370:13–22

Daugherty SL (2012) Incidence and prognosis of resistant hypertension in hypertensive patients. Hypertension 125(13):1635–1642

Drager L (2010) Characteristics and predictors of obstructive sleep apnea in patients with systemic hypertension. Am J Cardiol 105(8):1135–1139

Esler MD, Krum H, Sobotka PA, Schlaich MP, Schmieder RE, Bohm M (2010) Renal sympathetic denervation in patients with treatment-resistant hypertension (the SYMPLICITY HTN-2 Trial): a randomised controlled trial. Lancet 376:1903–1909

Fothersby M (1993) Effects of moderate sodium restriction on clinic and twenty-four-hour ambulatory blood pressure in elderly hypertensive subjects. J Hypertens 11

Gavras H (1981) Role of reactive hyperreninemia in blood pressure changes induced by sodium depletion in patients with refractory hypertension. Hypertension 3(4): 441–447, Jul–Aug

Grimson KS, Orgain ES, Anderson B, Broome RA, Longino FH (1949) Results of treatment of patients with hypertension by total thoracic and partial to total lumbar sympathectomy, splanchnicectomy and celiac ganglionectomy. Ann Surg 129:850–871

Guerrero M (2009) Clinical spectrum of pheochromocytoma. J Am Coll Surg 209(6):727–732

Hyun JM (2015) Clinical features of obstructive sleep apnea that determine its high prevalence in resistant hypertension. Yonsei Med K 56(5):1258–1265

Jamerson K et al (2008) Benazepril plus Amlodipine or Hydrochorothiazide for hypertension in high risk patients. N Engl J Med 359:2417–2428

James P et al (2014) Evidence-based guidelines for the management of high blood pressure in adults. Report from the panel members appointed to the Eighth Joint National Committee (JNC8). JAMA 311:284–427

Kaplan N et al (2010) Clinical hypertension. Lippincott, Philadelphia, Print

Khosla N (2009) Predictors of hyperkalemia risk following hypertension control with aldosterone blockade. Am J Nephrol 30(5):418–424

Krieger EM et al (2014) Resistant hypertension optimal treatment trial: a randomized controlled trial. Clin Cardiol 37(6):388

Lobo M (2015) Central arteriovenous anastomosis for the treatment of patients with uncontrolled hypertension. (the ROX CONTROL HTN study): a randomised controlled trial. Lancet 385: 1634–1641

Mantero F (2000) A survey on adrenal incidentaloma in Italy. Study Group on adrenal tumors of the Italian Society of Endocrinology. J Clin Endocrinol Metab 637

Moneva M (2002) Pathophysiology of adrenal hypertension. Semin Nephrol 22:44–53

Ohkubo T et al (2000) Prediction of stroke by ambulatory blood pressure monitoring versus screening blood pressure measurements in a general population: the Ohasama study. J Hypertens 18(7):847–854

Pepine CJ, Handberg-Thurmond E, Marks RG et al (1998) Rationale and design of the International Verapamil SR/Trandolapril Study (INVEST): an Internet-based randomized trial in coronary artery disease patients with hypertension. J Am Coll Cardiol 32 (5):1228–1237

Persell SD (2011) Prevalence of resistant hypertension in the United States, 2003–2008. Hypertension 57:1076–1080

Pimenta E et al (2012) Resistant hypertension: incidence, prevalence, and prognosis. Circulation 125 (13):1594–1596

Pisoni R (2009) Characterization and treatment of resistant hypertension. Curr Cardiol Rep 11:407–413

Prisant L (2004) Coarctation of the aorta: a secondary cause of hypertension. J Clin Hypertens 6:347–350

Rose BD (2001) Clinical physiology of acid–base and electrolyte disorders. McGraw Hill, New York, Print

Sacks F et al (2001) Effects on blood pressure of reduced dietary sodium and the Dietary Approaches to Stop Hypertension (DASH) diet. DASH-Sodium Collaborative Research Group. New Engl J Med 344(1):3–10

Salles GF et al (2008) Prognostic influence of office and ambulatory blood pressures in resistant hypertension. Arch Intern Med 168(21):2340–2346

Sarafidis P (2011) Epidemiology of resistant hypertension. J Clin Hypertens 13:523–528

Sharma A et al (2004) High prevalence and poor control of hypertension in primary care: a cross-sectional study. J Hypertens 22:479–486

Stein P (1981) A simplified diagnostic approach to pheochomocytoma. A review of the literature and report of one institution's experience. Medicine (Baltimore) 46–66

Tauzin-Fin P (2004) Effects of perioperative alpha block on haemodynamic control during laparoscopic surgery for phaeochromocytoma. Br J Anaestholy 92:512–517

The ALLHAT Officers and Coordinators for the ALLHAT Collaborative Research Group (2002) Major outcomes in high-risk hypertensive patients randomized to angiotensin-converting enzyme inhibitor or calcium channel blocker vs. diuretic: the antihypertensive and lipid-lowering treatment to prevent heart attack trial (ALLHAT). JAMA 288:2981–2997

The Astral Trial Investigators (2009) Revascularization versus medical therapy for renal-artery stenosis. N Engl J Med 361:1953–1962

Thomas G (2015) Prevalance and prognostic significance of apparent treatment resistant hypertension in chronic kidney disease: Report from the Chronic Renal Insufficiency Cohort Study. Hypertension 67(2):387–396

Ulick S et al (1992) Cortisol inactivation overload: a mechanism of mineralocorticoid hypertension in the ectopic adrenocorticotropin syndrome. J Clin Endocrinol Metab 74:963–967

Williams B et al (2015) Spironolactone versus placebo, bisoprolol, and doxazosin to determine the optimal treatment for drug-resistant hypertension (PATHWAY-2): a randomised, double-blind, crossover trial. Lancet 386:2059–2068

Yetman AT (1997) Balloon angioplasty of recurrent coarctation: a 12 year review. J Am Coll Cardiol 30 (3):811–816

Adv Exp Med Biol - Advances in Internal Medicine (2017) 2: 191–208
DOI 10.1007/5584_2016_170
© Springer International Publishing AG 2016
Published online: 14 December 2016

Renal Ultrasound (and Doppler Sonography) in Hypertension: An Update

Maria Boddi

Abstract

Ultrasound (US) allows the non-invasive evaluation of morphological changes of kidney structure (by means of B-Mode) and patterns of renal and extrarenal vascularization (by means of color-Doppler and contrast-enhanced US). In hypertensive subjects it offers a relevant contribution to the diagnosis of early renal damage, acute or chronic nephropathies and nephrovascular disease. However, morphological changes are often detected late and non-specific and in recent years evidence has increased regarding the clinical relevance of renal resistive index (RRI) for the study of vascular and renal parenchymal renal abnormalities. RRI is measured by Doppler sonography in an intrarenal artery, as the difference between the peak systolic and end-diastolic blood velocities divided by the peak systolic velocity. At first RRI was proved to be a marker of renal disease onset and progression; later the influence of systemic vascular properties on RRI was shown and authors claimed its use as an independent predictor of cardiovascular risk rather than of renal damage. Indeed, renal vascular resistance is only one of several renal (vascular compliance, interstitial and venous pressure), and extrarenal (heart rate, pulse pressure) determinants that concur to determine RRI individual values but not the most important one. The clinical relevance of RRI measurement as a surrogate endpoint of specific renal damage or/and as surrogate endpoint of atherosclerotic diffuse vascular damage is still debated.To summarize, from the literature: (a) In hypertensives with normal renal function and no albuminuria, especially in younger people, RRI is an early marker of renal damage that is especially useful when hypertension and diabetes concur in the same subjects. In these subjects RRI could improve current clinical scores used to stratify early renal damage. In older subjects RRI increases in accordance with the increase in systemic vascular stiffness and, because

M. Boddi (✉)
Experimental and Clinical Department, University of
Florence, Florence, Italy
e-mail: maria.boddi@unifi.it

of this close relationship, RRI is also a marker of systemic atherosclerotic burden and the role of renal determinants can weaken. The clinical relevance was not specifically investigated. (b) In transplant kidney and in chronic renal disease high (>0.80) RRI values can independently predict renal failure. The recent claim that systemic (pulse pressure) rather than renal hemodynamic determinants sustain this predictive role of RRI, does not significantly reduce this predictive role of RRI. (c) Doppler ultrasound allows diagnosis and grading of renal stenosis in both fibromuscolar dysplastic and atherosclerotic diseases. Moreover, by RRI assay Doppler ultrasound can indirectly measure the hemodynamic impact of renal artery stenosis on the homolateral kidney, by virtue of the stenosis-related decrease in pulse pressure. However, in elderly subjects with atherosclerotic renal artery stenosis coexisting renal diseases can independently increase RRI by the augmentation in renal vascular stiffness and tubulo-interstitial pressure and hidden changes due to renal artery stenosis.

Keywords

Renal resistive index • Ultrasonography • Hypertension • Renal disease • Renal artery stenosis

1   Introduction

The pathophysiological relationship between increased blood pressure and kidneys is complex. High blood pressure causes progressive renal damage but also vascular or parenchymal renal disease can sustain increase in blood pressure.

Ultrasound (US) has a key role in evaluating both morphological changes of kidney structure (by means of B-Mode) and patterns of renal and extrarenal vascularization (by means of color-Doppler and contrast-enhanced US), thus contributing to the diagnosis of early renal damage, acute or chronic nephropathies and nephrovascular disease in hypertensive patients. Maximum renal diameter is a morphological marker of CKD. It decreases contemporarily to Glomerular Filtration Rate (GFR) and a significant correlation of both renal diameter and cortical thickness with renal function has been demonstrated (Meola et al. 2016a). A direct correlation between the number of functional renal units, nephrons, renal mass, renal function and ultrasound-measured renal volume has also been reported. Kidney size was measured by US which compared with other radiologic methods gave results that came closest to the actual size of the kidney measured during surgery (Vegar Zubović et al. 2016). Ultrasound-measured volume of kidneys correlates well with the stage and the progression of CKD and can be used to evaluate CKD progression. However, ultrasound-detected morphological changes are late and not specific. In recent years increasing attention has been paid to the study of renal resistive index (RRI) obtained by Doppler arterial waveform analysis of intrarenal arteries as an independent marker of early renal damage when albuminuria and glomerular filtration rate are still normal, and as an independent predictor of renal failure progression in chronic renal disease (Radermacher et al. 2002; Ikee et al. 2005; Sugiura 2011; Bigè et al. 2012).

Infact, as well synthesized in the review by Viazzi et al. (Viazzi et al. 2014), not only does Doppler ultrasonography detect renal macroscopic vascular abnormalities that allows diagnosis and grading of renal artery stenosis, but it also identifies changes in blood flow at the micro-vascular level that reflect functional or structural changes within the kidneys. Specifically, acute functional changes in renovascular resistance physiologically induced by sympathetic activation or pharmacologically by ACE inhibitors (Bardelli et al. 1992; Jensen et al. 1994),acute increase in tubulo-interstitial pressure by hydronephrosis or acute kidney injury and chronic structural damage of arteriolar or tubule-interstitial rather than glomerular compartment do affect RRI.

Recent clinical and experimental evidence indicates that increased RRI in patients with primary hypertension with normal or reduced renal function may reflect and score changes in intrarenal perfusion because of arteriolar and/or tubule-interstitial renal damage that can occur independently of glomerular damage. Moreover,in hypertensive patients high RRI is also associated with worse systemic hemodynamics and atherosclerotic burden. Due to this relationship,RRI has been also proposed as a new independent marker and predictor of systemic cardiovascular risk in asymptomatic subjects. The clinical relevance and the possible therapeutic implications of this use need dedicated studies (Chirinos and Townsend 2014; O'Neill 2014). This review tries to give information on the knowledge of physiopathological renal and extra-renal determinants of RRI, necessary for the correct use of RRI ultrasound measurement in clinical practice when focused on the study of early and late renal damage in essential hypertension and in the diagnosis and grading of renal artery stenosis. Specifically, we want to show whether and when the measurement of RRI should be considered as a specific marker of renal damage to use together and in addition to Glomerular Filtration Rate (GFR) and microalbuminuria or as a parameter of systemic cardiovascular risk to use together and in addition to intima-media-thickness and other surrogate ultrasound endpoints for cardiovascular risk stratification of asymptomatic patients.

According to recent recommendations by the major societies for the study of hypertension (the American Heart Association, the American College of Cardiology and the Centers for Disease Control and Prevention, the American Society of Hypertension and the International Society of Hypertension, the Canadian Hypertension Educational Program, the European Society of Cardiology and the European Society of Hypertension, the National Institute for Health and Care Excellence, The French Society of Hypertension, the Taiwan and the Chinese Society of Hypertension) (James et al. 2014; Go et al. 2014; Weber et al. 2014; Dasgupta et al. 2014; Mancia et al. 2013; National Institute for Health and Care Excellence 2014; Blacher et al. 2014; Chiang et al. 2010; Liu 2010), the study of hypertensive patients by renal ultrasonography is mainly dedicated to patients with the clinical suspicion of secondary hypertension. This is because ultrasound can detect the presence of renal parenchymal disease, polycystic renal disease, and urinary tract obstruction. Specifically, when clinical characteristics point to renovascular hypertension, ultrasound screening is recommended to confirm or rule out the diagnosis of renal artery stenosis, grading the stenosis and investigating its hemodynamic impact on the homolateral kidney. At present, the ultrasound study of renal target-organ damage in essential hypertension has not been codified; and the determination of GFR and of albuminuria excretion rate are recommended.

This review wants to give strong support to the use of RRI for investigating early and late renal damage in hypertensive patients, as an independent predictor of renal failure and/or of cardiovascular risk. To have a high RRI selects subjects at increased risk of developing renal failure and of having cardiovascular events beyond the pattern of other current renal and ultrasound markers of risk.

2 Renal Resistive Index (RRI)

RRI, derived from the Doppler spectrum of intrarenal (segmental or interlobar) arteries, is obtained by the difference between maximum (peak systolic) and minimum (end-diastolic) flow velocity to maximum flow velocity (Fig. 1):

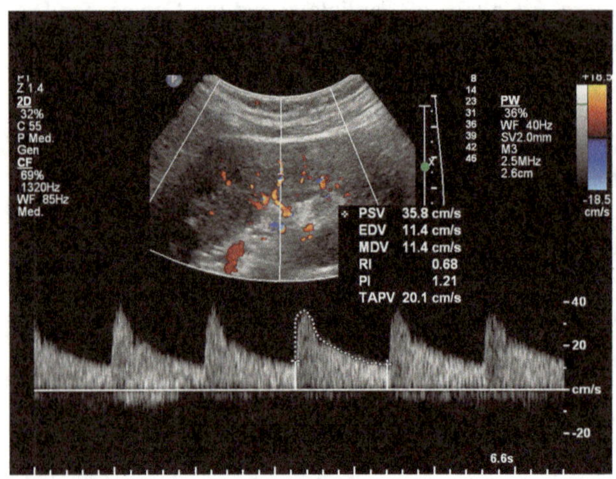
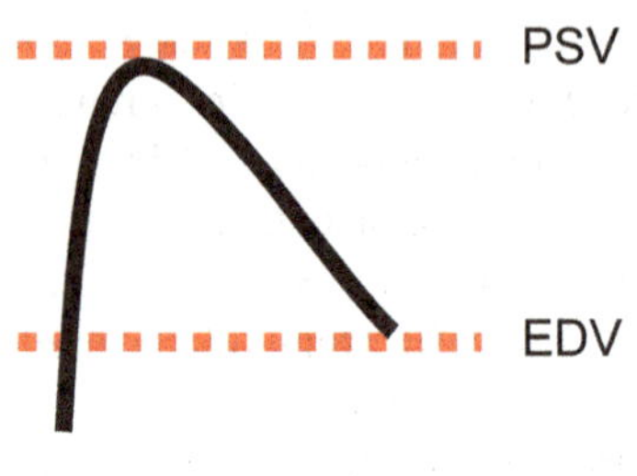

Fig. 1 RRI is measured by Doppler sonography in an intrarenal artery, as the difference between the peak systolic (PS) and end-diastolic (ED) blood velocities divided by the peak systolic velocity (PSV)

$$\mathrm{RRI} = \frac{(\text{peak systolic velocity (PSV)} - \text{end} - \text{diastolic velocity (EDS)})}{\text{Peak systolic velocity (PSV)}}$$

The morphology of Doppler spectrum of RRI is mainly determined by the velocity/time (V/t) curve that is assayed along the main renal artery, that can be defined as a "low resistance" curve. The systolic phase quickly increases to peak velocity and is followed by a progressive and gradual deceleration phase with a telediastolic velocity that does not decrease below 30–40 cm/sec. This Doppler spectrum is common and peculiar to all parenchymal flows, because a sufficient oxygen supply must be assured throughout the cardiac cycle (Meola et al. 2016b).

RRI was introduced in 1950 and initially proposed for the semi-quantitative assay of intra-renal vascular resistance by Pourcelot in (1974). He showed that the ratio was influenced by changes in vascular resistance distally to the point of RRI assay. The term RRI has been kept to the present time, even if the strict relationship between RRI and actual renal vascular resistance has become very weak (Chirinos and Townsend 2014; O'Neill 2014).

According to these findings RRI was initially used for the diagnosis and follow-up of acute and chronic renal disease (Radermacher et al. 2002; Viazzi et al. 2014) which are associated to dynamic and/or structural changes in intra-renal vessels. Later on RRI was proved to be a strong independent predictor of renal failure (Radermacher et al. 2002; Sugiura 2011). However, in the meantime growing evidence showed that RRI is the result of many intra and extra-renal determinants and that renal vascular resistance is only one of these, and not the most important (Boddi et al. 2015) (Fig. 2). Remarkably, in 1991 Gosling et al. (1991), and in 1999 Bude and Rubin (1999), clearly showed by in vitro experiments performed in simple artificial circuits, that RRI is dependent on both renal vascular compliance and resistance, becoming less dependent on resistance as compliance decreases. When compliance is zero, RRI is independent of changes in renal vascular resistance. Moreover, new experimental (Chirinos and Townsend 2014; Tublin et al. 2003) and clinical data (Chirinos and Townsend 2014; O'Neill 2014) were obtained showing that RRI was markedly affected by the changes in renal (renal interstitial and venous pressure) and systemic (pulse pressure) determinants of vascular compliance, and only scarcely by the chronic

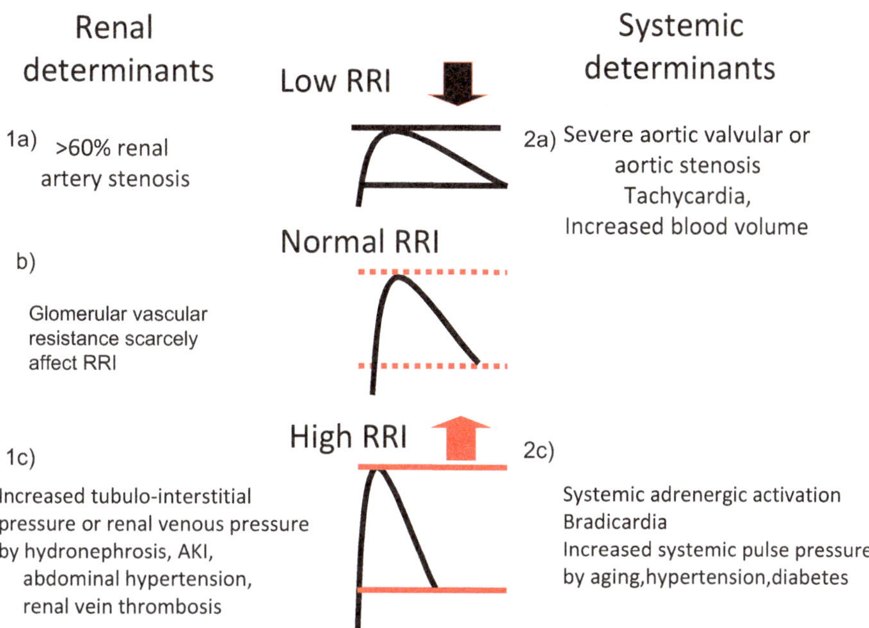

Fig. 2 Different renal and extrarenal systemic determinants concur to determine RRI. (**1a**) and (**2a**): renal and systemic determinants that decrease RRI. (**b**): glomerular resistance scarcely or not affect RRI. (**1c**) and (**2c**): renal and systemic determinants that increase RRI (Adapted by Boddi et al. 2015)

increase in renal vascular resistance. In chronic renal diseases and in transplant recipients, RRI mainly depends on systemic vascular compliance assayed as pulse pressure, rather than renal vascular properties (Chirinos and Townsend 2014; O'Neill 2014). In these patients the increase in RRI is strictly associated with the decrease in systemic vascular compliance assayed as pulse pressure that is negatively modulated by aging and traditional cardiovascular (CV) risk factors, among which hypertension plays a major role (Chirinos and Townsend 2014). According to this point of view, in hypertensive patients with and without renal function impairment, the increase in RRI predicts worse renal and general outcomes, as a marker of systemic atherosclerotic burden rather than of local renal damage. However, this statement is still a matter of debate and do not weaken the clinical relevance of RRI measurement for risk scoring.

On the contrary full agreement was reached on the clinical use of RRI as a specific marker of renal damage, in subjects affected by those renal pathologies that can promote the progression of renal damage in hypertensive patients, i.e. hydronephrosis, renal vein thrombosis, increased abdominal pressure and acute kidney injury. In all these conditions the acute and marked increase in renal tubule-interstitial and venous pressure due to hydrostatic or inflammatory edema leads to the direct increase in RRI values (Boddi et al. 2015).

3   RRI Threshold in Clinical Practice

Aging is associated with a progressive quantitative decrease of renal microvascular bed and with an increased thickness of tunica media of renal arterioles (Fig. 2). This determines a decrease in the lumen/vessel wall ratio. Both these changes result in a progressive increase in RRI (Boddi et al. 1996) that can be amplified by the contemporaneous increase in systemic arterial stiffness. The steep age-dependent rise in RRI values is specific to the renal vasculature and is not seen in other vascular beds. The age-related hypertrophic remodelling of the vessel wall of renal microvessels can be further amplified by hypertension and/or diabetes (Pontremoli et al. 1999a; Maestripieri et al. 2012). In healthy adults most authors use >0.70 as the cut-off limit for pathological RRI and do not establish normal values according to age. However, in healthy subjects >70 year, RRI >0.70 can be measured in the absence of renal diseases, whereas in subjects aged >40 year can be the first marker of renal damage that anticipates GRF reduction and the occurrence of albuminuria (Boddi et al. 1996). Further an emerging clinical issue is the evaluation of the actual renal function in elderly normal patients or diabetics, since the estimated values of GFR by math formula suffer of limits in these subgroups. So that, in elderly subjects with normal renal function or diabetics, RRI assessment might be considered an other non-invasive way to reveal early renal damage.

In a recent large multicentric family-based population study, age was confirmed as a determinant of RRI. Ponte et al. (2014) also showed that the relationship of RRI with age is nonlinear and that RRI increases sharply after the age of 40.

In the same multicentric study female sex was associated with higher RRI values due to hormone differences and the fact that RRI has a genetic tract was reported (Ponte et al. 2014); the clinical relevance of these findings must be investigated by dedicated studies.

In newborns and in children under the age of four, RRI > 0.70 can be found because of renal anatomical structure in this period and is not associated with renal pathologies (Bude et al. 1992).

4 Systemic and Renal Determinants of RRI

In any arterial vascular tract, Doppler waveform is the integrated result of what happens before and downstream from the point where the flow is assayed.

4.1 Systemic and Extrarenal Determinants

4.1.1 Stiffness-Related Systemic Pulse Pressure

The ratio of systolic to diastolic blood pressure (see RRI equation) is an inverse function of pulse pressure. Thus, for any given intra-renal vascular resistance an increase in systemic systolic arterial pressure promotes a higher peak renal velocity and/or a decrease in diastolic arterial pressure. That results in a lower end-diastolic velocity. As a direct consequence, in vivo any increase in systemic arterial stiffness that causes increased pulse pressure is associated with high RRI values, both in physiological (aging) and pathological (hypertension) conditions (Fig. 2c). Changes in pulse pressure can also be tonic or phasic, as during an infusion of L-NG-monomethyl argirine (L-NMMA), an inhibitor of endothelial NOS. Neither RRI under baseline conditions nor RRI during L-NMMA infusion were related with renal vascular resistance or renal perfusion, assayed by para-aminohippuric acid and insulin clearance (Raff et al. 2010). On the contrary, RRI changed according to variations of central pulse pressure.

The relationship between RRI and pulse pressure has also been investigated in recipients of kidney transplants where systemic pulse pressure is recipient-specific, whereas the compliance of interlobular arteries is donor specific; in these kidneys RRI correlated with the age of the recipient but not of the donor, with recipient pulse pressure but not parameters of allograft function and with RRI of other (i.e. splenic) districts of the recipient (Naesens et al. 2013). As a whole the findings observed in transplant recipients strongly support that RRI primarily reflects the properties of the systemic vasculature that can hidden or weaken the effects of local renal damage on intrarenal vasculature.

4.1.2 Stenosis-Related Pulse Pressure

Severe (>80 %) renal artery thoracic or sovrarenal abdominal aorta or valvular aortic stenosis all decrease pulse pressure in vascular districts distal to stenosis, and decrease RRI values (<0.60) as a result of low peak systolic velocity (Fig. 2, 2a). The dampened flow is revealed by the peculiar Doppler wave pattern characterized by a "tardus", slow, and "parvus", small pulsus (Figs. 2 and 3). The finding of low RRI in the homolateral kidney and the lateralization of RRI (delta > 0.05) is indirect but reliable proof of severe renal artery stenosis (Fig. 4). In fact the gradual reduction of renal perfusion pressure up to 40 % does not substantially change renal blood flow and glomerular filtration rate, thanks to the self-regulating mechanisms of intrarenal circulation. In these conditions RRI is not affected. This mechanism becomes ineffective when morphological renal arterial stenosis is >75 %, renal perfusion pressure falls >40 % and renal systolic pressure is <70–80 mm Hg (Textor and Wilcox 2001; Jacobson 1988). This renal stenosis is

defined hemodynamically significant, because it activates the renal renin angiotensin system (Meola et al. 2016b; Butterly and Schwab 2000) and demodulates Doppler waveform at intrarenal arteries. However, when distal renal vascular disease coexists due to chronic ischemic kidney, the hemodynamic effects of renal artery stenosis may be hidden. In these patients RRI is symmetrically high, not lateralized and the hemodynamic effect of arterial stenosis on renal parenchyma cannot be evaluated by Doppler ultrasound (Meola et al. 2016b; Boddi et al. 2015) (Fig. 4) (see also *Ultrasound diagnostics of renal artery stenosis, page 14*).

4.1.3 Heart Rate

Changes in heart rate can affect RRI independently from the other hemodynamic parameters because of changes in diastolic duration that modulate end-diastolic velocity. During

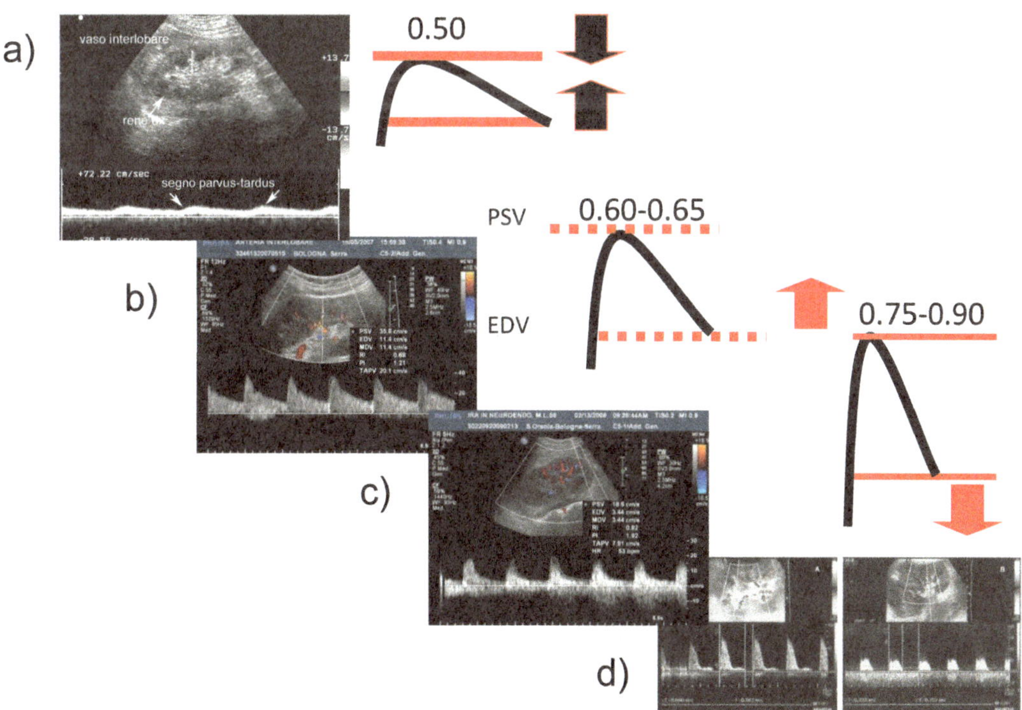

Fig. 3 Schematic representation of possible RRI changes. From the left to the right:(**a**) low RRI values (0.50) because of low peak systolic velocity (PSV) with peculiar Doppler wave pattern of post-stenotic flow characterized by a "tardus", slow, and "parvus", little pulsus; (**b**) normal Doppler wave pattern and PSV/EDV at interlobar arteries; (**c**, **d**) high RRI (0.75–0.90) due to high peak systolic (PSV) and decreased end-diastolic velocity (EDV) (Adapted by Boddi et al. 2015)

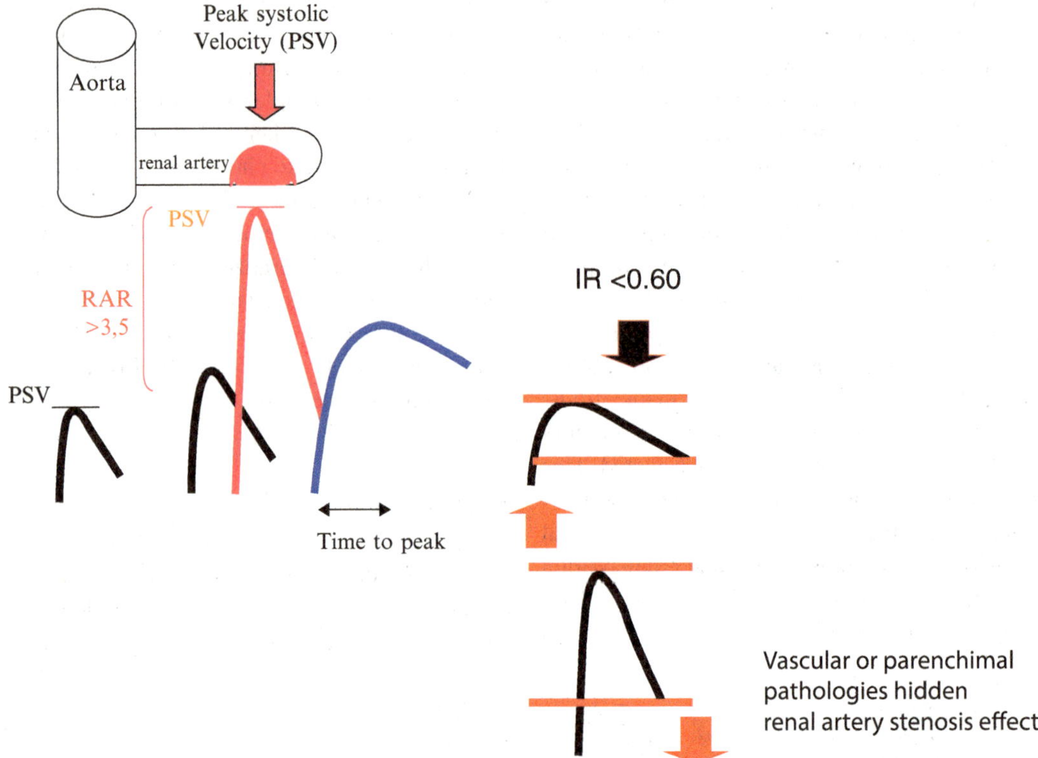

Fig. 4 Schematic representation of Doppler flow patterns assayed at and distal to a hemodynamically arterial renal stenosis; RRI is lateralized (delta > 0.05); when vascular or parenchimal nephropathies coexist, RRI values symmetrically increase and the hemodinamic effect of renal artery stenosis is hidden (Adapted from Boddi et al. 2015)

bradicardia diastolic duration increases and high RRI is measured. On the contrary during tachicardia diastolic duration shortens and RRI decreases (Fig. 2, 2a and c).

4.2 Renal Determinants

4.2.1 Renal Interstitial and Venous Pressure

The renal capillary wedge pressure (interstitial tissue plus venous pressure) is a major renal determinant of RRI. In ex vivo rabbit kidney model elevations in ureteral pressure were significantly correlated with increased RRI values, mean renal vascular resistance (pressure/flow) and decreased mean conductance (flow/pressure) (Tublin et al. 1999). In humans in vivo the acute increase of renal interstitial pressure by hydronephrosis or of venous pressure by venous thrombosis, or of both by abdominal hypertension, results in a linearly related increase in RRI (Fig. 2, 1c). Also renal hematoma can acutely increase the pressure of interstitial compartment and elevate RRI (Platt et al. 1989).

Most importantly, acute kidney injury (AKI) is associated with an acute increase in interstitial pressure because of sustained vasoconstriction and ischemic and inflammatory damage of the tubulo-interstial compartment by sustained hypoperfusion. In all these clinical conditions the occurrence, severity and progression of renal damage can be well monitored by changes in RRI values (Platt et al. 1989; Schnell et al. 2012; Dewitte 2013; Le Dorze et al. 2012; Darmon et al. 2011). Recently, in critical patients admitted for medical, surgical or trauma disease, high RRI values at admission were significantly and independently associated with in-ICU mortality and persistent AKI at ICU discharge (Boddi et al. 2016).

4.2.2 Histological Renal Parameters – RRI and the Tubulo-Interstitial Compartment

Twenty years ago Platt et al. showed that RRI was significantly higher in nephropathies with tubulo-interstitial and/or vascular injury than in isolated glomerulopathies (Platt et al. 1990). Glomerular arterial resistance, that accounts for about 20 % of total renal vascular resistance, scarcely concurs to the determination of RRI; and nephropathies characterized by prevalent glomerular involvement are not associated with increased RRI. RRI is not a marker of renal function (Fig. 2).

The studies on the relationship between tubular, interstitial and arterial damage and RRI in renal disease and in kidney transplants show conflicting results: according to Ikee et al., only arteriolosclerosis out of all histological parameters independently correlated with RRI in chronic renal disease (Ikee et al. 2005), whereas in renal transplants investigated at 3, 12 and 24 months after transplantation RRI was not associated with any renal allograft histological features. On the contrary, other Authors reported that high RRI values were related to more severe tubulo-interstitial damage score, and an association between RRI values and the extension of interstitial fibrosis was shown, probably due to the rise in pressure exerted by interstitial fibrosis on adjacent vessels. Remarkably, interstitial fibrosis closely correlated to renal function and long-term prognosis and could underline the role of RRI as an independent marker of renal and clinical outcome in patients with CKD (Sugiura 2011; Bigè et al. 2012).

The possible use of RRI as a marker of tubulo-interstitial nephropathy is supported by the findings that the detection of high RRI values allowed the early identification of both normotensive and hypertensive patients with chronic tubulo-interstitial nephropathy diagnosed by 99 mTc DMSA scintigraphy and signs of tubular dysfunction, when renal function was still preserved (Boddi et al. 2006). Moveover, in hypertensive patients with normal creatinine clearance and no albuminuria, high RRI values were associated with low grade inflammation (Protein C reactive >2 mg/dl) and hyperuricemia (>6.5 mg/dl) (Berni et al. 2012, 2010). Both sustain a tubulo-interstitial nephropathy. In hypertensive patients, serum uric acid strongly correlated with RRI, independently of renal function or albuminuria, but the altered intrarenal hemodynamics did not explain the pathophysiology of hyperuricemic renal damage (Geraci et al. 2016).

A generalized consensus was reached that tubulo-interstitial and not glomerular nephropathies affect RRI and that RRI does not measure renal function.

4.2.3 Role of Arterial Vascular Resistance

Based on early experimental animal data (Bude and Rubin 1999; Tublin et al. 1999), RRI was long considered to directly mirror intrarenal resistance, thus allowing a non-invasive glimpse into intrarenal (patho) physiology (Norris and Barnes 1984). Under physiological conditions RRI assay could detect phasic increase in renal vascular resistance induced by sympathetic activation obtained by cold pressor test or handgrip; in the same subjects the increase of blood volume by acute hydration resulted in an RRI decrease (Boddi et al. 1996). Repeated daily sessions of music-guided slow-breathing increased parasympathetic modulation and decreased RRI early in the study. These changes were being followed by a positive modulation of baroflex sensitivity and decrease in blood pressure (Modesti et al. 2015). In patients with heart failure high RRI values were associated with increased intrarenal vascular resistance due to neurohormonal hyperactivity and independently predicted heart failure progression (Ciccone et al. 2014). In septic shock Doppler ultrasonography and RRI measurements may help determine in each patient the optimal mean aortic pressure for renal blood flow and may be a relevant end-point to titrate the haemodynamic treatment by fluid and norepinephrine administration (Deruddre et al. 2007).Catheter-based renal sympathetic denervation in patients with resistant hypertension reduced RRI probably through a decrease in intraparenchymal resistance, not mediated by reduction in systolic blood pressure (Mahfoud et al. 2012). As a whole these findings sustain that the RRI can detect phasic changes in renal vascular resistance.

On the contrary, RRI changes during dynamic vasodilation caused by nytroglicerin or (L-NMMA) infusion were poorly associated with the concurring direct measurement of renal resistance by scintigraphy, even if the changes in RRI and in renal vascular resistance moved in the same direction. Rather, RRI changes were directly related to changes in pulse pressure (Raff et al. 2010). Increased RRI has been shown to correlate with systemic arterial stiffness measured by ambulatory blood pressure derived by Ambulatory Arterial Stiffness Index (Ratto et al. 2006). Moreover, a close relationship between RRI and other markers of systemic atherosclerotic burden, as intima-media thickness and ankle brachial index, was shown in hypertensive patients with chronic renal disease, independently of renal damage (Pontremoli et al. 1999b).

For many years the role of high RRI values as an independent marker of renal outcome in patients with CKD was mainly due to the assumption that RRI increase was determined above all by the progressive "tonic" increase in vascular resistance because of: (a) decrease in arterial compliance due to renal arteriosclerosis; (b) elevation of extra-vascular renal pressure exerted by interstitial fibrosis in adjacent vessels; (c) vasoconstriction secondary to hypoxia and to loss of capillaries associated with renal fibrosis. All these are associated with decline in renal function (Boddi et al. 2015).

In recent years evidence has been gathered around RRI being an independent marker of renal and cardiovascular outcomes, because it measures systemic and not renal hemodynamic parameters, and reflects systemic vascular disease (Granata et al. 2014). We agree with O Neill's title "Renal resistive index. A case of mistaken identity" (O'Neill 2014). However, there is no doubt that both phasic (sympathetic activation) and tonic (arteriolosclerotic) changes in renal arterial resistance can modulate RRI.

4.2.4 RRI and Subclinical Renal Damage in Hypertension

In clinical practice albuminuria is measured to define subclinical renal damage in hypertensive patients, and the combination of eGFR and albuminuria is a useful predictor of CV disease (Viazzi et al. 2014). In recent years RRI was also validated as a clinical marker of subclinical renal damage as well as a prognostic predictor of renal and CV outcomes to use in addition to the above mentioned markers in order to improve their performance.

In untreated patients with primary hypertension and normal renal function, high RRI (>0.70) highlights subclinical signs of renal damage and shows a direct relationship with the amount of urine albumin excretion (Miyoshi et al. 2016). Further RRI was proved to be a useful index to predict increase in urinary albumin excretion in patients with essential hypertension (Viazzi et al. 2014). With the progression of hypertensive renal damage, high RRI values are often associated with a mild reduction in glomerular filtration rate and increased albuminuria or both (Doi et al. 2012). In hypertensive patients high (>0.70) RRI predicts renal dysfunction evaluated at 12 months by Cystatin C determination (Okura et al. 2010). Evaluation of both eGFR and RRI instead of albuminuria could be another investigative option to identify essential hypertensive subjects without clinical evidence of renal damage and cardiovascular disease, predisposed to worse renal and CV outcomes.

In hypertensive patients undergoing chronic antihypertensive therapy with no microalbuminuria and normal renal function, higher RRI values were found in those with hyperuricemia or low grade inflammation (PCR >2 mg/dl), both associated with tubulo-interstitial inflammation and endothelial dysfunction (Berni et al. 2012). Remarkably, in experimental studies it was found that hyperuricemia causes glomerular hypertension, vasoconstriction and ischemia, a potent stimulus for tubulo-interstitial inflammation and fibrosis (Berni et al. 2010; Sanchez-Losada et al. 2005).

Dynamic evaluation of RRI in normoalbuminuric patients with newly diagnosed hypertension showed that the decrease in RRI induced by nytroglicerine was lower in hypertensives than in controls despite similar baseline RRI (Bruno et al. 2011). Reduced renal vasodilation was independently related to the increase of systemic arterial stiffness and suggests a role of systemic hemodynamic load in determining early renal microvascular alteration in hypertension. RRI determination could help to understand the intricate link between hypertension and subclinical renal damage, till now mainly supported by the relationship between hypertension and microalbuminuria. The unifying mechanism that accounts for the different roles of RRI as a marker of subclinical renal damage and a prognostic predictor of renal and cardiovascular outcomes was suggested by Hashimoto et al. (Hashimoto and Hito 2011) who recorded aortic pressures, aortic and peripheral pulse wave velocities and RRI in 133 hypertensive patients: (a) RRI depends strongly on aortic pulse pressure and aortic stiffness; (b) RRI correlates inversely with the femoral reverse-flow and diastolic forward-flow indices; and (c) RRI predicts urinary albumin excretion together with the aortic pulse pressure. In these hypertensive patients the altered renal hemodynamics due to increased central pulse pressure and aortic stiffness contributed to the development of renal microvascular damage marked by high RRI. Every 0.1 increase in renal RRI was associated with a 5.4-fold increase in the adjusted relative risk of albuminuria (Hashimoto and Hito 2011). According to these findings atherosclerosis increases systemic arterial stiffness, predisposes renal circulation to a greater hemodynamic load (pulse pressure) and results in higher renal microvascular resistance. Increased systemic arterial stiffness underlines the strict relationship between RRI and atherosclerotic damage such as left ventricular hypertrophy, carotid intima media thickness and ankle brachial index (Pontremoli et al. 1999a; Calabia et al. 2014; Geraci et al. 2015). On the other hand high RRI might contribute to systemic

arterial stiffening by renal dysfunction and activate a self-perpetuating process. Moreover, RRI proved to be an independent predictor of worse renal and CV outcomes in 426 patients with primary hypertension and no previous CV disease followed for a mean of 3.1 years (Doi et al. 2013). We can conclude that in hypertensive patients with normal renal function RRI is an early clinical marker of subclinical renal damage, that can anticipate the occurrence of microalbuminuria, but also signals systemic atherosclerotic burden. For both reasons high RRI is a good predictor of worse renal and cardiovascular outcomes.

The vast majority of RRI measurements reported in literature are carried out in hypertensives on different pharmacological combinations without a wash-out period; this could result in confounding factors for the study of determinants of RRI.Remarkably, scarce data are available in literature (Leoncini et al. 2002; Watanabe et al. 2006) about the effect of pharmacological therapy on RRI values; whether and how the decrease in RRI values could result in an improvement of renal damage and in renal and CV outcomes is unknown. This fact is mainly responsible for the limited use of RRI in clinical practice and need dedicated studi.

4.2.5 RRI and Renal Damage in Diabetes

RRI can detect early renal damage in patients with diabetes type 1 and 2: when renal function is normal and albuminuria is absent; increased RRI predicts the occurrence of albuminuria (Hamano et al. 2008; Nosadini et al. 2006). Most importantly, in patients without microalbuminuria RRI values >0.70 independently predicted the occurrence of diabetic nephropathy. In diabetic subjects with albuminuria and reduced creatinine clearance, RRI >0.80 predicts a worse renal outcome (Boddi et al. 2015).

Newly diagnosed Type 2 diabetic patients show higher baseline RRI and lower vasodilation induced by nytroglicerin than those observed in newly diagnosed hypertensive subjects (Bruno et al. 2011). Pulse pressure proved to be a strong predictor of impaired RRI decrease in hypertensives and diabetics, but only in diabetic subjects was impaired vasodilatation significantly related to glycated haemoglobin and systolic pressure. Indeed,in patients with diabetic nephropathy the postglomerular vessels were the major contributor to increased resistance, whereas the pathognomonic histological sign of hypertensive nephropathy is preglomerular arteriolar hyalinosis disease.

These findings suggest that in diabetic patients renal vasculature might be compromised even in the presence of early glucose metabolism impairment, as in pre-diabetic condition where systemic vascular dysfunction and increased arterial stiffness are already present.

Accordingly, in hypertensive patients with no albuminuria and normal renal function, the coexistence of diabetes was associated with higher RRI values despite similar PWV in hypertensives with and without diabetes (Maestripieri et al. 2012).

4.2.6 RRI and Renal Damage in Chronic Renal Disease

In 2002 Radermacher et al. reported that in patients with chronic renal disease of any cause, an increased (>0.80) RRI correlates with the rate of decline in renal function and predicts the course of the disease (Radermacher et al. 2002). During a mean 3 years of follow up in these patients proteinuria (>1 g/day) and creatinine clearance (<40 ml/min) were also important indicators of disease progression, but in terms of positive and negative prediction RRI demonstrated superior utility. High RRI values were not secondary to differences in pulse rate or in the use of antihypertensive medication (Radermacher et al. 2002). Sugiura and Wada (2011) showed that high (>0.70) RRI as well as proteinuria, low GFR and hypertension, are independent risk factors for the progression of CKD (follow-up 4 years) and reinforced the feeling that RRI could be used as an additional tool for predicting the progression of CKD. High RRI could identify patients at high risk of end stage renal disease, because the initial measurements of RRI in patients with various nephropathies at the time of renal biopsy is associated with severe interstitial fibrosis and arteriolosclerosis and a

worse glomerular filtration rate at 18 months (Bigè et al. 2012). In the high (>0.70) RRI group of 202 patients with CKD who underwent renal biopsies, RI ≥ 0.7, hypertension, proteinuria, and low eGFR at diagnosis were independent risk factors for predicting worse renal dysfunction.

In conclusion, according to the above reported findings RRI in CKD patients can be considered an independent predictor of renal failure, histological damage, and worse renal prognosis, as well as a possible determinant of the response to steroid therapy.

In middle aged and elderly hypertensive subjects Doi et al. (2013) confirmed the relationship between high RRI and worse cardiovascular and renal outcomes and that the combination of (<40 ml/min) eGFR and RRI was a powerful independent predictor of worse outcome, even when adjusted for traditional cardiovascular risk factors. The independent role of RRI in outcomes was maintained also for subjects with a GRF <60 mL/min. It is noteworthy that patients with both decreased eGFR and increased RRI had a significant burden of CV risk factors and a higher risk of the primary composite end points compared with those with either isolated decreased eGFR or increased RRI. Although both eGFR and increased RRI reflect renal dysfunction, the pathophysiological mechanisms leading to these abnormalities may, at least in part, be different. (Radermacher et al. 2002; Boddi et al. 2015; Doi et al. 2013).

Increased RI could be considered a marker of systemic atherosclerotic vessel damage, and compounded with reduced eGFR it may significantly increase the cardiovascular and renal risk. Data obtained from renal transplant recipients strongly supported that the predictive role of RRI for renal and CV outcome was the expression of systemic and not renal determinants (Chirinos and Townsend 2014; O'Neill 2014).

5   Resistant Hypertension

We have already mentioned that patients with treatment-resistant hypertension showed high

RRI (Mahfoud et al. 2012). In these patients renal denervation was proposed as an attractive opportunity but so far only invasive procedures have been tested with conflicting results. Recently an approach for delivering externally focused ultrasound specifically targeting the perirenal artery tissues has been proposed. The application of acoustic energy creates a thermal field which is capable of ablating renal nerves around the renal artery, up to 1 cm beyond the lumen. In 69 patients with treatment-resistant hypertension who underwent renal denervation with externally delivered focused ultrasound, a good reduction (24/10 mmHg) after 6 months was observed without major side effects (Neuzil et al. 2016). Further studies are needed to confirm these first promising results.

6 Ultrasound Diagnostics of Renal Artery Stenosis

Eligibility for ultrasound screening for renal artery stenosis is based on clinical criteria (Meola et al. 2016a, b; Schaberle et al. 2016). Screened subjects are mostly adults (especially elderly subjects) with atherosclerotic vascular disease involving multiple districts and stage 2 and 3 CKD without a documented history of renal disease. During a routine ultrasound examination a small kidney (length <9 cm) can suggest ischemic damage due to renal artery stenosis. The Doppler parameters used to define stenosis as hemodinamically significant are well standardized and can be divided into "major or direct" and "minor or indirect", or even "intrarenal or extrarenal" parameters. The criteria adopted by Zierler and Strandnes, published in the American Journal of Hypertension 1996 (Zierler et al. 1996), are still in use. Currently, RRI assay is the only Doppler parameter that provides information on the total vascular impedance of the parenchymal circle (Meola et al. 2016b; Schaberle et al. 2016).

Direct criteria are peak systolic velocity (PSV) and the ratio between PSV at renal stenosis and PSV in the aorta (Fig. 4); renal aortic ratio (RAR) a- PSV determines the degree of stenosis

according to the continuity equation, because PSV is inversely proportional to the cross-sectional area of stenosis. However, PSV is also influenced by current blood pressure, wall vessel compliance, tortuosity of renal arteries and chronic renal parenchymal damage. Hyperdynamic circle as observed in young people, hyperthyroidism and anemia, can also affect PSV. b-RAR compares the increased intrastenotic flow velocity in the renal arteries with the reference value measured in the aorta, and permits the decrease of the influence of the above mentioned systemic factors on PSV, measured at renal artery. Under physiological conditions the PSV along the main renal artery ranges between 60 and 120 cm/sec.

We want to remind readers that since eccentric stenosis results in a lower hemodynamic effect at the same angiographic diameter reduction, compared with concentric stenosis, (50 % of diameter reduction in concentric stenosis = 75 % of area reduction, whereas = 50 % in eccentric stenosis), PSV can rise twice as high at the same diameter reduction in eccentric stenosis. Compared with gold standard angiography, PSV measured by Color Duplex ultrasound shows sensitivities of 71–98 % and specificities of 62–98 %. Studies usually set the PSV cut-off value for >60 % renal artery stenosis at 180–200 cm/s, but they are determined by each author using receiver operating characteristics (ROC) curves, and different values are reported by different authors. It is to be noticed that selecting higher PSV cut-off values results in lower sensitivity and greater specificity in ROC curves compared with angiography (Meola et al. 2016b; Schaberle et al. 2016).

The combined use of PSV with RAR allows the increase in sensitivity and specificity of Doppler renal ultrasound to detect severe renal artery stenosis (Schaberle et al. 2016).

End-diastolic peak velocity was reported as stenosis criteria for the grading of carotid stenosis, but is markedly influenced by peripheral resistance which increases early in renal parenchymal damage and its use in the grading of renal artery stenosis is discussed.

We would like to point out that only >70–75 % RAS causes a relevant post-stenotic pressure drop, activating the renin angiotension system and requiring treatment. Only in high grade drop in post stenotic pressure can the severity of renal artery stenosis be calculated as validated for iliac arteries (Meola et al. 2016b; Schaberle et al. 2016).

Indirect criteria are based on the analysis of post-stenotic Doppler frequency spectra found distally to a >70 % renal artery stenosis, that depend also on intrarenal wall vessel and extravascular compliance and parenchyma function (Fig. 4) 1- RRI assayed in the kidney distally to renal artery stenosis shows a decreased difference between maximum and minimum flow velocity with a tardus-parvus spectrum and is lateralized with a difference in RRI >0.05 between the two kidneys, 2-Delayed acceleration time (AT) i.e. delay in the systolic rise from end diastole up to PSV on RRI spectral analysis. These ultrasound findings suggest that the ischemic kidney is protected by marked vasodilation, modulated by the self-regulating intrarenal mechanisms (Meola et al. 2016b; Zierler et al. 1996) which predict a good outcome of revascularization in terms of blood pressure control and recovery of renal function.

Renal artery stenosis due to fibromuscular dysplasia., usually discovered in young female, is characterized by specific renal vascular modifications and a normal renal function. For this kind of renal artery stenosis has been clearly shown the utility of doppler findings (PSV, RRI) in evaluating the severity of stenosis and the presence of intrarenal hemodynamic modifications before and after interventional procedures when compared to those obtained from the gold standard such as selective renal arteriography (Schaberle et al. 2016; Zierler et al. 1996).

In subjects with atherosclerotic renal artery stenosis, the typical post-stenotic criteria can be well evident in patients aged <60, with normal renal function, but not always in older patients with combined arteriolosclerosis and renal damage. These older subjects show high and symmetric RRI. The concurrence of chronic renal disease independently increasing RRI can hide the hemodynamic effect of renal artery stenosis and limit the information obtainable through Doppler ultrasound. Moreover, when parenchymal renal damage is asymmetrical as in pielonephritis, the bias for RRI measurement as marker of severe renal artery stenosis further increases (Boddi et al. 2015) (Fig. 4).

Recently, RRI >0.73 measured in the kidney controlateral to renal artery stenosis was the strongest predictor of renal function, worsening after renal revascularization also adjusted for male sex, regional angioplasty without stenting, obesity, pulse pressure >75 mmHg and serum creatinine >1.8 mg/dl (Bruno et al. 2014).

When hypoperfusion due to renal arterial stenosis persists for a long time and becomes chronic, damage of renal parenchyma develops, with a progressive reduction of renal volume and increase in interstitial and vascular resistance that results in high RRI (Bommart et al. 2010). High RRI (>0.75), especially when associated wih renal interpolar diameter < 9 cm and low renal volume, predicts a bad outcome of revascularization (Radermacher et al. 2001). An increased RRI value >80 is a strong predictor of renal functional decline in patients with renal artery stenosis, despite correction of the stenosis. As a whole data available in literature can be summarized as follows:

(a) Asymmetric low RRI distal to renal artery stenosis is a good marker of the hemodynamic impact of renal artery stenosis on renal parenchyma.

(b) When parenchymal disease concurs to renal artery stenosis and causes a symmetrical increase in RRI values, scarce or no information can be obtained on the hemodynamic impact of arterial stenosis on renal parenchyma.

(c) High asymmetric RRI values (≥0.80) distal to renal artery stenosis, with low interpolar diameter and volume of the ischemic kidney, are associated to bad outcome after revascularization.

(d) In subjectcs with renal artery stenosis and high symmetric RRI values can be also the mirror of systemic rather than renal parameters; in these subjects the predictive role of RRI for good revascularization outcome is under debate.

In the absence of direct or indirect signs of renal artery stenosis, increases in the intraparenchymal RRI (RI > 0.75 e/o > 0.80; PI > 1.50) associated with systemic atherosclerotic disease are indicative of microcirculatory damage related to nephroangiosclerosis or atheroembolic disease (Meola et al. 2016a).

7 Conclusions

The use of RRI in clinical practice is limited by the incomplete knowledge of all renal and extra-renal pathophysiological determinants that can concur to modulate RRI value in a different way in different subjects. In acute conditions such as hydronephrosis and AKI, renal determinants have a major role and RRI can directly monitor renal damage. In vascular and parenchymal nephropathies, the role of renal and extra-renal determinants must be analyzed singly, according to the subject's clinical characteristics and questions put to RRI by the internist, who searches for an early marker of targeted organ damage in hypertension or diabetes, or for an independent predictor of renal and CV outcome (Lennartz et al. 2016). To summarize, from the literature: (a) In hypertensives with normal renal function and no albuminuria, RRI is an early marker of renal damage and could improve current clinical scores used to stratify early renal damage. Especially in younger hypertensive and diabetics subjects. In older subjects RRI increases in accordance with the increase in systemic vascular stiffness and the role of renal determinants can weaken; because of this close relationship, RRI is also a marker of systemic atherosclerotic burden but the clinical relevance was not specifically investigated. (b) In transplant kidney and in chronic renal disease high (>0.80) RRI values can mark renal damge and independently predict renal failure. (c) Doppler ultrasound allows diagnosis and grading of renal stenosis in both fibromuscolar dysplastic and atherosclerotic diseases and can indirectly measure the hemodynamic impact of renal artery stenosis on the homolateral kidney. However, in elderly subjects with atherosclerotic renal artery stenosis coexisting renal diseases can independently increase RRI by the augmentation in renal vascular stiffness and tubulo-interstitial pressure and partially or completely hidden changes due to renal artery stenosis.

How and whether RRI assay could allow for improving the prediction of renal damage and of cardiovascular risk in asymptomatic subjects remains a matter of debate.

Aknowledgements I thank Ms. Susan Seeley for her precious help in revising the manuscript.

References

Bardelli M, Jensen G, Volkmann R, Caidahl K, Aurell M (1992) Experimental variations in renovascular resistance in normal man as detected by means of ultrasound. Eur J Clin Investig 22(9):619–624

Berni A, Boddi M, Fattori EB et al (2010) Serum uric acid levels and renal damage in hyperuricemic hypertensive patients treated with renin angiotensin system blockers. Am J Hypertens 23:675–680

Berni A, Ciani E, Bernetti M, Cecioni I, Berardino S, Poggesi L, Abbate R, Boddi M (2012) Renal resistive index and low-grade inflammation in patients with essential hypertension. J Hum Hypertens 26 (12):723–730

Bigè N, Levy PP, Callard P, Faintuch J-M, Chigot V, Jousselin V et al (2012) Renal arterial resistive index is associated with severe histological changes and poor renal outcome during chronic disease. BMC Nephrol 25(13):139. doi:10.1186/1471-2369-13-139

Blacher J, Halimi JM, Hanon O et al (2014) Management of hypertension in adults: the 2013 French society of hypertension guidelines. Fundam Clin Pharmacol 28:1–9

Boddi M, Sacchi S, Lammel RM, Mohseni R, Neri Serneri GG (1996) Age-related and vasomotor stimuli-induced changes in renal vascular resistance detected by Doppler ultrasound. Am J Hypertens 9 (5):461–466

Boddi M, Cecioni I, Poggesi L, Fiorentino F, Olianti K, Berardino S, La Cava G, Gensini GF (2006) Renal resistive index early detects chronic tubulointerstitial nephropathy in normo- and hypertensive patients. Am J Nephrol 26(1):16–21

Boddi M, Natucci F, Ciani E (2015) The internist and the renal resistive index: truths and doubts. Intern Emerg Med 10(8):893–905

Boddi M, Bonizzoli M, Chiostri M, Begliomini D, Molinaro A, Tadini Boninsegni L, Gensini GF, Peris A (2016) Renal resistive Index and mortality in critical patients with acute kidney injury. Eur J Clin Investig 46(3):242–251

Bommart S, Cliche A, Therasse E et al (2010) Renal artery revascularization: predictive value of kidney length and volume weighted by resistive index. AJR Am J Roentgenol 194(5):1365–1372

Bruno RM, Daghini E, Landini L et al (2011) Dynamic evaluation of renal resistive index in normoalbuminuric patients with newly diagnosed hypertension or type 2 diabetes. Diabetologia 54 (9):2430–2439

Bruno RM, Daghini E, Versari D, Sgrò M, Sanna M, Venturini L et al (2014) Predictive role of renal resistive index for clinical outcome after revascularization in hypertensive patients with atherosclerotic renal artery stenosis: a monocentric observational study. Cardiovasc Ultrasound 12:9. doi:10.1186/1476-7120-12-9

Bude RO, Rubin JM (1999) Relationship between the resistive index and vascular compliance and resistance. Radiology 211(2):411–417

Bude RO, Di Pietro MA, Platt JF, Rubin JM, Miesowicz S, Lundquist C (1992) Age dependency of the renal resistive index in healthy children. Radiology 184(2):469–473

Butterly DW, Schwab SJ (2000) Renal artery stenosis: the case for conservative management. Mayo Clin Proc 75 (5):435–436

Calabia J, Tourguet P, Garcia I et al (2014) The relationship between renal resistive index, arterial stiffness, and atherosclerotic burden: the link between macrocirculation and microcirculation. J Clin Hyperens (Greenwhich) 16(3):186–191

Chiang C-E, Wang T-D, Li Y-H et al (2010) 2010 guidelines of the Taiwan society of cardiology for the management of hypertension. J Formos Med Assoc 109:740–773

Chirinos JA, Townsend RR (2014) Systemic arterial hemodynamics and the "renal resistive index": what is in a name? J Clin Hypertens (Greenwich) 16 (3):170–171. doi:10.1111/jch.12276

Ciccone MM, Iacoviello M, Gesualdo L, Puzzovivo A, Antoncecchi V, Doronzo A, Monitillo F, Citarelli G, Paradies V, Favale S (2014) The renal arterial index: a marker of renal function with an independent and incremental role in predicting heart failure progression. Eur J Heart Fail 16(2):210–216

Darmon M, Schortgen F, Vargas F et al (2011) Diagnostic accuracy of Doppler renal resistive index for reversibility of acute kidney injury in critically ill patients. Intensive Care Med 37(1):68–76

Dasgupta K, RR Q, KB Z et al (2014) The 2014 Canadian Hypertension Education Program (CHEP) recommendations for blood pressure measurement, diagnosis, assessment of risk, prevention and treatment of hypertension. Can J Cardiol (30):485–501

Deruddre S, Cheisson G, Mazoit JX, Vicaut E, Benhamou D, Duranteau J (2007) Renal arterial resistance in septic shock: effects of increasing mean arterial pressure with norepinephrine on the renal resistive index assessed with Doppler ultrasonography. Intensive Care Med 33(9):1557–1562 Epub 2007 May 8

Dewitte A (2013) Jrenal Doppler in the management of the acute kidney injury in intensive care unit. J Crit Care 28(3):314. doi:10.1016/j.jcrc.2013.01.003

Doi Y, Iwashima Y, Yoshihara F, Kamide K, Takata H, Fujii T et al (2012) Association of renal resistive index with target organ damage in essential hypertension. Am J Hypertens 25(12):1292–1298

Doi Y, Iwashima Y, Yoshinhara F, Kamide K, Hayashi S, Kubota Y et al (2013) Response to renal resistive index and cardiovascular and renal outcomes in essential hypetension. Hypertension 61(2):e23

Geraci G, Mulè G, Mogavero M, Geraci C, D'Ignoti D, Guglielmo C (2015) Renal haemodynamics and severity of carotid atherosclerosis in hypertensive patients with and without impaired renal function. Nutr Metab Cardiovasc Dis 25(2):160–166

Geraci G, Mulè G, Mogavero M, Geraci C, Nardi E, Cottone S (2016) Association between uric acid and renal haemodinamics: pathophysiological implications for renal damage in hypertensive patients. J Clin Hypertens 2:1–8

Go AS, Bauman M, King SMC et al (2014) An effective approach to high blood pressure control: a science advisory from the American Heart Association, the American College of Cardiology, and the Centers for Disease Control and Prevention. Hypertension 63:878–885

Gosling RG, Lo PT, Taylor MG (1991) Interpretation of pulsatility index in feeder arteries to low-impedance vascular beds. Ultrasound Obstet Gynecol 1 (3):175–179

Granata A, Zanoli L, Clementi S, Fatuzzo P, Di Nicolò P, Fiorini F (2014) Resistive intrarenal index: myth or reality? Br J Radiol 87(1038):20140004

Hamano K, Nitta A, Ohtake T, Kobayashi S (2008) Associations of renal vascular resistance with albuminuria and other macroangiopathy in type 2 diabetic patients. Diabetes Care 31:1853–1857

Hashimoto J, Hito S (2011) Central pulse pressure and aortic stiffness determine renal haemodynamics: pathophysiological implication for microalbuminuria in hypertension. Hypertension 58(5):839–846

Ikee R, Kobayashi S, Hemmi N, Imakiire T, Kikuchi Y, Moriya H et al (2005) Correlation between the resistive index by Doppler ultrasound and kidney function and histology. Am J Kidney Dis 46(4):603–609

Jacobson HR (1988) Ischemic renal disease: an overlooked clinical entity. Kidney Int 34:729–743

James PA, Oparil S, Carter BL et al (2014) 2014 evidence-based guideline for the management of high blood pressure in adults: report from the panel members appointed to the eighth joint national committee (JNC 8). JAMA 311:507–520

Jensen G, Bardelli M, Volkmann R, Caidahl K, Rose G, Aurell M (1994) Renovascular resistance in primary hypertension: experimental variations detected by means of Doppler ultrasound. J Hypertens 12 (8):959–964

Le Dorze M, Bouglè A, Deruddre S, Duranteau J (2012) Renal Doppler ultrasound: a nex tool to asses renal perfusion in critical illness. Shock 37(4):360–365

Lennartz CS, Pickering JW, Seiler-Mußler S, Bauer L, Untersteller K, Emrich IE et al (2016) External validation of the kidney failure risk equation and re-calibration with addition of ultrasound parameters. Clin J Am Soc Nephrol 11(4):609–615. doi:10.2215/CJN.08110715.Epub

Leoncini G, Martinoli C, Viazzi F, Ravera M, Parodi D, Ratto E et al (2002) Changes in renal resistive index and urinary albumin excretion in hypertensive patients under long-term treatment with lisinopril or nifedipine GITS. Nephron 90(2):169–173

Liu LS (2010) Chinese guidelines for the management of hypertension. zhonghua Xin Xue Guan Bing Za Zhi 39:579–615

Maestripieri V, Pacciani G, Tassinari I et al (2012) Hypertensive patients with diabetes mellitus and normal arterial stifness show an early increase in renal resistive index. Eur Heart J 33(N 17/201):70–75

Mahfoud F, Cremers B, Janker J, Link B, Vonend O, Ukena C, Linz D, Schmieder R, Rump LC, Kindermann I, Sobotka PA, Krum H, Scheller B, Schlaich M, Laufs U, Böhm M (2012) Renal hemodynamics and renal function after catheter-based renal sympathetic denervation in patient with resistant hypertension. Hypertension 60(2):419–424

Mancia G, Fagard R, Narkiewicz K et al (2013) 2013 ESH/ESC guidelines for the management of arterial hypertension: the task force for the management of arterial hypertension of the European Society of Hypertension (ESH) and of the European Society of Cardiology (ESC). Eur Heart J 34:2159–2219

Meola M, Samoni S, Petrucci I (2016a) Imaging in chronic kidney disease. Contrib Nephrol 188:69–80

Meola M, Samoni S, Petrucci I (2016b) Clinical scenario in chronic kidney disease: vascular chronic disease. Contrib Nephrol 188:81–88

Miyoshi K, Okura T, Tanino A, Kukida M, Nagao T, Higaki J (2016) Usefulness of renal resistive index to predict an increase in urinary albumin excretion in patients with essential hypertension. J Hum Hypertens. Online Publication. doi:10.1038/jhh.2016.38

Modesti PA, Ferrari A, Bazzini C, Boddi M (2015) Time sequence of autonomic changes induced by daily slow-breatinghing sessions. Clin Auton Res 25 (2):95–104

Naesens M, Heylen L, Lerut E et al (2013) Intrarenal resistive index after renal transplantation. N Engl J Med 369(19):1797–1806. doi:10.56/NEJMoa1301064

National Institute for Health and Care Excellence (2014) Hypertension: clinical management of primary hypertension in adults (Clinical guideline 127). http://guidance.nice.org.uk/CG127. Accessed 19 June 2014

Neuzil P, Ormiston J, Brinton TJ, Starek Z, Esler M, Dawood O et al (2016) Externally delivered focused ultrasound for renal denervation. ACC Cardiovasc Interv 9(12):1292–1299. doi:10.1016/j.jcin.2016.04.013 Epub 2016 Jun 20

Norris CS, Barnes RW (1984) Renal artery flow velocity analysis: a sensitive measure of experimental and clinical renovascular resistance. J Surg Res 36 (3):230–236

Nosadini R, Velussi M, Brocco E et al (2006) Increased renal arterial resistance predicts the course of renal function in type 2diabetes with microalbuminuria. Diabetes 55:234–239

O'Neill WC (2014) Renal resistive index: a case of mistaken identity. Hypertension 64(59):915–917

Okura T, Jotoku M, Irita J, Enomoto D, Nagao T, Desilva VR, Yamane S, Pei Z, Kojima S, Hamano Y, Mashiba S, Kurata M, Miyoshi K, Higaki J (2010) Association between cystatin C and inflammation in patients with essential hypertension. Clin Exp Nephrol 14(6):584–588

Platt JF, Rubin JM, Ellis JH (1989) Distinction between obstructive and nonostructive pyelocaliectasis duplex Doppler sonography. AJR Am J Roentgenol 153 (5):997–1000

Platt JF, Ellis JH, Rubin JM, Di Pietro MA, Sedman AB (1990) Intrarenal arterial Doppler sonography in patients with nonobstructive renal disease: correlation of resistive index with biopsy findings. AJR Am J Roentgenol 154(6):1223–1227

Ponte B, Pruijm M, Ackermann D, Vuistiner P, Eisenberger U, Guessons I et al (2014) Reference values and factors associated with renal resistive index in a family-based population study. Hypertension 63(1):136–142

Pontremoli R, Viazzi F, Martinoli C, Ravera M, Nicolella C, Berruti V, Leoncini G, Ruello N, Zagami P, Bezante GP, Derchi LE, Deferrari G (1999a) Increased renal resistive index in patients with essential hypertension: a marker of target organ damage. Nephrol Dial Transplant 14(2):360–365

Pontremoli R, Viazzi F, Martinoli C, Ravera M, Nicolella C, Berruti V et al (1999b) Increased renal resistive index in patients with essential hypertension: a marker of organ damage. Nephrol Dial Transplant 14:360–365

Pourcelot L (1974) Applications Clinique de l'examen Doppler transcutane. In: Peronneau P (ed) Symposium: Velocimetric Ultrasonnordoppler. Inserm, Paris, pp 213–240

Radermacher J, Chavan A, Bleck J, Vitzthum A, Stoess B, MJ G et al (2001) Use of Doppler ultrasonography to predict the outcome of therapy for renal-artery stenosis. N Engl J Med 344(6):410–417

Radermacher J, Ellis S, Haller H (2002) Renal resistance index and progression of renal disease. Hypertension 2 (2 Pt2):699–703

Raff U, Ott C, John S, Schmidt BM, Fleischmann EH, Schmieder RE (2010) Nitric oxide and reactive hyperemia: role of location and duration of ischemia. Am J Hypertens 23(8):865–869. doi:10.1038/ajh.2010.72

Ratto E, Leoncini G, Viazzi F, Vaccaro V, Falqui V, Parodi A, Conti N, Tomolillo C, Deferrari G, Pontremoli R (2006) Ambulatory arterial stiffness index and renal abnormalities in primary hypertension. J Hypertens 24(10):2033–2038

Sanchez-Losada LG, Tapia E et al (2005) Mild hyperuricemia induces vasoconstriction and maintaings glomerular hypertension in normal and remnant kidney rat. Kidney Int 67(1):237–247

Schaberle W, Leyerer L, Schierlinq W, Pfister K (2016) Ultrasound diagnostics of renal artery stenosis: stenosis criteria, CEUS and recurrent in-stent-stenosis. Gefässchirurgie 21:4–13

Schnell D, Deruddre S, Harrois A et al (2012) Renal resistive index better predicts the occurrence of acute kidney injury than cystatin C. Shock 38(6):592–597

Sugiura T, Wada A (2011) Resistive index predicts renal prognosis in chronic kidney disease: results of a 4-year follow-up. Clin Exp Nephrol 15(1):114–120

Textor SC, Wilcox CS (2001) Renal artery stenosis: a common treatable cause of renal failure? Annu Rev Med 52:421–442

Tublin ME, Tessler FN, Murphy ME (1999) Correlation between renal vascular resistance, pulse pressure, and resistive index in isolated perfused kidneys. Radiology 213(1):258–564

Tublin ME, Bude RO, Platt JF (2003) The resistive index in renal Doppler sonography: where do we stand? Am J Roentgenol 180:885–892

Vegar Zubović S, Kristić S, Sefić Pašić I (2016) Relationship between ultrasonographically determined kidney volume and progression of chronic kidney disease. Med Glas (Zenica) 13(2):90–94

Viazzi F, Leoncini G, Derchi LE, Pontremoli R (2014) Ultrasound Doppler renal resistive index: a useful tool for the management of the hypertensive patient. J Hypertens 32:149–153

Watanabe S, Okura T, Kurata M, Irita J, Manabe S, Miyoshi K et al (2006) Valsartan reduces serum cystatin C and the renal vascular resistance in patients with essential hypertension. Clin Exp Hypertens 28 (5):451–461

Weber MA, Schiffrin EL, White WB et al (2014) Clinical practice guidelines for the management of hypertension in the community a statement by the American Society of Hypertension and the International Society of Hypertension. J Hypertens 32:3–15

Zierler RE, Bergelin RO, Davidson RC et al (1996) A prospective study of disease progression in patients with atherosclerotic renal artery stenosis. Am J Hypertens 9(11):1055–1061

Adv Exp Med Biol - Advances in Internal Medicine (2017) 2: 209–213
DOI 10.1007/5584_2016_89
© Springer International Publishing AG 2016
Published online: 22 November 2016

Atherosclerotic Renal Artery Stenosis

Robert Schoepe, Stephen McQuillan, Debbie Valsan, and Geoffrey Teehan

Abstract

Atherosclerotic Renal Artery Stenosis is a form or peripheral arterial disease that tends to affect older subjects with hyperlipidemia, history of tobacco use, and who have other coexistent forms of vascular insufficiency. An abdominal bruit on physical exam can be a helpful clue. Slowly progressive, it can lead to critical narrowing of the renal arteries which creates a cascade of events such as renin-angiotensin-aldosterone activation (RAAS), hypertension, acute pulmonary edema, and renal fibrosis. The hypertension is considered a secondary form and can even be resistant to multiple antihypertensives. The diagnosis can be made with imaging (duplex ultrasound CT scans, MRA, or angiography). Because of the unique circulation to the kidney, stenting and angioplasty are rarely curative. This was confirmed in three recent large clinical trials. Therapy consists of lipid and blood pressure control, and dual anti-platelet agents. Because the disease activates the RAAS system, ace inhibitors and angiotensin receptor blockers can be useful agents but carry the risk of ischemic nephropathy, a form of acute kidney injury related to reduced renal blood flow after challenge with these agents. As such these agents are used with caution. Little is known about optimal blood pressure agents or the effect of lifestyle modification.

Keywords

Hypertension • Peripheral arterial disease • Stenosis • Hyperlipidemia • Acute pulmonary edema • Renin-angiotensin-aldosterone • Ischemic nephropathy • Abdominal bruit

R. Schoepe, S. McQuillan, D. Valsan, and G. Teehan (✉)
Lankenau Medical Center, 100 Lancaster Avenue, Suite 130, 19096 Wynnewood, PA, USA
e-mail: gteehan1@gmail.com

1 Introduction

Atherosclerotic Renal Artery Stenosis is a common finding in secondary hypertension evaluations. Many clues can lead to its diagnosis including an abdominal bruit, history of tobacco use, peripheral arterial disease, flash pulmonary edema, and the development of acute kidney injury on agents blocking the renin-angiotensin system. It is an unusual form of peripheral arterial disease in that stenting and angioplasty do not seem to alter the clinical course of the disease as compared with peripheral interventions elsewhere (i.e. carotid and iliac arterial disease). This chapter will focus on the diagnosis of the disease and the therapeutic considerations in light of the vast array of available clinical trial data.

2 Epidemiology

Atherosclerotic renal artery stenosis (ARAS) commonly complicates chronic kidney disease (CKD) and end-stage renal disease (ESRD). As many as 5–15 % of patients who develop ESRD and 5–22 % of patients with CKD over 50 years old may have ARAS. It has an even higher prevalence in patients with other forms of atherosclerotic vascular disease. Among those with non-ESRD CKD, the absolute risk of cardiovascular outcomes is greater than the risk of developing ESRD. In the ESRD population the mortality rate is up to 50 % at 3 years (Rimmer 1993).

The degree of stenosis correlates inversely with survival. Patients with incidentally found moderate ARAS by angiogram often maintain stable renal function and may not be at any higher risk of ESRD than the general population up to 10 years after diagnosis (Leertouwer et al. 2001). Patients who go on to develop ESRD were generally diagnosed later in the course of the disease with worse renal function and had a faster rate of decline in their remaining renal function (Baboolal et al. 1998).

3 Pathogenesis

ARAS is due to atherosclerosis of the main blood vessels to the kidneys, the left and right renal arteries. Slowly developing, it follows the same mechanisms of other atherosclerotic vascular diseases such as coronary artery disease, carotid stenosis, and peripheral arterial disease. ARAS more commonly affects the proximal renal artery or the ostium and the aortic take-off, versus another form of renal arterial disease, fibromuscular dysplasia (FMD). FMD tends to occurs in younger patients, predominantly women, and affects the middle portion of the renal artery (Olin et al. 2012).

In ARAS over time the atherosclerotic plaques impair blood flow to the kidney. Only the renal cortex, the site of the glomerulus, appears to undergo significant ischemia (Gloviczki et al. 2011). Autoregulation, an early compensatory mechanism, sustains renal blood flow to a degree, but begins to fail once the stenosis reaches roughly 60 % (Herrmann et al. 2016). At this point, declining renal blood flow and tissue hypoxia leads to renin release and activation of the renin-angiotensin-aldosterone system (RAAS) causing retention of sodium and water and also peripheral vasoconstriction (Ritchie et al. 2014). This all leads to hypertension associated with ARAS. This cascade of events also leads to local release of cytokines, inflammation, and eventually fibrosis and deterioration of renal function (Gloviczki et al. 2011).

4 Clinical Presentation

The presentation of ARAS is often chronic and insidious. As the ARAS progresses past the critical threshold from moderate to severe, the renal function will be compromised. The glomerular filtration rate (GFR) falls out of proportion to an expected age-related decline. Urinalysis is usually bland (no hematuria nor proteinuria) as ARAS has an initial pre-renal effect and subsequent renal dysfunction occurs due to hypertensive changes and fibrosis which has an intrinsic renal effect. Hypertension that was once easily controlled but now resistant or acutely worsening can be a sign of worsening RAS and should be considered during work up for secondary hypertension (Rimmer 1993).

Classically, ARAS may present with hypertensive crisis and associated flash pulmonary edema. Worsening renal function after starting RAAS blockade, ischemic nephropathy, or renal function that is excessively sensitive to intravascular volume may be clues to the diagnosis (Textor and Wilcox 2000). Many advocate stopping RAAS blockade if the serum creatinine rises by more than 30 % after use of such agents. ARAS is almost always associated with other forms of atherosclerotic diseases. Common risk factors are hyperlipidemia, smoking, and age over 50. On physical exam it may be possible to auscultate an abdominal bruit due to turbulent flow past a stenosis in a renal artery. Imaging of the kidneys is especially useful as it may reveal asymmetric or smaller than expected kidneys (Rimmer 1993). Table 1 lists common attributes of ARAS.

5 Diagnosis

A hallmark of ARAS is an elevated plasma renin assay and serum aldosterone concentration. Once suspected, duplex ultrasonography, magnetic resonance angiography (MRA) and computed tomography angiography (CTA) can aid in diagnosis (Rimmer 1993).

Duplex ultrasonography is the least sensitive and specific modality but is a safe and reasonable first test. It is labor-intensive, time-consuming, operator dependent, and in certain patients, particularly the obese, it is of limited utility. The resistive index ([peak systolic velocity – end-diastolic velocity] divided by peak systolic velocity) when added to duplex Doppler ultrasonography may aid in diagnosing RAS. A higher resistive index is indicative of more extensive atherosclerotic burden distal to the main renal arteries. Controversy exists as to whether a lower resistive index (i.e. < 80 %) represents an opportunity for revascularization resulting in lowering blood pressure (Williams et al. 2007).

MRA confers the risk of gadolinium-induced nephrogenic systemic fibrosis, a syndrome linked to individuals with a GFR <30 ml/min. Using arteriography as the gold standard, MRA had excellent sensitivity and specificity (100, 96 % respectively) for the detection of stenosis of the main renal arteries, but was less helpful in accessory renal arteries (Textor 2004).

CTA requires a significant volume of contrast and may be contraindicated in those with advancing CKD. Multidetector, spiral CTA can provide excellent sensitivity (96 %) and specificity (97 %), but is probably just a bit inferior to MRA (Crutchley et al. 2009). Conventional intra-arterial angiography can confirm the diagnosis but also carries a contrast nephropathy risk as well as that of atheroemboli. Blood oxygen level-dependent MRI which can identify renal ischemia in a non-invasive way may be a promising imaging modality (Gloviczki et al. 2011).

6 Treatment

Several recent clinical trials have addressed the role of interventional therapies versus medical management. The success of percutaneous

Table 1 Features of atheroclerotic renal arterial disease (ARAS)

Age of onset (years)	50–60
Common lab findings	AKI after RAAS agent usage.
Preferred BP agents	Unknown but caution with RAAS agents.
Location of lesion	Typically ostial, proximal 1/3 of renal artery versus Fibromuscular Dysplasia which affects middle portion of renal artery
How diagnosed?	Duplex ultrasound, CT Angiography, MR Angiography
Risk factors	Hyperlipidemia, Age > 50, Tobacco use

Rimmer (1993), Ritchie et al. (2014) and Textor and Wilcox (2000)

interventions in other peripheral arterial sites has not been demonstrated in RAS. Three randomized trials, ASTRAL, CORAL, and STAR compared standard medical therapy to the same therapy plus intervention (stenting/angioplasty) (Levy and Creager 2009; Cooper et al. 2014; Bax et al. 2009). The trials found no improvement in renal function, clinically significant reduction in antihypertensive requirements, nor mortality benefit, while morbidity was not trivial among those stented. Percutaneous interventions are no longer the standard of care in the management of ARAS following these trials and as such Medicare claims data for such procedures fell dramatically following the publication of these trials (Bax et al. 2009). While there may be a benefit to revascularization in a smaller population of patients with recurrent flash pulmonary edema, severe resistant hypertension, or rapidly progressive CKD, this has been poorly studied.

The disappointing results in intervention trials have paved the way toward a newer paradigm in therapy of ARAS. In the absence of compelling data regarding who will respond to vascular interventions, we reserve stenting and angioplasty for those who have failed medical therapy and develop resistant or refractory hypertension and/or pulmonary edema. At that point there is little else to offer and we feel the risks of the procedure are justified.

Now, the most important goal is to optimize any potential risk factors present. This includes a comprehensive effort to control hypertension, hyperlipidemia, and limit platelet aggregation. Hyperlipidemia can be managed with a statin. Dual antiplatelet therapy may be employed depending on risk factors for bleeding (Cooper et al. 2014).

The control of hypertension associated with ARAS is complicated. As noted above, ARAS leads to increased activation of the RAAS system making it is a logical target to guide therapy. Angiotensin-converting enzyme inhibitors (ACEI) and angiotensin-receptor blockers (ARB) are key components for controlling the hyperactivation of the RAAS system, but confounded by the potential for ischemic

nephropathy. About 20 % of patients with ARAS will have an unacceptable deterioration in renal function (>30 % rise in serum creatinine) following initiation of RAAS blockade (Franklin and Ronald 1985). We do not advocate the use of RAAS agents without nephrology consultation. A subject with ARAS and treated with RAAS agents must have regular bloodwork (creatinine, blood urea nitrogen, and potassium) and must strictly avoid nonsteroidal agents that alter renal hemodynamics, as well as be mindful of developing volume depletion. Still, the benefits of RAAS blockade in delaying the progression of CKD and their particular mechanism of action make these agents a potentially valuable option.

Little data exists about the best agents to control blood pressure, but we can use the experiences in STAR, ASTRAL, and CORAL (Levy and Creager 2009; Cooper et al. 2014; Bax et al. 2009). Table 2 highlights the features of the trials and agents used. RAAS blocking agents were used quite commonly if not outright mandated for use. The CORAL trial provided an ARB (Candesartan) to all patients and also mandated the use of Hydrochlorothiazide, and the combination pill of Amlodipine and Atorvastatin. RAAS agents were used to a lesser degree (40–60 %) in the other trials. Both STAR and ASTRAL emphasized lipid control and antiplatelet agents as well.

As with all forms of resistant hypertension (RH), focusing on modifiable factors should supplement pharmacologic and/or interventional

Table 2 Clinical trials in renal artery stenosis (RAS)

Trial	Coral	Star	Astral
Year	2014	2009	2009
Number of patients	921	140	806
Mean age (Yrs)	69	69	70
Mean BP or SBP (mm Hg)	150	150	150/76
Primary endpoint P value	NS	NS	NS
Baseline GFR (ml/min)	58	46 (CrCl)	40
Mean # Drugs	*	2.9	2.8
% Taking ACEI or ARB	100	56–60	38–47

Levy and Creager (2009), Cooper et al. (2014) and Bax et al. (2009)

* Implies no data available on that parameter

therapies. The effect of lifestyle modification on RH is being investigated across a broad class of hypertensive diseases in the upcoming Triumph Trial and may shed light on the role of weight loss, sodium restriction, and exercise on the progression of ARAS (Blumenthal et al. 2015). In the CORAL trial some of the reassuring renal outcomes were attributed to addressing smoking, diabetes, and other non-hypertension factors.

7 Conclusions

ARAS is frequently identified in patients with high risk for peripheral arterial disease, diagnosed by duplex ultrasonography, CT angiography, MR angiography, or direct visualization. Therapy addresses blood pressure control, lipids, and utilizing anti-platelet therapy. The approach to interventional therapies is complex and we advocate a case-by-case basis to determine how to proceed. Modifying risk factors such as smoking, diabetes, sedentary lifestyle, and use of confounding agents like non-steroidals and sodium are non-pharmacologic adjuncts we expect to play a bigger role in the future.

References

Baboolal K, Evans C, Moore R (1998) Incidence of end-stage renal disease in medically treated patients with severe bilateral atherosclerotic renovascular disease. Am J Kidney Dis 31(6):971–977

Bax L et al (2009) Stent placement in patients with atherosclerotic renal artery stenosis and impaired renal function: a randomized trial. Ann Intern Med 150 (12):840–848

Blumenthal JA et al (2015) Lifestyle modificcation for resistant hypertension: the TRIUMPH randomized clinical trial. Am Heart J 170(5):986–994

Cooper C et al (2014) Stenting and medical therapy for atherosclerotic renal- artery stenosis. N Engl J Med 370:13–22

Crutchley TA, Pearce JD, Craven TE et al (2009) Clinical utility of the resistive index in atherosclerotic renovascular disease. J Vasc Surg 49:148

Franklin SS, Ronald DS (1985) Comparison of effects of enalapril plus hydrochlorothiazide versus standard triple therapy on renal function in renovascular hypertension. Am J Med 79.3:14–23, Web

Gloviczki ML, Glockner JF, Crane JA, Mckusick MA, Misra S, Grande JP, Lerman LO, Textor SC (2011) Blood oxygen level-dependent magnetic resonance imaging identifies cortical hypoxia in severe renovascular disease. Hypertension 58(6):1066–1072

Herrmann SMS, Saad A, Eirin A, Woollard J, Tang H, Mckusick MA, Misra S, Glockner JF, Lerman LO, Textor SC (2016) Differences in GFR and tissue oxygenation, and interactions between stenotic and contralateral kidneys in unilateral atherosclerotic renovascular disease. Clin J Am Soc Nephrol 11 (3):458–469

Leertouwer TC, Pattynama PMt, Van Den Berg-Huysmans A (2001) Incidental renal artery stenosis in peripheral vascular disease: a case for treatment? Kidney Int 59(4):1480–1483

Levy MS, Creager MA (2009) Revascularization versus medical therapy for renal-artery stenosis. The ASTRAL investigators. N Engl J Med 361:1953–1962, Vasc Med 15.4 (2010):343–345. Web

Olin JW, Froehlich J, Gu X, Bacharach JM, Eagle K, Gray BH, Jaff MR, Kim ES, Mace P, Matsumoto AH, McBane RD, Kline-Rogers E, White CJ, Gornik HL (2012) The United States registry for fibromuscular dysplasia: results in the first 447 patients. Circulation 125(25):3182

Rimmer JM (1993) Atherosclerotic renovascular disease and progressive renal failure. Ann Intern Med 118.9:712

Ritchie J, Green D, Chrysochou C, Chalmers N, Foley RN, Kalra PA (2014) High-risk clinical presentations in atherosclerotic renovascular disease: prognosis and response to renal artery revascularization. Am J Kidney Dis 63(2):186–197

Textor SC (2004) Pitfalls in imaging for renal artery stenosis. Ann Intern Med 141:730

Textor SC, Wilcox CS (2000) Ischemic nephropathy/azotemic renovascular disease. Semin Nephrol 20 (5):489–502. Web

Williams GJ, Macaskill P, Chan SF et al (2007) Comparative accuracy of renal duplex sonographic parameters in the diagnosis of renal artery stenosis: paired and unpaired analysis. AJR Am J Roentgenol 188:798

Adv Exp Med Biol - Advances in Internal Medicine (2017) 2: 215–237
DOI 10.1007/5584_2016_26
© Springer International Publishing AG 2016
Published online: 19 November 2016

Endocrine Hypertension: A Practical Approach

Joseph M. Pappachan and Harit N. Buch

Abstract

Elevated blood pressure resulting from few endocrine disorders (endocrine hypertension) accounts for a high proportion of cases of secondary hypertension. Although some features may be suggestive, many cases of endocrine hypertension remain silent until worked up for the disease. A majority of cases result from primary aldosteronism. Other conditions that can cause endocrine hypertension are: congenital adrenal hyperplasia, Liddle syndrome, pheochromocytomas, Cushing's syndrome, acromegaly, thyroid diseases, primary hyperparathyroidism and iatrogenic hormone manipulation. Early identification and treatment of the cause of endocrine hypertension may help to reduce morbidity and mortality related to these disorders. This article gives a comprehensive and practical approach to the diagnosis and management of endocrine hypertension.

Keywords

Endocrine hypertension • Primary aldosteronism • Congenital adrenal hyperplasia • Liddle syndrome • Pheochromocytoma • Cushing's syndrome • Acromegaly • Thyroid disease • Primary hyperparathyroidism

1   Introduction

Hypertension is a chronic condition with multi-system involvement and is associated with high morbidity and mortality. The prevalence of hypertension is approximately 40 % among adults over the age of 25 years and contributes to 45–50 % of deaths due to heart disease and stroke (World Health Organization. Obesity and overweight 2015). Although the prevalence of hypertension is high in the general population, only in around 10 % of cases an underlying specific cause can be identified (secondary hypertension), of which the majority are related to renal and endocrine disorders (Young 2015). If secondary hypertension is suspected, it is important

J.M. Pappachan (✉) and H.N. Buch
Department of Endocrinology & Diabetes, New Cross Hospital, The Royal Wolverhampton Hospital NHS Trust, Wolverhampton WV10 0QP, UK
e-mail: drpappachan@yahoo.co.in

to identify the cause, as treatment of the primary condition may lead to complete or partial cure of hypertension.

A multitude of endocrine disorders can present with secondary hypertension, collectively termed here as endocrine hypertension. Some of these disorders may present with unique clinical features while the others may be asymptomatic and identified during work-up of resistant hypertension (refractory to standard anti-hypertensive therapy), or a hypertension-related complication. Early diagnosis and appropriate management of the primary illness often result in marked improvement or cure of hypertension. In this chapter, we describe a comprehensive and practical approach to endocrine hypertension.

2 When to Suspect Endocrine Hypertension?

Secondary hypertension is suspected in patients who present with: hypertension at an early age, sudden onset of uncontrolled hypertension, loss of control over previously well-controlled blood pressure and a hypertensive emergency (Velasco and Vongpatanasin 2014; Weber et al. 2014; Thomas et al. 2015).

Endocrine hypertension is the second most common cause of secondary hypertension after renal disease, and forms a major aetiological factor for resistant hypertension. A diagnosis of endocrine hypertension may be obvious when patients present with typical clinical features of the underlying condition like acromegaly, Cushing syndrome, hyperthyroidism, hypothyroidism and features of virilisation in congenital adrenal hyperplasia (Young 2015). They may present with a typical history e.g. paroxysmal palpitations and orthostatic hypotension in phaeochromocytoma (Pappachan et al. 2014; Desai et al. 2009; Kiernan and Solórzano 2016). Occasionally routine laboratory tests in a patient with hypertension may raise the suspicion of an endocrine cause e.g. hypokalemia in mineralcorticoid excess (Thomas et al. 2015).

However, in a high proportion of patients, an endocrine cause may not be obvious, and all patients suspected to have secondary hypertension should be evaluated for an endocrine cause unless an alternative aetiology for hypertension is obvious from the initial clinical and laboratory picture.

3 Causes of Endocrine Hypertension

A number of endocrine conditions can result in hypertension although only a few of them are common in clinical practice. A detailed discussion of individual disorders, the clinicpathological features and diagnostic evaluation is elaborated below.

4 Primary Mineralocorticoid Excess

Mineralocorticoids are steroid hormones that control the water and salt balance in the body. Aldosterone is the principal endogenous mineralocorticoid hormone in the body although other hormones including glucocorticoids and sex steroids may exert mineralocorticoid effects. Aldosterone is synthesised by the zona glomerulosa cells of the adrenal cortex, and is under control of angiotensin II, plasma potassium levels, and to a lesser extent adrenocorticotrophin (ACTH).

Clinical conditions in which primary mineralocorticoid excess can occur are: overproduction of mineralocorticoid hormones as in primary aldosteronism (PA) and congenital adrenal hyperplasia (CAH), or increased effect of mineralocorticoid hormones as in Liddle syndrome, syndrome of apparent mineralocorticoid excess (AME), pseudohypoaldosteronism type 2 (Gordon syndrome) and Geller syndrome. These conditions are elaborated in the sections below.

4.1 Hypermineralocorticoidism

Overproduction of aldosterone occurs in PA or CAH, and these disorders are elaborated in the following sections.

4.1.1 Primary Aldosteronism (PA)

PA is one of the most common disorders that causes secondary hypertension and forms the majority of cases of endocrine hypertension. The disease accounts for 5–13 % of cases in people with age of onset of hypertension between 30 and 60 years (Thomas et al. 2015; Young 2007). About 10 % of cases in hypertension clinics, 4 % in the community (Hannemann and Wallaschofski 2012; Boulkroun et al. 2015), and nearly 20 % with resistant hypertension are estimated to be resulting from PA (Boulkroun et al. 2015). The variability in the reported incidence is related to the use of different definitions, biochemical tests and cut-offs. Nearly 60–65 % of cases of PA are from idiopathic hyperaldosteronism (IHA) and 30–35 % result from an aldosterone producing adrenal adenoma (APA) (Thomas et al. 2015; Young 2007). Roughly 5 % of cases of PA are familial (familial hyperaldosteronism type I, II and III [FH-I, II and III]) with clear genetic background (Zennaro et al. 2015a).

Pathophysiology

PA results from aldosterone over-production with a consequent suppression of plasma renin, and manifests with hypertension, retention of sodium, and over-excretion of potassium that may lead to hypokalemia (Funder et al. 2008). Although many of the complex molecular, cellular and genetic mechanisms involved in these pathways have been recently elucidated (Boulkroun et al. 2015; Zennaro et al. 2015a; Piaditis et al. 2015), they are beyond the scope of this chapter. Excess production of aldosterone in PA has multiple biologic and pleiotropic effects in human body that results in the manifestations and complications of the disease.

Aldosterone causes retention of sodium from the distal renal tubules and collecting ducts in exchange for hydrogen and potassium ions. The corresponding increase in the water absorption results in an increase in blood volume and blood pressure and the loss of hydrogen ions and potassium results in a state of hypokalemic metabolic alkalosis in some but not all patients (Thomas et al. 2015; Mulatero et al. 2004). A reduction of plasma renin levels is classical of PA. Apart from the usual complications related to essential hypertension, PA is found to be associated with elevated risk of cardiac hypertrophy and fibrosis, vascular endothelial dysfunction, albuminuria and nephrocalcinosis.

Clinical Presentation

Although the classical presentation of PA is with resistant hypertension and hypokalemia (sometimes symptomatic), it is not often observed in clinical practice (Thomas et al. 2015; Funder et al. 2008). The following categories of cases should be considered for screening: hypertension inadequately controlled with three or more anti-hypertensive medications, hypertension with an adrenal incidentaloma, hypertension in young adults, or those presumed to have secondary hypertension (Thomas et al. 2015; Young 2007). Apart from these categories, the 2008 American Endocrine Society Guidelines also suggest screening for: hypertensives with diuretic-induced hypokalemia, patients with family history of early-onset hypertension or stroke before 40 years of age and hypertensive patients with a first degree relative having PA (Thomas et al. 2015; Manolopoulou et al. 2015).

Diagnostic Approach

Initial Screening Patients with suspected PA should be tested with an estimation of plasma aldosterone and renin levels with the calculation of aldosterone to renin ratio (ARR). The assay should be ideally performed in the morning after the individual has been out of bed for 2 h and seated for 5–15 min (Thomas et al. 2015; Funder et al. 2008). Different laboratories use different units and cut off values for ARR depending on the assay, and a practical approach could be following the local guidelines. A recent study using a method-specific ARR cut-off of 1.2

(ng/dl)/(μIU/ml), determined with direct, automated chemi-luminescence immunoassays allowing the simultaneous measurement of plasma aldosterone and renin concentrations, provided 98.9 % sensitivity and 78.9 % specificity (Manolopoulou et al. 2015). These results have been reproduced by other studies but method-specific cut off needs to be derived. Different centres use renin activity or renin concentration, and the ratio cut-off is significantly affected by this and other laboratory-based variables. An absolute cut-off value for aldosterone concentration (also method-specific) is often used as an additional criterion to make ARR more specific. Aldosterone antagonists and beta-blockers should be withdrawn prior to the test as they disproportionately affect the ARR.

Confounders Several antihypertensive medications can interfere with the screening results to a varying extent because of interference with the renin-angiotensin-aldosterone (RAA) system causing high false-positive and false-negative rates, with betablockers and diuretics being the main culprits. Hypokalemia, and treatment with antihypertensive medications such as dihydropyridine group of calcium channel blockers, angiotensin convertase enzyme inhibitors and angiotensin II receptor blockers, can cause false negative results of ARR in patients with mild PA. Discontinuation of interfering medications for sufficient time period may be considered if feasible. For example, diuretics and aldosterone antagonists should be withdrawn 4 weeks prior to, and the other antihypertensives described above, 2 weeks prior to the intended ARR estimation (Funder et al. 2008). Antihypertensives such as verapamil (slow release), hydralazine and alpha-adrenergic blockers possess minimal effects on RAA system and are recommended for control of hypertension before ARR measurement if other antihypertensive drugs are to be discontinued (Thomas et al. 2015; Funder et al. 2008). However, in patients with severe hypertension resistant to conventional medications, switching to these drugs may not be easy, considering the anticipated hypertensive complications.

Biochemical Confirmation Although a raised ARR in a clinically relevant scenario is highly suggestive of PA, one of the four confirmatory tests is recommended by the American Endocrine Society Guidelines (Funder et al. 2008). These tests are: oral sodium loading with measurement of urinary aldosterone excretion, intravenous saline infusion with measurement of plasma aldosterone levels (levels suppressed in absence of PA), fludorcortisone suppression test and captopril challenge test. The latter two tests are not routinely used now, and severe uncontrolled hypertension and heart failure are relative contraindications to the former two (Thomas et al. 2015). The former two confirmatory tests may become necessary in cases with mild PA, where the ARR is only marginally elevated in the absence of severe hypertension or heart failure. A detailed description and interpretation of the confirmatory tests and results are beyond the scope of this chapter and are freely available to the readers in the full text of the American Endocrine Society Guidelines (Funder et al. 2008).

Adrenal Imaging Computed tomography (CT) scan of the adrenal glands is recommended in all cases of PA for localisation of the disease and to exclude the small possibility of an adrenocortical carcinoma (Thomas et al. 2015; Funder et al. 2008). Adrenal CT is preferred over magnetic resonance imaging (MRI) as an imaging modality for localisation purpose because it is more economical and has better spatial resolution. However, adrenal imaging had a low sensitivity of 58.6 % to detect unilateral disease (Lim et al. 2014).

Adrenal Venous Sampling (AVS) AVS is the gold standard test for detection of the source of aldosterone excess, and is recommended in most cases for lateralisation of the abnormal adrenal gland if a surgical cure is contemplated. The technical difficulty with the procedure, lack of availability in many centres and relatively higher complication rates (about 5 %) are the main concerns in the routine performance of AVS. A recent expert consensus statement recommends avoiding AVS in the following situations: age is < 40 years with marked PA in presence of a typical unilateral adrenal adenoma and normal appearance of the opposite adrenal on CT, suspicion of adrenocortical carcinoma from adrenal imaging, high risk cases for adrenalectomy, proven cases of FH-I and FH-III (Thomas et al. 2015; Rossi et al. 2014).

Tests for Familial Hyperaldosteronism (FH)
FH-I (GRA) is screened by a low-dose dexamethasone suppression test with serial measurements of blood pressure and plasma aldosterone levels (Mussa et al. 2012; Korah and Scholl 2015). Normalisation of blood pressure and suppression of aldosterone are characteristics of FH-I. In addition, urinary 18-oxocortisol and 18-hydroxycortisol are usually elevated in patients with FH-I (Mussa et al. 2012). In patients with FH-II, blood pressure is un-responsive to glucocorticoid challenge and aldosterone suppression is partial or absent (Mussa et al. 2012). Urinary 18-oxocortisol and 18-hydroxycortisol levels are normal/moderately elevated. Blood pressure is unresponsive/increases with a paradoxical increase in aldosterone levels occurs in cases of FH-III during dexamethasone suppression test (Mussa et al. 2012). The urinary 18-steroid metabolites are very high in FH-III. Genetic testing confirms the autosomal dominant gene mutations in all the three forms of FH (Korah and Scholl 2015; Zennaro et al. 2013).

Management of PA

Surgical Management Surgical management is possible only in selected cases of PA where there is a clear evidence of lateralisation of the aldosterone excess to the side of an adrenal adenoma as described above. A recent systematic review showed that adrenalectomy for unilateral disease was associated with normalization of blood pressure in about 42 % (range 20–72) and cure of PA in 96–100 % with a mean complication rate of 4.7 % among 1056 patients (Muth et al. 2015). Compared to medical therapy, use of fewer antihypertensive drugs, improvement of quality of life, and possibly all-cause mortality were observed after surgery, although without an observed benefit on cardiovascular complications.

Laparoscopic adrenalectomy is the preferred surgical procedure because of lower morbidity, shorter length of hospital stay and faster recovery compared to open adrenalectomy. Partial adrenalectomy may be an option in selected case of unilateral PA. Both hypertension and hypokalemia should be well controlled pre-operatively, and levels of plasma aldosterone and renin should be measured postoperatively to assess the biochemical response (Thomas et al. 2015; Funder et al. 2008). Withdrawal of potassium supplements and mineralocorticoid receptor (MR) antagonist are usually possible on the first postoperative day after successful surgery, with reduction/discontinuation of antihypertensive medications within 1–6 months in most cases. Bilateral adrenalectomy may be necessary in FH-III to control the disease (Mussa et al. 2012).

Medical Therapy Medical treatment is the option in a majority of cases of PA with bilateral disease and in cases not appropriate for adrenalectomy. MR antagonist spironolactone is the first line of treatment. With a starting dose of 12.5–25 mg, the dose is gradually up-titrated to optimise the dose (usually up to 100 mg daily) to get adequate control of BP and potassium levels. Eplerenone, a selective MR antagonist, is started at a dose of 25 mg once or twice daily. Caution must be taken in chronic kidney disease stage 3 and above while using these drugs. Amiloride/triamterene are useful alternative medications if MR antagonists are not tolerated/contra-indicated (Funder et al. 2008).

PA resulting from FH-I (GRA) should be managed with glucocorticoids in adults and MR antagonists in paediatric cases (because of the effect of steroids on growth retardation) until they reach adulthood. Starting dose of dexamethasone is 0.125–0.25 mg or prednisolone is 2.5–5 mg at night and the doses are titrated to partially suppress the ACTH levels to optimise the aldosterone levels and BP control (Funder et al. 2008). FH-II is managed with MR antagonists +/− amiloride to optimise BP control.

4.1.2 Congenital Adrenal Hyperplasia (CAH) with Mineralocorticoid Excess

CAH is the most common inborn error of adrenal gland function (Speiser 2015; Sahakitrungruang 2015; Miller and Auchus 2011). There are different forms of CAH depending on the type of genetic mutations and the related enzyme defect in the adrenocortical hormone synthesis that cause these disorders. Two types of enzyme defects cause mineralocorticoid excess in CAH, viz. 11-β-hydroxylase deficiency (11OHD) and 17-α-hydroxylase deficiency (Sahakitrungruang 2015).

About 5–8 % of cases of CAH among Caucasians and about 15 % among Middle-Eastern populations results from 11OHD (Sahakitrungruang 2015; Miller and Auchus 2011). The enzyme deficiency causes decreased cortisol production with accumulation of 11-deoxycortisol and 11-deoxycorticosterone (DOC; a mineralocorticoid precursor). The disease is transmitted as an autosomal recessive trait with more than 80 mutations described already (Zennaro et al. 2015b). Hypertension and varying degrees of virilisation and precocious puberty in both sexes are the results of 11OHD clinically.

17-α-hydroxylase deficiency results in a reduction of cortisol synthesis with overproduction of corticosterone, and deoxycorticosterone (mineralocorticoid). Hypertension, hypokalemia and sexual infantilism secondary to hypergonadotropic hypogonadism are the common clinical features of this disorder. Inheritance pattern is autosomal recessive with more than 90 gene mutations described to date (Zennaro et al. 2015b).

Diagnostic Approach to CAH (with Mineralocorticoid-Induced Hypertension)

Diagnosis of 11OHD is established by elevated baseline levels of DOC and 11-deoxycortisol with significant increase in the levels following ACTH challenge (Sahakitrungruang 2015; Zennaro et al. 2015b). Plasma renin and aldosterone levels will be low. Definitive diagnosis is proved with genetic testing for the mutation. 17-α-hydroxylase deficiency results in elevated levels of DOC, ACTH and gonadotropins with suppressed levels of androgens and estrogen (Zennaro et al. 2015b; Kim and Rhee 2015). Unlike the classical and non-classical forms of CAH, levels of 17-hydroxyprogesterone levels are low and the levels do not rise with ACTH challenge. Genetic testing establishes the diagnosis with identification of the related mutations.

Management

The mainstay of management in patients with 11OHD is glucocorticoids that normalise ACTH, the driving force for DOC overproduction, with improvement of hypertension (Zennaro et al. 2015b). Addition of MR antagonists such as spironolactone or eplerenone may be necessary in some cases to treat hypertension. Patients with 17-α-hydroxylase deficiency should be treated with glucocorticoids and sex steroids when necessary (Zennaro et al. 2015b; Kim and Rhee 2015). The genital abnormalities related to virilisation should be managed by appropriate surgical procedures.

Increased Mineralocortocoid Action

Even with normal levels of mineralocorticoid hormones, mineralocorticoid-related hypertension can result from rare genetic disorders from exaggerated actions of the hormone at the receptor/effecter-tissue levels. These disorders are briefly discussed in the following section.

4.1.3 Liddle Syndrome

This is an autosomal dominant genetic disorder associated with hypertension, hypokalemia, metabolic alkalosis, and low plasma renin and aldosterone levels. Because of similarity to the clinical presentation of PA, the condition is termed "pseudoaldosteronism" (Wang et al. 2015). Liddle syndrome results from gain-of-function mutations in genes encoding the subunits of epithelial sodium channel (ENaC) that cause increased sodium re-absorption and potassium loss from the kidney and hypertension

(Zennaro et al. 2015b; Wang et al. 2015; Melcescu et al. 2012).

Diagnosis is considered in hypertensives with a family history of early-onset hypertension, hypokalemia, low levels of renin and aldosterone, and prompt response to ENaC antagonists such as amiolride and triamterine without response to MR antagonists (Zennaro et al. 2015b; Wang et al. 2015; Melcescu et al. 2012). Confirmation of the diagnosis is by screening for mutations in the genes encoding the β and γ subunits ENaC. Patients are managed by a low sodium diet and ENaC antagonists.

4.1.4 Syndrome of Apparent Mineralocorticoid Excess (AME)

AME is an autosomal recessive disorder characterised by hypertension, hypokalemia, metabolic alkalosis with low levels of plasma renin and aldosterone levels (Zennaro et al. 2015b; Melcescu et al. 2012). It is caused by mutations in the HSD11B2 gene coding for the enzyme 11β-Hydroxysteroid dehydrogenase 2 (HSD11B2) on chromosome 16 (Zennaro et al. 2015b; Melcescu et al. 2012). This enzyme is responsible for the inter-conversion of cortisol to cortisone in aldosterone-selective tissues including kidneys liver, colon, salivary glands, lungs, placenta and some neural tissues. Around 40 different types of mutations are described in the gene already (Zennaro et al. 2015b).

Severe form of the disease is usually diagnosed in early childhood with hypertension, polyuria, polydypsia, hypokalemia, metabolic alkalosis and failure to thrive in presence of suppressed plasma renin and aldosterone levels (Zennaro et al. 2015b; Melcescu et al. 2012). Short stature, renal cysts and nephrocalcinosis may be present in some cases (Zennaro et al. 2015b; New et al. 2005). Milder forms may present during adult life. Biochemical diagnosis of AME is based on measurement of the ratio of urinary metabolites of cortisol to cortisone (high ratio in cases) (Zennaro et al. 2015b; New et al. 2005). Confirmation of the diagnosis is by genetic testing. Management is usually by MR antagonists +/− thiazide diuretics along with small doses of dexamethasone.

4.1.5 Pseudohypoaldosteronism Type 2 (Gordon Syndrome; Familial Hyperkalemic Hypertension)

This is a rare genetic disorder associated with hypertension, hyperkalemic-hyperchloremic metabolic acidosis, low renin and normal or elevated levels of aldosterone (Zennaro et al. 2015b; Melcescu et al. 2012). Multiple genetic mutations are identified (in the genes WNK1, WNK4, KLHL3 and CUL3) that modulate the thiazide-sensitive Na-Cl cotransporter in the kidney leading to increased re-absorption of sodium and chloride from the kidney with the resultant biochemical and clinical manifestations of the disease.

Diagnosis is based on the biochemical abnormalities described above and the genetic testing for different culprit gene mutations (Zennaro et al. 2015b; Melcescu et al. 2012). Management of the disease is with dietary sodium restriction and thiazide diuretics.

4.1.6 Geller Syndrome

This disorder results from a mutation activating the mineralocorticoid receptor (MR) that was first described by Geller et al. in 2000 (Geller et al. 2000). The index case presented with early-onset severe hypertension associated with low plasma renin and aldostereone, and exacerbation of hypertension during pregnancy. So far, only one family has been identified with a p. Ser810Leu mutation, located in the ligand binding domain of the MR (Zennaro et al. 2015b; Melcescu et al. 2012). Amiloride may be effective in the correction of the biochemical abnormalities and improvement of hypertension, but spironolactone has to be avoided as it is a potent agonist of the mutant receptor (Zennaro et al. 2015b).

A flow chart depicting the algorithm for work up and management of primary mineralocorticoid excess states is shown in Fig. 1.

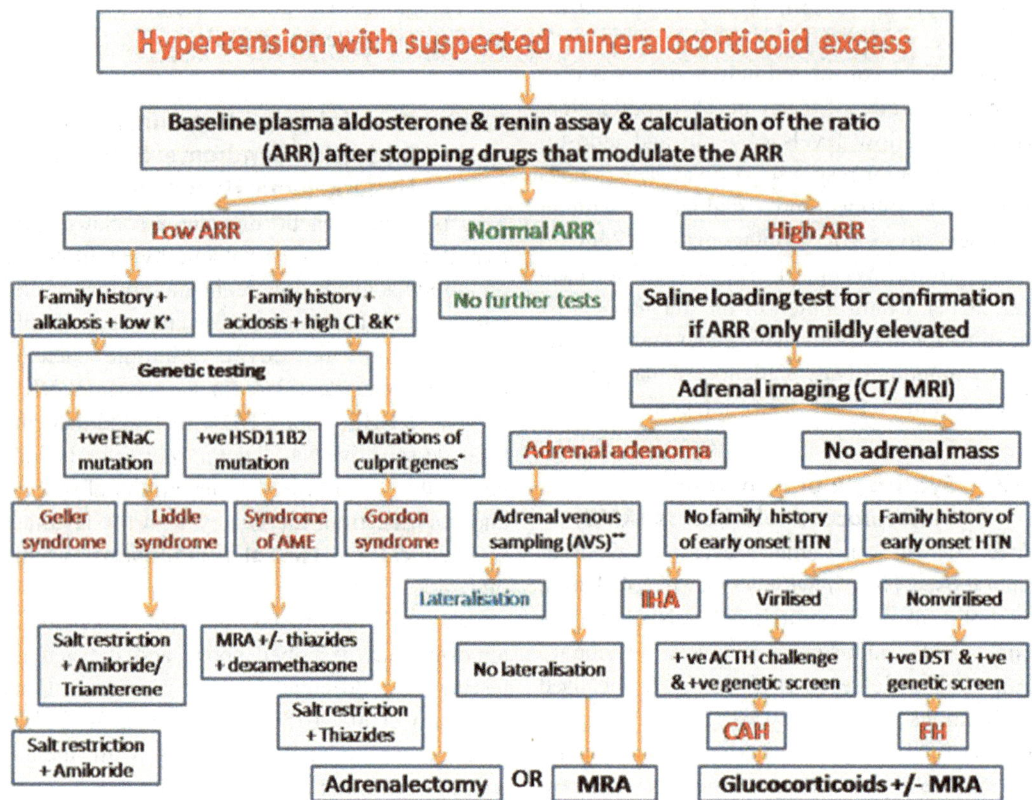

Fig. 1 An algorithm for diagnostic evaluation and management of primary mineralocorticoid excess states (*HTN* hypertension, *CT* computed tomography, *MRI* magnetic resonance imaging, K^+ potassium, Cl^- chloride, *ENaC* epithelial sodium channel, *HSD11B2* 11β-Hydroxysteroid dehydrogenase 2, *AME* apparent mineralocorticoid excess, *IHA* idiopathic hyperaldosteronism, *MRA* mineralocorticoid antagonist, *ACTH* Adrenocorticotropic hormone, *DST* dexamethasone suppression test, *CAH* congenital adrenal hyperplasia, *FH* familial hyperaldosteronism, *Culprit genes** WNK1, WNK4, KLHL3 and CUL3, *(AVS)*** adrenal venous sampling may be avoided in certain situations as mentioned in the text)

5   Pheochromocytomas and Paragangliomas

Pheochromocytomas (PCC) and paragangliomas (PGL) are rare neuroendocrine tumours arising from the chromaffin tissues of the embryonic neural crest cells that become the adrenal medulla and autonomic neural ganglia in adult life. With an estimated annual incidence of 2–8 per million, these tumors account for 0.2–0.6 % of hypertension in the community (Pappachan et al. 2014; Kasperlik-Zaluska et al. 2006). About 85 % of pheochromocytomas arise from the adrenal medulla (PCCs) and the remainder from the extra-adrenal autonomic ganglia (PGLs).

Pathophysiology

Increased production and release of catecholamines (epinephrine, norepinephrine and dopamine) by the tumors to circulation result in the clinico-pathological manifestations of PCCs and PGLs. Catecholamines cause intense vasospasm and hypertension through α-adrenergic effect, and vasodilatation, diaphoresis and tachycardia from the β-adrenergic effect (Pappachan et al. 2014). Severe orthostatic hypotension with syncopal episodes can occasionally result from unbalanced effects of α-

and β-adrenergic receptors in different vasculature in the body (Pappachan et al. 2014; Desai et al. 2009).

The paroxysmal nature of the catecholamine release may explain the episodic nature of symptoms in PCCs/PGLs. Recurrent surge of these hormones may cause a (reversible) form of cardiomyopathy called catecholaminergic cardiomyopathy (Pappachan et al. 2014; Desai et al. 2009). 10–15 % of PCCs and 20–50 % of PGLs can be malignant, and as there is no clear-cut histological criteria to determine malignancy in resected tumors, life-long follow up for recurrence in an appropriate clinical scenario is recommended by many authorities (Parenti et al. 2012; Tsirlin et al. 2014; Lenders et al. 2014). Several genetic mutations have been recently described in PCCs/PGLs (Pappachan et al. 2014) that may be associated with malignant potential and inheritance to successive generations, and the recent endocrine society guidelines in 2014 recommend appropriate testing and follow up algorithm of the disease (Lenders et al. 2014).

Clinical Features

Although the classical clinical presentation is with headaches, palpitations and sweating with hypertension, many of these tumours present with protean manifestations including prolonged periods of clinical silence. <1 % of resistant hypertension cases are related to PCCs/PGLs (Rimoldi et al. 2014). With the increasing use of cross sectional abdominal imaging for medical diagnostics, many cases of PCCs/PGLs are diagnosed in the recent years while evaluating adrenal incidentalomas. About 4 % of adrenal incidentalomas are reported to be PCCs (Kasperlik-Zaluska et al. 2006). Few multi-organ endocrine neoplastic syndromes such as Multiple Endocrine Neoplasia (MEN) 2A and 2B, Von Hippel-Lindau (VHL) disease and neurofibromatosis type 1 can have PCCs/PGLs as disease manifestations (Pappachan et al. 2014; Desai et al. 2009). Hypertensive crisis during emergency surgery, general anaesthesia or contrast radiography, unexplained heart failure,

drug-induced hypertensive crisis (with beta-blockers or monoamine oxidase inhibitors), and new-onset diabetes in an young lean hypertensive are some of the atypical clinical presentations of the disease (Pappachan et al. 2014).

Diagnostic Approach

Biochemical As in any other endocrine disease biochemical confirmation of the diagnosis is the first-line approach to the diagnosis of PCCs/PGLs. Plasma free metanephrines or urinary fractionated metanephrines is the screening investigation of choice for suspected cases with very high sensitivity and good specificity (Pappachan et al. 2014; Lenders et al. 2014). Intake of multiple medications and other chemicals before testing can interfere with the results reducing the positive predictive value of this screening assay. A detailed list of these medications can be found in the relevant literature (Pappachan et al. 2014; Lenders et al. 2014). Therefore, raised levels ≤ 3–4 times the laboratory reference range should be interpreted with caution to avoid un-necessary work up because of a false positive test. A clonidine suppression test may be useful in such situations (Lenders et al. 2014; Eisenhofer et al. 2003).

Anatomical Imaging Imaging studies for localisation should only be undertaken after the biochemical diagnosis is proven. CT scan and Magnetic Resonance Imaging (MRI) have excellent sensitivity and reasonable specificity for anatomical localisation of these tumours. Non-ionic contrast is preferred for CT scan because of the risk of hypertensive crisis (Lenders et al. 2014). MRI is preferred over CT in patients in whom where radiation needs to be avoided and in patients suspected to have metastatic disease (Pappachan et al. 2014; Lenders et al. 2014).

Functional Imaging Once the anatomical diagnosis is established with an initial imaging modality, functional imaging is usually recommended to prove the diagnosis, and to exclude the possibility of metastasis and multisite disease in cases of PGLs. ^{123}I-metaiodobenzylguanidine (MIBG) scitigraphy is the usual functional imaging modality utilized in most centers. The sensitivity and specificity of ^{123}I-MIBG scintigraphy is around 85 % in PCCs. A variety of different radio-pharmaceutical agents can be used for functional imaging in cases with a negative ^{123}I-MIBG scintigraphy (Pappachan et al. 2014; Lenders et al. 2014).

Genetic Testing The recommendations for genetic testing and the testing algorithm can be found in the 2014 Endocrine society guidelines (Lenders et al. 2014).

An algorithm for diagnostic work up of clinically suspected PCCs/PGLs is shown in Fig. 2.

Management Surgery is the preferred definitive management option for all cases of PCCs/PGLs unless contraindicated. Complete resection of the tumor often results in cure of the disease although improvement in hypertension depends on other factors too.

Peri-Operative Management

Prompt control of hypertension and appropriate preoperative preparation is a must as manipulation of the tumour during surgery results in hypertensive crisis because of the massive release of catecholamines to circulation. Adequate control of hypertension with non-selective α-adrenergic blockers such as phenoxybenzamine (10 mg BD to a maximum of 1 mg/kg/day) or α-1 selective agent doxazosin (2–32 mg/day) 10–14 days prior to the surgery along with liberal intake of fluids and salt to replenish volume depletion is recommended in

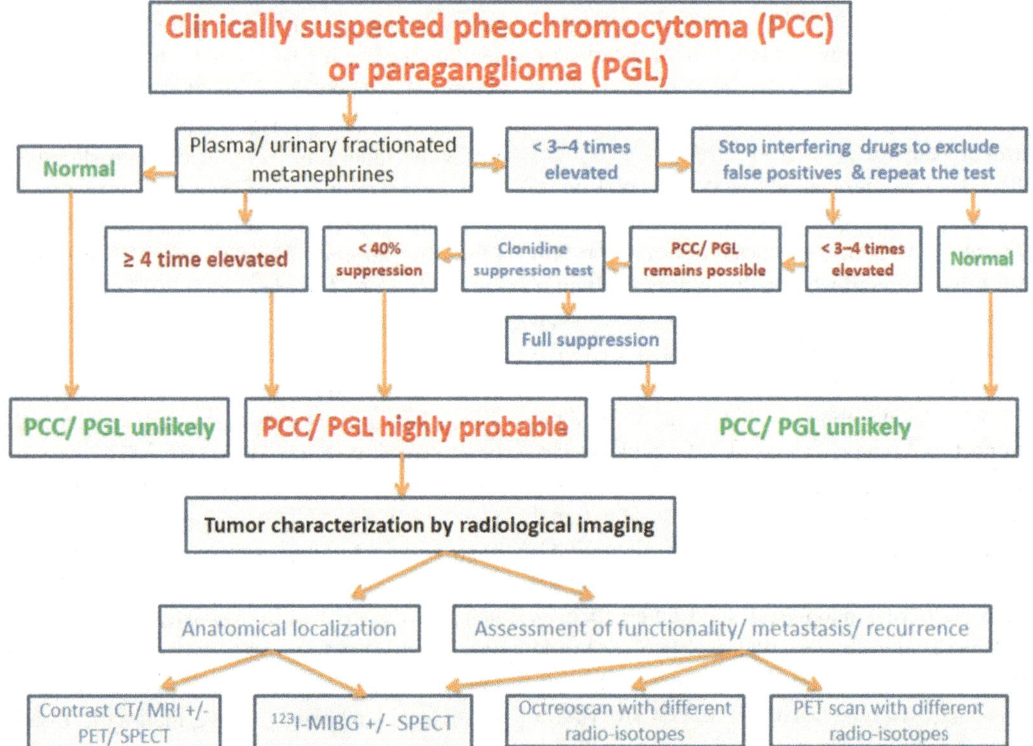

Fig. 2 Diagnostic evaluation of pheochromocytomas (PCCs) and paragangliomas (PGLs) (*CT* Computed tomography, *MRI* Magnetic resonance imaging, *PET* Positron emission tomography, *SPECT* Single photon emission computed tomography, *[123]I-MIBG* [123]Iodine-Meta-iodo-benzyl-guanidine. Reproduced with permission from Pappachan et al. (2014))

all cases (Pappachan et al. 2014; Lenders et al. 2014). Addition of a β-adrenergic blocker such as propranolol or atenolol to counteract the reflex tachycardia and postural hypotension associated with α-blockers may be necessary after few days of starting α-blockers. Other antihypertensive medications such as calcium channel antagonists and metyrosine may be necessary for optimal control of BP in some cases (Pappachan et al. 2014; Tsirlin et al. 2014; Lenders et al. 2014). The target BP control should be < 130/80 mm Hg while seated and > 90 mm systolic while standing and a heart rate 70–80 per minute (Pappachan et al. 2014; Tsirlin et al. 2014; Lenders et al. 2014). Appropriate modifications in these targets may be made in the presence of cardiovascular disease.

Operative Management Surgeon and anaesthetist with sufficient experience with the management of these rare tumors should perform the surgery to optimise safe outcomes. Laparoscopic adrenalectomy is the preferred surgery in most cases of PCCs. Large tumors, PGLs and suspected metastatic disease are indications for an open surgery (Pappachan et al. 2014; Tsirlin et al. 2014; Lenders et al. 2014). Intra-operative BP changes should be closely monitored with administration of intravenous α-adrenergic blockers (phentolamine or phenoxybenzamine) for hypertensive episodes during surgery, and intravenous crystalloids and vasopressors to manage the postoperative hypotension in an intensive care unit may be necessary to manage cases (Pappachan et al. 2014; Tsirlin et al. 2014).

Postoperative Care Withdrawal of the antihypertensive medications and hypoglycemic agents (if secondary diabetes was present pre-operatively) may be possible in some cases. Testing plasma (or urinary) metanephrines 10 days after the surgery to ensure complete removal of the tumor is recommended in all cases (Pappachan et al. 2014; Tsirlin et al. 2014; Lenders et al. 2014). Regular endocrine follow up of the patients with appropriate long-term care plan is also mandatory.

Follow Up The follow up care of patients with PCCs and PGLs is detailed in the 2014 guidelines of the Endocrine Society (Lenders et al. 2014).

An algorithm for management and follow up of PCCs/PGLs is shown in Fig. 3.

6 Glucocorticoid Excess (Cushing's Syndrome)

Glucocorticoids are hormones from the zona fasciculata of the adrenal cortex. Although physiological levels are critically important for homeostasis in normal subjects, excess production of glucocorticoids in the body (endogenous hypercortisolism) or prolonged administration of the hormone in high doses (iatrogenic hypercortisolism) result in a pathologic state known as Cushing's syndrome (CS) that is associated with protean manifestations including secondary hypertension. The disease is associated with excess morbidity, mortality and poor quality of life, and an early diagnosis and appropriate management may mitigate this natural history (Nieman 2015). The clinical picture of CS cases varies depending on the extent and duration of cortisol excess.

Pathophysiology

A majority of cases of CS results from an ACTH producing pituitary adenoma that is otherwise known as Cushing's disease. Ectopic production of ACTH accounts for a significant proportion of cases other than pituitary Cushing's, followed by cortisol-secreting adrenal adenomas and carcinomas, and adrenal nodular hyperplasia. Exogenous steroid administration for therapeutic purposes results in iatrogenic CS in many patients. Carney complex, a rare genetic disorder (autosomal dominant), characterized by pigmented skin and mucosal lesions, cardiac and cutaneous myxomas, and multiple endocrine and non-endocrine neoplasms is an uncommon cause of CS (Correa et al. 2015). Another rare cause for CS is ectopic CRH (corticotropin releasing hormone) producing tumors. Subclinical CS, results from alterations in the hypothalamus–pituitary–adrenal (HPA) axis without overt signs or symptoms of hypercortisolism (Di Dalmazi et al. 2015).

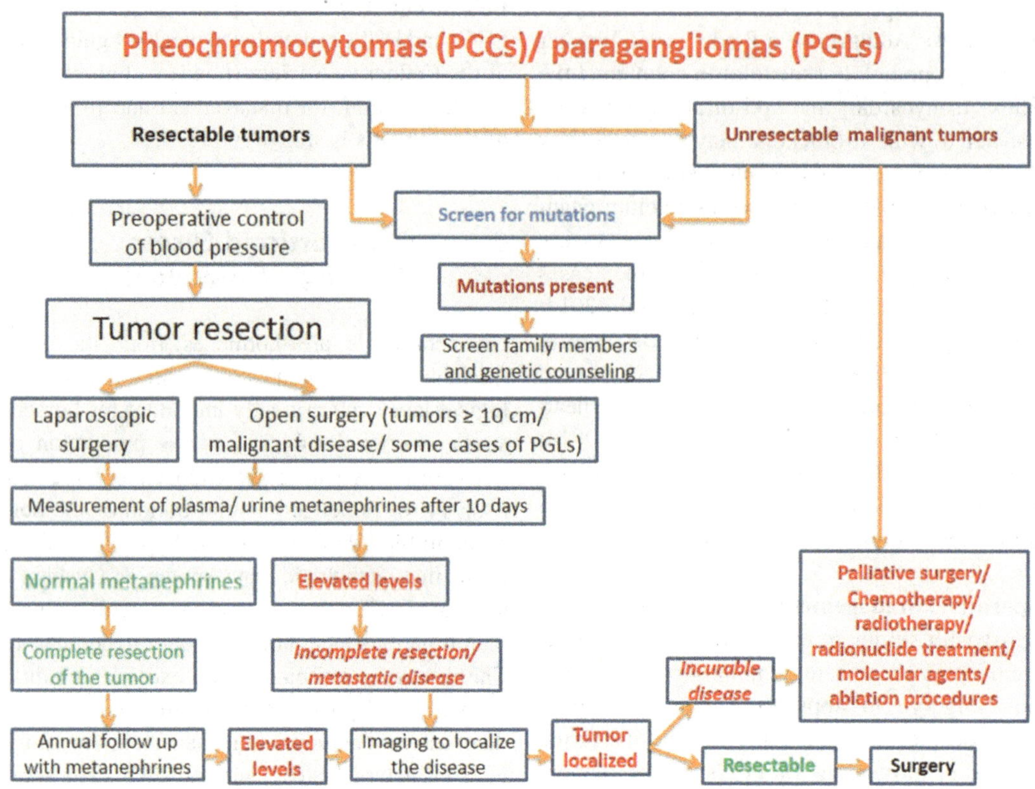

Fig. 3 Management and follow up care of pheochromocytomas (PCCs) and paragangliomas (PGLs) (Reproduced with permission from Pappachan et al. (2014))

Hypertension in CS may be multi-factorial, and the exact mechanisms still remain elusive. Several putative mechanisms have been identified including imbalance between vasodilatory and vasoconstrictor chemicals such as prostacyclin, nitric oxide and endothelins, the mineralocorticoid receptor activation (Di Dalmazi et al. 2015; Anagnostis et al. 2009; Mihailidou et al. 2009; De Leo et al. 2010; Rizzoni et al. 2009), endothelial abnormalities (Di Dalmazi et al. 2015; Anagnostis et al. 2009), and development of metabolic syndrome (Di Dalmazi et al. 2015; Anagnostis et al. 2009; Ferraù and Korbonits 2015).

Clinical Features

A wide variety of clinical manifestation may be seen in a classical case of overt CS (Nieman 2015). These include facial plethora, fragility of skin, acne, hirsutism, thinning of scalp hair, weight gain with truncal obesity, buffalo hump and supraclavicular fatty pad (due to ectopic fat distribution), labile mood and sometimes frank psychosis, menstrual irregularities, proximal myopathy, growth failure in children, sexual dysfunction (and even impotence), hypertension, hypokalaemia, glucose intolerance or frank diabetes, osteoporosis, metabolic syndrome, and susceptibility to infections due to suppressed immunity. However, these classical manifestations are less frequently observed these days because of wide availability of investigations and awareness of the disease among physicians. In up to 15 % of adults with CS, the clinical manifestations may occur only periodically, a condition known as cyclical Cushing's syndrome (Alexandraki et al. 2009).

Diagnostic Approach

Although the American Endocrine Society Guidelines on diagnostic evaluation of CS is slightly old (Nieman et al. 2008), most of the recommendations are still valid for work up of suspected cases. An exclusive meeting to discuss about CS, held in Germany in October 2014 with wide participation from global experts, compiled further evidence on the diagnostic and management algorithms of the disease (Reincke 2015). A detailed discussion of the diagnostic approach to CS can be found in these published literature and only a brief account is given here.

A thorough history of extraneous steroid administration should be obtained in all cases of clinically suspected CS before biochemical testing. The Endocrine society recommends testing for CS in patients with multiple clinical features described above, children with growth retardation with abnormal weight gain, illnesses uncommon in younger age-groups such as hypertension and osteoporosis, and adrenal adenomas (Nieman et al. 2008).

In suspected cases of CS, one of the following screening investigations should be performed initially: 24-hour urinary free cortisol (at least 2 samples), late night salivary cortisol, 1-mg overnight dexamethasone suppression test (DST) or low-dose DST (0.5 mg QDS for 48 h) (Nieman et al. 2008). Further evaluation by an endocrinologist is recommended in cases with at least one positive test and in those with negative screening tests and clinically suspected cyclical CS. Random plasma cortisol measurement has no value for screening cases of CS because of the marked variability of levels depending of many factors.

Confirmation of CS in suspected cases needs detailed endocrine work up. Measurement of corticotrophin (ACTH) levels is the next step in diagnosis. Suppressed level of ACTH indicate an adrenal/iatrogenic source of hypercortisolism. If adrenal source is suspected a contrast CT scan of the adrenal glands should be done. If ACTH levels are high or high normal, an MRI of pituitary should be done. A pituitary mass ≥ 1 cm may be an indication of Cushing's disease and pituitary surgery although controversy still remains among endocrinologists on size criteria (Florez et al. 2013). A high-dose DST (using 2 mg QDS for 48 h) and/or CRH stimulation tests is recommended by some centers if the pituitary mass is smaller or absent, in presence of raised ACTH levels. A suppressible cortisol with high-dose DST or 20 % rise in cortisol following CRH administration indicates pituitary-driven corticotrophin excess although overlap with ectopic source is well recognised. Bilateral inferior petrosal sinus sampling (BIPSS) with baseline and CRH-stimulated ACTH measurements is the next step. If BIPSS is negative, imaging of thorax and/or abdomen and pelvis should be performed to identify an ectopic source of ACTH. Finally, an octreotide scan may be necessary if all other confirmatory tests are negative. A useful algorithm for diagnostic work up of CS can be found in the full-test article (freely available) by Florez et al. (2013).

Management

Management of CS can be complex in many cases, and the mortality related to the disease is reported to be higher than in normal age-matched controls even in treated cases (Clayton et al. 2011; Graversen et al. 2012). Complete cure of the disease may not be always possible, and management of disease manifestations shall be the only options in such cases. Whenever feasible, surgical removal of the cause of excess cortisol/ACTH is the most appropriate and potentially curable management option.

Medical Therapy Even in curable cases, medical management should bridge the definitive surgery for adequate preparation of the patient. First-line agent widely used is metyrapone, a 11-β-hydroxylase enzyme inhibitor (dose range 1–4 g/day in divided doses). The drug has been found to be very effective for short- and long-term control of endogenous steroid excess in a recent multicenter study (Daniel et al. 2015). However, the drug can increase the adrenal synthesis of steroids with mineralocorticoid activity that worsens hypertension (Ferraù and Korbonits 2015). Other cortisol-lowering medications such as ketoconazole (Nieman 2002), mitotane (Donadille et al. 2010) and mifepristone (Fleseriu et al. 2012) also have beneficial effects on hypertension in CS, although careful monitoring for side effects of these agents is necessary. Recent guidelines from the Endocrine Society and recommendation from the European Medicines Agency suggest ketoconazole as highly effective option for medical management of CS when used judiciously (European Medicines Agency 2016; Nieman et al. 2015). Combination therapy with ketoconazole and metyrapone may be necessary to obtain rapid control hypercortisolism in some cases (Nieman et al. 2015). Pasireotide alone (Colao et al. 2012), or in combination with cabergoline and ketoconazole (Feelders et al. 2010) also have been reported to benefit treatment of hypertension in CS. Recently, retinoic acid (Pecori Giraldi et al. 2012) and LCI699 have been shown to be effective in treatment of CS and disease-related hypertension (Bertagna et al. 2014; Daniel and Newell-Price 2015). Along with medical measures to manage hypercortisolism, conventional antihypertensive treatment also needs to be administered for control of BP in patients with CS.

Surgery Transphenoidal hypophysectomy is the preferred surgical treatment in Cushing's disease although cure is not guaranteed in all cases owing to the difficulty in removal of the entire tumour tissue in some cases, especially small adenomas. Pituitary radiotherapy may be necessary in selected cases with residual tumour although associated with higher long-term complication rates including pan-hypopituitarism. Functional imaging of the pituitary with (11)C-methionine positron emission tomography-computed tomography (PET-CT) scan is recently reported to be an excellent tool to localise residual disease after previous hypophysectomy for targeted therapy (Koulouri et al. 2015).

Removal of the source of ectopic ACTH-driven CS may be easy if precise tumour localisation is possible pre-surgically.

Hypophysectomy with or without pituitary radiotherapy is usually associated with multiple pituitary hormone insufficiencies that necessitates lifelong hormone replacement with endocrine follow up. Sometimes bilateral adrenalectomy may be necessary for patients with intractable CS where source of ACTH excess is irremovable (Reincke et al. 2015). This surgery is reported to be relatively safe and highly effective in such cases. Patients need lifelong steroid and mineralocorticoid replacement and Nelson's syndrome is a possible consequence of this surgery in CS due to the growth of the pituitary adenoma in absence of feedback inhibition from corticosteroids.

---

7 Acromegaly

Acromegaly results from prolonged growth hormone (GH) excess in adults. GH exerts its hormonal effect in the body through the protein molecule Insulin-like Growth Factor-1 (IGF-1) secreted from liver. The classical cases of acromegaly with all the phenotypic features are less often encountered currently in clinical practice owing to better investigation facilities and heightened awareness of the disease among physicians that result in early diagnosis of the disease. The estimated prevalence of the disease is 30–60 cases/one million population and arterial hypertension is encountered in 40 % of the cases (Capatina and Wass 2015).

Pathophysiology

In over 95 % of cases, acromegaly results from a GH-secreting somatotroph adenoma of pituitary causing GH and IGF-1 overproduction (Melmed 2009; Katznelson et al. 2014). Majority of these are macroadenomas (size > 1 cm). Less than 5 % of cases results from a hypothalamic tumour or a neuroendocrine tumour secreting Growth Hormone Releasing Hormone (GHRH) or rarely GH overproduction from a hemopoeitic or abdominal tumor (Katznelson et al. 2014). GH-producing tumours may be a consequence of the genetic MEN-1 syndrome.

Overstimulation from the excess GH in circulation results in raised plasma levels of IGF-1 produced from liver that causes overgrowth of somatic tissues culminating in the clinical manifestations of acromegaly. Disfigurement of the facial skeleton and enlargement of limbs result from prolonged hyper-stimulation of IGF-1. The clinical manifestations of the disease are related to overgrowth of tissues and the metabolic abnormalities related to excess circulating IGF-1 levels.

Clinical Features

The disease affects most body organs and the common manifestations are headache, coarse facial features (frontal bossing and prognathism), enlargement of hands and feet, hypertension and diabetes, osteoarthritis, entrapment neuropathies, sleep apnoea, visual field defects and heart failure. A detailed account of the disease and its clinical features can be found in the recent article (available free in the web) by Capatina et al. (2015).

Diagnostic Approach

All patients with clinically suspected acromegaly and typical features should undergo testing for IGF-1 levels. Those with some of the features without a definite clinical picture may also need IGF-1 testing when some of disease-associated features such as sleep apnoea, type 2 diabetes, hypertension, carpel tunnel syndrome, debilitating arthritis or hyperhidrosis are present (Katznelson et al. 2014). IGF-1 levels also should be measured in patients with a pituitary mass to exclude the disease. Biochemical confirmation of acromegaly in patients with elevated or equivocal IGF-1 levels is by a glucose tolerance test to show lack of suppression of GH levels during hyperglycemia (Capatina and Wass 2015; Katznelson et al. 2014).

In biochemically confirmed cases, disease localisation should be done by an appropriate imaging study. An MRI of the pituitary detects a macroadenoma in about 77 % cases (Katznelson et al. 2014; Mestron et al. 2004), and a hyper-intense T2-weighted MRI signal may have prognostic significance (enhanced response to somatostatin receptor ligand [SRL] therapy) (Katznelson et al. 2014; Puig-Domingo et al. 2010). Visual field testing is recommended in all cases with a pituitary macroadenoma in the MRI. If pituitary imaging is negative, GHRH levels should be measured to exclude rare location of the disease in hypothalamus or other tissues with appropriate imaging when necessary (Capatina and Wass 2015).

Management

Surgery All resectable tumors in the pituitary should be removed through a transphenoidal hypophysectomy if possible. Some large tumors may need a trans-cranial or combined approach. Sometimes surgical de-bulking improves the medical treatment outcome later if complete removal of the tumor is impossible (Katznelson et al. 2014; Katznelson 2010). Repeated surgery may be necessary if initial procedure did not clear the entire tumor. Postoperative measurement of GH and IGF-1 levels give evidence for clearance of tumor during surgery and pituitary imaging is necessary for anatomical assessment. These are usually done after 12 weeks of surgery (Katznelson et al. 2014).

Medical Treatment Medical management becomes necessary when tumors are inoperable or when surgery is incomplete with residual disease. SRLs and pegvisomant are the two classes of drugs with good activity against acromegaly. 2 forms of SRLs are commercially available widely (Octreotide LAR [long acting release] and lanreotide depot/autogel). Pasereotide is a novel SRL with enhanced activity and confers better tumoral response to treatment (Capatina and Wass 2015; Katznelson et al. 2014; Colao et al. 2014). Pegvisomant possess better treatment response than SRLs in patients with acromegaly (Katznelson et al. 2014; van der Lely et al. 2012). Monitoring of response to treatment and dose adjustments are done with serial measurements of IGF-1 and pituitary imaging.

Mild disease may respond to dopamine agonists such as cabergoline. Combinations of different drug classes in different multi-drug regimes may be necessary in some cases for enhanced response to treatment (Capatina and Wass 2015; Katznelson et al. 2014). Pituitary radiotherapy may also be necessary in cases with residual disease when medical therapy fails to control the disease.

Management of multi-system manifestations of the disease such as diabetes, hypertension, entrapment neuropathy and heart disease should be as per the individual needs of the patient. In general, acromegaly cases are managed in a multi-disciplinary team environment involving endocrinologists, surgeons, biochemists and anaesthesiologists with significant expertise in the management of this uncommon disease.

8　Thyroid Diseases

Thyroid disorders are the second most common causes of endocrine disease after diabetes mellitus. Although not associated with severe hypertension, both hypothyroidism and hyperthyroidism can cause high BP in some patients.

8.1　Hypothyroidism

Hypothyroidism is a common endocrine disease with higher prevalence towards older age-groups. Subclinical hypothyroidism (without overt symptoms and signs) affects about 3-8 % of adult population that reaches around 10 % by the sixth decade of life (Hollowell et al. 2002; Fatourechi 2009). Overt hypothyroidism presents with multiple clinical features such as lethargy, constipation, cold intolerance, menstrual abnormalities, weight gain, dry skin, hair loss, hoarseness of voice, psychomotor retardation, neuropsychiatric abnormalities, bradycardia and in severe cases, myxedema and coma.

Bradycardia, mild hypertension, narrow pulse pressure, and muffling of heart sounds are the most common signs of overt hypothyroidism (Klein and Ojamaa 2001). Positive correlation between serum thyrotropin levels and hypertension was observed in children and adolescents, suggesting a linear relationship between even subclinical hypothyroidism and BP, in two large cohort studies among two populations with entirely different genetic backgrounds (Chen et al. 2012; Ittermann et al. 2012). High serum thyrotropin levels were positively associated with systolic and diastolic blood pressure, in children and adolescents with Odds ratios 1.12 and 1.19 respectively ($p < 0.05$ in both) (Ittermann et al. 2012). Appropriate control of hypothyroid state with thyroid hormone replacement results in normalisation of blood pressure as many of the other abnormalities related to the disease.

8.2　Hyperthyroidism

Hyperthyroidism results from excessive circulating levels of thyroid hormones. Primary hyperthyroidism from diseases of the thyroid gland is usually autoimmune. Subclinical hyperthyroidism, a state of suppressed thyrotropin levels and normal thyroid hormones, is seen in up to 1 % of men and 1.5 % of women older than 60 years (Ittermann et al. 2012; Helfand 2004). The clinical features of hyperthyroidism are mostly opposite to hypothyroidism, familiar to most physicians, and therefore, not described here.

Hyperthyroidism increases cardiac output by 50–300 % because of a decrease in systemic vascular resistance, an increase in heart rate, increase in left ventricular output, and an increase in the blood volume (Klein and Ojamaa 2001). Therefore, systolic hypertension with a widened pulse pressure (opposite to the hypothyroid state) is the usual clinical manifestation in hyperthyroidism. Prompt resolution of hypertension is usually observed in patients with hyperthyroidism after full control of the disease by medical or surgical intervention.

9 Primary Hyperparathyroidism

Primary hyperparathyroidism (PHPT) results from increase in secretion of parathyroid hormone (PTH) from the parathyroid glands. The estimated incidence of PHPT in the United States from 1993 to 2001 was approximately 22 cases per 100,000 person years (Wermers et al. 2006; Marcocci and Cetani 2011). Prevalence of PHPT can be as high as 2.1 % on older individuals (Lundgren et al. 1997). Many cases are asymptomatic, and the diagnosis is often made while investigating patients for the cause of mild hypercalcemia. Sometimes patients may present with severe hypercalcemia, renal stones, osteoporosis and fractures, acute kidney injury, and chronic renal impairment.

Frequent association between PHPT and hypertension is well documented even among patients with mild PHPT (Silverberg et al. 2009). Mean 24-h BP (both systolic and diastolic) obtained by ambulatory monitoring was significantly higher, with a higher prevalence of hypertension in 47 % of patients with PHPT compared to controls (Letizia et al. 2005). Plasma ionised calcium levels was found to be an independent risk factor for elevated BP in multiple linear regression model in this study. The probable mechanism of hypertension in PHPT is increased arterial stiffness in these patients. A recent large community-based cohort study indicated that plasma calcium levels were independently associated with higher arterial stiffness, and the PTH levels with arterial blood pressures (Hagström et al. 2015).

Generally, mild cases of PHPT are not treated by parathyroid surgery, and the follow up is with regular monitoring of calcium, renal function and bone mineral density assessments in the endocrine outpatient clinics. Hypertension is managed by conventional antihypertensive drugs as in a normal case. Thiazide diuretics should be avoided as antihypertensives because of the risk of worsening hypercalcemia. There is conflicting data on the improvement of hypertension in patients undergoing parathyroidectomy for PHPT with some studies showing benefit (Nainby-Luxmoore et al. 1982; Ringe 1984; Broulik et al. 2011), while others without a positive effect (Rapado 1986; Lind et al. 1991). Although improvement of the substantial cardiac and vascular dysfunction related to symptomatic PHPT was observed in patients after parathyroidectomy (Agarwal et al. 2013), PHPT-related hypertension is not an indication for surgery currently.

10 Iatrogenic Hormone Manipulation

Therapeutic administration of hormones for different medical conditions can result in development of/or worsening of hypertension. Glucocorticoid administration is the most common cause for drug-induced endocrine hypertension. Prevalence of Steroid-induced hypertension increases with age, and new-onset hypertension was observed in 22 % of cases receiving long-term steroids for giant-cell arteritis (Proven et al. 2003). Studies on the effect of hormone replacement on hypertension in post-menopausal women showed conflicting results with positive (Preston 2009), and negative effects (Akkad et al. 1997). Although testosterone can theoretically increase BP by the effects of vasoconstriction and stimulation of renin-angiotensin-aldosterone system (Kienitz and Quinkler 2008), testosterone replacement resulted in improvement of the parameters of metabolic syndrome including hypertension in hypogonadal men (Janjgava et al. 2014).

A classification of different endocrine disorders causing hypertension, their common clinical presentations, important diagnostic features and treatment are summarized in Table 1.

11 Conclusions

Endocrine hypertension is a cause of secondary hypertension in a significant proportion of cases. Some clinical characteristics of the patients may

Table 1 The causes of endocrine hypertension, their common clinical characteristics, diagnostic features & treatment

Clinical condition				Common clinical characteristics	Diagnostic features	Treatment
Primary mineralocorticoid Excess	*Hypermineralocorticoidism*	**Primary aldosteronism**	*Aldosterone producing adenoma (APA)*	Resistant HTN & adrenal adenoma	Raised ARR, CT – adrenal adenoma, AVS – lateralisation to side of adenoma	Adenoma removal/MR antagonist
			Idiopathic hyperaldosteronism	Resistant HTN	Raised ARR, CT adrenal – negative	MR antagonist
			Type 1 familial hyperaldosteronism (FH-I)	Resistant HTN and strong family history	Raised ARR; HTN & aldosterone suppressed by dexamethasone	Glucocorticoid therapy
		Congenital adrenal hyperplasia	*11-β-hydroxylase deficiency*	HTN, virilisation and precocious puberty	Elevated DOC & 11-deoxycortisol. Abnormal genes	Glucocorticoids; (MR antagonists in some cases)
			17-α-hydroxylase deficiency	Hypokalemia, HTN & sexual infantilism	High ACTH, DOC & gonadotropins, low androgens, estrogens. Abnormal genes	Glucocorticoids & sex steroids when necessary
	Increased minrealocorticoid action	**Liddle syndrome (pseudo-aldosteronism)**		HTN, hypokalemia & alkalosis with family history	Low aldosterone & rennin, ENaC gene mutation	Low sodium diet + amiloride or triamterine
		Syndrome of apparent mineralocorticoid excess (AME)		Hypokalemia, HTN, & alkalosis. Severe disease: growth failure and short stature in children	Low aldosterone & renin, high ratio of urine cortisol/cortisone metabolites & HSD11B2 gene mutation	MR antagonists +/– thiazide diuretics & small doses of dexamethasone
		Pseudohypoaldosteronism type 2 (Gordon syndrome)		HTN, hyperkalemic-hyperchloremic metabolic acidosis	low renin, normal or elevated aldosterone level, abnormal gene mutations	Dietary sodium restriction and thiazide diuretics
		Geller syndrome		Early onset HTN & worsening of HTN during pregnancy	Low plasma aldosterone & renin & activating mutation of MR	Sodium restriction & amiloride for HTN

Pheochromocytomas and paragangliomas (PCC & PGL)	Episodic symptoms with HTN. Adrenal incidentaloma	High plasma and urinary metanephrines. PCC or PGL on imaging	Tumor removal with surgical precautions. Long-term follow up
Glucocorticoid excess (Cushing's syndrome)	HTN with cushingoid appearance, diabetes, metabolic syndrome, infection susceptibility & osteoporosis	High plasma and urinary cortisol, ACTH – high in central & ectopic; low in adrenal Cushing's. Imaging evidence of source of high ACTH or adrenal disease.	Metyrapone, antihypertensives, surgery to remove ACTH source or adrenalectomy
Acromegaly	Coarse body features with facial & limb enlargement, HTN, diabetes, sleep apnoea, visual field defects & arthritis	High levels of insulin-like growth factor 1 & growth hormone (GH), lack of GH suppression on glucose tolerance test & pituitary adenoma on imaging	Pituitary adenoma removal by surgery if possible. GH suppression by SRL therapy & antihypertensives
Thyroid diseases *Hypothyroidism*	Diastolic HTN, weight gain & coarse features	High levels of thyrotrophin with low/ low-normal level of thyroid hormones	Thyroid hormone replacement
Hyperthyroidism	Systolic HTN with weight loss	Low levels of thyrotrophin with high/ high-normal level of thyroid hormones	Antithyroid drugs, thyroidectomy/radio-iodine therapy
Primary hyperparathyroidism	HTN, asymptomatic disease in many, fractures & osteoporosis, acute/ chronic renal failure	Hypercalcemia with raised parathyroid hormone level and parathyroid adenoma or hyperplasia	Parathyroidectomy in selected cases. Close monitoring & periodic evaluation in mild cases
Iatrogenic hormone manipulation	HTN with history of hormone treatment	History and blood pressure elevation	Antihypertensives and withdrawal of hormone if feasible

HTN hypertension, *ARR* aldosterone to renin ratio, *MR* mineralocorticoid receptor, *ENaC* epithelial sodium channel, *CT* computed tomography, *ACTH* adrenocorticotrophin help clinician to suspect an endocrine cause for hypertension. Primary aldosteronism is the most common cause for endocrine hypertension. The Endocrine society guidelines on individual diseases that cause endocrine hypertension may help clinician to appropriately evaluate and manage patients.

References

Agarwal G, Nanda G, Kapoor A, Singh KR, Chand G, Mishra A et al (2013) Cardiovascular dysfunction in symptomatic primary hyperparathyroidism and its reversal after curative parathyroidectomy: results of a prospective case control study. Surgery 154:1394–1403

Akkad AA, Halligan AW, Abrams K, al-Azzawi F (1997) Differing responses in blood pressure over 24 hours in normotensive women receiving oral or transdermal estrogen replacement therapy. Obstet Gynecol 89:97–103

Alexandraki KI, Kaltsas GA, Isidori AM, Akker SA, Drake WM, Chew SL et al (2009) The prevalence and characteristic features of cyclicity and variability in Cushing's disease. Eur J Endocrinol 160:1011–1018

Anagnostis P, Athyros VG, Tziomalos K, Karagiannis A, Mikhailidis DP (2009) The pathogenetic role of cortisol in the metabolic syndrome: a hypothesis. J Clin Endocrinol Metab 94:2692–2701

Bertagna X, Pivonello R, Fleseriu M, Zhang Y, Robinson P, Taylor A et al (2014) LCI699, a potent 11β-hydroxylase inhibitor, normalizes urinary cortisol in patients with Cushing's disease: results from a ulticentre, proof-of-concept study. J Clin Endocrinol Metab 99:1375–1383

Boulkroun S, Fernandes-Rosa FL, Zennaro MC (2015) Molecular and cellular mechanisms of aldosterone producing adenoma development. Front Endocrinol (Lausanne) 6:95

Broulik PD, Brouliková A, Adámek S, Libanský P, Tvrdoň J, Broulikova K et al (2011) Improvement of hypertension after parathyroidectomy of patients suffering from primary hyperparathyroidism. Int J Endocrinol 2011:309068

Capatina C, Wass JA (2015) 60 years of neuroendocrinology: acromegaly. J Endocrinol 226:T141–T160

Chen H, Xi Q, Zhang H, Song B, Liu X, Mao X et al (2012) Investigation of thyroid function and blood pressure in school-aged subjects without overt thyroid disease. Endocrine 41:122–129

Clayton RN, Raskauskiene D, Reulen RC, Jones PW (2011) Mortality and morbidity in Cushing's disease over 50 years in Stoke-on-Trent, UK: audit and meta-analysis of literature. J Clin Endocrinol Metab 96:632–642

Colao A, Petersenn S, Newell-Price J, Findling JW, Gu F, Maldonado M et al (2012) A 12-month phase 3 study of pasireotide in Cushing's disease. New Engl J Med 366:914–924

Colao A, Bronstein MD, Freda P et al (2014) Pasireotide versus octreotide in acromegaly: a head-to-head superiority study. J Clin Endocrinol Metab 99:791–799

Correa R, Salpea P, Stratakis C (2015) Carney complex: an update. Eur J Endocrinol 173:M85–M97

Daniel E, Newell-Price JD (2015) Therapy of endocrine disease: steroidogenesis enzyme inhibitors in Cushing's syndrome. Eur J Endocrinol 172:R263–R280

Daniel E, Aylwin S, Mustafa O, Ball S, Munir A, Boelaert K et al (2015) Effectiveness of metyrapone in treating Cushing's Syndrome: a retrospective multicenter study in 195 patients. J Clin Endocrinol Metab 100:4146–4154

De Leo M, Pivonello R, Auriemma RS, Cozzolino A, Vitale P, Simeoli C et al (2010) Cardiovascular disease in Cushing's syndrome: heart versus vasculature. Neuroendocrinology 92:50–54

Desai AS, Chutkow WA, Edelman E, Economy KE, Dec GW Jr (2009) Clinical problem-solving. A crisis in late pregnancy. N Engl J Med 361:2271–2277

Di Dalmazi G, Pasquali R, Beuschlein F, Reincke M (2015) Subclinical hypercortisolism: a state, a syndrome, or a disease? Eur J Endocrinol 173:M61–M71

Donadille B, Groussin L, Waintrop C, Abbas H, Tenenbaum F, Dugue MA (2010) Management of Cushing's syndrome due to ectopic adrenocorticotropin secretion with 1, ortho-1, para'-dichloro-diphenyl-dichloro-ethane: findings in 23 patients from a single center. J Clin Endocrinol Metab 95:537–544

Eisenhofer G, Goldstein DS, Walther MM et al (2003) Biochemical diagnosis of pheochromocytoma: how to distinguish true- from false-positive test results. J Clin Endocrinol Metab 88:2656–2666

European Medicines Agency (2016) Ketoconazole HRA recommended for approval in Cushing's syndrome. Available from URL: http://www.ema.europa.eu/ema/index.jsp?curl = pages/news_and_events/news/2014/09/news_detail_002174.jsp&mid = WC0b01ac058004d5c1. Assessed 02 Feb 2016

Fatourechi V (2009) Subclinical hypothyroidism: an update for primary care physicians. Mayo Clin Proc 84:65–71

Feelders RA, de Bruin C, Pereira AM, Romijn JA, Netea-Maier RT, Hermus AR et al (2010) Pasireotide alone or with cabergoline and ketoconazole in Cushing's disease. New Engl J Med 362:1846–1848

Ferraù F, Korbonits M (2015) Metabolic comorbidities in Cushing's syndrome. Eur J Endocrinol 173:M133–M157

Fleseriu M, Biller BM, Findling JW, Molitch ME, Schteingart DE, Gross C et al (2012) Mifepristone, a glucocorticoid receptor antagonist, produces clinical and metabolic benefits in patients with Cushing's syndrome. J Clin Endocrinol Metab 97:2039–2049

Florez JC, Shepard JA, Kradin RL (2013) Case records of the Massachusetts General Hospital. Case 17–2013. A 56-year-old woman with poorly controlled diabetes mellitus and fatigue. N Engl J Med 368:2126–2136

Funder JW, Carey RM, Fardella C, Gomez-Sanchez CE, Mantero F, Stowasser M et al (2008) Case detection, diagnosis, and treatment of patients with primary aldosteronism: an endocrine society clinical practice guideline. J Clin Endocrinol Metab 93:3266–3281

Geller DS, Farhi A, Pinkerton N, Fradley M, Moritz M, Spitzer A et al (2000) Activating mineralocorticoid receptor mutation in hypertension exacerbated by pregnancy. Science 289(5476):119–123

Graversen D, Vestergaard P, Stochholm K, Gravholt CH, Jørgensen JO (2012) Mortality in Cushing's syndrome: a systematic review and meta-analysis. Eur J Intern Med 23:278–282

Hagström E, Ahlström T, Ärnlöv J, Larsson A, Melhus H, Hellman P et al (2015) Parathyroid hormone and calcium are independently associated with subclinical vascular disease in a community-based cohort. Atherosclerosis 238:420–426

Hannemann A, Wallaschofski H (2012) Prevalence of primary aldosteronism in patient's cohorts and in population-based studies – a review of the current literature. Horm Metab Res 44:157–162

Helfand M, U.S. Preventive Services Task Force (2004) Screening for subclinical thyroid dysfunction in nonpregnant adults: a summary of the evidence for the U.S. Preventive Services Task Force. Ann Intern Med 140:128–141

Hollowell JG, Staehling NW, Flanders WD et al (2002) Serum TSH, T(4), and thyroid antibodies in the United States population (1988 to 1994): National Health and Nutrition Examination Survey (NHANES III). J Clin Endocrinol Metab 87:489–499

Ittermann T, Thamm M, Wallaschofski H, Rettig R, Völzke H (2012) Serum thyroid-stimulating hormone levels are associated with blood pressure in children and adolescents. J Clin Endocrinol Metab 97:828–834

Janjgava S, Zerekidze T, Uchava L, Giorgadze E, Asatiani K (2014) Influence of testosterone replacement therapy on metabolic disorders in male patients with type 2 diabetes mellitus and androgen deficiency. Eur J Med Res 19:56

Kasperlik-Zaluska AA, Roslonowska E, Slowinska-Srzednicka J, Otto M, Cichocki A, Cwikla J et al (2006) 1,111 patients with adrenal incidentalomas observed at a single endocrinological center: incidence of chromaffin tumors. Ann N Y Acad Sci 1073:38–46

Katznelson L (2010) Approach to the patient with persistent acromegaly after pituitary surgery. J Clin Endocrinol Metab 95:4114–4123

Katznelson L, Laws ER Jr, Melmed S, Molitch ME, Murad MH, Utz A et al (2014) Acromegaly: an

endocrine society clinical practice guideline. J Clin Endocrinol Metab 99:3933–3951

Kienitz T, Quinkler M (2008) Testosterone and blood pressure regulation. Kidney Blood Press Res 31:71–79

Kiernan CM, Solórzano CC (2016) Pheochromocytoma and paraganglioma: Diagnosis, genetics, and treatment. Surg Oncol Clin N Am 25:119–138

Kim SM, Rhee JH (2015) A case of 17 alpha-hydroxylase deficiency. Clin Exp Reprod Med 42:72–76

Klein I, Ojamaa K (2001) Thyroid hormone and the cardiovascular system. N Engl J Med 344:501–509

Korah HE, Scholl UI (2015) An update on familial hyperaldosteronism. Horm Metab Res 47 (13):941–946. [Epub ahead of print]

Koulouri O, Steuwe A, Gillett D, Hoole AC, Powlson AS, Donnelly NA et al (2015) A role for 11C-methionine PET imaging in ACTH-dependent Cushing's syndrome. Eur J Endocrinol 173:M107–M120

Lenders JW, Duh QY, Eisenhofer G, Gimenez-Roqueplo AP, Grebe SK, Murad MH et al (2014) Pheochromocytoma and paraganglioma: an endocrine society clinical practice guideline. J Clin Endocrinol Metab 99:1915–1942

Letizia C, Ferrari P, Cotesta D, Caliumi C, Cianci R, Cerci S et al (2005) Ambulatory Monitoring of Blood Pressure (AMBP) in patients with primary hyperparathyroidism. J Hum Hypertens 19:901–906

Lim V, Guo Q, Grant CS, Thompson GB, Richards ML, Farley DR et al (2014) Accuracy of adrenal imaging and adrenal venous sampling in predicting surgical cure of primary aldosteronism. J Clin Endocrinol Metab 99:2712–2719

Lind L, Jacobsson S, Palmer M, Lithell H, Wengle B, Ljunghall S (1991) Cardiovascular risk factors in primary hyperparathyroidism: a 15-year follow-up of operated and unoperated cases. J Intern Med 230:29–35

Lundgren E, Rastad J, Thrufjell E, Akerstrom G, Ljunghall S (1997) Population-based screening for primary hyperparathyroidism with serum calcium and parathyroid hormone values in menopausal women. Surgery 121:287–294

Manolopoulou J, Fischer E, Dietz A, Diederich S, Holmes D, Junnila R et al (2015) Clinical validation for the aldosterone-to-renin ratio and aldosterone suppression testing using simultaneous fully automated chemiluminescence immunoassays. J Hypertens 33:2500–2511

Marcocci C, Cetani F (2011) Clinical practice. Primary hyperparathyroidism. N Engl J Med 365:2389–2397

Melcescu E, Phillips J, Moll G, Subauste JS, Koch CA (2012) 11Beta-hydroxylase deficiency and other syndromes of mineralocorticoid excess as a rare cause of endocrine hypertension. Horm Metab Res 44:867–878

Melmed S (2009) Acromegaly pathogenesis and treatment. J Clin Invest 119:3189–3202

Mestron A, Webb SM, Astorga R et al (2004) Epidemiology, clinical characteristics, outcome, morbidity and mortality in acromegaly based on the Spanish Acromegaly Registry (Registro Espanol de Acromegalia, REA). Eur J Endocrinol 151:439–446

Mihailidou AS, Le Loan TY, Mardini M, Funder JW (2009) Glucocorticoids activate cardiac mineralocorticoid receptors during experimental myocardial infarction. Hypertension 54:1306–1312

Miller WL, Auchus RJ (2011) The molecular biology, biochemistry, and physiology of human steroidogenesis and its disorders. Endocr Rev 32:81–151

Mulatero P, Stowasser M, Loh KC, Fardella CE, Gordon RD, Mosso L et al (2004) Increased diagnosis of primary aldosteronism, including surgically correctable forms, in centers from five continents. J Clin Endocrinol Metab 89:1045–1050

Mussa A, Camilla R, Monticone S, Porta F, Tessaris D, Verna F et al (2012) Polyuric-polydipsic syndrome in a pediatric case of non-glucocorticoid remediable familial hyperaldosteronism. Endocr J 59:497–502

Muth A, Ragnarsson O, Johannsson G, Wängberg B (2015) Systematic review of surgery and outcomes in patients with primary aldosteronism. Br J Surg 102:307–317

Nainby-Luxmoore JC, Langford HG, Nelson NC, Watson RL, Barnes TY (1982) A case-comparison study of hypertension and hyperparathyroidism. J Clin Endocrinol Metab 55:303–306

New MI, Geller DS, Fallo F, Wilson RC (2005) Monogenic low renin hypertension. Trends Endocrinol Metab 16:92–97

Nieman LK (2002) Medical therapy of Cushing's disease. Pituitary 5:77–82

Nieman LK (2015) Cushing's syndrome: update on signs, symptoms and biochemical screening. Eur J Endocrinol 173:M33–M38

Nieman LK, Biller BM, Findling JW, Newell-Price J, Savage MO, Stewart PM et al (2008) The diagnosis of Cushing's syndrome: an Endocrine Society clinical practice guideline. J Clin Endocrinol Metab 93:1526–1540

Nieman LK, Biller BM, Findling JW, Murad MH, Newell-Price J, Savage MO et al (2015) Treatment of Cushing's syndrome: An Endocrine Society clinical practice guideline. J Clin Endocrinol Metab 100:2807–2831

Pappachan JM, Raskauskiene D, Sriraman R, Edavalath M, Hanna FW (2014) Diagnosis and management of pheochromocytoma: a practical guide to clinicians. Curr Hypertens Rep 16:442

Parenti G, Zampetti B, Rapizzi E et al (2012) Updated and new perspectives on diagnosis, prognosis, and therapy of malignant pheochromocytoma/paraganglioma. J Oncol 2012:872713

Pecori Giraldi F, Ambrogio AG, Andrioli M, Sanguin F, Karamouzis I, Corsello SM et al (2012) Potential role for retinoic acid in patients with Cushing's disease. J Clin Endocrinol Metab 97:3577–3583

Piaditis G, Markou A, Papanastasiou L, Androulakis II, Kaltsas G (2015) Progress in aldosteronism: a review of the prevalence of primary aldosteronism in pre-hypertension and hypertension. Eur J Endocrinol 172:R191–R203

Preston RA (2009) Comparative effects of conventional vs. novel hormone replacement therapy on blood pressure in postmenopausal women. Climacteric 12(Suppl 1):66–70

Proven A, Gabriel SE, Orces C, O'Fallon WM, Hunder GG (2003) Glucocorticoid therapy in giant cell arteritis: duration and adverse outcomes. Arthritis Rheum 49:703–708

Puig-Domingo M, Resmini E, Gomez-Anson B et al (2010) Magnetic resonance imaging as a predictor of response to somatostatin analogues in acromegaly after surgical failure. J Clin Endocrinol Metab 95:4973–4978

Rapado A (1986) Arterial hypertension and primary hyperparathyroidism. Incidence and follow-up after parathyroidectomy. Am J Nephrol 6(Suppl 1):49–50

Reincke M (2015) Improving outcome in Cushing's syndrome. Eur J Endocrinol 173:E3–E5

Reincke M, Ritzel K, Oßwald A, Berr C, Stalla G, Hallfeldt K, Reisch N et al (2015) A critical reappraisal of bilateral adrenalectomy for ACTH-dependent Cushing's syndrome. Eur J Endocrinol 173:M23–M32

Rimoldi SF, Scherrer U, Messerli FH (2014) Secondary arterial hypertension: when, who, and how to screen? Eur Heart J 35:1245–1254

Ringe JD (1984) Reversible hypertension in primary hyperparathyroidism—pre- and postoperative blood pressure in 75 cases. Klin Wochenschr 62:465–469

Rizzoni D, Porteri E, De Ciuceis C, Rodella LF, Paiardi S, Rizzardi N et al (2009) Hypertrophic ulticentre of subcutaneous small resistance arteries in patients with Cushing's syndrome. J Clin Endocrinol Metab 94:5010–5018

Rossi GP, Auchus RJ, Brown M, Lenders JW, Naruse M, Plouin PF et al (2014) An expert consensus statement on use of adrenal vein sampling for the subtyping of primary aldosteronism. Hypertension 63:151–160

Sahakitrungruang T (2015) Clinical and molecular review of atypical congenital adrenal hyperplasia. Ann Pediatr Endocrinol Metab 20:1–7

Silverberg SJ, Lewiecki EM, Mosekilde L, Peacock M, Rubin MR et al (2009) Presentation of asymptomatic primary hyperparathyroidism: proceedings of the third international workshop. J Clin Endocrinol Metab 94:351–365

Speiser PW (2015) Congenital adrenal hyperplasia. F1000Res; 4(F1000 Faculty Rev): 601.

Thomas RM, Ruel E, Shantavasinkul PC, Corsino L (2015) Endocrine hypertension: an overview on the current etiopathogenesis and management options. World J Hypertens 5:14–27

Tsirlin A, Oo Y, Sharma R, Kansara A, Gliwa A, Banerji MA (2014) Pheochromocytoma: a review. Maturitas 77:229–238

van der Lely AJ, Biller BM, Brue T et al (2012) Long-term safety of pegvisomant in patients with acromegaly: comprehensive review of 1288 subjects in ACROSTUDY. J Clin Endocrinol Metab 97:1589–1597

Velasco A, Vongpatanasin W (2014) The evaluation and treatment of endocrine forms of hypertension. Curr Cardiol Rep 16:528

Wang LP, Yang KQ, Jiang XJ, Wu HY, Zhang HM, Zou YB et al (2015) Prevalence of Liddle syndrome among young hypertension patients of undetermined cause in a Chinese population. J Clin Hypertens (Greenwich) 17:902–907

Weber MA, Schiffrin EL, White WB, Mann S, Lindholm LH, Kenerson JG et al (2014) Clinical practice guidelines for the management of hypertension in the community: a statement by the American Society of Hypertension and the International Society of Hypertension. J Clin Hypertens (Greenwich) 16:14–26

Wermers RA, Khosla S, Atkinson EJ, Achenbach SJ, Oberg AL, Grant CS et al (2006) Incidence of primary hyperparathyroidism in Rochester, Minnesota, 1993–2001: an update on the changing epidemiology of the disease. J Bone Miner Res 21:171–177

World Health Organization. Obesity and overweight. 2015. [assessed 30 November 2015]. Available from URL: http://apps.who.int/iris/bitstream/10665/79059/1/WHO_DCO_WHD_2013.2_eng.pdf?ua=1

Young WF (2007) Primary aldosteronism: renaissance of a syndrome. Clin Endocrinol (Oxf) 66:607–618

Young WF Jr (2015) Endocrine hypertension. In: Melmed S, Polonsky KS, Larsen PR, Kronenberg HM (eds) Williams textbook of endocrinology, 13th edn. Elsevier, New York, pp 556–588

Zennaro MC, Rickard AJ, Boulkroun S (2013) Genetics of mineralocorticoid excess: an update for clinicians. Eur J Endocrinol 169:R15–R25

Zennaro MC, Boulkroun S, Fernandes-Rosa F (2015a) An update on novel mechanisms of primary aldosteronism. J Endocrinol 224:R63–R77

Zennaro MC, Boulkroun S, Fernandes-Rosa F (2015b) Inherited forms of mineralocorticoid hypertension. Best Pract Res Clin Endocrinol Metab 29:633–645

Adv Exp Med Biol - Advances in Internal Medicine (2017) 2: 239–259
DOI 10.1007/5584_2016_76
© Springer International Publishing AG 2016
Published online: 26 November 2016

Phaeochromocytoma and Paraganglioma

P.T. Kavinga Gunawardane and Ashley Grossman

Abstract

Phaeochromocytomas and paragangliomas are relatively uncommon tumours which may be manifest in many ways, specifically as sustained or paroxysmal hypertension, episodes of palpitations, sweating, headache and anxiety, or increasingly as an incidental finding. Recent studies have shown that an increasing number are due to germline mutations. This review concentrates on the diagnosis, biochemistry and treatment of these fascinating tumours.

Keywords

Phaeochromocytomas • Paragangliomas • Review • Diagnosis • Treatment • Malignant

1 Introduction

Phaeochromocytomas are uncommon tumours originating from the neural crest- derived chromafin cells in the adrenal medulla. They commonly produce one or more catecholamines: adrenaline (epinephrine), noradrenaline (norepinephrine) or dopamine, and the excess secretion of these causes a wide array of clinical features, including hypertension. The highest prevalence of phaeochromocytoma is seen in the fourth and fifth decades, with an equal incidence in men and women.

Although the annual incidence of phaeochromocytoma is predicted to be approximately 0.8 per 100,000 person years (Beard et al. 1983), this number might be an under-estimation, as autopsy studies have indicated that over 50 % of phaeochromocytomas found at autopsy were not clinically suspected (Sutton et al. 1981). Even though it is considered to be a rare cause of hypertension, accounting for only approximately 0.2 %, phaeochromocytomas should be diagnosed early as they cause significant morbidity with at least a 10 % possibility of malignancy

P.T.K. Gunawardane
Oxford Centre for Diabetes, Endocrinology and Metabolism, University of Oxford, Oxford, UK

Ministry of Health, Colombo, Sri Lanka

A. Grossman (✉)
Oxford Centre for Diabetes, Endocrinology and Metabolism, University of Oxford, Oxford, UK
e-mail: endo@thelondonclinic.co.uk

and an even higher percentage of familial disease (Young 2011) (see below).

The great majority, some 95 %, of catecholamine-secreting tumours are in the abdomen, of which 90 % are intra-adrenal and 10 % are extra-adrenal and are referred to as paragangliomas (also known as extra-adrenal phaeochromocytomas). Approximately 10 % of catecholamine-secreting tumours are multiple (Bravo 1991).

2 Catecholamines and Their Receptors

Catecholamines exert many cardiovascular and metabolic effects including increasing heart rate, blood pressure, myocardial contractility and the velocity of cardiac conduction. Their action is via three main receptors: α, β, and dopaminergic. These receptors have several subtypes that have different physiological actions on the cardiovascular and central nervous systems (Table 1).

3 Clinical Presentation

The presentation of phaeochromocytomas can have a wide clinical spectrum from asymptomatic disease to non-specific symptoms leading all the way up to resistant hypertension and hypertensive crises. The clinical literature describes a classic clinical triad seen in phaeochromocytoma including headache, sweating and tachycardia. Although typical when present, this clinical triad is not commonly encountered in most patients with phaeochromocytomas.

Paroxysmal clinical features or 'spells' are a well-recognised consequence of episodic secretion and release of catecholamines. A spell can start with a sense of shortness of breath followed by palpitations and a throbbing headache. Peripheral vasoconstriction associated with such an episode leads to cold peripheries and facial pallor. Towards the end of the episode the patient may feel a sense of warmth and sweating. These can be either spontaneous or precipitated by postural change, medications (Table 2), exercise, or manoeuvres such as lifting and straining. The presentation of spells can be highly variable; however, they tend to be stereotypical for each patient. The frequency of episodes can vary as well, where some patients experience spells several times a day, while others only develop them very infrequently (Young 2011). It is important to bear in mind that these episodes are common and can be due to many other causes apart from

Table 1 Catecholamine receptors, their locations and main actions

Receptor		Location	Main action
α	$\alpha1$	Postsynaptic receptor	Vascular and smooth muscle contraction causing vasoconstriction and increases in blood pressure
	$\alpha2$	Presynaptic sympathetic nerve endings.	Inhibit release of noradrenaline causing suppression of central sympathetic outflow and decreased blood pressure
β	$\beta1$	Predominantly in cardiac tissue	Positive inotropic and chronotropic effects on the heart
			More responsive to isoproterenol (isoprenaline) than to adrenaline or noradrenaline
			Increase renin secretion
	$\beta2$	Bronchial, vascular smooth muscle	Bronchodilatation, vasodilatation in skeletal muscle
			Increase release of noradrenaline from sympathetic nerve terminals
	$\beta3$	Mainly in adipose tissue	Regulation of lipolysis and thermogenesis
D	D1	Cerebral, renal, mesenteric and coronary vessels	Local vasodilatation
	D2	Presynaptic sympathetic nerve endings in sympathetic ganglia and brain	Inhibit the release of noradrenaline, inhibits ganglionic transmission
			Inhibit prolactin release

Table 2 Commonly used medications that can precipitate hypertension/hypertensive crisis in phaeochromocytoma

Drugs	Example
Dopamine D2 receptor antagonists	Metoclopramide, sulpiride, chlorpromazine, prochlorperazine
β-Adrenergic receptor blockers	Propranolol, sotalol, timolol, nadolol, labetalol
Sympathomimetics	Ephedrine, fenfluramine, methylphenidate, phentermine
Opioid analgesics	Morphine, pethidine, tramadol
Noradrenaline reuptake inhibitors/tricyclic antidepressants	Amitriptyline, imipramine, including the newer SNRIs
Monoamine oxidase inhibitors	Tranylcypromine, moclobemide, phenelzine
Corticosteroids (rarely)	Dexamethasone, prednisone, hydrocortisone, betamethasone
Neuromuscular blocking agents	Succinylcholine, tubocurarine, atracurium

Table adapted from reference Lenders et al. (2014)

phaeochromocytoma. Facial flushing is described in many textbooks, but in our view is rarely seen. Concomitant swelling of the thyroid has been described (Nakamura et al. 2011).

Hypertension is one of the most common presenting features of catecholamine-secreting tumours. Several large retrospective case series have elaborated the prevalence of hypertension in patients with phaeochromocytomas to be between 51 % and 90 % (Baguet et al. 2004; Guerrero et al. 2009). The presentation of hypertension can be quite variable in phaeochromocytoma. It is usually stable and permanent; however, it can be paroxysmal with wide fluctuations, and resistant to treatment. Although uncommon, phaeochromocytoma can also present with postural symptoms with episodic *hypotension* due to extreme blood pressure fluctuations. This has been reported in patients with predominantly adrenaline-producing tumors, where the presentation can be with hypotension or even shock (Streeten and Anderson 1996; Bergland 1989). Hypotension in these patients could be due to the catecholamine-induced intravascular volume depletion, an abrupt decline of catecholamine levels due to tumour necrosis, hypercalcaemia, desensitisation of adrenoceptors, or acute cardiovascular events such as acute myocardial infarction, tachyarrhythmia or aortic/coronary artery dissection.

Several case series have elaborated the association between phaeochromocytoma and hypertension. In one series, approximately 50 % of the patients were discovered due to hypertension of which half of these had hypertension that was paroxysmal in nature. The series further elaborates that, when the reason for the discovery of phaeochromocytoma was permanent hypertension, it was symptomatic, severe, and treatment resistant (Baguet et al. 2004). Moreover, approximately 10 % of patients in the series presented with normal blood pressure, which was commonly seen in patients with adrenal incidentalomas or in those undergoing screening for familial phaeochromocytoma. However, it is important to bear in mind that, in phaeochromocytoma, patients with normal blood pressure can still have life-threatening paroxysms of hypertension. There appears to be a more pathological effect on cardiac function than the hypertension *per se* would impose (Stolk et al. 2013).

Therefore, hypertension is the initial presentation in most patients with catecholamine excess, and one should be alerted to the possibility of a phaeochromocytoma in patients with hypertension, especially if the hypertension is:

- Paroxysmal, resistant or young onset (<20 years)
- Paradoxical despite therapy (especially during treatment with β-blockers)
- New onset or worsening of hypertension with tricyclic anti-depressants and other medications (Table 2)
- Severe symptomatic hypotension when initiating therapy with α-blockers

Table 3 Frequency of common signs and symptoms in phaeochromocytoma

Symptom		Frequency (%)
Hypertension	Sustained	50
	Paroxysmal	30
	Orthostatic	12
Headache		60–90
Palpitations		50–70
Sweating		55–75
Pallor		40
Weight loss		20–40
Fatigue		25–40
Anxiety and panic		20–40
Hyperglycaemia		40
Fever		60

Table adapted from reference Young (2011) and Lenders et al. (2005)

- Severe hypertension or hypertensive crises following any procedure (eg. anaesthesia, surgery, or angiography)
- In pregnant patients with hypertension not typical of pregnancy-induced hypertension

With the widespread availability of imaging techniques, the detection of adrenal incidentalomas has increased over the last few decades. Approximately 5 % of all incidentally-detected adrenal tumours are found to be phaeochromocytomas, and some 25 % of all phaeochromocytomas are now being incidentally discovered during imaging studies for unrelated disorders (Young 2011; Lenders et al. 2005; Mantero et al. 2000).

Apart from hypertension and incidental discovery, phaeochromocytoma can present with a wide variety of clinical features (Table 3).

Cardiovascular complications are another well-recognised presentation in phaeochromocytoma. Apart from the cardiac emergencies such as myocardial infarction, cardiac arrhythmias and aneurysms, it can present with more long-standing cardiac complications such as dilated or hypertrophic cardiomyopathy and congestive heart failure (Liao et al. 2000).

Excess catecholamines can also affect the gastrointestinal system including inhibition of peristalsis causing constipation or even pseudo-obstruction or ileus. Moreover, vasoconstriction

of the mesenteric artery can lead to ischaemic enterocolitis and intestinal necrosis.

In the clinical evaluation of patients with phaeochromocytoma, it is important to always bear in mind the syndromic nature of phaeochromocytoma, and to actively seek out features such as Marfanoid body habitus, *café-au-lait* spots, axillary freckling, subcutaneous neurofibromas, mucosal neuromas on the tongue, retinal angiomas, iris hamartomas and multiple other clinical features suggestive of an underlying clinical syndrome.

In summary, patients with excess catecholamines can show a wide spectrum of clinical features and it is recommended that one considers the possibility of a phaeochromocytoma especially when patients exhibit certain clinical features (Lenders et al. 2014):

- Hyperadrenergic spells (episodic self-limiting non-exertional palpitations, diaphoresis, headache, pallor)
- A personal or family history of familial syndrome that predisposes to catecholamine-secreting tumors (e.g., MEN2, NF1, VHL, etc.)
- An adrenal incidentaloma
- Idiopathic dilated cardiomyopathy

4 Familial Phaeochromocytoma

In contrast to the conventional teaching of a 10 % familial tendency, recent studies have identified multiple genes in association with phaeochromocytoma, with up to 30 % or possibly more exhibiting a disease-causing germ-line mutation. Along with the well-recognised genetic disorders such as multiple endocrine neoplasia-2 (MEN-2), neurofibromatosis type 1 and Von-Hippel Lindau syndrome, nearly 21 genes have been identified in association with phaeochromocytoma. Most phaeochromocytomas due to syndromic causes present at a younger age than their sporadic counterparts, although part of this earlier identification my relate to genetic or biochemical screening.

Multiple endocrine neoplasia-2 is the one of the earliest syndromes to have been associated with phaeochromocytoma. Interestingly, only half of the patients with phaeochromocytoma with MEN2 exhibit clinical feature and fewer patients have hypertension (Pomares et al. 1998). This might relate to early diagnosis due to other syndromic associations or screening. MEN 2A (now known as MEN2) is characterised by medullary thyroid cancer in all patients, phaeochromocytoma in 40–50 % and primary hyperparathyroidism in 20 %. MEN2B (now known as MEN3) accounts for approximately 5 % of MEN syndromes and has a similar percentage of medullary carcinoma and phaeochromocytoma along with mucocutaneous neuromas; however, it is not associated with hyperparathyroidism. The genetic defect in MEN2 and MEN3 is in the *RET* proto-oncogene on chromosome 10, which is inherited in an autosomal dominant pattern with high penetrance. Several codon mutations in the RET gene have been associated with MEN2/3 and these are gain-of-function mutations: the great majority of MEN2 are associated with a mutation at codon 634 which codes for the extra-cellular domain of RET, while for MEN3 the dominant mutation at 918 codes for part of the intra-cellular domain. It has been hypothesised that the subtle changes in the clinical presentation is due to these genetic variations in the mutation (Mulligan and Ponder 1995). It is vital to identify phaeochromocytomas in these patients to avoid perioperative hypertensive crisis during thyroidectomy for medullary thyroid carcinoma. Phaeochromocytomas seen in MEN2 are frequently bilateral and almost invariably benign.

Neurofibromatosis type 1 (NF1) is another autosomal dominant disorder, characterized by neurofibromas, *café-au-lait* spots, freckling, Lisch nodules, phaeochromocytoma and paraganglioma: 2 % of patients with the NF1 gene present with solitary and benign pheochromocytoma. However, they can occasionally be bilateral or extra-adrenal (Walther et al. 1999). Insulinomas and somatostatinomas are also seen in this syndrome.

In von Hippel-Lindau (VHL) syndrome, phaeochromocytomas are more frequently bilateral with mediastinal, abdominal or pelvic paragangliomas. Other syndromic features of VHL include CNS hemangioblastoma, retinal angioma, clear cell renal cell carcinoma, pancreatic neuroendocrine tumours and middle ear tumours. As in MEN-2, VHL too has considerable genetic variability among kindreds with certain mutations causing a higher frequency (up to 20 %) of phaeochromocytoma, (Dluhy 2002). Interestingly, patients habouring the VHL mutation have a lower incidence of hypertension and have elevated normetanephrine, in contrast to patients with MEN-2, who show elevated metanephrine levels (Eisenhofer et al. 2001). Malignancy is rare but does occur.

Another important cause for familial catecholamine-hypersecreting tumours is succinate dehydrogenase (SDH) gene mutation. Several mutations in the SDH gene have been identified including SDHB, SDHC, SDHD, SDHAF2, and (very rarely) SDHA. Similar to the previously mentioned mutations, SDH mutations are also inherited in an autosomal dominant pattern. However, interestingly, SDHD and SDHAF2 have a paternal inheritance pattern due to maternal imprinting. In patients with SDH mutations causing paragangliomas/phaeochromocytomas, the type of catecholamine produced depends on its location. An SDH-induced paraganglioma is different from phaeochromocytoma in general in the fact that tissue expression of PMNT in these tumors is minimal, which means that the preferential catecholamine production is norepinephrine or dopamine and they produce normetanephrine, or normetanephrine and methoxytyramine, or rarely only methoxytyramine (Timmers et al. 2007). Interestingly, tumours only producing methoxytyramine are usually SDH tumors. Of abdominal paragangliomas, most secrete noradrenaline, often both noradrenaline and dopamine and rarely only dopamine. The rate of noradrenaline production is much lower in head-and-neck paragangliomas. Most mutations in the SDHD, SDHAF2 and SDHC are associated with non-catecholamine secreting, head-and-neck paragangliomas (Kantorovich et al. 2010). Although SDHB mutation commonly presents with extra-adrenal abdominal or thoracic disease, a primary presentation with an adrenal phaeochromocytoma is still evident in some patients. Approximately 1/3 of patients with SDHB mutations present with multifocal disease (Kantorovich et al. 2010). Moreover, carriers of SDHB mutations can develop early onset abdominal, pelvic, and thoracic catecholamine-secreting paragangliomas that are more likely to be malignant, possibly in up to 50 % of patients. SDHB carriers who develop malignant paragangliomas are more likely to develop other neoplasms including papillary thyroid tumours, renal cell carcinoma, neuroblastoma, or gastrointestinal stromal tumours (GIST) (Neumann et al. 2004). A link has also been shown between SDH mutation status and pituitary tumours (Galan and Kann 2013).

Apart from these more commonly known mutations, several new mutations have been identified in association with pheochromocytoma. TMEM127 is a recently identified germline mutation, inherited autosomal dominantly, commonly associated with benign unilateral adrenal phaeochromocytoma. However, there are few case studies of bilateral, malignant and extra-adrenal disease. Interestingly, the presentation of these patients is in the fifth decade, more in keeping with the onset of sporadic phaeochromocytoma rather than the familial form.

The *MAX* (Myc-associated factor X) gene is another more recently reported susceptibility gene, which is inherited as autosomal dominant and, similar to SDHD and SDHAF2, has a paternal inheritance pattern. The majority of patients with MAX mutations present at a younger age and tend to have bilateral or unilateral phaeochromocytoma with an increased potential to develop malignant disease and predominantly produce noradrenaline (Dénes et al. 2015; Comino-Mendez et al. 2011).

Several other mutations such as HIF2α, KIF1β, fumarate hydratase and PHD2 have been reported recently, although detailed studies have yet to be performed on their syndromic associations and characteristics of phaeochromocytoma. (eg. Carney–Stratakis syndrome- familial paraganglioma and Gastrointestinal Stromal Tumours (GIST),). Finally, the recently-described Pacak-Zhuang syndrome, which shows an association between paragangliomas, polycythaemia and retinal angiomas with somatic mutation of HIF-2α, most likely occurs as a mosaicism similar to the McCune-Albright syndrome (Zhuang et al. 2012).

Genetic screening plays a vital role in the management of phaeochromocytoma, not only to detect other associated life-threatening conditions in the index patient but also for the diagnosis and treatment family members with certain mutations (eg, medullary carcinoma of the thyroid with *RET* mutations). Moreover, genetics can alert the physician to the malignant potential of phaeochromocytomas, especially in patients harbouring certain mutations (eg, SDHB), and to actively seek for the presence of metastases. Similar to the genetic mutation offering clues regarding character of the tumour, certain characteristics such as tumour location, the presence of metastases and the type of catecholamine synthesised can give clues to the possible causative mutation. Therefore, genetic analysis has become an important tool in the investigatory armamentarium for the evaluation and management of this rare syndrome. Accordingly, recently-published major guidelines recommend that all patients diagnosed with phaeochromocytoma/paraganglioma should be engaged in shared decision making for genetic testing for a possible somatic or germ line mutation (Lenders et al. 2014). Due to cost factors, the Endocrine Society recommends prioritising certain genetic screening based on the clinical and biochemical features (Fig. 1). Nevertheless, in Oxford we screen routinely for a panel of 10 genes in almost all patients. It has been shown that even in older patients with single benign phaeochromocytomas and no family history or syndromic featues, nearly 10 % will still harbour a germline mutation (Brito et al. 2015).

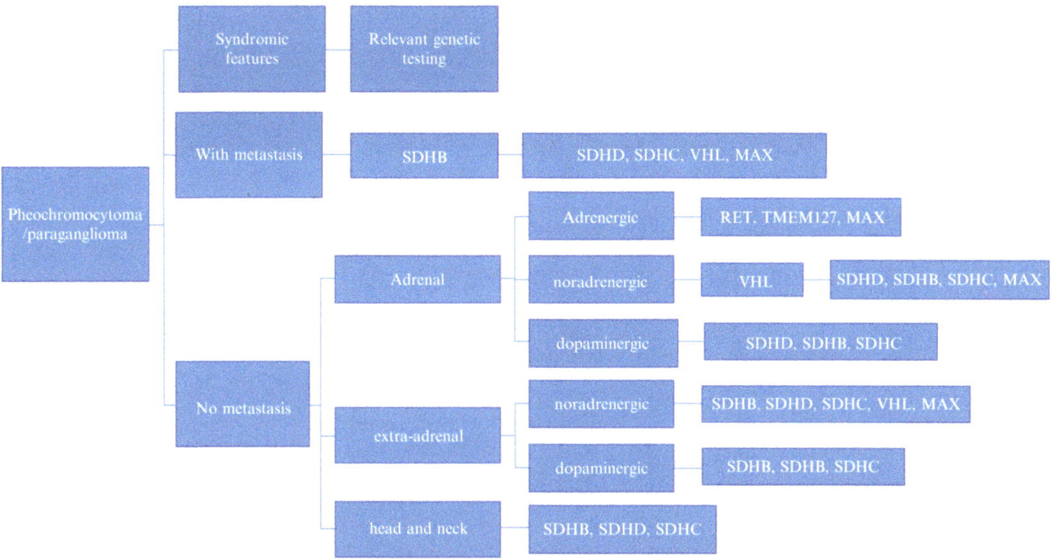

Fig. 1 Algorithm for genetic testing in patients diagnosed with pheochromocytoma (Adapted from reference Lenders et al. (2014))

5 Synthesis, Storage and Metabolism of Catecholamines

The measurement of catecholamines and/or their by-products is the key in diagnosing pheochromocytoma. Although in the past the direct measurement of catecholamines was commonly used in the diagnosis, it is now considered a poor screening tool due to its relatively low sensitivity.

All catecholamines have a similar chemical structure with a catechol ring (ortho-dihydroxybenzene) and an amine group (Fig. 2).

Tyrosine is the initial substrate in the formation of catecholamines and is either derived from food or is synthesised in the liver from phenylalanine (Fig. 3). It subsequently enters chromaffin cells by active transportation and undergoes hydroxylation and decarboxylation to form various types of catecholamines. The rate-limiting step in catecholamine synthesis is the conversion of tyrosine to DOPA, which is regulated by the enzyme tyrosine hydroxylase. In managing patients with catecholamine-secreting neoplasms, inhibition of this rate-limiting step by tyrosine hydroxylase inhibitors

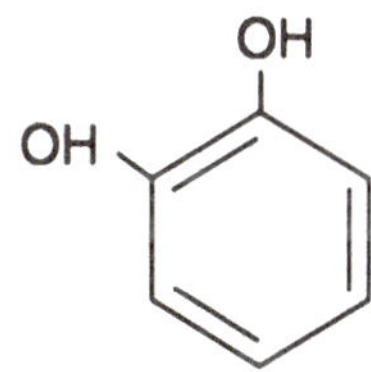
Fig. 2 Catechol ring (ortho-dihydroxybenzene)

(e.g. metyrosine) can inhibit the synthesis of catecholamines.

Subsequent to this rate-limiting step, dopamine is synthesised by further decarboxylation of DOPA by the enzyme, aromatic L-amino acid decarboxylase. It is then hydroxylated to form noradrenaline and stored as granules within the chromafin cells. It is subsequently released it to the cytoplasm of the chromaffin cells in the adrenal medulla, where phenylethanolamine N-methyltransferase (PNMT) converts it to adrenaline. Interestingly, PNMT is regulated by glucocorticoids and, due to the corticomedullary portal system in the adrenal gland, medullary PNMT-producing cells are exposed to high concentrations of cortisol, making the adrenal medulla the prime location for adrenaline-secreting adrenal tumours.

Once formed, these catecholamines are stored in electron-dense granules. Transport of

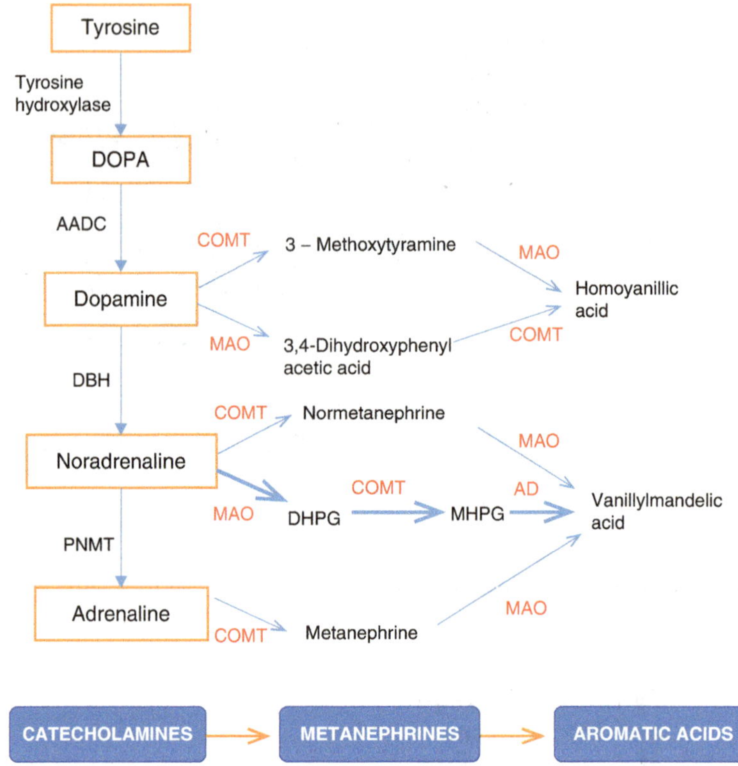

Fig. 3 Production of catecholamines (*AADC* aromatic L-amino acid decarboxylase, *DBH* dopamine B-hydroxylase, *PNMT* phenylethanolamine N-methyltransferase, *MHPG* 3-methoxy-4-hydroxyphenylglycol, *DHPG* 3,4-dihydroxyphenylglycol, *AD* aldehyde dehydrogenase)

substances into these granules is regulated by vesicular monoamine transporters (VMAT). Iodine-labelled MIBG (^{123}I or ^{131}I) is transported by VMAT into these storage granules and is a useful tool in localising (and treating) catecholamine-secreting pheochromocytoma/paraganglioma.

6 Biochemical Evaluation

Catecholamines have a short half-life, of approximately 10–100 s, in the plasma. The nerve terminals reuptake the catecholamines they produce themselves, while extra-neuronal catecholamines are metabolised by catechol-O-methyl-transferase (COMT) to form metanephrine and normetanephrine. Sympathetic nerves contain MAO, but not catechol-O-methyltransferase (COMT). Intraneuronal metabolism of norepinephrine leads to production of the deaminated metabolite, DHPG, but not the O-methylated metabolite, normetanephrine. Consequently, almost all of the DHPG in plasma has a neuronal source, whereas normetanephrine and metanephrine are derived exclusively from non-neuronal sources including chromaffin cells in the adrenal medulla (Eisenhofer et al. 2004). Normally the O-methylation pathway represents a minor route of catecholamine metabolism while deamination of noradrenaline within sympathetic nerves is the major pathway (Fig. 3). However, in patients with pheochromocytoma, intratumoral O-methylation pathway dominates catecholamine metabolism, leading to relatively large increases in production of the O-methylated metabolites compared with minor increases of the deaminated metabolites (Eisenhofer et al. 2004; Eisenhofer 2012).

Unfortunately, the short half-life of catecholamines makes it difficult to discriminate pathological overproduction from normal transient bursts of secretion during stress. Therefore, due to the short plasma half-life and intermittent nature of secretion, measurement of catecholamines can give a high rate of false positive results, while sampling between bouts of paroxysmal release will cause false negatives. Most authorities, including major guidelines, recommend that either free plasma metanephrines or fractionated urinary metanephrines as the investigations of choice for the diagnosis of phaeochromocytoma. The recommended laboratory techniques are liquid chromatography with mass spectrometric or an electrochemical detection method (Lenders et al. 2014) Although plasma free metanephrine and normetanephrine are nearly as rapidly cleared from the circulation as their catecholamine precursors, they are superior to catecholamines for diagnosis as these metabolites are produced continuously from catecholamines leaking from storage vesicles into the cytoplasm where COMT then leads to conversion to metanephrine and normetanephrine. This process is not only continuous, but also independent of exocytotic catecholamine secretion, which in phaeochromocytomas can be intermittent or only active with low rates of secretion.

Plasma fractionated metanephrines have a high sensitivity, 96–100 %, with a specificity of 85–89 %, and is especially useful in diagnosing patients who carry a higher risk for habouring a phaeochromocytoma. High-risk patients, who would benefit from initial plasma metanephrine measurment, are patients with resistant hypertension, typical spells, a past history of phaeochromocytoma, genetic syndromes or a family history of a genetic syndrome, or an adrenal incidentaloma suggestive of a phaeochromocytoma. Apart from these, plasma measurements can be useful in children where 24-h urine collection is difficult. Due to its high sensitivity, a normal plasma metanephrine result will exclude the presence of a phaeochromocytoma in the above-mentioned high-risk patients. The only exceptions are seen in preclinical early disease or tumours with selective dopamine hypersecretion (Sawka et al. 2003). The plasma sample should ideally be drawn from a supine patient (fully recumbent for at least 20–30 min) and appropriate supine cut-offs should be used in the interpretation. In fact, it has been recently indicated that with a 'seated sampling' the diagnostic accuracy of the plasma test is no better, if not worse, than the urinary test (Lenders et al. 2014; Därr et al. 2014).

Twenty-hour fractionated urinary metanephrines are another investigation frequently used by clinicians. Perry et al. demonstrated that 24-h urine fractionated metanephrines using mass spectrometry provide excellent sensitivity (97 %) and specificity (91 %) for the diagnosis of a phaeochromocytoma. Therefore, it can be used in patients with a lower index of clinical suspicion as it has a higher specificity than the plasma measurement (Perry et al. 2007). Urinary metanephrines should include a urinary creatinine measurement to verify adequacy of urine collection, and assessments of the utility of random urine samples are in process. However, it should be emphasised that in practice there is probably little difference in the utility of plasma or urinary collections, with appropriate cut-offs, and the assay employed will often depend on local resources and experience.

7　Interfering Medications

Although metanephrine and normetanephrine are the preferred biochemical substances for diagnosis in comparison to catecholamines, their levels can be altered by several medications due to their effect on the metabolising enzymes, COMT and MAO, and uptake pathways. Tricyclic antidepressants (TCA) are well recognised to interfere with the assessment of metanephrines, and it is recommended to taper off and withhold TCAs and other anti-psychotics (except highly selective serotonin reuptake inhibitors) for at least 2 weeks prior to metanephrine analysis (Neary et al. 2011) (Table 4).

8　Tumour Localisation

Once catecholamine excess is biochemically confirmed, tumor localisation can be initiated by way of imaging. While imaging is almost always followed by biochemical confirmation, in patients with high risk factors such as a past history or genetic predisposition to phaeochromocytoma (eg. SDH mutation) there might be justification to proceed with imaging in the

Table 4 Medications that may cause falsely elevated results for catecholamine and metanephrine levels

Medications that cause pharmacodynamics interference and elevate levels (affect all assays)
Tricyclic antidepressants
Levodopa
Antipsychotic agents
Drugs containing adrenergic receptor agonists (e.g., decongestants)
Serotonin and noradrenaline reuptake inhibitors (duloxetine, venlafaxine)
MAO inhibitors
Amphetamines
Prochlorperazine
Reserpine
Phenoxybenzamine (elevate plasma and urinary normetanephrine)
Ethanol
Illicit drugs (e.g., cocaine, heroin) and withdrawal from these, and possibly cannabis.
Medications that cause analytical interference with some assays- (LC-ECD)*
Acetaminophen (a.k.a Paracetamol, elevate plasma and urinary normetanephrine)
Labetalol, sotalol (elevate urinary meta/normetanephrine)
Buspirone (elevate plasma and urinary metanephrine)
Methyldopa (elevate plasma and urinary normetanephrine)
Sulphasalizine (elevate plasma and urinary normetanephrine)
Midodrine

**LC-ECD Liquid chromatography with electrochemical or fluorometric detection*

absence of compelling biochemical evidence. Some paragangliomas, especially in the head and neck region, can be biochemically silent and imaging with negative biochemistry is warranted in these instances as well.

As discussed previously, 90 % of phaeochromocytomas are adrenal in origin, while 10 % are extra-adrenal. Of these extra-adrenal phaeochromocytomas or paragangliomas, 80–95 % are within the abdomen and pelvis (superior and inferior para-aortic areas in the abdomen −75 %, urinary bladder- 10 %, thorax −10 %, head, neck, and pelvis −5 %) (Whalen et al. 1992). Therefore, CT scanning of the abdomen and pelvis following an adrenal protocol is the recommended initial imaging modality (Mantero et al. 2000). CT provides high tomographic resolution with a localisation sensitivity between 88 % and 100 %. On CT imaging, phaeochromocytomas can be homogeneous or heterogeneous, solid or cystic and with or without calcification. Phaeochromocytomas are notorious in being able to mimic the radiological features of adrenal carcinoma. Most (if not all) phaeochromocytomas have an attenuation greater than 10HU due to their lower fat content, while some can demonstrate very high attenuation due to haemorrhage (Sane et al. 2012; Blake et al. 2004).

The use of contrast agents during CT scanning has been an area of controversy for many years with concerns on risk of precipitating a hypertensive crisis; however, low-osmolar non-ionic contrast agents have been used safely in patients with phaeochromocytoma (Mukherjee et al. 1997), and this has more recently been confirmed (Baid et al. 2009). Phaeochromocytomas typically enhance avidly, indicating the rich capillary framework in the tumour, but nevertheless they can be heterogeneous with regions of absent enhancement due to cystic changes and necrosis. Contrast washout is useful in the evaluation of adrenal lesions, with an absolute contrast wash out of >60 % or a relative washout of >40 % at 15 min indicating a lipid-rich adenoma. Phaeochromocytoma, in its typical inconsistent nature, can have variable washout patterns, although the majority of phaeochromocytomas have a delayed contrast washout (Blake et al. 2004) (Fig. 4).

MRI is another useful tool in localising phaeochromocytomas. The most common MR imaging appearance of a phaeochromocytoma is of low signal intensity on T1 imaging and high signal intensity on T2-weighted imaging. They usually enhance avidly on T1-weighted imaging after gadolinium-enhancement. Although MRI lacks the superior spatial resolution of CT, it is useful to detect skull base and neck paragangliomas, for patients who cannot undergo CT scanning (metal clips, allergy to contrast, etc.), and for patients in whom exposure to radiation should be minimised (children, pregnant women, patients with known germline mutations undergoing regular screening) (Lenders et al. 2014; Jalil et al. 1998).

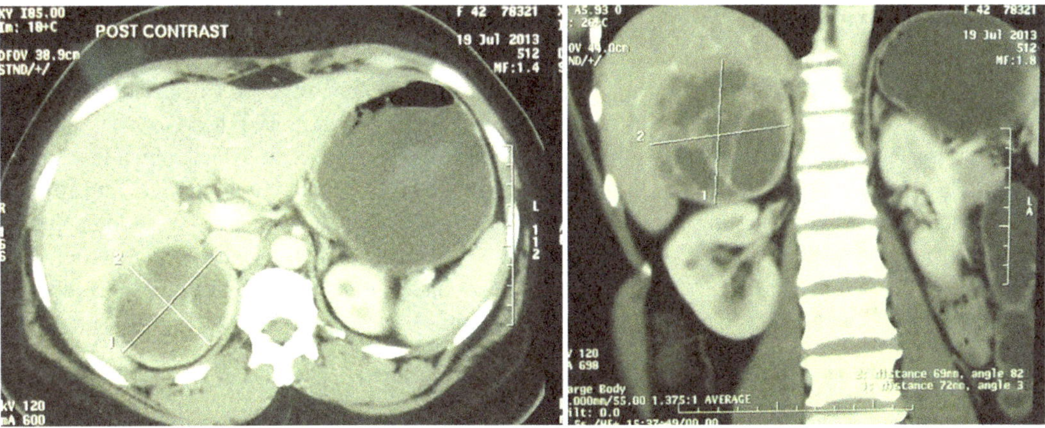

Fig. 4 Contrast enhanced CT scan of a young female presenting with hypertension showing a large, inhomogeneous, multiloculated mass with cystic and solid areas. A mass measuring 76 × 66 × 66 mm is seen in the right adrenal gland

Functional imaging is another widely used imaging modality for phaeochromocytomas. Meta-iodobenzylguanidine (MIBG) is a radiopharmaceutical agent that accumulates preferentially in catecholamine-producing cells and is transported into the electron-dense catecholamine storing granules via the transporter molecule VMAT. Radiolabelled MIBG is taken up by normal tissue innervated by the sympathetic system, such as heart, salivary glands, and tumours that express the neurohormonal transporters. ^{123}I-labelled MIBG has a sensitivity between 85 % and 88 % for phaeochromocytomas and between 56 % and 75 % for paragangliomas. Its specificity ranges from 70–100 % to 84–100 %, respectively (Berglund et al. 2001; Bhatia et al. 2008; Jacobson et al. 2010; Mozley et al. 1994). ^{123}I-MIBG allows better imaging when compared to ^{131}I-MIBG as its photon energy allows SPECT scanning which can greatly improve the sensitivity of the image. Therefore, ^{123}I MIBG remains the recommended agent for functional imaging in patients with phaeochromocytoma. Due to the fact that up to 50 % of normal adrenals take up MIBG asymmetrically, one should be aware of false positive results, especially when performed on a patient with normal biochemistry or after unilateral adrenalectomy (Jacobson et al. 2010). The major uses of MIBG imaging are confirmation that an adrenal lesion is a phaeochromocytoma, the identification

Table 5 Drugs that interfere with MIBG scanning

Tricyclic antidepressants
Prochlorperazine
Anti-psychotics
Cocaine
Amphetamines
Dopamine
Reserpine
Sympathomimetics
Labetalol
Ca^{++}-channel blockers (?increase uptake)

of metastases, and for assessing suitability for ^{131}I-MIBG therapy. ^{123}I-MIBG imaging gives a valuable hint on the response to ^{131}I MIBG treatment in patients with metastatic pheochromocytoma or paraganglioma. Apart from this, ^{123}I MIBG can be used to detect occult metastasis in patients with increased risk for metastatic phaeochromocytoma or paraganglioma (eg, a large primary tumour, recurrent disease, and extra-adrenal or multifocal disease) (Lenders et al. 2014).

Prior to ^{123}I MIBG imaging, thyroid uptake of radioactive iodine must be blocked with iodide, usually nowadays in the form of potassium iodide. It is also important to bear in mind that certain medications can impair the uptake of MIBG and should be withheld for 2 weeks (Table 5).

Apart from MIBG, recent studies have identified several other functional imaging modalities including PET scanning using ^{18}F-fluorodopamine, ^{18}F-fluorodihydroxy-phenylalanine (^{18}F-DOPA), or ^{18}F-fluoro-deoxy-glucose (FDG). This is especially used in paragangliomas or metastatic disease including SDH-related tumours (Timmers et al. 2009). However, few of these are generally available. ^{18}F-FDG-PET can also be of use when other localising imaging techniques are negative as it is highly sensitive to these tumours which demonstrate increase glycolysis compared to aerobic metabolism, especially tumours showing SDH mutations, or rapidly growing metastatic tumours (Mamede et al. 2006).

Other functioning imaging modalities now being considered for localization are ^{111}In-pentetreotide scintigraphy in combination with CT/MRI and ^{68}Ga-DOTA-NOC. As both phaeochromocytomas and paragangliomas express somatostatin receptors to some extent, these somatostatin receptor scintigraphic studies have been shown to localise malignant, metastatic and extra-adrenal lesions very effectively, and can indicate the possibility of peptide radio-receptor therapy (Naswa et al. 2012).

9 Treatment of Pheochromocytoma in Adults

9.1 Perioperative Medical Management

Once diagnosed and localised, the treatment of choice in phaeochromocytoma is surgical removal. Surgical mortality in patients with undiagnosed pheochromocytoma' who undergo any surgery without preoperative medical therapy is high due to lethal hypertensive crises, malignant arrhythmias, and multi-organ failure. Adrenalectomy itself can release high levels of circulating catecholamines during surgery, leading to hypertensive crises and arrhythmias, even in normotensive and asymptomatic patients. Therefore, all patients with a hormonally-active phaeochromocytoma/paraganglioma should undergo preoperative adrenergic blockade and the first choice should be an alpha-adrenergic receptor blocker (Lenders et al. 2014). Unfortunately, there are no randomised head-to-head clinical trials to compare as to which alpha-blocker is most suitable. Phenoxybenzamine is an irreversible, non-selective, non-competitive, α-adrenoceptor blocker, with a longer duration of action due to its irreversible action. This should be initiated at least 7–14 days prior to surgery to ensure adequate α-blockade. Phenoxybenzamine is started at a dose of 10 mg twice daily and titrated up gradually till the patient is normotensive with no paroxysms of tachycardia or hypertension. The dose can be titrated up by 10–20 mg daily dose increments, going up to a maximum tolerable dose, which is generally a total daily dose of 1 mg/kg. The common side effects of phenoxybenzamine are postural hypotension with reflex tachycardia and dizziness, syncope and nasal congestion. It can also lead to inhibition of ejaculation, miosis and lassitude. Although the irreversible, prolonged inhibition caused by phenoxybenzamine offers effective adrenergic blockade during adrenal surgery, the prolonged action can contribute to hypotension in the first 24 h after tumour removal (Pacak 2007).

Due to the aforementioned difficulty with phenoxybenzamine, selective α_1-adrenergic blockers such as prazosin, terazosin or doxazosin are used in some centres. Although there are no head-to-head comparison studies, some retrospective studies have demonstrated that selective α1-adrenergic blockers are associated with lower diastolic pressure preoperatively, a lower incidence of reactive tachycardia, lower intraoperative heart rate, and better postoperative recovery with lower incidence of sustained postoperative hypotension (Prys-Roberts and Farndon 2002). However, there are other studies demonstrating no significant benefit in selective α_1-adrenergic blockers over phenoxybenzamine (Kocak et al. 2002). If these are used, prazosin is administered at 2–5 mg two or three times a day, terazosin at 2–5 mg per day, and doxazosin in doses of 2–8 mg per day. Some centres initially use phenoxybenzamine and subsequently change over to prazosin to avoid post-operative hypotension (Malchoff et al. 2004).

Beta-adrenergic blockers are useful preoperatively to control tachycardia only after the administration of adequate alpha-adrenergic blockade. As shown in Table 1, α1 receptor stimulation causes vasoconstriction while β2-receptor stimulation can cause peripheral vasodilatation; β-receptor blockade prior to α-blockade will cause α1-induced severe vasoconstriction without compensatory β2-induced vasodilatation, leading to hypertensive crises. Propranolol and atenolol are recommended for pre-operative use and should be initiated at least 3–4 days after the initiation of alpha blockade (Lenders et al. 2014). Although labetalol and carvedilol have combined α- and β-adrenoceptor effects, they are not recommended as their alpha:beta inhibition ratio is 1:7. Therefore, if used alone they can precipitate a hypertensive crisis, due to poor α-receptor inhibition. Some centres only add in β-antagonists if there is significant tachycardia.

Another agent that can be used is a calcium channel blocker. These drugs block catecholamines and cause calcium influx into vascular smooth muscle, thereby controlling hypertension and tachycardia. Calcium channel blockers can be used as a supplement to an adrenoceptor blocker in patients with inadequate blood pressure control or as a replacement for patients with severe side-effects on adrenoceptor blockers.

Metyrosine is an inhibitor of tyrosine hydroxylase, which is the rate-limiting step in catecholamine synthesis (Fig. 2). It can be used in combination with α-blockers for a short period before surgery to further stabilise blood pressure and blood loss during surgery (Steinsapir et al. 1997), but it is of limited availability.

Apart from adrenoceptor blockade, in patients with phaeochromocytoma it is vital to ensure adequate intravascular volume repletion as catecholamine excess causes blood volume contraction which is only 60 % corrected by the use of α-adrenergic blockade (Grosse et al. 1990). This is crucial to avoid severe post-operative hypotension, especially as these patients respond poorly to inotropes, due to pre-operative alpha and beta-receptor blockade. Retrospective studies demonstrate that a pre-operative high-salt diet, subsequent to initiation of an α-blocker, can reverse the volume contraction and reduce the post-operative hypotension (Pacak 2007). Apart from the high salt diet, 1–2 l of intravenous normal saline can be used to replete intravascular volume 24 h prior to surgery. However, one must be cautious not to fluid overload patients with kidney or heart failure.

Although there are no randomised studies on the pre-operative target blood pressure, a target blood pressure of less than 130/80 mmHg and a resting heart rate of 70 bpm are considered reasonable by most authorities.

9.2 Adrenalectomy and Surgical Outcome

Minimally-invasive laparoscopic adrenalectomy is the procedure of choice in patients with solitary intra-adrenal phaeochromocytoma without obvious radiological features of malignancy. However, for larger tumours of >6–8 cm or with features of local invasion, open adrenalectomy may be necessary (Lenders et al. 2014; Assalia and Gagner 2004). Paragangliomas are more likely to be found in areas difficult to access laparoscopically and are more frequently malignant. Therefore, paragangliomas are more likely to require open resection. Partial cortex-sparing adrenalectomy can be considered in patients with hereditary phaeochromocytoma (eg. MEN-2, VHL) and in patients who had undergone previous unilateral adrenalectomy.

Surgery of any catecholamine-secreting tumor is a high-risk procedure and should ideally be performed in a centre with an experienced surgeon, endocrinologist, and a team of anaesthesiologists. The most crucial part in the management of these patients is the multidisciplinary approach with the involvement of the surgeon, endocrinologist, anaesthetists and the intensive care specialists. Depending on the experience of the surgeon, either transperitoneal or a retroperitoneal laparoscopic approach can be taken. It is vital to avoid fracture of the tumour during dissection to avoid seeding into the tumour bed and peritoneal cavity. Intact specimen bags should be used for the safe retrieval of the resected tumour and surgeons have successfully employed hand assistance or robot assistance for large, difficult to retrieve tumours (Brunaud et al. 2008). If cortical-sparing partial adrenalectomy is considered, devices such as ultrasonic shears can be used to minimise bleeding; 90 % of the patients who undergo cortical-sparing adrenalectomy remain glucocorticoid sufficient, especially so in patients with small tumours (Volkin et al. 2012). However, the disadvantage of cortical-sparing surgery is that inevitably there is some medullary tissue left behind which increases the rate of recurrence, with higher surgical complication risk during a second surgery.

As discussed above, patients should be satisfactorily blocked, as significant surges of catecholamines are inevitable during the surgery. Alpha and beta-adrenergic blockade should be continued until the morning of the surgery. Short-acting intravenous α- and β-adrenergic blocking agents should be available during surgery and agents such as fentanyl, ketamine and morphine should be avoided. Some anaesthetists use sodium nitroprusside to cause both arterial and venous dilatation and then fluid replace to maintain blood volume. Most anaesthetic gases can be used during surgery apart from halothane and desflurane. If bilateral adrenalectomy is planned, the patient should be on stress doses of hydrocortisone replacement peri-operatively. Cardiovascular and haemodynamic variables including intra-arterial pressure and heart rhythm must be monitored closely during and immediately follow surgery. If the patient has decreased cardiac reserve, monitoring of pulmonary capillary wedge pressure can be useful.

Acute hypertensive crises should be anticipated before or during surgery and should be treated with intravenous sodium nitroprusside, phentolamine or nicardipine. Sodium nitroprusside is a vasodilator and is ideal for intra-operative hypertension management due to its rapid onset and short duration of action. It should be initially started at a rate of 0.5–1.5 micrograms/kg/min, then increased in steps of 500 nanograms/kg/min every 5 min within range, 0.5–8 micrograms/kg/min. Intravenous phentolamine is a non-selective, short-acting α – adrenergic inhibitor, with a hypotensive response seen in 3–4 min following an intravenous bolus of 5 mg, which lasts for 10–15 min. Nicardipine is a dihydropyridine calcium channel blocker that relaxes vascular smooth muscle and dilates coronary and peripheral arteries. It can be used as an intravenous infusion to maintain blood pressure during surgery. For the management of tachyarrhythmias, intravenous lidocaine, esmolol or labetolol can be used (Memtsoudis et al. 2005).

Hypotension may occur during and after surgical resection of a phaeochromocytoma, and the mainstay of treatment should be intravenous fluids and colloids, and only if necessary intravenous pressor agents can follow. Postoperative hypotension is less frequent in patients with adequate preoperative volume expansion and α-adrenergic blockade. Hypoglycemia should be anticipated in the immediate postoperative period with regular monitoring of blood glucose. Fluids given intravenously should preferably be 5 % dextrose to avoid hypoglycaemia. Patients with congestive cardiac failure or poor cardiac reserve should have close haemodynamic monitoring post-operatively with minimum blood pressure and heart rate fluctuations.

Although blood pressure normalises in the majority, some patients remain hypertensive for up to 4–8 weeks post-operatively. Hypertension can be persistent in a few patients due to resetting of the baroreceptors, structural changes to the blood vessels due to long-standing hypertension, damage to polar renal vessels during surgery, and coexisting essential hypertension. In terms of the catecholamine cardiomyopathy, the alarming ECG changes frequently normalise, but there is recent evidence based on MRI imaging showing persisting decreases in sytolic and diastolic function due to fibrosis (Ferreira et al. 2016).

9.3   Postoperative Follow-Up

Two weeks following the surgery all patients should be retested with a 24-h urinary fractionated metanephrines. If the levels are within normal limits, surgery can be considered complete. However, elevated levels of metanephrines following surgery may indicate residual disease, which could be either residual adrenal disease or occult metastases.

All patients, including patients with normal metanephrines, should in our opinion have annual 24-h fractionated metanephrines evaluated for life. This is crucial to assess for metastatic disease, tumour recurrence in the adrenal bed and delayed appearance of multiple primary tumours. Several studies suggest a 10 % risk of tumour recurrence in the remnant adrenal gland (Yip et al. 2004). Moreover, higher recurrence rates should be expected in patients with familial disease, right-sided adrenal phaeochromocytoma, or paragangliomas (Young 2011; Amar et al. 2005). However, adrenal imaging is not routinely indicated, unless the metanephrines rise or in the follow-up of patients with a non-secretory primary lesion.

10 Histopathology

The typical histopathology of phaeochromocytomas and paragangliomas include chief cells with abundant granular cytoplasm and large vesicular nuclei and basophilic to amphophilic cells. However, some tumours may have scant cytoplasm with cellular and nuclear pleomorphism. Cytoplasmic hyaline globules and melanin-like pigment can be frequently seen. A prominent cell-nesting pattern called *zellballen* may be present with scattered ganglion cells. The chief cells are centrally located while Spindle shaped sustentacular or supporting cells are found periphery to the chief cell nests. Higher-grade tumours are characterized by a progressive loss in the ratio between chief cells and sustentacular cells with a decrease in the overall number of sustentacular cells (Barnes and Taylor 1990; Kliewer et al. 1989)

Immunohistochemical studies confirms the neuroendocrine origin of the tumour with positive staining of chief cells with chromogranin, synaptophysin and neuron-specific enolase (NSE). Moreover, sustentacular cells are negative for neuroendocrine markers and positive for molecular markers such as S100 acidic protein and GFAP. The absence of staining with certain molecular markers is of use when distinguishing phaeochromocytoma from other adrenal and renal tumours. For example, negative EMA staining in phaechromocytoma is useful to distinguish between renal cell tumours and negative staining with melan A, inhibin-α, calretinin, and keratin is helpful to distinguish between adrenocortical carcinoma. Further, phaeochromocytomas and paragangliomas are positive for chromogranin A and negative for melan A and keratin (Kliewer and Cochran 1989).

11 Malignant Phaeochromocytoma

Malignant phaeochromocytomas pose several challenges to the managing physician, starting from the diagnosis and leading up to the management. Identification of the malignant nature of a phaeochromocytoma remains a challenge as, unlike most malignant lesions, malignant phaeochromocytomas lack specific tumour and prognostic markers indicating malignancy: only the presence of metastases of chromaffin tissue at sites where no chromaffin tissue should be expected (eg. liver, bone, lymph nodes) establishes a definitive diagnosis of malignant phaeochromocytoma (Young 2011).

Several clinical, biochemical, radiological, genetic and histopathological clues can alert one to the potential of malignant disease in a patient with phaeochromocytoma. Malignant disease can present with features of catecholamine excess similar to benign phaeochromocytoma (eg. hypertension, funny spells etc.). However, malignancy can present with systemic and metastatic symptoms such as anorexia, weight loss and bone pain. If the malignant tumour is not well differentiated, the catecholamine production may not be complete, giving rise to absent or mild clinical features of catecholamine excess.

The anatomical site of the primary enterochromaffin tumour can give some idea of the possible malignant potential of a phaeochromocytoma. Some 10 % of phaeochromocytomas are malignant, while up to 35 % of mediastinal and abdominal paragangliomas are malignant. Head-and-neck paragangliomas have a lower overall risk of malignancy at 4 %, while vagal and carotid body paragangliomas have a risk of 10–15 % (Eisenhofer et al. 2012).

Apart from the anatomical site, the genetic background of the patient adds to the potential malignant risk of a pheochromocytoma. SDHB gene carries the highest malignancy rates and patients with paragangliomas with this mutation should undergo screening for distant metastatic disease as part of the preoperative evaluation; VHL and MEN-2 carry a low risk of malignancy, 5 % or less.

Biochemistry can be useful in the differentiation between benign and malignant pheochromocytoma, although it is of limited value. Due to poor differentiation of the catecholamine biosynthetic pathway, they often do not complete the catecholamine production all the way up to noradrenaline (Fig. 3): therefore, they produce high levels of dopamine and its metabolites, particularly 3–methoxytyramine. Therefore, predominant production of 3-methoxytyramine suggests a malignant rather than a benign phaeochromocytoma (Eisenhofer et al. 2012; Parenti et al. 2012). Few other biochemical substances have been suggested to be associated with phaeochromocytoma. Chromogranin A is a protein co-secreted with catecholamines and is elevated in the presence of catecholamine secreting tumours. However, malignancy has been associated with very high serum chromogranin A levels (Grossman et al. 2006).

Similar to clinical and biochemical features, imaging offers limited clues in distinguishing malignant from benign phaeochromocytoma. The typical malignant features of adrenal imaging such as attenuation greater than 10HU, delayed contrast washout and inhomogeneous consistency, are seen in both benign and malignant phaeochromocytoma. However, radiology can be helpful in assessing the size and the location of the lesion. Tumours that are greater than 5 cm in size and extra-adrenal in location carry a higher risk for malignant disease than tumours that are small or have an adrenal location: size matters (Korevaar and Grossman 2011).

Somatostatin analogues labelled with gallium-68 (^{68}Ga-DOTATOC), ^{111}In-

pentetreotide and ^{18}F-FDG are useful functional imaging modalities in identifying metastatic disease (Buchmann et al. 2007; Hofmann et al. 2001). Radiolabelled dopamine or dihydroxypheylalanine (DOPA), which is taken up by chromaffin cells, is another useful functional imaging modality, while PET with 6-[^{18}F]-fluoro-dopamine can detect metastatic phaeochromocytomas and paragangliomas with better sensitivity than ^{131}I-MIBG (Ilias et al. 2003).

Despite recent advances in histopathology and molecular markers, histological differentiation of benign and malignant phaeochromocytoma remains an area of difficulty as no single histological feature, by itself, is of significant value. Some evidence suggests that multifactorial analysis, combining several features, can be helpful in identifying significant metastatic risk. Several scoring systems have been proposed, considering growth patterns, invasion, cytology, mitotic activity and other tumour characteristics (Linnoila et al. 1990; Kimura et al. 2005). One of the most utilised scores is the "Pheochromocytoma of the Adrenal gland Scales Score" (PASS), proposed by Thompson et al. in 2002 (Table 6). Subsequent studies revealed that all malignant phaeochromocytomas had a PASS of

Table 6 Phaeochromocytoma of the adrenal gland scoring scale (PASS)

Feature	Value
Nuclear hyperchromasia	1
Profound nuclear pleomorphism	1
Capsular invasion	1
Vascular invasion	1
Extension into adipose tissue	2
Atypical mitotic figures	2
Greater than 3 of 10 mitotic figures high-power field	2
Tumor cell spindling	2
Cellular monotony	2
High cellularity	2
Central or confluent tumour necrosis	2
Large nests or diffuse growth (>10 % of tumour volume)	2
Total	**20**

Adopted from reference Thompson (2002)

>6 and a score of <4 suggested benign nature. Scores between 4 and 6 are indeterminate (Thompson 2002; Strong et al. 2008). Kimura has suggested a system bases on features of PAS but including Ki-67 as well as some non-histopathological criteria.

Several molecular markers associated with malignancy such as cyclooxygenase-2, secretogranin II-derived peptide, N-cadherin, vascular endothelial growth factor (VEGF), endothelin receptor type A (ETA), and type B (ETB) and telomerase have been identified. In particular, telomerase seem to be closely related to the malignant potential of paragangliomas (Parenti et al. 2012). Markers of proliferation such as Ki-67 based on the MIB-1 antibody can give additional information on the proliferative potential of the tumour. A Ki-67 of >2 % is considered a useful parameter predicting malignant potential (Liu et al. 2004). Recently, several micro-RNA expression studies have shown to act as biomarkers for differentiating benign and malignant phaeochromocytoma. Although promising, they need further evaluation with large cohort studies before the incorporation in to clinical practice (Parenti et al. 2012).

The treatment of malignant phaeochromocytoma can be a quite challenging and must be managed in a multidisciplinary setting. The prognosis can be variable with an overall 5-year survival rate of between 34 % and 60 %. The prognosis is worse in patients with lung and liver metastases rather than bone (Pacak et al. 2007). Surgical resection is the initial treatment with laparoscopic or open adrenalectomy with resection of locoregional lymph nodes. Surgical debulking is considered the mainstay of treatment for palliation, which can improve local or systemic symptoms related to catecholamine secretion and improves response to other therapeutic approaches. Liver metastases are treated with arterial or chemoembolisation as well as radiofrequency ablation (Maithel and Fong 2009).

Radio-metabolic treatment can be considered in patients with non-resectable lesions by using β-emitting isotopes coupled with MIBG or somatostatin analogues. ^{131}I-MIBG has been used for the treatment of malignant phaeochromocytoma over the last few decades and is usually preceded by diagnostic scintigraphy with ^{123}I-MIBG. About 60 % of metastatic sites are ^{131}I-MIBG avid with better responses seen in limited disease with soft-tissue metastases rather than diffuse disease with bone metastases (Loh et al. 1997). Radiolabelled somatostatin analogues are another form of treatment with the use of yttrium-90-DOTATOC (^{90}Y-DOTATOC) and lutetium-177- DOTA- TATE (^{177}Lu-DOTA- TATE). Both these can be used as potential treatment modalities if scintigraphy with either ^{111}In-pentetreotide or ^{68}Ga-DOTA-TOC shows high tumour uptake. Recent studies demonstrated that ^{68}Ga-DOTATATE PET/CT was significantly superior in detection rate to all other functional and anatomical imaging modalities and may represent the preferred future imaging modality in the evaluation of SDHB-related metastatic pheochromocytoma/paraganglioma (Janssen et al. 2015). Radionuclide treatment is low in toxicity with fewer side-effects compared to conventional cytotoxic agents and is useful in reducing the hormonal secretion and tumour bulk (Kwekkeboom et al. 2008; Forrer et al. 2008). Moreover, combination therapy with radiolabelled MIBG and somatostatin analogues can be considered as a future treatment option with lower toxicity and better efficacy (Sze et al. 2013).

The most used and effective anti-neoplastic chemotherapy regimen is a combination of cyclophosphamide, vincristine and dacarbazine (CVD). It is mainly considered in patients with locally advanced and/or metastatic lesion, unresectable tumours and disease resistant to the above mentioned treatment modalities (Andersen et al. 2011). Dacarbazine is an alkylating agent, which has the best chemotherapeutic effect on phaeochromocytoma. However, it remains unclear as to whether this combination regime prolongs survival. An oral alternative to dacarbazine, temozolomide has shown promise in a retrospective trial in the treatment of patients with malignant phaeochromocytoma/paraganglioma with SDHB mutation. The silencing of O-methylguanine-DNA methyltransferase

(MGMT) expression as a consequence of MGMT promoter hypermethylation in SDHB-mutated tumours has been considered as the possible mechanism of action of temozolomide (Hadoux et al. 2014). Neuroendocrine tumours have a rich vasculature and high levels of vascular endothelial growth factor (VEGF) expression. Therefore, agents inhibiting angiogenesis such as thalidomide has been evaluated for the treatment of malignant pheochromocytoma, in combination with temozolomide, but temozolomide alone is probably just as effective as the combination (Kulke et al. 2006). Molecular targeted therapy is another promising therapeutic option for malignant pheochromocytoma. Sunitinib, which is a potent inhibitor of multiple tyrosine kinase receptors, is an agent that has been considered patients with several studies showing a survival benefit. However, more data on the use of sunitinib will be released in the near future with the outcome of the First International Randomized Study in Malignant Progressive Pheochromocytoma and Paraganglioma (FIRST-MAPPP). Everolimus is an mTOR inhibitor which has not shown much efficacy when used on its own, but various animal and cell line studies have suggested that combinations of targeted therapy may be useful (Druce et al. 2009; Nölting et al. 2012; 2015).

Radiotherapy is another mode of treatment available for malignant pheochromocytoma. External beam radiotherapy is mainly considered for palliative treatment in pain management of bony metastases. It is important to bear in mind that adequate adrenergic blockade must be achieved prior to treatment as all these modalities can potentially precipitate a hypertensive crisis.

References

Amar L, Servais A, Gimeniz-Roqueplo AP et al (2005) Year of diagnosis, features at presentation, and risk of recurrence in patients with pheochromocytoma or secreting paraganglioma. J Clin Endocrinol Metab 90:2110–2116

Andersen KF, Altaf R, Krarup-Hansen A et al (2011) Malignant pheochromocytomas and paragangliomas—the importance of a multidisciplinary approach. Cancer Treat Rev 37(2):111–119

Assalia A, Gagner M (2004) Laparoscopic adrenalectomy. Br J Surg 91:1259–1274

Baguet JP, Hammer L, Mazzuco TL et al (2004) Circumstances of discovery of phaeochromocytoma: a retrospective study of 41 consecutive patients. Eur J Endocrinol 150:681

Baid SK, Lai EW, Wesley RA, Ling A, Timmers HJ, Adams KT, Kozupa A, Pacak K (2009) Brief communication: radiographic contrast infusion and catecholamine release in patients with pheochromocytoma. Ann Intern Med 150(1):27–32. Erratum in: Ann Intern Med. 2009 Feb 17;150(4):292

Barnes L, Taylor SR (1990) Carotid body paragangliomas. A clinicopathologic and DNA analysis of 13 tumors. Arch Otolaryngol Head Neck Surg 116

Beard CM, Sheps SG, Kurland LT et al (1983) Occurrence of pheochromocytoma in Rochester, Minnesota, 1950 through 1979. Mayo Clin Proc 58:802

Bergland BE (1989) Pheochromocytoma presenting as shock. Am J Emerg Med 7:44–48

Berglund AS, Hulthén UL, Manhem P, Thorsson O, Wollmer P, Törnquist C (2001) Metaiodobenzylguanidine (MIBG) scintigraphy and computed tomography (CT) in clinical practice. Primary and secondary evaluation for localization of phaeochromocytomas. J Intern Med 249:247–251

Bhatia KS, Ismail MM, Sahdev A et al (2008) 123I-metaiodobenzylguanidine (MIBG) scintigraphy for the detection of adrenal and extra-adrenal phaeochromocytomas: CT and MRI correlation. Clin Endocrinol (Oxf) 69:181–188

Blake MA et al (2004) Pheochromocytoma. An Imaging Chameleon. Radiographics 24:87–99

Bravo EL (1991) Pheochromocytoma: new concepts and future trends. Kidney Int 40:544

Brito JP, Asi N, Bancos I, Gionfriddo MR, Zeballos-Palacios CL, Leppin AL, Undavalli C, Wang Z, Domecq JP, Prustsky G, Elraiyah TA, Prokop LJ, Montori VM, Murad MH (2015) Testing for germline mutations in sporadic pheochromocytoma/paraganglioma: a systematic review. Clin Endocrinol (Oxf) 82(3):338–345. doi:10.1111/cen.12530, Epub 2014 Jul 7

Brunaud L, Ayav A, Zarnegar R et al (2008) Prospective evaluation of 100 robotic-assisted unilateral adrenalectomies. Surgery 144:995–1001

Buchmann I, Henze M, Engelbrecht S et al (2007) Comparison of ^{68}Ga-DOTATOC PET and ^{111}In-DTPAOC (Octreoscan) SPECT in patients with neuroendocrine tumours. Eur J Nucl Med Mol Imaging 34 (10):1617–1626

Comino-Mendez I, Gracia-Aznarez FJ, Schiavi F et al (2011) Exome sequencing identifies MAX mutations as a cause of hereditary pheochromocytoma. Nat Genet 43:663–777

Därr R, Pamporaki C, Peitzsch M, Miehle K, Prejbisz A et al (2014) Biochemical diagnosis of phaeochromocytoma using plasma-free normetanephrine,

metanephrine and methoxytyramine: importance of supine sampling under fasting conditions. Clin Endocrinol (Oxf) 80(4):478–486. doi:10.1111/cen.12327

Dénes J, Swords F, Rattenberry E, Stals K, Owens M, Cranston T, Xekouki P, Moran L, Kumar A, Wassif C, Fersht N, Baldeweg SE, Morris D, Lightman S, Agha A, Rees A, Grieve J, Powell M, Boguszewski CL, Dutta P, Thakker RV, Srirangalingam U, Thompson CJ, Druce M, Higham C, Davis J, Eeles R, Stevenson M, O'Sullivan B, Taniere P, Skordilis K, Gabrovska P, Barlier A, Webb SM, Aulinas A, Drake WM, Bevan JS, Preda C, Dalantaeva N, Ribeiro-Oliveira A Jr, Garcia IT, Yordanova G, Iotova V, Evanson J, Grossman AB, Trouillas J, Ellard S, Stratakis CA, Maher ER, Roncaroli F, Korbonits M (2015) Heterogeneous genetic background of the association of pheochromocytoma/paraganglioma and pituitary adenoma: results from a large patient cohort. J Clin Endocrinol Metab 100(3):E531–E541. doi:10.1210/jc.2014-3399, Epub 2014 Dec 12

Dluhy RG (2002) Pheochromocytoma-death of an axiom. N Engl J Med 346:1486

Druce MR, Kaltsas GA, Fraenkel M, Gross DJ, Grossman AB (2009) Novel and evolving therapies in the treatment of malignant phaeochromocytoma: experience with the mTOR inhibitor everolimus (RAD001). Horm Metab Res 41(9):697–702. doi:10.1055/s-0029-1220687, Epub 2009 May 7

Eisenhofer G (2012) Screening for pheochromocytomas and paragangliomas. Curr Hypertens Rep 14:130–137. doi:10.1007/s11906-012-0246-y

Eisenhofer G, Walther MM, Huynh TT et al (2001) Pheochromocytomas in von Hippel-Lindau syndrome and multiple endocrine neoplasia type 2 display distinct biochemical and clinical phenotypes. J Clin Endocrinol Metab 86:1999

Eisenhofer G, Kopin IJ, Goldstein DS (2004) Catecholamine metabolism: a contemporary view with implications for physiology and medicine. Pharmacol Rev 56:331–349

Eisenhofer G et al (2012) Plasma methoxytyramine: a novel biomarker of metastatic pheochromocytoma and paraganglioma in relation to established risk factors of tumour size, location and SDHB mutation status. Eur J Cancer 48(11):1739–1749

Ferreira VM, Marcelino M, Piechnik SK, Marini C, Karamitsos TD, Ntusi NAB, Francis JM, Robson MD, Arnold JR, Mihai R, Thomas JD, Herincs M, Hassan-Smith Z, Karavitaki N, Greiser A, Arlt W, Korbonits M, Grossman A, Wass J, Neubauer S (2016) Pheochromocytoma is characterized by catecholamine myocarditis, focal and diffuse fibrosis, and persistent subclinical systolic and diastolic dysfunction. J Am Coll Cardiol, in press

Forrer F, Riedweg I, Maecke HR, Mueller-Brand J (2008) Radiolabeled DOTATOC in patients with advanced paraganglioma and pheochromocytoma. Q J Nucl Med Mol Imaging 52(4):334–340

Galan SR, Kann PH (2013) Genetics and molecular pathogenesis of pheochromocytoma and paraganglioma. Clin Endocrinol (Oxf) 78(2):165–175

Grosse H, Schröder D, Schober O, Hausen B, Dralle H (1990) The importance of high-dose alpha-receptor blockade for blood volume and hemodynamics in pheochromocytoma [in German]. Anaesthesist 39:313–318

Grossman A, Pacak K, Sawka A et al (2006) Biochemical diagnosis and localization of pheochromocytoma: can we reach a consensus? Ann N Y Acad Sci 1073:332–347

Guerrero MA, Schreinemakers JM, Vriens MR et al (2009) Clinical spectrum of pheochromocytoma. J Am Coll Surg 209:727

Hadoux J, Favier J, Scoazec JY, Leboulleux S, Al Ghuzlan A et al (2014) SDHB mutations are associated with response to temozolomide in patients with metastatic pheochromocytoma or paraganglioma. Int J Cancer 135(11):2711–2720. doi:10.1002/ijc.28913

Hofmann M, Maecke H, Bo¨rner AR et al (2001) Biokinetics and imaging with the somatostatin receptor PET radioligand ^{68}Ga-DOTATOC: preliminary data. Eur J Nucl Med 28(12):1751–1757

Ilias I, Yu J, Carrasquillo JA et al (2003) Superiority of 6-[^{18}F]-fluorodopamine positron emission tomography versus [^{131}I]-metaiodobenzylguanidine scintigraphy in the localization of metastatic pheochromocytoma. J Clin Endocrinol Metab 88(9):4083–4087

Jacobson AF, Deng H, Lombard J, Lessig HJ, Black RR (2010) 123I-meta-iodobenzylguanidine scintigraphy for the detection of neuroblastoma and pheochromocytoma: results of a meta-analysis. J Clin Endocrinol Metab 95:2596–2606

Jalil ND, Pattou FN, Combemale F et al (1998) Effectiveness and limits of preoperative imaging studies for the localisation of pheochromocytomas and paragangliomas: a review of 282 cases. French Association of Surgery (AFC), and The French Association of Endocrine Surgeons (AFCE). Eur J Surg 164:23–28

Janssen I, Blanchet EM, Adams K et al (2015) Superiority of [68Ga]-DOTATATE PET/CT to other functional imaging modalities in the localization of SDHB-associated metastatic pheochromocytoma and paraganglioma. Clin Cancer Res 21(17):3888–3895. doi:10.1158/1078-0432.CCR-14-2751

Kantorovich V, King KS, Pacak K (2010) SDH-related pheochromocytoma and paraganglioma. Best Pract Res Clin Endocrinol Metab 24(3):415–424. doi:10.1016/j.beem.2010.04.001

Kimura N, Watanabe T, Noshiro T, Shizawa S, Miura Y (2005) Histological grading of adrenal and extra-adrenal pheochromocytomas and relationship to prognosis: a clinicopathological analysis of 116 adrenal pheochromocytomas and 30 extra-adrenal sympathetic paragangliomas including 38 malignant tumors. Endocr Pathol 16(1):23–32

Kliewer KE, Cochran AJ (1989) A review of the histology, ultrastructure, immunohistology, and molecular biology of extra-adrenal paragangliomas. Arch Pathol Lab Med 113:1209

Kliewer KE, Wen DR, Cancilla PA, Cochran AJ (1989) Paragangliomas: assessment of prognosis by histologic, immunohistochemical, and ultrastructural techniques. Hum Pathol 20:29

Kocak S, Aydintug S, Canakci N (2002) Alpha blockade in preoperative preparation of patients with pheochromocytomas. Int Surg 87:191–194

Korevaar TI, Grossman AB (2011) Pheochromocytomas and paragangliomas: assessment of malignant potential. Endocrine 40(3):354–365. doi:10.1007/s12020-011-9545-3, Epub 2011 Oct 25

Kulke MH, Stuart K, Enzinger PC, Ryan DP, Clark JW et al (2006) Phase II study of temozolomide and thalidomide in patients with metastatic neuroendocrine tumors. J Clin Oncol 24:401–406

Kwekkeboom DJ, De Herder WW, Kam BL et al (2008) Treatment with the radiolabeled somatostatin analog [177Lu- DOTA0, Tyr3]octreotate: toxicity, efficacy, and survival. J Clin Oncol 26(13):2124–2130

Lenders JW, Eisenhofer G, Mannelli M, Pacak K (2005) Phaeochromocytoma. Lancet 366:665–675

Lenders JWM, Duh QY et al (2014) Pheochromocytoma and paraganglioma: an endocrine society clinical practice guideline. J Clin Endocrinol Metab 99 (6):1915–1942

Liao WB, Liu CF, Chiang CW et al (2000) Cardiovascular manifestations of pheochromocytoma. Am J Emerg Med 18:622–625

Linnoila RI, Keiser HR, Steinberg SM, Lack EE (1990) Histopathology of benign versus malignant sympathoadrenal paragangliomas: clinicopathologic study of 120 cases including unusual histologic features. Hum Pathol 21(11):1168–1180

Liu TH, Chen YJ, Wu SF et al (2004) Distinction between benign and malignant pheochromocytomas. Zhonghua Bing Li Xue Za Zhi 33(3):198–202

Loh KC, Fitzgerald PA, Matthay KK, Yeo PPB, Price DC (1997) The treatment of malignant pheochromocytoma with iodine-131 metaiodobenzylguanidine (^{131}I-MIBG): a comprehensive review of 116 reported patients. J Endocrinol Investig 20(11):648–658

Maithel SK, Fong Y (2009) Hepatic ablation for neuroendocrine tumor metastases. J Surg Oncol 100 (8):635–638

Malchoff CD, MacGillivray D, Shichman S (2004) Pheochromocytoma treatment. In: Mansoor GA (ed) Secondary hypertension. Humana Press, Totowa, pp 235–249

Mamede M et al (2006) Discordant localization of 2-[18F]-fluoro-2-deoxy-D-glucose in 6-[18F]-fluorodopamine- and [123I]-metaiodobenzyl-guanidine-negative metastatic pheochromocytoma sites. Nucl Med Commun 27(1):31–36

Mantero F, Terzolo M, Arnaldi G et al (2000) A survey on adrenal incidentaloma in Italy. Study Group on Adrenal Tumors of the Italian Society of Endocrinology. J Clin Endocrinol Metab 85:637–644

Memtsoudis SG, Swamidoss C, Psoma M (2005) Anesthesia for adrenal surgery. In: Linos D, van Heerden JA (eds) Adrenal glands: diagnostic aspects and surgical therapy. Springer, New York, pp 287–297

Mozley PD, Kim CK, Mohsin J et al (1994) The efficacy of iodine-123- MIBG as a screening test for pheochromocytoma. J Nucl Med 35:1138–1144

Mukherjee JJ, Peppercorn PD, Reznek RH et al (1997) Pheochromocytoma: effect of nonionic contrast medium in CT on circulating catecholamine levels. Radiology 202:227–231

Mulligan LM, Ponder BA (1995) Genetic basis of endocrine disease: multiple endocrine neoplasia type 2. J Clin Endocrinol Metab 80:1989

Nakamura K, Ogata M, Ando T, Usa T, Kawakami A (2011) Paroxysmal thyroid swelling. A forgotten clinical finding of pheochromocytoma. J Clin Endocrinol Metab 96(12):3601–3602

Naswa N, Sharma P, Nazar AH, Agarwal KK, Kumar R, Ammini AC, Malhotra A, Bal C (2012) Prospective evaluation of 68Ga-DOTA-NOC PET-CT in phaeochromocytoma and paraganglioma: preliminary results from a single centre study. Eur Radiol 22 (3):710–719

Neary N, King KS, Pack K (2011) Drugs and pheochromocytoma—don't be fooled by every elevated metanephrine. N Engl J Med 364:23

Neumann HP, Pawlu C, Peczkowska M et al (2004) Distinct clinical features of paraganglioma syndromes associated with SDHB and SDHD gene mutations. JAMA 292:943

Nölting S, Garcia E, Alusi G, Giubellino A, Pacak K, Korbonits M, Grossman AB (2012) Combined blockade of signalling pathways shows marked anti-tumour potential in phaeochromocytoma cell lines. J Mol Endocrinol 49(2):79–96. doi:10.1530/JME-12-0028

Nölting S, Maurer J, Spöttl G, Aristizabal Prada ET, Reuther C, Young K, Korbonits M, Göke B, Grossman A, Auernhammer CJ (2015) Additive anti-tumor effects of lovastatin and everolimus in vitro through simultaneous inhibition of signaling pathways. PLoS ONE 10(12):e0143830. doi:10.1371/journal.pone.0143830, eCollection 2015

Pacak K (2007) Preoperative management of the pheochromocytoma patient. J Clin Endocrinol Metab 92:4069–4079

Pacak K, Eisenhofer G, Ahlman H et al (2007) Pheochromocytoma: recommendations for clinical practice from the First International Symposium. Nat Clin Pract Endocrinol Metab 3(2):92–102

Parenti G, Zampetti B, Rapizzi E, Ercolino T, Giachè V, Mannelli M (2012) Updated and new perspectives on diagnosis, prognosis, and therapy of malignant pheochromocytoma/paraganglioma. J Oncol 2012:872713, 10 pages. doi:10.1155/2012/872713

Perry CG, Sawka AM, Singh R, Thabane L, Bajnarek J, Young WF Jr (2007) The diagnostic efficacy of urinary fractionated metanephrines measured by tandem mass spectrometry in detection of pheochromocytoma. Clin Endocrinol (Oxf) 66:703–708

Pomares FJ, Cañas R, Rodriguez JM et al (1998) Differences between sporadic and multiple endocrine neoplasia type 2A phaeochromocytoma. Clin Endocrinol (Oxf) 48:195

Prys-Roberts C, Farndon JR (2002) Efficacy and safety of doxazosin for perioperative management of patients with pheochromocytoma. World J Surg 26:1037–1042

Sane T, Schalin-Jäntti C, Raade M (2012) Is biochemical screening for pheochromocytoma in adrenal incidentalomas expressing low unenhanced attenuation on computed tomography necessary? J Clin Endocrinol Metab 97(6):2077–2083. doi:10.1210/jc. 2012-1061, Epub 2012 Apr 6

Sawka AM, Jaeschke R, Singh RJ et al (2003) A comparison of biochemical tests for pheochromocytoma: measurement of fractionated plasma metanephrines compared with the combination of 24-hour urinary metanephrines and catecholamines. J Clin Endocrinol Metab 88:553–558

Steinsapir J, Carr AA, Prisant LM, Bransome ED Jr (1997) Metyrosine and pheochromocytoma. Arch Intern Med 157:901–906

Stolk RF, Bakx C, Mulder J, Timmers HJ, Lenders JW (2013) Is the excess cardiovascular morbidity in pheochromocytoma related to blood pressure or to catecholamines? J Clin Endocrinol Metab 98 (3):1100–1106. doi:10.1210/jc.2012-3669, Epub 2013 Feb 13

Streeten DH, Anderson GH Jr (1996) Mechanisms of orthostatic hypotension and tachycardia in patients with pheochromocytoma. Am J Hypertens 9 (8):760–769

Strong VE, Kennedy T, Al-Ahmadie H et al (2008) Prognostic indicators of malignancy in adrenal pheochromocytomas: clinical, histopathologic, and cell cycle/ apoptosis gene expression analysis. Surgery 143 (6):759–768

Sutton MG, Sheps SG, Lie JT (1981) Prevalence of clinically unsuspected pheochromocytoma. Review of a 50-year autopsy series. Mayo Clin Proc 56:354

Sze WC, Grossman AB, Goddard I, Amendra D, Shieh SC, Plowman PN, Drake WM, Akker SA, Druce MR (2013) Sequelae and survivorship in patients treated with (131)I-MIBG therapy. Br J Cancer 109 (3):565–572. doi:10.1038/bjc.2013.365, Epub 2013 Jul 16

Thompson LDR (2002) Pheochromocytoma of the adrenal gland scaled score (PASS) to separate benign from malignant neoplasms: a clinicopathologic and immunophenotypic study of 100 cases. Am J Surg Pathol 26(5):551–566

Timmers HJLM, Kozupa A, Eisenhofer G, Raygada M, Adams KT, Solis D, Lenders JWM, Pacak K (2007) Clinical presentations, biochemical phenotypes, and genotype-phenotype correlations in patients with succinate dehydrogenase subunit B-Associated pheochromocytomas and paragangliomas. J Clin Endocrinol Metab 92(3):779–786

Timmers HJ, Chen CC, Carrasquillo JA et al (2009) Comparison of 18F-fluoro-L-DOPA, 18F-fluoro-deoxyglucose, and 18F-fluorodopamine PET and 123I-MIBG scintigraphy in the localization of pheochromocytoma and paraganglioma. J Clin Endocrinol Metab 94:4757–4767

Volkin D, Yerram N, Ahmed F et al (2012) Partial adrenalectomy minimizes the need for long-term hormone replacement in pediatric patients with pheochromocytoma and von Hippel-Lindau syndrome. J Pediatr Surg 47:2077–2082

Walther MM, Herring J, Enquist E et al (1999) von Recklinghausen's disease and pheochromocytomas. J Urol 162:1582

Whalen RK, Althausen AF, Daniels GH (1992) Extra-adrenal pheochromocytoma. J Urol 147:1

Yip L, Lee JE, Shapiro SE et al (2004) Surgical management of hereditary pheochromocytoma. J Am Coll Surg 198:525–534

Young WF Jr (2011) Endocrine hypertension. In: Melmed S, Polonsky KS, Reed Larsen P, Kronenberg HM (eds) Williams textbook of endocrinology, 12th edn. Elsevier Saunders, Philadelphia

Zhuang Z, Yang C, Lorenzo F, Merino M, Fojo T, Kebebew E, Popovic V, Stratakis CA, Prchal JT, Pacak K (2012) Somatic HIF2A gain-of-function mutations in paraganglioma with polycythemia. N Engl J Med 367(10):922–930. doi:10.1056/ NEJMoa1205119

Adv Exp Med Biol - Advances in Internal Medicine (2017) 2: 261–277
DOI 10.1007/5584_2016_148
© Springer International Publishing AG 2016
Published online: 5 November 2016

Renal Denervation

Mohammed Awais Hameed and Indranil Dasgupta

Abstract

Sympathetic nervous system over-activity is closely linked with elevation of systemic blood pressure. Both animal and human studies suggest renal sympathetic nerves play an important role in this respect. Historically, modulation of sympathetic activity has been used to treat hypertension. More recently, catheter based renal sympathetic denervation was introduced for the management of treatment resistant hypertension. Sound physiological principles and surgical precedent underpin renal denervation as a therapy for treatment of resistant hypertension. Encouraging results of early studies led to a widespread adoption of the procedure for management of this condition. Subsequently a sham controlled randomised controlled study failed to confirm the benefit of renal denervation leading to a halt in its use in most countries in the world. However, critical analysis of the sham-controlled study indicates a number of flaws. A number of lessons have been learnt from this and other studies which need to be applied in future trials to ascertain the actual role of renal denervation in the management of treatment resistant hypertension before further implementation. This chapter deals with all these issues in detail.

Keywords

Sympathetic nervous system • Renal vascular resistance • Resistant hypertension • Renal angiography • Simplicity HTN-3 • Global Simplicity Registry

1 Role of the Sympathetic Nervous System in Hypertension

Roman scholar Cornelius Celsus (25 BC–50 AD) was probably the first person to observe the

M.A. Hameed and I. Dasgupta (✉)
Department of Nephrology, Heartlands Hospital, Birmingham, UK
e-mail: indranil.dasgupta@heartofengland.nhs.uk

relationship between sympathetic nervous system and elevated blood pressure by noting that exercise, passion and the presence of a doctor could all cause the pulse to increase in rate and tenseness (Freis 1995). The sympathetic nervous system is essential to the maintenance of systemic arterial pressure through changes in cardiac output, systemic vascular resistance, salt excretion and modulation of the renin angiotensin system in response to acute changes in blood pressure. Chronic activation of the sympathetic nervous system leads to increase in cardiac output and peripheral resistance, and retention of salt and water all of which play important roles in the development and maintenance of hypertension (Mark 1996). Increase in tubular sodium reabsorption, renin release and renal vascular resistance lead to shifting of the pressure natriuresis curve to the right and thus contributing to chronic elevation of blood pressure (Fig. 1).

It has been demonstrated in both animal models and humans that those with primary hypertension have higher sympathetic nerve activity (SNA) compared to those with normal blood pressure (Esler et al. 2003; Grassi et al. 1998; Yamada et al. 1989). Increased SNA causes vascular remodelling and smooth muscle hypertrophy leading to increased peripheral resistance (Oparil et al. 2003). These changes in the peripheral vasculature play important roles in the development and maintenance of chronic hypertension. Moreover, increased SNA in hypertension contributes to end organ damage as suggested by the correlation between left ventricular mass and reduced vascular compliance and elevated circulating noradrenaline (Marcus et al. 1994; Grassi et al. 1995). SNA overactivity may also be responsible for diastolic hypertension in young as indicated by the correlation between heart rate and diastolic blood pressure suggesting autonomic nervous system imbalance in the form of relative SNA overactivity (Kim et al. 1999). SNA overactivity has also been implicated in obesity related hypertension. Both the renal and cardiac sympathetic activities have been demonstrated to be increased in this situation (Esler 2000).

1.1 Mechanism of Sympathetic Stimulation in Hypertension

The mechanism of sympathetic stimulation in hypertension is complex but perhaps involves both baroreceptor and chemoreceptor pathways. Both central and peripheral baroreceptors are

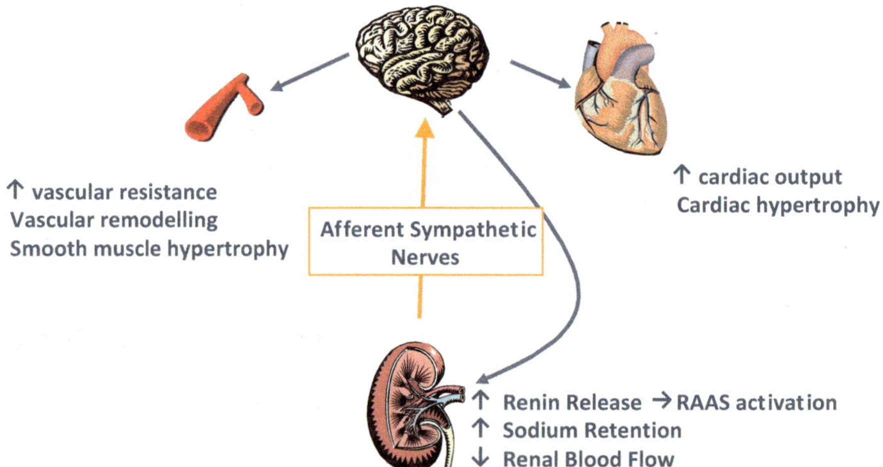

Fig. 1 Effects of sympathetic activation and the role of afferent renal sympathetic nerves in the development and control of hypertension (Reproduced with permission of Springer: The role of the kidney and the sympathetic nervous system in hypertension. Paediatric Nephrology 2015 (Thomas and Dasgupta 2015))

reset at higher blood pressures in hypertension; and returns to normal as blood pressure is lowered with treatment (Chapleau et al. 1988; Guo et al. 1983; Xie et al. 1990). Factors implicated in sympathetic stimulation are summarised in Box 1.

> **Box 1: Factors Implicated in Activation of Sympathetic Nervous System in Hypertension**
> - Abnormal sympathetic innervation and renal morphogenesis
> - Arterial baroreceptor resetting
> - Chemoreceptor stimulation to hypoxia and apnoea
> - Mental stress – recurrent stresses promotes increased vascular reactivity and maladaptive remodelling
> - Renal injury – stepwise relationship between declining renal function and SNA
> - Oxidative stress – experimental data show antioxidants reduce SNA
> - Reduced nitric oxide bioavailability – animal and human data showing ADMA correlates with SNA
> - Angiotensin II
> - Endothelin

Reproduced with permission of Springer: The role of the kidney and the sympathetic nervous system in hypertension. Paediatric Nephrology 2015 (Thomas and Dasgupta 2015).

1.2 Role of Renal Sympathetic Nerves in Hypertension

Renal nerves are the 'communication link between the central nervous system and the kidney'. The major structural and functional components of the kidney, the vessels, glomeruli, and tubules are innervated. In response to various stimuli, both mechanical and chemical, the efferent renal sympathetic nerves are activated. Activation of the efferent renal sympathetic nerves leads to reduction in renal blood flow and glomerular filtration rate, increase in renal tubular sodium and water reabsorption, and increase in renin release. Inhibition of these nerves has the functionally opposite effects. The afferent renal sympathetic nerves generally, in response to stretch, exert an inhibitory effect through facilitating sodium and water excretion. This reno-renal reflex plays an important role in maintaining sodium and water homeostasis in various physiological and pathological states. However, in states of kidney disease and injury the excitatory fibres in the afferent sympathetic nerves are stimulated which leads to increased peripheral and renal sympathetic nerve activity leading to peripheral vasoconstriction, increased cardiac output, renal vasoconstriction, increased renin release and tubular salt retention all of which contribute to elevation of systemic blood pressure. It is postulated that it is the activation of these fibres that contribute to initiation and maintenance of essential hypertension (DiBona and Sawin 1999; DiBona and Kopp 1995, 1997).

The evidence for the important role that the renal sympathetic nerve play in the pathogenesis and maintenance of hypertension come from animal experiments. There is a suggestion that the association between the SNS and the kidney starts in utero. In rodents, glial cell line-derived neurotrophic factor (GDNF) is essential to the normal development of renal sympathetic innervation and glomerular morphogenesis (Sainio et al. 1997). Deletion of a single GDNF gene in mice results in abnormal renal morphogenesis with the kidneys developing fewer, larger glomeruli and higher arterial pressures (~20 mmHg) compared to control animals with two copies of the gene (Cullen-McEwen et al. 2003). In spontaneously hypertensive rats (SHR), neonetal sympathectomy reduce blood pressure long-term (Gattone et al. 1990; Head 1989). This is further confirmed when kidneys from neonatally sympathectomised SHR are transplanted into untreated SHR. Mean arterial pressure is lower in these animals compared to the control group in which kidneys from hydralazine treated animals are transplanted into untreated SHR. This suggests that neonatal sympathectomy induces chronic changes to SHR kidney function leading to reduction of mean arterial pressure even when extrarenal sympathetic tone is restored (Grisk et al. 2002). It is suggested that it is the impairment of the reno-renal reflex mentioned above that contributes to the development of hypertension in SHR. Furthermore, there is a lot of evidence demonstrating renal denervation can delay development and attenuate several different types of experimental hypertension (Stella and Zancetti 1991).

Experiments in both rat models and humans have demonstrated that the SNS exhibits preferential activation of renal sympathetic fibres in response to baroreceptor unloading (Scislo et al. 1998; Johansson et al. 2003). In the human experiment enalaprilat, an intravenous angiotensin-converting enzyme inhibitor, was administered to healthy individuals. There was a minor drop in mean arterial pressure, but renal noradrenaline spillover increased to 26 % and 49 % in response to low and high dose enalaprilat respectively, whilst the cardiac and total body noradrenaline spillover remained constant. These findings suggest that in healthy individuals without activated renin angiotensin system, there is selective stimulation of renal sympathetic nerve activity in response to baroreceptor unloading (Johansson et al. 2003). Purported mediators of baroreflex resetting include angiotensin II and oxygen free radicals (Abboud 1974; Li et al. 1996).

1.3 Historical Treatments for Hypertension – Modulation of Sympathetic Activity

On the basis of the vasoconstrictor and cardioaccleratory properties of the sympathetic nervous system, a number of therapies have been developed in an attempt to modify the effect of the sympathetic nervous system on blood pressure (BP) control. Efficacy of these therapies further support the important role the SNA plays in hypertension. In 1923, Fritz Bruening performed the first surgical sympathectomy for hypertension based on the hypothesis that reduction of sympathetic outflow will lead to reduction in blood pressure (Freis 1990). This original concept was further developed by other surgeons such as Peet and Smithwick (Peet 1947; Smithwick and Thompson 1953) who performed more extensive operations termed splanchnicectomy which was offered to those with severe hypertension with evidence of cardiovascular damage. These procedures resulted in impressive reduction in blood pressure but were associated with significant surgical morbidities and complicated by orthostatic symptoms. With the availability of effective medical therapy these procedures were abandoned. However, the success of surgical sympathectomy in reducing high blood pressure led to the development of drugs producing chemical sympathectomy. A number of ganglion blocking agents were developed to treat hypertension like hexamethonium and tetraethylammonium chloride (Lyons et al. 1947; Paton and Zaimis 1948). These agents were the first pharmacological agents to block sympathetic outflow from the ganglion and also one of the earliest medical therapies for hypertension. Alpha-methyldopa a centrally acting anti-hypertensive agent which acts by inhibiting sympathetic outflow through binding to α_2 adrenoreceptors became available in the 1960s (Oates et al. 1960). Use of this drug is uncommon nowadays except in the context of hypertension in pregnancy. The role of sympathetic nervous system in the pathogenesis of hypertension is mediated by the alpha and beta adrenergic receptors. Beta-blockers were shown to be beneficial in the management of hypertension in 1964 (Prichard and Gillam 1964). The alpha-1 receptors present in the blood vessels are responsible for peripheral resistance. Selective alpha-1 receptor blockers were developed with a view to treating hypertension by reducing elevated total peripheral resistance (Nash 1990). However, in practice these agents have been found to have very modest blood pressure lowering effect (Heran et al. 2012).

Another example of sympathetic modulation to achieve blood pressure control is bilateral nephrectomy that used to be carried out in dialysis patients with refractory hypertension (Zazgornik et al. 1998). The improvement in blood pressure control in this situation is likely to be due to removal of the sympatho-excitatory effects of the damaged kidneys.

2 Catheter-Based Renal Denervation in Treatment Resistant Hypertension

A greater understanding of the role of the sympathetic nervous system in the pathogenesis and maintenance of primary hypertension and the lessons learnt from modulation of sympathetic activity in hypertension control has led to a number of novel device based therapies of which catheter based renal denervation (RDN) is the foremost. Initial encouraging results from clinical studies led to more than 10,000 procedures being carried out in treatment resistant hypertension (TRH) across the world in the last few years.

2.1 The Procedure

The renal nerves arise from T10 to L2 spinal segments, arborise around the renal artery and primarily lie within the adventitia of the artery. This presents an opportunity to ablate the renal sympathetic nerves percutaneously via the lumen of the main renal artery using a catheter connected to a radiofrequency generator. The access is gained through the common femoral artery which is punctured, under conscious sedation and local anaesthetic injection to the groin, using ultrasound guidance (Figs. 2 and 3). A guide sheath is introduced using a standard Seldinger technique. A renal angiogram is

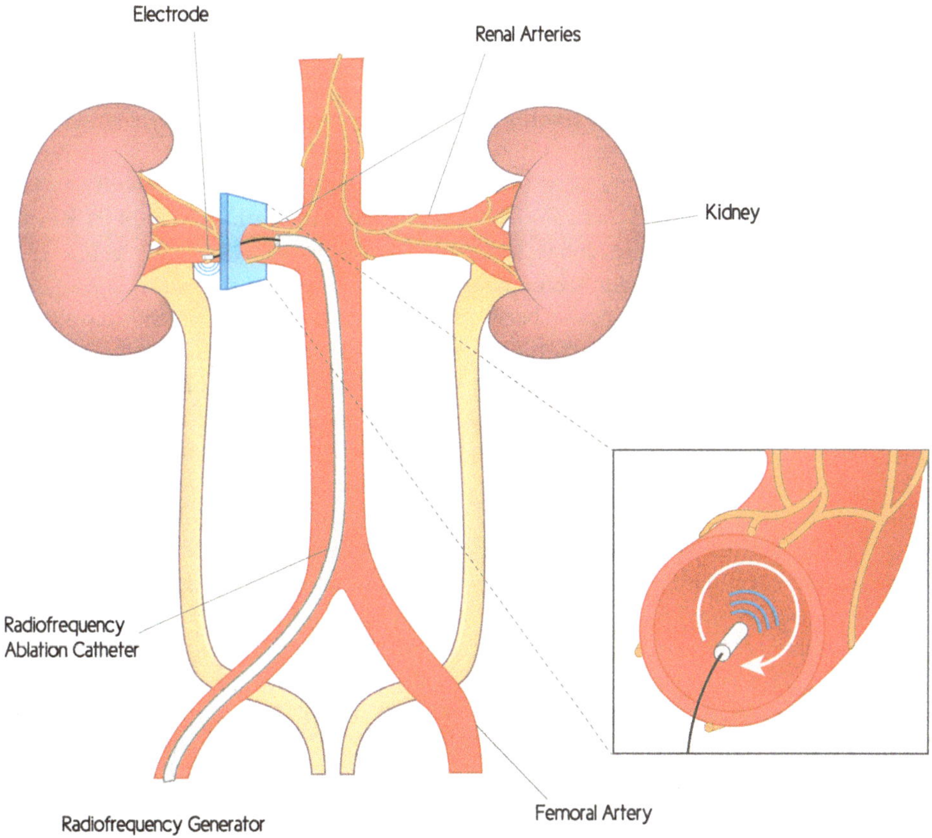

Fig. 2 Diagram demonstrating the radiofrequency renal denervation procedure

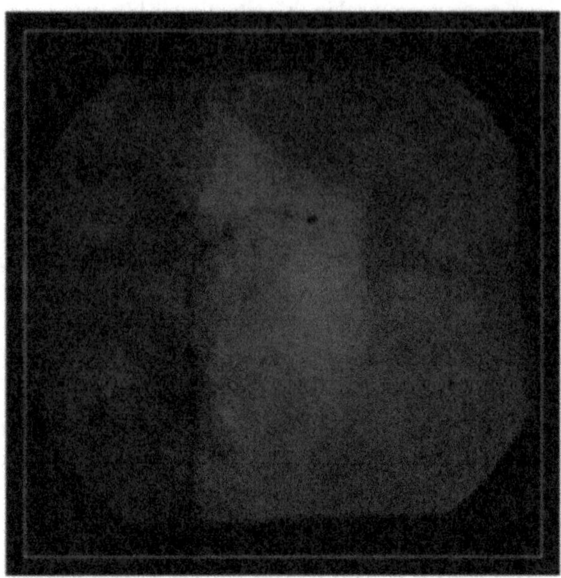

Fig. 3 Image showing renal denervation catheter in the left renal artery at the point of delivering radio-frequency ablation

performed using a non-ionic contrast agent to delineate the renal artery, ostia, bifurcation and accessory arteries. If the renal artery anatomy is suitable, a renal denervation catheter is positioned in the renal artery under fluoroscopic guidance at an initial position proximal to bifurcation of the renal artery. The early renal denervation catheters developed were unipolar with a flexible tip fitted with an electrode that can discharge radiofrequency waves when connected with a radiofrequency generator. More recently multipolar catheters of various designs have been developed. These are fitted with multiple electrodes capable of delivering multiple ablations simultaneously.

The treatment involves the delivery of relatively low power and precisely focused radiofrequency bursts through the wall of the renal artery to disrupt the surrounding renal nerves lying in the adventitia. Depending on the type of the catheter being used, unipolar or multipolar, it is repositioned after each treatment to ablate the sympathetic nerves in each quadrant of the renal artery in a helical pattern. Catheter tip temperature and impedance are constantly monitored during ablation, and radiofrequency energy delivery is regulated according to a predetermined algorithm. After a satisfactory treatment, a repeat selective renal arteriogram is taken to ensure patency of the renal artery post-ablation. The process is then repeated in the other renal artery and/or any accessory renal arteries. Following successful completion of the procedure a vascular closure device is deployed.

2.2 Pre-clinical and Proof of Principle Studies of Renal Denervation

The preclinical studies of catheter-based RDN were carried out in juvenile swine model. It was shown to be comparable to direct surgical RDN via renal artery transection and re-anastomosis. As proof of success, noradrenaline spillover rates were reduced by more than 85 % after denervation (Krum et al. 2009). In humans, bilateral renal denervation was demonstrated to reduce noradrenaline spillover, decrease renin activity, and increase renal plasma flow at 30 days after the procedure (Schlaich et al. 2009).

The proof-of-concept trial of RDN in humans (SYMPLICITY HTN-1), included 45 patients with treatment resistant hypertension with a clinic systolic blood pressure (BP) $\geq$160 mmHg who underwent RDN using the single electrode catheter (Symplicity catheter system, Ardian Inc. Mountain View, CA, USA; Medtronic Inc.,

Santa Rosa, CA, USA) (Krum et al. 2009). All patients were taking at least three anti-hypertensive agents of different classes including a diuretic. Significant reductions in office BP readings compared to baseline were observed, $-22/-11$ mmHg and $-27/-17$ mmHg at 6 month and 12 month after RDN respectively.

Serial estimated glomerular filtration rate (eGFR), renal angiography and magnetic resonance renal angiography (MRA) were used to assess safety of the procedure. The procedure was found to be safe with no significant change in renal function and no incidence of renal artery stenosis on the MRA at 6 months. Two patients experienced adverse events; one had renal artery dissection which occurred before any radio-frequency ablation could be applied to the artery and the second had a pseudoaneurysm at the femoral access site.

To assess physiological response of renal denervation, efferent sympathetic nervous system activity at the level of the kidneys was assessed by isotope dilution renal noradrenaline spillover testing in a subgroup of 10 patients. A mean reduction of noradrenaline spillover of 47 % (95 % confidence interval: 28–65 %) was observed 1 month after denervation. These observations, alongside the substantial reductions in clinic BP suggested successful targeting of efferent renal nerves. Therefore, this initial proof-of-concept study in human subjects demonstrated that the procedure was safe and was associated with a significant BP reduction at 1 year.

Furthermore, BP reduction following renal denervation was sustained. One hundred and fifty three patients undergoing open-label RDN, including the cohort of the proof of principle study, were followed up for 3 years. There was a mean reduction of 32/14 mmHg in office BP at 3 years with 93 % of the patients having a reduction in systolic BP of greater than ≥ 10 mmHg (Krum et al. 2014). The average number of BP-lowering medications prescribed at baseline and 36 months were similar. Sustained BP reduction suggested that re-growth of efferent nerve fibres had not occurred over time.

2.3 Further Clinical Studies Demonstrating Efficacy of Catheter Based Renal Denervation

An open-label, multicentre, randomised control trial (RCT) of renal denervation versus usual care in patients with TRH further supported the efficacy and safety of the procedure (SYMPLICITY HTN-2) (Esler et al. 2010). In this open labelled RCT, efficacy of RDN was compared against usual care; 106 patients were randomised to either RDN or a control arm. At 6 months, there was a 32/12 mmHg reduction in office BP in the RDN group, but no difference in office BP in the control arm, when compared with baseline BP. No procedural or device-based adverse events were observed.

Following these encouraging results a number of new catheter systems were developed and the efficacy tested in clinical trials. A meta-analysis of the early studies of renal denervation further supported the BP lowering benefits of this therapy (Davis et al. 2013). In the RCTs, there were reductions in mean office BP at 6 and 12 months of 28.9/11.0 mmHg and 25.4/10.0 mmHg respectively with RDN compared with medical therapy. Similar lowering in office BP was observed in uncontrolled studies; reductions of 25.0/10.0 mmHg and 22.8/10.6 mmHg respectively at 6 and 12 months post RDN compared with baseline.

2.3.1 Pitfalls of Early Studies of Renal Denervation

There were two main criticisms of early studies of catheter based renal denervation. Ambulatory blood pressure (ABP) readings were infrequently used for primary assessment of BP response. The few studies, which reported on the ABP, showed much lower BP reductions with a mean of 13.2/7.3 mmHg at 6 months after procedure compared with baseline (Davis et al. 2013). Secondly, there was absence of blinding due to the invasive nature of the procedure. Therefore, the placebo effect could not be excluded and the medication taking behaviour of the patient may have been altered by inclusion in a device-based trial.

2.4 The Sham Controlled Trial of Renal Denervation

Sham controlled trials are considered to be the most rigorous way of assessing efficacy of new surgical techniques or device-based interventions. As such, RDN was compared against a sham procedure where the patients randomised to the sham arm received a renal angiogram only (SYMPLICITY HTN-3) (Bhatt et al. 2014). This RCT included 535 patients with TRH across 88 centres in the USA and was designed to address the issues raised regarding the design of prior open-label RDN studies. The mean change in office systolic BP after 6 months were -14.1 mmHg and -11.7 mmHg respectively in the denervation and sham arms, an absolute difference of 2.4 mmHg between the groups. The primary efficacy end point, a difference of 5 mmHg between the groups in change of office systolic BP from baseline to 6 months, was not met. The secondary efficacy end point of a 2 mmHg difference between groups in change in 24-h ambulatory systolic BP was also not met; there was a reduction of 6.75 mmHg obtained in the denervation group and 4.79 mm Hg in the sham-procedure group. However, there was no difference between the groups in major safety end points, 1.4 % in denervation group versus 06 % in the sham group. Therefore, the sham-controlled study suggests that catheter based renal denervation is a safe procedure but does not lower BP effectively in patients with treatment resistant hypertension.

2.4.1 Critical Analysis of the Sham Controlled Study

Critical analysis of this study by the investigators and others suggest a number of factors which may have been associated with better BP response in some patients within this trial (Kandzari et al. 2015; Lobo et al. 2015a). Factors which have been shown to be associated with

favourable BP response within this trial include (Box 2):

> **Box 2: Factors Associated with Favourable Blood Pressure Response Observed in Clinical Studies of Renal Denervation**
> - Younger age (<65 years)
> - Non African American ethnic origin
> - Higher baseline office systolic blood pressure ($\geq$180 mmHg)
> - Concurrent use of aldosterone antagonists
> - Non-use of a vasodilator
> - Total number of ablations in both renal arteries ($\geq$12)
> - 4-quadrant ablation of renal arteries
> - Higher baseline eGFR ($\geq$60 ml/min/1.73m^2)

(a) Number of ablations: Consistently greater reductions in BP were observed in patients who received a higher number of renal artery ablations in the treatment group. An increased difference in office and ambulatory BPs with an increasing number of ablations was observed after patients in the two groups were propensity score matched for the baseline characteristics. This trend was shown to be statistically significant. Twelve or more ablations in both renal arteries were found to be predictive of a greater change in ambulatory systolic BP. There was no increase in safety events corresponding to the increasing number of renal artery ablations.

(b) Pattern of ablation: There was a trend towards an increasing BP response with delivery of ablations in a four-quadrant pattern to neither, one or both renal arteries. However, this was not statistically significant. In the treatment arm, only 19 (5 %) patients received four-quadrant ablations in both renal arteries.

(c) Younger age: The subgroup of patients <65 years in age was associated with office systolic BP change in the RDN group on univariate analysis but not in the multivariable model.

(d) Ethnicity: A significant difference in office SBP was observed in the non-American-African subgroup as compared with the African-American subgroup, but there was no significant difference observed in mean 24-h ambulatory BP or home BP.

(e) Higher baseline clinic systolic BP: Multivariable analysis of the overall group identified baseline office SBP $\geq$180 mmHg was a positive predictor of 6-month response of office BP reduction.

(f) Type of antihypertensive medications used: Multivariable analysis showed use of aldosterone antagonist to positively predict an increased 6 month change in office SBP. Conversely, use of vasodilators was found to be a negative predictor for change in office SBP at 6 months.

(g) Higher baseline eGFR: Baseline eGFR $\geq$60 mL/min/1.73 m^2 was shown to be an independent predictor of a greater change in ambulatory BP at 6 months.

Factors that may have contributed to the apparent ineffectiveness of RDN in the sham-controlled study are operator inexperience and medication adherence. The procedure-related predictors observed, four quadrant ablations and total number of ablations in both renal arteries, could be a consequence of operator inexperience of a relatively new procedure. In 88 centres in the US, where the study was conducted, 364 RDN procedures were carried out. One hundred and eleven interventionists performed at least one procedure, with approximately one third doing one procedure and only 26 operators doing more than five procedures suggesting the majority of interventionists were relatively inexperienced with the RDN procedure (Lobo et al. 2015a). The procedure had been unlicensed in the US prior to this trial so the learning curve of the operators fell within the period of the trial.

Adherence to prescribed antihypertensive medication was assessed by self-reported diary completed by the patient. This is an indirect method of assessing mediation adherence which does not prove actual ingestion, is open to manipulation and is likely to over-estimate adherence. It is important to assess adherence to prescribed antihypertensive medication in patients with TRH objectively as up to half may be completely or partially non-adherent (Hameed et al. 2016; Rosa et al. 2014). Inclusion in a clinical trial may result in a change in the subjects' pill-taking behaviour due to their awareness of being observed. This phenomenon is termed 'the Hawthorne effect'.

2.5 Results of Studies Published After the Sham Controlled Trial

Since the publication of SYMPLICITY HTN-3, a number of studies have been published which help us understand the role of RDN in the management of treatment resistant hypertension and give us a future direction. Some of the main studies are described here.

A prospective, open-label, multicentre registry was set up to assess the safety and efficacy of RDN (Global SYMPLICITY Registry) (Böhm et al. 2015). The results of nearly 1000 patients undergoing RDN around the world confirm the favourable safety profile of the procedure. The mean 6-month reduction in office and 24-h ambulatory systolic BP were 11.6 mmHg and 6.6 mmHg respectively. This was a real-world registry with more lenient inclusion criteria. The greatest reduction in clinic and 24-h ambulatory systolic BPs (20.3 mmHg and 8.9 mmHg respectively) were seen in patients with severe hypertension at baseline: office systolic BP $\geq$160 mmHg with a 24-h ambulatory systolic BP $\geq$135 mmHg and taking $\geq$3 antihypertensive medication.

The results of an open-label, multicentre RCT of stepped-care standardised antihypertensive treatment (SSAHT) with or without RDN for TRH was published (Denervation for Resistant Hypertension, DNERHTN) (Azizi et al. 2015). This was a rigorously designed trial which randomised patients to either RDN or to continue on SSAHT after confirmation of TRH by ABPM 4 weeks after having been commenced on SSAHT. There were 48 patients in the RDN group and 53 patients in the control group. Adherence to antihypertensive medications was assessed using a validated Morisky Medication Adherence Scale [MMAS-8] and 24-h ABPM was used to measure the primary efficacy of RDN in this trial.

The results showed a reduction of 15.4/ 9.7 mmHg and 9.5/6.6 mmHg in the 24-h ABPM for RDN and control groups respectively with a difference of 5.9/3.1 mmHg between the groups. There was a statistically significant reduction in 24-h ambulatory SBP in patients with proven TRH receiving RDN in addition to the standardised antihypertensive regimens as recommended by European and UK hypertension guidelines. Therefore, although this was an open-label study, this study addressed the two of the factors that may have affected the results of the sham-controlled study, i.e. use of ABP as primary measure of efficacy and more formal adherence testing.

However, another RCT compared RDN to intensified pharmacotherapy including spironolactone showed no significant difference in BP reductions (ambulatory and office) in the two groups (the PRAGUE-15 study) (Rosa et al. 2015). This was the first RCT to include patients with true TRH by excluding non-adherence using quantitative plasma drugs level measurements, white-coat hypertension, and secondary causes of hypertension. Unlike the previous RCT (Azizi et al. 2015), the antihypertensive regimen here was not standardised and spironolactone was added in the intensified pharmacotherapy arm of the study.

Another real world study (UK Renal Denervation Affiliation, UKRDA) involving 253 patients with true TRH reported a drop of 22/9 mmHg and 12/7 mmHg in clinic and ambulatory BP respectively at 11 months, which was independent of medication changes during follow-up and use of aldosterone antagonists (Sharp et al. 2016). Furthermore, patients in the two highest quartiles of daytime ambulatory systolic blood pressure at baseline (mean systolic ABP at baseline of 176 and 199 mmHg respectively) exhibited significant ambulatory blood pressure reductions (22 and 14 mmHg respectively), whilst those in the lowest quartile exhibited little response. Table 1 summarises

the major clinical studies of renal denervation to date, including their strengths and weaknesses.

2.6 Future Direction

Although sound physiological principles and surgical precedent underpin renal denervation as a therapy for treatment resistant hypertension, clinical studies so far have produced conflicting results. Further research is required before its implementation in routine clinical management of TRH. Lessons learnt from these studies are listed below which should be considered in future clinical research.

2.6.1 Appropriate Patient Selection

The results the clinical trials of renal denervation suggest younger patients (<65 years), those with normal kidney function, and those with higher baseline office BP (systolic $\geq$180 mmHg) respond best to RDN. Patients should have a thorough assessment to confirm the presence of true TRH with exclusion of white-coat effect, non-adherence and secondary causes of hypertension. Reliable methods are now available to test adherence to antihypertensives using urine samples (Lawson et al. 2016; Tomaszewski et al. 2014) which have confirmed that up to 50 % of patients with TRH are partially or completely non-adherent (Jung et al. 2013).

2.6.2 Medication Optimisation

Patients with TRH in the trials of RDN were on 4–5 antihypertensive agents on average. There is now good evidence from trials of pharmacological intervention to recommend the addition of an aldosterone receptor antagonist (AA) to the routine combination of a thiazide diuretic, a calcium channel-blocker and a renin angiotensin system blocking agents to treat TRH (Williams et al. 2015; Dahal et al. 2015). Post hoc analysis of SYMPLICITY HTN-3 also shows higher response rate to denervation in patients taking AAs (Kandzari et al. 2015). Any trials designed to test the efficacy of RDN should consider all patients to be started on a standardised regimen

Table 1 A table showing studies of renal denervation including their methods, primary outcomes, strengths and weaknesses

Study	Method	Number of patients	Primary outcome	Strength	Weaknesses
SYMPLICITY HTN-1 (Krum et al. 2014)	Single-arm, open-label, case-series	153	Change in clinic BP at 6 months post-RDN: −22/−10 mmHg (150) Change in clinic BP at 3 years post-RDN: −32/−14 mmHg (88)	First proof-of-concept study demonstrating safety and efficacy of RDN	No ABPM measurements
				Patients followed up for 3 years	
				Assessment of noradrenaline spillover	Lack of a comparator group
				RDN shown to be safe	
SYMPLICITY HTN-2 (Esler et al. 2010)	Open label, RCT, RDN vs usual treatment	106 (52 RDN; 56 control)	Difference in mean clinic BP at 6 months post-RDN between RDN and usual Rx: −33/−12 mmHg	Randomised controlled trial	Un-blinded
				Statistically powered to detect a difference between RDN and usual Rx.	
				RDN shown to be safe	
SYMPLICITY HTN-3 (Bhatt et al. 2014)	Single blinded, RCT, RDN vs sham procedure	535 (364 RDN; 171 Sham)	Difference in mean clinic systolic BP at 6 months post-RDN between RDN and Sham: −2.4 mmHg	Largest RCT of RDN	Change in ABPM not a primary endpoint.
				Sham comparator group	
				Confirms safety of RDN	Lack of operator experience resulting in inadequate ablation self-reported medication adherence assessment
Global SYMPLICITY Registry (Böhm et al. 2015)	Single-arm, open-label, case series	998	Change in Clinic and 24-h mean SBP at 6 months: −11.5 and −6.6 respectively.	Real-life use of RDN	Heterogonous inclusion criteria
				Analysis shows severe hypertension more likely to be responders	SYMPLICITY catheter only

(continued)

Table 1 (continued)

Study	Method	Number of patients	Primary outcome	Strength	Weaknesses
DNERHTN (Azizi et al. 2015)	Open label, RCT, RDN vs stepped-care standardised antihypertensive treatment (SSAHT)	106 (53 RDN, 53 SSAHT)	Difference in mean 24-h ambulatory BP at 6 months between RDN and SSAHT: −5.9/−3.1 mmHg	Change in ABPM is the primary outcome	Non-use of aldosterone antagonists
				Experienced operators	
				Standardised antihypertensive regimens used	Unblinded (No sham procedure)
				Validated questionnaire used for adherence assessment	
PRAGUE-15 (Rosa et al. 2015)	Open label, RCT, RDN vs intensified pharmacotherapy (PHAR)	106 (52 RDN; 54 PHAR)	Difference in mean 24-h ambulatory BP at 6 months between RDN and PHAR: −0.5/−1.1 mmHg	True resistant hypertension confirmed.	Unblinded (No sham procedure)
				Adherence confirmed using plasma antihypertensive drug level	
				Use of aldosterone	
				Change in ABPM is the primary outcome	
UK renal denervation affiliation report (Sharp et al. 2016)	Single-arm, open-label, case series	253	Change in mean daytime ABP after an average of 8.5 months following RDN: −12/−7 mmHg	Well characterised group of patients	No control/sham group for comparison
				High percentage of patients with ambulatory BP results	Retrospective registry
				Real-life use of RDN	
EnligHTN I (Thomas and Dasgupta 2015; Worthley et al. 2013)	Single-arm, open label, series	46	Change in clinic BP at 6 months post-RDN: −26/−10 mmHg	Multi-electrode catheter	Observational study
EnliHTN II (Lobo et el. 2015b)	Single-arm, open label, series	103	Change in clinic BP at 6 months post-RDN: −18/−8 mmHg	Multi-electrode catheter	Observational study
EnligHTN III (Worthley et al. 2015)	Single-arm, open label, series	39	Change in clinic BP at 6 months post-RDN: −25/−7 mmHg	Multi-electrode catheter	Observational study

of antihypertensives, as used in the DNERHTN, with 6–8 weeks of time to allow the medication to take their full affect before RDN is attempted. Adherence assessment, using a direct method such as urine drug analysis, should be made at each post RDN visit to allow the researchers to attribute any BP changes observed directly to RDN.

2.6.3 Appropriate Efficacy Assessment

Studies of denervation should be powered for difference in ABPM, as it is less sensitive to regression to the mean (O'Brien et al. 2013; Warren et al. 2010), rather than office BP.

2.6.4 Procedural Development

Failure of SYMPLICITY HTN-3 to meet its primary efficacy may be in part due to operator inexperience in RDN as highlighted above. Recently, Sakakura and colleagues have shown from autopsy examination of renal arteries of 20 patients with hypertension (Sakakura et al. 2014) that the distance from renal artery lumen to nerve location is shortest (mean 2.6 mm) in the distal arterial segments compared with the proximal (mean 3.4 mm) and middle segments (mean 3.1 mm), although the volume of renal nerves is higher in the proximal and mid-vessel. As radiofrequency waves do not penetrate deeper than 3 mm, it is possible that the variable responses seen between variable open-label studies and sham controlled study of RDN is related to the mechanism and technique by which ablations were delivered. In future studies, efforts should be made to deliver radiofrequency energies distally in the renal artery with a view to achieving more complete denervation of the kidney.

Multi-electrode catheters have now been developed to deliver radio-frequency ablations simultaneously to multiple points around the renal artery. Use of these catheters will help deliver four quadrant ablations and increase the number of ablations producing more complete denervation.

2.6.5 Need for a Test to Confirm Adequacy of Renal Denervation

Currently there is no simple way of assessing whether adequate denervation has taken place. Regional noradrenaline spillover and peroneal muscle sympathetic nerve activity are two methods which have been used to assess the effect of RDN on sympathetic activity (Esler et al. 1984a; Esler et al. 1984b; Vallbo et al. 1979). However, due to the invasive nature of these techniques and the expertise required to perform these tests, there is limited uptake of these tests in clinical trials let alone in routine clinical practice. Therefore, there is a need for a test which will allow confirmation of successful denervation, ideally whilst the patient is still on the table to allow the operator to make adjustments as necessary.

2.6.6 Identifying Predictors of Response

There is heterogeneity in the level of BP-response to RDN. It will be helpful to be able to predict which patients with TRH are more likely to respond to RDN. This will allow appropriate patient selection for selective use of the technique with greater success. Post hoc-analyses of clinical trials of RDN, Global Symplicity Registry and UKRDA have highlighted patient and procedure related predictors of response. Other studies have focussed upon physiological testing and biochemical markers of response to RDN. In a clinical trial of RDN the use of baroreflex sensitivity (BRS) has been tested as a predictive marker of response to RDN (Zuern et al. 2013). The results of this study show that cardiac BRS is a strong and independent predictor of response to RDN in patients with TRH. Another study examined the effect of RDN on angiogenic markers, and found intercellular cell adhesion molecule-1 [ICAM-1] and vascular cell adhesion molecule-1 [VCAM-1] and fms-like tyrosine kinase-1 [sFLT-1]) predict response to RDN (Dorr et al. 2014).

3 Ultrasound Renal Denervation

High frequency ultrasound renal denervation is a non-invasive form of renal denervation which is undergoing clinical trial at present. It is based on delivery of externally focused ultrasound to the renal nerves using Doppler based ultrasound image guidance to track and automatically correct for renal artery motion during treatment. The novel applicator used incorporates an anatomically customized phased-array ultrasound transducer to generate and focus therapeutic energy to the depth of the renal artery, and an ultrasound imaging transducer to facilitate locating, targeting and tracking the renal artery for treatment.

Following preliminary feasibility studies in an open animal model, studies were performed using the external applicator system in Yorkshire swine. There was a 71 % reduction in norepinephrine levels at 1 week following renal denervation which persisted for 6 weeks demonstrating the feasibility of targeted external ultrasound for renal sympathetic denervation in an animal model and supported further investigation in patients with hypertension (Brinton et al. 2011).

The proof of principle study of twenty-four patients with refractory hypertension demonstrated a 27 mmHg reduction in systolic blood pressure at 6 months after denervation treatment. This initial technique utilised external focused ultrasound navigated by a targeting catheter in the renal artery. In the second phase of the study, 13 patients with resistant hypertension underwent bilateral externally focused ultrasound utilizing a 5 F intravascular catheter for targeting and tracking. The procedure was well tolerated except one patient complained of back pain lasting 24 h. At 6 week follow up an 18 mmHg reduction in office systolic blood pressure was noted (Neuzil et al. 2013).

In the next stage, a fully non-invasive ultrasound renal denervation was studied on 23 patients with resistant hypertension with office systolic blood pressure greater than 160 mmHg taking more than 3 antihypertensive medications. At 6 weeks the investigators reported an average reduction of office systolic blood pressure of 23 mmHg. Six patients experienced back pain resolving with 24 h of the procedure (Ormiston et al. 2014).

This technology appears promising. Currently, an international multicentre phase 3 randomised controlled trial, in patients with treatment resistant hypertension, is underway, comparing targeted ultrasound renal denervation with sham treatment. If this study shows significant blood pressure reduction in the treatment arm, it may prove to be a useful non-invasive device-based therapy for treatment of treatment resistant hypertension.

4 Conclusion

Hypertension is one of the most preventable causes of premature morbidity and mortality in the world. Treatment-resistant hypertension is a major clinical problem that requires further treatment options. Catheter based renal denervation is a technology borne out of sound basic science and clinical precedent. Clinical studies of this technology in treatment resistant hypertension so far have produced conflicting results. Critical analysis of these studies suggest that there are a number of patient related and procedural factors which will need to be addressed in future studies before implementation of catheter based renal denervation in routine clinical practice. Non-invasive ultrasound renal denervation is an exciting innovation currently undergoing rigorous clinical trial before it becomes available in the clinic (Box 3).

Box 3: Factors to Be Considered for Future Research in Renal Denervation for Treatment Resistant Hypertension

- Appropriate patient selection
  - age ($<$65 years)
  - baseline office systolic BP at high end ($\geq$180 mmHg)
  - exclusion of white coat effect, secondary hypertension and nonadherence to antihypertensive medication
- Medication optimisation
  - standardised regimen of medication for at least 6 weeks before procedure
  - aldosterone antagonists
  - adherence testing at every visit following renal denervation using direct method, e.g. urine assay
- Use of 24 h ambulatory blood pressure to assess efficacy
- Improvement in procedural factors
  - use of multipolar catheters to achieve maximum number of ablations ($\geq$12)
  - distal ablations
- Need for a test to confirm adequacy of denervation at the time of procedure
- Identification of predictors of response to improve patient selection
  - Clinical
  - baro-reflex sensitivity
  - ?angiogenic markers

References

Abboud FM (1974) Effects of sodium, angiotensin, and steroids on vascular reactivity in man. Fed Proc 33:143–149

Azizi M, Sapoval M, Gosse P, Monge M, Bobrie G, Delsart P et al (2015) Optimum and stepped care standardised antihypertensive treatment with or without renal denervation for resistant hypertension (DENERHTN): a multicentre, open-label, randomised controlled trial. The Lancet 385(9981):1957–1965

Bhatt DL, Kandzari DE, O'Neill WW, D'Agostino R, Flack JM, Katzen BT et al (2014) A controlled trial of renal denervation for resistant hypertension. N Engl J Med 370(15):1393–1401

Böhm M, Mahfoud F, Ukena C, Hoppe UC, Narkiewicz K, Negoita M et al (2015) First report of the global SYMPLICITY registry on the effect of renal artery denervation in patients with uncontrolled hypertension. Hypertension 65(4):766–774

Brinton T, Anderson T, Zhang J, Gertner M (2011) Ultrasound mediated renal sympathetic denervation. Circulation 124:A12272 (Abstract)

Chapleau MW, Hajduczok G, Abboud FM (1988) Mechanisms of resetting of arterial baroreceptors: an overview. Am J Med Sci 295:327–334

Cullen-McEwen LA, Kett MM, Dowling J, Anderson WP, Bertram JF (2003) Nephron number, renal function, and arterial pressure in aged GDNF heterozygous mice. Hypertension 41:335–340

Dahal K, Kunwar S, Rijal J, Alqatahni F, Panta R, Ishak N et al (2015) The effects of aldosterone antagonists in patients with resistant hypertension: a meta-analysis of randomized and nonrandomized studies. Am J Hypertens 28(11):1376–1385

Davis MI, Filion KB, Zhang D, Eisenberg MJ, Afilalo J, Schiffrin EL et al (2013) Effectiveness of renal denervation therapy for resistant hypertension: a systematic review and meta-analysis. J Am Coll Cardiol 62 (3):231–241

DiBona GF, Kopp UC (1995) Neural control of renal function: role in human hypertension. In: Laragh JH, Brenner BM (eds) Hypertension: pathophysiology, diagnosis, and management, 2nd edn. Raven, New York, pp 1349–1358

DiBona GF, Kopp UC (1997) Neural control of renal function. Physiol Rev 77:75–197

DiBona GF, Sawin LL (1999) Functional significance of the pattern of renal sympathetic nerve activation. Am J Physiol 277:R346–R353

Dorr O, Liebetrau C, Mollmann H, Gaede L, Troidl C, Rixe J et al (2014) Soluble fms-like tyrosine kinase-1 and endothelial adhesion molecules (intercellular cell adhesion molecule-1 and vascular cell adhesion molecule-1) as predictive markers for blood pressure reduction after renal sympathetic denervation. Hypertension 63(5):984–990

Esler M (2000) The sympathetic system and hypertension. Am J Hypertens 13:99S–105S

Esler M, Jennings G, Korner P, Blombery P, Sacharias N, Leonard P (1984a) Measurement of total and organ-specific norepinephrine kinetics in humans. Am J Physiol 247:E21–E28

Esler M, Jennings G, Leonard P, Sacharias N, Burke F, Johns J et al (1984b) Contribution of individual organs to total noradrenaline release in humans. Acta Physiol Scand Suppl 527:11–16

Esler M, Lambert G, Brunner-La Rocca HP, Vaddadi G, Kaye D (2003) Sympathetic nerve activity and neurotransmitter release in humans: translation from pathophysiology into clinical practice. Acta Physiol Scand 177(3):275–284

Esler MD, Krum H, Sobotka PA, Schlaich MP, Schmieder RE, Böhm M (2010) Renal sympathetic denervation in patients with treatment-resistant hypertension (The Symplicity HTN-2 Trial): a randomised controlled trial. The Lancet 376(9756):1903–9

Freis ED (1990) Origins and development of antihypertensive treatment. In: Laragh JH, Brenner BM (eds) Hypertension: pathophysiology, diagnosis, and management, 2nd edn. Raven, New York, pp 2093–2094

Freis ED (1995) Historical development of antihypertensive treatment. In: Laragh JH, Brenner BM (eds) Hypertension: pathophysiology, diagnosis, and management, 2nd edn. Raven, New York, pp 2741–2751

Gattone VH, Evan AP, Overhage JM, Severs WB (1990) Developing renal innervation in the spontaneously hypertensive rat: evidence for a role of the sympathetic nervous system in renal damage. J Hypertens 8:423–428

Grassi G, Giannattasio C, Failla M, Pesenti A, Peretti G, Marinoni E et al (1995) Sympathetic modulation of radial artery compliance in congestive heart failure. Hypertension 26(2):348–354

Grassi G, Colombo M, Seravalle G, Spaziani D, Mancia G (1998) Dissociation between muscle and skin sympathetic nerve activity in essential hypertension, obesity, and congestive heart failure. Hypertension 31(1):64–67

Grisk O, Rose H-J, Lorenz G, Rettig R (2002) Sympathetic – renal interaction in chronic arterial pressure control. Am J Physiol Regul Integr Comp Physiol 283: R441–R450

Guo GB, Thames MD, Abboud FM (1983) Arterial baroreflexes in renal hypertensive rabbits. Selectivity and redundancy of baroreceptor influence on heart rate, vascular resistance, and lumbar sympathetic nerve activity. Circ Res 53:223–234

Hameed MA, Tebbit L, Jacques N, Thomas M, Dasgupta I (2016) Non-adherence to antihypertensive medication is very common among resistant hypertensives: results of a directly observed therapy clinic. J Hum Hypertens 30(2):83–9

Head RJ (1989) Hypernoradrenergic innervation: its relationship to functional and hyperplastic changes in the vasculature of the spontaneously hypertensive rat. Blood Vessels 26:1–20

Heran BS, Galm BP, Wright JM (2012) Blood pressure lowering efficacy of alpha blockers for primary hypertension. Cochrane Database Syst Rev 15(8): CD004643. doi:10.1002/14651858.CD004643.pub3

Johansson M, Rundqvist B, Petersson M, Lambert G, Friberg P (2003) Regional norepinephrine spillover in response to angiotensin-converting enzyme inhibition in healthy subjects. J Hypertens 21:1371–1375

Jung O, Gechter JL, Wunder C, Paulke A, Bartel C, Geiger H et al (2013) Resistant hypertension? Assessment of adherence by toxicological urine analysis. J Hypertens 31(4):766–774

Kandzari DE, Bhatt DL, Brar S, Devireddy CM, Esler M, Fahy M et al (2015) Predictors of blood pressure response in the SYMPLICITY HTN-3 trial. Eur Heart J 36(4):219–227

Kim JR, Kiefe CI, Liu K, Williams OD, Jacobs DR Jr, Oberman A (1999) Heart rate and subsequent blood pressure in young adults: the CARDIA study. Hypertension 33(2):640–646

Krum H, Schlaich M, Whitbourn R, Sobotka PA, Sadowski J, Bartus K et al (2009) Catheter-based renal sympathetic denervation for resistant hypertension: a multicentre safety and proof-of-principle cohort study. The Lancet 373(9671):1275–1281

Krum H, Schlaich MP, Sobotka PA, Böhm M, Mahfoud F, Rocha-Singh K et al (2014) Percutaneous renal denervation in patients with treatment-resistant hypertension: final 3-year report of the Symplicity HTN-1 study. The Lancet 383(9917):622–629

Lawson AJ, Shipman KE, George S, Dasgupta I (2016) A novel 'dilute-and-shoot' liquid chromatography-tandem mass spectrometry method for the screening of antihypertensive drugs in urine. J Anal Toxicol 40 (1):17–27

Li Z, Mao HZ, Abboud FM, Chapleau MW (1996) Oxygen-derived free radicals contribute to baroreceptor dysfunction in atherosclerotic rabbits. Circ Res 79:802–811

Lobo MD, de Belder MA, Cleveland T, Collier D, Dasgupta I, Deanfield J et al (2015a) Joint UK societies' 2014 consensus statement on renal denervation for resistant hypertension. Heart 101:10–16. doi:10.1136/heartjnl-2014-307029

Lobo M, Saxena M, Jain AJ, Walters D, Pincus M, Montarello J et al (2015b) 4a.09: safety and performance of the enlightn renal denervation system in patients with severe uncontrolled hypertension: 12 month results from the Enlightn Ii Study. J Hypertens 33(Suppl 1):e51

Lyons RH, Moe GK, Neligh RM, Hoobler SW, Campbell KN, Berry RL et al (1947) The effects of blockade of the autonomic ganglia in man with tetraethylammonium; preliminary observations on its clinical application. Am J Med Sci 213:315–323

Marcus R, Krause L, Weder AB, Dominguez-Meja A, Schork NJ, Julius S (1994) Sex-specific determinants of increased left ventricular mass in the Tecumseh Blood Pressure Study. Circulation 90(2):928–936

Mark AL (1996) The sympathetic nervous system in hypertension: a potential long-term regulator of arterial pressure. J Hypertens Suppl 14(5):S159–65

Nash DT (1990) Alpha-adrenergic blockers: mechanism of action, blood pressure control, and effects of lipoprotein metabolism. Clin Cardiol 13:764–772

Neuzil P, Whitbourn R, Starek Z, Esler M, Brinton T, Gertner M (2013) Optimized external focused ultrasound for renal sympathetic denervation – wave II trial. J Am Coll Cardiol 62(18_S1):B20–B20 (Abstract)

O'Brien E, Parati G, Stergiou G, Asmar R, Beilin L, Bilo G et al (2013) European Society of Hypertension position paper on ambulatory blood pressure monitoring. J Hypertens 31(9):1731–1768

Oates JA, Gillespie L Jr, Udenfiiend S, Sjoerdsma A (1960) Decarboxylase inhibition and blood pressure reduction by alpha-methyl-3,4-dihydroxy-DL-phenylalanine. Science 131:1890–1891

Oparil S, Zaman MA, Calhoun DA (2003) Pathogenesis of hypertension. Ann Intern Med 139(9):761–776

Ormiston J et al (2014) Non-invasive renal denervation using externally delivered focused ultrasound: early experience using Doppler-based image targeting and tracking for treatment. J Am Coll Cardiol 64/11(Suppl B): TCT–412. (Abstract)

Paton WDM, Zaimis EJ (1948) Clinical potentialities of certain bisquaternary salts causing neuromuscular and ganglionic block. Nature 162:810

Peet MM (1947) Results of bilateral supradiaphragmatic splanchnicectomy for arterial hypertension. N Engl J Med 236:270–276

Prichard BN, Gillam PM (1964) Use of propranolol (Inderal) in treatment of hypertension. Br Med J 2:725–732

Rosa J, Zelinka T, Petrak O, Strauch B, Somloova Z, Indra T et al (2014) Importance of thorough investigation of resistant hypertension before renal denervation: should compliance to treatment be evaluated systematically? J Hum Hypertens 28(11):684–688

Rosa J, Widimský P, Toušek P, Petrák O, Curila K, Waldauf P et al (2015) Randomized comparison of renal denervation versus intensified pharmacotherapy including spironolactone in true-resistant hypertension: six-month results from the Prague-15 study. Hypertension 65(2):407–413

Sainio K, Suvanto P, Davies J, Wartiovaara J, Wartiovaara K, Saarma M et al (1997) Glial-cell-line-derived neurotrophic factor is required for bud initiation from ureteric epithelium. Development 124:4077–4087

Sakakura K, Ladich E, Cheng Q, Otsuka F, Yahagi K, Fowler DR et al (2014) Anatomic assessment of sympathetic peri-arterial renal nerves in man. J Am Coll Cardiol 64(7):635–643

Schlaich MP, Sobotka PA, Krum H, Lambert E, Esler MD (2009) Renal sympathetic-nerve ablation for uncontrolled hypertension. N Engl J Med 361 (9):932–934

Scislo TJ, Augustyniak RA, O'Leary DS (1998) Differential arterial baroreflex regulation of renal, lumbar, and adrenal sympathetic nerve activity in the rat. Am J Physiol 275:R995–R1002

Sharp AS, Davies JE, Lobo MD, Bent CL, Mark PB, Burchell AE et al (2016) Renal artery sympathetic denervation: observations from the UK experience. Clin Res Cardiol:1–9. doi:10.1007/s00392-015-0959-4

Smithwick RH, Thompson JE (1953) Splanchnicectomy for essential hypertension; results in 1,266 cases. JAMA 152:1501–1504

Stella A, Zancetti A (1991) Role of renal affarents. Physiological Reviews 71(3):659–682

Thomas P, Dasgupta I (2015) The role of the kidney and the sympathetic nervous system in hypertension. Paediatric Nephrology 30(4):549–60. doi:10.1007/s00467-014-2789-4

Tomaszewski M, White C, Patel P, Masca N, Damani R, Hepworth J et al (2014) High rates of non-adherence to antihypertensive treatment revealed by high-performance liquid chromatography-tandem mass spectrometry (HP LC-MS/MS) urine analysis. Heart 100:855–61

Vallbo AB, Hagbarth KE, Torebjork HE, Wallin BG (1979) Somatosensory, proprioceptive, and sympathetic activity in human peripheral nerves. Physiol Rev 59:919–957

Warren RE, Marshall T, Padfield PL, Chrubasik S (2010) Variability of office, 24-hour ambulatory, and self-monitored blood pressure measurements. Br J Gen Pract 60(578):675–680

Williams B, MacDonald TM, Morant S, Webb DJ, Sever P, McInnes G et al (2015) Spironolactone versus placebo, bisoprolol, and doxazosin to determine the optimal treatment for drug-resistant hypertension (PATHWAY-2): a randomised, double-blind, crossover trial. The Lancet 386(10008):2059–2068

Worthley SG, Tsioufis CP, Worthley MI, Sinhal A, Chew DP, Meredith IT et al (2013) Safety and efficacy of a multi-electrode renal sympathetic denervation system in resistant hypertension: the EnligHTN I trial. Eur Heart J 34(28):2132–2140

Worthley SG, Wilkins GT, Webster MW, Montarello JK, Antonis PR, Whitbourn RJ, et al (2015) Safety and performance of the next generation EnligHTN™ renal denervation system in patients with drug-resistant, uncontrolled hypertension: The EnligHTN III first-in-human multicentre study. Clin Trials Reg Sci Cardiol 8(8):4–10

Xie PL, Chapleau MW, McDowell TS, Hajduczok G, Abboud FM (1990) Mechanism of decreased baroreceptor activity in chronic hypertensive rabbits. Role of endogenous prostanoids. J Clin Invest 86:625–630

Yamada Y, Miyajima E, Tochikubo O, Matsukawa T, Ishii M (1989) Age-related changes in muscle sympathetic nerve activity in essential hypertension. Hypertension 13(6 Pt 2):870–877

Zazgornik J, Biesenbach G, Janko O, Gross C, Mair R, Brücke P et al (1998) Bilateral nephrectomy: the best, but often overlooked, treatment for refractory hypertension in hemodialysis patients. J Am Hypertens 11:1364–1370

Zuern CS, Eick C, Rizas KD, Bauer S, Langer H, Gawaz M et al (2013) Impaired cardiac baroreflex sensitivity predicts response to renal sympathetic denervation in patients with resistant hypertension. J Am Coll Cardiol 62(22):2124–30

Adv Exp Med Biol - Advances in Internal Medicine (2017) 2: 279–306
DOI 10.1007/5584_2016_85
© Springer International Publishing AG 2016
Published online: 22 November 2016

Subclinical Kidney Damage in Hypertensive Patients: A Renal Window Opened on the Cardiovascular System. Focus on Microalbuminuria

Giuseppe Mulè, Antonella Castiglia, Claudia Cusumano, Emilia Scaduto, Giulio Geraci, Dario Altieri, Epifanio Di Natale, Onofrio Cacciatore, Giovanni Cerasola, and Santina Cottone

Abstract

The kidney is one of the major target organs of hypertension.

Kidney damage represents a frequent event in the course of hypertension and arterial hypertension is one of the leading causes of end-stage renal disease (ESRD).

ESRD has long been recognized as a strong predictor of cardiovascular (CV) morbidity and mortality. However, over the past 20 years a large and consistent body of evidence has been produced suggesting that CV risk progressively increases as the estimated glomerular filtration rate (eGFR) declines and is already significantly elevated even in the earliest stages of renal damage. Data was supported by the very large collaborative meta-analysis of the Chronic Kidney Disease Prognosis Consortium, which provided undisputable evidence that there is an inverse association between eGFR and CV risk. It is important to remember that in evaluating CV disease using renal parameters, GFR should be assessed simultaneously with albuminuria.

Indeed, data from the same meta-analysis indicate that also increased urinary albumin levels or proteinuria carry an increased risk of all-cause and CV mortality. Thus, lower eGFR and higher urinary albumin values are not only predictors of progressive kidney failure, but also of

G. Mulè (✉), A. Castiglia, C. Cusumano, E. Scaduto,
G. Geraci, D. Altieri, G. Cerasola, and S. Cottone
Dipartimento Biomedico di Medicina Interna,
e Specialistica (DIBIMIS), Cattedra di Nefrologia,
European Society of Hypertension Excellence Centre,
Università di Palermo, Via Monte San Calogero, 29,
90146 Palermo, Italy
e-mail: giuseppe.mule@unipa.it

E. Di Natale
Unit of Nephrology, Caltanissetta, Italy

O. Cacciatore
Long-term care Unit, Agrigento, Italy

all-cause and CV mortality, independent of each other and of traditional CV risk factors.

Although subjects with ESRD are at the highest risk of CV diseases, there will likely be more events in subjects with mil-to-moderate renal dysfunction, because of its much higher prevalence.

These findings are even more noteworthy when one considers that a mild reduction in renal function is very common in hypertensive patients.

The current European Society of Hypertension (ESH)/European Society of Cardiology (ESC) guidelines for the management of arterial hypertension recommend to sought in every patient signs of subclinical (or asymptomatic) renal damage. This was defined by the detection of eGFR between 30 mL/min/1.73 m^2 and 60 mL/min/1.73 m^2 or the presence of microalbuminuria (MAU), that is an amount of albumin in the urine of 30–300 mg/day or an albumin/creatinine ratio, preferentially on morning spot urine, of 30–300 mg/g.

There is clear evidence that urinary albumin excretion levels, even below the cut-off values used to define MAU, are associated with an increased risk of CV events. The relationships of MAU with a variety of risk factors, such as blood pressure, diabetes and metabolic syndrome and with several indices of subclinical organ damage, may contribute, at least in part, to explain the enhanced CV risk conferred by MAU. Nonetheless, several studies showed that the association between MAU and CV disease remains when all these risk factors are taken into account in multivariate analyses. Therefore, the exact pathophysiological mechanisms explaining the association between MAU and CV risk remain to be elucidated. The simple search for MAU and in general of subclinical renal involvement in hypertensive patients may enable the clinician to better assess absolute CV risk, and its identification may induce physicians to encourage patients to make healthy lifestyle changes and perhaps would prompt to more aggressive modification of standard CV risk factors.

Keywords

Arterial hypertension • Blood pressure • Glomerular filtration rate • Microalbuminuria • Proteinuria • Subclinical renal disease • Early kidney injury • Target organ damage • Cardiovascular disease • Cardiovascular risk assessment

1   Introduction

The kidney plays a dual role in arterial hypertension. On the one hand, even subtle renal dysfunction may cause elevation in blood pressure; on the other, systemic hypertension, whether primary or secondary, may cause renal disease or may accelerate the loss of kidney function in subjects with established parenchymal disease (Ruilope 2002).

Indeed, hypertension, along with diabetes, are the leading causes of chronic kidney disease (CKD) (Ruilope 2002; Gansevoort et al. 2013; Levin et al. 2013).

CKD is a worldwide public health problem, in view of both the number of patients and cost of treatment involved. Globally, CKD is the 12th most common cause of death and the 17th leading cause of disability (Gansevoort et al. 2013).

End-stage renal disease (ESRD) has long been recognized as an extremely powerful predictor of serious cardiovascular (CV) sequelae and death (Ruilope 2002; Gansevoort et al. 2013; Foley et al. 2005). However, over the past 20 years a large and consistent body of evidence has been produced suggesting that people with any stage of CKD have an increased risk of developing cardiovascular diseases (CVD) (Ruilope 2002; Gansevoort et al. 2013; Levin et al. 2013; Matsushita et al. 2010). It has been also shown that middle aged and elderly patients with mild-to-moderate CKD are more likely to die due to CKD than to reach ESRD (Gansevoort et al. 2013; Levin et al. 2013). Moreover, although people with ESRD are at the highest risk of a CVD, there will be more events in subjects with early stage CKD, because of its much higher prevalence (Ruilope 2002; Gansevoort et al. 2013).

Numerous studies in recent years have provided convincing evidence that there is a quantitative association between decreased estimated glomerular filtration rate (eGFR) and CV risk (Ruilope 2002; Gansevoort et al. 2013; Levin et al. 2013; Matsushita et al. 2010; Go et al. 2004; Hemmelgarn et al. 2010; Hallan et al. 2009; The Chronic Kidney Disease Prognosis Consortium 2011).

Studies that have assessed the relation between kidney function and CV risk generally fall into three categories: investigations conducted in general population cohorts, in cohorts at high risk for chronic kidney disease, and in CKD patients (Matsushita et al. 2010; Go et al. 2004; Hemmelgarn et al. 2010; Hallan et al. 2009; 2012; The Chronic Kidney Disease Prognosis Consortium 2011; Mafham et al. 2011; O'Hare et al. 2007; Moynihan et al. 2013; van der Velde et al. 2011; Astor et al. 2011; Nitsch et al. 2013; Mahmoodi et al. 2012; Fox et al. 2012).

Despite differences in the populations studied and adjustment for confounding variables, the results are surprisingly consistent.

A meta-analysis of 19 studies (including over 160,000 events) has shown that for each 20 mL/min/1.73 m^2 reduction in eGFR, the risk for major vascular events (which includes both non-fatal and fatal events) increases by approximately 50 % (hazard ratio (HR), 1.49; 95 % CI, 1.38–1.61) (Mafham et al. 2011). The Chronic Kidney Disease Prognosis Consortium has presented results from a collaborative meta-analysis of 21 general population cohorts, which included more than 1.2 million participants from 14 countries in North America, Europe, Asia, and Oceania. The meta-analysis demonstrated that, after adjustment for age, sex, ethnicity, diabetes, blood pressure (BP), total cholesterol level, smoking, and history of CVD, lower eGFR was associated with an increased risk for death from any CV cause as compared to the reference group (eGFR 90–104 mL/min/1.73 m^2). The hazard ratio for all-cause mortality at eGFRs of 60, 45, and 15 mL/min/1.73 m^2 were 1.18, 1.57, and 3.14 respectively when compared to an eGFR of 95 mL/min/1.73 m^2 (Matsushita et al. 2010).

The current threshold of eGFR <60 ml/min/1.73 m^2 used to define overt CKD (Levin et al. 2013) has been disputed for several reasons. Data obtained in the CKD prognosis consortium meta-analysis, about mortality and ESRD indicated that the risk of death and renal failure increased exponentially for eGFR values <75 ml/min per 1.73 m^2, suggesting that eGFR values in the range 60–74 ml/min per 1.73 m^2 could represent the early stages of kidney disease (Matsushita et al. 2010). On the other hand, the use of a single eGFR threshold for all age groups may potentially lead to an overdiagnosis of CKD in low-risk elderly individuals, assuming that some decline in kidney function may be regarded as a physiologic phenomenon associated with normal aging (O'Hare et al. 2007; Moynihan et al. 2013).

However, another important observation from the meta-analysis is that data were not significantly different between individuals aged <65 years and ≥65 years (Hallan et al. 2012), a finding which does not support the idea that kidney dysfunction is a physiologic change of aging.

Data from the same meta-analysis indicate that also a higher level of albuminuria carried an increased risk of all-causes and CV mortality. Albuminuria and eGFR were multiplicatively associated with all-cause mortality, without evidence for interaction. Thus, lower eGFR and higher albuminuria are risk factors for not only progressive kidney failure, but also for all-cause and CV mortality, independent of each other and of CV risk factors (Matsushita et al. 2010). Subsequently, the analysis of cohorts at risk for CKD (van der Velde et al. 2011) or with CKD (Astor et al. 2011) has demonstrated similar associations. In addition, a recent new evaluation of these cohorts assessed for the presence of a sex interaction in the associations of eGFR and urinary albumin excretion (UAE) with all-cause mortality, CV mortality, and ESRD (Nitsch et al. 2013). This study demonstrated that both sexes with reduced eGFR and increasing UAE. face an enhanced risk of all-cause mortality, CV mortality, and ESRD.

Importantly, the association of kidney disease measures with mortality or ESRD has also been consistently found in those with or without hypertension (Mahmoodi et al. 2012), diabetes (Fox et al. 2012) and also regardless of age (Hallan et al. 2012). Overall, the results of all these studies support the view that assessment of both proteinuria (and albuminuria) and eGFR level is needed in order to improve the identification of individuals at high risk of cardiovascular complications and to establish appropriate measures of prevention.

On the basis of these findings, the Kidney Disease: Improving Global Outcomes (KDIGO) clinical practice guideline for evaluation and management of chronic kidney disease (Levin et al. 2013) has recommended the following: (1) the assessment of both albuminuria (or proteinuria) and eGFR in general practice and (2) the classification of CKD stages by using both kidney parameters (Fig. 1).

This because integrating both eGFR and albuminuria into CKD staging paradigms provides more precise classification and more accurate prognostic information.

Assessment of subclinical (or asymptomatic) target organ damage is a key element in the evaluation of patients with arterial hypertension (Mancia et al. 2013). Subclinical organ damage at cardiac, vascular, and renal levels often precedes and predicts the development of morbid events (Mancia et al. 2013). It has been shown that a systematic in-depth search for multiple risk factors or organ damage significantly increases the likelihood of identifying high-risk individuals. According to recent hypertension guidelines (Mancia et al. 2013) reduced eGFR, in the range 60–30 ml/min per 1.73 m^2 and microalbuminuria (MAU) have been proposed as useful integrated markers of subclinical renal damage (Mancia et al. 2013).

In the following sections we describe some epidemiological, pathophysiological, and clinical aspects regarding microalbuminuria.

2 Microalbuminuria

2.1 History

The term "microalbuminuria" was first proposed in the early 1960s, when Professor Harry Keen's Group at Guy's Hospital developed a radioimmunoassay technique for measuring in the urine of patients with type 1 diabetes, very low concentrations of albumin, well below the detection threshold of commonly used methods (Keen and Chlouverakis 1963). However, it was not until the 1980s, that it became an official part of the medical lexicon, when Svendsen and coll (Svendsen et al. 1981) and Viberti and coll (Viberti et al. 1982) described MAU as the presence of albuminuria below the detection limit of a standard dipstick, but at a level, revealed by using sensitive immunological methods, that was highly predictive of future overt proteinuria in diabetic patients.

It was initially defined as an albumin excretion rate between 20 and 200 µg/min. Although the lower bound was chosen because 95 % of 'normal' individuals had excretion rates below that limit, it was recognized that risk of

Composite ranking for relative risks by glomerular filtration rate (GFR) and albuminuria			Albuminuria stages, description and range		
			A1	A2	A3
			Normal or high normal	Increased	Severely increased and nephrotic
			< 30 mg/g	30-299 mg/g	≥ 300 mg/g
			< 30 mg/day	30-299 mg/day	≥ 300 mg/day
			< 3 mg/mmol	3-29 mg/mmol	≥ 30 mg/mmol
GFR stages, description and range (ml/min per 1.73 m2)	G1	Normal or High	≥ 90	==*	↑	↑↑
	G2	Mildly decreased	60-89	==**	↑	↑↑
	G3a	Mildly to moderate decreased	45-59	↑	↑↑	↑↑↑
	G3b	Mildly to severely decreased	30-44	↑↑	↑↑↑	↑↑↑
	G4	Severely decreased	15-29	↑↑↑	↑↑↑	↑↑↑
	G5	Kidney failure	<15	↑↑↑	↑↑↑	↑↑↑

Fig. 1 Prognosis of CKD by GFR and Albuminuria categories as identified by 2012 Kidney Disease: Improving Global Outcomes (KDIGO) clinical practice guidelines for evaluation and management of chronic kidney disease (Modified from Ref. (Levin et al. 2013), (== low risk; ↑ moderate risk; ↑↑ high risk; ↑↑↑ very high risk. * The risk may be slightly increased in subjects with ACR in the high normal range ** The risk begins to rise in subjects with estimated GFR < 75 ml/min/1.73 m^2)

progression to nephropathy was elevated among diabetics in the 'high normal' range (The Chronic Kidney Disease Prognosis Consortium 2011; Svendsen et al. 1981; Viberti et al. 1982). Mogensen was the first to describe the importance of MAU not only as a renal risk factor but also as a powerful predictor of CV mortality in patients with type 2 diabetes (Mogensen and Christensen 1984; Mogensen 1984).

In recent years, however, it has received increased attention as a prognostic marker for CV and/or renal risk even in non-diabetic subjects (Ruilope 2002; Matsushita et al. 2010; Gerstein et al. 2001; Hillege et al. 2001; 2002; Arnlov et al. 2005; Ruggenenti and Remuzzi 2006; Yuyun et al. 2004; Cirillo et al. 1998; Pontremoli et al. 1997; Pedrinelli et al. 2002; Bramlage et al. 2007; Coresh et al. 2007; Agrawal et al. 1996; Cerasola et al. 2008; 2010; Leoncini et al. 2010).

Similar to the relationship between BP and risk of CV events, mounting evidence indicates a continuous relationship between albumin excretion and risk (Matsushita et al. 2010; Gerstein et al. 2001; Hillege et al. 2001; 2002; Arnlov et al. 2005; Ruggenenti and Remuzzi 2006).

2.2 Epidemiology

European studies report a 2.2–11.8 % prevalence of MAU in the general population (Hillege et al. 2001; Yuyun et al. 2004; Cirillo et al. 1998; Pontremoli et al. 1997; Pedrinelli et al. 2002; Bramlage et al. 2007; Coresh et al. 2007). Among the European epidemiological investigations performed in this field deserves to be mentioned the PREVEND (Prevention of Renal and Vascular End-stage Disease) study (Hillege et al. 2001) which involved 40,856 inhabitants of the city of Groningen (The Netherlands), aged 28–75 years. Microalbuminuria, defined as urinary albumin concentration 20–200 mg/L, was present in 7.2 % of population. After excluding the diabetic and hypertensive subjects MAU was still prevalent in 6.6 % of the individuals, and it was independently associated with age, gender, hypertension, diabetes, smoking, previous myocardial infarction and stroke. Cardiovascular risk factors were already elevated at levels of urinary albumin currently considered to be normal (10–20 mg/L or 15–30 mg per 24 h) (Hillege et al. 2001).

These percentages indicate that MAU is more often present in subjects with CV risk factors; however, in apparently healthy subjects MAU can frequently be encountered.

Data from the US National Health and Nutrition Examination Surveys (NHANES) showed an increase in prevalence of MAU (defined as a urinary albumin– creatinine ratio [ACR] of 30–300 mg/g) from 7.1 to 8.2 % during the survey periods 1988–1994 and 1999–2004. The increase was attributed to older age of the population, greater proportion of minority groups, prevalence of hypertension and diabetes and higher body mass index (Coresh et al. 2007).

In arterial hypertension, prevalence of MAU ranging from 5 to 60 % has been reported (Agrawal et al. 1996; Cerasola et al. 2008; 2010; Leoncini et al. 2010; Böhm et al. 2007; Meccariello et al. 2016). This wide range may be due to differences in ethnic groups, specimen collection, cut-off level of albumin excretion, analytical methods and influence of antihypertensive medications. The distribution of demographic and coexisting diseases may also contribute.

In the abovementioned large-scale population surveys, the NHANES III (Coresh et al. 2007) and the PREVEND study (Hillege et al. 2001),

MAU was detected respectively in 16 % and 11.5 % of people with hypertension.

The international, observational, practice based study i-SEARCH (Survey for Evaluating Microalbuminuria Routinely by Cardiologists in patients with Hypertension) was designed to assess the frequency with which MAU occurred in a very large group of hypertensive outpatients attending a cardiologist or internist. A total of 21,050 patients from 26 countries were included in the primary analysis. Overall, this study demonstrated a very high worldwide prevalence (58.4 %) of MAU in high-risk cardiovascular patients, but with a considerable variation across countries (Böhm et al. 2007).

The use of a semi-quantitative test, which tend to overestimate urine albumin concentration, may explain to some extent the unusually high prevalence of microalbuminuria reported in this large-scale study (Böhm et al. 2007), as well as in other ones (Bramlage et al. 2007; Agrawal et al. 1996). In a very recent study conducted in 1024 unselected hypertensive patients followed by 13 Italian general practitioners MAU was detected in 35 % of the overall population (Dworkin et al. 1983).

A lower frequency of MAU (22.7 %) was observed in the REDHY (REnal Dysfunction in HYpertension) study that was conducted in 1856 non-diabetic middle-aged subjects with arterial hypertension and without cardiovascular complications and known renal diseases (Cerasola et al. 2008; 2010). Moreover, in the I-DEMAND (Italy Developing Education and awareness on Microalbuminuria in patients with hyperteNsive Disease) study, an observational, cross-sectional investigation performed in 87 centers of specialized care (Internal Medicine, Cardiology, Nephrology, Diabetology) MAU was found in 27 % of the entire population, including 3534 patients, 37 % of whom had diabetes mellitus (Leoncini et al. 2010).

2.3 Pathophysiology

The presence of microalbuminuria implies dysfunction of the glomerular filtration barrier. It may result from haemodynamic-mediated mechanisms and/or functional or structural impairment of the glomerular barrier.

Microalbuminuria in essential hypertensive patients is the consequence of an increased transglomerular passage of albumin rather than the result of a decrease in the proximal tubule reabsorption of albumin. At least two mechanisms have been proposed for the greater albumin excretion rate (AER) in some patients with essential hypertension: increased glomerular hydrostatic pressure or increased permselectivity of the glomerular basement membrane (Mountokalakis 1997). Glomerular hydrostatic pressure is regulated by the relative vasoconstriction-vasodilatation of the afferent and efferent glomerular arterioles. The tone of these arterioles is regulated by different mechanisms, and their sensitivity to pressor/depressor substances also varies substantially (Dworkin et al. 1983).

A variety of endocrine, paracrine, and autocrine substances, as well as pharmacological agents, may influence intraglomerular hemodynamic independently of actions on systemic blood pressure (BP).

Normally, an elevation of systemic arterial pressure is associated with vasoconstriction of the glomerular afferent arterioles, which prevents transmission of the elevated hydrostatic pressure to the glomerulus and maintains the glomerular hydrostatic pressure unaltered (Hostetter et al. 1981). This protects the glomeruli from the potential damages of hypertension. If the autoregulatory adaptation of the glomerular afferent arterioles is defective, increased glomerular hydrostatic pressure may ensue. Alternatively, an exaggerated vasoconstriction of the efferent arterioles may increase intraglomerular hydrostatic pressure, even in the presence of normal systemic pressure (Hostetter et al. 1981).

A large body of experimental and clinical evidence supports the notion that derangements of these adaptive mechanisms are important determinants for the susceptibility to develop progressive renal disease (Mountokalakis 1997).

In 1992 our group, in order to verify if in essential hypertension (EH) MAU increase could be due to hemodynamic modifications or to glomerular structural changes, in a very small group of newly diagnosed essential hypertensives (n = 30; EHs) having 24-h AER > 16 µg/min (n =15) and in 15 EHs with 24-h AER < 16 µg/min, the day- and night-time behaviour of creatinine clearance (Ccr), as well as AER clearance (AER-C) and fractional clearance (AER-FC), and behaviour of BP were evaluated (Cottone and Cerasola 1992). Patients with 24-h AER > 16 µg/min showed hyperfiltering values of both 24-h and daytime creatinine clearance than the other group of EHs, while during the night period, there were no significant differences between the two groups. On the contrary, AER and both AER-C and AER-FC resulted markedly and significantly higher in the EHs with 24-h AER > 16 µg/min not only in the 24-h evaluation, but also during the night-time study notwithstanding the significant decrease in BP and in Ccr observed during the night. We concluded that these data, in the absence of correlations between BP and AER-FC seemed to demonstrate that among newly diagnosed essential hypertensives a subgroup of them could have early renal hemodynamic changes (Cottone and Cerasola 1992). These hemodynamic modifications, along with defects of the glomerular membrane permselectivity, led to increased microalbuminuria.

Hyperfiltration is probably mediated by abnormal transmission of systemic hypertension to the glomerulus through a disturbance in glomerular autoregulation and/or from progressive loss of functioning nephrons. Of the non-haemodynamics, functional abnormalities of the glomerular basal membrane have been claimed, although some evidence has been against this in hypertension.

More widely accepted, however, is that MAU reflects the kidney expression of a more generalised state of endothelial dysfunction (Deckert et al. 1989; Pedrinelli et al. 1994; Cottone et al. 2000; 2007).

With regard to systemic endothelial dysfunction, our group hypothesized that in EHs, plasma levels of pro-atherogenic adhesion molecules would be increased and related with AER. Thus, we studied biochemical markers of endothelial activation ICAM-1 and VCAM-1, and their relationship with AER in a group of individuals with uncomplicated EH (Cottone et al. 2007). One hundred patients with essential hypertension and no diabetes or ultrasonographic evidence of atherosclerosis were included in the study. EHs were first studied overall, than were divided into two subgroups: those with AER >20 μg/min (MAUs) and those with AER <20 μg/min (non-MAUs). Microalbuminuric hypertensives had greater levels of adhesion molecules than non- MAUs. In multiple regression models in hypertensive persons AER was independently associated with ICAM-1, and VCAM-1. These findings showed that in EH there is a very early activation of endothelial adhesion molecules favouring atherosclerosis.

A further interesting data emerging from that study was the significant difference of plasma concentrations of adhesion molecules when comparing non-MAU hypertensives with healthy controls. Indeed, it seemed that endothelial activation expressed by adhesion molecules would be earlier than microalbuminuria, confirming that microalbuminuria could be considered a marker of systemic endothelial dysfunction (Cottone et al. 2007). A study by Klausen (Klausen et al. 2004) demonstrated that in the general population urinary albumin excretion, below the MAU definition, was associated with increased coronary heart disease risk, independently of hypertension. Thus, the Authors hypothesize that MAU emerges later in the atherosclerotic process. Our findings, showing a pro-atherogenic endothelial activation in the presence of values of AER currently considered as 'normal' seemed to be in line with this finding.

Considering the role that inflammation plays in the development of endothelial changes that lead to atherosclerosis, studies on this issue were performed (Pedrinelli et al. 2004; Festa et al. 2000; Jager et al. 2002; Kshirsagar et al. 2008).

C-Reactive Protein (CRP), a well-known marker of inflammation, was positively associated with microalbuminuria in the large data set compiled from the National Health and Nutrition Examination Surveys (NHANES) 1999 through 2004 (Kshirsagar et al. 2008). In this study, including 12,831 US men and women, the multivariate analysis showed that an increase of one milligram per liter in CRP concentration was significantly associated with a 2 % increased odds of microalbuminuria (p = 0.0003) (Kshirsagar et al. 2008).

2.4 Methodology and Limitations

Microalbuminuria can be revealed by several methods based on immunologic detection (immunonephelometry, immunoturbidimetry, radioimmunoassay, enzyme-linked immunosorbent assay) (Miller et al. 2009). Among these there are also a variety of semiquantitative dipsticks, such as Clinitek Microalbumin Dipsticks and Micral-Test II test strips, which can be used for MAU screening. The reported sensitivity and specificity of these tests range from 80 to 97 % and 33 to 80 %, respectively (Miller et al. 2009).

Microalbuminuria has been defined as an AER higher than the threshold value obtained from studies assessing the risk for developing nephropathy in diabetes, that is an AER between 20 and 200 μg/min. It is now clear that its significance extends beyond nephropathy and it likely mirrors a more widespread vascular injury.

It should be noted that AER may also be expressed in terms of milligrams per day (mg/day), in which case the range for microalbuminuria is 30–300 mg/day (Levin et al. 2013; Mancia et al. 2013).

Indeed, there is growing evidence, arising from several prospective studies that urinary albumin excretion levels well below the current microalbuminuria threshold ("low-grade albuminuria") are also associated with an increased risk of incident cardiovascular disease and all-cause mortality (Matsushita et al. 2010; van der Velde et al. 2011; Astor et al. 2011; Nitsch et al. 2013; Mahmoodi et al. 2012; Fox et al. 2012; Hallan et al. 2012; Klausen et al. 2004; Redon and Williams 2002). Even in apparently healthy individuals (without diabetes or hypertension), such an association has been shown (Hillege et al. 2001). These epidemiological data prompted some authors to propose the adoption of a lower AER cut-off point for the detection of subjects with an enhanced cardiovascular risk (Redon and Williams 2002) and other ones (Ruggenenti and Remuzzi 2006) to abandon the terms of microalbuminuria and macroalbuminuria and replaced with 'urine albumin', because the use of arbitrary dichotomous categorisation does not reflect the continuously increasing risk associated with progression of urine albumin concentrations. Moreover, the term microalbuminuria may be confusing, since it should reflect small albumin molecules, and not small amounts of albumin (Ruggenenti and Remuzzi 2006).

Despite this criticism, the term microalbuminuria has become widely accepted in clinical practice.

Although 24-h urine collection is the gold standard for the detection of microalbuminuria, it has been suggested that screening can be more simply achieved by a timed urine collection or by untimed spot urine sample. In this latter case the confounding effect of variations in urine volume on the urine albumin concentration can be avoided normalizing the urinary albumin concentration to the urinary creatinine concentration (since creatinine excretion rate is considered constant) (Miller et al. 2009; Levey et al. 2009).

Indeed, the albumin/creatinine ratio (ACR) from spot urine, preferably that first voided in the morning, may be considered equivalent to the values during a 24-h urine collection (Miller et al. 2009; Levey et al. 2009).

Even if the ACR corrects for unknown urine volumes, it needs theoretically differentiation of males from females in whom creatininuria is lower because of reduced muscle mass (Miller et al. 2009; Cirillo et al. 2006; Mogensen et al. 1995), a fact not taken into account, by the KDIGO guidelines for evaluation of CKD (Levin et al. 2013) and by the 2013 ESH-ESC guidelines for management of arterial hypertension (Mancia et al. 2013), that for the definition of microalbuminuria do not recommend the use of gender-specific ACR thresholds, but a single

cut-off value, that for simplicity was arbitrarily rounded to 30 mg/g (Levin et al. 2013; Mancia et al. 2013) (Fig. 1).

For the same reasons described above, albumin excretion will be underestimated in a muscular man with a high rate of creatinine excretion and overestimated in a cachectic patient in whom muscle mass and creatinine excretion are markedly reduced (Miller et al. 2009; Cirillo et al. 2006).

A number of physiologic and pathologic factors must be taken into account when interpreting AER and ACR results. Albumin excretion is normally about 25 % higher during the day, and it can vary by 10–25 or more in day-to-day measurements. In addition to age and sex, body mass index and a high-protein meal can all affect the AER. Vigorous exercise can cause a transient increase in albumin excretion. As a result, patients should refrain from vigorous exercise in the 24 h prior to the test. Measurement can be further confounded by fever, congestive heart failure, urinary tract infection, and by some drugs (Mogensen et al. 1995). Because the limited reproducibility of AER and ACR measurements, most expert committees recommend that a presumptive indication of microalbuminuria should be confirmed by quantitative measurement of urinary albumin in at least two of three, preferably nonconsecutive, specimens (Mogensen et al. 1995). Even a single determination of elevated albumin concentration, however, can predict (albeit with reduced precision) renal and cardiovascular diseases (Gerstein et al. 2001; Hillege et al. 2002).

2.5 Microalbuminuria and Cardiovascular Risk Factors

There is a strong evidence of a close relationship of microalbuminuria with a variety of cardiovascular risk factors, such as hypertension, diabetes, aging, smoking, hyperlipidemia and metabolic syndrome.

The association of microalbuminuria with all these factors is so relevant that MAU may

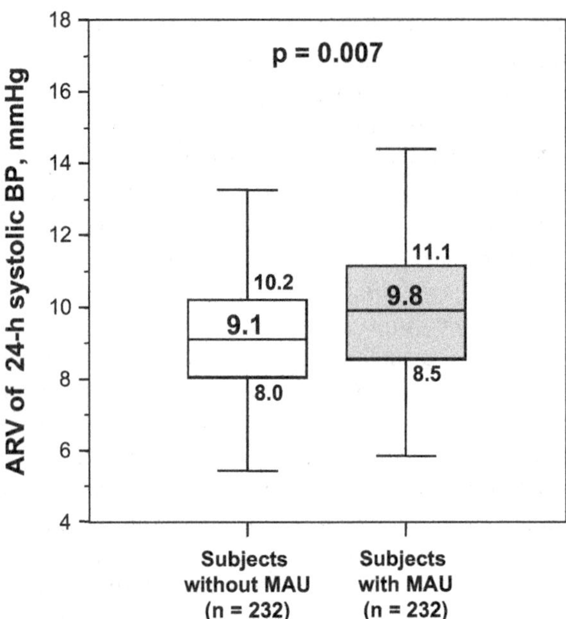

Fig. 2 Box plots showing average real variability (ARV) of 24-h systolic blood pressure (BP) in hypertensive patients with microalbuminuria and in those without it. In the Box and Whisker plots, the central boxes represent the values from the lower to upper quartile (25–75 percentile). The middle lines represent the medians. Lower and upper whiskers extend to 5th and 95th percentiles. This difference remained significant (P = 0.02), even after adjustment by ANCOVA for age, gender, average 24-h systolic BP, waist circumference, serum uric acid and diabetic status (Mulè et al. 2016)

legitimately be regarded as an integrated marker of cardiovascular risk (Pedrinelli et al. 2002).

Several studies have shown significant correlations between blood pressure values and AER (Cirillo et al. 1998; Bramlage et al. 2007; Coresh et al. 2007; Agrawal et al. 1996; Cerasola et al. 2008; 2010; Leoncini et al. 2010; Böhm et al. 2007; Cerasola et al. 1989; 1996; Hsu et al. 2009). There is also evidence that the relationship of BP with albuminuria is relatively continuous and graded, with even high-normal levels of BP associated with albuminuria (Hsu et al. 2009).

In general, the association of BP values with albuminuria becomes even closer when BP is recorded through ambulatory blood pressure monitoring (Cerasola et al. 1989; 1996; Palatini et al. 1995) which provides a more precise estimation of the real BP status. Ambulatory BP monitoring also allowed to show that there are no significant differences in AER between the white coat hypertensive and the normotensive subjects (Cerasola et al. 1995; Palatini et al. 1998) and that urinary albumin levels are higher in hypertensives in whom a blunted or absent nocturnal fall of BP occurs (non dippers) (Bianchi et al. 1994; Redon et al. 1994). In this context it is interesting to note that a clinical condition characterized by a non-dipping BP pattern, such as the obstructive sleep apnea syndrome, has been associated with microalbuminuria in patients with arterial hypertension (Tsioufis et al. 2008).

Very recently, in a group of more than 300 untreated hypertensive subjects, we reported a positive association of AER with average real variability (ARV) of 24-h systolic blood pressure (Fig. 2), a measure of short-term blood pressure variability endowed with prognostic implications (Mulè et al. 2016). This association was weakened, but still significant, taking into account the effect of the mean level of 24-h SBP and other potential confounders. Moreover, in the subset of patients with MAU and inverse relationship between ARV of 24-h SBP and eGFR was also found (Mulè et al. 2015a).

Accumulating data indicate that MAU clusters with several metabolic abnormalities

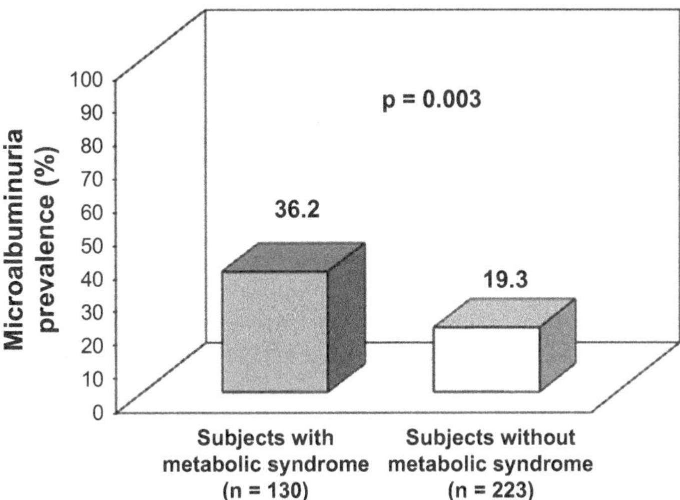

Fig. 3 Microalbuminuria prevalence in 353 non diabetic essential hypertensive patients divided on the basis of the presence or absence of metabolic syndrome, as defined by ATP III criteria (Mulè et al. 2005)

(Cirillo et al. 1998; Pontremoli et al. 1997; Cerasola et al. 2008; 2010; Leoncini et al. 2010; Campese et al. 1999; Cerasola and Cottone 1997; Pinto-Sietsma et al. 2003; Klausen et al. 2009; Mulè et al. 2006; Palaniappan et al. 2003; Andronico et al. 1998; Srinivasan et al. 2000; Alberti and Zimmet 1998; Jager et al. 1998; Chen et al. 2004; Mulè et al. 2005; Cuspidi et al. 2004; Klausen et al. 2007; Parving et al. 2006), including some phenotypes of the metabolic syndrome (MetS) and may be indeed a part of this syndrome (Alberti and Zimmet 1998).

We have previously shown, in a group of 353 essential hypertensive subjects that the prevalence of microalbuminuria and the levels of AER were higher in patients with MetS than in those without it (Mulè et al. 2005) (Fig. 3). Furthermore, although researchers have reported mixed results (Andronico et al. 1998; Srinivasan et al. 2000; Jager et al. 1998) on the association between MAU and hyperinsulinemia and insulin-resistance, multiple studies confirmed this relation (Andronico et al. 1998; Srinivasan et al. 2000). An investigation of 5659 men and women from the NHANES III, confirmed the association between MAU and the MetS, with the strongest association being with high fasting serum glucose and high BP (Palaniappan et al. 2003). A further analysis of the same study documented that the multivariate-adjusted odds ratios of microalbuminuria increased progressively with a higher number of components of the MetS, defined by the ATP III guidelines (Chen et al. 2004).

Similar results were obtained in patients with arterial hypertension (Mulè et al. 2005; Cuspidi et al. 2004).

In the general population of the Copenhagen City Heart Study not only the strong association between microalbuminuria and the MetS was confirmed, but interestingly it was also observed that MAU (even when defined by a very low cut-off value, that is > 5 µg/min) confers an increased risk of death and CV disease to a similar extent as the MetS and independently of it and of other confounding factors (Klausen et al. 2007).

A relationship between higher AER and cigarette smoking has been described in diabetic individuals (Parving et al. 2006; Gerstein et al. 2000) and in hypertensive people (Andronico et al. 2005), in subjects with increased CV risk (Gerstein et al. 2000) as well as in the general population (Pinto-Sietsma et al. 2000).

In the PREVEND study, current smokers had a higher median albumin excretion than nonsmokers and were more likely to have microalbuminuria. After adjustment for several potential confounding factors, persons who smoked 20 or fewer cigarettes/day and persons who smoked more than 20 cigarettes/day, when compared to nonsmokers, showed a relative risk of microalbuminuria of 1.92 [CI, 1.54–2.39] and

2.15 [CI, 1.52–3.03], respectively (Pinto-Sietsma et al. 2000).

However, overall, in the various studies, the link between smoking and MAU is not very strong and it seems unlikely that smoking may explain much of the excess CV risk associated with MAU.

Besides the associations reported between microalbuminuria and various conventional cardiovascular risk factors, significant correlations have been observed between increased AER and nontraditional risk factors for cardiovascular diseases.

For example, during the last decade, several cross-sectional investigations have documented that microalbuminuria is related to various inflammatory markers (Pedrinelli et al. 2004; Festa et al. 2000; Jager et al. 2002; Kshirsagar et al. 2008; Mulè et al. 2009) and to some markers of endothelial damage and dysfunction, including von Willebrand factor and adhesion molecules (sVCAM1 and sICAM1 and e-selectin) (Pedrinelli et al. 1994; Cottone et al. 2000; 2007).

2.6 Microalbuminuria and Kidney Dysfunction

The influence of glomerular filtration rate (GFR) on the microalbuminuria of hypertension merits a comment. The prevalence of microalbuminuria increases as the GFR decreases, although not always in parallel. Moreover, when GFR is < 60 ml/min/1.73 m^2, the probability of AER normalisation during antihypertensive treatment is clearly reduced (Pascual et al. 2006).

Changes in proteinuria have been suggested as a surrogate outcome for kidney disease progression to facilitate the conduct of clinical trials (Levey et al. 2009). The progression of CKD is often slow, and until late stages, it is often asymptomatic. Thus, end points for clinical trials may be long delayed from disease onset and the time that interventions may be effective. Surrogate end points may provide an opportunity to detect early evidence of effectiveness. Proteinuria is an accepted marker for kidney damage; is related to diagnosis, prognosis, and treatment in kidney disease; and has been suggested as a surrogate outcome for clinical trials of kidney disease progression (Pascual et al. 2006). A biomarker is a characteristic that is objectively measured and evaluated as an indicator of normal biological processes, pathogenic processes, or pharmacological responses to a therapeutic intervention (Biomarkers Definitions Working Group 2001). By definition, proteinuria and decreased GFR are biomarkers for CKD and potentially could be surrogate end points for kidney failure because in general, they precede the development of kidney failure.

An intermediate end point is a biomarker that is intermediate in the causal pathway between an intervention and a clinical end point. Decreased GFR also is an intermediate end point because it is on the causal pathway to kidney failure. Doubling of serum creatinine level is accepted as a surrogate end point because it reflects a large decrease in GFR and predicts the development of kidney failure. The increase in albumin excretion rate potentially could be a surrogate outcome for a large decrease in GFR in clinical trials.

Indeed, among the impressive number of data the PREVEND Study offered, the role of albumin excretion as a better marker than estimated GFR to identify individuals at risk for accelerated GFR loss is relevant. The 8592 patients who were included in this study were followed for a 4-year period. Among them, 134 patients with macroalbuminuria, 128 with erythrocyturia, and 103 with impaired renal function were identified. In the general population the prevalence of macroalbuminuria, erythrocyturia, and impaired renal function was calculated to be 0.6, 1.3, and 0.9 %, respectively (Halbesma et al. 2006). After a mean follow-up of 4.2 year, the macroalbuminuria group showed a -7.2 ml/min/1.73 m^2 estimated GFR loss compared with -2.3 ml/min/1.73 m^2 in the control group (difference $p < 0.001$). After exclusion of individuals with diabetes, the observed renal function decline in the macroalbuminuria group was 7.1 ml/min/1.73 m^2. It is interesting that eGFR fell by only 0.2 ml/min/1.73 m^2 (-0.4 %) in participants with impaired renal function. Participants who at baseline had both macroalbuminuria and impaired renal function (n =18) experienced a rate of renal function decline of 9.0 ml/min/1.73 m^2 (Halbesma et al. 2006).

More recently, it was analyzed whether screening for albuminuria in the general population identifies individuals at increased risk for renal replacement therapy or accelerated loss of renal function. In a general population-based cohort of 40,854 individuals aged 28–75 year, a first morning void for measurement of urinary albumin was collected. In a subset of 6, 879 individuals, 24-h urinary albumin excretion and estimated GFR at baseline and during 6 years of follow-up were measured. Linkage with the national renal replacement therapy registry identified 45 individuals who started renal replacement therapy during 9 year of follow-up. The quantity of albuminuria was associated with increased renal risk: the higher the level of albuminuria, the higher the risk of need for renal replacement therapy and the more rapid renal function decline. A urinary albumin concentration $\geq$ 20 mg/L identified individuals who started renal replacement therapy during follow-up with 58 % sensitivity and 92 % specificity. Of the identified individuals, 39 % were previously unknown to have impaired renal function. Restricting screening to high-risk groups (e.g., known hypertension, diabetes, cardiovascular disease, and older age) reduced the sensitivity of the test only marginally but failed to identify 45 % of individuals with micro- and macroalbuminuria. Therefore, individuals with elevated levels of urinary albumin are at increased risk for RRT and accelerated loss of renal function. Screening for albuminuria identifies patients at increased risk for progressive renal disease, 40–50 % of whom were previously undiagnosed or untreated (van der Velde et al. 2009).

In arterial hypertensive subjects a retrospective cohort analysis of 141 hypertensive individuals followed up for approximately 7 years was carried out several years ago (Bigazzi et al. 1998). During follow-up, the rate of clearance of creatinine from patients with microalbuminuria decreased more than did that from those with normal urinary albumin excretion (Bigazzi et al. 1998).

Similar associations between albuminuria and renal function decline have been described by Viazzi et al in a larger cohort of patients with essential hypertension. Subjects who developed a renal event had higher baseline albumin-to-creatinine ratio compared with subjects who did not develop a renal event (5.12 vs 4.42 mg/g; p < 0.001) (Viazzi et al. 2010).

2.7 Microalbuminuria and Subclinical Organ Damage

According to several studies microalbuminuria correlate with various cardiac abnormalities and diseases, including left ventricular (LV) hypertrophy and dysfunction, electrocardiographic abnormalities, and coronary atherosclerosis.

There is an extensive and highly consistent body of evidence showing that microalbuminuric patients exhibited a higher prevalence of left ventricular hypertrophy (LVH), assessed either by electrocardiography or echocardiography, compared to normoalbuminurics (Cerasola et al. 1989; 1996; 2004; Palatini et al. 1995; Pontremoli et al. 1999; Wachtell et al. 2002a; b; Tsioufis et al. 2002; Ratto et al. 2008; Smilde et al. 2005; Lieb et al. 2006).

Since the first description of our group in 1989 of a close relationship between LV mass and albumin excretion rate in hypertensive patients (Cerasola et al. 1989), the vast majority of the following reports supported the view that hypertensives with elevated AER had higher cardiac mass, indicating that early renal damage and LVH occur in a parallel fashion.

It is important to note that the association between left ventricular mass and AER not only reflects an abnormal pressor overload, but remains statistically significant after accounting for blood pressure values (Cerasola et al. 1996; 2004; Palatini et al. 1995; Pontremoli et al. 1999; Wachtell et al. 2002a; 2002b; Tsioufis et al. 2002; Ratto et al. 2008; Smilde et al. 2005). Further support to the blood pressure independent relationship of microalbuminuria with LVH arises from the observation that inappropriate left ventricular mass, that is the LV mass exceeding the compensatory needs for cardiac workload, is more strongly associated with microalbuminuria than do appropriate LV mass (Ratto et al. 2008).

Even if albumin excretion rate and LV mass are significantly and independently correlated, AER determination may add information on cardiovascular risk stratification beyond those provided by ultrasonographic detected LVH. Indeed, in a group of 312 essential hypertensive patients, we observed that a more intensive investigation for target organ damage, including ultrasound examination of the heart to detect LVH and microalbuminuria determination, beyond routine work-up alone, increases the proportion of hypertensive patients who should be classified as having a high absolute risk of cardiovascular morbidity and mortality. Overall, 26 % of patients changed risk category (mostly shifting from the medium- to high-risk stratum), a proportion that was significantly different from the percentage of patients reclassified after the addition to the routine work-up of either microalbuminuria (14 %) or echocardiography alone (16 %) (Cerasola et al. 2004). In some (Pontremoli et al. 1999), but not all studies (Wachtell et al. 2002a) microalbuminuric subjects showed a higher prevalence of concentric than eccentric LVH, being the former geometric pattern associated with a worse outcome than the latter.

Furthermore, patients with microalbuminuria showed subclinical impairment of systolic and diastolic LV (Pontremoli et al. 1999; Wachtell et al. 2002a). In the LIFE study, patients with microalbuminuria had significantly lower endocardial and midwall fractional shortening. On the other hand, patients with abnormal diastolic LV filling parameters had a significantly increased prevalence of microalbuminuria (Wachtell et al. 2002a).

Further data supporting the close association between elevated AER and cardiac abnormalities derive also from the cross-sectional relationship observed between MAU and silent myocardial ischemia, which can be evidenced by ST segment and T wave changes on an electrocardiogram (Diercks et al. 2000). Moreover, a significant and independent association between MAU and various ECG abnormalities (arrhythmias, intraventricular conduction defects, ventricular repolarization alterations and left-axis deviation) in the large observational I-DEMAND study, including 4121 hypertensive patients without overt cardiovascular disease, was found (Sciarretta et al. 2009).

Elevated AER was also directly associated with angiographic evidence of CAD. A study of 308 patients who underwent elective coronary angiography revealed that patients with angiographic evidence of CAD had significantly higher urinary albumin levels than disease-free individuals and that AER correlated with the severity of coronary atherosclerosis at angiography (Tuttle et al. 1999).

A significant association between microalbuminuria and several functional and structural changes of the arterial tree, beyond the coronary bed, has been described

Despite some conflicting results, several cross-sectional studies (Yokoyama et al. 2004; Bigazzi et al. 1995; Rodondi et al. 2007; Furtner et al. 2005; Geraci et al. 2016; Jørgensen et al. 2007), found that MAU was associated with higher thickness of the intima and media (IMT) layers of the carotid artery. In a wide population of hypertensive subjects with (n = 183) and without CKD (n = 280), we recently found greater values of carotid IMT in microalbuminuric patients when compared to normoalbuminuric ones (Geraci et al. 2016) (Fig. 4).

Moreover, in the Bruneck Study, a prospective population-based survey including 684 Caucasians adults, ACR was significantly and independently associated with the presence and severity of carotid and femoral atherosclerosis (Furtner et al. 2005). In addition, microalbuminuria predicts the development and progression of carotid atherosclerosis (Jørgensen et al. 2007).

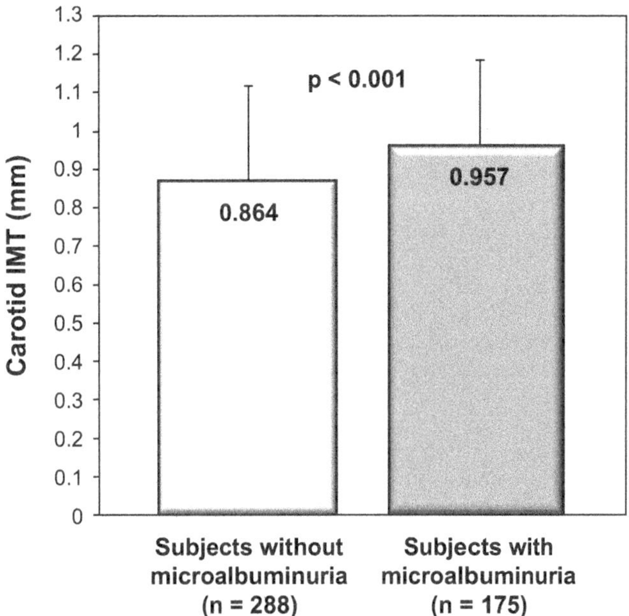

Fig. 4 Carotid intima-media thickness in hypertensive patients with and without microalbuminuria (Geraci et al. 2016). The data are given as means (the numbers inside the histograms) ± SD

Hence, it is not unexpected that microalbuminuria in several studies has been associated with a greater incidence of stroke (Gerstein et al. 2001; Hillege et al. 2002; Yuyun et al. 2004), and with cerebral small vessel disease (Ravera et al. 2002; Wada et al. 2007).

In addition, albumin excretion rate correlates with functional abnormalities of the vasculature, such as alterations of flow- and nitroglycerin-mediated brachial artery dilatation (Stehouwer et al. 2004; Malik et al. 2007) and impaired large artery elastic properties (Mulè et al. 2004; 2009; 2010; Smith et al. 2005; Hermans et al. 2007; Upadhyay et al. 2009; Munakata et al. 2009).

Large artery stiffness, especially aortic stiffness, assessed by pulse wave velocity (PWV) measurement is now well accepted as an independent predictor of cardiovascular morbidity and mortality. We demonstrated in a sample of 140 untreated nondiabetic essential hypertensive patients that microalbuminuria, was significantly associated with an augmented aortic stiffness, independently of low-grade inflammation, expressed by increased plasma level of high-sensitivity C-reactive, and of other potential confounding factors (Mulè et al. 2009). Our findings, which were replicated in a wider group of hypertensive patients (Mulè et al. 2010), are in line with previous observations of our group (Mulè et al. 2004) and of other authors (Yokoyama et al. 2004; Smith et al. 2005; Hermans et al. 2007; Upadhyay et al. 2009; Munakata et al. 2009) that reported significant relations of micro-albuminuria with different indices of reduced arterial distensibility in a variety of populations. At the level of renal vasculature, micro-albuminuria has been associated with increased intrarenal resistive index (RRI), a sonographic parameter, which is defined as the dimensionless ratio of the difference between maximum and minimum (end-diastolic) flow velocity to maximum flow velocity (Mulè et al. 2015b; Viazzi et al. 2015) (Fig. 5).

It is thought to indicate a greater intraparenchymal vascular impedance to blood flow and a greater risk of function worsening in the long term. However, accumulating evidence indicates that the RRI provides important information about the systemic vasculature as well (Geraci et al. 2015a; b; 2016; Mulè et al. 2015b; Viazzi et al. 2015; Morreale et al. 2016). Indeed, recent

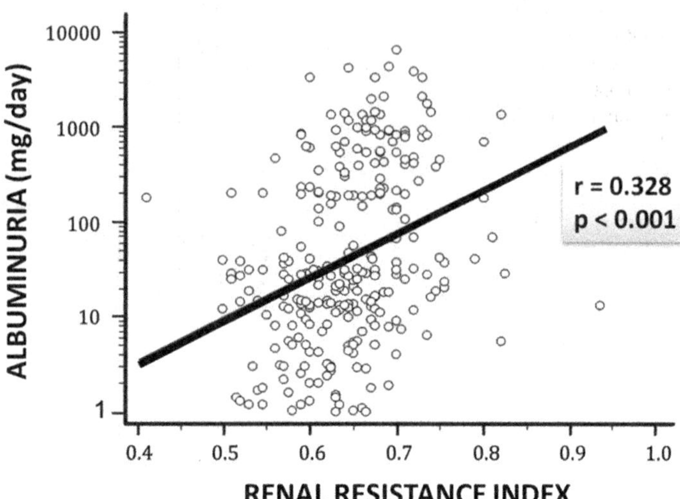

Fig. 5 Relationship between albuminuria (in logarithmic scale) and renal resistance index in hypertensive patients (Geraci et al. 2016)

data suggest that this parameter is not only expression of parenchymal perfusion, but may be also influenced by upstream vascular factors and indeed these factors appear to play a more important role than intrarenal resistance. Moreover, recent reports described significant associations of RRI with an enhanced cardiovascular risk (Mulè et al. 2015b; Viazzi et al. 2015).

Finally, an increased prevalence of retinal vascular changes has been reported in microalbuminuric hypertensive patients. Among 383 essential hypertensive subjects those with AER > 20 µg/min had a prevalence of hypertensive retinopathy of 69 %, significantly higher than that observed in subjects having AER < 11 µg/min (48 %) (Cerasola et al. 1996). There is also evidence, especially in type 1 diabetes, that MAU is a powerful predictor for the development of proliferative diabetic retinopathy and blindness (Newman et al. 2005).

2.8 Microalbuminuria as Predictor of Cardiovascular Morbidity and Mortality

It has long been recognised that microalbuminuria is an early sign of increased risk for developing overt nephropathy and cardiovascular disease in type 1 and type 2 diabetes (Viberti et al. 1982; Mogensen and Christensen 1984; Mogensen 1984; 2003). A meta-analysis evaluating the relationship between microalbuminuria and mortality in type 2 diabetes found that microalbuminuria doubled cardiovascular morbidity and mortality (odds ratio [OR], 2; 95 % CI, 1.4–2.7) and more than doubled the all-cause mortality rate (OR, 2.4; 95 % CI, 1.8–3.1) (Dinneen and Gerstein 1997). Subsequently, these results were confirmed in an observational analysis of the large Action in Diabetes and Vascular disease: preterAx and diamicroN-MR Controlled Evaluation (ADVANCE) study, involving 10,640 type 2 diabetes patients. During an average 4.3-years follow-up, the multivariable-adjusted hazard ratio for cardiovascular events was 2.48 (95 % confidence interval 1.74–3.52) for every 10-fold increase in baseline ACR, even taking into account the level of estimated glomerular filtration rate (Ninomiya et al. 2009a).

In the past decade, a large body of evidence has been published suggesting that the value of microalbuminuria as predictor of cardiovascular events and total mortality may be extended to nondiabetic subjects and to patients with essential hypertension (Ruilope 2002; Gansevoort et al. 2013; Matsushita et al. 2010; Hallan et al. 2009; The Chronic Kidney Disease Prognosis Consortium 2011; van der Velde et al. 2011; Astor et al. 2011; Nitsch et al. 2013; Mahmoodi et al. 2012; Fox et al. 2012; Gerstein et al. 2001; Hillege et al. 2002; Arnlov et al. 2005; Yuyun et al. 2004; Klausen et al. 2004; Brantsma et al. 2008).

In the large Netherlands cohort of the PREVEND study, after adjustment for cardiovascular risk factors, a twofold increase in urinary albumin concentration was associated with a 29 % increased risk of death from CVD (hazard ratio, 1.29; 95 % confidence interval [CI], 1.18–1.40; p < 0.001) (Hillege et al. 2002). Across the whole spectrum of urine albumin excretion, there was a continuous association between CVD and increasing albuminuria. The extended follow-up of the same study, limited to 8496 individuals, showed that baseline albuminuria remains a durable predictor of cardiovascular events up to 5 years after initial measurement and provides clues to determine optimal intervals between urinary albumin measurements for cardiovascular risk stratification (Brantsma et al. 2008).

Data from the NHANES III, spanning 13 years of follow-up in 14.586 adults, revealed that after adjustment for conventional CVD risk factors, C-reactive protein, and eGFR, a doubling of albuminuria was associated with a 6.3 % increase in CVD mortality and a 6.3 % increase in all-cause mortality, with similar results in patients with and without diabetes (Astor et al. 2008).

Likewise, in 1665 men and women of the Gubbio Population Study (aged 45–64 years), the highest sex-specific decile of urinary AER distribution was associated with an enhanced risk for incident cardiovascular disease, that was furtherly magnified by the concomitant presence of a high AER and a low estimated glomerular filtration rate (Cirillo et al. 2008).

The findings of these and other studies are supported by the results of two meta-analyses (Matsushita et al. 2010; Perkovic et al. 2008). The largest of these, the abovementioned Chronic Kidney Disease Prognosis Consortium study (Matsushita et al. 2010), used pooled individual data of more than 100.000 subjects with ACR measurements and 1.1 million participants with dipstick measurements from 21 general population cohorts. ACR was associated with risk of mortality linearly along its entire distribution, without threshold effects. Compared with ACR 0.6 mg/mmol, adjusted HRs for all-cause mortality were 1.20 (1.15–1.26) for ACR 1.1 mg/mmol, 1.63 (1.50–1.77) for 3.4 mg/mmol, and 2.22 (1.97–2.51) for 33.9 mg/mmol (Matsushita et al. 2010). A new recent analysis of the same data showed that there was a sex-related difference in the relationships between ACR and mortality (Nitsch et al. 2013). Compared with an ACR of 5 mg/mmol, the adjusted hazard ratio for all-cause mortality at urinary albumincreatinine ratio 30 was higher in women [1.69 (1.54–1.84)] than in men [1.43 (1.31–1.57); p for interaction <0.01] (Nitsch et al. 2013).

On the other hand, another meta-analysis involving 24,470 participants, documented a strong independent relationship between proteinuria and cerebrovascular events. Patients with proteinuria had a 70 % greater risk of stroke compared with those without (Ninomiya et al. 2009b).

Urinary excretion of excessive amounts of albumin and cognitive impairment may be regarded as manifestations of microvascular disease, respectively of the kidney and of the brain. Therefore, these conditions may share a common pathogenesis. The results of the following study seem to be in line with this hypothesis (Barzilay et al. 2011).

In a total of 28,384 subjects with vascular disease or diabetes mellitus participating in the Ongoing Telmisartan Alone and in Combination With Ramipril Global End Point Trial (ONTARGET) and in the Telmisartan Randomized Assessment Study in ACE [Angiotensin-Converting Enzyme]–Intolerant Subjects With Cardiovascular Disease (TRANSCEND) it has been demonstrated that microalbuminuria and macroalbuminuria are associated with increased odds or risk of cognitive decline (Barzilay et al. 2011). Compared with participants with normoalbuminuria, those with microalbuminuria were more likely to have a reduced Mini-Mental State Examination (MMSE) score (<24). On follow-up, participants with baseline albuminuria had increased odds of cognitive decline (decrease in MMSE score

$\geq$3 points) compared with those with normoalbuminuria (microalbuminuria: OR, 1.22; 95 % CI, 1.07–1.38; macroalbuminuria: 1.21; 0.94–1.55). Participants with baseline macroalbuminuria treated with an angiotensin-converting enzyme inhibitor and/or angiotensin receptor blocker had lower odds of MMSE decline than participants treated with placebo.

Even though MAU is closely related to several traditional and non traditional CV risk factors and to a variety of indices of preclinical organ damage, the epidemiological studies above described showed that the association between microalbuminuria and cardiovascular disease remains even when all these risk factors are taken into account in multivariate analyses.

Therefore, the exact pathophysiological mechanisms explaining the association between MAU and CV disease remain uncompletely understood.

It is doubtful whether MAU causes atherothrombosis or vice versa. The most likely hypothesis is that a common pathophysiologic process, such as endothelial dysfunction, low-grade inflammation, or increased transvascular leakage of macromolecules, underlies the association between MAU and CV disease. In the STENO hypothesis put forward by Deckert et al. (Deckert et al. 1989) albumin leakage into the urine is a reflection of widespread vascular damage. The kidney thus would become a window to the vasculature; leaky renal vessels reflecting the permeability of the vasculature in general, caused by some alterations such as a reduction in the density of heparan sulfate-proteoglycan, not only of the glomerular basement membrane but also of the vascular wall. Generalized endothelial dysfunction (i.e., affecting many endothelial functions) plays an important role in both the initiation and the progression of atherosclerosis and MAU has been repeatedly shown to be accompanied by abnormalities in various markers of endothelial cell function in patients with and without diabetes (Fig. 6). However, there are some inconsistencies in the literature, and although microalbuminuria, marker of endothelial dysfunction, and low-grade inflammation are interrelated, they all are independently associated with risk for cardiovascular death.

Therefore, further studies are needed to explore the nature of the link between microalbuminuria and cardiovascular risk.

2.9 Microalbuminuria as Therapeutic Target

While there is now a very large and highly consistent amount of data showing that MAU is a strong predictor of CV risk, it is less clear whether reducing levels of MAU or limiting the progression to macroalbuminuria translates to a reduction in CV risk.

Although both ACE inhibitors and angiotensin receptors blockers (ARBs) (Redon 1998; ACE Inhibitors in Diabetic Nephropathy Trialist Group 2001; Viberti et al. 2002) have been shown to significantly reduce AER in patients with hypertension and diabetes mellitus, as well as in those with previous history of CVD, none of these clinical trials were designed to primarily study the effect of reducing microalbuminuria on CVD and renal outcomes.

In clinical trials of patients with chronic kidney disease and macroproteinuria as a result of type 2 diabetes, such as Irbesartan Diabetic Nephropathy Trial (IDNT) (Lewis et al. 2001) and Reduction of Endpoints in NIDDM with the Angiotensin II Antagonist Losartan (RENAAL) (Brenner et al. 2001), it is evident that therapeutic strategies that are associated with reduction of proteinuria are associated with fewer cardiovascular and kidney disease end points. However, whether one can extrapolate these observations to microalbuminuric patients is unknown.

The Prevention of REnal and Vascular ENdstage Disease Intervention Trial (PREVEND IT) is the only randomized trial to study the effect of albuminuria lowering in microalbuminuric, otherwise healthy individuals, who were not receiving antihypertensive or lipid-lowering agents (Asselbergs et al. 2004). In this clinical trial, 864 patients from the PREVEND cohort were enrolled and

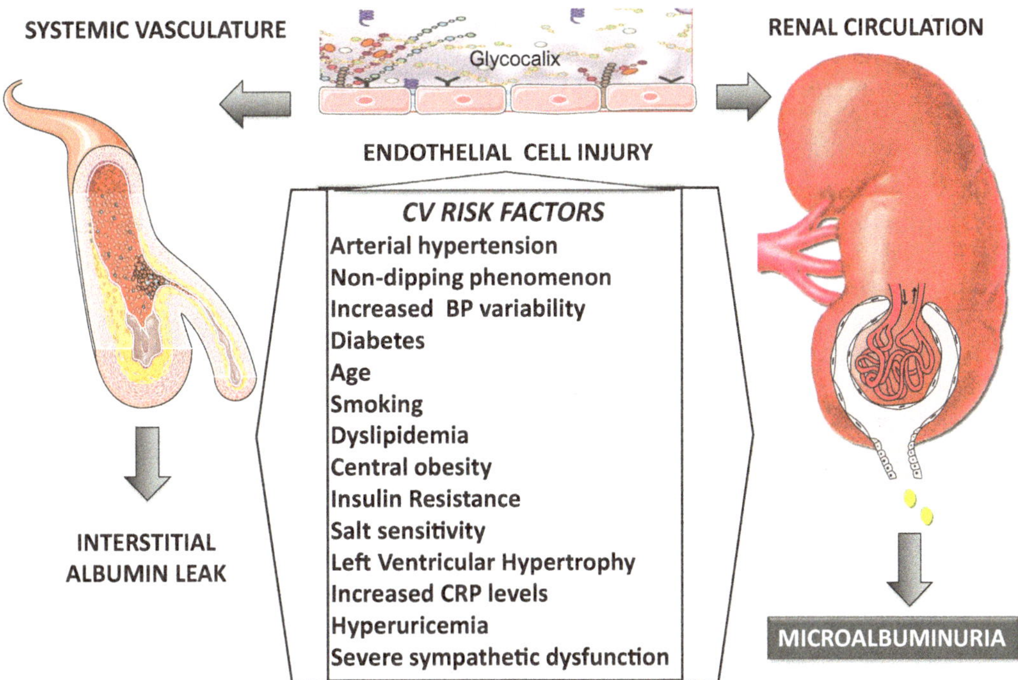

Fig. 6 Microalbuminuria as manifestation of systemic endothelial injury. Maladaptation of several endothelial functions, as a consequence of the deleterious effect of traditional and non traditional cardiovascular risk factors, is believed as an important effector mechanism in the development of albuminuria and of cardiovascular disease. A key mechanism that contributes to this process may be the loss of the glycocalyx—a proteoglycans-rich gel-like structure that lines the luminal endothelial surface. It mediates most of the regulatory functions of the endothelium and normally acts as a barrier against albumin filtration. Degradation of the glycocalyx in response to endothelial activation can lead to albuminuria and subsequent renal and vascular inflammation, thus providing a pathophysiological framework for the clinical association of albuminuria with renal and cardiovascular diseases

were randomized to receive fosinopril (20 mg/d) and/or pravastatin (40 mg/d) versus matching placebo in a 2 × 2 factorial design. The primary study end point was a composite of CVD mortality and hospitalization for nonfatal MI or myocardial ischemia, heart failure, peripheral vascular disease, or cerebrovascular accident. Participants were followed for a mean duration of 46 months. Median AER in these participants was 22.8 mg/d, and less than 5 % of participants were diabetic or had a previous CVD event. Fosinopril reduced albuminuria by 26 % (p < 0.001) and was associated with a 40 % reduction in the primary end point (p = 0.098) compared with placebo. Interestingly, a 90 % reduction (p = 0.03) in cerebrovascular events was observed in the group treated with fosinopril.

Adjustment for the blood pressure–lowering effect of fosinopril did not significantly change the primary outcome results (Asselbergs et al. 2004). On the other hand, pravastatin did not reduce albuminuria and was associated with a non significant 13 % reduction in the primary end point.

Although this was the first study that specifically targeted reducing albuminuria, it was essentially a primary prevention trial for cardiovascular disease (only 3.4 % of the participants had a history of CVD) and had an insufficient number of patients to be followed for a sufficient period of time to have enough events, so it was underpowered to determine a change in outcomes attributable to the antialbuminuric effect of fosinopril.

In the LIFE study, 8206 hypertensive patients with electrocardiographic evidence of left ventricular hypertrophy were randomized to either losartan or atenolol and observed for a median of 4.8 years. The treatment with the angiotensin receptor blocker resulted in a greater reduction in albuminuria compared with the beta blocker, despite equivalent decreases in blood pressure. Moreover, losartan reduced the incidence of the primary composite end point (nonfatal myocardial infarction and stroke and CV death) more than atenolol did. This effect of losartan on albuminuria accounted for about one fifth of its beneficial effect on the composite end point (Ibsen et al. 2004).

A prespecified secondary analysis of the same trial noted that a decrease of albuminuria levels in the first 12 month of treatment predicted a better long-term cardiovascular outcome, independently of in-treatment level of blood pressure, suggesting that therapeutic strategies that are associated with a reduction of albuminuria may be cardioprotective (Ibsen et al. 2005).

The Irbesartan in Patients With Type 2 Diabetes and Microalbuminuria (IRMA-2) study randomized 590 hypertensive patients with type 2 diabetes mellitus and microalbuminuria (urinary albumin excretion 20–200 μg/min) to irbesartan (150 mg/d or 300 mg/d) or placebo and observed them for a median duration of 2 years. Compared with placebo, irbesartan significantly reduced urinary albumin excretion at both doses, producing a mean reduction of 24 % with 150 mg/d and 38 % with 300 mg/d. Nonfatal CVD events tended to be slightly less frequent in the irbesartan 300 mg/d group than in the placebo group (4.5 % vs 8.7 %, p = 0.11) (Parving et al. 2001).

The Ongoing Telmisartan Alone and in Combination With Ramipril Global Endpoint Trial (ONTARGET), in which 25,600 people were enrolled with vascular disease comparing the effects on the incidence of CV events of ramipril with telmisartan versus the combination of telmisartan along with ramipril (Investigators et al. 2008), also provides little insight on the relationships between microalbuminuria reduction and CVD outcomes. In this very large study it was observed a greater decrease in proteinuria with the combination therapy, but no additional benefit on cardiovascular disease, and a faster decrease in GFR and increased risk of kidney failure and death. In this trial, the geometric mean baseline urine albumin-creatinine ratio was approximately 10 mg/g, with microalbuminuria and macroalbuminuria in only 13 % and 4 % of participants, respectively (Mann et al. 2008). However, even if the ONTARGET was not designed and powered to evaluate the associations between AER variations and CV end-points, when the study population changes in albuminuria were assessed regardless of randomization to specific drug, a greater reduction of urinary albumin under treatment was related to a lower incidence CV events (Schmieder et al. 2011).

Similar results were obtained in post hoc analyses of Action in Diabetes Mellitus and Vascular Disease (ADVANCE) (Zoungas et al. 2009). However, Avoiding Cardiovascular Events through Combination Therapy in Patients Living with Systolic Hypertension (ACCOMPLISH) (Bakris et al. 2010) does not confirm the potential prognostic value of AER changes. Likewise, a prospective study Olmesartan for the Delay or Prevention of Microalbuminuria in Type 2 Diabetes Mellitus (ROADMAP) (Haller et al. 2011) reported no association between changes in microalbuminuria and CV events during the double-blind period, although an observational follow-up concluded that development of microalbuminuria was a marker of cardiovascular events (Menne et al. 2014).

A single-center Spanish study (Pascual et al. 2014) including 2.835 patients showed that subjects in which microalbuminuria developed during a median follow-up of 4.7 years, or persisted from the beginning, had a significantly higher rate of events than if remained normoalbuminuric.

A recent meta-regression analysis by Savarese et al showed that a successfully reduced albuminuria was associated with lower risk of myocardial infarction and stroke (Fig. 7) (Savarese et al. 2014). However, this analysis included many heterogeneous studies wherein therapeutic intervention was not primarily aimed at reducing blood pressure, had a very short follow-up time

Fig. 7 Meta-regression analysis of 32 trials showing the association of albuminuria reduction with lower incidence of cardiovascular events in hypertensive and/or diabetic patients (Pascual et al. 2014) (Composite outcome: myocardial infarction, stroke, and cardiovascular death)

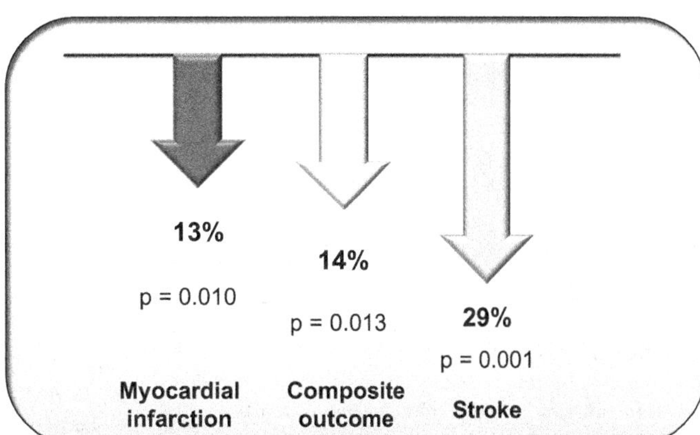

and did not include four trials specifically conducted on antihypertensive treatment. Similar conclusions were attained in another more recent meta-regression analysis showing a relationship between changes in albuminuria and CV risk, after adjustment for blood pressure variation under treatment. In studies reporting changes in CV events on the basis of albuminuria variations (six trials and 36,325 patients, mean follow-up 60 months, 3741 cardiovascular events), the overall adjusted relative risk of total CV events was 0.51 (95 % CI 0.38–0.59, P < 0.000) for albuminuria regression/no variation vs increase suggesting that urinary albumin excretion changes may be used in clinical practice as an intermediate endpoint of antihypertensive treatment (Viazzi et al. 2016). In the last European Society of Hypertension guidelines changes in albuminuria are regarded as potentially useful tool to monitor the effectiveness of treatment strategy in hypertensive patients, recognizing to this test the sensitivity to detect clinically meaningful changes over a timeframe of weeks or months (Mancia et al. 2013).

3　Conclusions

A large and highly consistent body of evidence supports the statements of recent guidelines for the management of hypertension (Mancia et al. 2013) and of KDIGO guidelines for evaluation and management of chronic kidney disease (Levin et al. 2013) that recommend to use both albuminuria and reduced GFR in all hypertensive subjects in order to provide more accurate prognostic information and therefore more precise risk stratification.

In particular, the powerful association between UAE and cardiovascular diseases, documented even below the current microalbuminuria threshold, reflects the underlying biological complexity of albumin excretion, in which subtle fluctuations signal important changes within the cardiovascular system.

In addition, it challenges our previous definition of normal, suggesting that albuminuria should be interpreted as a continuum rather than as threshold cut-off values.

Although there are some conflicting data, the great majority of studies and meta-analyses show that reducing albuminuria improves cardiovascular outcome. The simple search for subclinical renal damage in hypertensive patients may enable the clinician to better assess absolute cardiovascular.

Risk and make a more correct decision regarding therapeutic strategies. Identification of MAU and of a moderate reduction in eGFR may induce physicians to encourage patients to make healthy lifestyle changes, and perhaps would prompt to more aggressive modification of standard risk factors for cardiovascular diseases.

References

ACE Inhibitors in Diabetic Nephropathy Trialist Group (2001) Should all patients with type 1 diabetes mellitus and microalbuminuria receive angiotensin converting enzyme inhibitors? A meta-analysis of individual patient data. Ann Intern Med 134:370–379

Agrawal B, Berger A, Wolf K, Luft FC (1996) Microalbuminuria screening by reagent strip predicts cardiovascular risk in hypertension. J Hypertens 14:223–228

Alberti KG, Zimmet PZ (1998) Definition, diagnosis and classification of diabetes mellitus and its complications. Part 1: diagnosis and classification of diabetes mellitus: provisional report of a WHO consultation. Diabet Med 15:539–553

Andronico G, Ferrara L, Mangano M, Mulè G, Cerasola G (1998) Insulin, sodium-lithium countertransport, and microalbuminuria in hypertensive patients. Hypertension 31:110–113

Andronico G, Romé M, Lo Cicero A, Parsi R, Seddio G, Ferraro-Mortellaro R et al (2005) Renal plasma flow, filtration fraction and microalbuminuria in hypertensive patients: effects of chronic smoking. Nephrology (Carlton) 10:483–486

Arnlov J, Evans JC, Meigs JB, Wang TJ, Fox CS, Levy D et al (2005) Low-grade albuminuria and incidence of cardiovascular disease events in nonhypertensive and nondiabetic individuals: The Framingham Heart Study. Circulation 112:969–975

Asselbergs FW, Diercks GFH, Hillege HL, van Boven AJ, Janssen WM, Voors AA, et al. for the Prevention of Renal and Vascular Endstage Disease Intervention Trial investigators (2004) Effects of fosinopril and pravastatin on cardiovascular events in subjects with microalbuminuria. Circulation 110: 2809–2816

Astor BC, Hallan SI, Miller ER 3rd, Yeung E, Coresh J (2008) Glomerular filtration rate, albuminuria, and risk of cardiovascular and all-cause mortality in the US population. Am J Epidemiol 167:1226–1234

Astor BC, Matsushita K, Gansevoort RT, van der Velde M, Woodward M, Levey AS et al (2011) Lower estimated glomerular filtration rate and higher albuminuria are associated with mortality and end-stage renal disease. A collaborative meta-analysis of kidney disease population cohorts. Kidney Int 79:1331–1340

Bakris GL, Sarafidis PA, Weir MR, Dahlöf B, Pitt B, Jamerson K, ACCOMPLISH Trial Investigators et al (2010) Renal outcomes with different fixed-dose combination therapies in patients with hypertension at high risk for cardiovascular events (ACCOMPLISH): a prespecified secondary analysis of a randomised controlled trial. Lancet 375:1173–1181

Barzilay JI, Gao P, O'Donnell M et al (2011) Albuminuria and decline in cognitive function: the ONTARGET/ TRANSCEND studies. Arch Intern Med 171:142–150

Bianchi S, Bigazzi R, Baldari G, Sgherri GP, Campese VM (1994) Diurnal variation of blood pressure and microalbuminuria in essential hypertension. Am J Hypertens 7:23–29

Bigazzi R, Bianchi S, Nenci R, Baldari D, Baldari G, Campese VM (1995) Increased thickness of the carotid artery in patients with essential hypertension and microalbuminuria. J Hum Hypertens 9:827–833

Bigazzi R, Bianchi S, Baldari S, Campese VM (1998) Microalbuminuria predicts cardiovascular events and renal insufficiency in patients with essential hypertension. J Hypertens 16:1325–1333

Biomarkers Definitions Working Group (2001) Biomarkers and surrogate endpoints: Preferred definitions and conceptual framework. Clin Pharmacol Ther 69:89–95

Böhm M, Thoenes M, Danchin N, Bramlage P, La Puerta P, Volpe M (2007) Association of cardiovascular risk factors with microalbuminuria in hypertensive individuals: the i-SEARCH global study. J Hypertens 25:2317–2324

Bramlage P, Pittrow D, Lehnert H, Höfler M, Kirch W, Ritz E, Wittchen HU (2007) Frequency of albuminuria in primary care: a cross sectional study. Eur J Cardiovasc Prev Rehabil 14:107–113

Brantsma AH, Bakker SJ, de Zeeuw D, de Jong PE, Gansevoort RT (2008) Extended prognostic value of urinary albumin excretion for cardiovascular events. J Am Soc Nephrol 19:1785–1791

Brenner BM, Cooper ME, de Zeeuw D, Keane WF, Mitch WE, Parving HH et al (2001) Effects of losartan on renal and cardiovascular outcomes in patients with type 2 diabetes and nephropathy. N Engl J Med 345:861–869

Campese VM, Bianchi S, Bigazzi R (1999) Association between hyperlipidemia and microalbuminuria in essential hypertension. Kidney Int 56(Suppl 7):S10–S13

Cerasola G, Cottone S (1997) Microalbuminuria as a marker of vascular damage in hypertension: influence of blood pressure and metabolic patterns. Nutr Metab Cardiovasc Dis 7:92–95

Cerasola G, Cottone S, D'Ignoto G, Grasso L, Mangano MT, Andronico G (1989) Microalbuminuria as a predictor of cardiovascular damage in essential hypertension. J Hypertens 7(Suppl 6):S332–S333

Cerasola G, Cottone S, Nardi E, D'Ignoto G, Volpe V, Mulé G, Carollo C (1995) White-coat hypertension and cardiovascular risk. J Cardiovasc Risk 2:545–549

Cerasola G, Cottone S, Mulè G, Nardi E, Mangano MT, Andronico G, Contorno A et al (1996) Microalbuminuria, renal dysfunction and cardiovascular complication in essential hypertension. J Hypertens 14:915–920

Cerasola G, Mulè G, Nardi E, Cottone S, Andronico G, Mongiovì R et al (2004) Usefulness of microalbuminuria in cardiovascular risk stratification of essential hypertensive patients. Nephron Clin Pract 96:c23–c30

Cerasola G, Mulè G, Cottone S, Nardi E, Cusimano P (2008) Hypertension, microalbuminuria and renal dysfunction: the Renal Dysfunction in Hypertension (REDHY) study. J Nephrol 21:368–373

Cerasola G, Mulè G, Nardi E, Cusimano P, Palermo A, Arsena R et al (2010) Clinical correlates of renal dysfunction in hypertensive patients without cardiovascular complications: the REDHY study. J Hum Hypertens 24:44–50

Chen J, Muntner P, Hamm LL, Jones DW, Batuman V, Fonseca V et al (2004) The metabolic syndrome and chronic kidney disease in U.S. adults. Ann Intern Med 140:167–174

Cirillo M, Senigalliesi L, Laurenzi M, Alfieri R, Stamler J, Stamler R et al (1998) Microalbuminuria in nondiabetic adults: relation of blood pressure, body mass index, plasma cholesterol levels, and smoking: The Gubbio Population Study. Arch Intern Med 158:1933–1939

Cirillo M, Laurenzi M, Mancini M, Zanchetti A, De Santo NG (2006) Low muscular mass and overestimation of microalbuminuria by urinary albumin/creatinine ratio. Hypertension 47:56–61

Cirillo M, Lanti MP, Menotti A, Laurenzi M, Mancini M, Zanchetti A, De Santo NG (2008) Definition of kidney dysfunction as a cardiovascular risk factor: use of urinary albumin excretion and estimated glomerular filtration rate. Arch Intern Med 168:617–624

Coresh J, Selvin E, Stevens LA, Manzi J, Kusek JW, Eggers P et al (2007) Prevalence of chronic kidney disease in the United States. JAMA 298:2038–2047

Cottone S, Cerasola G (1992) Microalbuminuria fractional clearance and early renal permselectivity changes in essential hypertension. Am J Nephrol 12:326–329

Cottone S, Vadalà A, Mangano MT, Vella MC, Riccobene R, Neri AL et al (2000) Endothelium-derived factors in microalbuminuric and nonmicroalbuminuric essential hypertensives. Am J Hypertens 13:172–176

Cottone S, Mulè G, Nardi E, Lorito MC, Guarneri M, Arsena R, Cerasola G (2007) Microalbuminuria and early endothelial activation in essential hypertension. J Hum Hypertens 21:167–172

Cuspidi C, Meani S, Fusi V, Severgnini B, Valerio C, Catini E et al (2004) Metabolic syndrome and target organ damage in untreated essential hypertensives. J Hypertens 22:1991–1998

Deckert T, Feldt-Rasmussen B, Borch-Johnsen K, Jensen T, Kofoed-Enevoldsen A (1989) Albuminuria reflects widespread vascular damage. The Steno hypothesis. Diabetologia 32:219–226

Diercks GF, van Boven AJ, Hillege HL, Janssen WM, Kors JA, de Jong PE et al (2000) Microalbuminuria is independently associated with ischaemic electrocardiographic abnormalities in a large nondiabetic population. The PREVEND (Prevention of Renal and Vascular ENdstage Disease) study. Eur Heart J 21:1922–1927

Dinneen SF, Gerstein HC (1997) The association of microalbuminuria and mortality in non-insulin-dependent diabetes mellitus: a systematic overview of the literature. Arch Intern Med 157:1413–1418

Dworkin LD, Ichikawa I, Brenner BM (1983) Hormonal modulation of glomerular function. Am J Physiol 244:F95–F104

Festa A, D'Agostino R, Howard G, Mykkanen L, Tracy RP, Haffner SM (2000) Inflammation and microalbuminuria in nondiabetic and type 2 diabetic subjects: the Insulin Resistance Atherosclerosis Study. Kidney Int 58:1703–1710

Foley RN, Murray AM, Li S, Herzog CA, McBean AM, Eggers PW et al (2005) Chronic kidney disease and the risk for cardiovascular disease, renal replacement, and death in the United States Medicare population, 1998 to 1999. J Am Soc Nephrol 16:489–495

Fox CS, Matsushita K, Woodward M, Bilo HJG, Chalmers J, Heerspink HJL et al (2012) Associations of kidney disease measures with mortality and end-stage renal disease in individuals with and without diabetes: a meta-analysis. Lancet 380:1662–1673

Furtner M, Kiechl S, Mair A, Seppi K, Weger S, Oberhollenzer F et al (2005) Urinary albumin excretion is independently associated with carotid and femoral artery atherosclerosis in the general population. Eur Heart J 26:279–287

Gansevoort RT, Correa-Rotter R, Hemmelgarn BR, Jafar TH, Heerspink HJL, Mann JF et al (2013) Chronic kidney disease and cardiovascular risk: epidemiology, mechanisms, and prevention. Lancet 382:339–352

Geraci G, Mulè G, Geraci C, Mogavero M, D'Ignoto F, Morreale M et al (2015a) Association of renal resistive index with aortic pulse wave velocity in hypertensive patients. Eur J Prev Cardiol 22:415–422

Geraci G, Mulè G, Mogavero M, Geraci C, D'Ignoti D, Guglielmo C et al (2015b) Renal haemodynamics and severity of carotid atherosclerosis in hypertensive patients with and without impaired renal function. Nutr Metab Cardiovasc 25:160–166

Geraci G, Mulè G, Costanza G, Mogavero M, Geraci C, Cottone S (2016) Relationship between carotid atherosclerosis and pulse pressure with renal hemodynamics in hypertensive patients. Am J Hypertens 29:519–527

Gerstein HC, Mann JF, Pogue J, Dinneen SF, Hallé JP, Hoogwerf B et al (2000) Prevalence and determinants of microalbuminuria in high-risk diabetic and nondiabetic patients in the Heart Outcomes Prevention Evaluation Study. The HOPE Study Investigators. Diabetes Care 23(Suppl 2):B35–B39

Gerstein HC, Mann JF, Yi Q, Zinman B, Dinneen SF, Hoogwerf B, Halle JP et al (2001) Albuminuria and risk of cardiovascular events, death, and heart failure in diabetic and nondiabetic individuals. JAMA 286:421–426

Go A, Chertow G, Fan D, Mcculloch CE, Hsu C (2004) Chronic kidney disease and the risks of death, cardiovascular events, and hospitalization. New Eng J Med 351:1296–1305

Halbesma N, Kuiken DS, Brantsma AH, Bakker SJL, Wetzels JFM, de Zeeuw D et al (2006) Macroalbuminuria is a better risk marker than low estimated GFR to identify individuals at risk for accelerated GFR loss in population screening. J Am Soc Nephrol 17:2582–2590

Hallan SI, Ritz E, Lydersen S, Romundstad S, Kvenild K, Orth SR (2009) Combining GFR and albuminuria to classify CKD improves prediction of ESRD. J Am Soc Nephrol 20:1069–1077

Hallan SI, Matsushita K, Sang Y, Mahmoodi BK, Black C, Ishani A et al (2012) Age and association of kidney measures with mortality and end-stage renal disease. JAMA 308:2349–2360

Haller H, Ito S, Izzo JL Jr, Januszewicz A, Katayama S, Menne J, ROADMAP Trial Investigators et al (2011) Olmesartan for the delay or prevention of microalbuminuria in type 2 diabetes. N Engl J Med 364:907–917

Hemmelgarn BR, Manns BJ, Lloyd A, James MT, Klarenbach S, Quinn RR et al (2010) Relation between kidney function, proteinuria, and adverse outcomes. JAMA 303:423–429

Hermans MM, Henry R, Dekker JM, Kooman JP, Kostense PJ, Nijpels G et al (2007) Estimated glomerular filtration rate and urinary albumin excretion are independently associated with greater arterial stiffness: the Hoorn Study. J Am Soc Nephrol 18:1942–1952

Hillege HL, Janssen WM, Bak AA, Diercks GF, Grobbee DE, Crijns HJ et al (2001) Microalbuminuria is common, also in a nondiabetic, nonhypertensive population, and an independent indicator of cardiovascular risk factors and cardiovascular morbidity. J Intern Med 249:519–526

Hillege HL, Fidler V, Diercks GF, van Gilst WH, de Zeeuw D, van Veldhuisen DJ et al (2002) Urinary albumin excretion predicts cardiovascular and noncardiovascular mortality in general population. Circulation 106:1777–1782

Hostetter TH, Olson JL, Rennke HG, Venkatachalam MA, Brenner BM (1981) Hyperfiltration in remnant nephrons: A potential adverse response to renal ablation. Am J Physiol 241:F85–F93

Hsu CC, Brancati FL, Astor BC, Kao WH, Steffes MW, Folsom AR, Coresh J (2009) Blood pressure, atherosclerosis, and albuminuria in 10,113 participants in the Atherosclerosis Risk in Communities Study. J Hypertens 27:397–409

Ibsen H, Wachtell K, Olsen MH, Borch-Johnsen K, Lindholm LH, Mogensen CE et al (2004) Does albuminuria predict cardiovascular outcome on treatment with losartan versus atenolol in hypertension with left ventricular hypertrophy? A LIFE substudy. J Hypertens 22:1805–1811

Ibsen H, Olsen MH, Wachtell K, Borch-Johnsen K, Lindholm LH, Mogensen CE et al (2005) Reduction in albuminuria translates to reduction in cardiovascular events in hypertensive patients: Losartan

Intervention for Endpoint Reduction in Hypertension Study. Hypertension 45:198–202

Investigators ONTARGET, Yusuf S, Teo KK, Pogue J, Dyal L, Copland I, Schumacher H et al (2008) Telmisartan, ramipril, or both in patients at high risk for vascular events. N Engl J Med 358:1547–1559

Jager A, Kostense PJ, Nijpels G, Heine RJ, Bouter LM, Stehouwer CD (1998) Microalbuminuria is strongly associated with NIDDM and hypertension, but not with the insulin resistance syndrome: the Hoorn Study. Diabetologia 41:694–700

Jager A, van Hinsbergh VW, Kostense PJ, Emeis JJ, Nijpels G, Dekker JM, Heine RJ, Bouter LM, Stehouwer CD (2002) C-reactive protein and soluble vascular cell adhesion molecule-1 are associated with elevated urinary albumin excretion but do not explain its link with cardiovascular risk. Arterioscler Thromb Vasc Biol 22:593–598

Jørgensen L, Jenssen T, Johnsen SH, Mathiesen EB, Heuch I, Joakimsen O et al (2007) Albuminuria as risk factor for initiation and progression of carotid atherosclerosis in non-diabetic persons: the Tromsø Study. Eur Heart J 28:363–369

Keen H, Chlouverakis C (1963) An immunoassay method for urinary albumin at low concentrations. Lancet 2:913–914

Klausen K, Borch-Johnsen K, Feldt-Rasmussen B, Jensen G, Clausen P, Scharling H et al (2004) Very low levels of microalbuminuria are associated with increased risk of coronary heart disease and death independently of renal function, hypertension, and diabetes. Circulation 110:32–35

Klausen KP, Parving HH, Scharling H, Jensen JS (2007) The association between metabolic syndrome, microalbuminuria and impaired renal function in the general population: impact on cardiovascular disease and mortality. J Intern Med 262:470–478

Klausen KP, Parving HH, Scharling H, Jensen JS (2009) Microalbuminuria and obesity: impact on cardiovascular disease and mortality. Clin Endocrinol (Oxf) 71:40–45

Kshirsagar AV, Bomback AS, Bang H, Gerber LM, Vupputuri S, Shoham DA et al (2008) Association of C-reactive protein and microalbuminuria (from the National Health and Nutrition Examination Surveys, 1999 to 2004). Am J Cardiol 101:401–406

Leoncini G, Viazzi F, Agabiti Rosei E, Ambrosioni E, Costa FV, Leonetti G et al (2010) Chronic kidney disease in hypertension under specialist care: the I-DEMAND study. J Hypertens 28:156–162

Levey AS, Cattran D, Friedman A, Miller WG, Sedor J, Tuttle K et al (2009) Proteinuria as a surrogate outcome in CKD: report of a scientific workshop sponsored by the National Kidney Foundation and the US Food and Drug Administration. Am J Kidney Dis 54:205–226

Levin A, Stevens PE, Bilous RW, Coresh J, De Francisco ALM, de Jong PE, Kidney Disease: Improving Global Outcomes (KDIGO) CKD Work Group et al (2013)

KDIGO 2012 clinical practice guideline for the evaluation and management of chronic kidney disease. Kidney Int Suppl 3:4

Lewis EJ, Hunsicker LG, Clarke WR, Berl T, Pohl MA, Lewis JB et al (2001) Renoprotective effect of the angiotensin-receptor antagonist irbesartan in patients with nephropathy due to type 2 diabetes. N Engl J Med 345:851–860

Lieb W, Mayer B, Stritzke J, Doering A, Hense HW, Loewel H, Erdmann J et al (2006) Association of low-grade urinary albumin excretion with left ventricular hypertrophy in the general population: the MONICA/KORA Augsburg Echocardiographic Substudy. Nephrol Dial Transplant 21:2780–2787

Mafham M, Emberson J, Landray MJ, Wen C-P, Baigent C (2011) Estimated glomerular filtration rate and the risk of major vascular events and all-cause mortality: a meta-analysis. PLoS ONE 6:e25920

Mahmoodi BK, Matsushita K, Woodward M, Blankestijn PJ, Cirillo M, Ohkubo T et al (2012) Associations of kidney disease measures with mortality and end-stage renal disease in individuals with and without hypertension: a meta-analysis. Lancet 380:1649–1661

Malik AR, Sultan S, Turner ST, Kullo IJ (2007) Urinary albumin excretion is associated with impaired flow- and nitroglycerin-mediated brachial artery dilatation in hypertensive adults. J Hum Hypertens 21:231–238

Mancia G, Fagard R, Narkiewicz K, Redon J, Zanchetti A, Bhöm M (2013) et al; Task Force Members. 2013 ESH/ESC Guidelines for the Management of Arterial Hypertension. The Task Force for the Management of Arterial Hypertension of the European Society of Hypertension (ESH) and of the European Society of Cardiology (ESC). J Hypertens 31:1281–1357

Mann JF, Schmieder RE, McQueen M, Dyal L, Schumacher H, Pogue J, ONTARGET investigators et al (2008) Renal outcomes with telmisartan, ramipril, or both, in people at high vascular risk (the ONTARGET study): a multicentre, randomised, double-blind, controlled trial. Lancet 372:547–553

Matsushita K, van der Velde M, Astor BC, Woodward M, Levey AS, de Jong PE et al (2010) Association of estimated glomerular filtration rate and albuminuria with all-cause and cardiovascular mortality in general population cohorts: a collaborative meta-analysis. Lancet 375:2073–2081

Meccariello A, Buono F, Verrengia E, Orefice G, Grieco F, Romeo F et al (2016) Microalbuminuria predicts the recurrence of cardiovascular events in patients with essential hypertension. J Hypertens 34:646–665

Menne J, Ritz E, Ruilope LM, Chatzikyrkou C, Viberti G, Haller H (2014) The Randomized Olmesartan and Diabetes Microalbuminuria Prevention (ROADMAP) observational follow-up study: benefits of RAS blockade with olmesartan treatment are sustained after study discontinuation. J Am Heart Assoc 3:e000810

Miller WG, Bruns DE, Hortin GL, Sandberg S, Aakre KM, McQueen MJ et al (2009) Current issues in measurement and reporting of urinary albumin excretion. Clin Chem 55:24–38

Mogensen CE (1984) Microalbuminuria predicts clinical proteinuria and early mortality in maturity onset diabetes. N Engl J Med 310:356–360

Mogensen CE (2003) Microalbuminuria and hypertension with focus on type 1 and type 2 diabetes. J Intern Med 254:45–66

Mogensen CE, Christensen CK (1984) Predicting diabetic nephropathy in insulin-dependent patients. New Eng J Med 31:89–93

Mogensen CE, Vestbo E, Poulsen PL, Christiansen C, Damsgaard EM, Eiskjaer H et al (1995) Microalbuminuria and potential confounders. A review and some observations on variability of urinary albumin excretion. Diabetes Care 18:572–581

Morreale M, Mulè G, Ferrante A, D'ignoto F, Cottone S (2016) Association of renal resistive index with markers of extrarenal vascular changes in patients with systemic lupus erythematosus. Ultrasound Med Biol 42:1103–1110. doi:10.1016/j.ultrasmedbio.2015.12.025

Mountokalakis TD (1997) The renal consequences of hypertension. Kidney Int 51:1639–1653

Moynihan R, Glassock R, Doust J (2013) Chronic kidney disease controversy: how expanding definitions are unnecessarily labelling many people as diseased. BMJ 347:f4298

Mulè G, Cottone S, Vadalà A, Volpe V, Mezzatesta G, Mongiovì R et al (2004) Relationship between albumin excretion rate and aortic stiffness in untreated essential hypertensive patients. J Intern Med 256:22–29

Mulè G, Nardi E, Cottone S, Cusimano P, Volpe V, Piazza G et al (2005) Influence of metabolic syndrome on hypertension-related target organ damage. J Intern Med 257:503–513

Mulè G, Cottone S, Mongiovì R, Cusimano P, Mezzatesta G, Seddio G et al (2006) Influence of metabolic syndrome on aortic stiffness in never treated hypertensive patients. Nutr Metab Cardiovasc Dis 16:54–59

Mulè G, Cottone S, Cusimano P, Riccobene R, Palermo A, Geraci C et al (2009) The association of microalbuminuria with aortic stiffness is independent of C-reactive protein in essential hypertension. Am J Hypertens 22:1041–1047

Mulè G, Cottone S, Cusimano P, Palermo A, Geraci C, Nardi E et al (2010) Unfavourable interaction of microalbuminuria and mildly reduced creatinine clearance on aortic stiffness in essential hypertension. Int J Cardiol 145:372–375. http://dx.doi.org/10.1016/j.ijcard.2010.02.047

Mulè G, Calcaterra I, Costanzo M, Geraci G, Guarino L, Foraci L et al (2015a) Relationship between short-term blood pressure variability and subclinical renal damage in essential hypertensive patients. J Clin Hypertens (Greenwich) 17:473–480

Mulè G, Geraci G, Geraci C, Morreale M, Cottone S (2015b) The renal resistive index: is it a misnomer.

Intern Emerg Med 10:889–891. doi:10.1007/s11739-015-1323-1324

Mulè G, Calcaterra I, Costanzo M, Morreale M, Castiglia A, D'Ignoto F et al (2016) Average real variability of 24-h systolic blood pressure is associated with microalbuminuria in patients with primary hypertension. J Hum Hypertens 30:164–170

Munakata M, Miura Y, Yoshinaga K, J-TOPP study group (2009) Higher brachial-ankle pulse wave velocity as an independent risk factor for future microalbuminuria in patients with essential hypertension: the J-TOPP study. J Hypertens 27:1466–1471

Newman DJ, Mattock MB, Dawnay AB, Kerry S, McGuire A, Yaqoob M et al (2005) Systematic review on urine albumin testing for early detection of diabetic complications. Health Technol Assess 9:iii–vi, xiii–163

Ninomiya T, Perkovic V, de Galan BE, Zoungas S, Pillai A, Jardine M, et al on behalf of the ADVANCE Collaborative Group (2009) Albuminuria and kidney function independently predict cardiovascular and renal outcomes in diabetes. J Am Soc Nephrol 20:1813–1821

Ninomiya T, Perkovic V, Verdon C, Barzi F, Cass A, Gallagher M, Jardine M, Anderson C, Chalmers J, Craig JC, Huxley R (2009b) Proteinuria and stroke: a meta-analysis of cohort studies. Am J Kidney Dis 53:417–425

Nitsch D, Grams M, Sang Y, Black C, Cirillo M, Djurdjev O et al (2013) Associations of estimated glomerular filtration rate and albuminuria with mortality and renal failure by sex: a meta-analysis. BMJ 346:f324

O'Hare AM, Choi AI, Bertenthal D, Bacchetti P, Garg AX, Kaufman JS et al (2007) Age affects outcomes in chronic kidney disease. J Am Soc Nephrol 18:2758–2765

Palaniappan L, Carnethon M, Fortmann SP (2003) Association between microalbuminuria and the metabolic syndrome: NHANES III. Am J Hypertens 16:952–958

Palatini P, Graniero GR, Canali C, Santonastaso M, Mos L, Piccolo D et al (1995) Relationship between albumin excretion rate, ambulatory blood pressure and left ventricular hypertrophy in mild hypertension. J Hypertens 13:1796–1800

Palatini P, Mormino P, Santonastaso M, Mos L, Dal Follo M, Zanata G, Pessina AC (1998) Target-organ damage in stage I hypertensive subjects with white coat and sustained hypertension: results from the HARVEST study. Hypertension 31:57–63

Parving HH, Lehnert H, Brochner-Mortenson J, Gomis R, Andersen S, Arner P. for the Irbesartan in Patients with Type 2 Diabetes and Microalbuminuria Study Group (2001) The effect of irbesartan on the development of diabetic nephropathy in patients with type 2 diabetes. N Engl J Med 345: 870–878

Parving HH, Lewis JB, Ravid M, Remuzzi G, Hunsicker LG (2006) Prevalence and risk factors for microalbuminuria in a referred cohort of type II diabetic patients: a global perspective. Kidney Int 69:2057–2063

Pascual JM, Rodilla E, Miralles A, Gonzalez C, Redon J (2006) Determinants of urinary albumin excretion reduction in essential hypertension: a long-term follow-up study. J Hypertens 24:2277–2284

Pascual JM, Rodilla E, Costa JA, Garcia-Escrich M, Gonzalez C, Redon J (2014) Prognostic value of microalbuminuria during antihypertensive treatment in essential hypertension. Hypertension 64:1228–1234

Pedrinelli R, Giampietro O, Cammassi F, Melillo E, Dell'Olmo G, Catapano G (1994) Microalbuminuria and endothelial dysfunction in essential hypertension. Lancet 344:14–18

Pedrinelli R, Dell'Omo G, Di Bello V, Pontremoli R, Mariani M (2002) Microalbuminuria an integrated marker of cardiovascular risk in essential hypertension. J Hum Hypertens 16:79–89

Pedrinelli R, Dell'Omo G, Di Bello V, Pellegrini G, Pucci L, Del Prato S, Penno G (2004) Low-grade inflammation and microalbuminuria in hypertension. Arterioscler Thromb Vasc Biol 24:2414–2419

Perkovic V, Verdon C, Ninomiya T, Barzi F, Cass A, Patel A, Jardine M, Gallagher M, Turnbull F, Chalmers J, Craig J, Huxley R (2008) The relationship between proteinuria and coronary risk: a systematic review and meta-analysis. PLoS Med 5(10):e207

Pinto-Sietsma SJ, Mulder J, Janssen WM, Hillege HL, De Zeeuw D, De Jong PE (2000) Smoking is related to albuminuria and abnormal renal function in nondiabetic persons. Ann Int Med 133:585–591

Pinto-Sietsma SJ, Navis G, Janssen WM, de Zeeuw D, Gans RO, de Jong PE, PREVEND Study Group (2003) A central body fat distribution is related to renal function impairment, even in lean subjects. Am J Kidney Dis 41:733–741

Pontremoli R, Sofia A, Ravera M, Nicolella C, Viazzi F, Tirotta A et al (1997) Prevalence and clinical correlates of microalbuminuria in essential hypertension: the MAGIC Study. Microalbuminuria: A Genoa Investigation on Complications. Hypertension 30:1135–1143

Pontremoli R, Ravera M, Bezante GP, Viazzi F, Nicolella C, Berruti V et al (1999) Left ventricular geometry and function in patients with essential hypertension and microalbuminuria. J Hypertens 17:993–1000

Ratto E, Leoncini G, Viazzi F, Bezante GP, Falqui V, Parodi A et al (2008) Inappropriate left ventricular mass is associated with microalbuminuria independently of left ventricular hypertrophy in primary hypertension. J Hypertens 26:345–350

Ravera M, Ratto E, Vettoretti S, Viazzi F, Leoncini G, Parodi D et al (2002) Microalbuminuria and subclinical cerebrovascular damage in essential hypertension. J Nephrol 15:519–524

Redon J (1998) Renal protection by antihypertensive drugs: insights from microalbuminuria studies. J Hypertens 16:2091–2100

Redon J, Williams B (2002) Microalbuminuria in essential hypertension. Redefining the threshold. J Hypertens 20:353–355

Redon J, Liao Y, Lozano JV, Miralles A, Pasqual JM, Cooper RS (1994) Ambulatory blood pressure and microalbuminuria in essential hypertension: role of circadian variability. J Hypertens 12:947–953

Rodondi N, Yerly P, Gabriel A, Riesen WF, Burnier M, Paccaud F et al (2007) Microalbuminuria, but not cystatin C, is associated with carotid atherosclerosis in middle-aged adults. Nephrol Dial Transplant 22:1107–1114

Ruggenenti P, Remuzzi G (2006) Time to abandon microalbuminuria? Kidney Int 70:1214–1222

Ruilope LM (2002) The kidney as a sensor of cardiovascular risk in essential hypertension prevalence of mild renal insufficiency in essential hypertension. J Am Soc Nephrol Suppl 3: S165–S168.

Savarese G, Dei Cas A, Rosano G, D'Amore C, Musella F, Mosca S et al (2014) Reduction of albumin urinary excretion is associated with reduced cardiovascular events in hypertensive and/or diabetic patients. A meta-regression analysis of 32 randomized trials. Int J Cardiol 172:403–410

Schmieder RE, Mann JF, Schumacher H, Gao P, Mancia G, Weber MA et al (2011) ONTARGET Investigators. Changes in albuminuria predict mortality and morbidity in patients with vascular disease. J Am Soc Nephrol 22:1353–1364

Sciarretta S, Pontremoli R, Rosei EA, Ambrosioni E, Costa V, Leonetti G et al (2009) Independent association of ECG abnormalities with microalbuminuria and renal damage in hypertensive patients without overt cardiovascular disease: data from Italy-Developing Education and awareness on MicroAlbuminuria in patients with hypertensive Disease study. J Hypertens 27:410–417

Smilde TD, Asselbergs FW, Hillege HL, Voors AA, Kors JA, Gansevoort RT et al (2005) Mild renal dysfunction is associated with electrocardiographic left ventricular hypertrophy. Am J Hypertens 18:342–347

Smith A, Karalliedde J, De Angelis L, Goldsmith D, Viberti G (2005) Aortic pulse wave velocity and albuminuria in patients with type 2 diabetes. J Am Soc Nephrol 16:1069–1075

Srinivasan SR, Myers L, Berenson GS (2000) Risk variables of insulin resistance syndrome in African American and Caucasian young adults with microalbuminuria: the Bogalusa Heart Study. Am J Hypertens 13:1274–1279

Stehouwer CDA, Henry RMA, Dekker JM, Nijpels G, Heine RJ, Bouter LM (2004) Microalbuminuria is associated with impaired brachial artery, flow-mediated vasodilation in elderly individuals without and with diabetes: Further evidence for a link between microalbuminuria and endothelial dysfunction—The Hoorn Study. Kidney Int 66(Suppl 92):S42–S44

Svendsen PA, Oxenball B, Christiansen JS (1981) Microalbuminuria in diabetic patients: a longitudinal study. Acta Endocrinol Suppl (Copenh) 242:53–54

The Chronic Kidney Disease Prognosis Consortium (2011) Association of estimated glomerular filtration rate and albuminuria with mortality and end-stage renal disease: a collaborative meta-analysis of kidney disease cohorts. Kidney Int 79:1331–1340

Tsioufis C, Stefanadis C, Antoniadis D, Toutouza M, Kallikazaros I, Pitsavos C et al (2002) Microalbuminuria is associated with unfavorable left ventricular geometry patterns in untreated, non-diabetic, patients with essential hypertension. J Hum Hypertens 16:249–254

Tsioufis C, Thomopoulos C, Dimitriadis K, Amfilochiou A, Tsiachris D, Selima M et al (2008) Association of obstructive sleep apnea with urinary albumin excretion in essential hypertension: a cross-sectional study. Am J Kidney Dis 52:285–293

Tuttle KR, Puhlman ME, Cooney SK, Short R (1999) Urinary albumin and insulin as predictors of coronary artery disease: an angiographic study. Am J Kidney Dis 34:918–925

Upadhyay A, Hwang SJ, Mitchell GF, Vasan RS, Vita JA, Stantchev PI, Meigs JB, Larson MG, Levy D, Benjamin EJ, Fox CS (2009) Arterial stiffness in mild-to-moderate CKD. J Am Soc Nephrol 20:2044–2053

van der Velde M, Halbesma N, de Charro FT, Bakker SJ, de Zeeuw D, de Jong PE, Gansevoort RT (2009) Screening for albuminuria identifies individuals at increased renal risk. J Am Soc Nephrol 20:852–862

van der Velde M, Matsushita K, Coresh J, Astor BC, Woodward M, Levey AS et al (2011) Lower estimated glomerular filtration rate and higher albuminuria are associated with all-cause and cardiovascular mortality. A collaborative meta-analysis of high-risk population cohorts. Kidney Int 79:1341–1352

Viazzi F, Leoncini G, Conti N, Tomolillo C, Giachero G, Vercelli M et al (2010) Microalbuminuria is a predictor of chronic renal insufficiency in patients without diabetes and with hypertension: the MAGIC study. Clin J Am Soc Nephrol 5:1099–1106

Viazzi F, Leoncini G, Derchi LE, Pontremoli R (2015) Ultrasound Doppler renal resistive index: a useful tool for the management of the hypertensive patient. J Hypertens 32:149–153

Viazzi F, Muiesan ML, Schillaci G, Salvetti M, Pucci G, Bonino B et al (2016) Changes in albuminuria and cardiovascular risk under antihypertensive treatment: a systematic review and meta-regression analysis. J Hypertens 34:1689–1697. [Epub ahead of print] doi: 10.1097/HJH.0000000000000991

Viberti GC, Hill RD, Jarret RJ, Argyropoulos A, Mahmud U, Keen H (1982) Microalbuminuria as a predictor of clinical nephropathy in insulin-dependent diabetes mellitus. Lancet 1:1430–1432

Viberti GC, Wheelden NM, for the MicroAlbuminuria Reduction with VALsartan (MARVAL) Study Investigators (2002) Microalbuminuria reduction with valsartan in patients with type 2 diabetes mellitus: a blood pressure-independent effect. Circulation 106: 672–678

Wachtell K, Palmieri V, Olsen MH, Bella JN, Aalto T, Dahlof B et al (2002a) Urine albumin/creatinine ratio and echocardiographic left ventricular structure and function in hypertensive patients with electrocardiographic left ventricular hypertrophy: The LIFE study. Losartan Intervention for Endpoint Reduction. Am Heart J 143:319–326

Wachtell K, Olsen MH, Dahlöf B, Devereux RB, Kjeldsen SE, Nieminen MS et al (2002b) Microalbuminuria in hypertensive patients with electrocardiographic left ventricular hypertrophy: the LIFE study. J Hypertens 20:405–412

Wada M, Nagasawa H, Kurita K, Koyama S, Arawaka S, Kawanami T, Tajima K et al (2007) Microalbuminuria is a risk factor for cerebral small vessel disease in community-based elderly subjects. J Neurol Sci 255:27–34

Yokoyama H, Aoki T, Imahori M, Kuramitsu M (2004) Subclinical atherosclerosis is increased in type 2 diabetic patients with microalbuminuria evaluated by intima-media thickness and pulse wave velocity. Kidney Int 66:448–454

Yuyun MF, Khaw KT, Luben R, Welch A, Bingham S, Day NE, Wareham NJ (2004) Microalbuminuria, cardiovascular risk factors and cardiovascular morbidity in a British population: The EPIC-Norfolk Population-based Study. Eur J Cardiovasc Prev Rehabil 11:207–213

Zoungas S, de Galan BE, Ninomiya T, Grobbee D, Hamet P, Heller S, ADVANCE Collaborative Group et al (2009) Combined effects of routine blood pressure lowering and intensive glucose control on macrovascularand microvascular outcomes in patients with type 2 diabetes: new results from the ADVANCE trial. Diabetes Care 32:2068–2074

Adv Exp Med Biol - Advances in Internal Medicine (2017) 2: 307–325
DOI 10.1007/5584_2016_84
© Springer International Publishing AG 2016
Published online: 22 November 2016

Hypertension in Chronic Kidney Disease

Seyed Mehrdad Hamrahian and Bonita Falkner

Abstract

Hypertension, a global public health problem, is currently the leading factor in the global burden of disease. It is the major modifiable risk factor for heart disease, stroke and kidney failure. Chronic kidney disease (CKD) is both a common cause of hypertension and CKD is also a complication of uncontrolled hypertension. The interaction between hypertension and CKD is complex and increases the risk of adverse cardiovascular and cerebrovascular outcomes. This is particularly significant in the setting of resistant hypertension commonly seen in patient with CKD. The pathophysiology of CKD associated hypertension is multi-factorial with different mechanisms contributing to hypertension. These pathogenic mechanisms include sodium dysregulation, increased sympathetic nervous system and alterations in renin angiotensin aldosterone system activity. Standardized blood pressure (BP) measurement is essential in establishing the diagnosis and management of hypertension in CKD. Use of ambulatory blood pressure monitoring provides an additional assessment of diurnal variation in BP commonly seen in CKD patients. The optimal BP target in the treatment of hypertension in general and CKD population remains a matter of debate and controversial despite recent guidelines and clinical trial data. Medical therapy of patients with CKD associated hypertension can be difficult and challenging. Additional evaluation by a hypertension specialist may be required in the setting of treatment resistant hypertension by excluding pseudo-resistance and treatable secondary causes. Treatment with a combination of antihypertensive drugs, including appropriate diuretic choice, based on estimated glomerular filtration rate, is a key component of hypertension management in

S.M. Hamrahian (✉) and B. Falkner
Division of Nephrology, Department of Medicine, Sidney
Kimmel School of Medicine, Thomas Jefferson
University, 833 Chestnut Street, Suite 700, Philadelphia,
PA 19107, USA
e-mail: seyed.hamrahian@Jefferson.edu

CKD patients. In addition to drug treatment non-pharmacological approaches including life style modification, most important of which is dietary salt restriction, should be included in the management of hypertension in CKD patients.

Keywords

Hypertension • Blood pressure • Adults • Chronic kidney disease • Ambulatory blood pressure monitoring • White coat hypertension • Masked hypertension • Sodium • Salt • Resistant hypertension

1 Introduction and Epidemiology

Hypertension is a global public health issue and the major risk factor for heart disease, stroke and kidney failure resulting in premature death and disability (World Health Organization 2013). Over the last decade, hypertension has become the number one factor in the global burden of disease. Concurrently, there has been an increasing number of deaths and disability-adjusted life years related to poorly controlled blood pressure (BP) (Murray and Lopez 2013). Despite increased awareness and improved treatment of hypertension, the prevalence of hypertension is rising. Review of the 2011–2014 National Health and Nutrition Examination Survey (NHANES) data shows that nearly one-half (47 %) of adults aged 20 and over with hypertension had uncontrolled high BP in the United States (Yoon et al. 2015). These data include individuals with true resistant hypertension – defined as BP that remains above goal despite the concurrent use of three antihypertensive agents of different classes, including a diuretic, prescribed at optimal doses (Calhoun et al. 2008) without a secondary cause.

Chronic kidney disease (CKD) is another common and growing problem. CKD is defined as kidney damage for ≥3 months, due to structural or functional abnormalities of the kidney, with or without decreased glomerular filtration rate (GFR) or GFR <60 mL/min/1.73 m^2 for ≥3 months, with or without kidney damage. Renal parenchymal disease is both a common cause and complication of uncontrolled hypertension (Peralta et al. 2012). In other words hypertension is the most common comorbidity seen in patients with CKD. And its prevalence increases with declining renal function (Muntner et al. 2010). Additionally, CKD is recognized as a risk factor for cardiovascular disease, which makes treatment of hypertension even more important for CKD patients. Along the same line individuals with CKD are more likely to have resistant hypertension. The prevalence of resistant hypertension increases as GFR decreases, with resistant hypertension rates of >20 % described based on ambulatory blood pressure monitoring (ABPM) (De Nicola et al. 2013; Sakhuja et al. 2015).

In summary CKD interacts with hypertension on many levels. There is a bidirectional relationship between the two diseases. Hypertension, particularly resistant hypertension, can not only occur as the result of CKD, but it is also an important risk factor for CKD progression. Resistant hypertension is very common amongst patients with CKD and the prevalence appears to be proportional to the degree of renal dysfunction (Tanner et al. 2013). At some point it becomes difficult to determine which disease process precedes the other, as both diseases share similar risk factors including age, obesity, minority descent and comorbidities like diabetes or cardiovascular disease (Table 1). The interaction between hypertension and CKD is complex and increases the risk of adverse cardiovascular and cerebrovascular outcomes particularly in the setting of resistant hypertension.

Table 1 Patient's characteristic and risk factors for hypertension in CKD

Older age
High baseline BP
Obesity
Obstructive sleep apnea
Ethnic minorities
Diabetes
Excessive dietary salt ingestion
Heavy alcohol consumption
Smoking
Vascular atherosclerosis

2 Blood Pressure Measurement and Role of Ambulatory Blood Pressure Monitoring

Accurate BP measurement is an important factor in establishing the diagnosis and management of hypertension. A standardized approach to measuring BP improves the consistency and accuracy of the recorded readings. Inaccurate BP measurement techniques such as measuring the BP before the patient rests quietly for 5 min and use of inappropriately small cuff are the most common causes of falsely elevated BP readings (Pickering et al. 2005). Multiple readings taken at intervals of at least 1–2 min and then averaged is a better representation of a patient's BP. The BP should be measured in both arms to check for any major reading discrepancies, as between-arm BP differences are common even in healthy people. In hypertensive patients, a difference of 4–5 mmHg is not uncommon. A difference in systolic BP of over 10 mmHg requires vascular assessment, as heavily calcified or arteriosclerotic arteries, seen more commonly in patients with CKD, cannot be compressed fully for accurate BP readings. BP values between arms that are different by over 15 mmHg could indicate a heightened risk for vascular disease and death (Clark et al. 2012). In general, for management purposes it is recommended that the higher BP of the two arms be used.

Major causes of uncontrolled BP in patients with CKD include non-adherence to important lifestyle changes such as low salt diet, an inadequate or suboptimal treatment regimen including diuretics, and poor adherence to antihypertensive therapy, sometimes due to medication intolerance (Yiannakopoulou et al. 2005). Other possible causes of uncontrolled BP are previously undiagnosed but curable secondary hypertension; psychiatric causes; use of an interfering substance such as non-steroidal anti-inflammatory drugs (NSAIDs) or amphetamines; and drug interactions.

In general clinic BP measurements are the most common method of assessment to evaluate hypertension. Ambulatory blood pressure monitoring (ABPM) is a useful tool that adds additional clinical information on a patient's BP pattern including an assessment of nighttime BP and diurnal variation in BP. ABPM may also provide additional diagnostic information, such as white-coat hypertension and masked hypertension (Drawz et al. 2012). White-coat hypertension is defined as persistently elevated clinic BP readings while out-of-office BP values measured by 24-h ABPM are normal. This condition is a common cause of apparent resistant hypertension and should be ruled out to avoid over treatment with antihypertensive drugs (de la Sierra et al. 2011). Patients with CKD and white-coat effect have a much lower cumulative risk of progressing to end stage renal disease (ESRD), highlighting the importance of ABPM in CKD patients (Agarwal and Andersen 2006). Alternatively, masked hypertension is defined as normal, or near normal, office BP levels but out-of-office hypertension. Masked hypertension appears to be remarkably prevalent in CKD patients (Agarwal et al. 2016). Patients with masked hypertension are at increased risk for target organ damage and cardiovascular events (Fagard and Cornelissen 2007). CKD patients with this condition appear to have a higher cumulative risk of end stage renal disease (ESRD) compared to those with controlled ambulatory pressures (Agarwal 2006). ABPM provides additional information compared to home and office recordings with measures of BP variability and nocturnal BP measurements. The circadian BP rhythm and nocturnal BP are often abnormal in patients with CKD. Patients with CKD often loose the physiologic nocturnal 10–20 % fall in systolic and diastolic BP level. Patients with advanced CKD might even exhibit a rise in nocturnal BP, a phenomena called riser. The absence of nocturnal dip has been linked to increased risk of cardiovascular disease and target organ damage including progression of CKD (Kanno et al. 2013)· (Muxfeldt et al. 2009). Similarly there is a positive association between BP variability and the progression of renal damage and cardiovascular events (Ciobanu et al. 2013). When ABPM is not available, home BP measurement can provide some information on possible presence of white coat, masked, or resistant hypertension. Population studies both in general and in CKD (Cohen et al. 2014) demonstrate that home-measured BP is prognostically superior to office BP readings, correlates more closely with ABPM than office BP measurements, and is more predictive of adverse cardiovascular outcomes (Dolan et al. 2005; Niiranen et al. 2010). Therefore, out-of-office BP readings, ABPM or home BP measurement, should be used in management of hypertension.

3   Target Blood Pressure in Chronic Kidney Disease

The optimal BP level, whether systolic or diastolic, in the treatment of hypertension in general and CKD population remains a matter of debate and has become controversial despite recent guidelines and clinical trial data (James et al. 2014; SPRINT Research Group et al. 2015). In addition to prevention of cardiovascular events (McCullough et al. 2011), the goal in patients with CKD is to delay progression to ESRD with need for renal transplant or renal replacement therapy (Whaley-Connell et al. 2008).

Multiple trials in non-diabetics, including MDRD (Klahr et al. 1994), AASK (Wright et al. 2002), and REIN-2 (Ruggenenti et al. 2005) failed to show benefit from lower BP targets of <130/80 mmHg compared to <140/90 mmHg in slowing the progression of CKD to ESRD. A clinical trial on type 2 diabetics, that include a large number of diabetics with CKD, detected a small but statistically insignificant reduction in cardiovascular events among diabetics treated to the intensive systolic BP goal of <120 mmHg compared to goal BP of <140 mmHg (Cushman et al. 2010). In contrast, data from SPRINT (SPRINT Research Group et al. 2015) which excluded diabetics, but included 28 % of participants with reduced estimated GFR of 20–60 ml/min/1.73 m^2 showed a 25 % relative risk reduction in the cardiovascular events. There was no difference in rates of 50 % reduction of estimated GFR or ESRD between the intensive-BP treated group compared to standard-BP group. More patients without incident CKD had >30 % decline in estimated GFR with intensive treatment. Both ACCORD and SPRINT trials showed an increase in the risk of serious adverse events with the more intensive BP–lowering strategy. The benefit of BP target of less than 130/80 mm Hg in patients with CKD and proteinuria is supported based on post hoc analyses (Upadhyay et al. 2011). Hence, as depicted in Table 2, based on the limited clinical trial evidence almost all of the clinical practice guidelines for the management of BP in CKD without albuminuria or proteinuria recommend a goal BP of <140/90 mm Hg. The recommendation, based on expert opinion, is a lower BP target of <130/80 mm Hg for CKD patients with albuminuria or proteinuria.

The foundation of antihypertensive therapy in CKD patients should be based on the evidence-based strategy of using inhibitors of the renin angiotensin aldosterone system (RAAS) with diuretics, either thiazide or thiazide–type agents in the absence of significantly low GFR (<30 mL/min/1.73 m^2). Addition of other agents such as calcium channel blockers, or other drug classes should be considered as necessary to achieve a lower systolic BP level. It is important to balance the anticipated cardiovascular benefits of therapy in patients with higher cardiovascular risk with possible serious adverse effects of intensive targeted BP.

Table 2 Blood pressure targets and treatment recommendations in CKD

Guideline	BP target in CKD without Albuminuria or Proteinuria	BP target in CKD with Albuminuria or Proteinuria
JNC8 (James et al. 2014)	<140/90 mmHg	<140/90 mmHg
KDIGO (2012)	<140/90 mmHg	<130/80 mmHg
NICE (National Institute for Health and Care Excellence Hypertension clinical management of primary hypertension in adults; National Institute for Health and Care Excellence Chronic kidney disease)	<140/90 mmHg	<130/80 mmHg
CHEP (Dasgupta et al. 2014)	<140/90 mmHg	<140/90 mmHg
ESC/ESH (Mancia et al. 2013)	<140 mmHg	<130 mmHg
ASH/ISH (Weber et al. 2014b)	<140/90 mmHg	<140/90 mmHg
ISHIB (Flack et al. 2010)	<130/80 mmHg	<130/80 mmHg
ADA (American Diabetes Association 2013)	<140/80 mmHg	

Abbreviations: *ADA* American Diabetes Association, *ASH/ISH* American Society of Hypertension/International Society of Hypertension, *CHEP* Canadian Hypertension Education Program, *ESC/ESH* European Society of Cardiology/European Society of Hypertension, *ISHIB* International Society of Hypertension in Blacks, *KDIGO* Kidney Disease: Improving Global Outcomes, *NICE* National Institute for Heath and Care Excellence, *JNC8* USA Eighth Joint National Committee

4 Pathophysiology of Blood Pressure Regulation and Pathogenesis of Hypertension in Chronic Kidney Disease

The pathophysiology of CKD associated hypertension is complex because the kidney is not only the contributing organ, but is also a target organ of the hypertensive processes. Multiple mechanisms contribute to hypertension in CKD and their contributions might differ between patients.

Blood pressure is mainly regulated by four pathways. These include the sodium regulation, sympathetic nervous system (SNS) activity, humoral system – Renin Angiotensin Aldosterone System (RAAS), and auto-regulatory system. These pathways could have independent or interdependent effect on BP regulation. The pathological activity of one or multiple factors plus additional exogenous factors can influence BP and its management in patients with CKD. The endogenous pathologic factors in CKD include increased SNS (Klein et al. 2003) and RAAS activity plus endothelial dysfunction. Hypertension can cause and accelerate renal injury when impaired auto-regulation allows the transmission of high systemic pressures to the glomeruli, resulting in glomerulosclerosis (Bidani et al. 2013). Renal injury and loss of GFR in turn can cause hypertension due to impairment in sodium excretion and increased salt sensitivity (Koomans et al. 1982; Pimenta et al. 2009). Respectively, exogenous factors including high dietary sodium intake, and intervening medications like over-the-counters, such as NSAID (LeLorier et al. 2002) add to this complexity.

In general, GFR decreases with age and CKD accelerates the vascular ageing and atherosclerosis. This leads to increased arterial stiffness and increased risk of development of systolic hypertension in elderly patients with CKD (Briet et al. 2012). Similarly CKD is more common in patients with obesity and metabolic syndrome. The relationship between obesity and hypertension is well described (Hall 2003). However, the pathophysiology of obesity-induced hypertension is complex and not fully understood. Plausible mechanistic pathways of hypertension in CKD patients that are similar to obesity associated hypertension include impaired sodium excretion, increased SNS activity, and activation of the RAAS. There is also a high prevalence of obstructive sleep apnea (OSA) in CKD patients (Nicholl et al. 2012) and in patients with resistant hypertension, indicative of considerable overlap in these conditions. Although the exact unifying pathologic mechanism of this relationship is unclear, it appears to be linked with hyperaldosteronism and salt and volume retention (Gonzaga et al. 2010).

5 Sodium Regulation

The kidneys filter over 25,000 mmol of sodium per day excreting only less than 1 % of the filtered sodium load. Mismatch of input and output as the result of inadequate sodium excretion in the setting of CKD over time can result in volume mediated hypertension. Initial volume expansion increases cardiac filling and cardiac output; leading to a decrease in RAAS activation and results in increased sodium excretion. Loss of sodium regulation in the setting of CKD and low GFR is associated with a greater sensitivity of BP to salt. This leads to the increased prevalence of salt-sensitive hypertension seen in CKD. In addition increased sodium intake results in arterial vessel stiffness, decreased nitric oxide release, and the promotion of inflammatory processes all of which contribute to BP elevation (Hovater and Sanders 2012). Excessive salt intake also blunts the BP lowering effect of most classes of antihypertensive agents thus favoring development of resistant hypertension (Luft and Weinberger 1988). These effects are more pronounced in salt-sensitive patients, including the elderly, African Americans, and patients with CKD (Boudville et al. 2005). The American Heart Association recommends a sodium intake of 1500 mg per day in patients at high risk, including those with hypertension, diabetes, African descent, and CKD (American Heart Association Shaking the salt habit). Patients with CKD usually have co-morbidities and polypharmacy is not an unusual scenario. Several medications, some commonly used by this patient population, interfere with BP control and can contribute to treatment resistance (Grossman and Messerli 2012). Consequently, there can be blunting of the BP lowering effect of several antihypertensive drug classes,

Table 3 Pharmacological agents that can increase blood pressure

Nonsteroidal anti-inflammatory agents, including aspirin
Selective COX-2 inhibitors
Sympathomimetic agents (decongestants, diet pills, cocaine)
Stimulants (methylphenidate, dexmethylphenidate, dextroamphetamine, amphetamine, methamphetamine, modafinil)
Glucocorticoids with greater mineralocorticoid effect
Oral contraceptives
Cyclosporine
Erythropoietin
Natural licorice
Herbal compounds (ephedra or ma huang)

including diuretics, angiotensin converting enzyme inhibitors (ACE), angiotensin receptor blockers (ARBs), and beta blockers (Conlin et al. 2000) (Table 3).

Non-steroidal anti-inflammatory drugs (NSAIDs) have an inhibitory effect on renal prostaglandin production, especially prostaglandin E2 and prostaglandin I2. This effect can lead to sodium and fluid retention. These adverse effects are especially manifested in elderly patients, diabetics, and patients with CKD (Johnson et al. 1994). Use of immunosuppressive agents in patients with CKD as a result of primary glomerulopathy or tubule-interstitial disease is common and associated with adverse effects including hypertension. Glucocorticoids with greater mineralocorticoid effect (e.g. cortisol) can cause significant increases in BP by inducing sodium and fluid retention. In such cases, use of a mineralocorticoid receptor antagonist (spironolactone or eplerenone) can be an effective strategy to lower BP. Similarly, drugs like Calcineurin inhibitors induce a salt sensitive hypertension as a result of increased renal expression of the phosphorylated (active) form of the thiazide-sensitive NaCl co-transporter (NCC) (Hoorn et al. 2011). This phenotype is similar to familial hyperkalemic hypertension (also known as pseudo-hypoaldosteronism type II or Gordon's syndrome), which presents as hypertension, renal sodium and potassium retention, and renal tubular acidosis. Other agents that can add difficulty in BP management include decongestant and diet pills that contain sympathomimetic, amphetamine-like stimulants, oral contraceptives, and herbal preparations containing ephedra (or ma huang) (Mansoor 2001).

6 Sympathetic Nervous System Regulation

SNS activity is increased in CKD (Klein et al. 2003). Assessment of SNS activity and its contribution to BP regulation is imprecise, as circulating catecholamine levels provide only a rough estimate of SNS activity. Measurement of muscle sympathetic nerve activity is more precise, but remains a limited available diagnostic tool. The renal artery is highly innervated, with efferent renal nerves that originate from the central nervous system, and afferent renal nerves that originate from the kidneys. Stimulation of efferent renal nerves via β-1 adrenoreceptor stimulates renin secretion and activates the RAAS resulting in decreased urinary sodium excretion. Maximal stimulation of the efferent nerves can lead to an increase in renal vascular resistance (DiBona and Kopp 1997). Another well-described pathophysiology is the hypoxemia induced sustained increase in SNS activity seen in obstructive sleep apnea (OSA), which in turn raises BP through an increase in cardiac output, increase in peripheral resistance, and fluid retention (Somers et al. 1995). Accordingly, β-1 adrenergic blockers, ACE inhibitors, and ARBs are among the most effective antihypertensive agents in conditions with high SNS activity status including CKD and OSA.

7 Humoral System – Renin Angiotensin Aldosterone Regulation

Renin is secreted from the juxtaglomerular apparatus, which is the nephron site wherein there is contact between the afferent arteriole, and the distal convoluted tubule. While SNS stimulation induces renin secretion through the efferent renal nerves, renin secretion is also highly volume regulated (Davis and Freeman 1976). Volume depletion leads to renin secretion whereas volume overload and increased afferent arteriolar stretch suppress the renin secretion. In response to renin secretion, subsequent activation of RAAS causes vasoconstriction via angiotensin II effect. RAAS activation also increases sodium reabsorption by both angiotensin II in the proximal tubule and aldosterone in the distal nephron in exchange for the secretion of potassium. In addition to mineralocorticoid receptor stimulation aldosterone has a direct effect on the vasculature (Briet and Schiffrin 2013). Other factors like endothelins, oxidative stressors, and inflammatory mediators may also contribute to hypertension in CKD. Endothelins, such as ET-1, are potent vasoconstrictors. Oxidative stressors such as reactive oxygen species promote vasoconstriction, the release of renin, and increased urinary protein excretion (Araujo and Wilcox 2014). Inflammatory mediators or cytokines, such as TNF and IFNγ, further impair endothelial function (Crowley 2014). In addition, patients with CKD are at increased risk of vascular calcification and arterial stiffness which promote hypertension.

8 Chronic Kidney Disease and Resistant Hypertension

There is a strong association of CKD with greater prevalence of resistant hypertension, and greater risk of end-organ damage. Among CKD patients the severity of hypertension increases as GFR declines and sodium excretion decreases. Excess salt intake and subclinical volume overload are important contributors to the increased prevalence of resistant hypertension (Pimenta et al. 2009). As discussed earlier, a high dietary salt intake amplifies the consequences of impaired sodium excretion on BP. Therefore, a reduction in salt intake can have a synergistic effect on the actions of antihypertensive drugs that block the renin angiotensin aldosterone system in control of BP (Kwakernaak et al. 2014). Presence of significant proteinuria, commonly seen in CKD, may have an accentuating effect.

Aberrant filtration of plasminogen and its conversion within the urinary space to plasmin by urokinase-type plasminogen activator may increase sodium retention by activating the epithelial sodium channel (ENaC) and contributing further to volume overload status (Svenningsen et al. 2013). Similar results have been observed in patients with preeclampsia (Buhl et al. 2012). Overall, these findings stress the possible important role of amiloride use in the management of salt-sensitive hypertension associated with proteinuria or nephrotic syndrome.

The epidemic of obesity, a common finding in patients with CKD, with angiotensin-II independent release of aldosterone by adipocytes could be a reason for the increased occurrence of aldosterone mediated resistant hypertension (Ehrhart-Bornstein et al. 2003). Along the same line patients with CKD and Obesity are at high risk of developing OSA. The pathophysiology of OSA associated hypertension has not been fully elucidated, but in patients with resistant hypertension, it has been shown that aldosterone levels correlate with severity of OSA (Dudenbostel and Calhoun 2012). Blockade of aldosterone by mineralocorticoid receptor blockers reduces the severity of OSA and is an effective treatment strategy in the many patients who continue to have uncontrolled BP levels while taking three antihypertensive agents (Ziegler et al. 2011).

Patients with CKD have high prevalence of a blunted nocturnal BP decline and loss of the circadian BP pattern. During sleep in healthy individuals, there is a physiological BP decrease of 10–20 % of the average awake BP level. Patients with CKD often fail to show this nocturnal BP dip during the sleep period. These patients are referred to as non-dippers. In addition to the non-dipping phenomena as determined by ABPM, there may also be an increase in the sleep period BP levels, a pattern referred to as a riser. Other factors independently associated with elevated nighttime BP are proteinuria, older age, black race, and presence of diabetes (Drawz et al. 2016). There is a strong association between elevated nighttime BP and masked hypertension. Masked hypertension appears to have the same risk for cardiovascular events as sustained hypertension and is a well-established risk factor for target organ damage, such as LVH, vascular stiffness, and cardiovascular events (Hänninen et al. 2013). The loss of circadian rhythm and increased prevalence of the riser BP pattern, is associated with highest cardiovascular events risk among all possible BP patterns, and is 2.5-fold more prevalent in CKD, and up to five-fold more prevalent in end-stage renal disease (Mojón et al. 2013). The high prevalence of non dipping BP, rising BP at night and/or masked hypertension in patients with CKD reinforces the need to measure out-of-office BP for a full characterization of the burden of Hypertension. Hence, ABPM is an important useful tool in assessing the overall 24-h BP pattern and contributes substantially to the risk stratification of cardiovascular outcomes in the high risk CKD population.

9 Evaluation of Hypertension in Chronic Kidney Disease

Patients with CKD and hypertension have complex hypertension. Achieving optimal BP control is frequently challenging even for nephrologists or hypertension specialists.

The first step in evaluation of a patient with CKD and difficult to treat hypertension is to confirm the diagnosis of true treatment resistance hypertension and exclude pseudo-resistance due to inaccurate blood pressure measurement technique and treatment non-adherence (Burnier et al. 2013) (Fig. 1). Barriers to successful medication adherence include polypharmacy, drug costs, dosing inconvenience and adverse effects of drugs. Once the diagnosis is confirmed, possible factors that can contribute to treatment resistance should be considered.. These include life style factors such as obesity, physical inactivity, high dietary salt intake, excessive alcohol ingestion and use of substances with potential interference with antihypertensive medications such as over the counter medications or herbs. It is important to consider and screen for overlapping conditions such as obstructive sleep apnea and possibly hyperaldosteronism.

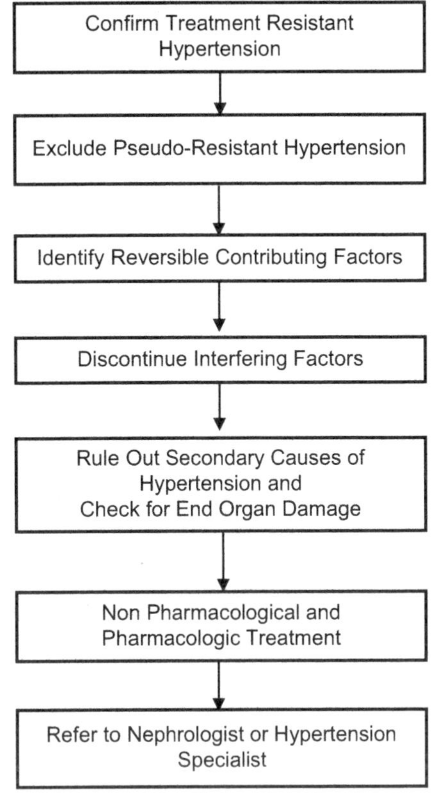

Fig. 1 A stepped sequence in evaluation and management of hypertension in patients with chronic kidney disease (See text for details for each step)

The medical history and physical examination should include information on duration, course, severity of the hypertension and if possible the chronologic relation to the established CKD diagnosis. It is important to inquire about presence of orthostatic complications (i.e. dizziness, fatigue, and vision blurring), prior regimens used, and any experienced side effect. History of snoring, witnessed apnea, and excessive daytime sleepiness indicates further evaluation for OSA. Presence of abdominal bruits in young female or carotid bruits in an elderly patient with known atherosclerotic disease increases the possibility of renal artery stenosis. Discrepancy between arm and thigh blood pressure readings is suggestive of aortic coarctation and features of Cushing's disease are suggested by central obesity, abdominal striae, moon face or prominent interscapular fat deposition.

Screening for target-organ damage including left ventricular hypertrophy (LVH $\geq$115 g/m^2 for men and $\geq$95 g/m^2 for women), retinopathy, microalbuminuria (increased urinary albumin excretion of $\geq$30–299 mg/g of creatinine), macroalbuminuria (increased urinary albumin excretion of $\geq$300 mg/g of creatinine), and degree of CKD by estimated GFR are essential to assess the overall increased risk of cardiovascular complications such as myocardial infarction, heart failure, stroke and further deterioration of renal function. The risk increases both with the degree and the duration of uncontrolled BP and CKD. The relationship between cardiovascular disease and target organ damage including CKD can be bidirectional. Uncontrolled BP can cause cardiovascular and renal structural and functional alterations, and contribute to development of LVH, aortic stiffness, microvascular disease. Overall, CKD can render hypertension more difficult to control (Muiesan et al. 2013).

Alternatively, the clinical findings of great discrepancy between higher clinic BP measurements and lower out-of office BP measurements particularly in a patient with orthostatic symptoms and no sign of target organ damage requires investigation for possible white-coat hypertension and overtreatment. Out-of-office BP measurements done by the patient, using a manual or automated blood pressure monitor, or the use of 24-h ABPM, as a more accurate alternative, can be used to document the presence and/or significance of any white-coat effect. 24-h ABPM also allows the assessment for absence of a nocturnal dipping, presence of a riser pattern, or significantly increased pulse pressure suggestive of vascular remodeling and vascular stiffness (Muxfeldt and Salles 2008). Hence, in accordance with the recent U.S. Preventive Services Task Force statement (Siu 2015) and evidence based data (Persu et al. 2014) it is recommended to confirm a diagnosis of hypertension or resistant hypertension with ABPM.

Basic laboratory evaluation of a hypertensive individual with CKD includes a routine metabolic profile, and urinalysis. Evaluation for a renal vascular lesion should be considered, particularly in a young female patient, whose presentation may suggest the presence of fibromuscular dysplasia or an older patient at increased risk of atherosclerotic disease in whom there has been a recent deterioration in renal function following therapy with ACE-inhibitors or ARBs, or history of flash pulmonary edema. When a renal vascular lesion is suspected, a duplex ultrasound study is required to rule out renal artery stenosis (Rimoldi et al. 2014). Although duplex ultrasound results depend on the level of training and experience of operator, they are preferred modality over computer tomographic angiography in patients with CKD in view of increased risk of contrast induced acute kidney injury. The gold standard diagnostic renal arteriograms in the absence of suspicious noninvasive imaging are not recommended. The presence of persistent and otherwise unexplained hypokalemia requires measurement of both plasma renin activity and aldosterone concentration to rule out hyperaldosteronism. However, with low GFR and reduced potassium excretion, hypokalemia may be absent. In patients already taking antihypertensive drugs it can be difficult to interpret renin and aldosterone levels. Suppressed renin level without elevated aldosterone concentration is suggestive of inappropriate volume expansion commonly seen in patients with CKD.

10   Non-pharmacologic Therapy

Treatment of hypertension in patients with CKD starts with non-pharmacological approaches. The modification of lifestyle factors – restriction of dietary salt, weight loss, regular exercise, and decreased alcohol ingestion, factors that contribute to treatment resistance is of high importance. Also included in this approach in CKD patients is discontinuation of any potentially interfering substances, like NSAIDs, as clinically allowable. Although the benefit of dietary modification interventions has not been extensively studied in patients with hypertension and CKD, the data

on their benefits in general hypertensive population is compelling.

Compliance in adhering to a low salt diet in hypertensive patients, particularly in salt sensitive patients like African-Americans, elderly, and individuals with CKD is associated with significant reductions in systolic and diastolic BP (Vollmer et al. 2001). High salt diet blunts the effect of ACE inhibitors (Singer et al. 1991) and sodium reduction enhances the antiproteinuric effect of ARBs (Kwakernaak et al. 2014) which is an important renal protective effect of RAAS blockaders. Accordingly, dietary salt restriction to less than 100 mEq (2300 mg) of sodium/24-h is recommended by most clinical practice guidelines. Additionally ingestion of a diet rich in fruits and vegetables, with close monitoring of the potassium levels in CKD patients, reduces systolic and diastolic BP compared to a usual diet in hypertensive patients (Appel et al. 1997).

Long-term weight loss, although difficult to achieve and to maintain, is clearly associated with modest improvement of BP level. Successful reduction in excess body weight may also lead to a reduction in the number of antihypertensive medications (Aucott et al. 2005). Similarly, data from meta-analysis including both normotensive and hypertensive cohorts show regular aerobic exercise results in mild reduction of both systolic and diastolic BP (Whelton et al. 2002). Based on these observational data, patients should be encouraged to maintain an ideal weight and exercise for at least a minimum of 30 min on most days of the week.

High alcohol consumption is associated with increased risk of treatment resistant hypertension (Wildman et al. 2005; Aguilera et al. 1999). Alcohol intake should be limited to no more than 28 g of ethanol per day for men and 14 g per day for women as moderation in alcohol intake significantly improves BP control.

To improve and maximize patient adherence to prescribed medication, it is important to avoid complex dosing regimens and high out-of-pocket costs. The medication regimen should be simplified by using long-acting drugs, if possible, and include antihypertensive drugs from different classes in order to provide a combination of pharmacological effects. A treatment strategy that reduces the number of tablets taken per day and the number of doses per day, as well as minimizing adverse effects facilitate drug treatment adherence. Encouraging patient involvement in their care by requesting frequent home BP measurements also can enhance medication adherence (Ogedegbe and Schoenthaler 2006).

11   Pharmacologic Therapy

The goal of pharmacologic therapy should be to achieve and maintain BP control using the least number of medications with minimal adverse effects. Individualization of treatment should consider etiologies and comorbidities that commonly co-exist among subgroups of patients. It is also important to consider the high cardiovascular disease risk status, age, sex, ethnicity, any disease associated target organ damage, and risk of drug–drug interactions. As an example, RAAS activation is often absent in elderly patients and in patients of African origin. For these patient sub-groups RAAS blockade for the treatment of treatment resistant hypertension may be less effective.

The standard recommended medical treatment regimen for hypertension is A + C + D. A = angiotensin-converting enzyme inhibitor or angiotensin-receptor blocker; C = calcium channel blocker; D = thiazide-like diuretic (James et al. 2014; Weber et al. 2014a). The 'A + C + D' combination is well tolerated and acts on different BP regulatory systems with increased renal sodium excretion and inhibition of both the RAAS and the SNS activity. There is strong evidence that combination regimens reduce cardiovascular events in hypertensive individuals (Dahlof et al. 2005; Patel et al. 2007; Chalmers et al. 2014).

Resistant hypertension is commonly present in patients with CKD, especially with advanced CKD. Therefore a combination drug regimen that blocks different regulatory pathways is necessary to reduce BP level. Loss of GFR is associated with a slower rate of sodium excretion. The subsequent development of volume overload status plays a key factor in the pathogenesis of resistant hypertension in CKD, and diuretics are essential in achieving BP control. When sodium excretion cannot keep pace with constant sodium intake in patients with CKD, dietary salt restriction in conjunction with diuretics is required to maintain euvolemia. Lack of or underuse of diuretics in patients with CKD is a common cause of treatment resistant hypertension. Appropriate diuretic choice, based on estimated GFR, is a crucial component in hypertension management in CKD patients (Sica 2008).

Modification of an antihypertensive regimen by adding a diuretic, increasing the dose of the diuretic, or changing the class of prescribed diuretic based on GFR can significantly improve BP control (Tamargo et al. 2014a, b). Thiazides, unlike the thiazide-like compound indapamide, appear to have a small vasodilatory effect at high concentrations (Pickkers et al. 1998). In general the long-acting thiazide-like diuretic chlorthalidone (Ernst et al. 2006) is the most potent thiazide diuretic and can be used unless the GFR is very low. With a GFR less than 30 ml/min/1.73 m^2 loop diuretics should be used. Loop diuretics are more potent natriuretic agents. KDIGO guideline (Kidney Disease: Improving Global Outcomes (KDIGO) CKD Work Group 2013) recommends a switch from thiazide diuretic to loop diuretic at CKD Stage 4 (<30 mL/min/1.73 m^2). This recommendation however has been challenged recently, based on few small studies that reported efficacy of thiazide – type diuretics at GRF below 30 ml/min/ 1.73 m^2 (Cirillo et al. 2014). However, individuals with advanced CKD with or without albuminuria may require even higher doses of loop diuretics to achieve natriuresis and BP reduction. To avoid counter-regulatory rebound sodium reabsorption and volume retention in patients with CKD the diuretics should be dosed more frequently if short acting drugs are used (Shankar and Brater 2003). Use of long acting diuretics such as chlorthalidone or

Table 4 Properties of common diuretics

Drug class	Site of action	Drugs	Usual PO dose – mg	Dosing interval
Thiazide-type	Na-Cl cotransporter in distal convoluted tubule	HCTZ	12.5–50	Daily
		Chlorothalidone	6.25–25	
		Metolazone	2.5–10	
		Indapamide	1.25–5	
Loop agents	Na-K-2Cl cotransporter in thick ascending limb of the loop of Henle	Furosemide	20–80	Twice a day
		Bumetanide	0.5–2.0	Twice a day
		Torsemide	5–20	Daily
		Ethacrynic acid[a]	25	
Aldosterone antagonists	Cortical collecting tubule	Spironolactone	25–50	Daily
		Eplerenone	50	
Epithelial Na-Channel Blocker	Cortical collecting tubule	Amiloride	5–10	Daily

[a]Management of edema associated with renal disease in the setting of sulfa allergy

torsemide can avoid the rebound sodium absorption seen in patients using diuretics with short half-life. Moreover, the sequential blockade of sodium channels along the nephron with both a thiazide and loop diuretic is very effective, but this combination of diuretics requires frequent serum creatinine and electrolytes monitoring (Izzo 2012). In addition use of diuretics might correct the non-dipping BP during sleep, a phenomena commonly seen in patient with CKD (Uzu and Kimura 1999) (Table 4).

ACE inhibitors or ARBs if tolerated, are the important classes of drugs that are recommended in many guidelines for use in hypertensive CKD patients with or without proteinuria. Both ACE inhibitors and ARBs are recommended for CKD patients because of their efficacy, relatively low side effect profile, reno-protective effects and reduced risk for cardiovascular and renal events (Maione et al. 2011). RAAS blockers exert their reno-protective effect by reducing the intraglomerular pressure and thereby decreasing proteinuria (Anderson and Brenner 1988). A concurrent reduction in GFR and associated rise in serum creatinine of up to 30 % is physiologic and is associated with a better renal outcome (Holtkamp et al. 2011). The physiologic GFR drop is not an indication for drug cessation, unless there is complication of persistent hyperkalemia refractory to treatment. A greater

increase in serum creatinine, if observed following initiation of ACE-inhibition or ARB therapy, could be due to volume contraction, use of nephrotoxic agents such as NSAIDs, or bilateral renal artery stenosis, which would require further investigation. Although a combination of an ACE inhibitor with an ARB could improve BP control in difficult to treat hypertension, this combination is associated with significant adverse effects (ONTARGET Investigators et al. 2008) including risk of severe hyperkalemia, hypotension and acute renal failure (Fried et al. 2013). Similar findings are seen with aliskiren, a direct renin inhibitor used with ACE inhibitor or ARB (Parving et al. 2012). Therefore a combination of RAAS agents should be avoided.

Dihydropyridine calcium channel blockers (CCBs) in contrast to non-dihydropyridine CCBs that have an antiproteinuric effect are very effective antihypertensive drugs (Bakris et al. 2004). Due to the higher precapillary arterial dilatation effect of the drug, patients may experience lower extremity edema that is refractory to diuretics, but improves or resolves with the use of an ACE inhibitor or ARB. The combination of CCB with an ACEI might be more effective in slowing the progression of CKD, particularly in black patients (Bakris et al. 2010; Weir et al. 2012).

Uncontrolled BP despite use of combination regimen of A + C + D (i.e. office BP > 140/90 mmHg and/or 24 h ABPM > 130/80 mmHg) requires search for pathogenic mechanism and possibly additional antihypertensive agent. Mineralocorticoid receptor antagonist (MRA) or aldosterone antagonists are the most important drug of choice for patients uncontrolled on multidrug regimens and low-renin status as the result of volume expansion or possible aldosterone escape phenomenon (Eide et al. 2004). Addition of low dose spironolactone of 12.5–50 mg daily is suggested as the fourth line of therapy and could effectively lower both systolic and diastolic BP (Williams et al. 2015). The MRA effect is independent of patient's baseline plasma aldosterone or 24-h urinary aldosterone level, plasma renin activity, or plasma aldosterone/renin ratio (Nishizaka et al. 2003). The most common adverse effect of spironolactone, the breast tenderness with or without breast enlargement, is particularly seen in men and at higher doses of 50–100 mg/day. Use of an aldosterone antagonist combined with an ACE inhibitor or ARB though not contraindicated requires careful monitoring of serum potassium and creatinine levels. Similarly, the risk of hyperkalemia is increased in patients taking NSAIDs, or with co-morbidities particularly like diabetes and/or CKD. Use of MRA should be restricted to patients with GFR > 30 mL/min/1.73 m^2 and plasma potassium concentrations of <4.5 mmol/L.

Amiloride is a diuretic that functions as an indirect aldosterone antagonist by blocking the epithelial sodium channel in the distal collecting duct of the kidney. Amiloride has been shown to be an effective add-on therapy in patients with uncontrolled hypertension or patients with significant proteinuria (Muxfeldt and Salles 2008). Beta-Blockers, as the fifth drug of choice, are more often used when there is a coexisting cardiac disease such as ischemic heart disease or heart failure (Rosendorff et al. 2015). If indicated, the more effective beta-blocking drugs are the drugs with combined alpha and beta antagonist activity. However, in a clinical condition of increased SNS activity and/or arterial stiffness, use of an alpha-blocker like doxazosin may have a favorable effect on BP and vascular remodeling. The main side effect of this drug is dizziness. Centrally acting agent, clonidine, can be very effective, but requires frequent dosing. The drug has a significant adverse effect profile and using a dose of over 0.6 mg per day is associated with rebound hypertension if doses are frequently missed. Potent vasodilators such as hydralazine or minoxidil have a higher incidence of adverse effects including lower extremity edema, and tachycardia.

Finally, an important factor in management of hypertension in CKD is the concept of chronotherapy. Intake of at least one of the hypertensive agents at bedtime is associated with a better 24-h mean BP control and, in particular, could induce the desired nocturnal dip in non-dippers, which could be beneficial in reducing cardiovascular event risk (Hermida et al. 2011a, b).

12 Device Interventions

Device-based interventions like carotid baroreceptor stimulation and renal denervation (RDN) have been used for the treatment of drug resistant hypertension with high SNS activity. Carotid baroreceptor stimulation decreases central neural sympathetic outflow through electrical activation of the sympatho-inhibitory area thus lowering arterial pressure (Lohmeier and Iliescu 2015). Baroreceptor stimulation requires surgical implantation and the BP-lowering effect may be attenuated if the hypertension is associated with hyperaldosteronism (Lohmeier et al. 2015) and angiotensin II-induced hypertension.

In contrast the renal arteries are highly innervated with both afferent and efferent nerves. Denervation of the renal arteries as a potential treatment for patients with resistant hypertension has been investigated. Using a catheter-based radiofrequency method, renal denervation may become a plausible treatment option in management of difficult to control resistant hypertension. However, to date, the RDN studies have had conflicting results (Krum et al. 2009; Esler et al. 2010; Bhatt et al. 2014).

Although the intervention in patients with CKD at baseline has shown positive results and the procedure is safe and well tolerated (Hering et al. 2012; Ott et al. 2015), subsequent studies are needed to determine the effectiveness of RDN for hypertension management.

13 Prognosis

The long-term prognosis of individuals with difficult to treat hypertension compared to patients with controlled hypertension has not been adequately determined. Patients with resistant hypertension are more likely to have target-organ damage, including carotid intima–media thickening, LVH, impaired renal function and microalbuminuria (Cuspidi et al. 2001). Respectively these patients have an unfavorable prognosis and are more likely to experience the combined outcome of death, myocardial infarction, congestive heart failure, stroke or CKD over time compared to those who have achieved goal blood pressure (Daugherty et al. 2012). Furthermore this risk increases if patients have CKD (De Nicola et al. 2013).

14 Summary

Hypertension is a global public health problem and is currently the number one factor in the global burden of disease. It is the major modifiable risk factor for heart disease, stroke and kidney failure. Renal parenchymal disease is both a common cause and also a complication of uncontrolled hypertension. The interaction between hypertension and CKD is complex and increases the risk of adverse cardiovascular and cerebrovascular outcomes. This is particularly significant in the setting of resistant hypertension commonly seen in patient with CKD. The pathophysiology of CKD associated hypertension is multi-factorial with different mechanisms contributing to hypertension. These include sodium dysregulation, increased sympathetic nervous system and renin angiotensin aldosterone system activity plus disturbance in auto-

regulatory system. Standardized blood pressure measurement is an important factor in establishing the diagnosis and management of hypertension in CKD. Use of ambulatory blood pressure monitoring provides an assessment of diurnal variation in BP commonly seen in CKD patients. The optimal BP target in the treatment of hypertension in general and CKD population remains a matter of debate and controversial despite recent guidelines and clinical trial data. Medical therapy of patients with CKD associated hypertension can be difficult, challenging, and even frustrating. Evaluation by a hypertension specialist may be required in the setting of commonly seen treatment resistant hypertension by excluding pseudo-resistance and treatable secondary causes. Use of combination regimen including appropriate diuretic choice, based on estimated glomerular filtration rate, is a crucial and key component of hypertension management in CKD patients. In addition to drug treatment non-pharmacological approaches including life style modification, most important of which is dietary salt restriction, should be included in the management of hypertension in CKD patients.

References

Agarwal R (2006) Hypertension diagnosis and prognosis in chronic kidney disease with out-of-office blood pressure monitoring. Curr Opin Nephrol Hypertens 15:309–313

Agarwal R, Andersen MJ (2006) Prognostic importance of ambulatory blood pressure recordings in patients with chronic kidney disease. Kidney Int 69:1175–1180

Agarwal R, Pappas MK, Sinha AD (2016) Masked uncontrolled hypertension in CKD. J Am Soc Nephrol 27:924–932

Aguilera MT, de la Sierra A, Coca A, Estruch R, Fernandez-Sola J, Urbano-Marquez A (1999) Effect of alcohol abstinence on blood pressure: assessment by 24-hour ambulatory blood pressure monitoring. Hypertension 33:653–657

American Diabetes Association (2013) Standards of medical care in diabetes—2013. Diabetes Care 36:S11–S66

American Heart Association: Shaking the salt habit. http://www.heart.org/HEARTORG/Conditions/

HighBloodPressure/PreventionTreatmentofHighBlood Pressure/Shaking-the-Salt-Habit

Anderson S, Brenner BM (1988) Therapeutic benefit of converting-enzyme inhibition in progressive renal disease. Am J Hypertens 1:380S–383S

Appel LJ, Moore TJ, Obarzanek E, Vollmer WM, Svetkey LP, Sacks FM et al (1997) A clinical trial of the effects of dietary patterns on blood pressure. DASH Collaborative Research Group. N Engl J Med 336:1117–1124

Araujo M, Wilcox CS (2014) Oxidative stress in hypertension: role of the kidney. Antioxid Redox Signal 20:74–101

Aucott L, Poobalan A, Smith WC, Avenell A, Jung R, Broom J (2005) Effects of weight loss in overweight/obese individuals and long-term hypertension outcomes: a systematic review. Hypertension 45:1035–1041

Bakris GL, Weir MR, Secic M, Campbell B, Weis-McNulty A (2004) Differential effects of calcium antagonist subclasses on markers of nephropathy progression. Kidney Int 65:1991–2002

Bakris GL, Sarafidis PA, Weir MR, Dahlöf B, Pitt B, Jamerson K et al (2010) Renal outcomes with different fixed-dose combination therapies in patients with hypertension at high risk for cardiovascular events (ACCOMPLISH): a prespecified secondary analysis of a randomised controlled trial. Lancet 375:1173–1181

Bhatt DL, Kandzari DE, O'Neill WW, D'Agostino R, Flack JM, Katzen BT et al (2014) A controlled trial of renal denervation for resistant hypertension. N Engl J Med 370:1393–1401

Bidani AK, Polichnowski AJ, Loutzenhiser R, Griffin KA (2013) Renal microvascular dysfunction, hypertension and CKD progression. Curr Opin Nephrol Hypertens 22:1–9

Boudville N, Ward S, Benaroia M, House AA (2005) Increased sodium intake correlates with greater use of antihypertensive agents by subjects with chronic kidney disease. Am J Hypertens 18:1300–1305

Briet M, Schiffrin EL (2013) Vascular actions of aldosterone. J Vasc Res 50:89–99

Briet M, Boutouyrie P, Laurent S, London GM (2012) Arterial stiffness and pulse pressure in CKD and ESRD. Kidney Int 82:388–400

Buhl KB, Friis UG, Svenningsen P, Gulaveerasingam A, Ovesen P, Frederiksen-Møller B et al (2012) Urinary plasmin activates collecting duct ENaC current in preeclampsia. Hypertension 60:1346–1351

Burnier M, Wuerzner G, Struijker-Boudier H, Urquhart J (2013) Measuring, analyzing, and managing drug adherence in resistant hypertension. Hypertension 62:218–225

Calhoun DA, Jones D, Textor S, Goff DC, Murphy TP, Toto RD et al (2008) Resistant hypertension: diagnosis, evaluation, and treatment. A scientific statement from the American Heart Association Professional Education Committee of the Council for High Blood Pressure Research. Hypertension 51:1403–1419

Chalmers J, Arima H, Woodward M, Mancia G, Poulter N, Hirakawa Y et al (2014) Effects of combination of perindopril, indapamide, and calcium channel blockers in patients with type 2 diabetes mellitus: results from the Action in Diabetes and Vascular Disease: Preterax and Diamicron Controlled Evaluation (ADVANCE) trial. Hypertension 63:259–264

Ciobanu AO, Gherghinescu CL, Dulgheru R, Magda S, Dragoi Galrinho R, Florescu M et al (2013) The impact of blood pressure variability on subclinical ventricular, renal and vascular dysfunction, in patients with hypertension and diabetes. Maedica 8:129–136

Cirillo M, Marcarelli F, Mele AA, Romano M, Lombardi C, Bilancio G (2014) Parallel-group 8-week study on chlorthalidone effects in hypertensives with low kidney function. Hypertension 63:692–697

Clark CE, Taylor RS, Shore AC, Ukoumunne OC, Campbell JL (2012) Association of a difference in systolic blood pressure between arms with vascular disease and mortality: a systematic review and metaanalysis. Lancet 379:905–914

Cohen DL, Huan Y, Townsend RR (2014) Home blood pressure monitoring in CKD. Am J Kidney Dis 63:835–842

Conlin PR, Moore TJ, Swartz SL, Barr E, Gazdick L, Fletcher C et al (2000) Effect of indomethacin on blood pressure lowering by captopril and losartan in hypertensive patients. Hypertension 36:461–465

Crowley SD (2014) The cooperative roles of inflammation and oxidative stress in the pathogenesis of hypertension. Antioxid Redox Signal 20:102–120

Cushman WC, Evans GW, Byington RP, Goff DC Jr, Grimm RH Jr, Cutler JA et al (2010) Effects of intensive blood-pressure control in type 2 diabetes mellitus. N Engl J Med 362:1575–1585

Cuspidi C, Macca G, Sampieri L, Michev I, Salerno M, Fusi V et al (2001) High prevalence of cardiac and extracardiac target organ damage in refractory hypertension. J Hypertens 19:2063–2070

Dahlof B, Sever PS, Poulter NR, Wedel H, Beevers DG, Caulfield M et al (2005) Prevention of cardiovascular events with an antihypertensive regimen of amlodipine adding perindopril as required versus atenolol adding bendroflumethiazide as required, in the Anglo-Scandinavian Cardiac Outcomes Trial-Blood Pressure Lowering Arm (ASCOT-BPLA): a multicentre randomized controlled trial. Lancet 366:895–906

Dasgupta K, Quinn RR, Zarnke KB, Rabi DM, Ravani P, Daskalopoulou SS et al (2014) The 2014 Canadian Hypertension Education Program recommendations for blood pressure measurement, diagnosis, assessment of risk, prevention, and treatment of hypertension. Can J Cardiol 30:485–501

Daugherty SL, Powers JD, Magid DJ, Tavel HM, Masoudi FA, Margolis KL et al (2012) Incidence and prognosis of resistant hypertension in hypertensive patients. Circulation 125:1635–1642

Davis JO, Freeman RH (1976) Mechanisms regulating renin release. Physiol Rev 56:1–56

de la Sierra A, Segura J, Banegas JR, Gorostidi M, de la Cruz JJ, Armario P et al (2011) Clinical features of 8295 patients with resistant hypertension classified on the basis of ambulatory blood pressure monitoring. Hypertension 57:898–902

De Nicola L, Gabbai FB, Agarwal R, Chiodini P, Borrelli S, Bellizzi V et al (2013) Prevalence and prognostic role of resistant hypertension in chronic kidney disease patients. J Am Coll Cardiol 61:2461–2467

DiBona GF, Kopp UC (1997) Neural control of renal function. Physiol Rev 77:75–197

Dolan E, Stanton A, Thijs L, Hinedi K, Atkins N, McClory S et al (2005) Superiority of ambulatory over clinic blood pressure measurement in predicting mortality: the Dublin outcome study. Hypertension 46:156–161

Drawz PE, Abdalla M, Rahman M (2012) Blood pressure measurement: clinic, home, ambulatory, and beyond. Am J Kidney Dis 60:449–462

Drawz PE, Alper AB, Anderson AH, Brecklin CS, Charleston J, Chen J et al (2016) Masked hypertension and elevated nighttime blood pressure in CKD: prevalence and association with target organ damage. Clin J Am Soc Nephrol 11:642–652

Dudenbostel T, Calhoun DA (2012) Resistant hypertension, obstructive sleep apnea and aldosterone. J Hum Hypertens 26:281–287

Ehrhart-Bornstein M, Lamounier-Zepter V, Schraven A, Langenbach J, Willenberg HS, Barthel A et al (2003) Human adipocytes secrete mineralocorticoid-releasing factors. Proc Natl Acad Sci U S A 100:14211–14216

Eide IK, Torjesen PA, Drolsum A, Babovic A, Lilledahl NP (2004) Low-renin status in therapy-resistant hypertension: a clue to efficient treatment. J Hypertens 22:2217–2226

Ernst ME, Carter BL, Goerdt CJ, Steffensmeier JJ, Phillips BB, Zimmerman MB et al (2006) Comparative antihypertensive effects of hydrochlorothiazide and chlorthalidone on ambulatory and office blood pressure. Hypertension 47:352–358

Esler MD, Krum H, Sobotka PA, Schlaich MP, Schmieder RE, Bohm M (2010) Renal sympathetic denervation in patients with treatment-resistant hypertension. (The Symplicity HTN-2 Trial) a randomized controlled trial. Lancet 376:1903–1909

Fagard RH, Cornelissen VA (2007) Incidence of cardiovascular events in white-coat, masked and sustained hypertension versus true normotension: a meta-analysis. J Hypertens 25:2193–2198

Flack JM, Sica DA, Bakris G, Brown AL, Ferdinand KC, Grimm RH Jr et al (2010) Management of high blood pressure in Blacks: an update of the International Society on Hypertension in Blacks consensus statement. Hypertension 56:780–800

Fried LF, Emanuele N, Zhang JH, Brophy M, Conner TA, Duckworth W et al (2013) Combined angiotensin inhibition for the treatment of diabetic nephropathy. N Engl J Med 369:1892–1903

Gonzaga CC, Gaddam KK, Ahmed MI, Pimenta E, Thomas SJ, Harding SM et al (2010) Severity of obstructive sleep apnea is related to aldosterone status in subjects with resistant hypertension. J Clin Sleep Med 6:363–368

Grossman E, Messerli FH (2012) Drug-induced hypertension: an unappreciated cause of secondary hypertension. Am J Med 125:14–22

Hall JE (2003) The kidney, hypertension, and obesity. Hypertension 41:625–633

Hänninen MR, Niiranen TJ, Puukka PJ, Kesäniemi YA, Kähönen M, Jula AM (2013) Target organ damage and masked hypertension in the general population: the Finn-Home study. J Hypertens 31:1136–1143

Hering D, Mahfoud F, Walton AS, Krum H, Lambert GW, Lambert EA et al (2012) Renal denervation in moderate to severe CKD. J Am Soc Nephrol 23:1250–1257

Hermida RC, Diana E, Ayala DE, Mojón A, Fernández JR (2011a) Bedtime dosing of antihypertensive medications reduces cardiovascular risk in CKD. J Am Soc Nephrol 22:2313–2321

Hermida RC, Ayala DE, Mojon A, Fernandez JR (2011b) Decreasing sleep-time blood pressure determined by ambulatory monitoring reduces cardiovascular risk. J Am Coll Cardiol 58:1165–1173

Holtkamp FA, de Zeeuw D, Thomas MC, Cooper ME, de Graeff PA, Hillege HJ et al (2011) An acute fall in estimated glomerular filtration rate during treatment with losartan predicts a slower decrease in long-term renal function. Kidney Int 80:282–287

Hoorn EJ, Walsh SB, McCormick JA, Fürstenberg A, Yang CL, Roeschel T et al (2011) The calcineurin inhibitor tacrolimus activates the renal sodium chloride cotransporter to cause hypertension. Nat Med 17:1304–1309

Hovater MB, Sanders PW (2012) Effect of dietary salt on regulation of TGF-beta in the kidney. Semin Nephrol 32:269–276

Izzo JL (2012) Value of combined thiazide-loop diuretic therapy in chronic kidney disease: heart failure and reninangiotensin-aldosterone blockade. J Clin Hypertens 14:344

James PA, Oparil S, Carter BL, Cushman WC, Dennison-Himmelfarb C, Handler J et al (2014) 2014 evidence-based guideline for the management of high blood pressure in adults: report from the panel members appointed to the Eighth Joint National Committee (JNC 8). JAMA 311:507–520

Johnson AG, Nguyen TV, Day RO (1994) Do nonsteroidal anti-inflammatory drugs affect blood pressure? Meta-Analysis Ann Intern Med 121:289–300

Kanno A, Kikuya M, Asayama K, Satoh M, Inoue R, Hosaka M et al (2013) Night-time blood pressure is associated with the development of chronic kidney disease in a general population: the Ohasama Study. J Hypertens 31:2410–2417

Kidney Disease: Improving Global Outcomes (KDIGO) Blood Pressure Work Group (2012) KDIGO clinical practice guideline for the management of blood pressure in chronic kidney disease. Kidney Int Suppl 2:337–414

Kidney Disease: Improving Global Outcomes (KDIGO) CKD Work Group (2013) KDIGO 2012 clinical practice guideline for the evaluation and management of chronic kidney disease. Kidney Int Suppl 3:1–150

Klahr S, Levey AS, Beck GJ, Caggiula AW, Hunsicker L, Kusek JW et al (1994) The effects of dietary protein restriction and blood-pressure control on the progression of chronic renal disease. Modification of Diet in Renal Disease Study Group. N Engl J Med 330:877–884

Klein IH, Ligtenberg G, Neumann J, Oey PL, Koomans HA, Blankestijn PJ (2003) Sympathetic nerve activity is inappropriately increased in chronic renal disease. J Am Soc Nephrol 14:3239–3244

Koomans HA, Roos JC, Boer P, Geyskes GG, Mees EJ (1982) Salt sensitivity of blood pressure in chronic renal failure. Evidence for renal control of body fluid distribution in man. Hypertension 4:190–197

Krum H, Schlaich M, Whitbourn R, Sobotka PA, Sadowski J, Bartus K et al (2009) Catheter-based renal sympathetic denervation for resistant hypertension: a multicentre safety and proof-of-principle cohort study. Lancet 373:1275–1281

Kwakernaak AJ, Krikken JA, Binnenmars SH, Visser FW, Hemmelder MH, Woittiez AJ et al (2014) Effects of sodium restriction and hydrochlorothiazide on RAAS blockade efficacy in diabetic nephropathy: a randomised clinical trial. Lancet Diabetes Endocrinol 2:385–395

LeLorier J, Bombardier C, Burgess E, Moist L, Wright N, Cartier P et al (2002) Practical considerations for the use of nonsteroidal anti-inflammatory drugs and cyclo-oxygenase-2 inhibitors in hypertension and kidney disease. Can J Cardiol 18:1301–1308

Lohmeier TE, Iliescu R (2015) The baroreflex as a long-term controller of arterial pressure. Physiology 30:148–158

Lohmeier TE, Liu B, Hildebrandt DA, Cates AW, Georgakopoulos D, Irwin ED (2015) Global- and renal-specific sympathoinhibition in aldosterone hypertension. Hypertension 65:1223–1230

Luft FC, Weinberger MH (1988) Review of salt restriction and the response to antihypertensive drugs: satellite symposium on calcium antagonists. Hypertension 11:I-229–32

Maione A, Navaneethan SD, Graziano G, Mitchell R, Johnson D, Mann JF et al (2011) Angiotensin-converting enzyme inhibitors, angiotensin receptor blockers and combined therapy in patients with micro- and macroalbuminuria and other cardiovascular risk factors: a systematic review of randomized controlled trials. Nephrol Dial Transplant 26:2827–2847

Mancia G, Fagard R, Narkiewicz K, Redón J, Zanchetti A, Böhm M et al (2013) 2013 ESH/ESC Guidelines for the management of arterial hypertension: the Task Force for the management of arterial hypertension of the European Society of Hypertension (ESH) and of the European Society of Cardiology (ESC). J Hypertens 31:1281–1357

Mansoor GA (2001) Herbs and alternative therapies in the hypertension clinic. Am J Hypertens 14:971–975

McCullough PA, Steigerwalt S, Tolia K, Chen SC, Li S, Norris KC et al (2011) Cardiovascular disease in chronic kidney disease: data from the Kidney Early Evaluation Program (KEEP). Curr Diab Rep 11:47–55

Mojón A, Ayala DE, Piñeiro L, Otero A, Crespo JJ, Moyá A et al (2013) Comparison of ambulatory blood pressure parameters of hypertensive patients with and without chronic kidney disease. Chronobiol Int 30:145–158

Muiesan ML, Salvetti M, Rizzoni D, Paini A, Agabiti-Rosei C, Aggiusti C et al (2013) Resistant hypertension and target organ damage. Hypertens Res 36:485–491

Muntner P, Anderson A, Charleston J, Chen Z, Ford V, Makos G et al (2010) Hypertension awareness, treatment, and control in adults with CKD: results from the Chronic Renal Insufficiency Cohort (CRIC) Study. Am J Kidney Dis 55:441–451

Murray CJ, Lopez AD (2013) Measuring the global burden of disease. N Engl J Med 369:448–457

Muxfeldt ES, Salles GF (2008) Pulse pressure or dipping pattern: which one is a better cardiovascular risk marker in resistant hypertension? J Hypertens 26:878–884

Muxfeldt ES, Cardoso CR, Salles GF (2009) Prognostic value of nocturnal blood pressure reduction in resistant hypertension. Arch Intern Med 169:874–880

National Institute for Health and Care Excellence. Chronic kidney disease. http://www.nice.org.uk/guidance/cg182/evidence/cg182-chronic-kidney-disease

National Institute for Health and Care Excellence. Hypertension: clinical management of primary hypertension in adults. http://www.nice.org.uk/guidance/cg127/resources/guidancehypertension

Nicholl DD, Ahmed SB, Loewen AH, Hemmelgarn BR, Sola DY, Beecroft JM et al (2012) Declining kidney function increases the prevalence of sleep apnea and nocturnal hypoxia. Chest 141:1422–1430

Niiranen TJ, Hänninen MR, Johansson J, Reunanen A, Jula AM (2010) Home measured blood pressure is a stronger predictor of cardiovascular risk than office blood pressure: the Finn-Home study. Hypertension 55:1346–1351

Nishizaka MK, Zaman MA, Calhoun DA (2003) Efficacy of low-dose spironolactone in subjects with resistant hypertension. Am J Hypertens 16:925–930

Ogedegbe G, Schoenthaler A (2006) A systematic review of the effects of home blood pressure monitoring on medication adherence. J Clin Hypertens 8:174–180

ONTARGET Investigators, Yusuf S, Teo KK, Pogue J, Dyal L, Copland I et al (2008) Telmisartan, ramipril, or both in patients at high risk for vascular events. N Engl J Med 358:1547–1559

Ott C, Mahfoud F, Schmid A, Toennes SW, Ewen S, Ditting T et al (2015) Renal denervation preserves renal function in patients with chronic kidney disease and resistant hypertension. J Hypertens 33:1261–1266

Parving HH, Brenner BM, McMurray JJ, de Zeeuw D, Haffner SM, Solomon SD et al (2012) Cardiorenal end points in a trial of aliskiren for type 2 diabetes. N Engl J Med 367:2204–2213

Patel A, MacMahon S, Chalmers J, Neal B, Woodward M, Billot L et al (2007) Effects of a fixed combination of perindopril and indapamide on macrovascular and microvascular outcomes in patients with type 2 diabetes mellitus (the ADVANCE trial): a randomized controlled trial. Lancet 370:829–840

Peralta CA, Norris KC, Li S, Chang TI, Tamura MK, Jolly SE et al (2012) Blood pressure components and end-stage renal disease in persons with chronic kidney disease: the Kidney Early Evaluation Program (KEEP). Arch Intern Med 172:41–47

Persu A, O'Brien E, Verdecchia P (2014) Use of ambulatory blood pressure measurement in the definition of resistant hypertension: a review of the evidence. Hypertens Res 37:967–972

Pickering TG, Hall JE, Appel LJ, Falkner BE, Graves J, Hill MN et al (2005) Recommendations of blood pressure measurement in humans and experimental animals. Part 1: blood pressure measurement in humans. A statement for professionals from the subcommittee of professional and public education of the American Heart Association Council on High Blood Pressure Research. Circulation 111:697–716

Pickkers P, Hughes AD, Russel FG, Thien T, Smits P (1998) Thiazide-induced vasodilation in humans is mediated by potassium channel activation. Hypertension 32:1071–1076

Pimenta E, Gaddam KK, Oparil S, Aban I, Husain S, Dell'Italia LJ et al (2009) Effects of dietary sodium reduction on blood pressure in subjects with resistant hypertension: results from a randomized trial. Hypertension 54:475–481

Rimoldi SF, Scherrer U, Messerli FH (2014) Secondary arterial hypertension: when, who, and how to screen? Eur Heart J 35:1245–1254

Rosendorff C, Lackland DT, Allison M, Aronow WS, Black HR, Blumenthal RS et al (2015) Treatment of hypertension in patients with coronary artery disease: a scientific statement from the American Heart Association, American College of Cardiology, and American Society of Hypertension. Hypertension 65:1372–1407

Ruggenenti P, Perna A, Loriga G, Ganeva M, Ene-Iordache B, Turturro M et al (2005) Blood-pressure control for renoprotection in patients with non-diabetic chronic renal disease (REIN-2): multicentre, randomised controlled trial. Lancet 365:939–946

Sakhuja A, Textor SC, Taler SJ (2015) Uncontrolled hypertension by the evidence-based guideline: results from NHANES 2011–2012. J Hypertens 33:644–651

Shankar SS, Brater DC (2003) Loop diuretics: from the Na-K-2Cl transporter to clinical use. Am J Physiol Renal Physiol 284:F11–F21

Sica DA (2008) The kidney and hypertension: causes and treatment. J Clin Hypertens 10:541–548

Singer DR, Markandu ND, Sugden AL, Miller MA, MacGregor GA (1991) Sodium restriction in hypertensive patients treated with a converting enzyme inhibitor and a thiazide. Hypertension 17:798–803

Siu AL (2015) U.S. Preventive Services Task Force. Screening for high blood pressure in adults: U.S. Preventive Services Task Force Recommendation Statement. Ann Intern Med 163:778–786

Somers VK, Dyken ME, Clary MP, Abboud FM (1995) Sympathetic neural mechanisms in obstructive sleep apnea. J Clin Invest 96:1897–1904

SPRINT Research Group, Wright JT Jr, Williamson JD, Whelton PK, Snyder JK, Sink KM et al (2015) A randomized trial of intensive versus standard blood pressure control. N Engl J Med 373:2103–2116

Svenningsen P, Friis UG, Versland JB, Buhl KB, Møller Frederiksen B, Andersen H et al (2013) Mechanisms of renal NaCl retention in proteinuric disease. Acta Physiol 207:536–545

Tamargo J, Segura J, Ruilope LM (2014a) Diuretics in the treatment of hypertension. Part 1: thiazide and thiazide-like diuretics. Expert Opin Pharmacother 15:527–547

Tamargo J, Segura J, Ruilope LM (2014b) Diuretics in the treatment of hypertension. Part 2: loop diuretics and potassium-sparing agents. Expert Opin Pharmacother 15:605–621

Tanner RM, Calhoun DA, Bell EK, Bowling CB, Gutiérrez OM, Irvin MR et al (2013) Prevalence of apparent treatment-resistant hypertension among individuals with CKD. Clin J Am Soc Nephrol 8:1583–1590

Upadhyay A, Earley A, Haynes SM, Uhlig K (2011) Systematic review: blood pressure target in chronic kidney disease and proteinuria as an effect modifier. Ann Intern Med 154:541–548

Uzu T, Kimura G (1999) Diuretics shift circadian rhythm of blood pressure from nondipper to dipper in essential hypertension. Circulation 100:1635–1638

Vollmer WM, Sacks FM, Ard J, Appel LJ, Bray GA, Simons-Morton DG et al (2001) Effects of diet and sodium intake on blood pressure: subgroup analysis of the DASH-sodium trial. Ann Intern Med 135:1019–1028

Weber MA, Schiffrin EL, White WB, Mann S, Lindholm LH, Kenerson JG et al (2014a) Clinical practice guidelines for the management of hypertension in the community: a statement by the American Society of Hypertension and the International Society of Hypertension. J Clin Hypertens 16:14–26

Weber MA, Schiffrin EL, White WB, Mann S, Lindholm LH, Kenerson JG et al (2014b) Clinical practice guidelines for the management of hypertension in the community a statement by the American Society of Hypertension and the International Society of Hypertension. J Hypertens 32:3–15

Weir MR, Bakris GL, Weber MA, Dahlof B, Devereux RB, Kjeldsen SE et al (2012) Renal outcomes in hypertensive Black patients at high cardiovascular risk. Kidney Int 81:568–576

Whaley-Connell AT, Sowers JR, Stevens LA, McFarlane SI, Shlipak MG, Norris KC et al (2008) CKD in the United States: Kidney Early Evaluation Program (KEEP) and National Health and Nutrition Examination Survey (NHANES) 1999–2004. Am J Kidney Dis 51:S13–S20

Whelton SP, Chin A, Xin X, He J (2002) Effect of aerobic exercise on blood pressure: a meta-analysis of randomized, controlled trials. Ann Intern Med 136:493–503

Wildman RP, Gu D, Muntner P, Huang G, Chen J, Duan X et al (2005) Alcohol intake and hypertension subtypes in Chinese men. J Hypertens 23:737–743

Williams B, MacDonald TM, Morant S, Webb DJ, Sever P, McInnes G et al (2015) Spironolactone versus placebo, bisoprolol, and doxazosin to determine the optimal treatment for drug-resistant hypertension (PATHWAY-2): a randomised, double-blind, cross-over trial. Lancet 386:2059–2068

World Health Organization (2013) A global brief on hypertension: silent killer, global public health crisis. World Health Day 2013. World Health Organization, Geneva, pp 1–39

Wright JT Jr, Bakris G, Greene T, Agodoa LY, Appel LJ, Charleston J et al (2002) Effect of blood pressure lowering and antihypertensive drug class on progression of hypertensive kidney disease: results from the AASK trial. JAMA 288:2421–2431

Yiannakopoulou EC, Papadopulos JS, Cokkinos DV, Mountlkalakis TD (2005) Adherence to antihypertensive treatment: a critical factor for blood pressure control. Eur J Cardiovasc Prev Rehabil 12:243–249

Yoon SS, Fryar CD, Carroll MD (2015) Hypertension prevalence and control among adults: United States, 2011–2014, NCHS data brief, no 220. National Center for Health Statistics, Hyattsville

Ziegler MG, Milic M, Sun P (2011) Antihypertensive therapy for patients with obstructive sleep apnea. Curr Opin Nephrol Hypertens 20:50–55

Adv Exp Med Biol - Advances in Internal Medicine (2017) 2: 327–340
DOI 10.1007/5584_2016_88
© Springer International Publishing AG 2016
Published online: 22 November 2016

Hypertension in the Hemodialysis Patient

Musab Hommos and Carrie Schinstock

Abstract

Hypertension is common yet difficult to manage in the hemodialysis patients population. This chapter discusses various aspects of this problem including its prevalence, distinctive pathophysiology, methods of diagnosis and pharmacological and non pharmacological treatment approaches. The topic is relevant to any health care provider taking care of hemodialysis patients.

Keywords

Sodium balance • Extracellular volume • Sympathetic nervous system • Renin-angiotensin system • Aldosterone • Arterial stiffness • Hyperparathyroidism • Ambulatory blood pressure monitoring • Blood pressure target

1 Introduction

Hypertension is common among hemodialysis patients, and unfortunately it can be difficult to manage. In part this is related to the unique variability in BP that the dialysis patient experiences and the complexity of getting reliable BP readings. Distinctive pathophysiologic mechanisms also contribute to hypertension in this population and are challenging to recognize and measure. Not surprisingly, the optimal targets for BP control are also unclear in the dialysis population. The aim of this review is to discuss in detail the prevalence, pathophysiology, diagnosis, and management of BP in the hemodialysis population. The topics are not only relevant to a practicing nephrologist, but also for the general internist who sees dialysis patients in the hospital or clinic.

2 Prevalence of Hypertension Among Hemodialysis Patients

Hypertension is very common in hemodialysis patients and the reported prevalence internationally is between approximately 50–90 % (Agarwal et al. 2003, 2009; Salem 1995; Harper et al. 2009; Liu et al. 2014). Part of the wide variation in prevalence is explained by the different definitions of hypertension used in studies.

M. Hommos and C. Schinstock (✉)
Division of Nephrology and Hypertension, Mayo Clinic, 200 First Street SW, Rochester, MN, USA 55905
e-mail: Schinstock.carrie@mayo.edu

For example, hypertension has been defined as pre-dialysis systolic blood pressure (SBP) $\geq$ 150 mmHg, diastolic blood pressure (DBP) $\geq$ 85 mmHg or by the use of antihypertensive medications. Other studies used pre-dialysis mean arterial blood pressure (BP), average BP from 24 h ambulatory BP monitoring and pre-dialysis BP of > 140/90 to define hypertension (Salem 1995; Agarwal 2011).

Gender (Agarwal et al. 2003; Salem 1995) and ethnicity (Agarwal et al. 2003) do not appear to influence the prevalence of hypertension, but, hypertension is more common among patients who have diabetes or hypertension as the etiology of their ESRD (Agarwal et al. 2003). Other factors that have been associated with hypertension among hemodialysis patients include erythropoietin use (Agarwal 2011), younger age (Agarwal et al. 2003; Salem 1995) and lower BMI (Agarwal 2011; Levin et al. 2010). Interestingly, erythropoietin use also reported to be associated with blunted circadian rhythm (Liu et al. 2014).

3 Pathophysiology of Hypertension in Hemodialysis Patients

Multiple factors contribute to inadequate BP control in hemodialysis patients. The following section describes some of the most well studied etiologic factors.

3.1 Positive Sodium Balance and Extracellular Volume Expansion

Impaired renal function leads to impaired salt and water excretion. The resulting increase in extracellular volume raises BP. Agarwal et al. (2009) showed that reduction in dry weight of 1 kg over 8 weeks resulted in drop in ambulatory SBP of 6.6 mmHg and DBP of 3.3 mmHg. The authors of that study reported a drop in SBP of only 2 mmHg immediately post dialysis suggesting that immediate post dialysis BP is a poor indicator of overall BP load and thus may not be reliable indicator of degree of extracellular volume expansion. Weight gain between dialysis sessions has also been correlated with pre-dialysis BP and the number of antihypertensive medications (Lopez-Gomez et al. 2005). For every 1 % increase in weight gain between dialysis sessions, there was 1 mmHg increase in pre-dialysis and intra-dialysis SBP (Inrig et al. 2007a). Using bioimpedance analysis spectroscopy, Fagugli et al. (2003) showed that extracellular water was associated with ambulatory blood pressure and left ventricular mass index. Another bioimpedance based study showed a significantly higher extracellular volume in hypertensive patients as compared to normotensive patients. All patients with excessive extracellular volume had hypertension, but not all hypertensive patients had excessive extracellular volume (Chen et al. 2002).

Integral to the control of extracellular volume is the maintenance of sodium balance: neutral intake and output of sodium. Most hemodialysis patients are oligo or anuric and therefore, the removal of sodium is largely dependent on hemodialysis. Further complicating the issue, hemodialysis patients on average have a higher intake of sodium than what is even recommended for the general population. The average sodium intake is 2.2–4.2 g of sodium per day, despite a recommended sodium restriction of 2 g or less per day (Maduell and Navarro 2001; Mc Causland et al. 2012).

Besides the oral intake of sodium, the dialysate sodium concentration is probably the main determinant of overall sodium balance. In an attempt to minimize symptoms of dialysis disequilibrium after the widespread use of high flux dialyzers, many nephrologists began prescribing a higher dialysate sodium concentration. The use of a higher dialysate sodium concentration (time averaged concentration of 147 mmol/L vs 138 mmol/L) was associated with increased weight gain between dialysis sessions and increased ambulatory BP (Song et al. 2002). A higher dialysate sodium concentration has also been associated with the use of more antihypertensives and the need to use more classes of medications (Davenport 2006). Just lowering dialysate sodium from 140 to 135 mmol/L over 8 weeks combined with dietary sodium restriction to less than 2.3 g per day has been shown to result in a decrease in mean BP from 108 to 98 mmHg and the reduced use of antihypertensives (Krautzig et al. 1998).

3.2 Sympathetic Nervous System Dysregulation

Although poorly understood, patients with chronic kidney disease appear to have increased sympathetic nervous system activity, which is a likely contributor to hypertension. Converse et al. (1992) compared postganglionic sympathetic nerve discharge among hemodialysis patients, patients who had undergone bilateral nephrectomy, and to normal subjects. In this study, hemodialysis patients with native kidneys had a 2.5 times higher rate of sympathetic nerve discharge and a higher BP as compared to post-nephrectomy patients and normal subjects. These findings did not correlate with plasma norepinephrine or renin, (Converse et al. 1992) and thus, these levels can't be used as a surrogate marker of sympathetic activity. Kidney transplant patients have persistently elevated muscle sympathetic nerve activity despite the correction of uremia with transplantation, (Hausberg et al. 2002) which suggests that uremia is not the cause of increased sympathetic activity (Hausberg et al. 2002). Recent evidence has shown that patients on hemodialysis have an increase in sympathetic nerve density in the internal area of the peri-adventitial tissue compared to nondialysis patients (Mauriello et al. 2015).

Supporting that idea, sympathetic activity decreases after native kidney nephrectomy. Short daily hemodialysis also leads to a reduction in sympathetic hyperactivity and reduced blood pressure (Zilch et al. 2007).

3.3 Renin Angiotensin Aldosterone System

As discussed above, most hemodialysis patients are volume expanded. The normal hormonal response to volume expansion is a suppression of the renin angiotensin system, but this may not occur in hemodialysis patients. One study showed that hemodialysis patients whose BP does not improve with euvolemia have increased plasma renin activity as compared to those hemodialysis patients whose BP improves with volume control. Moreover, BP control improved after nephrectomy in that study (Weidmann et al. 1971). More support for the role of inappropriately increased renin angiotensin system in the hypertension of hemodialysis patients is the effectiveness of aliskiren (a direct renin inhibitor) for BP control in this population (Morishita et al. 2012). Whether the elevated renin activity is driven by parenchymal kidney disease or secondary to renal artery stenosis is unclear.

3.4 Arterial Stiffness

The loss of arterial elasticity leading to arterial stiffness is known to result in an increase in systolic BP and pulse pressure in the general population. This phenomena is accelerated in ESRD (Utescu et al. 2013) and is associated with left ventricular hypertrophy, end organ damage, and a higher mortality (Fortier et al. 2015).

3.5 Hyperparathyroidism

Hyperparathyroidism, a common complication of chronic kidney disease, is also correlated with increased BP likely because of increased intracellular calcium. The use of active vitamin D analogues in a non-dialysis chronic kidney disease population was shown to reduce PTH and mean BP (Raine et al. 1993). Although none of the patients in the above described study were on hemodialysis, the data can likely be extrapolated to the hemodialysis population. Further supporting that notion, a case series in hemodialysis patients showed a drop in SBP following parathyroidectomy for secondary hyperparathyroidism. This drop in BP correlated with decrease in calcium (Goldsmith et al. 1996).

3.6 Other Potential Factors

Several other potential factors may be uniquely associated with elevated BP in the dialysis population including: reduced renalase, increased asymmetric dimethylarginine and dysregulated nitric oxide, increased endothelin, and exogenous erythropoietin.

Renalase is a flavin adenine dinucleotide-dependent amine oxidase known for metabolizing catecholamines (especially dopamine) in vitro. Its gene expression is the highest in the kidney, and the concentration of renalase is markedly reduced in patients with ESRD. Supporting the role for renalase in reducing BP, the injection of renalase into rats led to an immediate short term decrease in BP, heart rate and cardiac output (Xu et al. 2005).

Nitric oxide is a potent vasodilator that is produced by nitric oxide synthase. *Asymmetric dimethylarginine*, a potent inhibitor of nitric oxide, may be increased in hemodialysis patients (Vallance et al. 1992; Cooke 2000). In a rat model, the plasma level of asymmetric dimethylarginine was correlated with systolic BP (Matsuguma et al. 2006).

Plasma endothelin, a known potent vasoconstrictor is also shown to be elevated in ESRD patients with hypertension when compared to normotensive ESRD patients, although it is unclear if this elevation have a pathophysiological role in vivo (Shichiri et al. 1990).

Anemia treatment with exogenous *erythropoietin* is nearly ubiquitous in the hemodialysis population. The impact of erythropoietin on BP appears to be dose dependent and is associated with an increase in SBP up to 5–8 mmHg and DBP up to 4–6 mmHg. The proposed mechanism is enhanced adrenergic sensitivity and increased circulating endothelin-1 levels. A thorough review on the subject can be found in a review paper by Krapf et al. (2009).

4   Varied Methods of BP Measurement

As mentioned earlier, various BP measurement methods and thresholds have been utilized to define hypertension. BP can vary depending on the method and time of measurement in the general population, but this variation is especially pronounced in hemodialysis patients (Fagugli

et al. 2009). It is important to understand the advantages and disadvantages of the varied settings in which BP is obtained in the dialysis patients to individualize patient management.

4.1   Pre and Post Dialysis Readings

Immediate pre and post dialysis readings, which are obtained routinely during hemodialysis, tend to over- and under estimate interdialytic BP (Coomer et al. 1997; Agarwal et al. 2006a). Pre-dialysis SBP has been shown to overestimate mean SBP by 10 mmHg when compared to average SBP obtained by a 48 h ambulatory BP monitor. At the same time, the post dialysis SBP underestimated ambulatory BP by 7 mmHg. Thus, it is not surprising that in-center BP readings do not correlate well with markers of end organ damage like left ventricular hypertrophy (Agarwal et al. 2006b).

Pre and post dialysis BP readings are unreliable for several reasons. First, major volume shifts occur during the dialysis procedure leading to rapidly fluctuating BP. Also, the unreliability is related to the medications taken on hemodialysis days. It is not uncommon for hemodialysis patients to hold antihypertensives on the hemodialysis days to blunt the hypotension that can occur with volume removal. Another important consideration when interpreting BP measurements from the dialysis unit is how the BP was actually obtained. Because of various hemodialysis accesses and vascular issues, it is not uncommon for ankle or wrist BPs to be taken. These measurements are inherently unreliable.

BP measurements that are taken immediately pre or post hemodialysis also miss important aspects of BP control including diurnal variation, nocturnal hypertension and masked hypertension which are common among hemodialysis patients and have prognostic significance (Agarwal et al. 2011). However, BP monitoring in the dialysis unit remains important despite their limitations. These measurements are easily performed and widely available. These readings are important for the adjustment of the ultrafiltration target and are key to the detection of dialysis related complications such as hypotension/hypertension during the dialysis procedure, dialyzer reaction, and myocardial infarction among other complications.

Multiple studies utilizing in-center BP readings showed a U shape association between BP and mortality in hemodialysis patients (Lacson and Lazarus 2007; Li et al. 2006; Port et al. 1999; Stidley et al. 2006; Zager et al. 1998). For example, one group observed increased mortality when pre-dialysis SBP was <160 mmHg and >200 mmHg with significant increase in mortality seen in patients with pre-dialysis SBP <120 mmHg (Li et al. 2006). Another group found increased mortality in incident hemodialysis patients with SBP < 120 mmHg in first 2 years and in patients with SBP > 150 mmHg who survived more than 3 years on hemodialysis (Stidley et al. 2006).

A similar U shape relationship between diastolic BP and mortality has been reported in the general population (Boutitie et al. 2002). This is logical from a pathophysiologic perspective because low BP may lead to impaired organ perfusion and function. Observational studies suggest a shift in the systolic BP threshold on this U curve toward higher BP for unclear reasons. This could be related to the inherent limitations of pre and post dialysis BP measurement discussed above, but is likely because dialysis patients have marked vascular calcifications that lead to higher BP and impaired autoregulation. Alternatively, it is possible that low BP is just a marker of serious comorbidities that carry high risk of mortality such as development of heart failure (Foley et al. 1996).

4.2 Ambulatory BP Monitoring

Important aspects to consider when evaluating the BP of a dialysis patient and determining its impact on end organ damage are the following: BP load between dialysis sessions, diurnal variability, BP consistency, and reproducibility. The use of ambulatory BP monitoring is the optimal method for evaluating these aspects and is better correlated with end organ damage than single pre and post dialysis readings (Agarwal

et al. 2006b). In a prospective study, elevated 24 h pulse pressure and elevated nocturnal systolic BP were predictors of CV mortality (Amar et al. 2000). Alborzi et al. (2007) showed that when in-center pre and post dialysis BP was not predictive of total mortality, ambulatory BP was predictive of mortality with 50 % higher death rate for a 22.3 and 13.8 mmHg increase in systolic and diastolic BP, respectively. When patients were divided into quartiles based on their home and ambulatory SBP, patients with ambulatory SBP 115–125 mmHg and home SBP 125–144 mmHg had the lowest all-cause and cardiovascular mortality.

Forty-eight hour ambulatory BP monitoring is the gold standard because it will capture both dialysis and non-dialysis days (Fagugli et al. 2009). The disadvantage of ambulatory monitoring is its expense, inconvenience, and availability. 24 h BP monitoring, especially on non-dialysis days, appears to correlate well with 48 h ambulatory BP and can be done as an alternative (Fagugli et al. 2009; Peixoto et al. 2000) Additionally, because BP fluctuates frequently in the dialysis population, it is impractical to do 48 h monitoring whenever a change has been made in management.

4.3 Home BP Monitoring

A more readily available and less expensive alternative to ambulatory monitoring is home monitoring. Average home BP readings done on non-dialysis days correlates well with ambulatory readings and the presence of LVH (Agarwal et al. 2006b; Alborzi et al. 2007; Moriya et al. 2008). To get a representative sample of home readings, we recommend 3 readings per day over 1 week.

In summary, ambulatory and home BP monitoring correlate best with left ventricular hypertrophy and have better prognostic value in hemodialysis patients, but are sometimes cumbersome and expensive. Given the advantages and disadvantages of the various methods Table 1, we recommend reviewing the home BP readings in combination with pre and post

Table 1 Advantages and disadvantages of various blood pressure measurement methods

Method	Advantage	Disadvantage
In-center blood pressure	Readily available Help in adjusting rate of ultrafiltration Has a role in detecting hemodialysis related complications (e.g. dialyzer reaction)	Unreliable Does not represent interdialytic BP load Poor correlation with markers of end organ damage like LVH Miss nocturnal hypertension and masked hypertension
Ambulatory blood pressure monitoring	Reflect BP load in the interdialytic period Characterize diurnal variation in blood pressure Diagnose masked hypertension and nocturnal hypertension Correlate better with end organ damage	Expensive Not widely available Cumbersome for the patient
Home blood pressure monitoring	Easy to perform and widely available Reflect BP load in interdialytic period Better correlation with end organ damage	Require patient education and calibration of home devices Need to average multiple readings for a reliable result

dialysis readings. If there is an unexplained discrepancy, ambulatory monitoring is a consideration. Ambulatory monitoring should also be considered for difficult to control hypertension or unexplained end organ damage.

5   Targets for BP Control in the Hemodialysis Population

The optimal BP correlates with less end organ damage, fewer cardiovascular events, and lower mortality in the absence of symptomatic hypotension or medication adverse effects. Debate exists about BP targets in the general population and the optimal targets are less clear in the dialysis population. A paucity of large well-designed prospective studies of hypertension exist in the hemodialysis population, and most recommendations are extrapolated from the general population. The factors that complicate the design of hypertension studies in the hemodialysis population include the heterogeneous patient population, rapid extracellular volume shifts, and varied methods of BP measurement (dialysis readings versus ambulatory readings). Hemodialysis patients also have a shorter lifespan in general which also makes it difficult to show long term benefits of BP lowering.

Because hemodialysis specific studies are limited, the question is whether we can adopt BP goals derived from studies on general population (e.g. JNC and AHA recommendations). In short, the answer is not known. The international group KDIGO (Kidney Disease Improving Global Outcomes) has not recommended specific BP targets in ESRD patients, but they endorse the superiority of home BP measurement on nondialysis days and ambulatory measurements over in-center pre and post dialysis readings (Levin et al. 2010). However, KDOQI (Kidney Disease Outcomes Quality Initiative) recommends predialysis BP to be <140/90 mmHg and postdialysis BP to be <130/80 mmHg (K/DOQI Workgroup 2005). However, KDOQI acknowledges that ambulatory and self-measured home BP may correlate better with BP load on nondialysis days. Strikingly, using the KDOQI BP targets, more than two thirds of hemodialysis patients have uncontrolled BP.

6   Treatment

6.1   Nonpharmacological Therapy

6.1.1   Fluid and Sodium Restriction
By targeting some of the factors involved in the pathophysiology of hypertension in hemodialysis

patients, BP control can be improved to reduce medication burden. Because extracellular volume status is a major contributor to hypertension, the main components of nonpharmacological therapy are fluid and sodium restriction. Sodium restriction appears to be more important than fluid restriction (Tomson 2001; Ahmad 2004; Maduell and Navarro 2000). This may be because sodium consumption often leads to thirst and subsequent fluid intake. Also, because dialysis patients have less means to excrete sodium, fluid retention follows sodium retention to maintain serum osmolality.

In one study, sodium intake accounted for all of the weight gain between dialysis sessions in non-diabetic patients and half of the weight gain in diabetic patients (Ramdeen et al. 1998). Additionally, strict sodium restriction combined with intensive ultrafiltration lead to normalized BP over 3 months and a reduction in left ventricular hypertrophy over 12 months (Ozkahya et al. 2002). The goal sodium intake in hemodialysis patients has not been rigorously studied, but limiting sodium intake to less than 2 g per day is currently recommended. Modeling studies suggest that a stricter limit of 1200 mg of sodium a day could result in substantial reduction of cardiovascular events in general population and this may be extended to hemodialysis patients (Bibbins-Domingo et al. 2010).

6.1.2 Lower Dialysate Sodium Concentration

Higher dialysate sodium used to be viewed as a tool to improve hemodynamic stability during dialysis, (Cybulsky et al. 1985) but multiple studies have shown that higher dialysate sodium can lead to increased thirst, interdialytic weight gain, (Daugirdas et al. 1985; Barre et al. 1988) higher BP, and more antihypertensives use (Song et al. 2002; Davenport 2006). The use of sodium modeling to reduce intradialytic hypotension could also result in positive sodium balance and should be used with caution (Sang et al. 1997). It is critical to individualize sodium prescription and avoid hypertonic dialysate sodium. It has been suggested to use patient's pre-dialysis average sodium level as guide for dialysis sodium

prescription. This approach may result in better BP control and less interdialytic thirst and its ramifications (Santos and Peixoto 2008; de Paula et al. 2004).

6.1.3 Dry Weight Adjustment

Dry weight can be defined as the weight where a patient has only physiological extracellular volume (Raimann et al. 2008). In addition to fluid restriction, increased fluid removal at hemodialysis to establish a new dry weight can lead to improved BP. A reduction in dry weight of 1 kg over 8 weeks resulted in drop in ambulatory SBP of 6.6 mmHg and DBP of 3.3 mmHg (Agarwal et al. 2009). Unfortunately, this strategy is complicated because of the difficulty in establishing the dry weight and the other factors that lead to increased BP (cardiac output and vascular resistance). Also attempting to lower dry weight can lead to hypotension if fluid is removed too rapidly to allow for equilibration among tissues or if extracellular volume is reduced to the point of hypovolemia. Hypotension during dialysis is problematic because it can lead to symptoms such as cramping and headache, which often requires the discontinuation of ultrafiltration and possibly fluid administration. Symptomatic hypotension and orthostatic hypotension can affect quality of life and increase the risk of AV fistula clotting. Dry weight adjustment should be gradual and may require a tapering off of some antihypertensives. For unclear reasons, a lag time between dry weight reduction and reduced BP has been observed (Agarwal et al. 2009; Charra et al. 1998). Lack of appreciation of this phenomenon may result in adjusting dry weight too frequently leading to eventual hypotension.

Despite its importance, determining the dry weight in hemodialysis patients is mainly based on clinical judgment. Absence of edema does not correlate with euvolemia and is not a good marker of volume status in hemodialysis patients (Agarwal et al. 2008). Recent studies suggest that tools such as bioimpedance plethysmography, pre and postdialysis ANP levels, monitoring blood volume during dialysis using Crit-Line and measurement of IVC collapsibility are tools to estimate dry weight (Onofriescu et al. 2014;

Joffy and Rosner 2005; Rodriguez et al. 2005; Kraemer et al. 2006). With the exception of bioimpedance plethysmography, none of these methods were compared to clinical assessment alone.

6.1.4 Increased Frequency and Duration of Dialysis

Observational studies suggest that frequent dialysis can result in lower BP, fewer antihypertensives, and even a regression in left ventricular mass (Chan et al. 2002, 2005; Woods et al. 1999; Culleton et al. 2007). Whether this is result of improved volume control or result of removal of "uremic" toxins it is unclear. Similar findings were reported by frequent hemodialysis network study. In this study, hemodialysis patients were randomized to either conventional dialysis three times weekly or greater than 3 sessions per week. Patients who received more frequent dialysis had an increased drop in SBP, fewer antihypertensives, and improved left ventricular mass (Group et al. 2010). An added benefit of more frequent or longer dialysis sessions is the ability to do more gradual ultrafiltration which is better tolerated (Katzarski et al. 1999).

6.2 Pharmacological Therapy

Despite all of the potential nonpharmacological methods for BP reduction in the dialysis patient, antihypertensives remain an important tool in controlling BP. One meta-analyses found cardiovascular benefit from lowering BP using antihypertensives in hemodialysis patients, (Agarwal and Sinha 2009) and another reported reduction in cardiovascular events, all-cause mortality and cardiovascular mortality when various antihypertensives were used in dialysis patients (Heerspink et al. 2009). With the exception of diuretics, all other groups of antihypertensive can and have been used in dialysis patients. Thiazide diuretics are unlikely to work in a dialysis patient because they need tubular function to be active. However, loop diuretics may be very effective in a patient with residual kidney function to minimize weight gain between dialysis sessions, but it is unlikely to be beneficial in an anuric patients (Hayashi et al. 2008).

Few studies have been done to compare the efficacy of different antihypertensive in hemodialysis patients. K/DOQI guidelines consider ACEIs and ARBs as the agents of choice in treatment of hypertension in patients with significant residual kidney function (K/DOQI Workgroup 2005). Outside of this recommendation, the choice of medication should depend on other compelling indications and patient's comorbidities.

6.2.1 Angiotensin Converting Enzyme Inhibitors (ACEI) and Angiotensin II Receptors Blockers (ARB)

K/DOQI guidelines consider ACEIs and/or ARBs antihypertensive of choice in hemodialysis patients with residual kidney function since these two classes of medications may help preserve residual kidney function while on dialysis. However, there are few randomized controlled studies that looked into ACEI/ARB specifically in hemodialysis patients, and the results are conflicting. In one meta-analysis examining the cardiovascular effect of ACEI/ARB in hemodialysis patients, there was a reduction in LV mass but this did not translate into a reduction in the risk of fatal or non-fatal CV events (Tai et al. 2010). This meta-analysis was limited by small number of patients, short follow-up, and the studies included (988 patients from 8 RCTs). A more recent observational study had comparable results: ACEI/ARB were not associated with a reduction in the composite of all-cause mortality or hospitalization for myocardial infarction (MI), stroke, heart failure (HF), or coronary revascularization when compared to calcium channel blockers in hemodialysis patients (Bajaj et al. 2012). In contrast, other studies did show a reduction in fatal and non-fatal CVD with use of ARB, (Suzuki et al. 2008) and reduction in mortality among patients younger than age of 65 years with use of ACEI (Efrati et al. 2002).

Despite the conflicting results mentioned above, ACEI and ARB remain effective antihypertensives with probable survival and CV benefit in hemodialysis patient. They also play an important role in management of patients with cardiovascular comorbidities, especially systolic dysfunction where ACEI/ARB is associated with improved survival.

There are important side effect to monitor when using ACEI/ARB. Hyperkalemia is a potential dangerous complication and ACEI may exacerbate anemia. Although use of AN69 dialyzer has become very rare in US, it is important to note that anaphylactic reactions have been observed when patients are on ACEI and this dialyzer is used (Horl and Horl 2004). It is also important to remember pharmacokinetics of various ACEI and ARB before using them in hemodialysis patients. Some ACEI are removed by hemodialysis, while ARB are note removed by hemodialysis. Removal of medications during the dialysis session is a potential cause of hypertension during or after the dialysis session itself (Table 2).

6.2.2 Calcium Channel Blockers

Dihydropyridine and non-dihydropyridine calcium channel blockers can also be used for BP control in hemodialysis patient. A small prospective study showed a trend toward lower cardiovascular mortality in patients treated with amlodipine and a reduction in composite of all-cause mortality and cardiovascular events. (Tepel et al. 2008) Amlodipine was effective in reducing systolic BP in the treated group.

6.2.3 Beta Blockers

Beta blockers have an important role in the management of hemodialysis patients with cardiovascular comorbidities, including systolic heart failure and coronary artery disease. Among patients on hemodialysis with LVH, atenolol administered three times a week after dialysis was shown to be more effective in lowering BP, decreasing risk of serious cardiovascular events and all cause hospitalizations when compared to lisinopril dosed three times a week (Agarwal et al. 2014). It is again important to consider

Table 2 Pharmacokinetics of select antihypertensives use in dialysis patients (Inrig 2010a)

Drug	Removed by hemodialysis
ACEIs	
Captopril	Yes
Lisinopril	Partial
Enlapril	Partial
Fosinopril	Minimal
ARBs	No
Calcium channel blockers	
Amlodipine	No
Diltiazem	Partial
Nifedipine	No
B blockers	
Atenolol	Yes
Metoprolol	Yes
Carvedilol	No
Labetalol	No
Hydralazine	No
Minoxidil	Partial
Clonidine	No

pharmacokinetics of various b-blockers. Atenolol for example is primarily removed by the kidney itself and actually requires dose reduction in hemodialysis patients (Table 2). Given its longer half-life in hemodialysis patients, it may be a good option to use in patients with poor compliance since it can be dosed three times a week after dialysis. On the other hand, carvedilol does not require dose adjustment in hemodialysis patients and its alpha 1-adrenergic blocking activity may improve BP control beyond other b-blockers, but could also potentiate symptoms of postural hypotension.

6.2.4 Other Antihypertensives

Hydralazine and clonidine can be used for BP control in hemodialysis patients but both medications require multiple dosing during the day and may lead to reduced compliance especially in hemodialysis patients who already have large pill burden. An alternative option is transdermal clonidine patch which requires dosing once a week. Minoxidil is another potent vasodilator that can be dosed once a day but should be combined with beta blocker to prevent reflex tachycardia.

6.3 Treatment of Patients Non-adherent to Medications

Poor adherence to medications in hemodialysis patients is well recognized and likely contributes to uncontrolled BP. One study reported that only 48 % of hemodialysis patients were adherent to their treatment.(Neri et al. 2011) Multiple strategies have been suggested to help improve compliance with antihypertensives in hemodialysis patients, but the most important is to simplify the medication regimen. For example, use of longer acting formulations such as transdermal clonidine patch reduces pill burden. Directly observed therapy using other long acting antihypertensive such as atenolol and certain ACE inhibitors have also been utilized with some success.(Zheng et al. 2007) Other strategies include counseling, education and the exploration of social, financial and mental health issues that may be limiting compliance with medications.

7 Intradialytic Hypertension

Increase in BP during dialysis, or intradialytic hypertension, does not have a standard definition. Some studies defined it as increase in SBP > 10 mmHg from pre to post dialysis (Inrig et al. 2009). Intradialytic hypertension has been observed in 13 % of hemodialysis patients and has been associated with a higher risk of hospitalization and death than if BP decreases (Inrig et al. 2007b). In incident hemodialysis patients, intradialytic hypertension was associated with decreased 2 year survival in patients with predialysis SBP < 120 mmHg (Inrig et al. 2009). The pathogenesis of this phenomena is not well understood but some of the suggested mechanisms include altered balance of nitric oxide and endothelin-1, (Chou et al. 2006) removal of certain antihypertensives and administration of erythropoietin stimulating agents (Inrig 2010b). Treatment of this condition remains a challenge because its pathophysiology is not well understood. Any treatment strategy should include review of patient's interdialytic

BP control, dialysis sodium prescription, and dry weight. Additionally, a thorough review of the pharmacokinetics and timing of medications in relation to dialysis is needed. Carvedilol may have modest improvement in intradialytic and interdialytic BP control (Inrig et al. 2012). Another strategy is to use dialysate sodium concentration that is 5 mEq/L lower than serum sodium (Inrig et al. 2015).

8 Conclusion and Guidelines Recommendations

In summary, hypertension is common among hemodialysis patients and its control is complicated by the limitations of various blood pressure measurement methods. The only published guidelines that include exact blood pressure goal is K/DOQI clinical practice guidelines, which recommend pre-dialysis BP < 140/90 mmHg and post dialysis < 130/80 mmHg (K/DOQI Workgroup 2005). However, given the evidence of U shape relationship between blood pressure and outcomes in hemodialysis patients, we recommend individualizing BP goals and relying on combination of average home readings, in-center readings and ambulatory blood pressure monitoring. When treating blood pressure in hemodialysis patients, non-pharmacological approach including sodium restriction, probing dry weight and lowering dialysate sodium, and pharmacological approach utilizing ACEI/ARB as first line therapy especially in patients with residual kidney function should be utilized. Intradialytic hypertension remains a challenging area to manage and require review of dialysis prescription and patient medications.

References

Agarwal R (2011) Epidemiology of interdialytic ambulatory hypertension and the role of volume excess. Am J Nephrol 34(4):381–390

Agarwal R, Sinha AD (2009) Cardiovascular protection with antihypertensive drugs in dialysis patients:

systematic review and meta-analysis. Hypertension 53 (5):860–866

Agarwal R, Nissenson AR, Batlle D, Coyne DW, Trout JR, Warnock DG (2003) Prevalence, treatment, and control of hypertension in chronic hemodialysis patients in the United States. Am J Med 115 (4):291–297

Agarwal R, Peixoto AJ, Santos SF, Zoccali C (2006a) Pre- and postdialysis blood pressures are imprecise estimates of interdialytic ambulatory blood pressure. Clin J Am Soc Nephrol 1(3):389–398

Agarwal R, Brim NJ, Mahenthiran J, Andersen MJ, Saha C (2006b) Out-of-hemodialysis-unit blood pressure is a superior determinant of left ventricular hypertrophy. Hypertension 47(1):62–68

Agarwal R, Andersen MJ, Pratt JH (2008) On the importance of pedal edema in hemodialysis patients. Clin J Am Soc Nephrol 3(1):153–158

Agarwal R, Alborzi P, Satyan S, Light RP (2009) Dry-weight reduction in hypertensive hemodialysis patients (DRIP): a randomized, controlled trial. Hypertension 53(3):500–507

Agarwal R, Sinha AD, Light RP (2011) Toward a definition of masked hypertension and white-coat hypertension among hemodialysis patients. Clin J Am Soc Nephrol 6(8):2003–2008

Agarwal R, Sinha AD, Pappas MK, Abraham TN, Tegegne GG (2014) Hypertension in hemodialysis patients treated with atenolol or lisinopril: a randomized controlled trial. Nephrol Dial Transplant 29(3):672–681

Ahmad S (2004) Dietary sodium restriction for hypertension in dialysis patients. Semin Dial 17(4):284–287

Alborzi P, Patel N, Agarwal R (2007) Home blood pressures are of greater prognostic value than hemodialysis unit recordings. Clin J Am Soc Nephrol 2 (6):1228–1234

Amar J, Vernier I, Rossignol E, Bongard V, Arnaud C, Conte JJ et al (2000) Nocturnal blood pressure and 24-hour pulse pressure are potent indicators of mortality in hemodialysis patients. Kidney Int 57 (6):2485–2491

Bajaj RR, Wald R, Hackam DG, Gomes T, Perl J, Juurlink DN et al (2012) Use of angiotensin-converting enzyme inhibitors or angiotensin receptor blockers and cardiovascular outcomes in chronic dialysis patients: a population-based cohort study. Arch Intern Med 172(7):591–593

Barre PE, Brunelle G, Gascon-Barre M (1988) A randomized double blind trial of dialysate sodiums of 145 mEq/L, 150 mEq/L, and 155 mEq/L. ASAIO Trans 34(3):338–341

Bibbins-Domingo K, Chertow GM, Coxson PG, Moran A, Lightwood JM, Pletcher MJ et al (2010) Projected effect of dietary salt reductions on future cardiovascular disease. N Engl J Med 362(7):590–599

Boutitie F, Gueyffier F, Pocock S, Fagard R, Boissel JP (2002) J-shaped relationship between blood pressure and mortality in hypertensive patients: new insights from a meta-analysis of individual-patient data. Ann Intern Med 136(6):438–448

Chan CT, Floras JS, Miller JA, Richardson RM, Pierratos A (2002) Regression of left ventricular hypertrophy after conversion to nocturnal hemodialysis. Kidney Int 61(6):2235–2239

Chan CT, Jain V, Picton P, Pierratos A, Floras JS (2005) Nocturnal hemodialysis increases arterial baroreflex sensitivity and compliance and normalizes blood pressure of hypertensive patients with end-stage renal disease. Kidney Int 68(1):338–344

Charra B, Bergstrom J, Scribner BH (1998) Blood pressure control in dialysis patients: importance of the lag phenomenon. Am J Kidney Dis 32(5):720–724

Chen YC, Chen HH, Yeh JC, Chen SY (2002) Adjusting dry weight by extracellular volume and body composition in hemodialysis patients. Nephron 92(1):91–96

Chou KJ, Lee PT, Chen CL, Chiou CW, Hsu CY, Chung HM et al (2006) Physiological changes during hemodialysis in patients with intradialysis hypertension. Kidney Int 69(10):1833–1838

Converse RL Jr, Jacobsen TN, Toto RD, Jost CM, Cosentino F, Fouad-Tarazi F et al (1992) Sympathetic overactivity in patients with chronic renal failure. N Engl J Med 327(27):1912–1918

Cooke JP (2000) Does ADMA cause endothelial dysfunction? Arterioscler Thromb Vasc Biol 20 (9):2032–2037

Coomer RW, Schulman G, Breyer JA, Shyr Y (1997) Ambulatory blood pressure monitoring in dialysis patients and estimation of mean interdialytic blood pressure. Am J Kidney Dis 29(5):678–684

Culleton BF, Walsh M, Klarenbach SW, Mortis G, Scott-Douglas N, Quinn RR et al (2007) Effect of frequent nocturnal hemodialysis vs conventional hemodialysis on left ventricular mass and quality of life: a randomized controlled trial. JAMA 298 (11):1291–1299

Cybulsky AV, Matni A, Hollomby DJ (1985) Effects of high sodium dialysate during maintenance hemodialysis. Nephron 41(1):57–61

Daugirdas JT, Al-Kudsi RR, Ing TS, Norusis MJ (1985) A double-blind evaluation of sodium gradient hemodialysis. Am J Nephrol 5(3):163–168

Davenport A (2006) Audit of the effect of dialysate sodium concentration on inter-dialytic weight gains and blood pressure control in chronic haemodialysis patients. Nephron Clin pract 104(3):c120–c125

de Paula FM, Peixoto AJ, Pinto LV, Dorigo D, Patricio PJ, Santos SF (2004) Clinical consequences of an individualized dialysate sodium prescription in hemodialysis patients. Kidney Int 66(3):1232–1238

Efrati S, Zaidenstein R, Dishy V, Beberashvili I, Sharist M, Averbukh Z et al (2002) ACE inhibitors and survival of hemodialysis patients. Am J Kidney Dis 40(5):1023–1029

Fagugli RM, Pasini P, Quintaliani G, Pasticci F, Ciao G, Cicconi B et al (2003) Association between extracellular water, left ventricular mass and hypertension in haemodialysis patients. Nephrol Dial Transplant 18 (11):2332–2338

Fagugli RM, Ricciardi D, Rossi D, De Gaetano A, Taglioni C (2009) Blood pressure assessment in haemodialysis patients: comparison between pre-dialysis blood pressure and ambulatory blood pressure measurement. Nephrology 14(3):283–290

Foley RN, Parfrey PS, Harnett JD, Kent GM, Murray DC, Barre PE (1996) Impact of hypertension on cardiomyopathy, morbidity and mortality in end-stage renal disease. Kidney Int 49(5):1379–1385

Fortier C, Mac-Way F, Desmeules S, Marquis K, De Serres SA, Lebel M et al (2015) Aortic-brachial stiffness mismatch and mortality in dialysis population. Hypertension 65(2):378–384

Goldsmith DJ, Covic AA, Venning MC, Ackrill P (1996) Blood pressure reduction after parathyroidectomy for secondary hyperparathyroidism: further evidence implicating calcium homeostasis in blood pressure regulation. Am J Kidney Dis 27(6):819–825

Group FHNT, Chertow GM, Levin NW, Beck GJ, Depner TA, Eggers PW et al (2010) In-center hemodialysis six times per week versus three times per week. N Engl J Med 363(24):2287–2300

Harper J, Nicholas J, Ford D, Casula A, Williams AJ (2009) UK Renal Registry 11th annual report (December 2008): Chapter 11 Blood pressure profile of prevalent patients receiving dialysis in the UK in 2007: national and centre-specific analyses. Nephron Clin Pract 111(Suppl 1):c227–c245

Hausberg M, Kosch M, Harmelink P, Barenbrock M, Hohage H, Kisters K et al (2002) Sympathetic nerve activity in end-stage renal disease. Circulation 106 (15):1974–1979

Hayashi SY, Seeberger A, Lind B, Gunnes S, Alvestrand A, do Nascimento MM et al (2008) Acute effects of low and high intravenous doses of furosemide on myocardial function in anuric haemodialysis patients: a tissue Doppler study. Nephrol Dial Transplant 23(4):1355–1361

Heerspink HJ, Ninomiya T, Zoungas S, de Zeeuw D, Grobbee DE, Jardine MJ et al (2009) Effect of lowering blood pressure on cardiovascular events and mortality in patients on dialysis: a systematic review and meta-analysis of randomised controlled trials. Lancet 373(9668):1009–1015

Horl MP, Horl WH (2004) Drug therapy for hypertension in hemodialysis patients. Semin Dial 17(4):288–294

Inrig JK (2010a) Antihypertensive agents in hemodialysis patients: a current perspective. Semin Dial 23 (3):290–297

Inrig JK (2010b) Intradialytic hypertension: a less-recognized cardiovascular complication of hemodialysis. Am J Kidney Dis 55(3):580–589

Inrig JK, Patel UD, Gillespie BS, Hasselblad V, Himmelfarb J, Reddan D et al (2007a) Relationship between interdialytic weight gain and blood pressure among prevalent hemodialysis patients. Am J Kidney Dis 50(1):108–118, 18 e1–4

Inrig JK, Oddone EZ, Hasselblad V, Gillespie B, Patel UD, Reddan D et al (2007b) Association of intradialytic blood pressure changes with hospitalization and mortality rates in prevalent ESRD patients. Kidney Int 71(5):454–461

Inrig JK, Patel UD, Toto RD, Szczech LA (2009) Association of blood pressure increases during hemodialysis with 2-year mortality in incident hemodialysis patients: a secondary analysis of the Dialysis Morbidity and Mortality Wave 2 Study. Am J Kidney Dis 54 (5):881–890

Inrig JK, Van Buren P, Kim C, Vongpatanasin W, Povsic TJ, Toto R (2012) Probing the mechanisms of intradialytic hypertension: a pilot study targeting endothelial cell dysfunction. Clin J Am Soc Nephrol 7(8):1300–1309

Inrig JK, Molina C, D'Silva K, Kim C, Van Buren P, Allen JD et al (2015) Effect of low versus high dialysate sodium concentration on blood pressure and endothelial-derived vasoregulators during hemodialysis: a randomized crossover study. Am J Kidney Dis 65(3):464–473

Joffy S, Rosner MH (2005) Natriuretic peptides in ESRD. Am J Kidney Dis 46(1):1–10

K/DOQI Workgroup (2005) K/DOQI clinical practice guidelines for cardiovascular disease in dialysis patients. Am J Kidney Dis 45(4 Suppl 3):S1–S153

Katzarski KS, Charra B, Luik AJ, Nisell J, Divino Filho JC, Leypoldt JK et al (1999) Fluid state and blood pressure control in patients treated with long and short haemodialysis. Nephrol Dial Transplant 14 (2):369–375

Kraemer M, Rode C, Wizemann V (2006) Detection limit of methods to assess fluid status changes in dialysis patients. Kidney Int 69(9):1609–1620

Krapf R, Hulter HN (2009) Arterial hypertension induced by erythropoietin and erythropoiesis-stimulating agents (ESA). Clin J Am Soc Nephrol 4(2):470–480

Krautzig S, Janssen U, Koch KM, Granolleras C, Shaldon S (1998) Dietary salt restriction and reduction of dialysate sodium to control hypertension in maintenance haemodialysis patients. Nephrol Dial Transplant 13 (3):552–553

Lacson E Jr, Lazarus JM (2007) The association between blood pressure and mortality in ESRD-not different from the general population? Semin Dial 20 (6):510–517

Levin NW, Kotanko P, Eckardt KU, Kasiske BL, Chazot C, Cheung AK et al (2010) Blood pressure in chronic kidney disease stage 5D-report from a kidney disease: improving global outcomes controversies conference. Kidney Int 77(4):273–284

Li Z, Lacson E Jr, Lowrie EG, Ofsthun NJ, Kuhlmann MK, Lazarus JM et al (2006) The epidemiology of systolic blood pressure and death risk in hemodialysis patients. Am J Kidney Dis 48(4):606–615

Liu W, Ye H, Tang B, Song Z, Sun Z, Wen P et al (2014) Profile of interdialytic ambulatory blood pressure in a cohort of Chinese patients. J Hum Hypertens 28 (11):677–683

Lopez-Gomez JM, Villaverde M, Jofre R, Rodriguez-Benitez P, Perez-Garcia R (2005) Interdialytic weight gain as a marker of blood pressure, nutrition, and survival in hemodialysis patients. Kidney Int Suppl 93:S63–S68

Maduell F, Navarro V (2000) Dietary salt intake and blood pressure control in haemodialysis patients. Nephrol Dial Transplant 15(12):2063

Maduell F, Navarro V (2001) Assessment of salt intake in hemodialysis. Nefrologia 21(1):71–77

Matsuguma K, Ueda S, Yamagishi S, Matsumoto Y, Kaneyuki U, Shibata R et al (2006) Molecular mechanism for elevation of asymmetric dimethylarginine and its role for hypertension in chronic kidney disease. J Am Soc Nephrol 17(8):2176–2183

Mauriello A, Rovella V, Anemona L, Servadei F, Giannini E, Bove P et al (2015) Increased sympathetic renal innervation in hemodialysis patients is the anatomical substrate of sympathetic hyperactivity in end-stage renal disease. J Am Heart Assoc 4(12)

Mc Causland FR, Waikar SS, Brunelli SM (2012) Increased dietary sodium is independently associated with greater mortality among prevalent hemodialysis patients. Kidney Int 82(2):204–211

Morishita Y, Watanabe M, Hanawa S, Iimura O, Tsunematsu S, Ishibashi K et al (2012) Long-term effects of aliskiren on blood pressure and the renin-angiotensin-aldosterone system in hypertensive hemodialysis patients. Int J Nephrol Renov Dis 5:45–51

Moriya H, Oka M, Maesato K, Mano T, Ikee R, Ohtake T et al (2008) Weekly averaged blood pressure is more important than a single-point blood pressure measurement in the risk stratification of dialysis patients. Clin J Am Soc Nephrol 3(2):416–422

Neri L, Martini A, Andreucci VE, Gallieni M, Rey LA, Brancaccio D et al (2011) Regimen complexity and prescription adherence in dialysis patients. Am J Nephrol 34(1):71–76

Onofriescu M, Hogas S, Voroneanu L, Apetrii M, Nistor I, Kanbay M et al (2014) Bioimpedance-guided fluid management in maintenance hemodialysis: a pilot randomized controlled trial. Am J Kidney Dis 64(1):111–118

Ozkahya M, Toz H, Qzerkan F, Duman S, Ok E, Basci A et al (2002) Impact of volume control on left ventricular hypertrophy in dialysis patients. J Nephrol 15 (6):655–660

Peixoto AJ, Santos SF, Mendes RB, Crowley ST, Maldonado R, Orias M et al (2000) Reproducibility of ambulatory blood pressure monitoring in hemodialysis patients. Am J Kidney Dis 36(5):983–990

Port FK, Hulbert-Shearon TE, Wolfe RA, Bloembergen WE, Golper TA, Agodoa LY et al (1999) Predialysis blood pressure and mortality risk in a national sample of maintenance hemodialysis patients. Am J Kidney Dis 33(3):507–517

Raimann J, Liu L, Tyagi S, Levin NW, Kotanko P (2008) A fresh look at dry weight. Hemodial Int 12 (4):395–405

Raine AE, Bedford L, Simpson AW, Ashley CC, Brown R, Woodhead JS et al (1993) Hyperparathyroidism, platelet intracellular free calcium and hypertension in chronic renal failure. Kidney Int 43 (3):700–705

Ramdeen G, Tzamaloukas AH, Malhotra D, Leger A, Murata GH (1998) Estimates of interdialytic sodium and water intake based on the balance principle: differences between nondiabetic and diabetic subjects on hemodialysis. ASAIO J 44(6):812–817

Rodriguez HJ, Domenici R, Diroll A, Goykhman I (2005) Assessment of dry weight by monitoring changes in blood volume during hemodialysis using Crit-Line. Kidney Int 68(2):854–861

Salem MM (1995) Hypertension in the hemodialysis population: a survey of 649 patients. Am J Kidney Dis 26 (3):461–468

Sang GL, Kovithavongs C, Ulan R, Kjellstrand CM (1997) Sodium ramping in hemodialysis: a study of beneficial and adverse effects. Am J Kidney Dis 29 (5):669–677

Santos SF, Peixoto AJ (2008) Revisiting the dialysate sodium prescription as a tool for better blood pressure and interdialytic weight gain management in hemodialysis patients. Clin J Am Soc Nephrol 3(2):522–530

Shichiri M, Hirata Y, Ando K, Emori T, Ohta K, Kimoto S et al (1990) Plasma endothelin levels in hypertension and chronic renal failure. Hypertension 15 (5):493–496

Song JH, Lee SW, Suh CK, Kim MJ (2002) Time-averaged concentration of dialysate sodium relates with sodium load and interdialytic weight gain during sodium-profiling hemodialysis. Am J Kidney Dis 40 (2):291–301

Stidley CA, Hunt WC, Tentori F, Schmidt D, Rohrscheib M, Paine S et al (2006) Changing relationship of blood pressure with mortality over time among hemodialysis patients. JASN 17(2):513–520

Suzuki H, Kanno Y, Sugahara S, Ikeda N, Shoda J, Takenaka T et al (2008) Effect of angiotensin receptor blockers on cardiovascular events in patients undergoing hemodialysis: an open-label randomized controlled trial. Am J Kidney Dis 52(3):501–506

Tai DJ, Lim TW, James MT, Manns BJ, Tonelli M, Hemmelgarn BR et al (2010) Cardiovascular effects of angiotensin converting enzyme inhibition or angiotensin receptor blockade in hemodialysis: a meta-analysis. Clin J Am Soc Nephrol 5(4):623–630

Tepel M, Hopfenmueller W, Scholze A, Maier A, Zidek W (2008) Effect of amlodipine on cardiovascular events in hypertensive haemodialysis patients. Nephrol Dial Transplant 23(11):3605–3612

Tomson CR (2001) Advising dialysis patients to restrict fluid intake without restricting sodium intake is not based on evidence and is a waste of time. Nephrol Dial Transplant 16(8):1538–1542

Utescu MS, Couture V, Mac-Way F, De Serres SA, Marquis K, Lariviere R et al (2013) Determinants of progression of aortic stiffness in hemodialysis patients: a prospective longitudinal study. Hypertension 62(1):154–160

Vallance P, Leone A, Calver A, Collier J, Moncada S (1992) Accumulation of an endogenous inhibitor of nitric oxide synthesis in chronic renal failure. Lancet 339(8793):572–575

Weidmann P, Maxwell MH, Lupu AN, Lewin AJ, Massry SG (1971) Plasma renin activity and blood pressure in terminal renal failure. N Engl J Med 285(14):757–762

Woods JD, Port FK, Orzol S, Buoncristiani U, Young E, Wolfe RA et al (1999) Clinical and biochemical correlates of starting "daily" hemodialysis. Kidney Int 55(6):2467–2476

Xu J, Li G, Wang P, Velazquez H, Yao X, Li Y et al (2005) Renalase is a novel, soluble monoamine oxidase that regulates cardiac function and blood pressure. J Clin Invest 115(5):1275–1280

Zager PG, Nikolic J, Brown RH, Campbell MA, Hunt WC, Peterson D et al (1998) "U" curve association of blood pressure and mortality in hemodialysis patients. Medical Directors of Dialysis Clinic, Inc. Kidney Int 54(2):561–569

Zheng S, Nath V, Coyne DW (2007) ACE inhibitor-based, directly observed therapy for hypertension in hemodialysis patients. Am J Nephrol 27(5):522–529

Zilch O, Vos PF, Oey PL, Cramer MJ, Ligtenberg G, Koomans HA et al (2007) Sympathetic hyperactivity in haemodialysis patients is reduced by short daily haemodialysis. J Hypertens 25(6):1285–1289

Adv Exp Med Biol - Advances in Internal Medicine (2017) 2: 341–353
DOI 10.1007/5584_2016_87
© Springer International Publishing AG 2016
Published online: 5 November 2016

Unique Considerations When Managing Hypertension in the Transplant Patient

Donald Mitema and Carrie Schinstock

Abstract

For the select fortunate recipients of organ transplants, transplantation affords the rare opportunity for a new life. Given the scarcity of organs for transplantation, it is imperative that the health of transplant recipients be optimized in order to fully benefit from this gift of life. Unfortunately, hypertension is highly prevalent in the transplant population and it is considered a major cardiovascular risk factor contributing to mortality and morbidity in this population. In this chapter, we expound on the epidemiology, unique pathophysiology, evaluation, and management of hypertension as it pertains to the solid organ transplant recipient. In addition, a brief commentary is made on the subject of hypertension following living kidney donation, and practical aspects of management of hypertension in the solid organ recipient are summarized at the end of the chapter.

Keywords

Post-transplant hypertension • Blood pressure in solid organ transplant recipients • Hypertension • Calcineurin inhibitors

1   Introduction

For the select fortunate recipients of organ transplants, transplantation affords the rare opportunity for a new life. Given the scarcity of organs for transplantation, it is imperative that the health of transplant recipients be optimized in order to fully benefit from this gift of life. Car-diovascular disease is a major cause of death of a functioning graft in all of solid organ transplan-tation, and thus management of its risk factors are of utmost importance. Hypertension is a major cardiovascular risk factor and highly prev-alent in the transplant population. In spite of this, there remains a lack of consensus regarding the definition of hypertension in transplant recipients as well as the general population. Despite its importance, a paucity of evidence exists to

D. Mitema and C. Schinstock (✉)
William J. von Liebig Transplant Center, Mayo Clinic, Rochester, MN, USA
e-mail: Schinstock.carrie@mayo.edu

guide its management in the transplant population. In this review, we review the epidemiology, pathophysiology, and management of hypertension in the solid organ transplant population and discuss diagnostic and therapeutic considerations.

1.1 Epidemiology of Hypertension in the Transplant Population

Hypertension is strikingly prevalent across organ transplant recipients. It is estimated that hypertension is prevalent in 75–90 % of kidney transplant recipients (Campistol et al. 2004; Kasiske et al. 2004; Dobrowolski et al. 2016). Data from the International Society for Heart and Lung Transplantation (ISHLT) Registry shows that of 116,104 heart transplant recipients transplanted between 1995 and 2013, 72 % of recipients had hypertension within 1 year post-transplant. This increases up to 92 % at 5 years post-transplantation (Lund et al. 2014). In liver transplant recipients, the prevalence of hypertension ranges from 65 to 80 %

(Stegall et al. 1995; Sheiner et al. 2000; Guillaud et al. 2014), with similar rates noted in lung transplant recipients (Silverborn et al. 2005).

In the modern era of transplantation, calcineurin inhibitors (CNIs) are part of a standard immunosuppressive regimen for most patients (Textor et al. 2000; Hoorn et al. 2012; Azzi et al. 2013). Despite the benefits of CNIs from an immunosuppressive standpoint, they are known to exacerbate hypertension. Besides CNIs, there are multiple other factors that should be considered when managing hypertension in the transplant patient.

2 Hypertension in Select Settings

2.1 Hypertension Immediately Post-transplant

Blood pressure immediately post-transplant fluctuates and can be difficult to manage (Fig. 1). Unique considerations include

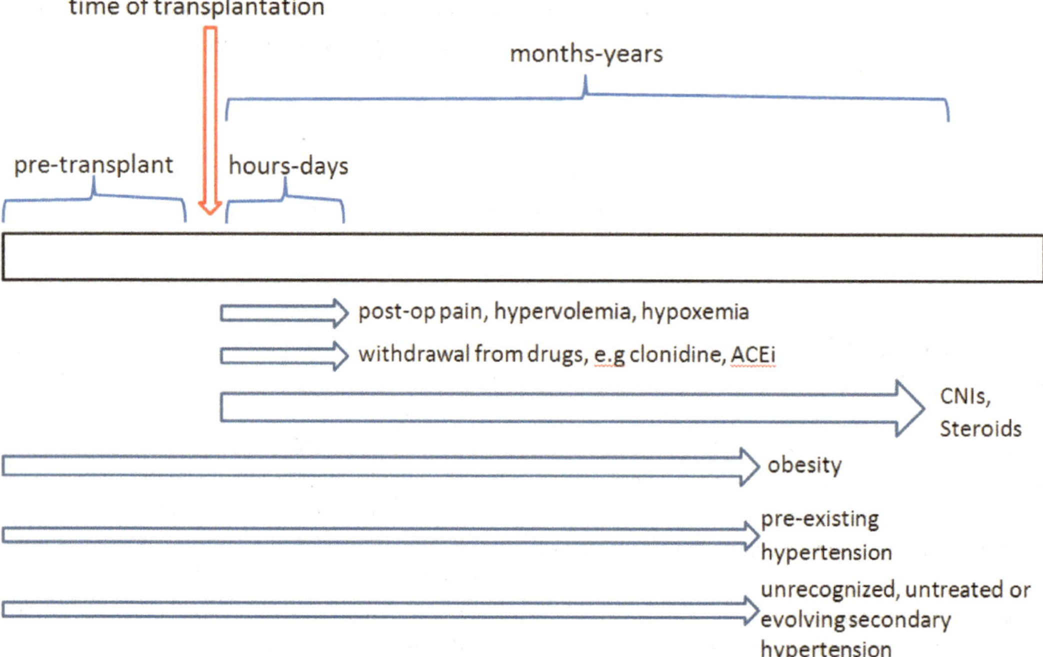

Fig. 1 Timeline for development of hypertension after solid organ transplant. The etiology of hypertension can differ depending on its timing post-transplantation. Recognizing the potential causes for hypertension in the post-transplant period is important for optimal blood pressure management

postoperative pain, hypervolemia, hypoxemia, anxiety, and discontinuation of oral anti-hypertensive medications (pre-transplant ACE inhibitors, ARB, or clonidine) or withdrawal (for example, clonidine). Not only can medication discontinuation lead to elevated blood pressure, the initiation of common immunosuppressants such as CNIs (tacrolimus or cyclosporine) and steroids commonly leads to elevated blood pressure.

Bladder distension is a less commonly recognized source of hypertension in a postsurgical patient. In a physiologic study evaluating the response to bladder distension in sixteen healthy volunteers, it was noted that an increase in the measured sympathetic outflow was noted when the urge to urinate was most pronounced. With this, there was also a concomitant increase in blood pressure from $125 \pm 2/74 \pm 2$ mmHg to $140 \pm 4/84 \pm 3$ mmHg (Fagius and Karhuvaara 1989). This effect of elevated blood pressure with bladder distension is especially a consideration in non-kidney transplant recipients because they are less likely to have their bladder routinely drained immediately post-surgery. Even if voiding was not a problem pre-transplant, this should be a consideration because several medications, particularly opioids, impair bladder emptying.

Liver transplant recipients have distinctive reasons to develop hypertension post-transplant. Prior to transplant, these patients are vasodilated and have decreased systemic vascular resistance and increased cardiac output. After liver transplantation, this pathophysiology reverses leading to increased systemic vascular resistance and later reduced cardiac output. This process is augmented by CNI mediated vasoconstriction, resulting in increasing blood pressure within weeks to months following liver transplantation (Hryniewiecka and Żegarska 2011). This phenomenon can be striking. Mean blood pressure can rise by up to 40–50 mmHg following liver transplantation (Textor 1993).

2.2 Chronic Hypertension Post-transplant

2.2.1 Contributing Factors Across All Solid Organ Transplant Recipients

Chronic hypertension is common in general population so it is not surprising that hypertension is widespread among transplant recipients who often have multiple medical comorbidities and are on medications known to aggravate hypertension (i.e. CNIs and steroids). Nevertheless, recognizing potentially modifiable factors that could contribute to hypertension is essential for optimal patient management and to reduce medication burden and side effects (Fig. 2). Obesity, non-steroidal anti-inflammatory drug (NSAID) use, alcohol consumption, excess sodium, sleep apnea, renal artery stenosis (especially a consideration for kidney transplant recipients), primary hyperaldosteronism, pheochromocytoma, and hypothyroidism are some of the most common modifiable factors that can lead to hypertension (Dalby et al. 2001). These potentially modifiable factors can easily be overlooked in transplant recipients who have complicated medical histories.

2.2.2 The Effect of Calcineurin Inhibitors (CNIs) on Blood Pressure

It is difficult to quantify the true effect of CNIs on the prevalence of hypertension, since the definition of high blood pressure has changed over time and the use of CNI-based maintenance immunosuppressive regimens is ubiquitous. What is striking, however, is the high prevalence of hypertension, across different organ transplants in immunosuppression regimens that primarily include CNIs. In one study, kidney transplant who were on belatacept based (non-CNI) immunosuppression needed fewer antihypertensive medications (median 2 drugs) compared with those on CNI based regimens (median 4 drugs) 10 years after follow up (Grannas et al. 2014). In liver transplant patients who typically are not hypertensive pre-

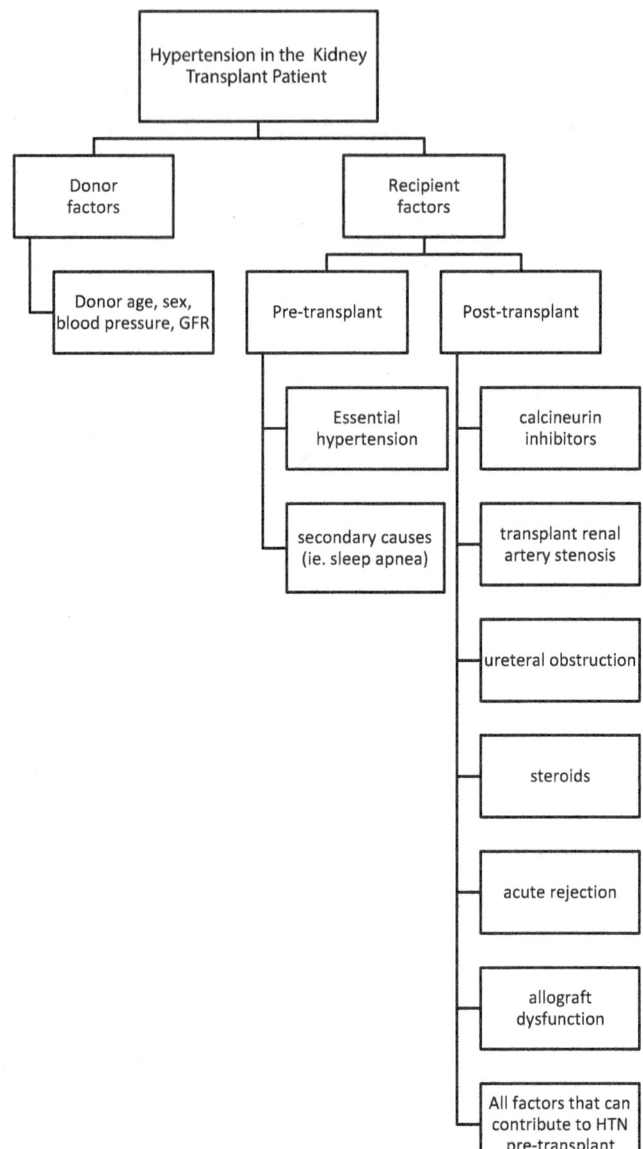

Fig. 2 Causative Factors Leading to Hypertension in Kidney Transplant Recipients

transplant, the prevalence of hypertension has been noted to rise to as high as 65–85 % of recipients post-transplant. Similar increases have been quoted for cardiac transplant patients (increase from 10 % pre-transplant to 71–100 % post-transplant), kidney transplant recipients (45–55 % pre-transplant, increasing to 67–86 post-transplant), and even bone marrow transplant recipients (5–10 % pre-transplant, increasing to 33–60 % post-transplant) (Textor et al. 1994). CNIs may have several physiologic effects on blood pressure. They can impair vascular tone by causing vasoconstriction and/or impairing vasodilatation. Cyclosporine (CSA) in particular is known to cause acute vasoconstriction of the renal vessels, mediated by increased levels of endothelin in the pre-glomerular vessels (Meyer-Lehnert et al. 1997; Haug et al. 1995). Thromboxane has also been implicated in promoting vasoconstriction, though experimental data has shown mixed results (Nasser et al. 2014). Other studies suggest that CNIs are associated with impaired vasodilation, which occurs because CNIs can activate protein kinase C leading to reduced nitric oxide production (Vaziri et al. 1998) by the vascular endothelium (Oriji and Keiser 1999). Calcium channel blockers may have a role to play in ameliorating some of these deleterious effects (Sanchez-Lozada et al. 2000; Chander and Chopra 2005).

Some data suggests that CNIs alter the renin/angiotensin system, but this is controversial. Some studies suggest that CNIs suppress renin secretion (Bantle et al. 1987), while others suggest that CNIs directly increases renin secretion (Kurtz et al. 1988; Saraswat et al. 2014). Similar heterogeneity is noted with regards to angiotensin. In one study, CNIs are associated with the up-regulation of angiotensin II receptors and calcium responses in human vascular smooth muscle cells (Avdonin et al. 1999) whereas other studies have noted a downregulation of angiotensin receptors in the kidney (Nishiyama et al. 2003). In addition to the aforementioned mechanisms, CNIs have been shown to promote a sodium-avid state by increasing sodium reabsorption in the proximal tubule (Epting et al. 2006) and the loop of Henle (Ciresi et al. 1992; Esteva-Font et al. 2007).

Chronic administration of CNIs has been associated with obliterative arteriolopathy, ischemic glomeruli, and striped fibrosis of the renal interstitium (Naesens et al. 2009). Given the kidneys central role in blood pressure control, it is logical that renal dysfunction resulting from CNIs could also aggravate hypertension.

In systemic vasculature, CNI use is associated with increased arterial stiffness (Martínez-Castelao et al. 2005), which would not only lead to hypertension, but cardiovascular risk in general. Sirolimus (Joannidès et al. 2011) and belatacept (Melilli et al. 2015) are both associated with reduced vascular stiffness and hypertension as compared to CNIs. The similar changes in blood pressure have been noted with other CNIs, including tacrolimus, although the hypertensive effect of cyclosporine is higher than that seen with tacrolimus (Radermacher et al. 1998).

2.2.3 The Effect of Corticosteroids on Blood Pressure in Transplant Recipients

Corticosteroids may mediate hypertension by stimulating mineralocorticoid receptors and promoting sodium reabsorption. The impact of corticosteroids on hypertension is most pronounced in the early post-transplant period when solid organ transplant recipients often receive high doses of corticosteroids as part of their induction therapy. However, kidney transplant recipients maintained on corticosteroids long term tend have higher blood pressure than those in steroid avoidance or withdrawal programs (Knight and Morris 2010). In a meta-analysis of 34 studies including 5637 kidney transplant recipients, there was a reduced incidence of hypertension in the steroid avoidance or withdrawal group, compared with those on steroids (RR 0.90, CI 0.85–0.94, P < 0.0001) (Knight and Morris 2010).

2.2.4 Unique Causes of Hypertension in Kidney Transplant Recipients

Because the kidney has a role in blood pressure control, any factor (donor or recipient related) that is associated with a lower GFR, is indirectly associated with hypertension post-transplant. Examples of donor related factors associated with hypertension post-transplant include: increased donor age (Ducloux et al. 2002), and presence of donor hypertension (Guidi et al. 1996).

Studies have shown that recipients of kidneys from hypertensive donors are prescribed more anti-hypertensive medications than recipients of kidneys from normotensive donors (Guidi et al. 1996). In the study by Guidi et al., this effect was mainly restricted to recipients without a family history of hypertension (Guidi et al. 1996). Recipients of kidneys from expanded criteria donors [defined as older kidney donors (≥60 years) or donors who are aged 50–59 years and have two of the following three features: hypertension, terminal serum creatinine >1.5 mg/dl, or death from cerebrovascular accident] also have higher rates of hypertension at 3 years and 5 years post transplantation than recipients of kidneys from standard criteria donors (Blanca et al. 2012; Wlodarczyk et al. 2003). Recipients of kidneys from older donors also have lower graft function after transplantation (Noppakun et al. 2011) and therefore the donor related factors associated with hypertension may simply be related to reduced renal allograft function, but this remains unclear.

Certain donor genetic variants such as single-nucleotide polymorphisms within the genes that encode for ABCC2, ABCB1 and CYP3A5, and APOL-1 have been indirectly associated with higher rates of post-transplant hypertension likely resulting from their association with reduced allograft function. Specifically, polymorphisms in ABCC2 are associated with delayed graft function and certain CYP3A5 mutations (Joy et al. 2007), and ABCB1 polymorphisms (Hauser et al. 2005) are associated with CNI toxicity. The APOL-1 gene variant which has been associated with kidney disease in African Americans is also associated with early graft failure in recipients of kidneys from donors with this gene variant (Thomas et al. 2013; Weir et al. 2015; Reeves-Daniel et al. 2011).

Just as renal artery stenosis in a non-transplant patient is associated with hypertension; renal artery stenosis of the transplant renal artery (TRAS) is associated with hypertension. Although the prevalence of TRAS is 1–23 % of renal transplant recipients, it is thought to contribute to hypertension in between 1 and 5 % of kidney transplant recipients (Fervenza et al. 1998; Bruno et al. 2004). It may become apparent at any time post transplantation, though presentation between 3 months and 2 years is typical. The stenosis most often occurs near the anastomosis and is a result of the technical aspects of the transplant surgery itself (Willicombe et al. 2014) such as vessel torsion, use of vascular clamps, perfusion pump cannulation injury, disproportionate vessel size, or a reaction to suture material. Less commonly the stenosis is diffuse along the transplant renal artery, in which case immune based mechanisms have been proposed as a potential etiology (Wong et al. 1996). In fact, the presence of de novo class II donor-specific antibodies has been associated with development of post-anastomosis TRAS (Willicombe et al. 2014).

The typical presentation of transplant renal artery stenosis is worsening or refractory hypertension and/or graft function, with notable edema from a sodium-avid state. An audible bruit in the correct clinical context may be useful in the diagnosis, though it is neither sensitive nor specific. Doppler ultrasound often demonstrates an increase in the peak systolic velocity >2.5 m/s, and a "tardus parvus" waveform abnormality in the intra-renal vessels. The gold standard for diagnosis, however, remains renal angiography (and if possible, carbon dioxide angiography should be utilized, in order to avoid iodinated contrast). Treatment options include conservative therapy, angioplasty with or without stent placement, versus surgical correction. Treatment decisions are determined on a case by case basis are are reviewed elsewhere (Bruno et al. 2004; Buturović-Ponikvar 2003; Chen et al. 2015). The effects of treatment on blood pressure have been mixed (Touma et al. 2014; Ali et al. 2015).

Other potential kidney transplant specific factors that could lead to hypertension include increased cold ischemia time and/or delayed graft function and other causes of impairment in allograft function such as acute and chronic rejection, medication induced nephrotoxicity, BK nephropathy, recurrent disease in the allograft, and ureteral obstruction (Weir et al. 2015; Mangray and Vella 2011; Cosio et al. 1999). Whenever a kidney transplant recipient has an abrupt change in blood pressure, these conditions should be a consideration. Not uncommonly, a change in blood pressure is the first signal of impending allograft dysfunction from rejection or recurrent disease.

2.2.5 Unique Contributors to Hypertension in Cardiac Transplant Recipients

Cardiac transplant patients experience inadequate adaptation of the renin-angiotensin system in the setting of fluid retention, which could contribute to the incidence and severity of hypertension in this population (Braith et al. 1996). Pharmacologic suppression of the RAS system eliminated avid salt and fluid retention in heart transplant recipients, improving blood pressure and overall fluid homeostasis (Braith et al. 2003).

3 Hypertension Following Living Kidney Donation

A paucity of data exists about the effect that living kidney donation has on blood pressure. Many live donors have not been followed prospectively, and it is hard to distinguish the effect of donation on blood pressure because hypertension is prevalent in the general population. In addition, the lack of appropriate control groups makes it challenging to make inferences about the effect of living kidney donation on blood pressure. A meta-analysis that included 5145 kidney donors revealed that factors associated with higher blood pressure post-kidney donation included older age at the time of donation, age, male sex, increased BMI, and a lower pre-donation glomerular filtration rate (Boudville et al. 2006). Recently, a prospective controlled trial evaluating live kidney donor outcomes 3 years post-donation revealed no difference in blood pressure as measured by ambulatory blood pressure monitoring at 36 months (Kasiske et al. 2015). A retrospective, matched-cohort study with a median follow up of 10.9 years demonstrated a higher incidence (11 %) of gestational hypertension or preeclampsia in living kidney donors than in matched non-donors (5 %), but maternal and fetal outcomes did not differ significantly between the two groups (Garg et al. 2015).

4 Hypertension Management for the Transplant Patient

4.1 Blood Pressure Measurement and Diagnosis

As in the general population, before acting on a blood pressure measurement; the provider must consider the circumstances and make sure that the measurement is reliable. Appropriate blood pressure measurement techniques are imperative to avoid falsely low or high readings as over or under-treatment of hypertension can lead to adverse outcomes. Furthermore, white coat hypertension and masked hypertension needs to be identified to avoid the unique risks in these situations (Griffin and Schinstock 2015).

Home and ambulatory blood pressure monitoring are useful adjuncts to in-office blood pressure readings. Several studies have suggested that office blood pressure readings are unreliable in both the general and the renal transplant population (Kooman et al. 2001; Stenehjem et al. 2006). In fact, home blood pressure readings correlate better with ambulatory blood pressure readings than office readings (Agena et al. 2011; Sberro-Soussan et al. 2012). When office blood pressures are compared with ambulatory blood pressure readings one can further identify patients with "white coat hypertension", in whom office blood pressures are typically higher than the 24 h readings, and patients with "masked hypertension", in which the opposite occurs: blood pressures in the office appear normal, whereas those at home are high. Additionally, ambulatory blood pressure readings are able to identify the nocturnal blood pressure patterns, stratifying patients into those with normal nocturnal dipping, versus those with a "non-dipping" pattern or even "reverse dipping". We recommend monitoring ambulatory blood pressures at the 1 year annual visit post transplantation, whenever feasible. In a study evaluating 24 h ambulatory blood pressures at 1 year post kidney transplantation, it was noted that the lack of nocturnal fall in SBP is related to poor allograft function, high chronic vascular score on biopsy, and high resistive index irrespective of allograft fibrosis (Wadei et al. 2007).

4.2 Goals of Therapy

Currently, there are no specific high quality evidence based recommendations for blood pressure targets in transplant recipients. As in the general population, there remains some debate regarding optimal blood pressure targets. According to the Eighth Report of the Joint National Committee on the Evidence-Based Guideline for Management of High Blood Pressure in Adults (James et al. 2014), blood pressure of greater than 140/90 is still felt to be a reasonable definition of high blood pressure, although the recently published SPRINT trial (SPRINT Research Group et al. 2015) suggests that certain patients (including some high risk patients with CKD) may do better with even lower blood pressures. In kidney transplant recipients, the Kidney Disease Outcomes Quality Initiative (KDOQI) commentary on the 2012 KDIGO guidelines stipulate that a target blood pressure of <130/80 in kidney transplant recipients is not guided by evidence, and in the absence of data to support the benefits of a BP goal <140/90 mmHg in transplant recipients, it is better to individualize BP goal decisions, taking into account risk and benefit profiles (Taler et al. 2013).

Excluding hypertensive emergencies when treatment is indicated for acute management of hypertension, the main goal of treatment is to reduce target organ damage and cardiovascular risk over the long term. Compared with End Stage Renal Disease (ESRD), kidney transplant recipients have an improved cardiovascular risk profile (Wolfe et al. 1999). However, the transplant in and of itself does not eliminate this risk (Ojo 2006), and death from cardiovascular disease remains the most common reason for decreased patient survival (Ojo et al. 2000). In addition to this, it is important to take into consideration that reduced allograft function in and of itself may confer increased cardiovascular risk. In a large retrospective analysis of 58,900 adult renal transplant recipients registered in the United States Renal Data System, it was noted that serum creatinine values at 1 year after transplantation were strongly associated with the risk for cardiovascular death (Meier-Kriesche et al. 2003). While the following text describes pharmacologic options in the management of hypertension after transplantation, it should be noted that other aspects of cardiovascular risk such as glycemic control and lipid status should also be addressed (Cosio et al. 2005) in tandem with lifestyle modification.

4.3 Pharmacological Therapy

An optimal antihypertensive treatment regimen for a transplant patient does not exist and initial anti-hypertensive therapy should be tailored based on the patient's underlying comorbidities and preferences. We recommend using medications the patient used prior to transplantation unless there are particular drug-drug interactions or adverse effects. Special considerations for transplant patients are described below.

4.3.1 Calcium Channel Blockers

Calcium channel blockers are classified into non-dihydropyridine calcium channel blockers (examples include verapamil and diltiazem) and dihydropyridine calcium channel blockers (examples include amlodipine, nifedipine, and nicardipine). The dihydropyridine calcium channel blockers have a higher selectivity for vascular smooth muscle compared with myocardial tissue. In the transplant population on CNIs, non-dihydropyridine calcium channel blockers need to be used with caution because they can lead to increased CNI levels due to the inhibition of CYP3A4 activity (Hooper et al. 2012; Hooper et al. 2011). Dihydropyridine calcium channel blockers such as nifedipine have been shown to have an antagonistic effect to CSA mediated vasoconstriction at the level of the endothelium, favoring their use in this population (Sanchez-Lozada et al. 2000; Chander and Chopra 2005; Ruggenenti et al. 1993; Cross et al. 2009; Mehrens et al. 2000; Kuypers et al. 2004).

In the general population, there is some concern for increased risk of myocardial infarction with high doses of short acting dihydropyridine calcium channel blockers such as nifedipine (Psaty et al. 1995), and longer acting agents such as amlodipine appear to be safer. In the renal transplant population, one study has shown that dihydropyridine calcium channel antagonists were associated with an increased risk for ischemic heart disease in this population (relative risk, 2.26; 95 % confidence interval, 1.24–4.12; P = 0.008), and this association was independent of other antihypertensive agents and risk factors (Kasiske et al. 2000). On the other hand, a prospective randomized (but non-blinded or placebo controlled) study in the cardiac transplant population suggested that diltiazem (selected in the study protocol due to its antihypertensive effects) may attenuate the usual reduction in the coronary artery diameter during the first year after cardiac transplantation and may inhibit the development of visually evident coronary artery disease (Schroeder et al. 1993).

4.3.2 Renin Angiotensin Aldosterone (RAS) Blockade

RAS blockade is a potentially attractive option in the management of hypertension in the transplant population. RAS blockade reduces intraglomerular pressures and proteinuria, but it may also play a role in retarding fibrosis of the renal allograft by reducing TGF-Beta expression (Campistol et al. 1999; Holgado et al. 2001; Mas et al. 2004). From a cardiovascular health prospective, RAS blockade may reverse left ventricular hypertrophy and improve remodeling of the heart (Klingbeil et al. 2000).

Data regarding the long term effects of ACE inhibitors on patient and graft survival has been mixed. In a retrospective cohort study of 2031 Austrian renal transplant recipients, 10 year patient survival rates were 74 % in the ACEI/ARB group but only 53 % in the no ACEI/ARB group. 10 year actual graft survival rate was 59 % in ACEI/ARB patients but only 41 % in nonusers (P = 0.002)(Heinze et al. 2006). However, in separate analyses, ACEI/ARB was not associated with improved transplant outcomes (Opelz et al. 2006; Opelz and Döhler 2014). Not unexpectedly, the use of ACEI/ARB is associated with reduced GFR (Cross et al. 2009), but it remains unclear whether this is an expected hemodynamic effect that is reversible with discontinuation of the drug or a lasting effect.

From a practical standpoint, it is advised to closely monitor renal function within several days of initiating or changing the dose of ACEi or ARB therapy in order to detect (i) acute drops in GFR beyond the acceptable 30 % threshold, and/or (ii) significant hyperkalemia. An abrupt rise in serum creatinine should raise the possibility of transplant renal artery stenosis.

4.3.3 Beta Blockade

Beta blockers are commonly used in transplant patients because they have relatively few drug interactions and they do not affect renal allograft function. The potential side effects that are particularly important in transplant recipients includes hyperkalemia (McCauley et al. 2002) deleterious lipid metabolism (more notable in metoprolol than carvedilol)(Bakris et al. 2004), and masking of hypoglycemic symptoms. In a study on cardiac transplant patients, it was noted that carvedilol, but not metoprolol, was associated with a significant increase in CSA levels, presumably by inhibiting P-glycoprotein (P-gp), a membrane protein that regulates CSA absorption (Bader et al. 2005).

4.3.4 Diuretics

Loop diuretics are commonly used in the early postoperative period where they may be useful to control hypertension mediated by hypervolemia. Although diuretics may counter CNI-mediated proximal tubule and/or loop of Henle sodium avidity, in our experience we generally favor calcium channel blockers, RAS blockers, and beta blockers over diuretics dueto their favorable cardio-metabolic profile and lower risk of hypovolemia.

5   Conclusions

Hypertension is prevalent in all of solid organ transplantation, but there is a paucity of evidence of to guide therapy. This is unfortunate because transplant patients are at high risk for cardiovascular disease, and hypertension management is essential. The contributors to hypertension are similar to that affecting the general population, but there are unique aspects to not overlook. Calcineurin inhibitors and steroids, which are commonly used in transplant patients exacerbates hypertension and have pertinent drug-drug interactions with common antihypertensives. To ultimately improve hypertension management in these patients, further research is needed.

6 Some Practical Points Regarding Management of Blood Pressure in Transplant Recipients

1. Whenever possible, use ambulatory blood pressure measurements and/or home monitoring to guide therapy.
2. Treatment decisions should be individualized to each patient.
3. In kidney transplant recipients in the immediate post-transplant period, we suggest allowing slightly higher blood pressures to maintain renal perfusion. Hypotension should be avoided in these circumstances.
4. In the long-term management of hypertension in transplant recipients, it is reasonable to treat these patients as one would the general population, taking into account their cardiovascular risk profile and drug interactions (e.g. Non-Dihydropyridine calcium channel blockers need to be used cautiously since their use can result in elevated CNI levels).

References

Agena F, Prado Edos S, Souza PS, da Silva GV, Lemos FB, Mion D Jr et al (2011) Home blood pressure (BP) monitoring in kidney transplant recipients is more adequate to monitor BP than office BP. Nephrol Dial Transplant 26(11):3745–3749

Ali A, Mishler D, Taber T, Agarwal D, Yaqub M, Mujtaba M et al (2015) Long-term outcomes of transplant recipients referred for angiography for suspected transplant renal artery stenosis. Clin Transpl 29 (9):747–755

Avdonin PV, Cottet-Maire F, Afanasjeva GV, Loktionova SA, Lhote P, Ruegg UT (1999) Cyclosporine A up-regulates angiotensin II receptors and calcium responses in human vascular smooth muscle cells. Kidney Int 55(6):2407–2414

Azzi JR, Sayegh MH, Mallat SG (2013) Calcineurin inhibitors: 40 years later, can't live without …. J Immunol 191(12):5785–5791

Bader FM, Hagan ME, Crompton JA, Gilbert EM (2005) The effect of β-blocker use on cyclosporine level in cardiac transplant recipients. J Heart Lung Transplant 24(12):2144–2147

Bakris GL, Fonseca V, Katholi RE et al (2004) Metabolic effects of carvedilol vs metoprolol in patients with type 2 diabetes mellitus and hypertension: a randomized controlled trial. JAMA 292 (18):2227–2236

Bantle JP, Boudreau RJ, Ferris TF (1987) Suppression of plasma renin activity by cyclosporine. Am J Med 83 (1):59–64

Blanca L, Jimenez T, Cabello M, Sola E, Gutierrez C, Burgos D et al (2012) Cardiovascular risk in recipients with kidney transplants from expanded criteria donors. Transplant Proc 44(9):2579–2581

Boudville N, Ramesh Prasad GV, Knoll G, Muirhead N, Thiessen-Philbrook H, Yang RC et al (2006) Meta-analysis: risk for hypertension in living kidney donors. Ann Intern Med 145(3):185–196

Braith RW, Mills RM Jr, Wilcox CS, Convertino VA, Davis GL, Limacher MC et al (1996) Fluid homeostasis after heart transplantation: the role of cardiac denervation. J Heart Lung Transplant 15(9):872–880

Braith RW, Mills RM, Wilcox CS, Davis GL, Hill JA, Wood CE (2003) High-dose angiotensin-converting enzyme inhibition restores body fluid homeostasis in heart-transplant recipients. J Am Coll Cardiol 41 (3):426–432

Bruno S, Remuzzi G, Ruggenenti P (2004) Transplant renal artery stenosis. J Am Soc Nephrol 15 (1):134–141

Buturović-Ponikvar J (2003) Renal transplant artery stenosis. Nephrol Dial Transplant 18(suppl 5):v74–v77

Campistol JM, Inigo P, Jimenez W, Lario S, Clesca PH, Oppenheimer F et al (1999) Losartan decreases plasma levels of TGF-beta1 in transplant patients with chronic allograft nephropathy. Kidney Int 56 (2):714–719

Campistol JM, Romero R, Paul J, Gutierrez-Dalmau A (2004) Epidemiology of arterial hypertension in renal transplant patients: changes over the last decade. Nephrol Dial Transplant 19(3):iii62–66

Chander V, Chopra K (2005) Nifedipine attenuates changes in nitric oxide levels, renal oxidative stress, and nephrotoxicity induced by cyclosporine. Ren Fail 27(4):441–450

Chen W, Kayler LK, Zand MS, Muttana R, Chernyak V, DeBoccardo GO (2015) Transplant renal artery stenosis: clinical manifestations, diagnosis and therapy. Clin Kidney J 8(1):71–78

Ciresi DL, Lloyd MA, Sandberg SM, Heublein DM, Edwards BS (1992) The sodium retaining effects of cyclosporine. Kidney Int 41(6):1599–1605

Cosio FG, Pelletier RP, Sedmak DD, Pesavento TE, Henry ML, Ferguson RM (1999) Renal allograft survival following acute rejection correlates with blood pressure levels and histopathology. Kidney Int 56 (5):1912–1919

Cosio FG, Kudva Y, van der Velde M, Larson TS, Textor SC, Griffin MD et al (2005) New onset hyperglycemia and diabetes are associated with increased cardiovascular risk after kidney transplantation. Kidney Int 67 (6):2415–2421

Cross NB, Webster AC, Masson P, O'Connell PJ, Craig JC (2009) Antihypertensives for kidney transplant recipients: systematic review and meta-analysis of randomized controlled trials. Transplantation 88 (1):7–18

Dalby MCD, Burke M, Radley-Smith R, Banner NR (2001) Pheochromocytoma presenting after cardiac transplantation for dilated cardiomyopathy. J Heart Lung Transplant 20(7):773–775

Dobrowolski LC, van Huis M, van der Lee JH, Peters Sengers H, Lilien MR, Cransberg K et al (2016) Epidemiology and management of hypertension in paediatric and young adult kidney transplant recipients in The Netherlands. Nephrol Dial Transplant 10

Ducloux D, Motte G, Kribs M, Abdelfatah AB, Bresson-Vautrin C, Rebibou JM et al (2002) Hypertension in renal transplantation: donor and recipient risk factors. Clin Nephrol 57(6):409–413

Epting T, Hartmann K, Sandqvist A, Nitschke R, Gordjani N (2006) Cyclosporin A stimulates apical Na+/H+ exchange in LLC-PK1/PKE20 proximal tubular cells. Pediatr Nephrol 21(7):939–946

Esteva-Font C, Ars E, Guillen-Gomez E, Campistol JM, Sanz L, Jimenez W et al (2007) Ciclosporin-induced hypertension is associated with increased sodium transporter of the loop of Henle (NKCC2). Nephrol Dial Transplant 22(10):2810–2816

Fagius J, Karhuvaara S (1989) Sympathetic activity and blood pressure increases with bladder distension in humans. Hypertension 14(5):511–517

Fervenza FC, Lafayette RA, Alfrey EJ, Petersen J (1998) Renal artery stenosis in kidney transplants. Am J Kidney Dis 31(1):142–148

Garg AX, Nevis IF, McArthur E, Sontrop JM, Koval JJ, Lam NN et al (2015) Gestational hypertension and preeclampsia in living kidney donors. N Engl J Med 372(2):124–133

Grannas G, Schrem H, Klempnauer J, Lehner F (2014) Ten years experience with belatacept-based immunosuppression after kidney transplantation. J Clin Med Res 6(2):98–110. Epub 2014 Feb 6 doi: 10.14740/jocmr1697w

Griffin BR, Schinstock CA (2015) Thinking beyond new clinical guidelines: update in hypertension. Mayo Clin Proc 90(2):273–279

Guidi E, Menghetti D, Milani S, Montagnino G, Palazzi P, Bianchi G (1996) Hypertension may be transplanted with the kidney in humans: a long-term historical prospective follow-up of recipients grafted with kidneys coming from donors with or without hypertension in their families. J Am Soc Nephrol 7 (8):1131–1138

Guillaud O, Boillot O, Sebbag L, Walter T, Bouffard Y, Dumortier J (2014) Cardiovascular risk 10 years after liver transplant. Exp Clin Transplant 12(1):55–61

Haug C, Duell T, Voisard R, Lenich A, Kolb HJ, Mickley V et al (1995) Cyclosporine A stimulates endothelin release. J Cardiovasc Pharmacol 26(3):S239–S241

Hauser IA, Schaeffeler E, Gauer S, Scheuermann EH, Wegner B, Gossmann J et al (2005) ABCB1 genotype of the donor but not of the recipient is a major risk factor for cyclosporine-related nephrotoxicity after renal transplantation. J Am Soc Nephrol 16 (5):1501–1511

Heinze G, Mitterbauer C, Regele H, Kramar R, Winkelmayer WC, Curhan GC et al (2006) Angiotensin-converting enzyme inhibitor or angiotensin II Type 1 receptor antagonist therapy is associated with prolonged patient and graft survival after renal transplantation. J Am Soc Nephrol 17(3):889–899

Holgado R, Anaya F, Del Castillo D (2001) Angiotensin II type 1 (AT1) receptor antagonists in the treatment of hypertension after renal transplantation. Nephrol Dial Transplant 1:117–120

Hooper DK, Carle AC, Schuchter J, Goebel J (2011) Interaction between tacrolimus and intravenous nicardipine in the treatment of post-kidney transplant hypertension at pediatric hospitals. Pediatr Transplant 15(1):88–95

Hooper DK, Fukuda T, Gardiner R, Logan B, Roy-Chaudhury A, Kirby CL et al (2012) Risk of tacrolimus toxicity in CYP3A5 nonexpressors treated with intravenous nicardipine after kidney transplantation. Transplantation 93(8):806–812

Hoorn EJ, Walsh SB, McCormick JA, Zietse R, Unwin RJ, Ellison DH (2012) Pathogenesis of calcineurin inhibitor–induced hypertension. J Nephrol 25 (3):269–275

Hryniewiecka E, Żegarska J (2011) Pączek L. Arterial hypertension in liver transplant recipients. Transplant Proc 43(8):3029–3034

James PA, Oparil S, Carter BL et al (2014) 2014 evidence-based guideline for the management of high blood pressure in adults: Report from the panel members appointed to the eighth joint national committee (jnc 8). JAMA 311(5):507–520

Joannidès R, Monteil C, De Ligny BH, Westeel PF, Iacob M, Thervet E et al (2011) Immunosuppressant regimen based on sirolimus decreases aortic stiffness in renal transplant recipients in comparison to cyclosporine. Am J Transplant 11(11):2414–2422

Joy MS, Hogan SL, Thompson BD, Finn WF, Nickeleit V (2007) Cytochrome P450 3A5 expression in the kidneys of patients with calcineurin inhibitor nephrotoxicity. Nephrol Dial Transplant 22(7):1963–1968

Kasiske BL, Chakkera HA, Roel J (2000) Explained and unexplained ischemic heart disease risk after renal transplantation. J Am Soc Nephrol 11(9):1735–1743

Kasiske BL, Anjum S, Shah R, Skogen J, Kandaswamy C, Danielson B et al (2004) Hypertension after kidney transplantation1. Am J Kidney Dis 43(6):1071–1081

Kasiske BL, Anderson-Haag T, Israni AK, Kalil RS, Kimmel PL, Kraus ES et al (2015) A prospective controlled study of living kidney donors: three-year follow-up. Am J Kidney Dis 66(1):114–124

Klingbeil AU, Muller HJ, Delles C, Fleischmann E, Schmieder RE (2000) Regression of left ventricular hypertrophy by AT1 receptor blockade in renal transplant recipients. Am J Hypertens 13(12):1295–1300

Knight SR, Morris PJ (2010) Steroid avoidance or withdrawal after renal transplantation increases the risk of acute rejection but decreases cardiovascular risk. A meta-analysis. Transplantation 89(1):1–14

Kooman JP, Christiaans MH, Boots JM, van Der Sande FM, Leunissen KM, van Hooff JP (2001) A comparison between office and ambulatory blood pressure measurements in renal transplant patients with chronic transplant nephropathy. Am J Kidney Dis 37 (6):1170–1176

Kurtz A, Della Bruna R, Kuhn K (1988) Cyclosporine A enhances renin secretion and production in isolated juxtaglomerular cells. Kidney Int 33(5):947–953

Kuypers DR, Neumayer HH, Fritsche L, Budde K, Rodicio JL, Vanrenterghem Y (2004) Calcium channel blockade and preservation of renal graft function in cyclosporine-treated recipients: a prospective randomized placebo-controlled 2-year study. Transplantation 78(8):1204–1211

Lund LH, Edwards LB, Kucheryavaya AY, Benden C, Christie JD, Dipchand AI et al (2014) The registry of the international society for heart and lung transplantation: Thirty-first Official Adult Heart Transplant Report—2014; Focus Theme: Retransplantation. J Heart Lung Transplant 33(10):996–1008

Mangray M, Vella JP (2011) Hypertension after kidney transplant. Am J Kidney Dis 57(2):331–341

Martínez-Castelao A, Sarrias X, Bestard O, Gil-Vernet S, Scrón D, Cruzado JM et al (2005) Arterial elasticity measurement in renal transplant patients under anticalcineurin immunosuppression. Transplant Proc 37(9):3788–3790

Mas VR, Alvarellos T, Maluf DG, Ferreira-Gonzalez A, Oliveros L, Maldonado RA et al (2004) Molecular and clinical response to angiotensin II receptor antagonist in kidney transplant patients with chronic allograft nephropathy. Transpl Int 17(9):540–544

McCauley J, Murray J, Jordan M, Scantlebury V, Vivas C, Shapiro R (2002) Labetalol-induced hyperkalemia in renal transplant recipients. Am J Nephrol 22 (4):347–351

Mehrens T, Thiele S, Suwelack B, Kempkes M, Hohage H (2000) The beneficial effects of calcium channel blockers on long-term kidney transplant survival are independent of blood-pressure reduction. Clin Transpl 14(3):257–261

Meier-Kriesche H-U, Baliga R, Kaplan B (2003) Decreased renal function is a strong risk factor for cardiovascular death after renal transplantation1,2. Transplantation 75(8):1291–1295

Melilli E, Bestard-Matamoros O, Manonelles-Montero A, Sala-Bassa N, Mast R, Grinyó-Boira JM et al (2015) Arterial stiffness in kidney transplantation: a single center case–control study comparing belatacept versus calcineurin inhibitor immunosuppressive based regimen. Nefrologia 35(1):58–65

Meyer-Lehnert H, Bokemeyer D, Friedrichs U, Backer A, Kramer HJ (1997) Cellular mechanisms of cyclosporine A-associated side-effects: role of endothelin. Kidney Int Suppl 61(31):S27–S31

Naesens M, Kuypers DR, Sarwal M (2009) Calcineurin inhibitor nephrotoxicity. Clin J Am Soc Nephrol 4 (2):481–508

Nasser SA, Elmallah AI, Sabra R, Khedr MM, El-Din MM, El-Mas MM (2014) Blockade of endothelin ET (A), but not thromboxane, receptors offsets the cyclosporine-evoked hypertension and interrelated baroreflex and vascular dysfunctions. Eur J Pharmacol 727:52–59

Nishiyama A, Kobori H, Fukui T, Zhang GX, Yao L, Rahman M et al (2003) Role of angiotensin II and reactive oxygen species in cyclosporine A-dependent hypertension. Hypertension 42(4):754–760

Noppakun K, Cosio FG, Dean PG, Taler SJ, Wauters R, Grande JP (2011) Living donor age and kidney transplant outcomes. Am J Transplant 11(6):1279–1286

Ojo AO (2006) Cardiovascular complications after renal transplantation and their prevention. Transplantation 82(5):603–611

Ojo AO, Hanson JA, Wolfe RA, Leichtman AB, Agodoa LY, Port FK (2000) Long-term survival in renal transplant recipients with graft function. Kidney Int 57 (1):307–313

Opelz G, Döhler B (2014) Cardiovascular death in kidney recipients treated with renin–angiotensin system blockers. Transplantation 97(3):310–315

Opelz G, Zeier M, Laux G, Morath C, Dohler B (2006) No improvement of patient or graft survival in transplant recipients treated with angiotensin-converting enzyme inhibitors or angiotensin II type 1 receptor blockers: a collaborative transplant study report. J Am Soc Nephrol 17(11):3257–3262

Oriji GK, Keiser HR (1999) Nitric oxide in cyclosporine A-induced hypertension: role of protein kinase C. Am J Hypertens 12(11 Pt 1):1091–1097

Psaty BM, Heckbert SR, Koepsell TD et al (1995) THe risk of myocardial infarction associated with antihypertensive drug therapies. JAMA 274(8):620–625

Radermacher J, Meiners M, Bramlage C, Kliem V, Behrend M, Schlitt HJ et al (1998) Pronounced renal vasoconstriction and systemic hypertension in renal transplant patients treated with cyclosporin A versus FK 506. Transpl Int 11(1):3–10

Reeves-Daniel AM, DePalma JA, Bleyer AJ, Rocco MV, Murea M, Adams PL et al (2011) The APOL1 gene and allograft survival after kidney transplantation. Am J Transplant 11(5):1025–1030

Ruggenenti P, Perico N, Mosconi L, Gaspari F, Benigni A, Amuchastegui CS et al (1993) Calcium channel blockers protect transplant patients from cyclosporine-induced daily renal hypoperfusion. Kidney Int 43(3):706–711

Sanchez-Lozada LG, Gamba G, Bolio A, Jimenez F, Herrera-Acosta J, Bobadilla NA (2000) Nifedipine prevents changes in nitric oxide synthase mRNA levels induced by cyclosporine. Hypertension 36(4):642–647

Saraswat MS, Addepalli V, Jain M, Pawar VD, Patel RB (2014) Renoprotective activity of aliskiren, a renin inhibitor in cyclosporine A induced hypertensive nephropathy in dTG mice. Pharmacol Rep 66 (1):62–67

Sberro-Soussan R, Rabant M, Snanoudj R, Zuber J, Bererhi L, Mamzer M-F et al (2012) Home and office blood pressure monitoring in renal transplant recipients. J Transplant 2012:702316

Schroeder JS, Gao S-Z, Alderman EL, Hunt SA, Johnstone I, Boothroyd DB et al (1993) A preliminary study of Diltiazem in the prevention of coronary artery disease in heart-transplant recipients. N Engl J Med 328(3):164–170

Sheiner PA, Magliocca JF, Bodian CA, Kim-Schluger L, Altaca G, Guarrera JV et al (2000) Long-term medical complications in patients surviving > or = 5 years after liver transplant. Transplantation 69 (5):781–789

Silverborn M, Jeppsson A, Martensson G, Nilsson F (2005) New-onset cardiovascular risk factors in lung transplant recipients. J Heart Lung Transplant 24 (10):1536–1543

SPRINT Research Group, Wright JT Jr, Williamson JD, Whelton PK, Snyder JK, Sink KM, Rocco MV, Reboussin DM, Rahman M, Oparil S, Lewis CE, Kimmel PL, Johnson KC, Goff DC Jr, Fine LJ, Cutler JA, Cushman WC, Cheung AK, Ambrosius WT (2015) A randomized trial of intensive versus standard blood-pressure control. N Engl J Med 373(22):2103–2116

Stegall MD, Everson G, Schroter G, Bilir B, Karrer F, Kam I (1995) Metabolic complications after liver transplantation. Diabetes, hypercholesterolemia, hypertension, and obesity. Transplantation 60(9):1057–1060

Stenehjem AE, Gudmundsdottir H, Os I (2006) Office blood pressure measurements overestimate blood pressure control in renal transplant patients. Blood Press Monit 11(3):125–133

Taler SJ, Agarwal R, Bakris GL, Flynn JT, Nilsson PM, Rahman M et al (2013) KDOQI US commentary on the 2012 KDIGO clinical practice guideline for management of blood pressure in CKD. Am J Kidney Dis: the official journal of the National Kidney Foundation 62(2):201–213

Textor SC (1993) De novo hypertension after liver transplantation. Hypertension 22(2):257–267

Textor SC, Canzanello VJ, Taler SJ, Wilson DJ, Schwartz LL, Augustine JE et al (1994) Cyclosporine-induced hypertension after transplantation. Mayo Clin Proc 69 (12):1182–1193

Textor SC, Taler SJ, Canzanello VJ, Schwartz L, Augustine JE (2000) Posttransplantation hypertension related to calcineurin inhibitors. Liver Transpl 6(5):521–530

Thomas B, Taber DJ, Srinivas TR (2013) Hypertension after kidney transplantation: a pathophysiologic approach. Curr Hypertens Rep 15(5):458–469

Touma J, Costanzo A, Boura B, Alomran F, Combes M (2014) Endovascular management of transplant renal artery stenosis. J Vasc Surg 59(4):1058–1065

Vaziri ND, Ni Z, Zhang YP, Ruzics EP, Maleki P, Ding Y (1998) Depressed renal and vascular nitric oxide synthase expression in cyclosporine-induced hypertension. Kidney Int 54(2):482–491

Wadei HM, Amer H, Taler SJ, Cosio FG, Griffin MD, Grande JP et al (2007) Diurnal blood pressure changes one year after kidney transplantation: relationship to Allograft function, histology, and resistive index. J Am Soc Nephrol 18(5):1607–1615

Weir MR, Burgess ED, Cooper JE, Fenves AZ, Goldsmith D, McKay D et al (2015) Assessment and management of hypertension in transplant patients. J Am Soc Nephrol 26(6):1248–1260

Willicombe M, Sandhu B, Brookes P, Gedroyc W, Hakim N, Hamady M et al (2014) Postanastomotic transplant renal artery stenosis: association with de novo class II donor-specific antibodies. Am J Transplant 14(1):133–143

Wlodarczyk Z, Glyda M, Koscianska L, Kolodziejczyk J, Sulikowska B, Manitius J (2003) Prevalence of arterial hypertension following kidney transplantation – a multifactorial analysis. Ann Transplant 8(2):43–46

Wolfe RA, Ashby VB, Milford EL, Ojo AO, Ettenger RE, Agodoa LYC et al (1999) Comparison of mortality in all patients on dialysis, patients on dialysis awaiting transplantation, and recipients of a first cadaveric transplant. N Engl J Med 341(23):1725–1730

Wong W, Fynn SP, Higgins RM, Walters H, Evans S, Deane C et al (1996) Transplant renal artery stenosis in 77 patients – does it have an immunological cause? Transplantation 61(2):215–219

Adv Exp Med Biol - Advances in Internal Medicine (2017) 2: 355–374
DOI 10.1007/5584_2016_168
© Springer International Publishing AG 2016
Published online: 22 November 2016

Evidence-Based Revised View of the Pathophysiology of Preeclampsia

Asif Ahmed, Homira Rezai, and Sophie Broadway-Stringer

Abstract

Preeclampsia is a life-threatening vascular disorder of pregnancy due to a failing stressed placenta. Millions of women risk death to give birth each year and globally each year, almost 300,000 lose their life in this process and over 500,000 babies die as a consequence of preeclampsia. Despite decades of research, we lack pharmacological agents to treat it. Maternal endothelial oxidative stress is a central phenomenon responsible for the preeclampsia phenotype of high maternal blood pressure and proteinuria. In 1997, it was proposed that preeclampsia arises due to the loss of VEGF activity, possibly due to elevation in anti-angiogenic factor, soluble Flt-1 (sFlt-1). Researchers showed that high sFlt-1 and soluble endoglin (sEng) elicit the severe preeclampsia phenotype in pregnant rodents. We demonstrated that heme oxygenase-1 (HO-1)/carbon monoxide (CO) pathway prevents placental stress and suppresses sFlt-1 and sEng release. Likewise, hydrogen sulphide (H_2S)/cystathionine-γ-lyase (Cth) systems limit sFlt-1 and sEng and protect against the preeclampsia phenotype in mice. Importantly, H_2S restores placental vasculature, and in doing so improves lagging fetal growth. These molecules act as the inhibitor systems in pregnancy and when they fail, preeclampsia is triggered. In this review, we discuss what are the hypotheses and models for the pathophysiology of preeclampsia on the basis of Bradford Hill causation criteria for disease causation and how further *in vivo* experimentation is needed to establish 'proof of principle'. Hypotheses that fail to meet the Bradford Hill causation criteria include abnormal spiral artery remodelling and inflammation and should be considered associated or consequential to the disorder. In contrast, the protection against cellular stress hypothesis that states that the protective pathways mitigate cellular stress by limiting elevation of anti-angiogenic factors or oxidative stress

A. Ahmed (✉), H. Rezai, and S. Broadway-Stringer
Aston Medical Research Institute, Aston Medical School,
Aston University, Birmingham B4 7ET, UK
e-mail: asif.ahmed@aston.ac.uk

and the subsequent clinical signs of preeclampsia appear to fulfil most of Bradford Hill causation criteria. Identifying the candidates on the roadmap to this pathway is essential in developing diagnostics and therapeutics to target the pathogenesis of preeclampsia.

Keywords

Preeclampsia • sFlt-1 • HO-1 • Inflammation • Hypoxia • Activin A • Gasotransmitter • microRNA • Oxidative stress • Angiogenic factors

1   Introduction

It is believed that in 400 B. C, Hippocrates was the first to state that convulsion during pregnancy was a sign of bad pregnancy, which resulted in imbalance in the 'humours' (Bell 2010). Today preeclampsia is still being debated as the "disease of theories" reported as a 'two-stage model'. The first stage being asymptomatic, characterized by an abnormal formation of the placenta and the release of placental factors into the maternal circulation. The second stage is symptomatic resulting in hypertension and proteinuria that can eventually culminate in angiospasm in the brain to cause eclampsia (Hladunewich et al. 2007). Preeclampsia is characterised as *de novo* hypertension (bp $\geq$140/90) and proteinuria ($\geq$300 mg/24 h) occurring after 20 weeks of pregnancy, however, neither are specific to the pathophysiology of preeclampsia (Brown et al. 2001). The prevalence of preeclampsia ranges from 5 to 8 % of pregnancies depending on the geographical location and affects 8.5 million pregnancies globally, accounting for over 70 000 maternal deaths and 500 000 infant deaths per year (Ramma and Ahmed 2014; Lowe et al. 2009).

The causes of preeclampsia remain largely unknown. Recent studies, however, have shed new light on factors originating in the placenta likely to cause the condition due to an imbalance in 'autacoids' factors (Ahmed and Ramma 2015). Preeclampsia still lacks a reliable means of diagnosis and prediction with no effective therapy or pharmacological agents available to treat the disease. The only solution is the early delivery of the pregnancy. If left untreated, preeclampsia can be life threatening and may progress to eclampsia with complications of HELLP syndrome (Elevated liver enzymes, haemolysis, and low platelets), placental abruption, acute renal failure and pulmonary oedema (Arulkumaran and Lightstone 2013). Although maternal symptoms appear to be largely resolved with the delivery of the baby, data are accumulating that preeclampsia is associated with long-term maternal cardiovascular and other complications such as renal diseases (Smith et al. 2001; Saxena et al. 2010; Garovic and Hayman 2007; Veerbeek et al. 2016).

As Steve Jobs once said "You can only connect the dots looking backwards". To gain a deeper insight into the pathophysiology of preeclampsia, we need to identify the "dots" critical in the pathogenesis of preeclampsia in order to discover the roadmap. What are the intersections that connect the dots to make up the roadmap of the preeclampsia phenotype? To discover the 'roadmaps' that connect the dots of preeclampsia, proof-of-principle experimentation that goes beyond association-type approaches need to be undertaken. Studies focused on *in vitro* experimentations to make bold claims of links to preeclampsia are misrepresenting the facts and provide limited insight into the mechanisms. Therefore, *in vitro* studies *per se,* should not be considered as representative vehicles for 'proof of principle'. Animal models which mimic the "preeclampsia phenotype", are better vehicles to connect and test the 'dots'. Even though animals rarely get preeclampsia, many phenotypes of the disorder can be modelled in rodents. In such a system, it is possible to test whether a potential cause can be reversed, ultimately leading to the rectification of symptoms and establishment of

Table 1 Bradford-Hill causation criteria

Criterion	Explanaion
Temporality	The cause always precedes the effect
Dose response	An increase in exposure results in an increase in the risk
Strength	The stronger the association, the more likely it is that there is a causal relationship between the associated factors
Consistency	The results can be replicated by different people or in different studies
Specificity	A single cause will result in a specific effect
Coherence	There must be coherence between the epidemiology and the experimental findings.
Plausibility	The cause can be linked to the effect through a plausible mechanism

'proof of principle'. Any hypotheses put forward for investigation should be critically analysed using the Bradford Hill causation criteria (Hill 1965), rather than claiming the 'cause and effect' status without it (Ramma and Ahmed 2011).

In this review, we discuss what are the hypotheses and models for the pathophysiology of preeclampsia. A revised view is presented to test the evidence for the role of circulating factors such as soluble fms-like tyrosine kinase-1 (sFlt-1) and inhibin, inflammation, oxidative stress and gasotransmitters on the basis of the Bradford Hill causation criteria for disease causation (see Table 1).

2   Evaluating the Current Hypothesis of Preeclampsia

Decades of research into placental histopathology of preeclampsia established certain dogmas. These now need to be challenged if we are to find therapies apart from prematurely delivering the baby. These dogmas include (i) abnormal spiral artery remodelling (Khong et al. 1986; Feinberg et al. 1991; Brosens et al. 2002; Burton et al. 2009) and (ii) failed trophoblast invasion (Zhou et al. 1997); accepted as the early primary defect causing preeclampsia. It is further claimed that the failure of trophoblast remodelling of spiral arteries precedes abnormal placentation to cause the secretion of placental factors into the maternal circulation that lead to (iii) aberrant maternal systemic inflammation, (iv) oxidative stress and (v) angiogenic imbalance (Redman and Sargent 2009; Maynard et al. 2008). These ultimately lead to the manifestation of clinical signs and symptoms of preeclampsia. A closer scrutiny based on the Bradford Hill criteria has brought many of the established dogmas into question.

3   Role of Inflammation in Abnormal Spiral Artery Remodelling

Evidence to support any mechanistic understanding of the processes of abnormal spiral artery remodelling or trophoblast invasion is lacking apart from association and descriptive studies. The two separate processes are highly interrelated and it is accepted that spiral artery remodelling involves the maternal immune system and the placenta. Recent studies established that spiral artery remodelling may be a common underlying contributing factor of abnormal placentation, but it is not specific to preeclampsia (Lyall et al. 2013).

Uterine natural killer cells (uNK), part of the innate immune response, differ from the classical natural killer cells in the peripheral blood. One possible role of the uNK cells is to maintain immunological tolerance for the semi-allogeneic fetus by antagonising the T_H17 subset of T cells through the secretion of Interferon-gamma (IFN-γ) (Fu et al. 2013). Loss of this regulation is linked to spontaneous abortion with a rise in T_H17 cells and local inflammation (Fu et al. 2013). However, the uNK also accumulate around uterine spiral arteries and are abundant in early pregnancy (Robson et al. 2012). Robson and co-workers showed that uNK-conditioned media containing secreted factors, IFN-γ, VEGF-C (Vascular Endothelial Growth Factor C), angiopoietin-1 and angiopoietin-2, impact upon vascular smooth muscle cell separation and extra cellular matrix remodelling *In vitro* studies (Robson et al. 2012), speculating that similar changes occur during spiral artery remodelling.

There is contrasting data on the levels of uNK in preeclampsia; immunohistochemistry and flow cytometry showed an increase in uNK levels (Stallmach et al. 1999; Bachmayer et al. 2006) whereas a reduced population was detected in placental bed biopsies from preeclampsia (Williams et al. 2009). These associations need to be supported by mechanistic *in vivo* experimentation. Therefore, more studies are necessary to establish the role of uNK in spiral artery remodelling and trophoblast invasion during preeclampsia. Furthermore, it is not clear whether the immunological alteration that occurs early in pregnancy contributes to the onset of preeclampsia or whether activation and elevation of pro-inflammatory mediators are a consequence of the disease (Ramma and Ahmed 2011; Cheng and Sharma 2016). Indeed immune deficient $Rag2^{-/-}/\gamma_c^{-/-}$ double-knockout mice that lack spiral artery remodelling remain normotensive and do not develop proteinuria, fetal growth restriction or other preeclampsia-like phenotype (Burke et al. 2010).

Interestingly, a temporal relationship between excessive inflammation and the onset of preeclampsia does not exist, evident from the lack of changes seen in the levels of pro-inflammatory cytokines before the onset of the disorder (Djurovic et al. 2002; Kronborg et al. 2011; Carty et al. 2012). Moreover, the level of inflammation does not correlate with the severity of the disorder, supported by the absence of significant quantitative differences in serum TNF-α and IL-6 (Ozler et al. 2012). Pregnant women with increased levels of IL-6 have normal angiogenic status with no symptoms of hypertension or proteinuria (Ramma et al. 2012). Finally, corticosteroid treatment in women with severe preeclampsia did not resolve the condition and only transiently reduced the levels of IL-6 and C-reactive protein along with improving the clinical manifestations for approximately 48 h (Nayeri et al. 2014). Thus, it can be said that treatment of inflammation does not remove the stimulus of the disorder.

4 Hypoxia and Spiral Artery Remodelling

Extravillous trophoblast cells become invasive, allowing the transformation of vessels to accommodate the increase in maternal blood flow (Carter et al. 2015). Oxygen levels were reported to be a regulating factor for this differentiation as Genbacev and colleagues demonstrated that at 2 % oxygen tension, trophoblasts maintained their proliferative state *in vitro*, whereas in 20 % oxygen they acquire an invasive phenotype (Genbacev et al. 1996). Therefore, hypoxia must be prolonged for the failure of trophoblast invasion to occur and must precede abnormal spiral artery remodelling (Huppertz et al. 2014). This is in mark contrast to the argument proposed by the Two Stage model where failure of trophoblast invasion leads to failed spiral artery remodelling, which leads to placental hypoxia (Roberts and Hubel 2009; Redman and Sargent 2005).

During the hypoxic conditions of the placenta, HIF-1α expression is high and is found to positively regulate trophoblast invasion though Transforming Growth Factor-β3 (TGFβ3) signalling *in vitro*. Inhibition of HIF-1α in hypoxic explants inhibited TGFβ3 expression leading to markers of an invasive trophoblast phenotype (Caniggia et al. 2000). In normal pregnancy, HIF-1a levels decrease in line with the increase in the placental oxygen tension throughout gestation (Rajakumar and Conrad 2000a; b). Interestingly these same authors showed that when placental villous explants obtained from women with preeclampsia were exposed to hypoxia (2 % oxygen) HIF-1a was not up-regulated as was the case in normal placental tissue indicating that something other than hypoxia affects the relative high levels of HIF-1a in preeclamptic placenta (Rajakumar et al. 2003a; b). These are at best loss association studies and collectively question the significance of hypoxia as a trigger for the pathogenesis of preeclampsia.

Recent studies challenge the view that abnormal spiral artery remodelling leads to the hypoxia during preeclampsia. Immunohistochemical analysis using Hypoxyprobe™-1 to detect cellular hypoxia showed that oxygen delivery to the placenta is not impaired in Rag2$^{-/-}$Il2rg$^{-/-}$ double knock-out pregnant mice, which fail to undergo normal physiological spiral arterial remodelling (Leno-Duran et al. 2010). In fact, it is known that 'hypoxia' is key to normal placentation during the first trimester of pregnancy, and increase in oxygen tension above 20 mmHg, through the dissolution of trophoblast plugs in the spiral arteries, can result in spontaneous abortion (Huppertz et al. 2014). Based on the above evidences, hypoxia as an initial stimulus for the causation of preeclampsia can be disputed. Levels of sFlt-1 are elevated in preeclamptic placental explants compared to normal placental explants, when cultured under atmospheric conditions (Ahmad and Ahmed 2004), demonstrating that sFlt-1 elevated before the onset of preeclampsia is not increased due to placental hypoxia. Thus, the Two Stage model of failed remodelling of spiral arteries leading to hypoxia and subsequent alteration in the downstream factors in preeclampsia is a misconception (Ahmed and Ramma 2015). The availability of materials limits the study of human spiral artery remodelling with no standard practice to follow for placenta collection. Animal models such as the murine 'reduced uterine placenta perfusion' model can generate the symptoms of preeclampsia through placental perfusion (Burke and Karumanchi 2013), however, this does not prove ischemia and hypoxia are key elements on the roadmap to preeclampsia phenotype.

5 Role of sFLT-1 in Preeclampsia

The most prominent factor linked to the pathogenesis of preeclampsia is the 'loss of VEGF activity' as proposed originally in 1997 (Ahmed 1997). Several groups showed elevated levels of naturally occurring anti-angiogenic molecule, sFlt-1, in women with preeclampsia, which is strongly linked to the clinical sign of hypertension through antagonising VEGF and PlGF (He et al. 1999; Ahmad and Ahmed 2001; Maynard et al. 2003; Levine et al. 2004).

Soluble Flt-1 is a splice variant of *flt-1* gene and belongs to the vascular endothelial growth receptor (VEGFR) family. Several isoforms of sFlt-1 have been identified (Thomas et al. 2009) with sFlt-1e15a thought to make up at least 80 % of placental sFlt-1 while sFlt-1i13 makes up ~15 % (Jebbink et al. 2011). The amount of sFlt-1e15a, coupled with its placental specificity, is considered as the main isoform responsible for the preeclampsia phenotype (Palmer et al. 2016). Recent *in vivo* studies reveal that mice injected with adenovirus to full length human sFlt-e15a, have increased levels of creatinine/albumin in the urine and elevated mean arterial pressure (Szalai et al. 2014).

The administration of sFlt-1 into mouse models induces hypertension and proteinuria as well as other clinical manifestations of preeclampsia (Maynard et al. 2003). Furthermore, reduction in sFlt-1 levels in preeclamptic women using 'dextran sulfate' apheresis, reduced proteinuria and stabilised blood pressure (Thadhani et al. 2011; 2016). Loss of VEGF activity causing preeclampsia-like syndrome comes from human cancer chemotherapy patients receiving anti-VEGF treatment (Cross et al. 2012). Two patients treated with bevacizumab, (VEGF neutralising antibody), developed a preeclampsia-like syndrome characterised by hypertension, proteinuria, liver enzyme elevation and central nervous system irritability (Cross et al. 2012). Interestingly, VEGF increased sFlt-1 mRNA expression and release in cultured endothelial cells. Furthermore, adenovirus overexpression of VEGF-A in mice resulted in an eight-fold increase in circulating sFlt-1 levels (Ahmad et al. 2011). Following these observations *in vivo*, it is reasonable to state that the 'loss of VEGF activity' may play a central role in the pathogenesis of preeclampsia.

Hypoxic conditions induce VEGF expression (Shweiki et al. 1992) and the same relationship exists for sFlt-1 (Ahmad and Ahmed 2004; Palmer et al. 2016). Further contradicting the 'hypoxia hypothesis' as contributing to preeclampsia pathogenesis. However, hypoxia may affect cell types differently *in vitro*; an increase in sFlt-1 secretion and mRNA expression in cytotrophoblasts exposed to 8 % or 2 % oxygen concentration is not seen in endothelial cells and villous fibroblasts (Nagamatsu et al. 2004). Interestingly, endothelial cells incubated with VEGF-A revealed an increase in sFlt-1 mRNA expression and secretion, which was then replicated *in vivo*, using adenovirus overexpression of VEGF-A in mice, resulting in an 8-fold increase in circulating sFlt-1 levels (Ahmad et al. 2011).

An important growth factor in placental development appears to be placenta growth factor (PlGF) that is also antagonised by sFlt-1. It is dramatically decreased before the onset of pre-eclampsia and remains suppressed during the disorder in relation to the severity (Levine et al. 2004, 2006). The temporal relationship between PlGF levels and the onset of preeclampsia signifying a clear role of PlGF in preeclampsia, however, this remains unknown and unproven.

6 Role of Soluble Endoglin in Preeclampsia

Membrane glycoprotein, endoglin is a co-receptor for TGFβ signalling. Its cleaved isoform, soluble endoglin (sEng), is increased along with sFlt-1 before the onset of clinical symptoms of preeclampsia (Levine et al. 2006). Transgenic mice that express sEng (*Sol.eng$^+$*) exhibit symptoms of hypertension, small pup size, proteinuria and renal damage, which mimic the signs of preeclampsia (Valbuena-Diez et al. 2012).

An increase in sEng, blocking the TGFβ downstream signalling, results in a reduction in endothelial nitric oxide synthase (NOS3) activity (Venkatesha et al. 2006). This ultimately leads to a decrease in the vasodilator, NO. As TGFβ1 and TGFβ3 are also anti-inflammatory cytokines, sEng levels may influence the polarisation of different T cell subsets, mainly Tregs and T_H17 cells, both of which are found to be decreased and increased respectively in pre-eclamptic patients when compared to normotensive pregnancy controls (Darmochwal-Kolarz et al. 2012). This dysregulation of signaling may lead to the exacerbation of the inflammatory response seen in preeclampsia and would suggest that a rise in

sEng precedes the immune response. However, *in vivo* studies regarding the relationship between sEng and T cell populations are needed to support any associative link.

7 The Role of Anti-angiogenic Factors in Endothelial Dysfunction

Maternal endothelial dysfunction is central to the hypertensive phenotype and other clinical manifestations of preeclampsia. Endothelial cell surface adhesion molecules are markers of endothelial activation (Farzadnia et al. 2013). These markers are elevated in preeclampsia, soluble E-selectin was significantly higher at 12–16 weeks' gestation in women who subsequently developed preeclampsia (Carty et al. 2012). A recent study also revealed soluble VCAM-1 and ICAM-1 levels to be elevated in severe preeclampsia compared to normotensive pregnancy controls (Farzadnia et al. 2013). Both of these adhesion molecules are key to identifying endothelial activation (Farzadnia et al. 2013). However, no significant differences were seen in both adhesion molecules between normal and mild preeclamptic pregnancy.

Soluble Flt-1 and sEng are factors thought to induce endothelial dysfunction in preeclampsia. It was reported that *in vitro*, sFlt-1 alone does not cause endothelial dysfunction but works in concert with pro-inflammatory cytokines (TNF-α) to sensitise and amplify endothelial dysfunction (Cindrova-Davies et al. 2011). However, sFlt-1 alone does induces endothelial dysfunction *in vivo* (Bergmann et al. 2010). This contrast in results, demonstrates potential false positive nature of *in vitro* studies *per se*. In vitro studies should refrain from over claims unless further support for the argument comes from *in vivo* studies used to complete 'proof of principle'.

Inhibition of TGFβ signaling using an adenovirus to overexpress sEng in mice, increased leukocyte rolling, demonstrating a chemokinetic response (Walshe et al. 2009). Soluble VCAM-1 and E-selectin expression also increased correlating with a decrease in leukocyte velocity.

Thus, this study shows sEng to be involved in the activation of endothelial cells, ready for an immunological response (Walshe et al. 2009). Overexpression of sFlt-1 and sEng together in mice demonstrates a synergistic approach to induce endothelial dysfunction, ultimately resulting in severe vascular damage, hypertension, proteinuria, fetal growth restriction and HELPP syndrome (Venkatesha et al. 2006). In a separate rodent study, it was also found to cause focal vasospasm, and increased vascular permeability leading to brain odema, which is associated with eclampsia (Maharaj et al. 2008). Therefore, given the evidence for their temporal relationship with preeclampsia, sFlt-1 and sEng elevation may lie close to the root cause of endothelial dysfunction in preeclampsia, further supports to the possibility of these two anti-angiogenic factors being important 'dots' on the roadmap of preeclampsia development.

8 Oxidative Stress

Oxidative stress reflects on the imbalance of oxidative substances, such as reactive oxygen species (ROS) over the innate anti-oxidants that make up the endogenous defence system. Oxidative stress acts through several mechanisms such as DNA damage, inhibition of protein synthesis, protein nitration and mitochondrial modification (Sanchez-Aranguren et al. 2014). An increase in oxidative stress in the placenta and maternal circulation is found in preeclampsia at which point, multiple factors converge leading to endothelial dysfunction, systemic inflammation and more oxidative stress (Alpoim et al. 2016; Tjoa et al. 2006). Measurement of mitochondrial dysfunction using oxygen consumption rate revealed dysfunction in trophoblast mitochondrion isolated from preeclamptic patients (Maloyan et al. 2012; Muralimanoharan et al. 2012).

The placental syncytiotrophoblast is sensitive to exposure to high oxygen and low anti-oxidant levels from the mother, and so oxidative stress is present in normal pregnancy (Myatt and Webster 2009). It is argued that the inadequate trophoblast invasion resulting in placental hypoxia, causes the formation of free radicals and a reduction in anti-oxidant molecules and thus increases oxidative stress in preeclampsia. However, this description of events is not supported by temporal evidence as discussed earlier in this review. Similar to hypoxia, failed trophoblast invasion and abnormal spiral artery remodelling are dispelled as causational factors, so the process by which oxidative stress produces free radicals needs to be identified. Do the answers lie with mitochondrial dysfunction, identified in the trophoblast cells of the preeclamptic placenta (Maloyan et al. 2012; Muralimanoharan et al. 2012)? What cannot be ruled out is that oxidative stress is part of the final common pathway to a preeclampsia phenotype. Superoxide can react with NO to produce peroxynitrite, leading to a reduction in the bioavailability of NO, thereby reducing vasodilation while promoting the production of vasoconstrictors (Sankaralingam et al. 2006). This is plausible and needs to be tested in vivo using mouse models, which produce the preeclampsia phenotype. Furthermore, many proteins are nitrated in the presence of NO and superoxide which can lead to either loss or gain of protein function (Peluffo and Radi 2007). Indeed, placental peroxynitrite expression is increased in preeclampsia (Myatt et al. 1996) and tyrosine nitration is increased in cardiovascular disease (Peluffo and Radi 2007).

The natural oxidative stress already present during pregnancy may be intensified by the decreased anti-oxidant levels (enzymatic and non-enzymatic) observed in the circulation of women with preeclampsia. However, there was no correlation found between the level of enzymatic anti-oxidant and the severity of the disease (Llurba et al. 2004). A systematic review showed that supplementation of anti-oxidant does not reduce the risk of preeclampsia (Salles et al. 2012), ruling oxidative stress as a secondary phenomenon to the pathogenesis of preeclampsia.

9 Protective and Stress Model

Pregnancy can be viewed as a 'journey in a car' with the accelerator and brake system controlling the movement and progression of the vehicle towards a successful birth. Getting in a car and getting to your destination is equivalent to a successful pregnancy outcome. If the car breaks down, it can be viewed as pregnancy complication but if the brakes fail altogether, the system crashes that's preeclampsia. What are the brakes in pregnancy that hold back the fuel for the accelerator? The fuel for the accelerator includes inflammation, oxidative stress and anti-angiogenic factors, while the brakes work to maintain control of the car through regulating the amount of fuel in the accelerator pathway. In this review we demonstrate that it is the failure in the braking system, representing the protective pathways, that causes the car to loose control until the system crashes, manifesting itself as preeclampsia. Identifying the braking systems (the protective pathways) and discovering how to enhance their effects, may restore balance leading to a possible prevention or cure of preeclampsia.

10 Gasotransmitters

Gaseous signalling molecules, NO, CO and H_2S, have potential to be part of the 'braking' system based on their roles in angiogenesis, cytoprotection and regulation of vascular tone. Numerous studies show NO, CO and H_2S as well as their related enzymes promote placental blood vasodilation *in vitro* and *in vivo* (Gude et al. 1990; Myatt et al. 1991; Learmont and Poston 1996; Ahmed et al. 2000; Bainbridge et al. 2002; Zhao et al. 2008; Cindrova-Davies et al. 2013; Wang et al. 2013) suggesting a role in the pathophysiology of preeclampsia (Fig. 1).

11 HO/CO System

Heme oxygenase (HO) is the rate-limiting enzyme responsible for the degradation of heme in the endoplasmic reticulum to generate equimolar amount of biliverdin, free iron and carbon monoxide (CO) (Tenhunen et al. 1969). Biliverdin is rapidly reduced to bilirubin, a potent antioxidant, by the cytosolic enzyme biliverdin reductase. Atmospheric CO is lethal; cellular CO is a potent vasodilator with anti-apoptotic properties (Dulak et al. 2008).

HO exists in two main isoforms; HO-2 (36 kDa) is constitutively expressed in several tissues around the body with high concentrations in the brain and vascular endothelium. Reduced HO-2 immunostaining at the maternal-placental interface reported to be associated with reduction in trophoblasts' invasion in preeclampsia and linked to abnormal placentation (Lyall et al. 2000). In mammalian tissues, the inducible

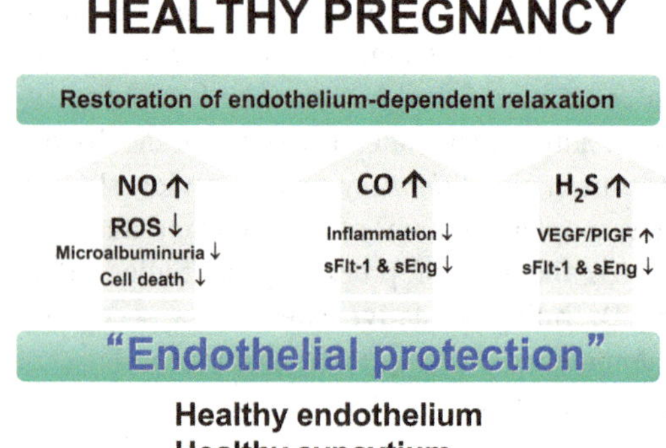

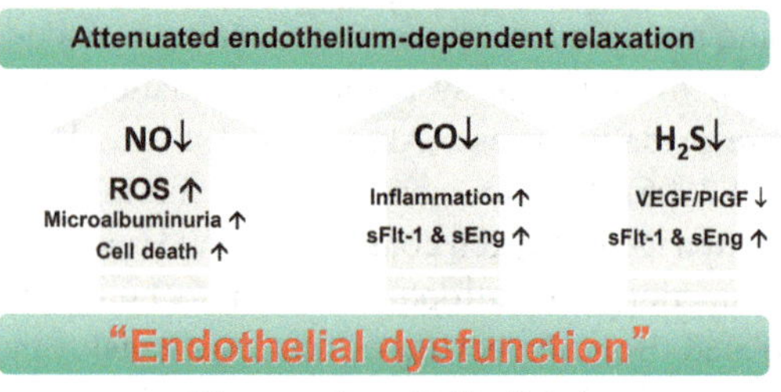

Fig. 1 Schematic diagram illustrating the molecules involved in the pathogenesis of preeclampsia. The upstream events consist of decrease in nitric oxide (NO), carbon monoxide (CO) and hydrogen sulphide (H_2S) leads to increase in microalbuminuria, cell death, inflammation, elevation in soluble Flt-1 (sFlt-1) and soluble Endoglin (sEng) and decrease in placenta growth factor (PlGF). These biochemical changes lead to generation of reactive oxygen species (ROS) and endothelial dysfunction that contributes to the pathogenesis of preeclampsia

isoform, HO-1, is found in the spleen and liver in high concentration but can be identified throughout the body. HO-1 expression is thought to be induced mainly by its substrate, heme, but can also be regulated by other stimuli such as peroxynitrite, cytokines, hypoxia, hypothermia, endotoxins, and metalloprphyrins (Sikorski et al. 2004). HO-1, via its products, inhibits inflammation, oxidative stress and is anti-apoptotic (Dulak et al. 2008). Indeed, deficiency in HO-1 results in severe endothelial damage marked by an increase in thrombomodulin and von Willebrand factor (Yachie et al. 1999).

12 HO/CO Pathway in Pregnancy

The HO-1/CO axis plays a crucial role in the maintenance of uterine quiescence during normal pregnancy (Acevedo and Ahmed 1998) and acts on the utero-placental circulation (Ahmed et al. 2000; Lyall et al. 2000). Placental HO protects human placenta from cellular damage and reduced HO-1 expression is associated with preeclampsia (Ahmed et al. 2000). HO-1 deficient mice that develop hypertension at the beginning of pregnancy (Linzke et al. 2014) further support the role of HO-1 in preeclampsia. Preeclamptic pregnant women also have decreased concentrations of CO compared to healthy pregnant women in their exhaled breath signifying a decrease in HO-1 enzymatic activity (Baum et al. 2000). Deletion of the *HO-1* gene leads to pregnancy complications including intrauterine growth restriction and fetal lethality as well as hypertension (Zenclussen et al. 2014). Furthermore, a recent murine study showed that treating HO-1-deficient animals with CO normalised the number of uNK and angiogenic factor expression as well as restoring spiral artery remodelling (Venditti et al. 2014) that was reported as deficient spiral artery remodelling in HO-1-deficient animals (Zenclussen et al. 2014). However, defect of spiral artery remodelling may be a generalised phenomenon rather than specific to preeclampsia, pointed out earlier in this review

as it fails to meet most of the Bradford Hill criteria. More importantly, human studies using fetal placenta cells (chorionic villous sampling, CVS) showed HO-1 mRNA expression to be reduced in women before the onset of preeclampsia (Alpoim et al. 2016; Farina et al. 2008) and so meets one of the key Bradford Hill causation criterion for disease causation.

When the first link between sFlt-1 and HO-1 was established (Cudmore et al. 2007), the significance of HO-1 in preeclampsia gained traction and other researchers entered the field. Adenoviral HO-1 expression or COP-releasing donors inhibited VEGF-mediated sFlt-1 release and IFN-γ and TNF-α-induced sEng release in cultured endothelial cells (Cudmore et al. 2007). Likewise, knockdown of HO-1 increased sFlt-1 release. In addition, a clinical study showed HO-1 mRNA levels to increase in samples of villous trophoblast, obtained from women between 6 and 11 weeks of gestation undergoing elective abortion, while the mRNA expression of sFlt-1 was decreased with gestational age (Miyagami et al. 2013). It is no surprise therefore that human trophoblast cells from patients with preeclampsia cultured with CO had reduced ability to secret sFlt-1 (Zenclussen et al. 2014). Indeed, women who smoke have reduced circulating sFlt-1 levels (Levine et al. 2006), we would argue this is due to an increase in CO levels. Despite a recent paper challenging the ability of Hmox1 to inhibit sFlt-1 production (Tong et al. 2015) an overwhelming number of studies show that a number of drugs that inhibit sFlt-1 do so via up-regulation of HO-1 (Onda et al. 2015; McCarthy et al. 2011); sildenafil suppresses sFlt-1 from trophoblast via HO-1 (Jeong et al. 2014). In addition, HO-1 induction attenuates ischemia-induced hypertension in pregnant rats (George et al. 2011) and proteinase-activated receptor-2 mediated sFlt-1 release (Al-Ani et al. 2010). Moreover, diastolic blood pressures and plasma sFlt-1 levels were significantly elevated in HO-1$^{+/-}$ pregnant mice (Zhao et al. 2009). HO-1 mRNA expression is also decreased in women destined to develop preeclampsia (Farina et al. 2008) and an Hmox1 promoter polymorphism is associated with preeclampsia (Kaartokallio et al. 2014) indicating HO activity is reduced in preeclampsia. Collectively, these studies show that HO-1 acts as a negative regulator of sFlt-1 and sEng (Cudmore et al. 2011) and support the argument that partial loss of HO-1 activity early in gestation maybe the cause of preeclampsia. In vivo proof-of-principle experiments are needed to validate this theory.

13   The Cth/H$_2$S System

Hydrogen sulfide (H$_2$S) is a gaseous signaling molecule promotes vasodilatation (Zhao et al. 2001), exhibits cytoprotective anti-inflammatory properties (Zanardo et al. 2006), protects against reperfusion injury induced cellular damage (Elrod et al. 2007) or lethal hypoxia (Blackstone and Roth 2007) and stimulates angiogenesis (Papapetropoulos et al. 2009). H$_2$S production is regulated by three enzymes; cystathionine γ-lyase (Cth, also known as CSE), cystathionine β synthase (CBS), and 3-mercaptopyruvate sulfurtransferase (MST) and is generated from the substrates cystathionine, homocysteine, cysteine, and mercaptopyruvate respectively (Wang et al. 2015). CBS is most abundant in the brain whereas Cth is primarily responsible for endogenous H$_2$S production in vasculature (Wang et al. 2015). Administration of the Cth selective inhibitor (DL-propargylglycine, PAG) leads to elevated blood pressure and vascular remodelling in rats (Yan et al. 2004), and mice lacking Cth develop age-dependent hypertension, severe hyperhomocysteinaemia, and endothelial dysfunction (Wang et al. 2015).

14   Cth/H$_2$S Pathway in Pregnancy

H$_2$S is produced by the placenta and other uterine tissues (Patel et al. 2009) and Cth and CBS both localise to the endothelium in chorionic and stem villi of the placenta (Holwerda et al. 2012). In normal vasculature, H$_2$S is vasodilatory (Leffler et al. 2006) and as expected perfusion of normal placenta with a H$_2$S donor causes vasorelaxation of pre-constricted vasculature *in vitro* (Cindrova-Davies et al. 2013). A dysregulation in H$_2$S levels in preeclampsia was reported due to reduced plasma H$_2$S levels in the maternal circulation and reduced expression of Cth in the placenta of these patients (Wang et al. 2013).

Recent studies regarding Cth and CBS expression levels in preeclampsia are inconsistent. Holwerda and colleagues observed in placental villous tissue from early onset preeclampsia, no changes in Cth expression, but a decrease in CBS expression using immunohistochemistry, mRNA and protein expression (Holwerda et al. 2012). In contrast, Cth immunoreactivity was reduced in placenta from pregnancies with severe early-onset growth-restriction and preeclampsia (Cindrova-Davies et al. 2013; Wang et al. 2013). Real-time PCR confirmed reduced Cth mRNA in preeclamptic women and was associated with decreased levels of plasma H$_2$S (Wang et al. 2013). These are observational studies and provide little insight into the contribution this enzyme system makes in preeclampsia.

Interestingly, the Cth pathway shows similar capabilities to the HO-1 system. Endothelial Cth knockdown by siRNA increased the release of sFlt-1 and sEng, while adenoviral-mediated Cth overexpression inhibited their release from endothelial cells (Wang et al. 2013). Furthermore, inhibition of Cth activity by administration of PAG to pregnant mice induced hypertension, liver damage, elevated sFlt-1 and sEng and promoted abnormal labyrinth vascularisation in the placenta as well as decreased fetal growth (Wang et al. 2013). These symptoms were reversed when the inhibitor was supplemented with GYY4137, a slow releasing H$_2$S-generating compound, demonstrating that the effect of PAG was due to inhibition of H$_2$S production (Wang et al. 2013). These findings strongly support a link between H_2S and the anti-angiogenic factors and implicate H2S/Cth as a player on the roadmap of preeclampsia phenotype.

Treatment with H_2S donor, SG-1002, offers cardio protection via upregulation of the VEGF–Akt–NOS3–NO pathway (Kondo et al. 2013). This is further supported by the uncoupling of eNOS in Cth KO mice, reducing the bioavailability of NO (Polhemus et al. 2014). This phenotype can be rescued with the restoration of H_2S levels. Heart failure patients with decreased levels of NO and H_2S, treated with SG-1002, showed an increase in NO bioavailability and plasma H_2S levels (Polhemus et al. 2014). This was also replicated in healthy individuals, illustrating the potential for exogenous H_2S to reverse some of the damaging changes in preeclampsia (Ahmed and Wang 2014, patent WO2014132083 A2). Interestingly, H_2S is known to stimulate VEGF and exposure of vascular smooth muscle cells to H_2S, up-regulates HIF-1α and VEGF protein levels and increased HIF-1α binding activity under hypoxic condition (Liu et al. 2010). Recently, VEGF receptor-2 was reported as the direct target of H_2S and VEGF receptor inhibitor suppressed angiogenesis induced by H_2S (Tao et al. 2013), suggesting that H_2S promotes angiogenesis via VEGF receptor activation. Studies regarding the impact of H_2S/Cth in preeclampsia indirectly support the original idea that loss of VEGF activity (Ahmed 1997) may be the major initiator of preeclampsia.

In preeclampsia, the maternal circulating level of PlGF is decreased well before the onset of the symptoms (Levine et al. 2004; 2006), and Cth dysregulation offers an explanation. Inhibition of Cth activity in early (first trimester) human placental explants obtained from termination of pregnancy results in a marked reduction in PlGF production (Wang et al. 2013). Administration of PlGF in lentiviral sFlt-1-infected non-pregnant mice depresses the level of sFlt-1 and ameliorates hypertension, glomerular endotheliosis and proteinuria (Kumasawa et al. 2011). Furthermore, mice deficient in PlGF ($PlGF^{-/-}$) and treated with an adenovirus containing sFlt-1 developed severe hypertension and proteinuria and H_2S releasing agent. GYY4137, reduced these symptoms (personal communication, Dr Shakil Ahmed). Therefore, Cth/H_2S activity may be upstream to PlGF and could be an earlier biomarker as well as a key regulator that keep the level of PlGF and VEGF activity sufficiently high to counteract antagonism by sFlt-1.

15 The NOS3/NO System

Nitric oxide (NO) is synthesized from the non-essential amino acid L-arginine by one of the three isoforms of NO synthase (NOS); NOS1 (neuronal), NOS2 (inducible), and NOS3 (endothelial). NO produced by NOS3 is important for the relaxation of smooth muscle cells and subsequently the promotion of vasodilation. It is critical for neovascularisation (Bussolati et al. 2001; Ahmad et al. 2006). Loss of NOS3 activity is an established contributor to endothelial dysfunction (Heitzer et al. 2001), a key sign associated with preeclampsia. In endothelial cells, NOS3 exists in a homodimeric complex that is stabilized by the cofactor tetrahydrobiopterin (BH4). Decreased availability of BH4 results in "uncoupling" of NOS3 activity and an increase in superoxide (d'Uscio et al. 2001; Bendall et al. 2005).

16 NOS3/NO Pathway in Pregnancy

Blocking the production of NO by administering a NOS-inhibiting agent produces virtually all the symptoms of preeclampsia in pregnant mice and rats, suggesting that the NOS pathway is a key player in this disorder (Lowe 2000). A meta-analysis showed that genetic variations in the *NOS3* gene contribute to an increased risk for preeclampsia (Dai et al. 2013). In non-pregnancy mice lacking NOS3, the sFlt-induced preeclampsia phenotype is aggravated (Li et al. 2012). Indeed, BH4 doubled NOS3 activity in a concentration dependent manner in homogenates of first trimester and term placenta (Kukor et al. 2000) and uncoupled NOS3 and oxidative stress in a rat model of pregnancy-induced hypertension (Mitchell et al. 2007). However, BH4 concentrations in preeclamptic placenta were reported to be comparable with those of normal placenta (Kukor et al. 2000). A nested case-control study of screening for pre-eclampsia revealed that asymmetric dimethylarginine (ADMA), an endogenous inhibitor of NO formation, normally increases during pregnancy but the concentrations in the second trimester were significantly elevated in pregnancies that later developed preeclampsia (Rizos 2012, #5348).

Reduced availability of the NOS3 substrate L-arginine is also linked to impaired endothelial NO production. Twenty years earlier, it was reported that blood pressure in men could be reduced through intravenous administration of L-arginine as well as improving renal plasma flow and decreased renal vascular resistance (Higashi 1995, #5535). In small clinical trials, L-arginine supplementation used in complicated pregnancy was without conclusive outcomes. L-arginine supplementation reduced the risk of preeclampsia in high-risk women (Vadillo-Ortega et al. 2011), while showed little or no beneficial effects (Staff et al. 2004). As L-arginine supplementation increases the levels of asymmetric dimethylarginine and arginase, direct and indirect competitive inhibitors of endothelial NOS (Jabecka et al. 2012), high expression of these enzymes can induce the uncoupling of NOS as a source of superoxide in the vasculature. A number of studies suggested that L-arginine supplementation could lead to a further increase in peroxynitrite (Xia et al. 1996; Sankaralingam et al. 2010). Indeed, long-term L-arginine supplementation is harmful both in animal models (Chen et al. 2003) and in patients with cardiovascular diseases (Schulman et al. 2006). Finally, there is still an absence of a solid mechanistic model for impact of L-arginine in preeclampsia.

17 Activin A and Inhibin A in Preeclampsia

Activin A and inhibin A are members of TGFβ superfamily. The main function of activin A is in trophoblast proliferation while both molecules have opposing effects on follicle stimulating hormone (FSH) production from the pituitary (Muttukrishna et al. 1997; Caniggia et al. 1997). They are elevated before the onset of the pre-eclamptic phenotype. An eight-fold and ten-fold increased serum concentration in activin A and inhibin A respectively was reported in women with preeclampsia compared to normal pregnancy (Muttukrishna et al. 2000). The more severe the preeclampsia, the higher the levels of inhinin A (Kang et al. 2008) supporting a dose-response correlation. However, the mechanism by which the interaction between activin A and inhibin A is not clear. Perhaps it contributes to the pathogenesis of preeclampsia potentially through decreasing protective factors or increasing ROS activity and is an area worthy of further investigation.

18 Role of microRNA in Preeclampsia

Micro RNA's (miRNA) are small, non-coding, single stranded RNA molecules that target specific mRNA. By annealing to their mRNA partner, they can manipulate the expression pattern of the mRNA (Lagos-Quintana et al. 2002). A large number of miRNAs are now being discovered in pregnancy. Pro-angiogenic miRNA-126 correlated with VEGF expression and was decreased in preeclampsia pregnancies (Hong et al. 2014). Another miRNA found to be reduced in endothelial cells from preeclampsia patients is miRNA-155, believed to down-regulate angiogenic factors, possibly contributing to the angiogenic imbalance seen in preeclampsia (Zhang et al. 2010). MiRNA-155 also linked to endothelial NOS3 modulation (Li et al. 2014) and trophoblast function (Dai et al. 2011). Exact role of these miRNA in pregnancy and preeclampsia remains to be defined in mechanistic and in vivo models as well as in clinical studies. MicroRNAs are not only found in the placenta but also in the maternal circulation and may be potentially important as diagnostic targets for preeclampsia (Mouillet et al. 2011).

19 Biochemical Markers to Predict Preeclampsia

Identified risk factors are used to screen pregnant women at high risk of developing preeclampsia. These include age, obesity, diabetes mellitus, renal disease, multiple pregnancy and history of preeclampsia in earlier pregnancies. Indeed, none of these alone can predict preeclampsia sufficiently, but combining these pre-dispositions with possible biomarkers may lead to effective diagnosis and potential predictions of disease onset (Bartsch et al. 2016). Both sFlt-1 and PlGF have been proposed as highly selective biomarkers for diagnosis of preeclampsia (Levine et al. 2006; Chappell et al. 2013). Placental protein 13 is another biomarker, which when combined with Doppler ultrasound pulsatility index showed a prediction rate of 90 % in first trimester of pregnancy (Nicolaides et al. 2005). However, ideal biomarkers needs to detected in plasma without the need of a sophisticated ultrasound or an obstetrician input. Biomarkers used to predict preeclampsia must precede the onset of preeclampsia, correlate with the severity of the disease and must show a high (>90 %) sensitivity and specificity and be overall low cost to existing management systems and ideally replace them.

20 Future Perspective and Conclusion

Despite substantial advances in the scientific and technological field, we have failed to provide effective treatment and diagnostic means for patients with preeclampsia. There is a vast amount of information but we are no closer to solving the enigma of preeclampsia. In order to identify suitable diagnosis, treatment and prevention strategies for preeclampsia, the roadmap of preeclampsia phenotype needs to be discovered and manipulated to illustrate a causation link. This review can only stress that any hypothesis proposed should be analyzed based on the Bradford Hill causation criteria in order to make claims for a given set of molecules to be implicated as a contributor in the causation of preeclampsia.

Both sFlt-1 and sEng are increased before the onset of symptoms. They both impact on VEGF and NO signaling pathways ultimately resulting in hypertension and other clinical symptoms. It is also evident that by removing these molecules, symptoms can improve. This cannot be said to be true for the "excessive inflammation" hypothesis seen during preeclampsia as corticosteroid treatment only transiently reduced symptoms. Both sFlt-1 and HO-1 pathways fit the disorder criteria to a greater extent, as there is a correlation between the levels of expression within the disorder progression as well as their regulatory relationship. Recent studies involving activin A and inhibin A expression also show a relationship between expression and severity. However, more in vivo research is needed to pinpoint the roles these molecules in roadmap of preeclampsia phenotype.

Limitations within the research field, as well as the dogma's compiled for the disorder, have blocked or created false intersections between the 'dots' of preeclampsia. *In vitro* studies should not be considered as the only means to demolish these roadblocks. There are now many mouse models, which rely on a number of different techniques to produce a preeclamptic phenotype. These *in vivo* models are and should be used to gather 'proper' evidence with regards to 'connecting the dots looking backwards' in order to answer; what 'dots' are inside the black box of causation? (Fig. 2) and how do the intersections between them fit together? Only by taking this approach can we hope to control and abolish this major disorder of pregnancy.

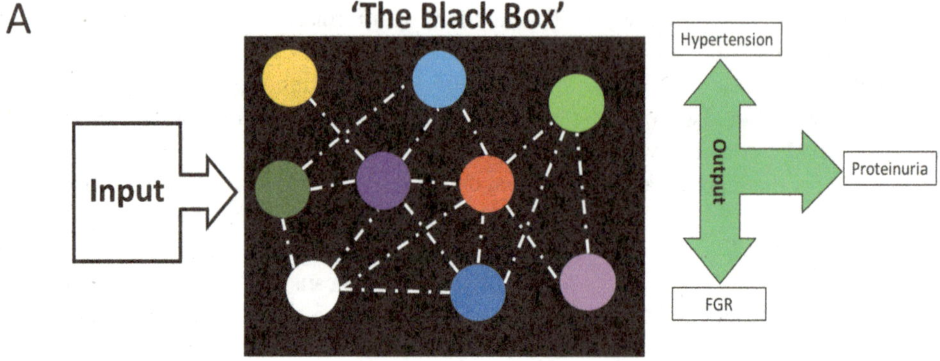

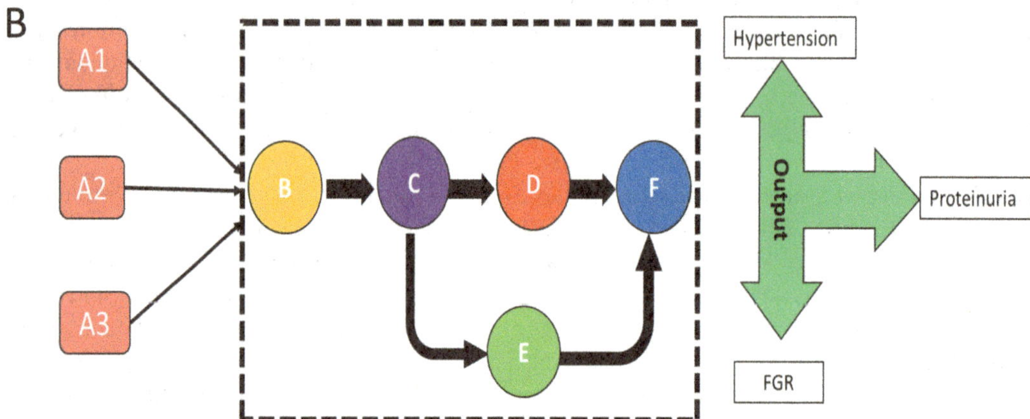

Fig. 2 The black box model. (**a**) Schematic representation for the roadmap of preeclampsia. An input equates to agents challenging pregnancy. These trigger series of factors denoted as *dots* in "the black box" and interconnected temporarily by "association studies" until the intersections are confirmed and established as solid connections using in vivo 'proof of principle' experimentations. (**b**) The schematic representation of preeclampsia roadmap pathway established by connecting the 'dots looking back' based on in vivo experimentations by gain or loss of the preeclampsia phenotype by manipulation of these *dots*

References

Acevedo CH, Ahmed A (1998) Hemeoxygenase-1 inhibits human myometrial contractility via carbon monoxide and is upregulated by progesterone during pregnancy. J Clin Invest 101(5):949–955

Ahmad S, Ahmed A (2001) Regulation of soluble VEGFR-1 by VEGF and oxygen and its elevation in pre-eclampsia and fetal growth restriction. Placenta 22 (8–9):A.7

Ahmad S, Ahmed A (2004) Elevated placental soluble vascular endothelial growth factor receptor-1 inhibits angiogenesis in preeclampsia. Circ Res 95 (9):884–891

Ahmad S, Hewett PW, Wang P, Al-Ani B, Cudmore M, Fujisawa T et al (2006) Direct evidence for endothelial vascular endothelial growth factor receptor-1 function in nitric oxide-mediated angiogenesis. Circ Res 99 (7):715–722

Ahmad S, Hewett PW, Al-Ani B, Sissaoui S, Fujisawa T, Cudmore MJ et al (2011) Autocrine activity of soluble Flt-1 controls endothelial cell function and angiogenesis. Vasc Cell 3(1):15

Ahmed A (1997) Heparin-binding angiogenic growth factors in pregnancy. Trophoblast Res 10:215–258

Ahmed A, Ramma W (2015) Unravelling the theories of pre-eclampsia: are the protective pathways the new paradigm? Br J Pharmacol 172(6):1574–1586

Ahmed A, Rahman M, Zhang X, Acevedo CH, Nijjar S, Rushton I et al (2000) Induction of placental heme oxygenase-1 is protective against TNFalpha- induced cytotoxicity and promotes vessel relaxation. Mol Med 6(5):391–409

Al-Ani B, Hewett PW, Cudmore MJ, Fujisawa T, Saifeddine M, Williams H et al (2010) Activation of proteinase-activated receptor 2 stimulates soluble vascular endothelial growth factor receptor 1 release via epidermal growth factor receptor transactivation in endothelial cells. Hypertension 55(3):689–697

Alpoim PN, Godoi LC, Pinheiro Mde B, Freitas LG, Carvalho M, Dusse LM (2016) The unexpected beneficial role of smoking in preeclampsia. Clin Chim Acta 459:105–108

Arulkumaran N, Lightstone L (2013) Severe pre-eclampsia and hypertensive crises. Best Pract Res Clin Obstet Gynaecol 27(6):877–884

Bachmayer N, Rafik Hamad R, Liszka L, Bremme K, Sverremark-Ekstrom E (2006) Aberrant uterine natural killer (NK)-cell expression and altered placental and serum levels of the NK-cell promoting cytokine interleukin-12 in pre-eclampsia. Am J Reprod Immunol 56(5–6):292–301

Bainbridge SA, Farley AE, McLaughlin BE, Graham CH, Marks GS, Nakatsu K et al (2002) Carbon monoxide decreases perfusion pressure in isolated human placenta. Placenta 23(8–9):563–569

Bartsch E, Medcalf KE, Park AL, Ray JG (2016) High risk of pre-eclampsia identification G. Clinical risk factors for pre-eclampsia determined in early pregnancy: systematic review and meta-analysis of large cohort studies. BMJ 353:i1753

Baum M, Schiff E, Kreiser D, Dennery PA, Stevenson DK, Rosenthal T et al (2000) End-tidal carbon monoxide measurements in women with pregnancy-induced hypertension and preeclampsia. Am J Obstet Gynecol 183(4):900–903

Bell MJ (2010) A historical overview of preeclampsia-eclampsia. J Obstet Gynecol Neonatal Nurs 39 (5):510–518

Bendall JK, Alp NJ, Warrick N, Cai S, Adlam D, Rockett K et al (2005) Stoichiometric relationships between endothelial tetrahydrobiopterin, endothelial NO synthase (eNOS) activity, and eNOS coupling in vivo: insights from transgenic mice with endothelial-targeted GTP cyclohydrolase 1 and eNOS overexpression. Circ Res 97(9):864–871

Bergmann A, Ahmad S, Cudmore M, Gruber AD, Wittschen P, Lindenmaier W et al (2010) Reduction of circulating soluble Flt-1 alleviates preeclampsia-like symptoms in a mouse model. J Cell Mol Med 14 (6B):1857–1867

Blackstone E, Roth MB (2007) Suspended animation-like state protects mice from lethal hypoxia. Shock 27 (4):370–372

Brosens JJ, Pijnenborg R, Brosens IA (2002) The myometrial junctional zone spiral arteries in normal and abnormal pregnancies: a review of the literature. Am J Obstet Gynecol 187(5):1416–1423

Brown MA, Lindheimer MD, de Swiet M, Van Assche A, Moutquin JM (2001) The classification and diagnosis of the hypertensive disorders of pregnancy: statement from the International Society for the Study of Hypertension in Pregnancy (ISSHP). Hypertens Pregnancy 20(1):IX–XIV

Burke SD, Karumanchi SA (2013) Spiral artery remodeling in preeclampsia revisited. Hypertension 62(6):1013–1014

Burke SD, Barrette VF, Bianco J, Thorne JG, Yamada AT, Pang SC et al (2010) Spiral arterial remodeling is not essential for normal blood pressure regulation in pregnant mice. Hypertension 55(3):729–737

Burton GJ, Woods AW, Jauniaux E, Kingdom JC (2009) Rheological and physiological consequences of conversion of the maternal spiral arteries for uteroplacental blood flow during human pregnancy. Placenta 30(6):473–482

Bussolati B, Dunk C, Grohman M, Kontos CD, Mason J, Ahmed A (2001) Vascular endothelial growth factor receptor-1 modulates vascular endothelial growth factor-mediated angiogenesis via nitric oxide. Am J Pathol 159(3):993–1008

Caniggia I, Lye SJ, Cross JC (1997) Activin is a local regulator of human cytotrophoblast cell differentiation. Endocrinology 138(9):3976–3986

Caniggia I, Mostachfi H, Winter J, Gassmann M, Lye SJ, Kuliszewski M et al (2000) Hypoxia-inducible factor-1 mediates the biological effects of oxygen on human trophoblast differentiation through TGFbeta(3). J Clin Invest 105(5):577–587

Carter AM, Enders AC, Pijnenborg R (2015) The role of invasive trophoblast in implantation and placentation of primates. Philos Trans R Soc Lond B Biol Sci 370 (1663):20140070

Carty DM, Anderson LA, Freeman DJ, Welsh PI, Brennand JE, Dominiczak AF et al (2012) Early pregnancy soluble E-selectin concentrations and risk of preeclampsia. J Hypertens 30(5):954–959

Chappell LC, Duckworth S, Seed PT, Griffin M, Myers J, Mackillop L et al (2013) Diagnostic accuracy of placental growth factor in women with suspected pre-eclampsia: a prospective multicenter study. Circulation 128(19):2121–2131

Chen J, Kuhlencordt P, Urano F, Ichinose H, Astern J, Huang PL (2003) Effects of chronic treatment with L-arginine on atherosclerosis in apoE knockout and apoE/inducible NO synthase double-knockout mice. Arterioscler Thromb Vasc Biol 23(1):97–103

Cheng SB, Sharma S (2016) Preeclampsia and health risks later in life: an immunological link. Semin Immunopathol

Cindrova-Davies T, Sanders DA, Burton GJ, Charnock-Jones DS (2011) Soluble FLT1 sensitizes endothelial cells to inflammatory cytokines by antagonizing VEGF receptor-mediated signalling. Cardiovasc Res 89(3):671–679

Cindrova-Davies T, Herrera EA, Niu Y, Kingdom J, Giussani DA, Burton GJ (2013) Reduced cystathionine gamma-lyase and increased microRNA-21 expression are associated with increased vascular resistance in growth-restricted pregnancies: hydrogen sulfide as a placental vasodilator. Am J Pathol

Cross SN, Ratner E, Rutherford TJ, Schwartz PE, Norwitz ER (2012) Bevacizumab-mediated interference with VEGF signaling is sufficient to induce a preeclampsia-like syndrome in nonpregnant women. Rev Obstet Gynecol 5(1):2–8

Cudmore M, Ahmad S, Al-Ani B, Fujisawa T, Coxall H, Chudasama K et al (2007) Negative regulation of soluble Flt-1 and soluble endoglin release by heme oxygenase-1. Circulation 115(13):1789–1797

Cudmore MJ, Ahmad S, Sissaoui S, Ramma W, Ma B, Fujisawa T et al (2011) Loss of Akt activity increases circulating soluble endoglin release in preeclampsia: identification of inter-dependency between Akt-1 and heme oxygenase-1. Eur Heart J

D'Uscio LV, Baker TA, Mantilla CB, Smith L, Weiler D, Sieck GC et al (2001) Mechanism of endothelial dysfunction in apolipoprotein E-deficient mice. Arterioscler Thromb Vasc Biol 21(6):1017–1022

Dai Y, Diao Z, Sun H, Li R, Qiu Z, Hu Y (2011) MicroRNA-155 is involved in the remodelling of human-trophoblast-derived HTR-8/SVneo cells induced by lipopolysaccharides. Hum Reprod 26(7):1882–1891

Dai B, Liu T, Zhang B, Zhang X, Wang Z (2013) The polymorphism for endothelial nitric oxide synthase gene, the level of nitric oxide and the risk for pre-eclampsia: a meta-analysis. Gene 519(1):187–193

Darmochwal-Kolarz D, Kludka-Sternik M, Tabarkiewicz J, Kolarz B, Rolinski J, Leszczynska-Gorzelak B et al (2012) The predominance of Th17 lymphocytes and decreased number and function of Treg cells in pre-eclampsia. J Reprod Immunol 93(2):75–81

Djurovic S, Clausen T, Wergeland R, Brosstad F, Berg K, Henriksen T (2002) Absence of enhanced systemic inflammatory response at 18 weeks of gestation in women with subsequent pre-eclampsia. Bjog 109(7):759–764

Dulak J, Deshane J, Jozkowicz A, Agarwal A (2008) Heme oxygenase-1 and carbon monoxide in vascular pathobiology: focus on angiogenesis. Circulation 117(2):231–241

Elrod JW, Calvert JW, Morrison J, Doeller JE, Kraus DW, Tao L et al (2007) Hydrogen sulfide attenuates myocardial ischemia-reperfusion injury by preservation of mitochondrial function. Proc Natl Acad Sci U S A 104(39):15560–15565

Farina A, Sekizawa A, De Sanctis P, Purwosunu Y, Okai T, Cha DH et al (2008) Gene expression in chorionic villous samples at 11 weeks' gestation from women destined to develop preeclampsia. Prenat Diagn 28(10):956–961

Farzadnia M, Ayatollahi H, Hasan-Zade M, Rahimi HR (2013) A comparative study of serum level of Vascular Cell Adhesion Molecule-1 (sVCAM-1), Intercellular Adhesion Molecule-1(ICAM-1) and high sensitive C–Reactive Protein (hs-CRP) in normal and pre-eclamptic pregnancies. Iran J Basic Med Sci 16(5):689–693

Feinberg RF, Kliman HJ, Cohen AW (1991) Preeclampsia, trisomy 13, and the placental bed. Obstet Gynecol 78(3 Pt 2):505–508

Fu B, Li X, Sun R, Tong X, Ling B, Tian Z et al (2013) Natural killer cells promote immune tolerance by regulating inflammatory TH17 cells at the human maternal-fetal interface. Proc Natl Acad Sci U S A 110(3):E231–E240

Garovic VD, Hayman SR (2007) Hypertension in pregnancy: an emerging risk factor for cardiovascular disease. Nat Clin Pract Nephrol 3(11):613–622

Genbacev O, Joslin R, Damsky CH, Polliotti BM, Fisher SJ (1996) Hypoxia alters early gestation human cytotrophoblast differentiation/invasion in vitro and models the placental defects that occur in preeclampsia. J Clin Invest 97(2):540–550

George EM, Cockrell K, Aranay M, Csongradi E, Stec DE, Granger JP (2011) Induction of heme oxygenase 1 attenuates placental ischemia-induced hypertension. Hypertension 57(5):941–948

Gude NM, King RG, Brennecke SP (1990) Role of endothelium-derived nitric oxide in maintenance of low fetal vascular resistance in placenta. Lancet 336(8730):1589–1590

He H, Venema VJ, Gu X, Venema RC, Marrero MB, Caldwell RB (1999) Vascular endothelial growth factor signals endothelial cell production of nitric oxide and prostacyclin through flk-1/KDR activation of c-Src. J Biol Chem 274(35):25130–25135

Heitzer T, Schlinzig T, Krohn K, Meinertz T, Munzel T (2001) Endothelial dysfunction, oxidative stress, and risk of cardiovascular events in patients with coronary artery disease. Circulation 104(22):2673–2678

Higashi Y (1995) Intravenous administration of L-arginine inhibits angiotensin- converting enzyme in humans. J Clin Endocrinol Metab 80(7):2198–2202

Hill AB (1965) The environment and disease: association or causation? Proc R Soc Med 58:295–300

Hladunewich M, Karumanchi SA, Lafayette R (2007) Pathophysiology of the clinical manifestations of pre-eclampsia. Clin J Am Soc Nephrol 2(3):543–549

Holwerda KM, Bos EM, Rajakumar A, Ris-Stalpers C, van Pampus MG, Timmer A et al (2012) Hydrogen sulfide producing enzymes in pregnancy and pre-eclampsia. Placenta

Hong F, Li Y, Xu Y (2014) Decreased placental miR-126 expression and vascular endothelial growth factor levels in patients with pre-eclampsia. J Int Med Res 42(6):1243–1251

Huppertz B, Weiss G, Moser G (2014) Trophoblast invasion and oxygenation of the placenta: measurements versus presumptions. J Reprod Immunol 101–102:74–79

Jabecka A, Ast J, Bogdaski P, Drozdowski M, Pawlak-Lemaska K, Cielewicz AR et al (2012) Oral

L-arginine supplementation in patients with mild arterial hypertension and its effect on plasma level of asymmetric dimethylarginine, L-citruline, L-arginine and antioxidant status. Eur Rev Med Pharmacol Sci 16 (12):1665–1674

Jebbink J, Keijser R, Veenboer G, van der Post J, Ris-Stalpers C, Afink G (2011) Expression of placental FLT1 transcript variants relates to both gestational hypertensive disease and fetal growth. Hypertension 58(1):70–76

Jeong JH, Kim HG, Choi OH (2014) Sildenafil inhibits advanced glycation end products-induced sFlt-1 release through upregulation of heme oxygenase-1. J Menop Med 20(2):57–68

Kaartokallio T, Klemetti MM, Timonen A, Uotila J, Heinonen S, Kajantie E et al (2014) Microsatellite polymorphism in the heme oxygenase-1 promoter is associated with nonsevere and late-onset preeclampsia. Hypertension 64(1):172–177

Kang JH, Farina A, Park JH, Kim SH, Kim JY, Rizzo N et al (2008) Down syndrome biochemical markers and screening for preeclampsia at first and second trimester: correlation with the week of onset and the severity. Prenat Diagn 28(8):704–709

Khong TY, De Wolf F, Robertson WB, Brosens I (1986) Inadequate maternal vascular response to placentation in pregnancies complicated by pre-eclampsia and by small-for-gestational age infants. Br J Obstet Gynaecol 93(10):1049–1059

Kondo K, Bhushan S, King AL, Prabhu SD, Hamid T, Koenig S et al (2013) H(2)S protects against pressure overload-induced heart failure via upregulation of endothelial nitric oxide synthase. Circulation 127 (10):1116–1127

Kronborg CS, Gjedsted J, Vittinghus E, Hansen TK, Allen J, Knudsen UB (2011) Longitudinal measurement of cytokines in pre-eclamptic and normotensive pregnancies. Acta Obstet Gynecol Scand 90 (7):791–796

Kukor Z, Valent S, Toth M (2000) Regulation of nitric oxide synthase activity by tetrahydrobiopterin in human placentae from normal and pre-eclamptic pregnancies. Placenta 21(8):763–772

Kumasawa K, Ikawa M, Kidoya H, Hasuwa H, Saito-Fujita T, Morioka Y et al (2011) Pravastatin induces placental growth factor (PGF) and ameliorates pre-eclampsia in a mouse model. Proc Natl Acad Sci U S A 108(4):1451–1455

Lagos-Quintana M, Rauhut R, Yalcin A, Meyer J, Lendeckel W, Tuschl T (2002) Identification of tissue-specific microRNAs from mouse. Curr Biol 12 (9):735–739

Learmont JG, Poston L (1996) Nitric oxide is involved in flow-induced dilation of isolated human small fetoplacental arteries. Am J Obstet Gynecol 174 (2):583–588

Leffler CW, Parfenova H, Jaggar JH, Wang R (2006) Carbon monoxide and hydrogen sulfide: gaseous messengers in cerebrovascular circulation. J Appl Physiol (1985) 100(3):1065–1076

Leno-Duran E, Hatta K, Bianco J, Yamada AT, Ruiz-Ruiz C, Olivares EG et al (2010) Fetal-placental hypoxia does not result from failure of spiral arterial modification in mice. Placenta 31(8):731–737

Levine RJ, Maynard SE, Qian C, Lim KH, England LJ, Yu KF et al (2004) Circulating angiogenic factors and the risk of preeclampsia. N Engl J Med 350 (7):672–683

Levine RJ, Lam C, Qian C, Yu KF, Maynard SE, Sachs BP et al (2006) Soluble endoglin and other circulating antiangiogenic factors in preeclampsia. N Engl J Med 355(10):992–1005

Li F, Hagaman JR, Kim HS, Maeda N, Jennette JC, Faber JE et al (2012) eNOS deficiency acts through endothelin to aggravate sFlt-1-induced pre-eclampsia-like phenotype. J Am Soc Nephrol 23(4):652–660

Li X, Li C, Dong X, Gou W (2014) MicroRNA-155 inhibits migration of trophoblast cells and contributes to the pathogenesis of severe preeclampsia by regulating endothelial nitric oxide synthase. Mol Med Rep 10(1):550–554

Linzke N, Schumacher A, Woidacki K, Croy BA, Zenclussen AC (2014) Carbon monoxide promotes proliferation of uterine natural killer cells and remodeling of spiral arteries in pregnant hypertensive heme oxygenase-1 mutant mice. Hypertension 63 (3):580–588

Liu X, Pan L, Zhuo Y, Gong Q, Rose P, Zhu Y (2010) Hypoxia-inducible factor-1alpha is involved in the pro-angiogenic effect of hydrogen sulfide under hypoxic stress. Biol Pharm Bull 33(9):1550–1554

Llurba E, Gratacos E, Martin-Gallan P, Cabero L, Dominguez C (2004) A comprehensive study of oxidative stress and antioxidant status in preeclampsia and normal pregnancy. Free Radic Biol Med 37 (4):557–570

Lowe DT (2000) Nitric oxide dysfunction in the pathophysiology of preeclampsia. Nitric Oxide 4 (4):441–458

Lowe SA, Brown MA, Dekker GA, Gatt S, McLintock CK, McMahon LP et al (2009) Guidelines for the management of hypertensive disorders of pregnancy 2008. Aust N Z J Obstet Gynaecol 49(3):242–246

Lyall F, Barber A, Myatt L, Bulmer JN, Robson SC (2000) Hemeoxygenase expression in human placenta and placental bed implies a role in regulation of trophoblast invasion and placental function. FASEB J 14 (1):208–219

Lyall F, Robson SC, Bulmer JN (2013) Spiral artery remodeling and trophoblast invasion in preeclampsia and fetal growth restriction: relationship to clinical outcome. Hypertension 62(6):1046–1054

Maharaj AS, Walshe TE, Saint-Geniez M, Venkatesha S, Maldonado AE, Himes NC et al (2008) VEGF and TGF-beta are required for the maintenance of the choroid plexus and ependyma. J Exp Med 205 (2):491–501

Maloyan A, Mele J, Muralimanohara B, Myatt L (2012) Measurement of mitochondrial respiration in trophoblast culture. Placenta 33(5):456–458

Maynard SE, Min JY, Merchan J, Lim KH, Li J, Mondal S et al (2003) Excess placental soluble fms-like tyrosine kinase 1 (sFlt1) may contribute to endothelial dysfunction, hypertension, and proteinuria in preeclampsia. J Clin Invest 111(5):649–658

Maynard S, Epstein FH, Karumanchi SA (2008) Preeclampsia and angiogenic imbalance. Annu Rev Med 59:61–78

McCarthy FP, Drewlo S, Kingdom J, Johns EJ, Walsh SK, Kenny LC (2011) Peroxisome proliferator-activated receptor-{gamma} as a potential therapeutic target in the treatment of preeclampsia. Hypertension 58 (2):280–286

Mitchell BM, Cook LG, Danchuk S, Puschett JB (2007) Uncoupled endothelial nitric oxide synthase and oxidative stress in a rat model of pregnancy-induced hypertension. Am J Hypertens 20(12):1297–1304

Miyagami S, Koide K, Sekizawa A, Ventura W, Yotsumoto J, Oishi S et al (2013) Physiological changes in the pattern of placental gene expression early in the first trimester. Reprod Sci 20(6):710–714

Mouillet JF, Chu T, Sadovsky Y (2011) Expression patterns of placental microRNAs. Birth Defects Res A Clin Mol Teratol 91(8):737–743

Muralimanoharan S, Maloyan A, Mele J, Guo C, Myatt LG, Myatt L (2012) MIR-210 modulates mitochondrial respiration in placenta with preeclampsia. Placenta 33(10):816–823

Muttukrishna S, Knight PG, Groome NP, Redman CW, Ledger WL (1997) Activin A and inhibin A as possible endocrine markers for pre-eclampsia. Lancet 349 (9061):1285–1288

Muttukrishna S, North RA, Morris J, Schellenberg JC, Taylor RS, Asselin J et al (2000) Serum inhibin A and activin A are elevated prior to the onset of pre-eclampsia. Hum Reprod 15(7):1640–1645

Myatt L, Webster RP (2009) Vascular biology of preeclampsia. J Thromb Haemost 7(3):375–384

Myatt L, Brewer A, Brockman DE (1991) The action of nitric oxide in the perfused human fetal-placental circulation. Am J Obstet Gynecol 164(2):687–692

Myatt L, Rosenfield RB, Eis AL, Brockman DE, Greer I, Lyall F (1996) Nitrotyrosine residues in placenta. Evidence of peroxynitrite formation and action. Hypertension 28(3):488–493

Nagamatsu T, Fujii T, Kusumi M, Li Z, Yamashita T, Osuga Y et al (2004) Cytotrophoblasts up-regulate soluble Fms-like tyrosine kinase-1 (sFlt-1) expression under reduced oxygen: an implication for the placental vascular development and the pathophysiology of pre-eclampsia. Endocrinology

Nayeri UA, Buhimschi IA, Laky CA, Cross SN, Duzyj CM, Ramma W et al (2014) Antenatal corticosteroids impact the inflammatory rather than the antiangiogenic profile of women with preeclampsia. Hypertension

Nicolaides KH, Spencer K, Avgidou K, Faiola S, Falcon O (2005) Multicenter study of first-trimester screening for trisomy 21 in 75 821 pregnancies: results and estimation of the potential impact of individual risk-orientated two-stage first-trimester screening. Ultrasound Obstet Gynecol 25(3):221–226

Onda K, Tong S, Nakahara A, Kondo M, Monchusho H, Hirano T et al (2015) Sofalcone upregulates the nuclear factor (erythroid-derived 2)-like 2/heme oxygenase-1 pathway, reduces soluble fms-like tyrosine kinase-1, and quenches endothelial dysfunction: potential therapeutic for preeclampsia. Hypertension 65(4):855–862

Ozler A, Turgut A, Sak ME, Evsen MS, Soydinc HE, Evliyaoglu O et al (2012) Serum levels of neopterin, tumor necrosis factor-alpha and Interleukin-6 in preeclampsia: relationship with disease severity. Eur Rev Med Pharmacol Sci 16(12):1707–1712

Palmer KR, Tong S, Tuohey L, Cannon P, Ye L, Hannan NJ et al (2016) Jumonji domain containing protein 6 is decreased in human preeclamptic placentas and regulates sFLT-1 splice variant production. Biol Reprod 94(3):59

Papapetropoulos A, Pyriochou A, Altaany Z, Yang G, Marazioti A, Zhou Z et al (2009) Hydrogen sulfide is an endogenous stimulator of angiogenesis. Proc Natl Acad Sci U S A 106(51):21972–21977

Patel P, Vatish M, Heptinstall J, Wang R, Carson RJ (2009) The endogenous production of hydrogen sulphide in intrauterine tissues. Reprod Biol Endocrinol 7:10

Peluffo G, Radi R (2007) Biochemistry of protein tyrosine nitration in cardiovascular pathology. Cardiovasc Res 75(2):291–302

Polhemus DJ, Calvert JW, Butler J, Lefer DJ (2014) The cardioprotective actions of hydrogen sulfide in acute myocardial infarction and heart failure. Scientifica (Cairo) 2014:768607

Rajakumar A, Conrad KP (2000a) Expression, ontogeny, and regulation of hypoxia-inducible transcription factors in the human placenta. Biol Reprod 63 (2):559–569

Rajakumar A, Conrad KP (2000b) Expression, ontogeny, and regulation of hypoxia-inducible transcription factors in the human placenta. Biol Reprod 63 (2):559–569

Rajakumar A, Doty K, Daftary A, Harger G, Conrad KP (2003a) Impaired oxygen-dependent reduction of HIF-1α and -2α proteins in pre-eclamptic placentae. Placenta 24(2–3):199–208

Rajakumar A, Doty K, Daftary A, Harger G, Conrad KP (2003b) Impaired oxygen-dependent reduction of HIF-1alpha and -2alpha proteins in pre-eclamptic placentae. Placenta 24(2–3):199–208

Ramma W, Ahmed A (2011) Is inflammation the cause of pre-eclampsia? Biochem Soc Trans 39(6):1619–1627

Ramma W, Ahmed A (2014) Therapeutic potential of statins and the induction of heme oxygenase-1 in preeclampsia. J Reprod Immunol 101–102:153–160

Ramma W, Buhimschi IA, Zhao G, Dulay AT, Nayeri UA, Buhimschi CS et al (2012) The elevation in circulating anti-angiogenic factors is independent of markers of neutrophil activation in preeclampsia. Angiogenesis

Redman CW, Sargent IL (2005) Latest advances in understanding preeclampsia. Science 308(5728):1592–1594

Redman CW, Sargent IL (2009) Placental stress and pre-eclampsia: a revised view. Placenta 30(Suppl A): S38–S42

Rizos D, Eleftheriades M, Batakis E, Rizou M, Haliassos A, Hassiakos D et al (2012) Levels of asymmetric dimethylarginine throughout normal pregnancy and in pregnancies complicated with preeclampsia or had a small for gestational age baby. J Mater Fetal Neonatal Med 25(8):1311–1315

Roberts JM, Hubel CA (2009) The two stage model of preeclampsia: variations on the theme. Placenta 30 (Suppl A):S32–S37

Robson A, Harris LK, Innes BA, Lash GE, Aljunaidy MM, Aplin JD et al (2012) Uterine natural killer cells initiate spiral artery remodeling in human pregnancy. FASEB J 26(12):4876–4885

Salles AM, Galvao TF, Silva MT, Motta LC, Pereira MG (2012) Antioxidants for preventing preeclampsia: a systematic review. ScientificWorldJournal 2012:243476

Sanchez-Aranguren LC, Prada CE, Riano-Medina CE, Lopez M (2014) Endothelial dysfunction and pre-eclampsia: role of oxidative stress. Front Physiol 5:372

Sankaralingam S, Arenas IA, Lalu MM, Davidge ST (2006) Preeclampsia: current understanding of the molecular basis of vascular dysfunction. Expert Rev Mol Med 8(3):1–20

Sankaralingam S, Xu H, Davidge ST (2010) Arginase contributes to endothelial cell oxidative stress in response to plasma from women with preeclampsia. Cardiovasc Res 85(1):194–203

Saxena AR, Karumanchi SA, Brown NJ, Royle CM, McElrath TF, Seely EW (2010) Increased sensitivity to angiotensin II is present postpartum in women with a history of hypertensive pregnancy. Hypertension 55 (5):1239–1245

Schulman SP, Becker LC, Kass DA, Champion HC, Terrin ML, Forman S et al (2006) L-arginine therapy in acute myocardial infarction: the Vascular Interaction with Age in Myocardial Infarction (VINTAGE MI) randomized clinical trial. JAMA 295(1):58–64

Shweiki D, Itin A, Soffer D, Keshet E (1992) Vascular endothelial growth factor induced by hypoxia may mediate hypoxia-initiated angiogenesis. Nature 359:843–848

Sikorski EM, Hock T, Hill-Kapturczak N, Agarwal A (2004) The story so far: molecular regulation of the heme oxygenase-1 gene in renal injury. Am J Physiol Renal Physiol 286(3):F425–F441

Smith GC, Pell JP, Walsh D (2001) Pregnancy complications and maternal risk of ischaemic heart disease: a retrospective cohort study of 129,290 births. Lancet 357(9273):2002–2006

Staff AC, Berge L, Haugen G, Lorentzen B, Mikkelsen B, Henriksen T (2004) Dietary supplementation with L-arginine or placebo in women with pre-eclampsia. Acta Obstet Gynecol Scand 83(1):103–107

Stallmach T, Hebisch G, Orban P, Lu X (1999) Aberrant positioning of trophoblast and lymphocytes in the feto-maternal interface with pre-eclampsia. Virchows Arch 434(3):207–211

Szalai G, Xu Y, Romero R, Chaiworapongsa T, Xu Z, Chiang PJ et al (2014) In vivo experiments reveal the good, the bad and the ugly faces of sFlt-1 in pregnancy. PLoS One 9(11):e110867

Tao BB, Liu SY, Zhang CC, Fu W, Cai WJ, Wang Y et al (2013) VEGFR2 functions as an H2S-targeting receptor protein kinase with its novel Cys1045-Cys1024 disulfide bond serving as a specific molecular switch for hydrogen sulfide actions in vascular endothelial cells. Antioxid Redox Signal 19(5):448–464

Tenhunen R, Marver HS, Schmid R (1969) Microsomal heme oxygenase. Characterization of the enzyme. J Biol Chem 244(23):6388–6394

Thadhani R, Kisner T, Hagmann H, Bossung V, Noack S, Schaarschmidt W et al (2011) Pilot study of extracorporeal removal of soluble fms-like tyrosine kinase 1 in preeclampsia. Circulation 124(8):940–950

Thadhani R, Hagmann H, Schaarschmidt W, Roth B, Cingoez T, Karumanchi SA et al (2016) Removal of soluble fms-like tyrosine kinase-1 by dextran sulfate apheresis in preeclampsia. J Am Soc Nephrol 27 (3):903–913

Thomas CP, Andrews JI, Raikwar NS, Kelley EA, Herse F, Dechend R et al (2009) A recently evolved novel trophoblast-enriched secreted form of fms-like tyrosine kinase-1 variant is up-regulated in hypoxia and pre-eclampsia. J Clin Endocrinol Metab 94(7):2524–2530

Tjoa ML, Cindrova-Davies T, Spasic-Boskovic O, Bianchi DW, Burton GJ (2006) Trophoblastic oxidative stress and the release of cell-free feto-placental DNA. Am J Pathol 169(2):400–404

Tong S, Kaitu'u-Lino TJ, Onda K, Beard S, Hastie R, Binder NK et al (2015) Heme oxygenase-1 is not decreased in preeclamptic placenta and does not negatively regulate placental soluble fms-like tyrosine kinase-1 or soluble endoglin secretion. Hypertension 66(5):1073–1081

Vadillo-Ortega F, Perichart-Perera O, Espino S, Avila-Vergara MA, Ibarra I, Ahued R et al (2011) Effect of supplementation during pregnancy with L-arginine and antioxidant vitamins in medical food on pre-eclampsia in high risk population: randomised controlled trial. BMJ 342:d2901

Valbuena-Diez AC, Blanco FJ, Oujo B, Langa C, Gonzalez-Nunez M, Llano E et al (2012) Oxysterol-induced soluble endoglin release and its involvement in hypertension. Circulation 126(22):2612–2624

Veerbeek JH, Brouwers L, Koster MP, Koenen SV, van Vliet EO, Nikkels PG et al (2016) Spiral artery remodeling and maternal cardiovascular risk: the spiral artery remodeling (SPAR) study. J Hypertens 34(8):1570–1577

Venditti CC, Casselman R, Young I, Karumanchi SA, Smith GN (2014) Carbon monoxide prevents hypertension and proteinuria in an adenovirus sFlt-1 preeclampsia-like mouse model. PLoS One 9(9): e106502

Venkatesha S, Toporsian M, Lam C, Hanai J, Mammoto T, Kim YM et al (2006) Soluble endoglin contributes to the pathogenesis of preeclampsia. Nat Med 12(6):642–649

Walshe TE, Dole VS, Maharaj AS, Patten IS, Wagner DD, D'Amore PA (2009) Inhibition of VEGF or TGF-{beta} signaling activates endothelium and increases leukocyte rolling. Arterioscler Thromb Vasc Biol 29(8):1185–1192

Wang K, Ahmad S, Cai M, Rennie J, Fujisawa T, Crispi F et al (2013) Dysregulation of hydrogen sulfide producing enzyme cystathionine gamma-lyase contributes to maternal hypertension and placental abnormalities in preeclampsia. Circulation 127(25):2514–2522

Wang R, Szabo C, Ichinose F, Ahmed A, Whiteman M, Papapetropoulos A (2015) The role of H2S bioavailability in endothelial dysfunction. Trends Pharmacol Sci 36(9):568–578

Williams PJ, Bulmer JN, Searle RF, Innes BA, Robson SC (2009) Altered decidual leucocyte populations in the placental bed in pre-eclampsia and foetal growth restriction: a comparison with late normal pregnancy. Reproduction 138(1):177–184

Xia Y, Dawson VL, Dawson TM, Snyder SH, Zweier JL (1996) Nitric oxide synthase generates superoxide and nitric oxide in arginine-depleted cells leading to peroxynitrite-mediated cellular injury. Proc Natl Acad Sci U S A 93(13):6770–6774

Yachie A, Niida Y, Wada T, Igarashi N, Kaneda H, Toma T et al (1999) Oxidative stress causes enhanced endothelial cell injury in human heme oxygenase-1 deficiency. J Clin Invest 103(1):129–135

Yan H, Du J, Tang C (2004) The possible role of hydrogen sulfide on the pathogenesis of spontaneous hypertension in rats. Biochem Biophys Res Commun 313 (1):22–27

Zanardo RC, Brancaleone V, Distrutti E, Fiorucci S, Cirino G, Wallace JL (2006) Hydrogen sulfide is an endogenous modulator of leukocyte-mediated inflammation. FASEB J 20(12):2118–2120

Zenclussen ML, Linzke N, Schumacher A, Fest S, Meyer N, Casalis PA et al (2014) Heme oxygenase-1 is critically involved in placentation, spiral artery remodeling, and blood pressure regulation during murine pregnancy. Front Pharmacol 5:291

Zhang Y, Diao Z, Su L, Sun H, Li R, Cui H et al (2010) MicroRNA-155 contributes to preeclampsia by down-regulating CYR61. Am J Obstet Gynecol 202(5):466 e1–7

Zhao W, Zhang J, Lu Y, Wang R (2001) The vasorelaxant effect of H(2)S as a novel endogenous gaseous K (ATP) channel opener. Embo J 20(21):6008–6016

Zhao H, Wong RJ, Doyle TC, Nayak N, Vreman HJ, Contag CH et al (2008) Regulation of maternal and fetal hemodynamics by heme oxygenase in mice. Biol Reprod 78(4):744–751

Zhao H, Wong RJ, Kalish FS, Nayak NR, Stevenson DK (2009) Effect of heme oxygenase-1 deficiency on placental development. Placenta 30(10):861–868

Zhou Y, Damsky CH, Fisher SJ (1997) Preeclampsia is associated with failure of human cytotrophoblasts to mimic a vascular adhesion phenotype. One cause of defective endovascular invasion in this syndrome? J Clin Invest 99(9):2152–2164

Adv Exp Med Biol - Advances in Internal Medicine (2017) 2: 375–393
DOI 10.1007/5584_2016_150
© Springer International Publishing AG 2016
Published online: 13 December 2016

Hypertension in Pregnancy

Roopa Malik and Viral Kumar

Abstract

Hypertensive disorders of pregnancy remain an unresolved and unpreventable problem in obstetrics. They remain one of the leading member of deadly triad causing maternal mortality, the other two being hemorrhage and sepsis which are preventable. The incidence of hypertensive disorders worldwide is 12 %. We have discussed various terminologies used to describe hypertension during pregnancy, risk factors, etiopathogenesis, pathophysiology, management guidelines, complications and long term consequences of hypertensive disorders of pregnancy in this chapter.

Keywords

Preeclampsia • Eclampsia • Pregnancy • Hypertension

In spite of extensive research, what causes pregnancy induced hypertension remains unsolved problem in obstetrics. Preeclampsia complicates 12 % of pregnancies worldwide (Walker 2000; ACOG Committee on Obstetric Practice 2002). It remains one of the members of deadly triad-along with hemorrhage and sepsis-that leads to maternal mortality.

R. Malik (✉)
Department Obstetrics and Gynaecology, PGIMS, University of Health Sciences, Rohtak, Haryana, India
e-mail: drroopa.sangwan@gmail.com

V. Kumar
Department of Internal Medicine, PGIMS, University of Health Sciences, Rohtak, Haryana, India
e-mail: drviralsangwan@yahoo.com

1 Classification of Hypertensive Disorders of Pregnancy

As per report of American College of Obstetricians and Gynecologists Task Force on Hypertension in Pregnancy four categories have been described (American College of Obstetricians and Gynecologists, Task Force on Hypertension in Pregnancy 2013).

1. Gestational hypertension (BP elevation after 20 weeks of gestation in absence of proteinuria or any of the severe features of preeclampsia listed below)
2. Preeclampsia- eclampsia (BP elevation after 20 weeks of gestation with proteinuria or any

of the severe features of preeclampsia listed below)

3. Chronic hypertension (of any cause that predates pregnancy)
4. Chronic hypertension with superimposed pre-eclampsia (chronic hypertension in association with preeclampsia)

Importantly, this classification differentiates preeclampsia syndrome from other hypertensive disorders because it is potentially more ominous.

1.1 Gestational Hypertension

Diagnosis of gestational hypertension is made when blood pressure rises >140/90 mm Hg for the first time after 20 weeks period of gestation, but in whom proteinuria is not identified. Almost half of these women progress to develop pre-eclampsia syndrome. The blood pressure generally returns to normal by 12 weeks postpartum.

1.2 Preeclampsia Syndrome

Preeclampsia is a pregnancy specific syndrome that can affect virtually every organ system of body. Although preeclampsia has been defined traditionally as hypertension with proteinuria (National High Blood Pressure Education 2000). It has been now appreciated that overt proteinuria may not be a feature in some women with preeclampsia syndrome (Sibai and Stella 2009). Proteinuria reflects the endothelial leak which characterizes the preeclampsia syndrome.

Abnormal protein excretion has been defined as excretion of $\geq$300 mg/dl of protein in a 24-h urine collection. Alternatively, a timed excretion that is extrapolated to this 24-h urine value or a protein/creatinine ratio of at least 0.3 (each measured as mg/dl). The dipstick method is discouraged for diagnostic use in presence of other methods. 1+ is considered as cutoff for the diagnosis of proteinuria.

The diagnosis of severe preeclampsia is no longer dependent the presence of proteinuria. Massive proteinuria (>5 g) has been eliminated from consideration of preeclampsia as severe (American College of Obstetricians and Gynecologists, Task Force on Hypertension in Pregnancy 2013).

1.3 Indicators of Preeclampsia Severity

Criteria listed in Table 1 are used to classify preeclampsia syndrome as severe or non severe. Many use "mild" or "severe" classification system; the Task force (2013) discourages the use of term "mild preeclampsia".

Some symptoms are considered to be ominous. Headaches or visual disturbances such as scotoma can be premonitory symptoms of eclampsia. Epigastric pain or right upper quadrant pain accompanies hepatocellular necrosis, ischemia, and edema that stretches Glisson's capsule. This characteristic pain is frequently associated with elevated serum hepatic

Table 1 Indicators of severity of preeclampsia

Criteria	Needed
1. Hypertension	Systolic $\geq$160 or diastolic $\geq$110 on two occasions at least 4 h apart while patient is on bed rest (unless antihypertensive therapy is initiated before this time
2. Thrombocytopenia	Platelet count <100,000
3. Impaired liver function	Elevated liver transaminases to twice the normal values, severe persistent right upper quadrant or epigastric pain unresponsive to medication and not accounted for by alternative diagnoses, or both.
4. New development of renal insufficiency	Elevated serum creatinine greater than 1.1 mg/dl, or doubling of serum creatinine in absence of other renal disease.
5. Pulmonary edema	
6. New onset cerebral or visual disturbances	

Fig. 1 Massive vulval edema in a woman with severe preeclampsia

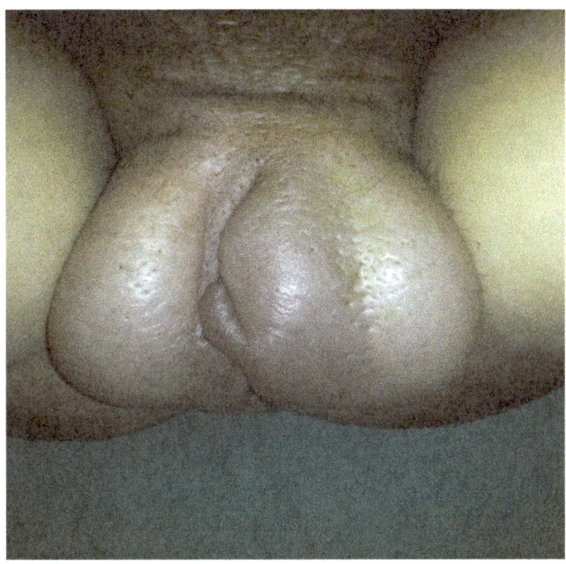

transaminases. Thrombocytopenia signifies platelet activation, aggregation and microangiopathic hemolysis. Other features of severe preeclampsia include renal or cardiac involvement. Importantly, fetal growth restriction has been removed as a finding indicative of severe preeclampsia.

1.4 Eclampsia

Preeclampsia when complicated with convulsions and/or coma is called eclampsia. Seizures are generalized tonic clonic type. They may occur before, during and after onset of labour and termed as antepartum, intapartum or postpartum eclampsia. Postpartum usually tend to occur within 48 h of delivery. However in 10 % of cases fits can occur after 48 h of delivery, termed as delayed postpartum eclampsia (Sibai 2005).

1.5 Chronic Hypertension

Chronic hypertension is defined as presence of hypertension of any cause antedating pregnancy or before 20th week of pregnancy and its presence beyond 12 weeks after delivery. The condition poses a difficult problem regarding diagnosis and management because there is fall in blood pressure during the second and early third trimesters in both normotensive and chronically hypertensive women. Even a careful search for systemic changes of hypertension may turn futile, as many of these do not have ventricular, retinal or renal changes.

1.6 Preeclampsia Superimposed on Chronic Hypertension

If baseline hypertension is accompanied by worsening, new-onset proteinuria or other symptoms listed in Table 1, then superimposed preeclampsia is diagnosed. Superimposed preeclampsia tend to occur earlier in pregnancy, more severe and often accompanied by fetal – growth restriction (Fig. 1).

2 Incidence

The incidence varies markedly with race and ethnicity e.g. in Maternal-Fetal Medicine Units (MFMU) Network study, the incidence of preeclampsia was 5 % in white, 9 % in Hispanic, and 11 % in African-American women (Myatt et al. 2012a, b). Staff and coworkers reported incidence in nulliparous women as 3–10 % (Staff et al. 2014) and somewhat lower in multiparous 1.4–4 % (Roberts et al. 2011). Incidence of eclampsia has decreased over the years in areas where prenatal care is readily available. In countries with adequate resources, incidence averages 1 in 2000 deliveries (Royal College of Obstetricians and Gynaecologists 2006).

3   Risk Factors

Hypertensive disorders are more likely to develop in women with following characteristics

- Are exposed to chorionic villi for the first time- young or elderly primigravida
- Are exposed to superabundance of chorionic villi – multiple pregnancy, hydatidiform mole
- Have preexisting conditions of endothelial activation or inflammation such as diabetes or renal or cardiovascular disease
- Are genetically predisposed to hypertension developing during pregnancy – family history of preeclampsia or hypertension, race and ethnicity
- Obesity – BMI >35 kg/m^2
- Hereditary thrombophilias – antiphospholipid antibody syndrome, protein C, protein S deficiency, Factor V Leiden mutation

Ironically, smoking has consistently been associated with a reduced risk for hypertension during pregnancy, possible mechanism may be upregulation of placental adrenomedullin expression, which regulates volume homeostasis.

4   Etiopathogenesis

Various theories have been proposed to explain pathogenesis of preeclampsia. Those currently considered important include:

1. **Abnormal trophoblastic invasion of uterine vessels –** Normal implantation is characterized by extensive remodeling of spiral arterioles within decidua basalis as well as myometrium. Endovascular trophoblasts replace the vascular endothelial and muscular lining to result in low resistance vessels. In preeclampsia, however, there is incomplete invasion, only the decidual vessels but not myometrial vessels are lined with trophoblasts resulting in high resistance vessels. Mc Mohan et al have provided evidence that decreased soluble antiangiogenic factors may be involved in faulty endovascular remodelling (McMohan et al. 2014). Nelson et al. in their study on 1200 women reported that vascular lesions including spiral arterioles narrowing, atherosis, and infarcts were common in placentas of women diagnosed with preeclampsia before 34 weeks (Nelson et al. 2014).

   Abnormally narrow spiral arterioles likely impair placental blood flow. Diminished perfusion and a hypoxic environment lead to release of placental micro particles that incite an inflammatory response.

2. **Immunological maladaptation between maternal, fetal and placental tissues-**
   Maternal immune system produces blocking antibodies against fetal and placental antigens in normal pregnancy which prevents immune rejection of fetus. Immune dysregulation is another theory cited to account for preeclampsia syndrome. Some of the factors associated with dysregulation include "Human leukocyte antigen (HLA), Natural killer (NK)- cells receptor haplotypes, and possibly shared susceptibility genes with diabetes and hypertension.

   Immune dysregulation may explain an increased risk in the first pregnancy and when paternal antigenic load is increased e.g. in molar pregnancy. Conversely, women previously exposed to paternal antigens, such as a prior pregnancy with same partner, are immunized against preeclampsia and hence protected.

3. **Endothelial Cell Activation -**
   Inresponse to placental factors released by ischemic changes, a cascade of events begins. Cytokines released from activated leukocytes such as tumour necrosis factor-α (TNF-α) and

interleukins (IL) contribute to oxidative stress associated with preeclampsia. It is characterized by reactive oxygen species and free radicals that lead to formation of self- propagating lipid peroxides which in turn generate highly toxic radicals that injure endothelial cells, modify nitric oxide production, and interfere with prostaglandin balance.

4. **Maternal genetic predisposition -**

Preeclampsia is a multifactorial, polygenic disorder. Ward and Taylor cite a 20–40 % risk of preeclampsia in daughters of preeclamptic mothers; 11–37 % in sisters of preeclamptic mothers and 22–47 % for twins (Ward and Taylor 2014).

Various genes with possible association with preeclampsia syndrome are listed in Table 2.

5. **Nutritional factors**

Role of antioxidants like vit C, vit E and Calcium have been evaluated in various studies in causation of preeclampsia. According to Task force 2013, supplementation with antioxidants vitamins C or E showed no benefits. Also, there is no role of calcium supplementation in population without deficiency of dietary calcium (American College of Obstetricians and Gynecologists, Task Force on Hypertension in Pregnancy 2013).

Table 2 Genes with possible association with preeclampsia syndrome

Gene	Function affected
MTHFR	Methylene tetrahydrofolate reductase
F5	Factor V leiden
AGT	Angiotensinogen
HLA	Human Leukocyte antigens
NOS3	Endothelial nitric oxide
F2	Prothrombin (factor II)
ACE	Angiotensin converting enzyme
CTLA4	Cytotoxic T-lymphocyte associated protein
LPL	Lipoprotein lipase
SERPINE 1	Serine peptidase inhibitor

Data from Buurma et al. (2013), Staines- Urias et al. (2012), Ward and Taylor (2014)

4.1 Pathogenesis

4.1.1 Vasospasm

Endothelial activation causes vascular constriction with increased resistance and subsequent hypertension. At the same time, endothelial damage causes interstitial leakage through which blood constituents, including platelets and fibrinogen are deposited subendothelially. With diminished blood flow ischemia of surrounding tissues causes necrosis, hemorrhage, and end organ disturbance.

4.1.2 Endothelial Cell Injury

Intact endothelium has anticoagulant properties, and endothelial cells blunt response of smooth muscle to agonists by releasing nitric oxide. In preaclampsia, placental factors are secreted into maternal circulation and provoke dysfunction of endothelium. Damaged endothelium produces less nitric oxide and secretes substances that promote coagulation and increase sensitivity to vasopresssors.

Pregnant women normally develop refractoriness to infused vasopressors. Women with preeclampsia, however have increased reactivity to infused norepinephrine and angiotensin II.

Similarly, in normal pregnancy vascular responsiveness is decreased due to endothelial prostacyclin (PGI2) production. Its synthesis is decreased in preeclampsia. At the same time thromboxane A2, a potent vasoconstrictor, secretion is increased by platelets and PGI2: TXA2 ratio decreases which favors increased sensitivity to infused angiotensin II and ultimately, vasoconstriction.

Nitric oxide, a potent vasodilator is synthesized by endothelial cells. Inhibition of nitric oxide synthesis in preeclampsia, increases mean arterial blood pressure, decreases heart rate, and reverses pregnancy associated refractoriness to vasopressors.

Endothelin 1 (Et 1) levels are increased in pregnancy but even more in preeclamptic women likely as a result of endothelial activation.

4.1.3   Angiogenic and Antiangiogenic Proteins

Angiogenic imbalance is another hypothesis to describe pathogenesis of preeclampsia. Trophoblasts of women destined to develop preeclampsia over produces anti angiogenic peptides that enter maternal circulation:

1. **Soluble Fms-like tyrosine kinase-1 (sFlt-1)** is a variant of Flt-1 receptor for placental growth factor (PIGF) and vascular endothelial growth factor (VEGF). Increased sFlt 1 levels inactivate and decrease PIGF and VEGF concentration leading to endothelial dysfunction.
2. **Soluble endoglin (sEng)**, a placenta derived molecule that blocks endoglin which is a surface coreceptor for TGFβ family. It inhibits various TGFβ isoforms from binding to endothelial receptors resulting in decreased endothelial nitric oxide dependent vasodilatation.

5   Pathophysiology

5.1   Cardiovascular System

Normal cardiovascular function is severely compromised in preeclampsia. Following changes are observed

1. Increased cardiac afterload caused by hypertension
2. Pathologically diminished hypervolemia of pregnancy
3. Endothelial activation causing interendothelial extravasation of intravascular fluid into extravascular space, especially lungs.

5.2   Myocardial Function

There is a ventricular remodellingas evidenced by diastolic dysfunction as an adaptive response to maintain normal contractility with increased afterload in preeclampsia. When combined with underlying ventricular dysfunction like concentric hypertrophy from chronic hypertension-

further diastolic dysfunction may cause cardiogenic pulmonary edema.

5.3   Ventricular Function

Both normal pregnant women and women with preeclampsia syndrome can have normal or slightly hyperdynamic ventricular function. Left ventricular filling pressures are dependent on the volume of intravenous fluids infused. Specifically, aggressive hydration results in overtly hyperdynamic ventricular function accompanied by elevated capillary wedge pressures resulting in pulmonary edema. This was compounded by endothelial- epithelial leak and decreased serum oncotic pressures from low serum albumin concentration.

5.4   Blood Volume

Hemoconcentration is a hallmark of eclampsia. Normal expected hypervolemia is severely curtailed with eclampsia. It results from generalized vasoconstriction that follows endothelial activation and leakage of plasma into interstitial space due to increased permeability. This vasospasm and endothelial leakage may persist for variable duration after delivery as endothelium is restored to normalcy. As this takes place, vasoconstriction reverses, the blood volume increases and hematocrit usually falls.

Women with preeclampsia are thus,

1. Unduly sensitive to vigorous fluid therapy resulting in pulmonary edema.
2. Are sensitive to blood loss at delivery considered normal for a normotensive woman.

5.5   Hematological Changes

5.5.1   Platelet Abnormalities

Thrombocytopenia
Overt thrombocytopenia defined by a platelet count <100,000/uL indicates severe disease.

Lower the platelet count higher the fetal and maternal morbidity and mortality. In most cases delivery is advisable as thrombocytopenia continues to worsen. After delivery platelet count declines for first 24 h but returns to normal thereafter within 3–5 days. Other causes like thrombotic microangiopathy should be ruled out if these do not reach a nadir until 48–72 h after delivery.

Other Platelet Abnormalities

Platelet bound and circulating platelet- bind ableimmunoglobulin are increased suggesting surface alteration. Platelet aggregation is decreased, compared with normal increase as in normal pregnancy, as a result of immunological processes or platelet deposition at the site of endothelial damage. Importantly, neonatal thrombocytopenia does not develop despite severe maternal thrombocytopenia so maternal thrombocytopenia is not a fetal indication of cesarean delivery.

Hemolysis

It is seen as elevated serum lactate dehydrogenase levels and decreased haptoglobin levels, schizocytosis, spherocytosis, and reticulocytosis in peripheral blood film. These changes result from microangiopathic hemolysis caused by endothelial disruption with platelet adherence and fibrin deposition. Erythrocytic membrane changes, increased adhesiveness, and aggregation may also promote hypercoagulable state.

Coagulation Changes

Increased intravascular coagulation and intravascular destruction are commonly found in preeclampsia syndrome. There is increased factor VII consumption, increased fibrinopeptides A and B, D dimers, and decreased anti thrombin III and protein C and S levels. Unless there is placental abruption, plasma fibrinogen levels do not differ remarkably from levels in normal pregnancy. Routine laboratory assessments of coagulation, including prothrombin time, activated partial thromboplastin time, and plasma fibrinogen levels are unnecessary in management of preeclampsia.

5.5.2 Fluid and Electrolyte changes

In preeclampsia the volume of extracellular fluid is much greater than that in normal pregnant women. The mechanism is thought to be endothelial injury. In addition, these women have decreased plasma oncotic pressure as a result of proteinuria.

Following a convulsion, serum pH and bicarbonate are lowered due to lactic acidosis and compensatory respiratory loss of carbon dioxide.

5.5.3 Kidney

As a result of preeclampsia renal perfusion and glomerular filtration are reduced but not much less than normal nonpregnant values. The mechanism may be due to increased renal afferent arteriolar resistance and to some extent reduced plasma volume.

Morphological changes include glomerular endotheliosis blocking filtration barrier. As already discussed these women are sensitive to intravenous fluid therapy due to risk of pulmonary edema, intensive fluid therapy for oliguria is not indicated except in diminished urine output due to hemorrhage or fluid loss from vomiting or fever.

Plasma uric acid concentration is typically elevated likely due to enhanced tubular reabsorption, increased placental urate production compensatory to increased oxidative stress.

Detection of proteinuria adds to diagnosis of preeclampsia. Proteinuria may develop late e.g. Zwart et al. did not find proteinuria in 17 % of women by the time of seizures (Zwart et al. 2008). Various methods for its estimation have already been discussed previously.

Rarely acute tubular necrosis occurs as a result of preeclampsia alone but more commonly it is induced by severe obstetrical hemorrhage for which adequate blood replacement is not given. Rarely, irreversible renal cortical necrosis develops.

5.5.4 Liver

Symptomatic involvement is considered to be a sign of severe disease. It typically manifests as moderate to severe right upper quadrant or epigastric pain and tenderness. Such women commonly have elevated levels of serum aminotransferases namely aspartate (AST) or alanine transferase (ALT). Asymptomatic elevations of serum transaminases- ALT and AST- are also considered markers for severe preeclampsia. Values seldom exceed 500 U/L but have been reported to be greater than 2000 U/L.

The characteristic lesions are periportal hemorrhage in liver periphery. Sheehan and Lynch described some degree of hepatic infarction accompanied hemorrhage in almost half of the women who died of eclampsia (Sheehan and Lynch 1973). Constellation of hemolysis, hepatocallular necrosis and thrombocytopenia was termed as HELLP syndrome by Weinstein in 1985 (Weinstein 1985).

Hemorrhagic infarction may extend to form a hepatic hematoma which in turn may extend to form a hepatic hematoma that may extend to form sub capsular rupture. Computed tomography (CT) scanning or magnetic resonance (MR) imaging may be used to identify these. Management usually consists of observation and conservative approach unless hemorrhage is ongoing where prompt surgical intervention may be lifesaving.

5.5.5 Brain

Cerebrovascular Pathophysiology

Auto regulation is the mechanism by which cerebral blood flow remains relatively constant despite alterations in cerebral perfusion pressure. This mechanism protects brain from hyper perfusion when mean arterial pressures increase to as high as 160 mm Hg, which is far greater thanthose seen in most women with eclampsia. Therefore, it was theorized that auto regulation must be altered by pregnancy.

Two theories have been proposed for the cerebrovascular changes seen in eclampsia. In the first, in response to acute and severe hypertension, cerebrovascular overregulation leads to vasospasm, diminished blood flow results in ischemia, cytotoxic edema and eventually tissue infarction. The second theory proposes that sudden elevations in systemic blood pressure exceed normal cerebrovascular autoregulatory capacity. Regions of forced vasodilation and vasoconstriction develop, especially in arterial bound zones. At the capillary level, disruption of end-capillary pressure causes increased hydrostatic pressure, hyperperfusion, and extravasation of plasma and red cells through endothelial tight-junction openings, leading to vasogenic edema. Very few eclamptic women have mean arterial pressures that exceed limits of autoregulation.

Most likely mechanism is the combination of the two. Thus, preeclampsia associated cell leak develops at a blood pressure levels much lower than those usually causing vasogenic edema and is coupled with a loss of upper-limit of autoregulation. To conclude eclampsia occurs when cerebral hyperperfusion forces capillary fluid interstitially because of endothelial damage, which leads to perivascular edema.

Manifestations

There are several neurological manifestations of preeclampsia syndrome, signifying severe involvement and immediate attention.

Headache and Scotomas

Fifty to Sixty percent of women have headaches and 20–30 % have visual changes preceding eclampsia (Sibai 2005). These are usually unresponsive to analgesic, but show improvement with magnesium sulphate therapy.

Convulsions

Diagnostic of eclampsia, convulsions may extend causing status and significant brain injury.

Visual Symptoms

Scotomas, blurred vision and diplopia are more common in severe preeclampsia and eclampsia. These usually improve with magnesium sulphate therapy. Blindness is less common and usually reversible. It is caused due to lesions at three levels visual cortex, lateral geniculate nuclei or the retina.

Occipital blindness- also called amaurosis- usually resolves completely in all cases except rarely when cerebral infarction is the cause leading to total or partial visual defects. Affected women have evidence of extensive vasogenic edema on imaging studies.

Retinal lesions- It may be due to serous retinal detachment, rarely by retinal infarction termed as, *Purtscher retinopathy*, or due to retinal artery occlusion where there may be permanent visual loss.

Direct evidence of vasoconstriction may be obtained by ophthalmologic examination. The most common findings in women with severe preeclampsia are an increase in vein to artery ratio and segmental vasospasm. Women without severe features usually have a normal fundoscopic examination. Papilloedema is not a common finding in preeclampsia and it suggests the possibility of brain tumour causing an increase in intracranial pressure. The presence of hemorrhages, exudates or extensive arteriolar changes suggests chronic hypertension.

Cerebral Edema

Widespread cerebral edema may develop which may be clinically evident ranging from lethargy, confusion, and blurred vision to coma. These women are susceptible to sudden and severe blood pressure elevations resulting in transtentorial herniation. Consideration for treatment with mannitol and dexamethasone should be given.

Posterior Reversible Leukoencephalopathy Syndrome (PRES)

Reversible posterior leukoencephalopathy syndrome is a recently proposed clinic-neuroradiological entity characterized by seizures, disorders of consciousness, visual abnormalities and headache associated with predominantly white matter changes on computerized tomography head and magnetic resonance imaging. This is a rare encephalopathy condition, where the diagnosis depends on clinical and radiological features. It is rare but now being recognized more often. The lesions of posterior leukoencephalopathy are best visualized with magnetic resonance imaging however computed tomography can also be used satisfactorily to detect hypo dense lesions of posterior leukoencephalopathy. T2 weighted MR images characteristically show diffuse hyper intensity selectively involving the parieto-occipital white matter, occasionally the lesions also involve grey matter. They may also involve other brain areas. In most cases these lesions are reversible (Fig. 2).

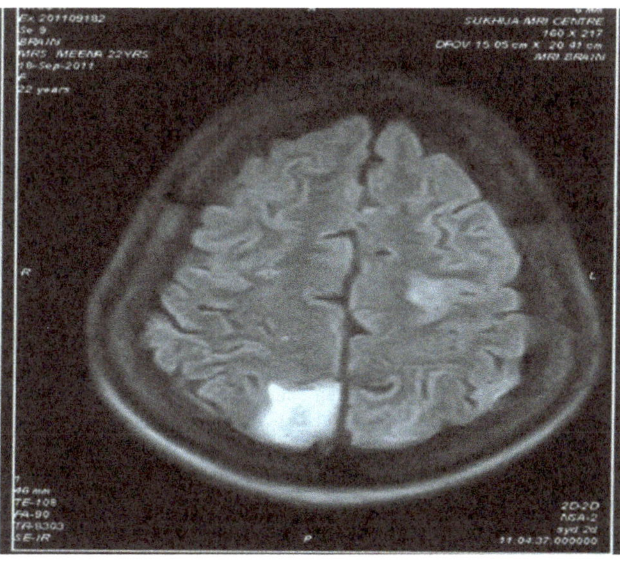

Fig. 2 MR Imaging showing posterior reversible encephalopathy syndrome in a woman with severe preeclampsia, she presented with cortical blindness which resolved following cesarean section

5.6 Prediction and Prevention

A good test for predicting women who will develop preeclampsia should be simple, rapid, noninvasive, inexpensive, easy to perform, and should not expose the patient to discomfort or risk. The technology should be widely available and the results reproducible and reliable, with a high likelihood ratio for a positive test and a low likelihood ratio for a negative result and good sensitivity and specificity. Ideally, it should provide an opportunity for intervention to prevent development of the disease, or at least result in better maternal and/or fetal outcomes.

The ability to predict preeclampsia is currently of limited benefit because neither the development of the disorder nor its progression from the mild to the severe spectrum of disease can be prevented in most patients, nor there is cure except delivery. Nevertheless, the accurate identification of women at risk, early diagnosis, and prompt and appropriate management may improve maternal outcome, and possibly perinatal outcome, as well. Various biological, biochemical and biophysical markers have been proposed to predict its development. Attempts have been made to identify markers of faulty placentation, impaired placental perfusion, endothelial cell activation and dysfunction, and activation of coagulation.

Currently, there are no clinically available tests that perform well in distinguishing women who will develop preeclampsia from those who will not. A detailed medical history to evaluate for risk factors is currently the best and only recommended screening approach for preeclampsia; it should remain the method of screening for preeclampsia until studies show that aspirin or other interventions reduce the incidence of preeclampsia for women at high risk based on first-trimester predictive tests (Table 3).

5.7 Prevention

Various methods have been studied worldwide to prevent onset of preeclampsia, some of these are listed in Table 4. In general, none have been proved to be beneficial convincingly. Of the mentioned strategies, calcium supplementation may have a role in preeclampsia prevention in calcium deficient women (Staff et al. 2014). Low dose aspirin in the doses of 50–150 mg daily

Table 3 Tests for prediction of development of preeclampsia

Related to	*Examples*
Placental perfusion/vascular resistance	Roll-over test, isometric handgrip or cold pressor test, pressor response to aerobic exercise, angiotensin-II infusion, midtrimester mean arterial pressure, platelet angiotensin-II binding, renin, 24- h ambulatory blood pressure monitoring, uterine artery or fetal transcranial Doppler velocimetry
Fetal-placental unit endocrine dysfunction	Human chorionic gonadotropin (HCG), alpha-fetoprotein (AFP), estriol, pregnancy associated protein A (PPAP A), inhibin A, activin A, placental protein 13, corticotrophin – releasing hormone, A disintegrin, ADAM-12, kisspeptin
Renal dysfunction	Serum uric acid, microalbuminuria, urinary calcium or kallikrein, microtransferrinuria, N-acetyl-β-glucosaminidase, cystatin C, podocyturia
Endothelial dysfunction/ oxidant stress	Platelet count and activation, fibronectin, endothelial adhesion molecules, prostaglandins, prostacyclin, MMP-9, thromboxane, C- reactive protein, cytokines, endothelin, neurokinin B, homocystein, lipids, insulin resistance, antiphopholipid antibodies, plasminogen activator inhibitor (PAI), leptin, p-selectin, angiogenic factors such as placental growth factors (PIGF), vascular endothelial growth factor (VEGF), fms- like tyrosine kinase receptor-1 (sFlt −1), endoglin
Others	Antithrombin III (AT 3), atrial natriuretic peptide (ANP), β2-microglobulin, haptoglobin, transferring, 25- hydroxyvitamin D, genetic markers, cell-free DNA, serum and urine proteomics and metabolomic markers, hepatic aminotransferases

ADAM 12 ADAM metallopeptidase domain 12, *MMP* matrix metalloproteinase
Adapted from Conde-Augudelo et al. (2014)

Table 4 Methods evaluated in various studies to prevent preeclampsia

Bed rest	
Dietary manipulation	Low sodium diet, calcium or fish oil supplementation
Exercise	Physical activity, stretching excercises
Cardiovascular drugs	Diuretics, antihypertensive drugs, statins
Antioxidants	Ascorbic acid (vitamin C), α- tocopherol (vitamin E), vitamin D
Antithrombotic agents	Low dose asprin, asprin/dipyridamole, aspirin + heparin, aspirin + ketanserin

have shown promising results in some of the trials like the Paris Collaborative Group performed meta-analysis including 31 randomized controlled trials (Askie et al. 2007). For women assigned to receive antiplatelet agents, the relative risk for development of preeclampsia, superimposed preeclampsia, preterm delivery and any adverse pregnancy outcome was significantly decreased by 10 %. The 2013 Task Force recommended use of low does aspirin in some high- risk women to prevent preeclampsia (American College of Obstetricians and Gynecologists, Task Force on Hypertension in Pregnancy 2013). Regarding usage of both low dose aspirin and heparin for prevention of preeclampsia, there is still insufficient evidence to support its use (Staff et al. 2014). Rest all methods have shown no benefit in reducing the risk of preeclampsia.

6 Management

The basic management goals for any pregnancy complicated with preeclampsia are:

1. Termination of pregnancy with least possible trauma to mother and fetus
2. Birth of an infant who subsequently thrives and
3. Complete restoration of health to the mother

Frequent antenatal visits during third trimester aids in early diagnosis and timely management of preeclampsia. This frequency should be increased in women in whom preeclampsia is suspected like women with new-onset diastolic blood pressure >80 mm Hg but <90 mm Hg or with sudden weight gain more than 2 pounds per week.

6.1 Hospitalization

There is no role of domiciliary treatment in an established case of preeclampsia. Hospitalization is considered necessary at least initially for new onset hypertension, especially if there is persistent or worsening hypertension or development of proteinuria. However, in some centers cases of mild preeclampsia are managed in day care centers. It is essential that she should be warned against the ominous symptoms such as headache, visual disturbance, vomiting, epigastric pain or scanty urine.

6.2 Evaluation

- Detailed physical examination followed by daily scrutiny for clinical findings such as headache, visual disturbance, epigastric pain and decreased urine output.
- Daily maternal weight
- Daily fetal kick count
- Blood pressure every 4 hrly in sitting position with appropriate size cuff except during night
- Analysis for proteinuria or urine protein-creatinine ratio twice weekly
- Complete hemogram including platelet count, liver transaminases and plasma creatinine levels. Frequency of testing depends on severity of preeclampsia. Task force recommends weekly testing in women with preeclamsia without severe features (American College of Obstetricians and Gynecologists, Task Force on Hypertension in Pregnancy 2013). Some recommend serum uric acid and lactate dehydrogenase levels and coagulation studies. However, value of these tests has been called to question (Conde-Augudelo et al. 2014).

- Evaluation of fetal well being with gravidogram and sonography.

Goals of management include early identification of worsening preeclampsia and timely delivery.

Restricted physical activity throughout the day is likely to be beneficial but as Task force, 2013 has recommended absolute bed rest is not desirable. There is no role of fluid and salt restriction. Ample proteins and calories should be included in diet.

Further management depends on

1. Preeclampsia severity
2. Gestational age of fetus
3. Condition of cervix.

6.3 Timing of Delivery

The treatment of preeclampsia is termination of pregnancy. The prime objective of management of preeclampsia is to avoid convulsions, to prevent serious maternal complications and to deliver a healthy newborn. When the fetus is preterm, the tendency is to gain some time hoping that a few more weeks in utero will reduce the risk of neonatal death and serious morbidity due to prematurity. Such a policy is justifiable only in cases of mild preeclampsia. Assessments of fetal and maternal well-being are performed repeatedly while conservative treatment. Tests for fetal well being include the non stress test and biophysical profile. If evidence of fetal growth restriction is suspected on clinical examination fetoplacental assessment that includes umbilical artery Doppler velocimetry as an adjunct antenatal test is recommended by task force (American College of Obstetricians and Gynecologists, Task Force on Hypertension in Pregnancy 2013).Measurement of lecithin-sphingomyelin (L/S) ratio in amniotic fluid may provide evidence of lung maturity. The task force recommends expectant management with fetal and maternal monitoring in women with mild preeclampsia without any severe features and no indication of delivery at less than 37 weeks

of gestation. Delivery rather than continued observation is suggested in mild preeclampsia when gestation is more than 37 weeks(American College of Obstetricians and Gynecologists, Task Force on Hypertension in Pregnancy 2013).

With severe preeclampsia that does not improve with hospitalization delivery is usually advisable for well being of both mother as well as fetus. This is true even when the cervix is unfavorable. Task force recommends delivery after initial maternal stabilization in women with severe preeclampsia at or beyond 34 weeks of gestation, and in those with unstable maternal or fetal conditions irrespective of gestational age. Expectant management is also not recommended in women with severe preeclampsia before fetal viability i.e. 23 weeks. For women with slightly more advanced gestation, 24–32 weeks, however the decision is less clear. Serious maternal complications like placental abruption, HELLP syndrome, pulmonary edema, eclampsia, acute renal failure are common in such an approach.

The decision of delivery is not based on amount of proteinuria or change in amount of proteinuria.

6.4 Corticosteroids

Corticosteroids can be administered and delivery deferred for 48 h if maternal and fetal condition remain stable for women with severe preeclampsia and a viable fetus at 34 weeks or less of gestation with any of the following:

1. Preterm premature rupture of membranes
2. Labor
3. Low platelet count ($<100,000$)
4. Persistently elevated liver enzymes (twice or more the upper normal values)
5. Fetal growth restriction
6. Severe oligohydramnios (AFI < 5 cm)
7. Reversed end-diastolic flow on Doppler studies
8. New onset renal dysfunction or increasing renal dysfunction

Table 5 Magnesium sulphate dosage schedule for severe preeclampsia and eclampsia

Continuous Intravenous (IV) Infusion
4–6 g loading dose as 20 % solution administered over 15–20 min.
Followed by 2 g/h in 100 ml of iv maintenance infusion. Some recommend 1 g/h.
Monitor for magnesium toxicity:
Assess deep tendon reflexes periodically
Respiratory rate, >12/min
Urine output the previous 4 h exceeded 100 ml
Some measure serum magnesium level at 4–6 h, maintain between 4 and 7 mEq/L (4.8–8.4 mg/dl)
Measure serum magnesium levels if serum creatinine ≥1.0 mg/dl.
Intermittent Intramuscular Injections
4 g of magnesium sulphate as a 20 % solution intravenously at a rate not exceeding 1 g/min
Followed by 10 g of 50 % magnesium sulphate solution, half (5 g) in each buttock deep intramuscular. If convulsion persists after 15 min, give upto 2 g more iv as 20 % solution and if women is large upto 4 g may be given slowly.
Thereafter every 4 h, give 5 g of 50 % solution injected deep intramuscularly in alternate buttocks, only after ensuring no magnesium toxicity. Check for magnesium toxicity as mentioned above.
To be discontinued 24 h after delivery or last fit whichever is later.

Corticosteroids may be administered if the fetus is viable and at 34 weeks or less of gestation, but delivery not delayed after initial maternal stabilization regardless of gestational age for women with severe preeclampsia that is complicated with any of the following

1. Uncontrolled severe hypertension
2. Eclamsia
3. Pulmonary edema
4. Abruption placentae
5. Disseminated intravascular coagulation
6. Evidence of nonreassuring fetal status
7. Intrapartum fetal demise

For women with HELLP syndrome with gestational age 32–34 weeks, if maternal and fetal condition permits delivery may be delayed for 24–48 h to complete a course of corticosteroids for fetal benefit. For women before gestational age of fetal viability and after 34 weeks or more, delivery should be undertaken shortly after initial maternal stabilization.

6.5 Eclampsia

Preeclampsia complicated with generalized tonic clonic convulsions is termed as eclampsia. In recent years, the incidence of postpartum eclampasia has risen, this may be presumably due to improved access to prenatal care, earlier detection of preeclampsia, and prophylactic use of magnesium sulphate. Maternal mortality rate approximates 1 % in women with eclampsia even in developed countries (Thorton et al. 2013).

Eclamptic seizures may rarely continue unabated-status epilepticus, or when convulsions are infrequent woman be regain some consciousness after each attack or very rarely may pass on to comatose state. Importantly, other diagnoses should be considered in women with convulsions more than 48 h postpartum or in women with focal neurological deficits, prolonged coma, or atypical eclampsia (Sibai 2012) (Table 5).

6.6 Antihypertensive Therapy

Severe hypertension can cause cerebrovascular hemorrhage, hypertensive encephalopathy, after load congestive heart failure, placental abruption and eclamptic seizures in women with preeclamsia.

Because of these dangerous sequels, National High Blood Pressure Education Program Working Group (National High Blood Pressure Education Program 2000) and the Task Force 2013 (American College of Obstetricians and Gynecologists, Task Force on Hypertension in Pregnancy 2013) recommend treatment to lower systolic blood pressure to or below 160 mm of Hg and diastolic pressures to or below 110 mm of Hg.

Several drugs are available to rapidly lower dangerously elevated blood pressure namely labetalol, hydralazine and nifedepin.

Name	Dose	Mechanism of action	Side effects
Hydralazine	5 mg intravenously initial dose followed by 5–10 mg doses at 15–20 min intervals until a satisfactory response (American College of Obstetricians and Gynecologists 2002).	Arterial dilator	Maternal tachycardia, palpitations and hypotension and fetal heart decelerations.
Labetalol	10 mg intravenously initial dose followed by 20 mg at 10 min interval followed by 40 mg and another 40 mg at 10 min interval. If salutary response not achieved, then 80 mg can be given, maximum 220 mg per treatment cycle.	α 1 and β blocker	Maternal hypotension, bradycardia and fetal heart declerations.
Nifedepin	10 mg oral initial dose to be repeated at every 30 min intervals if necessary, max dose 120 mg/day (National High Blood Pressure Education Program 2000)	Ca channel blocker	Maternal tachycardia, hypotension, fetal bradycardia

6.7 Alpha Methyl Dopa

For women with preeclampsia α Methyl Dopa, a centrally acting antihypertensive agent can be used. It is metabolized to alpha-methylnorepinephrine in the brain and activates central alpha-2 adrenergic receptors which appear to inhibit sympathetic nervous system output and lower blood pressure. It is metabolized in the liver and is excreted in urine. Usual dosage is 500–2000 mg per day in 2–4 divided dosage. Onset of action is 12–24 h after oral intake.

Use of angiotensin-converting enzyme inhibitors, angiotensin receptor blockers, renin inhibitors and mineralocorticoid receptor antagonists is not recommended.

6.8 Diuretics

Loop diuretics can further compromise placental perfusion which is already reduced compared to normal pregnancy therefore not used to lower blood pressure. Antepartum use is restricted solely to treat pulmonary edema.

6.9 Fluid Therapy

Lactated Ringer solution should be administered at a rate of 60–80 ml per hour. Infusion of larger amounts increases risk of pulmonary and cerebral edema except unless there is unusual fluid loss from vomiting, diarrhea, or post partum hemorrhage. For labor analgesia with neuraxial analgesia, crystalloid solutions are infused slowly in graded amounts.

6.10 Invasive Hemodynamic Monitoring

American College of Obstetricians and Gynaecologists (2013) recommends against routine invasive monitoring. It notes that such monitoring should be reserved only for severely preeclamptic women with accompanying severe cardiac disease, renal disease, or both or in cases of refractory hypertension, oliguria, and pulmonary edema.

6.11 Magnesium Sulphate

The largest comparative study, MAGnesium-Sulphate for Prevention of Eclampsia, reported by MAGPIE Trial Collaboration Group, 2002 that included 10,000 women with severe preeclampsia from 33 countries were randomly allocated to treatment with magnesium sulphate or placebo (Magpie Trial Collaboration Group 2002). Women with magnesium had 58-% lower risk of eclampsia than those given placebo.

The 2013 Task Force recommends that women with either eclampsia or severe preeclampsia should be given magnesium sulphate prophylaxis. At the same time, it also suggests that all women with "mild" preeclampsia do not need magnesium sulphate prophylaxis. For women with preeclampsia undergoing cesarean delivery continued intraoperative administration of magnesium sulphate to prevent eclampsia is recommended (American College of Obstetricians and Gynecologists, Task Force on Hypertension in Pregnancy 2013).

6.12 Route of Delivery

The route of delivery should be determined by fetal gestation, presentation, cervical status, and maternal and fetal condition. Vaginal route of delivery is attempted initially as serious morbidity is less common during purperium following vaginal route. Following seizure, labour often ensues spontaneously or can be induced successfully even in women remote from term. Labour induction is carried out, usually with preinduction cervical ripening with a prostaglandin. Whenever it appears that induction will not succeed or attempts have failed, cesarean delivery is indicated.

6.13 Blood Loss at Delivery

Hemoconcentration is a constant feature of severe preeclampsia-eclampsia. Women with severe preeclampsia are much less tolerant to even normal blood loss than are normotensive pregnant women. It is important to recognize that appreciable fall in blood pressure soon after delivery most often means excessive blood loss and not sudden resolution of vasospasm and endothelial damage. If identified, hemorrhage should be treated promptly with careful crystalloid and blood transfusion.

6.14 Anaesthesia and Analgesia

General anaesthesia has been disregarded as favored anaesthesia in women with preeclampsia as tracheal intubation may be particularly difficult and thus hazardous in women with tracheal edema. Moreover, stimulation of trachea can cause sudden severe hypertension, in turn; can cause pulmonary edema, cerebral edema, or intracranial hypertension (American College of Obstetrician and Gynecologists 2002). The use of conduction neuraxial analgesia (either spinal or epidural) has proven ideal but the problem with this method included hypotension and diminished uterine perfusion caused by sympathetic blockade. Slow induction epidural analgesia with dilute solutions of anaesthetic agents to counter need for rapid infusion of large volumes of crystalloid or colloid to correct maternal hypotension can mitigate pulmonary edema.

6.15 Lactation and Contraception

Preeclampsia itself is not itself a contraindication for breastfeeding, the use of antihypertensive drugs may be an issue for lactating women. Methyldopa is excreted in human milk in concentrations that probably do not cause any harm to the breastfed baby. However, methyl dopa should be avoided in women at risk of depression. Labetalol, is excreted only in small amounts therefore can be safely given during puerperium. Beta blockers, propanalol, atenolol and metoprolol are excreted in very less amount but baby should be monitored for symptoms of beta blockade. Calcium channel blockers, nifedepine and verapamil although excreted in very small amounts and are unlikely to be harmful. Ace inhibitors enalapril and captopril can be used when first choice agents cannot be used or are ineffective. Vasodilators like hydralazine can be used during puerperium. Diuretics should be avoided in preeclamptic breastfeeding women or expressing milk (Breastfeeding 2011). Exclusive breast feeding is recommended in patients of preeclamsia. Magnesium sulphate therapy is not a contraindication to breast feeding. Bromocriptine should be avoided for milk suppression. The best contraceptive strategy is only-progestin contraception or non-hormonal contraceptive use. The advice for contraception should be guided by the persistence of hypertension in postpartum period. Women in whom blood pressure has returned to normal in postpartum period, there seems to be no reason of denying her the benefits of combined oral contraceptives provided adequate and continuing supervision is available. Women with thrombophilia including antiphospholipid antibody syndrome should avoid estrogen containing contraceptives.

6.16 Persistent Severe Postpartum Hypertension

The potential problem of antihypertensive therapy causing severe compromise of uteroplacental perfusion and thus fetal well-being is obviated by delivery. Oral regimens using other antihypertensive agents can be given for example, labetalol or another β- blocker, nifedepine or other Ca channel blocker, and thiazide or furosemide diuretic. Refractory hypertension is likely due to mobilization of pathological interstitial fluid and redistribution into intravenous compartment, underlying chronic hypertension, or usually both. For women in whom gestational hypertension, preeclampsia, or superimposed preeclampsia is diagnosed task

force suggests that blood pressure be monitored for72 h postpartum and again 7–10 days after delivery or earlier with symptoms (American College of Obstetricians and Gynecologists, Task Force on Hypertension in Pregnancy 2013). Parentral magnesium sulphate should be administered in women with postpartum severe hypertension.

6.17 Counseling for Future pregnancy

Women who have had either gestational hypertension or preeclampsia are at greater risk to develop hypertension in future pregnancy and this risk increases if preeclampsia is early onset in index pregnancy (Bramham et al. 2011). The risk of subsequent preterm delivery and fetal growth restriction is increased even in subsequent normotensive pregnancies (Connealy et al. 2013) and the converse also holds true i.e. preterm birth and fetal growth restriction in first pregnancy significantly increases the risk of preeclampsia in second pregnancy.

Preconceptional counseling and assessment, modifiable activities like weight loss, increased physical activity should be encouraged. Preexisting hypertension and diabetes should be brought to best possible control. Folic acid supplementation and consideration for low-dose aspirin in upcoming pregnancy should be done.

7 Long-Term Consequences

7.1 Cardiovascular Consequences

The Working Group concluded that hypertension attributable to pregnancy should resolve within 12 weeks of delivery (National High Blood Pressure Education Program 2000). Persistence beyond this time is considered to be chronic hypertension. Current evidences suggest that the risk for long term cardiovascular morbidity is significantly increased in preeclamptic women.

In a Swedish population study of more than 40,000 nulliparas delivered between 1973 and 1982, increased incidence of ischemic heart disease was found with prior pregnancy associated hypertension (Wikstrom et al. 2005). The risk in later life was increased for hypertension, ischemic heart disease, stroke, venous thromboembolism, and all- causemortality. As emphasized by several investigators, other cofactors or co morbidities are related to acquisition of these long term adverse outcomes (Gastric et al. 2012; Spaan et al. 2012). Lifestyle modification (maintenance of a healthy weight, increased physical activity and smoking cessation) are recommended. In women with h/o recurrent and early onset preeclampsia yearly BP, fasting blood glucose and BMI should be done.

7.2   Renal Squeals

In a Norwegian study, although absolute risk of renal failure was small, preeclampsia was associated with a fourfold increased risk (Vikse et al. 2008). Women with recurrent preeclampsia had an even greater risk.

7.3   Neurological Squeals

Until recently it was believed that eclamptic seizures have no significant long term squeals. But now, it has been seen that it is not always the case. Aukes et al., 2009have reported long term persistence of brain white-matter lesions that were incurred during eclamptic seizures (Aukes et al. 2009). These investigators later also observed these white matter lesions in preeclamptic women without convulsions (Aukes et al. 2012). Aukes and colleagues (2007) reported that formerly eclamptic women had subjectively impaired cognitive functioning, impaired sustained attention compared to their normotensive controls (Aukes et al. 2007). Because there were no studies done before these women suffered preeclampsia or eclampsia, the investigators concluded that cause versus effect of these white-matter lesions remains unknown.

8   Chronic Hypertension and Superimposed Preeclampsia

Referral to a physician with expertise in treating hypertension to direct the workup is suggested. Women with poorly controlled BP, home BP monitoring are suggested. Weight loss and extremely low sodium (<100 mEq/d) diet should not be used for managing chronic hypertension in pregnancy. For women accustomed to exercises and in whom BP is well controlled moderate exercises can be continued throughout the pregnancy. Indications of starting antihypertensive therapy and goals of treatment are same as in preeclampsia. Choice of antihypertensive therapy is same uncomplicated chronic hypertension as in preeclampsia. Use of angiotensin receptor blockers, renin inhibitors, and mineralocorticoid receptor antagonists is not recommended unless there is compelling reason such as presence of proteinuric renal disease. Use of corticosteroids for fetal lung maturity in women at less than 34 weeks of gestation is recommended. Administration of daily low dose aspirin (60–80 mg) beginning in late first trimester for prevention of adverse pregnancy outcomes such as early onset preeclampsia, preterm delivery and intrauterine growth retardation is recommended. Ultrasonography and Doppler velocimetry as an adjunct test to screen for fetal growth restriction is recommended. Termination of pregnancy before 38 weeks is not recommended in uncomplicated cases. Indications of preterm termination are same as in preeclampsia. For women with superimposed preeclampsia with severe features treatment should be done in facilities with maternal and fetal intensive care resources. And expectant management beyond 34 weeks of gestation is not recommended (American College of Obstetricians and Gynecologists, Task Force on Hypertension in Pregnancy 2013).

References

ACOG Committee on Obstetric Practice (2002) Diagnosis and management of preeclampsia and eclampsia. ACOG Practice Bulletin No. 33. American College of Obstetricians and Gynaecologists. ObstetGynecol 99:159–167

American College of Obstetrician and Gynecologists (2002) Obstetric analgesia and anaesthesia. Practice bulletin No. 36, July 2002, Reaffirmed 2013d.

American College of Obstetricians and Gynecologists (2002) Diagnosis and management of preeclampsia-eclampsia. Practice Bulletin No. 33. January 2002, Reaffirmed 2012b.

American College of Obstetricians and Gynecologists, Task Force on Hypertension in Pregnancy (2013) Hypertension in pregnancy. Report of the ACOG Task Force on Hypertension in Pregnancy. Obstetrics and Gynaecology 122:1122

Askie LM, Henderson-Smart DJ, Stewart LA (2007) Antiplatelet agents for the prevention of preeclampsia: a meta-analysis of individual data. Lancet 369:179

Aukes AM, Wessel I, Dubois AM et al (2007) Self reported cognitive functioning in formerly eclamptic women. Am J Obstet Gynecol 197(4):365.e1

Aukes AM, de Groot JC, Aarnoudse JG et al (2009) Brain lesions several years after eclampsia. Am J Obstet Gynecol 200(5):504.e1

Aukes AM, de Groot JC, Weigman MJ et al (2012) Long-term cerebral imaging after preeclampsia. BJOG 119 (9):1117

Bramham K, Briley AL, Seed P et al (2011) Adverse maternal and perinatal outcomes in women with previous preeclampsia: a prospective study. Am J Obstet Gynecol 204(6):512.e1

Breastfeeding (2011) Hypertension in pregnancy: the management of hypertensive disorders during pregnancy. Nice clinical guidelines, No 107. RCOG

Buurma AJ, Turner RJ, Driessen JH et al (2013) Genetic variants in preeclampsia: a meta analysis. Hum Reprod Update 19(3):289

Committee Opinion No. 638 (2015) First-trimester risk assessment for early-onset preeclampsia. Obstet Gynecol 126(3):e25-7

Conde-Augudelo A, Romero R, Roberts JM (2014) Tests to predict preeclampsia. In: Taylor RN, Roberts JM, Cunningham FG (eds) Chesley's hypertensive disorders in pregnancy, 4th edn. Academic Press, Amsterdem

Connealy B, Carrreno C, Kase B et al (2013) A history of prior preeclampsia is a major risk factor for preterm birth. Abstract No. 619. Am J Obstet Gynecol 208 (1 Suppl):S264

Gastric MD, Gandhi SK, Pantazopoulos J et al (2012) Cardiovascular outcomes after preeclampsia or eclampsia complicated by myocardial infarction or stroke. Obstet Gynecol 120(4):823

Magpie Trial Collaboration Group (2002) Do women with preeclampsia, and their babies, benefit from magnesium sulphate? The Magpie Trial: a randomized placebo-controlled trial. Lancet 359:1877

McMohan K, Karumanchi SA, Dammann O et al (2014) Does soluble fms-like tyrosine kinase-1 regulate placental invasion? Insight from the invasive placenta. Am J Obstet Gynaecol 10:66.e1

Myatt L, Clifton RG, Roberts JM et al (2012a) First trimester prediction of preeclampsia in nulliparous women at low risk. Obstet Gynecol 119:6

Myatt L, Clifton RG, Roberts JM et al (2012b) The utility of uterine artery Doppler velocimetry in prediction of preeclampsia in a low risk population. Obstet Gynecol 120(4):815

National High Blood Pressure Education Program (2000) Working group report on high blood pressure in pregnancy. Am J Obstet Gynecol 183:51

Nelson DB, Ziadie MS, McIntire DD et al (2014) Placental pathology suggesting that preeclampsia is more than one disease. Am J Obstet Gynaecol 210:66.e1

Roberts CL, Ford JB, Algert CS et al (2011) Population based trends in pregnancy hypertension and preeclampsia: an international comparative study. BMJ Open 1(1):e000101

Royal College of Obstetricians and Gynaecologists (2006) The management of severe preeclampsia. RCOG Guideline 10A:1

Sheehan HL, Lynch JB (eds) (1973) Cerebral lesions. In: Patholgyof toxemia of pregnancy. Williams & Wilkins, Baltimore

Sibai BM (2005) Diagnosis, prevention, and management of eclampsia. Obstet Gynecol 105:402

Sibai BM (2012) Etiology and management of postpartum hypertension-preeclampsia. Am J Obstet Gynecol 206 (6):470

Sibai BM, Stella CL (2009) Diagnosis and management of atypical preeclampsia-eclampsia. Am J Obstet Gynecol 200:481.e1

Spaan JJ, Sep SJS, Lope van Balen V et al (2012) Metabolic syndrome as a risk factor for hypertension after preeclampsia. Obstet Gynecol 120(2 Pt 1):311

Staff AC, Sibai BM, Cunningham FG (2014) Prevention of preeclampsia and eclampsia. In: Taylor RN, Roberts JM, Cunningham FG (eds) Chesley's hypertensive disorders in pregnancy. Acedemic Press, Amsterdam

Stains-Urias E, Paez MC, Doyle P et al (2012) Genetic association studies in preeclampsia; systemic meta-analyses and field synopsis. Int J Epidemiol 41 (6):1764

Thorton C, Dahlen H, Korda A et al (2013) The incidence of preeclampsia and eclampsia and associated maternal mortality in Australia from population-linked datasets: 2000–2008. Am J Obstet Gynecol 208(6):476.e1

Vikse BE, Irgens LM, Leivestad T et al (2008) Preeclampsia and the risk of end-stage renal disease. N Engl J Med 359:800

Walker JJ (2000) Pre-eclampsia. Lancet 356:1260–5

Ward K, Taylor RN (2014) Genatic factors in etiology of preeclampsia. In: Taylor RN, Roberts JM, Cunningham FG (eds) Chesley's hypertensive disorders in pregnancy, 4th edn. Acedemic Press, Amsterdam

Weinstein L (1985) Preeclampsia- eclampsia with hemolysis, elevated liver enzymes and thrombocytopenia. Obstet Gynecol 66:657

Wikstrom AK, Haglund B, Olovsson M et al (2005) The risk of maternal ischemic heart disease after gestational hypertensive disease. BJOG 112:1486

Zwart JJ, Richters A, Ory F et al (2008) Eclampsia in The Netherlands. Obstet Gynecol 112:820

Adv Exp Med Biol - Advances in Internal Medicine (2017) 2: 395–407
DOI 10.1007/5584_2016_81
© Springer International Publishing AG 2016
Published online: 9 October 2016

Chronic Hypertension and Pregnancy

Luís Guedes-Martins

Abstract

Chronic hypertension is frequently encountered during pregnancy and needs to be distinguished from other hypertensive complications of pregnancy, such as preeclampsia and gestational hypertension. The prevalence of this pregnancy complication is attributable to the increased prevalence of obesity and maternal age at childbearing. Women with chronic arterial hypertension are at increased risk for several pregnancy complications, including superimposed preeclampsia, caesarean delivery, preterm delivery <37 weeks gestation, birth weight <2500 g, neonatal unit admission, and perinatal death. Therefore, specialized attention should be given to these women as part of family planning before conception to provide counseling about the pregnancy risks, to inform about surveillance of fetal well-being, to determine the timing of delivery, and to optimize BP control before, during, and after birth.

Keywords

Chronic arterial hypertension • Blood pressure • Pregnancy

Abbreviations

L. Guedes-Martins (✉)
Department of Experimental Biology, Faculty of Medicine, University of Porto, 4200-319 Porto, Portugal

Instituto de Investigação e Inovação em Saúde, Universidade do Porto, 4200-319 Porto, Portugal

Departamento da Mulher e da Medicina Reprodutiva, Centro Hospitalar do Porto EPE, Largo Prof. Abel Salazar, 4099-001 Porto, Portugal
e-mail: luis.guedes.martins@gmail.com

ACE	Angiotensin converting enzyme
ACOG	American College of Obstetricians and Gynecologists
ARB	angiotensin II receptor blockers
BP	blood pressure
CHIPS	Control of Hypertension in Pregnancy Study
cHT	chronic arterial hypertension

CI	confidence interval
DASH	Dietary Approaches to Stop Hypertension
FDA	Food and Drug Administration
HT	Hypertension
JNC-8	Eighth Joint National Committee
NHBPEP	National High Blood Pressure Education Program's
OR	odds ratio
PE	preeclampsia
RR	relative risk
SGA	Small for gestational age.

1 Definition and Epidemiology

Hypertensive disorders are important medical conditions during pregnancy and are a major cause of maternal and perinatal morbidity and mortality. In general, hypertension (HT) complicates 8–10 % of pregnancies and can lead to serious maternal and fetal complications (Zetterström et al. 2005, 2006; Lawler et al. 2007; Heshmati et al. 2013; Seely and Ecker 2014).

During pregnancy, four major hypertensive disorders are recognized: (1) preeclampsia-eclampsia; (2) gestational hypertension; (3) chronic hypertension; and (4) chronic hypertension with superimposed preeclampsia (Table 1). All hypertensive subtypes can lead to serious perinatal complications, although preeclampsia is that with the highest maternal and fetal risks (Leon et al. 2016; Lecarpentier et al. 2013; Sibai et al. 2011; Livingston et al. 2003; Sibai 2002).

Chronic arterial hypertension (cHT) complicates approximately 2–5 % of pregnancies (Lawler et al. 2007; Seely and Ecker 2014; Savitz et al. 2014) and, in pregnant women, is defined as blood pressure (BP) $\geq$ 140 mmHg systolic and/or 90 mmHg diastolic before pregnancy or developing before 20 weeks of gestation, use of antihypertensive medications before pregnancy, or persistence of hypertension for more than 12 weeks after delivery (The

Table 1 The American College of Obstetricians and Gynecologists (ACOG) classification of hypertension during pregnancy (The American College of Obstetricians and Gynecologists 2013)

Classification	Definition
Preeclampsia/Eclampsia	Occurrence of new-onset hypertension plus new-onset proteinuria. In the absence of proteinuria, PE is diagnosed as HT in association with thrombocytopenia (<100.000/microliter), impaired liver function (elevated blood levels of liver transaminases to twice the normal concentration), the new development of renal insufficiency (elevated serum creatinine greater than 1.1 mg/dL or a doubling of serum creatinine in the absence or other renal disease), pulmonary edema, or new-onset cerebral or visual disturbances.
	Eclampsia is the convulsive phase of the disorder and is among the more severe manifestations of the disease.
Chronic arterial hypertension (of any cause)	High BP known to predate conception or detected before 20 weeks of gestation.
Chronic hypertension with superimposed preeclampsia	Women with HT only in early gestation who develop proteinuria after 20 weeks of gestation and women with proteinuria before 20 weeks of gestation who have: (1) a sudden exacerbation of hypertension; (2) sudden manifestation of other signs and symptoms, such as an increase in liver enzymes to abnormal levels; (3) platelet levels below 100.000/microliter; (4) right upper quadrant pain and severe headaches; (5) pulmonary congestion or edema; (6) renal insufficiency; and (7) sudden, substantial, and sustained increases in protein excretion. In the presence of organ dysfunction, this is considered to be superimposed preeclampsia with severe features.
Gestational hypertension	New-onset elevations of BP after 20 weeks of gestation, often near term, in the absence of proteinuria. Failure of BP to normalize postpartum requires changing the diagnosis to chronic hypertension.

BP blood pressure, *HT* hypertension, *PE* preeclampsia

American College of Obstetricians and Gynecologists 2013).

Hypertension affects a substantial proportion of the adult population worldwide at progressively younger ages. Genetic, environmental, and behavioral factors influence the development of HT, which is considered a major causal risk factor for the development of cardiovascular disease, such as heart disease, vascular disease (including stroke), and renal disease (Danaei et al. 2011).

The prevalence of hypertension among adults 18 years of age and older in the United States was 30 %, or is present in nearly 1 in 3 adults. In particular, African American women have a prevalence of hypertension that is among the highest in the world, and its onset occurs at younger ages (Danaei et al. 2011; Centers for Disease Control and Prevention (CDC) 2011; Ezzati et al. 2008; Roger et al. 2011). Therefore, HT affects millions of persons worldwide, and less than half of those with hypertension have their condition controlled (Centers for Disease Control and Prevention (CDC) 2011). Approximately 80 % of hypertensive individuals were aware of their elevated BP, 70 % of them were receiving antihypertensive therapy, but only 48 % had a BP of <140/90 mmHg (Ezzati et al. 2008).

Age is among the strongest risk factors for hypertension (Singh et al. 2012). With an aging population, the overall prevalence of hypertension increases sharply (Roger et al. 2011). In addition, numerous studies have demonstrated the important role of weight gain in BP elevation (and weight reduction in BP lowering), noting that the increasing population weight is also one of the major determinants of increasing BP (Danaei et al. 2011; Centers for Disease Control and Prevention (CDC) 2011; Ezzati et al. 2008; Roger et al. 2011). Thus, the progressive increase in the female population weight and the age at which a woman becomes pregnant are two major problems that converge to contribute to the higher incidence of chronic hypertension during pregnancy.

2 Cardiovascular Changes During Pregnancy

Cardiovascular changes related to normal pregnancy begin early, prior to full placentation (Guedes-Martins et al. 2014, 2015a, b). Those changes include an increase in cardiac output, blood volume expansion, peripheral vasodilation and blood pressure reduction.

As in normotensive gestations (Strevens et al. 2001; Gaillard et al. 2011), in chronic hypertensive pregnant women the shapes of BP trajectories are characterized by a decrease until mid-pregnancy followed by an increase late in pregnancy, when it rises to return to prepregnancy values (Guedes-Martins et al. 2015c). This BP decrease begins early in the first trimester, and the physiological decrease in blood pressure, approximately 10 mmHg, is noted until the third trimester, at which time the BP profile tends to return to the patient's standard (typical of the non-pregnant state).

As a result, some hypertensive women become normotensive during pregnancy, which can delay the diagnosis of disease or confuse it with the occurrence of a hypertensive condition related to pregnancy itself (e.g., preeclampsia, gestational hypertension). Consequently, in such cases the diagnosis of chronic hypertension can only be performed after 12 weeks postpartum if the blood pressure values are not normalized (The American College of Obstetricians and Gynecologists 2013).

3 Chronic Hypertension and Pregnancy Outcomes

Chronic hypertension is a disease that can be well tolerated during pregnancy, and in some cases, cHT pregnancies have a normal outcome without maternal and fetal complications. However, specialized attention should be given to these pregnant women because cHT is an established risk factor for poor obstetrical outcomes.

Adverse outcomes are particularly observed in women with cHT with uncontrolled severe hypertension, in those with target organ damage, and in those who are noncompliant with prenatal visits. In addition, adverse outcomes are substantially increased in women who develop superimposed preeclampsia, which complicates 17–25 % of cHT pregnancies (vs. a 3–5 % preeclampsia frequency described for the general population) (Sibai 2002).

Superimposed preeclampsia is the most prevalent complication in pregnant women with chronic hypertension. Chappel and colleagues (2008) presented prospective contemporaneous data on the outcome of pregnancies in women with chronic hypertension. In their study (Chappell et al. 2008), indices of maternal and perinatal morbidity and mortality were determined using prospectively collected data for 822 women with chronic hypertension. The incidence of superimposed preeclampsia was 22 % with early onset preeclampsia ($\leq$34 weeks gestation) accounting for nearly half (44 %) of these cases (Chappell et al. 2008). Delivering an infant <10th customized birthweight percentile complicated 48 % (87/180) of those with superimposed preeclampsia and 21 % (137/642) of those without (relative risk [RR] 2.30; 95 % confidence intervals [$CI_{95\%}$] 1.85–2.84) (Chappell et al. 2008). Delivery at <37 weeks gestation occurred in 51 % of those with superimposed preeclampsia (98 % of these iatrogenic) and 15 % of those without (66 % iatrogenic) (RR 3.52; 95 % $CI_{95\%}$ 2.79–4.45) (Chappell et al. 2008). The results obtained by Chappell and colleagues suggests that the prevalence of infants born small for gestational age and preterm is considerably higher than background rates and is increased further in women with superimposed preeclampsia (Chappell et al. 2008). The results were similar to that reported by three previous, robust, observational studies of women with chronic hypertension (Rey and Couturier 1994; McCowan et al. 1996; Sibai et al. 1998). Nevertheless, even without superimposed preeclampsia, women with cHT have significantly higher

Table 2 Adverse pregnancy outcomes for women with chronic hypertension

Superimposed preeclampsia
Caesarean delivery
Pre-term delivery (<37 weeks)
Birth weight < 2500 g
Neonatal intensive care
Perinatal death

Bramham et al. (2014)

frequencies of perinatal death and small-for-gestational-age newborns than do normotensive women (Rey and Couturier 1994).

As a corollary, an extensive systematic review reporting meta-analyzed data from 55 studies of approximately 800,000 pregnancies (Bramham et al. 2014) showed that adverse outcomes of cHT pregnancy are common, and that review emphasized a need for adequate antenatal surveillance (Table 2).

Bramham and colleagues (2014) reported that women with chronic hypertension had high pooled incidences of superimposed pre-eclampsia (25.9 %, $CI_{95\%}$ 21.0–31.5 %), caesarean delivery (41.4 %, $CI_{95\%}$ 35.5–47.7 %), preterm delivery <37 weeks gestation (28.1 % $CI_{95\%}$ 22.6–34.4 %), birth weight <2500 g (16.9 %, $CI_{95\%}$ 13.1–21.5 %), neonatal intensive care unit admission (20.5 %, $CI_{95\%}$ 15.7–26.4 %), and perinatal death (4.0 %, $CI_{95\%}$ 2.9–5.4 %). In their systematic review, the incidences of adverse outcomes showed significantly higher risks in those with cHT: the relative risks were 7.7 ($CI_{95\%}$ 5.7–10.1) for superimposed pre-eclampsia compared with pre-eclampsia, 1.3 ($CI_{95\%}$ 1.1–1.5) for caesarean delivery, 2.7 ($CI_{95\%}$ 1.9–3.6) for preterm delivery <37 weeks gestation, 2.7 ($CI_{95\%}$ 1.9–3.8) for birth weight <2500 g, 3.2 ($CI_{95\%}$ 2.2–4.4) for neonatal intensive care unit admission, and 4.2 ($CI_{95\%}$ 2.7–6.5) for perinatal death (Bramham et al. 2014). These results should guide counseling, adequate drug treatment, and pre-pregnancy optimization of women affected by cHT (The American College of Obstetricians and Gynecologists 2013; Bramham et al. 2014).

4 Prepregnancy Care of Women with Chronic Hypertension

The American College of Obstetricians and Gynecologists (2013) recommends preconception explanation of the risks associated with chronic hypertension and education about the signs and symptoms of preeclampsia. The presence of diabetes, obesity, kidney disease, history of early preeclampsia, uncontrolled hypertension, and secondary hypertension are considered risk factors for the development of superimposed preeclampsia (The American College of Obstetricians and Gynecologists 2013). However, some evidence suggests that in women with chronic hypertension, a history of preeclampsia does not increase the rate of superimposed preeclampsia, but is associated with an increased rate of delivery at <37 weeks (Sibai et al. 2011). The ACOG and the National Institute for Health and Care Excellence guidelines guidance (2015) also recommends pre-conception discontinuation of medications with known fetal adverse effects, in particular angiotensin-converting enzyme (ACE) inhibitors, angiotensin receptor blockers, mineralocorticoid antagonists, and statins.

The Report of the National High Blood Pressure Education Program Working Group on High Blood Pressure in Pregnancy advises for the assessment for ventricular hypertrophy, retinopathy and renal disease in women with history of hypertension for more than several years because target organ damage, especially renal disease, can progress during pregnancy (Report of the National High Blood Pressure Education Program Working Group on High Blood Pressure in Pregnancy 2000). In women with severe hypertension of long duration (more than 4 years), assessment of left ventricular function with echocardiography or electrocardiography is considered good clinical practice (The American College of Obstetricians and Gynecologists 2013). This recommendation is also enhanced by the Canadian (Magee et al. 2014), Australasian and JNC 8 evidence guidelines for the management of high blood pressure in adults (James et al. 2014), reinforcing the importance of looking for signs and symptoms of secondary hypertension in women with cHT who seek preconception counseling. Particularly, the presence of resistant hypertension, hypokalemia (potassium levels less than 3.0 mEq/L), elevated serum creatinine level (greater than 1.1 mg/dL) and family history of kidney disease are important suggestive findings of secondary hypertension. Additionally, if the urinalysis is positive for protein, then a 24-h urine collection for protein analysis or measurement of spot urine protein-to-creatinine ratio can be assessed (Côté et al. 2008). This analysis might assist in the diagnosis of superimposed preeclampsia and can provide prognostic information about the development of fetal growth restriction when prepregnancy proteinuria is found (Seely and Ecker 2014; Sibai et al. 1998). The baseline concentrations of serum creatinine, electrolytes, uric acid, liver enzymes, and platelet count should be documented before conception to use as comparators if superimposed preeclampsia is suspected (The American College of Obstetricians and Gynecologists 2013). The ACOG task force recommendation (The American College of Obstetricians and Gynecologists 2013) also suggests referral to a physician with expertise in treating hypertension if secondary hypertension is suspected.

5 Management of the Pregnant with Chronic Arterial Hypertension

For the general population with cHT, the use of home BP monitoring in daily clinical practice is a useful instrument as an aid to achieving targets and monitoring responses to medication (Maldonado et al. 2009). For pregnant women with chronic hypertension and poorly controlled BP, the use of home BP monitoring is suggested, particularly in the second half of pregnancy when most superimposed preeclampsia occurs (The American College of Obstetricians and Gynecologists 2013). In particular, ambulatory BP monitoring can be of special interest for women with suspected white coat hypertension, avoiding overtreatment of BP and unnecessary adverse effects of treatment when not indicated

(The American College of Obstetricians and Gynecologists 2013; James et al. 2014).

Mild to moderate hypertension during pregnancy is a common finding. In daily clinical practice, antihypertensive drugs are often used in the belief that lowering blood pressure will prevent progression to more severe disease and thereby improve the outcome, reducing maternal morbidity by limiting episodes of severe hypertension (Seely and Ecker 2014; Abalos et al. 2014). However, it remains unclear whether antihypertensive drug therapy for mild to moderate hypertension during pregnancy is worthwhile (Abalos et al. 2014). In addition, overly aggressive antihypertensive treatment might decrease fetoplacental perfusion, increase the risk of fetal growth restriction (Seely and Ecker 2014; von Dadelszen et al. 2000), and reproduce fetal effects of diseases related to placental bed dysfunction.

Recently, the Control of Hypertension in Pregnancy Study (CHIPS) was designed to compare tight control (the use of antihypertensive therapy to normalize BP) with less-tight control of non-proteinuric, non-severe hypertension in pregnancy with respect to perinatal and maternal outcomes (Magee et al. 2015). CHIPS was an open, international, randomized, multicenter trial involving 987 women. The primary outcome was a composite of pregnancy loss (defined as miscarriage, ectopic pregnancy, pregnancy termination, stillbirth, or neonatal death) or high-level neonatal care (defined as greater-than-normal newborn care) for more than 48 h until 28 days of life or until discharge home, whichever was later. The secondary outcome was serious maternal complications occurring up to 6 weeks postpartum or until hospital discharge, whichever was later (Martin et al. 2005). This randomized trial showed that less-tight control of maternal hypertension in pregnancy compared with tight control resulted in no significant difference in the risk of adverse perinatal outcomes, as assessed by the rates of perinatal death or high-level neonatal care for more than 48 h (primary outcome) (Brown et al. 2000). Additionally, less-tight (vs. tight) control did not significantly increase the risk of overall serious maternal complications (secondary outcome).

However, with respect to the mothers, the CHIPS findings are consistent with a meta-analysis of previous trials that showed that less-tight versus tight control increases the incidence of severe maternal hypertension (but not pre-eclampsia) (Abalos et al. 2014; Magee et al. 2015), which is considered a risk factor for acute stroke during and outside of pregnancy (James et al. 2014; Martin et al. 2005). The treatment of severe hypertension (systolic BP more than 160 mmHg and/or diastolic BP more than 110 mmHg) is always recommended because it is believed to reduce the risk of maternal stroke and coronary events and to limit episodes of severe hypertension. However, the exact goal ranges for BP targets during pregnancy in women with chronic hypertension are not established.

The ACOG recommends antihypertensive therapy for pregnant women with persistent chronic hypertension with systolic BP of 160 mmHg or higher or diastolic BP of 105 mmHg or higher (The American College of Obstetricians and Gynecologists 2013). For pregnant women with chronic hypertension treated with antihypertensive medication, the ACOG suggests that BP levels be maintained between 120 mmHg systolic and 80 mmHg diastolic, and 160 mmHg systolic and 105 mmHg diastolic. The NHBPEP (Report of the National High Blood Pressure Education Program Working Group on High Blood Pressure in Pregnancy 2000) working group considers tapering antihypertensive medications and reinstituting or increasing the dose of antihypertensive drugs if BP is >150–160 mmHg systolic or >100–110 mmHg diastolic. Additionally, the JNC-8 suggests continuing medication if there is target-organ damage or a previous requirement for multiple antihypertensive agents for BP control, and if medication is stopped, instituting pharmacological treatment if BP is >150–160 mmHg systolic or >100–110 mmHg diastolic (James et al. 2014). The Society of Obstetricians and Gynaecologists of Canada (Magee et al. 2014) recommends treatment if BP is >159 mmHg systolic or >109 mmHg diastolic to reduce maternal risk with a target of <156 mmHg systolic and <106 mmHg diastolic in patients without cardiovascular risk factors. Finally, the Australasian Society for the Study of Hypertension in Pregnancy (Brown et al. 2000) suggests antihypertensive therapy in cases of BP >170 mmHg systolic or >110 mmHg diastolic with a recommended target of 120–140 mmHg systolic and 80–90 mmHg diastolic.

For women who enter pregnancy and receive antihypertensive therapy prior to conception, there are scarce or absent data to guide decisions regarding continuing or discontinuing therapy (The American College of Obstetricians and Gynecologists 2013).

6 Antihypertensive Agents in Pregnancy

The more commonly used antihypertensive agents with an acceptable safety profile in pregnancy and their Food and Drug Administration (FDA) classification are illustrated in Table 3.

Table 3 Antihypertensive medications used in pregnancy

Agent	FDA class	Dose	Contraindications	Potential side effects and comments
Methyldopa	B	250–1500 mg orally twice daily	Hypersensitivity to methyldopa or any component of the formulation; active hepatic disease (e.g.,, acute hepatitis, active cirrhosis); hepatic disorders previously associated with use of methyldopa; concurrent use of MAO inhibitors.	Only a mild antihypertensive agent and has a slow onset of action (3–6 h); Sedative effect at high doses.
Labetalol	C	100–1200 mg orally twice daily	Hypersensitivity to labetalol or any component of the formulation; severe bradycardia; heart block greater than first degree (except in patients with a functioning artificial pacemaker); cardiogenic shock; bronchial asthma; uncompensated cardiac failure; conditions associated with severe and prolonged hypotension.	Has both alpha- and beta-adrenergic blocking activity and might preserve uteroplacental blood flow to a greater extent than traditional beta-blockers; Hepatotoxicity.
Nifedipine	C	30–90 mg orally daily, as sustained release tablet	Hypersensitivity to nifedipine or any component of the formulation; concomitant use with strong CYP3A4 inducers (e.g.,, rifampin); cardiogenic shock.	There is a small risk of an acute, precipitous fall in blood pressure, which may result in a reduction in uteroplacental perfusion and headache.
Thiazide diuretics	C	Varies according to drug used	Hypotension; Hypersensitivity to sulfur-containing medications; Gout; Renal failure; Lithium therapy; Hypokalemia.	Volume depletion; Hypokalemia; Hyperglycemia.
Clonidine	C	0.1–0.3 mg/ 24 h patch applied once every 7 days	Hypersensitivity to clonidine hydrochloride.	Rebound hypertension if it is stopped suddenly; Particularly useful for patients who cannot take an oral antihypertensive drug.

FDA (Food and Drug Administration) classification of drugs in pregnancy: *Category A*, adequate and well-controlled studies have failed to demonstrate a risk to the fetus in the first trimester of pregnancy, and there is no evidence of risk in later trimesters; *Category B*, animal reproduction studies have failed to demonstrate a risk to the fetus, and there are no adequate and well-controlled studies in pregnant women; Category C, animal reproduction studies have shown an adverse effect on the fetus, and there are no adequate and well-controlled studies in humans, but potential benefits might warrant use of the drug in pregnant women despite potential risks; *Category D*, there is positive evidence of human fetal risk based on adverse reaction data from investigational or marketing experience or studies in humans, but potential benefits might warrant use of the drug in pregnant women despite potential risks; *Category X*, studies in animals or humans have demonstrated fetal abnormalities, and/or there is positive evidence of human fetal risk based on adverse reaction data from investigational or marketing experience, and the risks involved in use of the drug in pregnant women clearly outweigh potential benefits; *Category N*, the FDA has not classified the drug

Methyldopa has been widely used in pregnancy, seems safe to use, and is probably preferable to other drugs from the point of view of the neonate and child (Cockburn et al. 1982). For infants born to mothers with chronic hypertension, compared with those with mothers are treated by methyldopa alone, those whose mothers are treated by beta-blockers appear to be at increased risk of being small for gestational age (SGA) and being hospitalized during infancy (Xie et al. 2014). Methyldopa, a centrally acting alpha-2 adrenergic agonist, is considered a first-line drug for the treatment of hypertension in pregnancy (Seely and Ecker 2014), with no apparent adverse effects on uteroplacental hemodynamics (Montan et al. 1993), birth weight, neonatal complications, and development at 1 year after delivery (Mutch et al. 1977).

Beta-blockers are also commonly used during the first trimester of pregnancy, and data concerning the risks of congenital anomalies in offspring have not been summarized. Based on a 2013 systematic review of 13 population-based case control cohort studies examining the risk of congenital malformations, first-trimester oral β-blocker use showed no increased odds of all or major congenital anomalies (OR = 1.00; $CI_{95\%}$ 0.91–1.10). However, in analyses examining organ-specific malformations, increased odds of cardiovascular defects (OR = 2.01; $CI_{95\%}$ 1.18–3.42), cleft lip/palate (OR = 3.11; $CI_{95\%}$ 1.79–5.43), and neural tube defects (OR = 3.56; $CI_{95\%}$ 1.19–10.67) were observed. The effects on severe hypospadias were non-significant. The authors concluded that causality is difficult to interpret given the small number of heterogeneous studies and possibility of biases. Additionally, given the frequency of this exposure in pregnancy, further research is needed (Yakoob et al. 2013). Labetalol is a beta-blocker with alpha-blocking activity commonly used in pregnancy, with no significant differences in perinatal outcomes when compared with placebo or methyldopa (Sibai et al. 1990).

Calcium channel blockers are considered to be safe for use in pregnancy although they are a class of drugs that has not been extensively studied in pregnant women with chronic hypertension (The American College of Obstetricians and Gynecologists 2013). Oral nifedipine, the most commonly prescribed calcium channel blocker, is also a suitable option for the treatment of hypertension in pregnancy/postpartum (Firoz et al. 2014).

Diuretics, generally considered second-line drugs for the treatment of hypertension in pregnancy, can be especially useful in women with salt-sensitive hypertension (The American College of Obstetricians and Gynecologists 2013). Dose adjustments to minimize the adverse effects and risks, such as hypokalemia and intravascular volume depletion, are recommended (The American College of Obstetricians and Gynecologists 2013).

Clonidine has a similar mechanism of action as methyldopa and appears to be a safe antihypertensive agent in pregnancy (Horvath et al. 1985; Rothberger et al. 2010). Clonidine is particularly useful for patients who cannot take an oral antihypertensive drug because it is available as a transdermal patch (Table 3).

Angiotensin converting enzyme (ACE) inhibitors, angiotensin II receptor blockers (ARB) and direct renin inhibitors are contraindicated during pregnancy. When maternal exposure is in the second and third trimester, they are associated with renal abnormalities, adverse pregnancy outcomes, oligohydramnios, fetal growth restriction, skull hypoplasia, and fetal death, and first trimester exposure has been associated with fetal cardiac abnormalities (Cooper et al. 2006).

Hydralazine, labetalol, and calcium channel blockers are among the medications that were recommended for urgent lowering of BP in pregnant women with chronic hypertension (The American College of Obstetricians and Gynecologists 2013; Duley et al. 2013). Based on the results of a recent, robust Cochrane systematic review, evidence is inadequate to demonstrate the superior safety or efficacy of any of these medications (Duley et al. 2013). The authors state that until better evidence is available, the choice of antihypertensive should depend on the clinician's experience and familiarity with a particular drug, on what is known about adverse effects, and on the patient's preferences (Duley et al. 2013).

Nitroprusside is the agent of resort for urgent control of refractory severe hypertension. It is recommended that its use should be limited to emergency situations during a short period of time. Although under suspicion (Sass et al. 2007), at present there is insufficient evidence for definitive conclusions about any direct association between sodium nitroprusside use and fetal demise (Magee et al. 2014; Sass et al. 2007).

A systematic review with the purpose to establish which antihypertensive medications are safe for use while breastfeeding indicated that ACE inhibitors, methyldopa, beta-blockers with high protein binding, and some calcium channel blockers all appear to be safe treatments of hypertension in a nursing mother (Beardmore et al. 2002).

7 Lifestyle Modification and Blood Pressure Control of Women with Chronic Hypertension

There are no large randomized trials that have evaluated the benefits of limited weight gain or implementation or continuation of the DASH diet during pregnancy with chronic hypertension. However, the ACOG recommends that weight loss and extremely low-sodium diets (<100 mEq/d) should not be used for managing chronic hypertension in pregnancy. In addition, for women with chronic hypertension who are accustomed to exercising, and in whom BP is well controlled, it is suggested that moderate exercise should be continued during pregnancy (The American College of Obstetricians and Gynecologists 2013).

8 Prevention of Superimposed Preeclampsia

There does not appear to be any benefit for the prevention of preeclampsia from routine calcium supplementation (Levine et al. 1997) or the use of antioxidants (Rumbold et al. 2005) for women with chronic hypertension. However, there is some evidence that low-dose aspirin initiated in early pregnancy is an efficient method of reducing the incidence of preeclampsia (Duley et al. 2007; Bujold et al. 2010; Askie et al. 2007). Therefore, for women with chronic hypertension who are at a greatly increased risk of adverse pregnancy outcomes (history of early onset preeclampsia and preterm delivery at <34 weeks of gestation or preeclampsia in more than one prior pregnancy), the ACOG recommends initiating the administration of daily low-dose aspirin (60–80 mg) beginning in the late first trimester. Further information is required to assess which women are most likely to benefit when treatment is best started, and at what dose (Duley et al. 2007).

9 Fetal Surveillance and Timing of Delivery for Women with Chronic Hypertension

In general, more frequent prenatal visits are usual in daily clinical practice with the objective of following BP profile, urine protein, fundal height and maternal/fetal well-being (Seely and Ecker 2014). However, there is no consensus on the most appropriate fetal surveillance tests or the interval and timing of testing for women with chronic hypertension (The American College of Obstetricians and Gynecologists 2013). Notwithstanding, because these pregnancies are more likely to be complicated by fetal growth restriction, the ACOG suggests the use of ultrasonography (instead of fundal height) to screen for fetal growth abnormalities, and if evidence of fetal growth restriction is found, fetoplacental assessment to include umbilical artery Doppler velocimetry is recommended (The American College of Obstetricians and Gynecologists 2013). For women with chronic hypertension and no additional maternal or fetal complications, delivery before 38 weeks of gestation is not recommended by the ACOG (The American College of Obstetricians and Gynecologists 2013).

10 Women with Chronic Hypertension in the Postpartum Hypertension

Postpartum hypertension can be related to preexisting cHT, preeclampsia, persistence of gestational hypertension, or it could develop secondary to other causes (Sibai 2012). The exact incidence of postpartum hypertension is difficult to determine (Sibai 2012). However, despite the few data regarding hypertensive disorders that are diagnosed in the postpartum period, the reported prevalence of de novo postpartum hypertension or preeclampsia ranges from 0.3 to 27.5 % (Sibai 2012; Podymow and August 2010).

There are scarce data describing the etiology, differential diagnosis, and management of postpartum hypertension-preeclampsia (Sibai 2012). In daily clinical practice the differential diagnosis is extensive, and varies from benign (mild gestational or essential hypertension) to life-threatening such as severe preeclampsia-eclampsia, pheochromocytoma, and cerebrovascular accidents (Sibai 2012). Because delivery does not eliminate the risk for preeclampsia and its complications, efforts should be directed at the continued monitoring, reporting, and evaluating of the symptoms of preeclampsia during the postpartum period (Matthys et al. 2004). HT or exacerbation of hypertension postpartum may be due to either undiagnosed cHT (women with limited medical care prior to or early in pregnancy), or due to exacerbation of HT after delivery in those with superimposed preeclampsia.

Evaluation and management of women with postpartum HT should be guided by obtaining a detailed history, careful physical examination, selective laboratory and imaging studies, and response to initial treatment (Sibai 2012).

Women with cHT will usually require treatment with antihypertensive agents in the postpartum period, even if they were not treated during pregnancy (The American College of Obstetricians and Gynecologists 2013; National Institute for Health and Care Excellence guidelines [CG107], Hypertension in Pregnancy 2015; Report of the National High Blood Pressure Education Program Working Group on High Blood Pressure in Pregnancy 2000). Additionally, good clinical practice suggests that women with chronic hypertension should be encouraged to breastfeed, although there are no studies that have assessed either maternal or children outcomes in this patient population exposed to antihypertensive medications in breast milk (The American College of Obstetricians and Gynecologists 2013). Methyldopa, propranolol, labetalol, captopril, and channel blockers are considered safe, and concentrations in breast milk are low (The American College of Obstetricians and Gynecologists 2013). The concentration of diuretics in breast milk is also low but these agents may reduce the quantity of milk production (The American College of Obstetricians and Gynecologists 2013; National Institute for Health and Care Excellence guidelines [CG107], Hypertension in Pregnancy 2015; Report of the National High Blood Pressure Education Program Working Group on High Blood Pressure in Pregnancy 2000; Magee et al. 2014; James et al. 2014).

11 Conclusion

Chronic hypertension is frequently encountered during pregnancy and needs to be distinguished from other hypertensive complications of pregnancy, such as preeclampsia and gestational hypertension. Women with chronic arterial hypertension are at increased risk for several pregnancy complications, including superimposed pre-eclampsia, caesarean delivery, preterm delivery <37 weeks gestation, birth weight <2500 g, neonatal intensive care unit admission, and perinatal death. Therefore, specialized attention should be given to these women as part of family planning before conception, to provide counseling regarding the pregnancy risks, to inform about surveillance of fetal well-being, to determine the timing of delivery, and to optimize BP control before, during, and after birth.

Competing Financial Interests The author declares no conflicts of interest.

References

Abalos E, Duley L, Steyn DW (2014) Antihypertensive drug therapy for mild to moderate hypertension during pregnancy. Cochrane Database Syst Rev 2, CD002252. doi:10.1002/14651858.CD002252. pub3

Askie LM, Duley L, Henderson-Smart DJ, Stewart LA, PARIS Collaborative Group (2007) Antiplatelet agents for prevention of pre-eclampsia: a meta-analysis of individual patient data. Lancet 369 (9575):1791–1798

Beardmore KS, Morris JM, Gallery ED (2002) Excretion of antihypertensive medication into human breast milk: a systematic review. Hypertens Pregnancy 21 (1):85–95

Bramham K, Parnell B, Nelson-Piercy C, Seed PT, Poston L, Chappell LC (2014) Chronic hypertension and pregnancy outcomes: systematic review and meta-analysis. BMJ 348:g2301. doi:10.1136/bmj.g2301

Brown MA, Hague WM, Higgins J, Lowe S, McCowan L, Oats J, Peek MJ, Rowan JA, Walters BN, Austalasian Society of the Study of Hypertension in Pregnancy (2000) The detection, investigation and management of hypertension in pregnancy: full consensus statement. Aust N Z J Obstet Gynaecol 40(2):139–155

Bujold E, Roberge S, Lacasse Y, Bureau M, Audibert F, Marcoux S, Forest JC, Giguère Y (2010) Prevention of preeclampsia and intrauterine growth restriction with aspirin started in early pregnancy: a meta-analysis. Obstet Gynecol 116(2 Pt 1):402–414. doi:10.1097/AOG.0b013e3181e9322a

Centers for Disease Control and Prevention (CDC) (2011) Vital signs: prevalence, treatment, and control of hypertension – United States, 1999–2002 and 2005–2008. MMWR Morb Mortal Wkly Rep 60 (4):103–108

Chappell LC, Enye S, Seed P, Briley AL, Poston L, Shennan AH (2008) Adverse perinatal outcomes and risk factors for preeclampsia in women with chronic hypertension: a prospective study. Hypertension 51 (4):1002–1009. doi:10.1161/HYPERTENSIONAHA. 107.107565

Cockburn J, Moar VA, Ounsted M, Redman CW (1982) Final report of study on hypertension during pregnancy: the effects of specific treatment on the growth and development of the children. Lancet 1 (8273):647–649

Cooper WO, Hernandez-Diaz S, Arbogast PG, Dudley JA, Dyer S, Gideon PS, Hall K, Ray WA (2006) Major congenital malformations after first-trimester exposure to ACE inhibitors. N Engl J Med 354 (23):2443–2451

Côté AM, Brown MA, Lam E, von Dadelszen P, Firoz T, Liston RM, Magee LA (2008) Diagnostic accuracy of urinary spot protein:creatinine ratio for proteinuria in hypertensive pregnant women: systematic review. BMJ 336(7651):1003–1006

Danaei G, Finucane MM, Lin JK, Singh GM, Paciorek CJ, Cowan MJ, Farzadfar F, Stevens GA, Lim SS, Riley LM, Ezzati M, Global Burden of Metabolic Risk Factors of Chronic Diseases Collaborating Group (Blood Pressure) (2011) National, regional, and global trends in systolic blood pressure since 1980: systematic analysis of health examination surveys and epidemiological studies with 786 country-years and 5 · 4 million participants. Lancet 377 (9765):568–577. doi:10.1016/S0140-6736(10)62036-3

Duley L, Henderson-Smart DJ, Meher S, King JF (2007) Antiplatelet agents for preventing pre-eclampsia and its complications. Cochrane Database Syst Rev 2, CD004659

Duley L, Meher S, Jones L (2013) Drugs for treatment of very high blood pressure during pregnancy. Cochrane Database Syst Rev 7, CD001449. doi:10.1002/14651858.CD001449.pub3

Ezzati M, Oza S, Danaei G, Murray CJ (2008) Trends and cardiovascular mortality effects of state-level blood pressure and uncontrolled hypertension in the United States. Circulation 117(7):905–914. doi:10.1161/CIRCULATIONAHA.107.732131

Firoz T, Magee LA, MacDonell K, Payne BA, Gordon R, Vidler M, von Dadelszen P, Community Level Interventions for Pre-eclampsia (CLIP) Working Group (2014) Oral antihypertensive therapy for severe hypertension in pregnancy and postpartum: a systematic review. BJOG 121(10):1210–1218. doi:10.1111/1471-0528.12737

Gaillard R, Bakker R, Willemsen SP, Hofman A, Steegers EA, Jaddoe VW (2011) Blood pressure tracking during pregnancy and the risk of gestational hypertensive disorders: the Generation R Study. Eur Heart J 32 (24):3088–3097. doi:10.1093/eurheartj/ehr275

Guedes-Martins L, Saraiva J, Gaio R, Macedo F, Almeida H (2014) Uterine artery impedance at very early clinical pregnancy. Prenat Diagn 34(8):719–725. doi:10.1002/pd.4325

Guedes-Martins L, Gaio R, Saraiva J, Cerdeira S, Matos L, Silva E, Macedo F, Almeida H (2015a) Reference ranges for uterine artery pulsatility index during the menstrual cycle: a cross-sectional study. PLoS One 10(3), e0119103. doi:10.1371/journal.pone.0119103

Guedes-Martins L, Saraiva JP, Gaio AR, Reynolds A, Macedo F, Almeida H (2015b) Uterine artery Doppler in the management of early pregnancy loss: a prospective, longitudinal study. BMC Pregnancy Childbirth 15:28. doi:10.1186/s12884-015-0464-9

Guedes-Martins L, Carvalho M, Silva C, Cunha A, Saraiva J, Macedo F, Almeida H, Gaio AR (2015c) Relationship between body mass index and mean arterial pressure in normotensive and chronic hypertensive pregnant women: a prospective, longitudinal study. BMC Pregnancy Childbirth 15:281. doi:10.1186/s12884-015-0711-0

Heshmati A, Mishra G, Koupil I (2013) Childhood and adulthood socio-economic position and hypertensive disorders in pregnancy: the Uppsala birth cohort multigenerational study. J Epidemiol Community Health 67(11):939–946. doi:10.1136/jech-2012-202149

Horvath JS, Phippard A, Korda A, Henderson-Smart DJ, Child A, Tiller DJ (1985) Clonidine hydrochloride – a safe and effective antihypertensive agent in pregnancy. Obstet Gynecol 66(5):634–638

James PA, Oparil S, Carter BL, Cushman WC, Dennison-Himmelfarb C, Handler J, Lackland DT, LeFevre ML, MacKenzie TD, Ogedegbe O, Smith SC Jr, Svetkey LP, Taler SJ, Townsend RR, Wright JT Jr, Narva AS, Ortiz E (2014) 2014 evidence based guideline for the management of high blood pressure in adults: report from the panel members appointed to the Eighth Joint National Committee (JNC 8). JAMA 311(5):507–520. doi:10.1001/jama.2013.284427

Lawler J, Osman M, Shelton JA, Yeh J (2007) Population-based analysis of hypertensive disorders in pregnancy. Hypertens Pregnancy 26(1):67–76

Lecarpentier E, Tsatsaris V, Goffinet F, Cabrol D, Sibai B, Haddad B (2013) Risk factors of superimposed preeclampsia in women with essential chronic hypertension treated before pregnancy. PLoS One 8(5), e62140. doi:10.1371/journal.pone.0062140

Leon MG, Moussa HN, Longo M, Pedroza C, Haidar ZA, Mendez-Figueroa H, Blackwell SC, Sibai BM (2016) Rate of gestational diabetes mellitus and pregnancy outcomes in patients with chronic hypertension. Am J Perinatol 33:745

Levine RJ, Hauth JC, Curet LB, Sibai BM, Catalano PM, Morris CD, DerSimonian R, Esterlitz JR, Raymond EG, Bild DE, Clemens JD, Cutler JA (1997) Trial of calcium to prevent preeclampsia. N Engl J Med 337(2):69–76

Livingston JC, Maxwell BD, Sibai BM (2003) Chronic hypertension in pregnancy. Minerva Ginecol 55(1):1–13

Magee LA, Pels A, Helewa M, Rey E, von Dadelszen P, Canadian Hypertensive Disorders of Pregnancy (HDP) Working Group (2014) Diagnosis, evaluation, and management of the hypertensive disorders of pregnancy. Pregnancy Hypertens 4(2):105–145. doi:10.1016/j.preghy.2014.01.003

Magee LA, von Dadelszen P, Rey E, Ross S, Asztalos E, Murphy KE, Menzies J, Sanchez J, Singer J, Gafni A, Gruslin A, Helewa M, Hutton E, Lee SK, Lee T, Logan AG, Ganzevoort W, Welch R, Thornton JG, Moutquin JM (2015) Less-tight versus tight control of hypertension in pregnancy. N Engl J Med 372(5):407–417. doi:10.1056/NEJMoa1404595

Maldonado J, Pereira T, Estudo AMPA (2009) Self-measurement of blood pressure in arterial hypertension- preliminary results from the AMPA study. Rev Port Cardiol 28(1):7–21

Martin JN Jr, Thigpen BD, Moore RC, Rose CH, Cushman J, May W (2005) Stroke and severe preeclampsia and eclampsia: a paradigm shift focusing on systolic blood pressure. Obstet Gynecol 105(2):246–254

Matthys LA, Coppage KH, Lambers DS, Barton JR, Sibai BM (2004) Delayed postpartum preeclampsia: an experience of 151 cases. Am J Obstet Gynecol 190(5):1464–1466

McCowan LM, Buist RG, North RA, Gamble G (1996) Perinatal morbidity in chronic hypertension. Br J Obstet Gynaecol 103(2):123–129

Montan S, Anandakumar C, Arulkumaran S, Ingemarsson I, Ratnam SS (1993) Effects of methyldopa on uteroplacental and fetal hemodynamics in pregnancy-induced hypertension. Am J Obstet Gynecol 168(1 Pt 1):152–156

Mutch LM, Moar VA, Ounsted MK, Redman CW (1977) Hypertension during pregnancy, with and without specific hypotensive treatment. II. The growth and development of the infant in the first year of life. Early Hum Dev 1(1):59–67

National Institute for Health and Care Excellence guidelines [CG107], Hypertension in Pregnancy: diagnosis and management. 2015

Podymow T, August P (2010) Postpartum course of gestational hypertension and preeclampsia. Hypertens Pregnancy 29(3):294–300

Report of the National High Blood Pressure Education Program Working Group on High Blood Pressure in Pregnancy (2000). Am J Obstet Gynecol 183(1):S1–S22

Rey E, Couturier A (1994) The prognosis of pregnancy in women with chronic hypertension. Am J Obstet Gynecol 171(2):410–416

Roger VL, Go AS, Lloyd-Jones DM, Adams RJ, Berry JD, Brown TM, Carnethon MR, Dai S, de Simone G, Ford ES, Fox CS, Fullerton HJ, Gillespie C, Greenlund KJ, Hailpern SM, Heit JA, Ho PM, Howard VJ, Kissela BM, Kittner SJ, Lackland DT, Lichtman JH, Lisabeth LD, Makuc DM, Marcus GM, Marelli A, Matchar DB, McDermott MM, Meigs JB, Moy CS, Mozaffarian D, Mussolino ME, Nichol G, Paynter NP, Rosamond WD, Sorlie PD, Stafford RS, Turan TN, Turner MB, Wong ND, Wylie-Rosett J, American Heart Association Statistics Committee and Stroke Statistics Subcommittee (2011) Heart disease and stroke statistics – 2011 update: a report from the American Heart Association. Circulation 123(4):e18–e209. doi:10.1161/CIR.0b013e3182009701

Rothberger S, Carr D, Brateng D, Hebert M, Easterling TR (2010) Pharmacodynamics of clonidine therapy in pregnancy: a heterogeneous maternal response impacts foetal growth. Am J Hypertens 23(11):1234–1240. doi:10.1038/ajh.2010.159

Rumbold A, Duley L, Crowther C, Haslam R (2005) Antioxidants for preventing pre-eclampsia. Cochrane Database Syst Rev 4, CD004227

Sass N, Itamoto CH, Silva MP, Torloni MR, Atallah AN (2007) Does sodium nitroprusside kill babies? A systematic review. Sao Paulo Med J 125(2):108–111

Savitz DA, Danilack VA, Engel SM, Elston B, Lipkind HS (2014) Descriptive epidemiology of chronic hypertension, gestational hypertension, and pre-eclampsia in New York State, 1995–2004. Matern Child Health J 18(4):829–838. doi:10.1007/s10995-013-1307-9. PubMed PMID: 23793484

Seely EW, Ecker J (2014) Chronic hypertension in pregnancy. Circulation 129(11):1254–1261. doi:10.1161/CIRCULATIONAHA.113.003904

Sibai BM (2002) Chronic hypertension in pregnancy. Obstet Gynecol 100(2):369–377

Sibai BM (2012) Etiology and management of postpartum hypertension preeclampsia. Am J Obstet Gynecol 206 (6):470–475

Sibai BM, Mabie WC, Shamsa F, Villar MA, Anderson GD (1990) A comparison of no medication versus methyldopa or labetalol in chronic hypertension during pregnancy. Am J Obstet Gynecol 162 (4):960–966

Sibai BM, Lindheimer M, Hauth J, Caritis S, VanDorsten P, Klebanoff M, MacPherson C, Landon M, Miodovnik M, Paul R, Meis P, Dombrowski M (1998) Risk factors for preeclampsia, abruptio placentae, and adverse neonatal outcomes among women with chronic hypertension. National Institute of Child Health and Human Development Network of Maternal-Fetal Medicine Units. N Engl J Med 339(10):667–671

Sibai BM, Koch MA, Freire S, Silva JL P e, Rudge MV, Martins-Costa S, Moore J, Santos Cde B, Cecatti JG, Costa R, Ramos JG, Moss N, Spinnato JÁ 2nd (2011) The impact of prior preeclampsia on the risk of superimposed preeclampsia and other adverse pregnancy outcomes in patients with chronic hypertension.

Am J Obstet Gynecol 204(4):345.e1-6. doi:10.1016/j.ajog.2010.11.027

Singh GM, Danaei G, Pelizzari PM, Lin JK, Cowan MJ, Stevens GA, Farzadfar F, Khang YH, Lu Y, Riley LM, Lim SS, Ezzati M (2012) The age associations of blood pressure, cholesterol, and glucose: analysis of health examination surveys from international populations. Circulation 125(18):2204–2211. doi:10.1161/CIRCULATIONAHA.111.058834

Strevens H, Wide-Swensson D, Ingemarsson I (2001) Blood pressure during pregnancy in a Swedish population; impact of parity. Acta Obstet Gynecol Scand 80(9):824–829

The American College of Obstetricians and Gynecologists, Task Force on Hypertension in Pregnancy. Washington, 2013

von Dadelszen P, Ornstein MP, Bull SB, Logan AG, Koren G, Magee LA (2000) Fall in mean arterial pressure and fetal growth restriction in pregnancy hypertension: a meta-analysis. Lancet 355 (9198):87–92

Xie RH, Guo Y, Krewski D, Mattison D, Walker MC, Nerenberg K, Wen SW (2014) Beta blockers increase the risk of being born small for gestational age or of being institutionalised during infancy. BJOG 121 (9):1090–1096. doi:10.1111/1471-0528.12678

Yakoob MY, Bateman BT, Ho E, Hernandez-Diaz S, Franklin JM, Goodman JE, Hoban RA (2013) The risk of congenital malformations associated with exposure to β-blockers early in pregnancy: a meta-analysis. Hypertension 62(2):375–381. doi:10.1161/HYPERTENSIONAHA.111.00833

Zetterström K, Lindeberg SN, Haglund B, Hanson U (2005) Maternal complications in women with chronic hypertension: a population-based cohort study. Acta Obstet Gynecol Scand 84(5):419–424

Zetterström K, Lindeberg SN, Haglund B, Hanson U (2006) Chronic hypertension as a risk factor for offspring to be born small for gestational age. Acta Obstet Gynecol Scand 85(9):1046–1050

Adv Exp Med Biol - Advances in Internal Medicine (2017) 2: 409–417
DOI 10.1007/5584_2016_82
© Springer International Publishing AG 2016
Published online: 9 October 2016

Superimposed Preeclampsia

Luís Guedes-Martins

Abstract

Superimposed preeclampsia refers to women with chronic arterial hypertension (primary or secondary) who develop preeclampsia (PE). Because hypertension affects 5–15 % of pregnancies, it is itself a matter of concern. However, this concern should be permanent, given the increased risk of the hypertension worsening and, particularly, the appearance of superimposed PE. The search for factors that underlie or promote the development of this disorder has been the subject of intense research. However, despite the wealth of knowledge, the cause or causes remain to be determined.

Keywords

Preeclampsia • Superimposed preeclampsia • Hypertension • Pregnancy

Abbreviations

ACOG	American College of Obstetricians and Gynecologists
eNOS	endothelial nitric oxide synthase
IUGR	intra-uterine growth restriction
LR	likelihood ratio
NO	nitric oxide
PE	preeclampsia
PI	pulsatility index
PlGF	placental growth factor
sFlt-1	soluble fms-like tyrosine kinase
sPE	superimposed preeclampsia
UtA	uterine artery
−ve	negative
+ve	positive
VEGF	vascular endothelial growth factor.

L. Guedes-Martins (✉)
Department of Experimental Biology, Faculty of Medicine, University of Porto, 4200-319 Porto, Portugal

Instituto de Investigação e Inovação em Saúde, Universidade do Porto, 4200-319 Porto, Portugal

Departamento da Mulher e da Medicina Reprodutiva, Centro Hospitalar do Porto EPE, Largo Prof. Abel Salazar, 4099-001 Porto, Portugal
e-mail: luis.guedes.martins@gmail.com

1   Introduction

Hypertension is a serious human disorder that if left untreated, can lead to dire consequences, most often affecting target organs, such as the heart, brain, kidney and retina (Edwards et al. 2014; Leow 2015). Not unexpectedly, when a woman is diagnosed with hypertension and becomes pregnant, greater care is taken due to the additional effect of hypertension on the placenta and the fetus (Bramham et al. 2014; Seely and Ecker 2014).

According to the Report of the Working Group on Research on Hypertension During Pregnancy, from the 2001 Meeting at the National Heart, Lung, and Blood Institute, "hypertension during pregnancy is categorized as: preeclampsia (PE)/eclampsia, gestational hypertension, the continued presence of chronic hypertension, and preeclampsia superimposed upon chronic hypertension" (National Heart, Lung and Blood Institute 2001). This report further defines and emphasizes the relevance of these entities, in particular, the previous existence of hypertension and the precise point at which women suffering from hypertension have a significant risk "of superimposed PE (25 % risk), preterm delivery, fetal growth restriction or demise, abruptio placentae, congestive heart failure and renal failure. In addition, the outcome for mother and infant is worse than the outcome with de novo PE" (National Heart, Lung and Blood Institute 2001).

2 From Hypertension to Preeclampsia

Hypertension is defined as systolic blood pressure of at least 140 mmHg and diastolic blood pressure of 90 mmHg on at least two occasions; these measurements should be taken at least 4 h (but not more than 7 days) apart. The situation is considered severe if the systolic blood pressure is at least 160 mmHg and/or if the diastolic pressure is at least 110 mmHg on two occasions at least 4 h apart (Sibai and Stella 2009). Usually, the criteria to diagnose PE is beyond hypertension and includes the presence of proteinuria, defined primarily as a concentration of $\geq$30 mg/ dL (1+ in the dipstick) in at least 2 random urine specimens that were collected $\geq$4 h apart (but within a 7-day interval) or 0.3 g in a 24-h period

(Sibai et al. 2005). In the absence of proteinuria, PE is diagnosed as hypertension in association with thrombocytopenia ($<$100,000/µl), impaired liver function (elevated blood levels of liver transaminases to twice the normal concentration), the new development of renal insufficiency (elevated serum creatinine greater than 1.1 mg/ dL or a doubling of serum creatinine in the absence of other renal disease), pulmonary edema, or new-onset cerebral or visual disturbances (American College of Obstetricians and Gynecologists 2013).

Because hypertension affects 5–15 % of pregnancies (Lain and Roberts 2002; Anumba et al. 2010), it is itself a matter of concern. However, this concern should be permanent, given the increased risk of the hypertension worsening and, particularly, the appearance of superimposed PE. Compared to severe hypertension, the likelihood of preterm delivery and abruptio placenta in severe PE can increase to 50 %, and fetal death might supervene (Sibai and Stella 2009).

Understandably, the search for factors that underlie or promote the development of this disorder has been the subject of intense research. However, despite the wealth of knowledge, the cause or causes remain to be determined (Karumanchi et al. 2005). Thus, it is imperative to continue investigations into the factors responsible for hypertension.

A personal history of PE, the presence of hypertension, parity, obesity, black ancestry, insulin-dependent diabetes, collagen disorder, thrombotic abnormalities, twin pregnancy, hydatidiform molar disease and extremes of reproductive age are all factors that increase the risk of PE (Lain and Roberts 2002; Karumanchi et al. 2005). These data suggest that the cause or causes of hypertension are mostly of maternal origin and that the fetal structures are a target. Consequently, efforts to understand the unwanted effects of hypertension in pregnancy should emphasize the maternal side prior to the placental side.

In Western countries as a whole, the age at which women deliver their first child has steadily increased (Istance and Theisens 2008; Mathews and Hamilton 2009). This decision, likely the result of economic or educational reasons, has important medical implications because of the expected age-related reduction of natural fecundity (Menken et al. 1986) and the increased use of assisted reproductive technologies (de Mouzon et al. 2010).

Thus, older age, in contrast with younger age, is an increasingly relevant modulating factor of pregnancy outcome. Indeed, pregnancy in older women carries the enhanced risk for the occurrence of pregnancy disorders or serious complications, which include abortion, fetal death, preterm delivery, pre-eclampsia, intrauterine growth restriction and abruptio placenta (Oyelese and Ananth 2006; Balasch and Gratacós 2011). Furthermore, older women, compared to younger women, are more prone to suffer from hypertension (Hajjar et al. 2006), enhancing the risks associated with pregnancy. Therefore, due to the increased incidence and severity of consequences, one should pay closer attention to hypertensive, reproductive-age women in the clinical management of pregnancies (Jacobsson et al. 2004; van Katwijk and Peeters 1998).

It is also important that such clinical problems be studied with a biomedical approach. In fact, these conditions reflect disordered local gene expression that might be unveiled through the application of molecular biology techniques.

It is recognized that most of these complications of pregnancy result from abnormalities in the uterine placental bed transformation (Brosens et al. 2011). Yet, despite the amount of information known about the structural features observed in the myometrium, decidua and spiral arteries, the local regulation that leads to normal placentation or its derangement remains unknown.

3 Superimposed Preeclampsia: General Aspects

Superimposed preeclampsia refers to the development of PE following chronic arterial hypertension (primary or secondary) during pregnancy (American College of Obstetricians and Gynecologists 2013).

Chronic hypertension is a recognized risk factor for preeclampsia, and superimposed preeclampsia is associated with important maternal-fetal morbidity and mortality (American College of Obstetricians and Gynecologists 2013; Ferrer et al. 2000). Approximately 10–40 % of women with chronic arterial hypertension develop preeclampsia, either with or without underlying chronic hypertension, and experience worse perinatal outcomes (Ray et al. 2001). In addition, the risk of superimposed preeclampsia is significantly influenced by diagnostic criteria, the type of underlying hypertension, and the severity of hypertension (American College of Obstetricians and Gynecologists 2013; Ferrer et al. 2000; Ray et al. 2001). The Task Force on Hypertension in Pregnancy developed by the American College of Obstetricians and Gynecologists (2013) proposes that superimposed preeclampsia be stratified into two groups 'to guide management': (1) superimposed preeclampsia (sPE) and (2) superimposed preeclampsia with severe features (American College of Obstetricians and Gynecologists 2013).

After 20 weeks of gestation (with chronic arterial hypertension) when a sudden increase in blood pressure (BP) or escalation of antihypertensive drugs to control BP is noted, and new onset proteinuria or a sudden increase in proteinuria (in a pregnant women with known proteinuria early in pregnancy) is detected, sPE is likely be present (Bramham et al. 2014; American College of Obstetricians and Gynecologists 2013).

Superimposed preeclampsia with severe features is defined by the American College of Obstetricians and Gynecologists (2013) when any of the following criteria are present: (1) Severe range BP despite escalation of antihypertensive therapy; (2) Thrombocytopenia (platelet count <100.000/microliter); (3) Elevated liver transaminases (two times the upper limit of normal concentration for a particular laboratory); (4) New-onset and worsening renal insufficiency; (5) Pulmonary edema; and, (6) Persistent cerebral or visual disturbances.

4 Prediction of Preeclampsia/ Superimposed Preeclampsia

There is continuing research for improved tests to predict and/or diagnose preeclampsia.

In general, it is agreed that the increased blood flow to the uterus during pregnancy is accommodated through the close relationship between the maternal and fetal circulations. In the non-pregnant state, the uterine artery (UtA) Doppler waveform exhibits a rapid rise and fall in systolic flow velocity that is followed by a notch in early diastole (Steer et al. 1995). This peculiar feature typically fades during the pregnancy; the prevalence of bilateral notching is 46.3 % between 11 and 14 weeks, 16.5 % between 15 and 24 weeks, and 5 % between 25 and 41 weeks (Gómez et al. 2008). As a consequence of notch disappearance, the mean diastolic velocity rises, which results in a pulsatility index (PI) value reduction (Fig. 1).

Due to the value of UtA impedance assessments employing Doppler ultrasound, the reference ranges for the mean PI during the normal menstrual cycle (Guedes-Martins et al. 2015) and from 6 to 41 weeks in uneventful

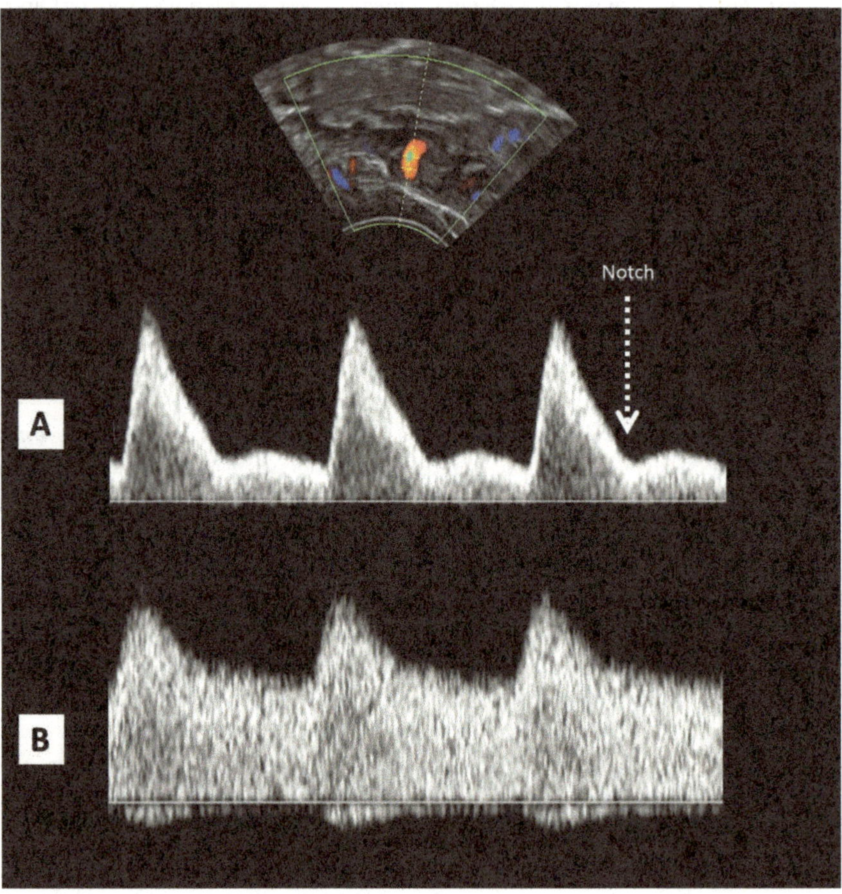

Fig. 1 UtA waveforms. Spectral analysis of normal blood flow velocity waveforms obtained before pregnancy (**a**) and at 20 weeks (**b**) of gestation. In non-pregnant women and during the first half of a normal pregnancy, the flow velocity waveforms from the main UtA are characterized by a well-defined protodiastolic notch (**a**). End-diastolic flow increases in the main UtA and its branches during the second half of the menstrual cycle, and this increase continues as pregnancy advances (Guedes-Martins et al. 2014a, b, 2015). The presence of early diastolic notches remains relevant, particularly if bilateral, to adverse pregnancy outcome, even with normal UtA resistance values

pregnancies were established and clearly revealed a general progressive gestational age-related decrement (Gómez et al. 2008; Guedes-Martins et al. 2014a). This trend has been attributed to the major changes in the placental bed that modify the properties of the UtA from a resistance vessel into a capacitance vessel (Osol and Mandala 2009).

Beyond the reference ranges for an uneventful pregnancy, a number of studies at different gestational ages have shown that UtA impedance is able to provide important predictive information about serious obstetrical disorders, such as PE. Notably, in women with gestational hypertension just before term, the incidence of elevated UtA impedance was found to be as high as 68 % and to rise to 89 % when associated with PE (Frusca et al. 2003). Other studies also observed a high incidence of abnormal UtA-PI, although at lower values, likely reflecting the different criteria for inclusion (Li et al. 2005; Meler et al. 2010).

In a group of unselected pregnant women at 22–24 weeks of gestation (Papageorghiou et al. 2001), the enhanced UtA-PI was reported to show a 69 % sensitivity for the appearance of PE with intra-uterine growth restriction (IUGR) in subsequent weeks, a value that increased to 83 % when the criteria included protodiastolic notch persistence. However, although the detection rate of PE as a result of enhanced UtA-PI was already shown to be superior to the patient's epidemiological data detection rate (Papageorghiou et al. 2005), additional conditions had to be met. In fact, other reports indicated that the correlation between abnormal UtA impedance at 22 weeks and the establishment of PE was significant only in situations in which the fetal outcome was poor, including IUGR and preterm birth (van den Elzen et al. 1995; Aardema et al. 2004). More recently, top-decile PI values and the presence of bilateral notching were considered to have a good predictive value for an enhanced risk of stillbirth resulting from placental causes (Smith et al. 2007). As a corollary of these studies, an extensive systematic review of 74 studies including 79,547 women (Cnossen et al. 2008) with the

intended purpose of evaluating the use of UtA Doppler velocimetry for the prediction of PE, concluded that UtA Doppler ultrasonography was more accurate for the prediction of PE when performed in the second trimester rather than in the first trimester. In addition, the prediction of the overall risk of PE and the risk of severe PE is significantly different in pregnant women with a low risk than in those with a high risk of developing the disease. In the group of low-risk patients, the overall risk of PE was best predicted by the presence of a second-trimester elevation of PI accompanied by UtA notching [sensitivity 23 %, specificity 99 %, positive likelihood ratio (+ve LR) 7.5, −ve LR 0.59]. Also in this low-risk group, the risk of severe PE was best predicted by either the second trimester PI (sensitivity 78 %, specificity 95 %, +ve LR 15.6, −ve LR 0.23) or bilateral notching (sensitivity 65 %, specificity 95 %, +ve LR 13.4, −ve LR 0.37). In contrast, in women at a high risk of developing PE, the overall risk of PE was best predicted by the presence of a second-trimester elevation of PI accompanied by UtA notching (sensitivity 19 %, specificity 99 %, +ve LR 21, −ve LR 0.82). Additionally, the risk of severe PE in high-risk patients was best predicted by second-trimester elevated RI (sensitivity 80 %, specificity 78 %, + ve LR 3.7, −ve LR 0.26). These findings supported the recommendation to employ PI and notching assessment in daily clinical practice (Cnossen et al. 2008).

This progressive increase in the maternal-placental blood flow during gestation is mainly due to vasodilation in part related to increased levels of 17β-estradiol, progesterone, and relaxin (Sprague et al. 2009; Vodstrcil et al. 2012). Additionally, the UtA diameter doubles in size after 20 weeks of pregnancy (Konje et al. 2001). Because blood flow within a vessel increases in proportion to the fourth power of the radius, this slight diameter increase in the UtA produces a significant blood flow capacity increase (Palmer et al. 1988; Mandala and Osol 2012) with a concomitant Doppler velocimetry increment. The downstream fall in vascular resistance leads to circumferential vessel growth, a process that nitric oxide (NO) appears to play a key role in regulating. NO is generated in the endothelium by endothelial nitric oxide synthase (eNOS) and is essential for proper endothelial function and the regulation of vascular tone. For instance, estrogen, placental growth factor (PlGF), and vascular endothelial growth factor (VEGF) augment eNOS and, consequently, NO production (Sprague et al. 2009; Mandala and Osol 2012; Grummer et al. 2009). In addition, increased soluble fms-like tyrosine kinase 1 (sFlt-1) levels inactivate and decrease circulating PlGF and VEGF concentrations and have been recognized as an important factor in PE pathogenesis (Karumanchi et al. 2005). To reverse this trend, the relative vascular insensitivity to infused angiotensin II and norepinephrine (Rosenfeld et al. 2012) also serves to increase the uteroplacental blood supply.

Abnormal UtA-PI and elevated levels of sFlt-1, reduced levels of PlGF, and an increased sFlt-1:PlGF ratio have been reported as potential predictive markers for the development of preeclampsia (Cnossen et al. 2008; Seely and Solomon 2016). However, these markers are not validated for clinical use in cases of superimposed preeclampsia.

5   Evaluation and Management of Women with Superimposed Preeclampsia

The surveillance of a pregnant woman with the diagnosis of sPE should be performed as an inpatient. This aspect is of particular importance because the failure of diagnosis or inadequate treatment of the disease is an important cause of poor obstetric outcomes, including fetal death. It is particularly important to look for signs and symptoms of severe preeclampsia, such as neurologic symptoms, epigastric or right upper quadrant pain, and nausea and vomiting (American College of Obstetricians and Gynecologists 2013).

Serial BP measurements, assessment of proteinuria from a 24-h urine collection, and laboratory evaluation (complete blood count with platelets, liver enzymes, lactic dehydrogenase, serum creatinine, and acid uric concentration) are needed. Ideally, the ACOG recommends that these laboratory results should be compared with baseline information obtained in early pregnancy. In addition, fetal growth and well-being should be assessed when sPE is suspected (American College of Obstetricians and Gynecologists 2013), and once the diagnosis of sPE is established, acute lowering of severe hypertension can be performed by oral or intravenous medications (See chapter 'Chronic Hypertension and Pregnancy').

For women with sPE who receive expectant management at less than 34 weeks of gestation, the American College of Obstetricians and Gynecologists recommends the administration of corticosteroids for fetal lung maturation (American College of Obstetricians and Gynecologists 2013; National Institutes of Health Consensus Development Panel 2001). Until then, there is only one randomized trial of glucocorticoids given to hypertensive women for fetal lung maturation (Amorim et al. 1999). This double-blind randomized trial enrolled 218 pregnant women with severe preeclampsia and gestational age between 26 and 34 weeks. One hundred ten women received betamethasone (12 mg administered intramuscularly, repeated after 24 h and then once a week), and 108 received placebo. The frequency of respiratory distress syndrome was significantly reduced in the corticosteroid group (23 %) compared to the placebo group (43 %), with a relative risk of 0.53 ($CI_{95\%}$ 0.35–0. 82). The relative risks of intraventricular hemorrhage, patent ductus arteriosus, and perinatal infection were also significantly decreased in the corticosteroid group: 0.35 ($CI_{95\%}$ 0.15–0.86), 0.27 ($CI_{95\%}$ 0.08–0.95), and 0.39 ($CI_{95\%}$ 0.39–0.97), respectively. There was no significant difference in the frequency of stillbirth, but the neonatal mortality rate was lower in the corticosteroid group (14 %) than in the placebo group (28 %), with a relative risk of 0.5 ($CI_{95\%}$ 0.28–0.89). Amorim and colleagues (1999) concluded that antenatal corticosteroid therapy with betamethasone for the acceleration of fetal lung maturity is a safe and efficient treatment in patients with severe preeclampsia between 26 and 34 weeks gestation.

Although the expectant management of preterm superimposed preeclampsia among women with chronic arterial hypertension is considered a reasonable management strategy, it is associated with some maternal morbidity (Samuel et al. 2011) and with a frequency of eclampsia development estimated in the range of 0–2.5 % (Samuel et al. 2011; Chappell et al. 2008). In this context, for women with chronic hypertension and sPE with severe features, ACOG recommends the administration of intra-partum parenteral magnesium sulfate to prevent eclampsia (American College of Obstetricians and Gynecologists 2013) and immediate delivery after maternal stabilization. The ACOG task force also reinforces that for women with sPE with severe features, expectant management beyond 34 weeks of gestation is not recommended. In fact, termination of pregnancy is the only cure for preeclampsia.

6 Conclusion

The development of sPE is the most prevalent complication in pregnancy in women with chronic hypertension, and it is an important cause of bad birth outcomes, such as preterm birth, caesarean delivery, placental abruption, and fetal growth abnormalities. Because worsening chronic hypertension is managed differently from preeclampsia, it is imperative to distinguish these two entities. In addition to the fact that the diagnosis can be really difficult to achieve, there are no known tests capable of early prediction of the disease. Future research is necessary to search for improved tests to both predict and diagnose sPE.

Competing Financial Interests The author declares no conflicts of interest.

References

Aardema MW, Saro MC, Lander M, De Wolf BT, Oosterhof H, Aarnoudse JG (2004) Second trimester Doppler ultrasound screening of the uterine arteries differentiates between subsequent normal and poor outcomes of hypertensive pregnancy: two different pathophysiological entities? Clin Sci (Lond) 106 (4):377–382

American College of Obstetricians and Gynecologists; Task Force on Hypertension in Pregnancy (2013) Hypertension in pregnancy. Report of the American College of Obstetricians and Gynecologists' Task Force on Hypertension in Pregnancy. Obstet Gynecol 122(5):1122–1131

Amorim MM, Santos LC, Faúndes A (1999) Corticosteroid therapy for prevention of respiratory distress syndrome in severe preeclampsia. Am J Obstet Gynecol 180(5):1283–1288

Anumba DO, Lincoln K, Robson SC (2010) Predictive value of clinical and laboratory indices at first assessment in women referred with suspected gestational hypertension. Hypertens Pregnancy 29(2):163–179

Balasch J, Gratacós E (2011) Delayed childbearing: effects on fertility and the outcome of pregnancy. Fetal Diagn Ther 29(4):263–273

Bramham K, Parnell B, Nelson-Piercy C, Seed PT, Poston L, Chappell LC (2014) Chronic hypertension and pregnancy outcomes: systematic review and meta-analysis. BMJ 348:g2301

Brosens I, Pijnenborg R, Vercruysse L, Romero R (2011) The "Great Obstetrical Syndromes" are associated with disorders of deep placentation. Am J Obstet Gynecol 204(3):193–201

Chappell LC, Enye S, Seed P, Briley AL, Poston L, Shennan AH (2008) Adverse perinatal outcomes and risk factors for preeclampsia in women with chronic hypertension: a prospective study. Hypertension 51 (4):1002–1009. doi:10.1161/HYPERTENSIONAHA. 107.107565

Cnossen JS, Morris RK, ter Riet G, Mol BW, van der Post JA, Coomarasamy A, Zwinderman AH, Robson SC, Bindels PJ, Kleijnen J, Khan KS (2008) Use of uterine artery Doppler ultrasonography to predict pre-eclampsia and intrauterine growth restriction: a systematic review and bivariable meta-analysis. CMAJ 178(6):701–711

de Mouzon J, Goossens V, Bhattacharya S, Castilla JA, Ferraretti AP, Korsak V, Kupka M, Nygren KG, Nyboe Andersen A, European IVF-monitoring (EIM) Consortium, for the European Society of Human Reproduction and Embryology (ESHRE) (2010) Assisted reproductive technology in Europe, 2006: results generated from European registers by ESHRE. Hum Reprod 25(8):1851–1862

Edwards EW, DiPette DJ, Townsend RR, Cohen DL (2014) Top 10 landmark studies in hypertension. J Am Soc Hypertens 8(6):437–447

Ferrer RL, Sibai BM, Mulrow CD, Chiquette E, Stevens KR, Cornell J (2000) Management of mild chronic hypertension during pregnancy: a review. Obstet Gynecol 96(5 Pt 2):849–860

Frusca T, Soregaroli M, Platto C, Enterri L, Lojacono A, Valcamonico A (2003) Uterine artery velocimetry in patients with gestational hypertension. Obstet Gynecol 102(1):136–140

Gómez O, Figueras F, Fernández S, Bennasar M, Martínez JM, Puerto B, Gratacós E (2008) Reference ranges for uterine artery mean pulsatility index at 11–41 weeks of gestation. Ultrasound Obstet Gynecol 32(2):128–132

Grummer MA, Sullivan JA, Magness RR, Bird IM (2009) Vascular endothelial growth factor acts through novel, pregnancy-enhanced receptor signalling pathways to stimulate endothelial nitric oxide synthase activity in uterine artery endothelial cells. Biochem J 417 (2):501–511

Guedes-Martins L, Saraiva J, Gaio R, Macedo F, Almeida H (2014a) Uterine artery impedance at very early clinical pregnancy. Prenat Diagn 34(8):719–725

Guedes-Martins L, Cunha A, Saraiva J, Gaio R, Macedo F, Almeida H (2014b) Internal iliac and uterine arteries Doppler ultrasound in the assessment of normotensive and chronic hypertensive pregnant women. Sci Rep 4:3785

Guedes-Martins L, Gaio R, Saraiva J, Cerdeira S, Matos L, Silva E, Macedo F, Almeida H (2015) Reference ranges for uterine artery pulsatility index during the menstrual cycle: a cross-sectional study. PLoS One 10(3), e0119103

Hajjar I, Kotchen JM, Kotchen TA (2006) Hypertension: trends in prevalence, incidence, and control. Annu Rev Public Health 27:465–490

Istance D, Theisens H (2008) Ageing OECD societies in trends shaping education 2008. Centre for Educational Research and Innovation. Organization for Economic Co-Operation and Development, OECD, pp 13–20

Jacobsson B, Ladfors L, Milsom I (2004) Advanced maternal age and adverse perinatal outcome. Obstet Gynecol 104(4):727–733

Karumanchi SA, Maynard SE, Stillman IE, Epstein FH, Sukhatme VP (2005) Preeclampsia: a renal perspective. Kidney Int 67(6):2101–2113

Konje JC, Kaufmann P, Bell SC, Taylor DJ (2001) A longitudinal study of quantitative uterine blood flow with the use of color power angiography in appropriate for gestational age pregnancies. Am J Obstet Gynecol 185(3):608–613

Lain KY, Roberts JM (2002) Contemporary concepts of the pathogenesis and management of preeclampsia. JAMA 287(24):3183–3186

Leow MK (2015) Environmental origins of hypertension: phylogeny, ontogeny and epigenetics. Hypertens Res 38:299

Li H, Gudnason H, Olofsson P, Dubiel M, Gudmundsson S (2005) Increased uterine artery vascular impedance is related to adverse outcome of pregnancy but is present in only one-third of late third-trimester pre-eclamptic women. Ultrasound Obstet Gynecol 25 (5):459–463

Mandala M, Osol G (2012) Physiological remodelling of the maternal uterine circulation during pregnancy. Basic Clin Pharmacol Toxicol 110(1):12–18

Mathews TJ, Hamilton BE (2009) Delayed childbearing: more women are having their first child later in life. NCHS data brief, no 21. Hyattsville, MD. National Center for Health Statistics 21:1–8

Meler E, Figueras F, Mula R, Crispi F, Benassar M, Gómez O, Gratacós E (2010) Prognostic role of uterine artery Doppler in patients with preeclampsia. Fetal Diagn Ther 27(1):8–13

Menken J, Trussell J, Larsen U (1986) Age and infertility. Science 233(4771):1389–1394

National Institutes of Health Consensus Development Panel (2001) Antenatal corticosteroids revisited: repeat courses – National Institutes of Health Consensus Development Conference Statement, August 17–18, 2000. Obstet Gynecol 98(1):144–150

National Heart, Lung and Blood Institute (2001) Report of the working group on research on hypertension during pregnancy. http://www.nhlbi.nih.gov/resources/hyperten_preg/

Osol G, Mandala M (2009) Maternal uterine vascular remodeling during pregnancy. Physiology (Bethesda, Md) 24:58–71

Oyelese Y, Ananth CV (2006) Placental abruption. Obstet Gynecol 108(4):1005–1016

Palmer RM, Ashton DS, Moncada S (1988) Vascular endothelial cells synthesize nitric oxide from L-arginine. Nature 333(6174):664–666

Papageorghiou AT, Yu CK, Bindra R, Pandis G, Nicolaides KH, Fetal Medicine Foundation Second Trimester Screening Group (2001) Multicenter screening for pre-eclampsia and fetal growth restriction by transvaginal uterine artery Doppler at 23 weeks of gestation. Ultrasound Obstet Gynecol 18 (5):441–449

Papageorghiou AT, Yu CK, Erasmus IE, Cuckle HS, Nicolaides KH (2005) Assessment of risk for the development of pre-eclampsia by maternal characteristics and uterine artery Doppler. BJOG 112 (6):703–709

Ray JG, Burrows RF, Burrows EA, Vermeulen MJ (2001) MOS HIP: McMaster outcome study of hypertension in pregnancy. Early Hum Dev 64(2):129–143

Rosenfeld CR, DeSpain K, Word RA, Liu XT (2012) Differential sensitivity to angiotensin II and norepinephrine in human uterine arteries. J Clin Endocrinol Metab 97(1):138–147

Samuel A, Lin C, Parviainen K, Jeyabalan A (2011) Expectant management of preeclampsia superimposed on chronic hypertension. J Matern Fetal Neonatal Med 24(7):907–911. doi:10.3109/14767058.2010.535874

Seely EW, Ecker J (2014) Chronic hypertension in pregnancy. Circulation 129(11):1254–1261

Seely EW, Solomon CG (2016) Improving the prediction of preeclampsia. N Engl J Med 374(1):83–84. doi:10.1056/NEJMe1515223

Sibai BM, Stella CL (2009) Diagnosis and management of atypical preeclampsia-eclampsia. Am J Obstet Gynecol 200(5):481.e1-7

Sibai B, Dekker G, Kupferminc M (2005) Pre-eclampsia. Lancet 365(9461):785–799

Smith GC, Yu CK, Papageorghiou AT, Cacho AM, Nicolaides KH, Fetal Medicine Foundation Second Trimester Screening Group (2007) Maternal uterine artery Doppler flow velocimetry and the risk of stillbirth. Obstet Gynecol 109(1):144–151

Sprague BJ, Phernetton TM, Magness RR, Chesler NC (2009) The effects of the ovarian cycle and pregnancy on uterine vascular impedance and uterine artery mechanics. Eur J Obstet Gynecol Reprod Biol 144 (Suppl 1):S170–S178

Steer CV, Williams J, Zaidi J, Campbell S, Tan SL (1995) Intra-observer, interobserver, interultrasound transducer and intercycle variation in colour Doppler assessment of uterine artery impedance. Hum Reprod 10(2):479–481

van den Elzen HJ, Cohen-Overbeek TE, Grobbee DE, Quartero RW, Wladimiroff JW (1995) Early uterine artery Doppler velocimetry and the outcome of pregnancy in women aged 35 years and older. Ultrasound Obstet Gynecol 5(5):328–333

van Katwijk C, Peeters LL (1998) Clinical aspects of pregnancy after the age of 35 years: a review of the literature. Hum Reprod Update 4(2):185–194

Vodstrcil LA, Tare M, Novak J, Dragomir N, Ramirez RJ, Wlodek ME, Conrad KP, Parry LJ (2012) Relaxin mediates uterine artery compliance during pregnancy and increases uterine blood flow. FASEB J 26 (10):4035–4044

Adv Exp Med Biol - Advances in Internal Medicine (2017) 2: 419–426
DOI 10.1007/5584_2016_99
© Springer International Publishing AG 2016
Published online: 5 November 2016

Hypertension Is a Risk Factor for Several Types of Heart Disease: Review of Prospective Studies

Yoshihiro Kokubo and Chisa Matsumoto

Abstract

Many prospective cohort studies have demonstrated that hypertension is a strong risk factor for total mortality and cardiovascular disease (CVD). Heart disease includes coronary heart disease (CHD), heart failure, atrial fibrillation, valvular disease, sudden cardiac death (SCD), sick sinus syndrome (SSS), cardiomyopathy, and aortic aneurysms. Most of the epidemiologic prospective studies of heart disease focused on coronary/ischemic heart disease. Here we comprehensively reviewed the association between hypertension and the above-mentioned heart diseases. We found that CHD, heart failure, atrial fibrillation, aortic valvular disease, SCD, SSS, left ventricular hypertrophy, and abdominal aortic aneurysms were all associated with hypertension. Those relations tended to be stronger in men. The prevention of hypertension and lowering one's blood pressure may help reduce the risk of developing heart disease.

Keywords

Heart disease • Hypertension • Prospective studies • Epidemiology • Risk factors

Y. Kokubo (✉)
Department of Preventive Cardiology, National Cerebral and Cardiovascular Center, 5-7-1, Fujishiro-dai, Suita, Osaka 565-8565, Japan
e-mail: ykokubo@hsp.ncvc.go.jp

C. Matsumoto
Department of Clinical Epidemiology, Hyogo College of Medicine, Nishinomiya, Hyogo, Japan

1   Introduction

Many prospective cohort studies have demonstrated that hypertension is a strong risk factor for total mortality and cardiovascular disease (CVD) (Heerspink et al. 2009). The management and prevention of hypertension are important to reduce the risk of CVD. Accumulating evidence suggests the importance of reducing blood pressure not only toward preventing CVD but also in the management of other diseases, such as brain–cardiorenal crosstalk and noncardiovascular diseases including dementia, cancer, oral health disorders, and osteoporosis (Kokubo and Iwashima 2015).

Risk factors for heart disease include not only hypercholesterolemia and smoking but also hypertension. Previous reviews concerning hypertension focused mainly on CVD. In the present review, we broaden the range of studies to comprehensibly examine the association between hypertension and heart disease, which disease includes CVD/coronary heart disease (CHD), heart failure, atrial fibrillation, aortic valve disease, sudden cardiac death (SCD), sick sinus syndrome (SSS), left ventricular hypertrophy (LVH), and thoracic and abdominal aortic aneurysms (TAA/AAA).

2 Coronary Heart Disease (CHD) and Cardiovascular Disease (CVD)

Hypertension is the largest risk factor for CVD (Wilson et al. 1998; Eshak et al. 2012). The population-attributable fractions (PAF) of combined prehypertension with hypertension for CVD were approximately 30–60 % (Kokubo et al. 2008; Ikeda et al. 2009). The prevention of hypertension and the improvement of blood pressure (BP) are essential and fundamental steps toward the prevention of CVD (Table 1).

The Framingham Heart Study showed that high-normal BP and hypertension (stage 1, stage 2, and higher) increased the risk of CHD in both men [relative risk (RR, 95 % confidence intervals, CI) = 1.31 (0.98–1.76), 1.67 (1.28–2.18), and 1.84 (1.37–2.49)] and women [RR (95 % CI) = 1.30 (0.86–1.98), 1.73 (1.19–2.52), and 2.12 (1.42–3.17)] (Wilson et al. 1998). The Suita Study, a Japanese urban cohort study, showed that high-normal BP and hypertension stage 1 and stage 2 or higher increased the risk of myocardial infarction (MI) in men [hazard ratios, HRs (95 % CI) = 2.65 (1.20–5.85), 2.72 (1.26–5.84), and 3.89 (1.76–8.56), respectively], and that hypertension stage 2 or higher was increased risk of MI

in women [HR (95 % CI) = 5.24 (1.85–14.85)] (Kokubo et al. 2008).

A meta-analysis of individual data for one million adults examined in 61 prospective studies showed that throughout the range of usual systolic blood pressure (SBP) values decreasing to ≤115 mmHg, the slope of the association between CHD mortality (plotted on a doubling scale) and the usual SBP levels were approximately constant within each age range, although the relative strength of the association was weaker for CHD than for stroke mortality in middle age (Lewington et al. 2002) (Table 2). In addition, for the association between CHD mortality and usual diastolic blood pressure (DBP) values decreasing to ≤75 mmHg, age-specific HRs associated with 10-mmHg differences in usual DBP are equivalent to those associated with 20-mmHg differences in usual SBP values.

The Japan Arteriosclerosis Longitudinal Study Group provided a meta-analysis of 16 cohort studies that included 48,224 Japanese men and women (40–89 years old) at baseline and an average 8.4-year follow-up (Miura et al. 2009). Higher SBP, pulse pressure, and mean BP were increased risks of MI in men, but not in women. The incidence of MI was 1.2 and 0.5 per 1000 person-years in the men and women, respectively. Due to the small sample size of women, the association between higher BP values and incident MI may not be observed in women.

3 Heart Failure

In the First National Health and Nutrition Examination Survey Epidemiologic (NHANES I) Follow-up Study, during the average follow-up of 19 years, 10.1 % of the Congestive heart failure (CHF) cases were documented. The incidence of CHF was significantly associated with coronary heart disease [RR (95 % CI) = 8.11 (6.95–9.46), PAF = 61.6 %], cigarette smoking [RR (95 % CI) = 1.59 (1.39–1.83), PAF = 17.1 %], hypertension [RR (95 % CI) = 1.40 (1.24–1.59), PAF = 10.1 %], in descending order of the PAF values (He et al. 2001).

Table 1 Review of studies of hypertension as a risk factor for heart disease

Disease	Population	No. of subjects	Age (years)	Design	Results
MI	Framingham Heart Study (Wilson et al. 1998)	M, 2489	48.6 ± 11.7	Prospective study	Men: normal BP: RR = 1.0 (ref), high normal BP: RR = 1.31 (0.98–1.76), HTN stage 1: RR = 1.67 (1.28–2.18), HTN stages 2–4: RR = 1.84 (1.37–2.49)
		W, 2856			Women: normal BP: RR = 1.0 (ref), high normal BP: RR = 1.30(0.86–1.98), HTN stage 1: RR = 1.73 (1.19–2.52), HTN stages 2–4: RR = 2.12 (1.42–3.17)
					*adjusted for total cholesterol
	Suita Study (Kokubo et al. 2008)	5494	30–79	Prospective study	Men: Optimal: HR = 1(ref), normal BP: 2.14 (0.94–4.86), high-normal BP: HR = 2.65 (1.20–5.85), HTN stage 1: HR = 2.72 (1.26–5.84), HTN stage ≥2: HR = 3.89 (1.76–8.56)
					Women: Optimal: HR = 1(ref), normal BP: HR = 1.44 (0.42–4.90), high-normal BP: HR = 2.27 (0.78–6.57), HTN stage 1: HR = 1.69 (0.56–5.10), HTN stage ≥2: HR = 5.24 (1.85–14.85)
HF	NHANES (He et al. 2001)	13,643	M, 52.2 ± 15.2 W, 48.1 ± 15.4	Prospective study	HTN: RR = 1.50 (1.34–1.68)
	Framingham Heart Study (Lee et al. 2007)	3362	62	Prospective study	SBP per 1-SD increment: HR = 1.31 (1.11–1.55)
Af	Framingham Heart study (Benjamin et al. 1994)	M, 2090	55–94	Prospective study	Men: HTN (1.5:1.2–2.0),
		W, 2641			Women: HTN (1.4:1.1–1.8)
	Southern Community Cohort Study (Lipworth et al. 2012)	8836	≥65	prospective study	HTN: HR = 1.29 (1.07–1.55)
AS	Cardiovascular Health Study (CHS) (Stewart et al. 1997)		≥65	Prospective study	HTN: OR = 1.23 (1.1–1.4)
MR	Framingham Heart Study (Singh et al. 1999)	M, 1696	54 ± 10	Prospective study	HTN: OR = 1.6 (1.2–2.0)
		W, 1893			
SCD	Nurses' Health Study (Albert et al. 2003)	121,701 women	30–55	Prospective study	HTN: OR = 2.49 (1.87–3.32)
SSS	ARIC & CHS (Jensen et al. 2014)	20,572	ARIC: 54 CHS: 73	Prospective study	HTN: OR = 1.56 (1.09–2.25)
LVH	Framingham Heart & Offspring Study (Verdecchia et al. 1996)	274	≥50	Prospective study	Men: HTN: OR = 2.58 (0.97–6.86)
					Women: HTN: OR = 5.94 (3.06–11.53)
AAA	Southern Community Cohort (Jahangir et al. 2015)	18,782	64.5	Prospective study	Normal BP: HR = 1.0 (ref), high BP: HR = 1.44 (1.04–2.01)

MI myocardial infarction, *HF* heart failure *Af* atrial fibrillation, *AS* aortic sclerosis, *MR* mitral regurgitation, *SCD* sudden cardiac death, *SSS* sick sinus syndrome, *LVH* left ventricular hypertrophy, *AAA* abdominal aortic aneurysm, *CHD* ischemic heart disease, *HTN* hypertension, *BP* blood pressure, *SBP* systolic blood pressure, *DBP* diastolic blood pressure, *MBP* mean blood pressure, *PP* pulse pressure, *M* men, *W* women, *HR* hazard ratio, *ref* reference, *OR* odds ratio, *SD* standard deviation

Table 2 Meta-analysis of studies of hypertension as a risk factor for heart disease

Disease	Population	No. of subjects	Results
CHD mortality	61 prospective studies (Lewington et al. 2002)	12.7 million person-years	Usual SBP: decreasing to ≤115 mmHg
			Age 40–49: HR = 0.49 (0.45–0.53)
			Age 50–59: HR = 0.50 (0.49–0.52)
			Age 60–69: HR = 0.54 (0.53–0.55)
			Age 70–79: HR = 0.60 (0.58–0.61)
			Age 80–89: HR = 0.67 (0.64–0.70)
			Usual DBP: decreasing to ≤75 mmHg
			Age 40–49: HR = 0.47 (0.43–0.51)
			Age 50–59: HR = 0.52 (0.50–0.55)
			Age 60–69: HR = 0.56 (0.54–0.58)
			Age 70–79: HR = 0.62 (0.60–0.64)
			Age 80–89: HR = 0.70 (0.65–0.74)
MI	16 Japanese cohort studies (Miura et al. 2009)	407,213 person-years	Men:
			SBP per 1-SD increment: HR = 1.23 (1.06–1.44)
			DBP per 1-SD increment: HR = 1.17 (0.99–1.39)
			PP per 1-SD increment: HR = 1.17 (1.01–1.36)
			MBP per 1-SD increment: HR = 1.22 (1.04–1.44)
			Women:
			SBP per 1-SD increment: HR = 1.25 (0.99–1.58)
			DBP per 1-SD increment: HR = 1.18 (0.92–1.52)
			PP per 1-SD increment: HR = 1.18 (0.95–1.47)
			MBP per 1-SD increment: HR = 1.25 (0.98–1.59)

Abbreviations are explained in the Table 1 footnote

In the Framingham Heart Study, during 67,240 person-years of follow-up, 518 incidence of heart failure were observed. Recent SBP [HR (95 % CI) per 1-SD increment = 1.31 (1.11–1.55)], pulse pressure [HR (95 % CI) per 1-SD increment = 1.33 (1.14–1.54)], and body mass index (BMI) [HR (95 % CI) per unit increase = 1.15 (1.08–1.23)] were associated with heart failure risk even after adjusting for current measures (Lee et al. 2007). Therefore, the presence of hypertension and higher SBP increased risk of heart failure.

4   Atrial Fibrillation

Atrial fibrillation (AF) is one of the most frequent types of arrhythmia and is a risk factor for mortality, CVD (Emdin et al. 2016), and ischemic stroke (Lip et al. 2012). In the Framingham Heart Study, hypertension was revealed to provide 1.5- and 1.4-increased risks of AF in men and women, respectively.(Benjamin et al. 1994) The

Women's Health Study showed that systolic high-normal BP and grades 1, 2 and 3 hypertension increased the risk of incident AF compared to systolic optimal BP [adjusted HRs (95 %c CI) = 1.28 (1.00–1.63), 1.56 (1.22–2.01), and 2.74 (1.77–4.22); P for trend <0.0001, respectively], and that diastolic high-normal BP and grade 2 and 3 hypertension increased the risk of incident AF compared to diastolic BP <65 mmHg [adjusted HRs (95 % CI) = 1.53 (1.05–2.23) and 2.15 (1.21–3.84); P for trend = 0.004] (Conen et al. 2009). A cohort study of Norwegian men also showed that high-normal BP was associated with incident AF (Grundvold et al. 2012). The Southern Community Cohort study showed that hypertension and diabetes increased the risk of AF, especially in blacks and women (Lipworth et al. 2012).

These associations were also confirmed in a recent Japanese cohort study (Kokubo et al. 2015). In that study, systolic and diastolic hypertension and pulse pressure are risk factors for incident AF. Compared to normal BP with normal weight, systolic prehypertension with overweight was shown to be associated with an increased risk of incident AF (P for interaction between SBP and body mass index = 0.04). In this study, Arterial stiffness, increased left atrial size, and left ventricular hypertrophy are important mediators of the relationship between BP and incident AF (Brignole et al. 2013). Higher SBP and body weight may mutually exacerbate hypertension and left ventricular hypertrophy, and consequently, these two factors may cooperatively increase the risk of AF.

5 Valve Disease

Aortic valve disease, manifested as aortic valve stenosis and regurgitation is one of the problematic heart disease in aging society. In the Cardiovascular Health Study, aortic valve sclerosis was present in 26 % and aortic valve stenosis in 2 % of the study cohort. The independent clinical factors associated with degenerative aortic valve disease included age (a two-fold increased risk for each 10-year increase in age), male gender (a two-fold excess risk), present smoking (a 35 % increase in risk), a history of hypertension (a 20 % increase in risk) (Stewart et al. 1997).

For mitral valve disease and tricuspid valve disease, in the Framingham Heart Study, the clinical determinant risk factors for mitral regurgitation were age (odds ratio [OR] = 1.3/ 9.9 years, 95 %CI = 1.2–1.5), hypertension (OR = 1.6, 95 %CI = 1.2–2.0), and BMI [OR (95 % CI) = 0.8 (0.7–0.9) per 4.3 kg/m^2]; the clinical determinant risk factors for tricuspid regurgitation were age [OR (95 % CI) = 1.5 (1.3–1.7) per 9.9 years], BMI [OR (95 % CI) = 0.7 (0.6–0.8) per 4.3 kg/m^2], and female gender [OR (95 % CI) = 1.2 (1.0–1.6)], and those for aortic regurgitation were age [OR (95 % CI) = 2.3 (2.0–2.7) per 9.9 years] and male gender [OR (95 % CI) = 1.6 (1.2–2.1)] (Singh et al. 1999). In that study of a U.S. general population, hypertension was a risk factor only for mitral regurgitation.

6 Sudden Cardiac Death (SCD)

The Nurses' Health Study Cohort showed that all of the cardiac risk factors examined—especially smoking, diabetes, and hypertension—were associated with the risk of SCD (Albert et al. 2003). Multivariable-adjusted risk factors associated with SCD included diabetes (a 2.9-fold increased risk), hypertension (a 2.5-fold increased risk), smoking (2.8-, 2.4-, and 4.1-fold increased risks in individuals who smoke <15, 15–24, and ≥25 cigarettes/day), and obesity (a 1.6-fold increased risk). The incident SCD in a Japanese general population living in rural areas was 0.13 per 1000 person-years.

7 Sick Sinus Syndrome (SSS)

Sick sinus syndrome (SSS) is the name for a group of heart rhythm problems (arrhythmias) in which the sinus node does not work properly. Typical symptoms of SSS are syncope, dizziness, palpitations, exertional dyspnea, easy fatigability from chronotropic incompetence, heart failure, and angina (Jensen et al. 2014). The joint study of the ARIC (Atherosclerosis Risk In Communities) study and the CHS (Cardiovascular Health Study) showed that the standardized incidence of SSS in white and black individuals is 0.9 and 0.7 per 1000 person-years, respectively, (Jensen et al. 2014) and the incident SSS was associated with prevalent hypertension [OR (95 % CI) = 1.56 (1.09–2.25)]. Older age, hypertension, heart failure, and history of CVD were associated with SSS in the ARIC and CHS (Sanders et al. 2004).

8 Left Ventricular Hypertrophy (LVH)

Left ventricular hypertrophy (LVH), the thickening of the myocardium of the left ventricle of the heart, is a strong BP-independent risk factor for cardiovascular morbidity and mortality in general populations (Schmieder and Messerli

2000). The Framingham Heart and Offspring Study showed that LV mass, but not its geometric pattern, provides important prognostic information independent of conventional risk markers including office and ambulatory BP values in hypertensive subjects with established LV hypertrophy (Verdecchia et al. 1996).

9 Thoracic and Abdominal Aortic Aneurysms (TAA/AAA)

Approximately 60 % of the instances of thoracic aortic aneurysms (TAAs) has been observed at the aortic root and/or the ascending aorta, 40 % at the descending aorta, and 10 % at the arch (Isselbacher 2005). An ascending TAA in particular most often results from cystic medial degeneration, where it appears as smooth muscle cell dropout and elastic fiber degeneration. Cystic medial degeneration accelerates with aging and hypertension (Guo et al. 2001).

Abdominal aortic aneurysms (AAAs) are much more common than TAAs. The risk factors of AAA are age, male sex, hypertension, hyperlipidemia, atherosclerosis, and smoking (Lederle et al. 1997; Lederle et al. 2001).

The Southern Community Cohort Study showed that incident AAA in black and white populations was 1.53 and 4.01 per 1000 person-years, respectively. The risk factors for incident AAA were female sex [HR (95 % CI) = 0.48 (0.36–0.65)], blacks [HR (95 % CI) = 0.51 (0.37–0.69)], smoking [former: HR (95 % CI) = 1.91 (1.27–2.87); current: HR (95 % CI) = 5.55 (3.67–8.40)], and a history of hypertension [HR (95 % CI) = 1.44 (1.04–2.01)] (Jahangir et al. 2015). Smoking is the strongest risk factor for AAA, whereas hypertension is a moderate but significant increased risk for AAA in the U.S. population. In an Asian population, the incident AAA in men and women >70 years old were 0.78 and 0.19 per 1000 person-years, respectively (Yii 2003). The prevalence of smoking and hypertension was ≥40% among AAA patients. The incidence of AAA was higher in Westerners compared to Asians. Smoking and hypertension were risk factors for AAA in both Westerners and Asians.

10 Clinical Implications

Hypertension is a risk factor for heart disease; not only CHD, but also heart failure, atrial fibrillation, aortic valvular disease, SCD, SSS, LVH, and AAA. The prevention of hypertension may reduce the risk of these heart diseases. In order to reduce higher BP, lifestyle modification is very important. The various guidelines issued by the Japanese Society of Hypertension, the American College of Cardiology/American Heart Association, and the European Society of Hypertension/European Society of Cardiology are essentially the same in stating that there are seven points of lifestyle modification that will help reduce and prevent hypertensions: eating sufficient amounts of vegetables and fruits, reducing salt and saturate fatty acid intakes, increasing fish intake, moderating one's alcohol intake, quitting smoking, engaging in regular exercise, and maintaining a normal weight (Shimamoto et al. 2014; Eckel et al. 2014; Mancia et al. 2013). The prevention of hypertension and lifestyle modifications may also reduce the risk of heart diseases and hypertension-related diseases such as dementia, chronic kidney disease, cancer, and periodontal disease (Kokubo and Iwashima 2015; Kokubo 2014).

Source of Funding This work was supported by the Intramural Research Fund of the National Cerebral and Cardiovascular Center, by the Japan Agency for Medical Research and development, AMED (15gk0210001h0101), and by a Grant-in-Aid for Scientific Research (B, No. 16H05252) and Challenging Exploratory Research (No. 16K15365) in Japan.

References

Albert CM, Chae CU, Grodstein F et al (2003) Prospective study of sudden cardiac death among women in the United States. Circulation 107:2096–2101

Benjamin EJ, Levy D, Vaziri SM, D'Agostino RB, Belanger AJ, Wolf PA (1994) Independent risk factors for atrial fibrillation in a population-based cohort. The Framingham Heart Study. JAMA 271:840–844

Brignole M, Auricchio A, Baron-Esquivias G et al (2013) 2013 ESC guidelines on cardiac pacing and cardiac resynchronization therapy: the task force on cardiac pacing and resynchronization therapy of the European Society of Cardiology (ESC). Developed in collaboration with the European Heart Rhythm Association (EHRA). Eur Heart J 34:2281–2329

Conen D, Tedrow UB, Koplan BA, Glynn RJ, Buring JE, Albert CM (2009) Influence of systolic and diastolic blood pressure on the risk of incident atrial fibrillation in women. Circulation 119:2146–2152

Eckel RH, Jakicic JM, Ard JD et al (2014) 2013 AHA/ACC guideline on lifestyle management to reduce cardiovascular risk: a report of the American College of Cardiology/American Heart Association Task Force on Practice Guidelines. Circulation 129: S76–S99

Emdin CA, Wong CX, Hsiao AJ et al (2016) Atrial fibrillation as risk factor for cardiovascular disease and death in women compared with men: systematic review and meta-analysis of cohort studies. BMJ 532: h7013

Eshak ES, Iso H, Kokubo Y et al (2012) Soft drink intake in relation to incident ischemic heart disease, stroke, and stroke subtypes in Japanese men and women: the Japan Public Health Centre-based study cohort I. Am J Clin Nutr 96:1390–1397

Grundvold I, Skretteberg PT, Liestol K et al (2012) Upper normal blood pressures predict incident atrial fibrillation in healthy middle-aged men: a 35-year follow-up study. Hypertension 59:198–204

Guo D, Hasham S, Kuang SQ et al (2001) Familial thoracic aortic aneurysms and dissections: genetic heterogeneity with a major locus mapping to 5q13-14. Circulation 103:2461–2468

He J, Ogden LG, Bazzano LA, Vupputuri S, Loria C, Whelton PK (2001) Risk factors for congestive heart failure in US men and women: NHANES I epidemiologic follow-up study. Arch Intern Med 161:996–1002

Heerspink HJ, Ninomiya T, Zoungas S et al (2009) Effect of lowering blood pressure on cardiovascular events and mortality in patients on dialysis: a systematic review and meta-analysis of randomised controlled trials. Lancet 373:1009–1015

Ikeda A, Iso H, Yamagishi K, Inoue M, Tsugane S (2009) Blood pressure and the risk of stroke, cardiovascular disease, and all-cause mortality among Japanese: the JPHC study. Am J Hypertens 22:273–280

Isselbacher EM (2005) Thoracic and abdominal aortic aneurysms. Circulation 111:816–828

Jahangir E, Lipworth L, Edwards TL et al (2015) Smoking, sex, risk factors and abdominal aortic aneurysms: a prospective study of 18 782 persons aged above 65 years in the Southern Community Cohort Study. J Epidemiol Community Health 69:481–488

Jensen PN, Gronroos NN, Chen LY et al (2014) Incidence of and risk factors for sick sinus syndrome in the general population. J Am Coll Cardiol 64:531–538

Kokubo Y (2014) Prevention of hypertension and cardiovascular diseases: a comparison of lifestyle factors in Westerners and East Asians. Hypertension 63:655–660

Kokubo Y, Iwashima Y (2015) Higher blood pressure as a risk factor for diseases other than stroke and ischemic heart disease. Hypertension 66:254–259

Kokubo Y, Kamide K, Okamura T et al (2008) Impact of high-normal blood pressure on the risk of cardiovascular disease in a Japanese urban cohort – the Suita study. Hypertension 52:652–659

Kokubo Y, Watanabe M, Higashiyama A et al (2015) Interaction of blood pressure and body mass index with risk of incident atrial fibrillation in a Japanese urban cohort: the Suita study. Am J Hypertens 28:1355–1361

Lederle FA, Johnson GR, Wilson SE et al (1997) Prevalence and associations of abdominal aortic aneurysm detected through screening. Aneurysm Detection and Management (ADAM) Veterans Affairs Cooperative Study Group. Ann Intern Med 126:441–449

Lederle FA, Johnson GR, Wilson SE, Aneurysm D, Management Veterans Affairs Cooperative S (2001) Abdominal aortic aneurysm in women. J Vasc Surg 34:122–126

Lee DS, Massaro JM, Wang TJ et al (2007) Antecedent blood pressure, body mass index, and the risk of incident heart failure in later life. Hypertension 50:869–876

Lewington S, Clarke R, Qizilbash N, Peto R, Collins R (2002) Age-specific relevance of usual blood pressure to vascular mortality: a meta-analysis of individual data for one million adults in 61 prospective studies. Lancet 360:1903–1913

Lip GY, Tse HF, Lane DA (2012) Atrial fibrillation. Lancet 379:648–661

Lipworth L, Okafor H, Mumma MT et al (2012) Race-specific impact of atrial fibrillation risk factors in blacks and whites in the southern community cohort study. Am J Cardiol 110:1637–1642

Mancia G, Fagard R, Narkiewicz K et al (2013) 2013 ESH/ESC Guidelines for the management of arterial hypertension: the Task Force for the management of arterial hypertension of the European Society of Hypertension (ESH) and of the European Society of Cardiology (ESC). J Hypertens 31:1281–1357

Miura K, Nakagawa H, Ohashi Y et al (2009) Four blood pressure indexes and the risk of stroke and myocardial infarction in Japanese men and women: a meta-analysis of 16 cohort studies. Circulation 119:1892–1898

Sanders P, Morton JB, Kistler PM et al (2004) Electrophysiological and electroanatomic characterization of the atria in sinus node disease: evidence of diffuse atrial remodeling. Circulation 109:1514–1522

Schmieder RE, Messerli FH (2000) Hypertension and the heart. J Hum Hypertens 14:597–604

Shimamoto K, Ando K, Fujita T et al (2014) The Japanese Society of Hypertension guidelines for the management of hypertension (JSH 2014). Hypertens Res 37:253–387

Singh JP, Evans JC, Levy D et al (1999) Prevalence and clinical determinants of mitral, tricuspid, and aortic regurgitation (the Framingham Heart Study). Am J Cardiol 83:897–902

Stewart BF, Siscovick D, Lind BK et al (1997) Clinical factors associated with calcific aortic valve disease. Cardiovascular health study. J Am Coll Cardiol 29:630–634

Verdecchia P, Schillaci G, Borgioni C et al (1996) Prognostic value of left ventricular mass and geometry in systemic hypertension with left ventricular hypertrophy. Am J Cardiol 78:197–202

Wilson PW, D'Agostino RB, Levy D, Belanger AM, Silbershatz H, Kannel WB (1998) Prediction of coronary heart disease using risk factor categories. Circulation 97:1837–1847

Yii MK (2003) Epidemiology of abdominal aortic aneurysm in an Asian population. ANZ J Surg 73:393–395

Adv Exp Med Biol - Advances in Internal Medicine (2017) 2: 427–445
DOI 10.1007/5584_2016_86
© Springer International Publishing AG 2016
Published online: 22 November 2016

The Relationship Between Aortic Root Size and Hypertension: An Unsolved Conundrum

Giuseppe Mulè, Emilio Nardi, Massimiliano Morreale,
Antonella Castiglia, Giulio Geraci, Dario Altieri,
Valentina Cacciatore, Margherita Schillaci,
Francesco Vaccaro, and Santina Cottone

Abstract

Thoracic aortic aneurysms rupture and dissection are among the most devastating vascular diseases, being characterized by elevated mortality, despite improvements in diagnostic imaging and surgical techniques.

An increased aortic root diameter (ARD) represents the main risk factor for thoracic aortic dissection and rupture and for aortic valve regurgitation.

Even though arterial hypertension is commonly regarded as a predisposing condition for the development of thoracic aorta aneurysms, the role of blood pressure (BP) as determinant of aortic root enlargement is still controversial. The use of different methods for indexation of ARD may have in part contributed to the heterogeneous findings obtained in the investigations exploring the relationships between ARD and BP. Indeed, the best methods for ARD indexation, as well as the normal values of aortic root size, are still a matter of debate.

Several non-hemodynamic factors influence ARD, including age, gender, and anthropometric variables, such as height, weight and their derivatives body surface area (BSA) and body mass index. Of these factors, anthropometric variables have the greatest impact.

Several studies documented an association between ARD enlargement, assessed by echocardiography, and some indices of hypertensive target

G. Mulè (✉), E. Nardi, M. Morreale, A. Castiglia,
G. Geraci, D. Altieri, V. Cacciatore, M. Schillaci,
F. Vaccaro, and S. Cottone
Dipartimento Biomedico di Medicina Interna,
e Specialistica (DIBIMIS), Cattedra di Nefrologia,
European Society of Hypertension Excellence Centre,
Università di Palermo, Palermo, Italy
e-mail: giuseppe.mule@unipa.it

organ damage such as left ventricular hypertrophy, diastolic dysfunction, and carotid intima–media thickening. Recently, we found that ARD, expressed either as absolute values or normalized for BSA (ARD/BSA) or height (ARD/H), was significantly greater in hypertensive subjects with chronic kidney disease (CKD) when compared to their counterparts with normal renal function. Moreover, at univariate analyses estimated glomerular filtration rate (eGFR) showed significant inverse correlations with ARD not indexed and with ARD/BSA and ARD/H. Taking into account the effect of age, sex, duration of hypertension and other potentially confounding factors, in multiple regression analyses, only the association of GFR with ARD/H and that between GFR and ARD/BSA remained statistically significant. The receiver-operating characteristic curve analysis revealed that an estimated GFR of about 50 ml/min/1.73 m^2 represents the better threshold to distinguish hypertensive patients with dilated aortic root from those with a normal one.

Some population-based studies showed that an enlarged ARD might predict an adverse prognosis, even in absence of aneurysmatic alterations.

In the Cardiovascular Health Study, a dilated aortic root was independently associated with an increased risk for stroke, cardiovascular and total mortality in both sexes and with incident congestive heart failure only in men. The relationship between ARD and heart failure has been observed also in the Framingham Heart Study. More recently, the PAMELA (Pressioni Arteriose Monitorate E Loro Associazioni) study demonstrated an independent relationship of ARD/H with incident cardiovascular morbidity and mortality.

Although the relationship between BP and aortic root size is still a matter of debate, increasing evidence seems to support the notion that aortic root dilatation, even in absence of aneurysmatic alterations, may be regarded as an hypertensive organ damage paralleling other preclinical markers whose unfavourable prognostic significance is firmly established. Future studies are needed to assess whether or not antihypertensive therapy is able to reduce aortic root dimension and the increased risk associated with its enlargement.

Keywords

Arterial hypertension • Blood pressure • Thoracic aorta • Aneurysm • Aortic root • Echocardiography • Glomerular filtration rate • Chronic kidney disease • Target organ damage • Cardiovascular disease

1   Introduction

The aorta represents a complex organ system which begins in the aortic ring adjacent to the aortic root with the origin of the two major coronary arteries, and ends at the iliac bifurcation. The size of the aorta decreases with distance from the aortic valve in a tapering fashion.

The gross anatomy of the aorta may be divided into the following segments: the aortic root; the sinotubular junction; the ascending aorta; the aortic arch; the isthmus and descending

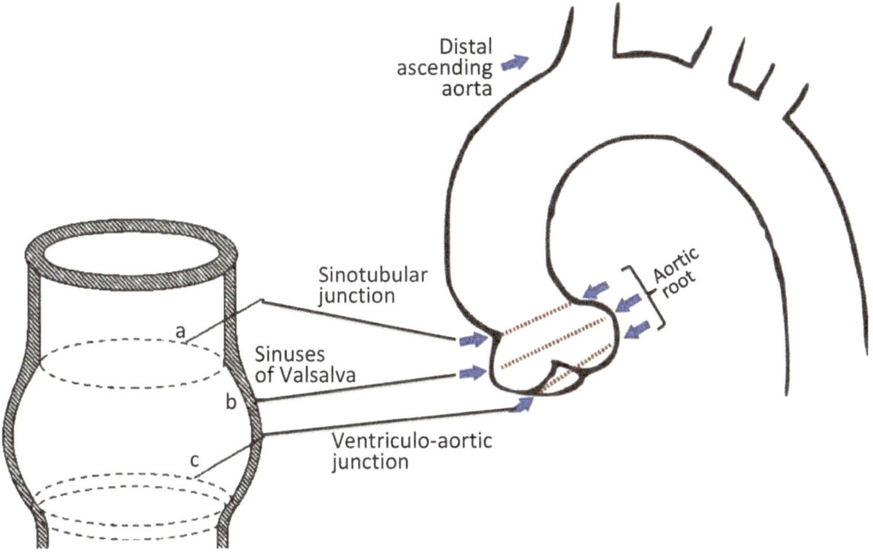

Fig. 1 Diagrammatical representation of the ascending aorta and in particular of the aortic root. (*a*: sinotubular junction; *b*: the sinuses of Valsalva; *c*: Ventriculo-aortic junction, also called basal ring or surgical annulus)

aorta; and the abdominal aorta. The aortic root is a geometrically complex structure that extends from the basal attachments of the aortic valve leaflets within the LV outflow tract to their distal attachment at the tubular portion of the aorta (the sinotubular junction), including principally the sinuses of Valsalva (SoV) (Fig. 1) (Erbel et al. 2014).

The aorta as an organ can be regarded as an elastic reservoir, storing kinetic energy during systole which is delivered during diastole, in order to convert the high velocity (around 1 m/s) pulsatile flow at the level of the ascending aorta to a low velocity (around 0.01 cm/s) steady flow necessary to cellular exchanges. This systolic-diastolic interplay has been defined "windkessel" effect by analogy with an old-fashioned hand-pumped fire engine (in German "windkessel" pump), that firemen used to obtain a constant water stream (Fig. 2).

The windkessel effect helps in damping the fluctuation in blood pressure during the cardiac cycle and assists in the maintenance of coronary perfusion during diastole when cardiac ejection ceases.

In addition to the conductance and pumping functions, the aorta plays an important role in the control of systemic vascular resistance and heart rate, via pressure-responsive receptors located in the ascending aorta and aortic arch. An increase in aortic pressure results in a decrease in heart rate and systemic vascular resistance, whereas a decrease in aortic pressure results in an increase in heart rate and systemic vascular resistance (Erbel et al. 2014).

2 Thoracic Aortic Aneurysm and Dissection

Acute dissection (AD) is one of the most devastating diseases of the aorta. This condition is often lethal, even when emergency surgery can be performed. Indeed, it is regarded as one of the most dramatic life-threatening vascular emergencies, characterized by elevated mortality despite improvements in diagnostic imaging and surgical techniques (Erbel et al. 2014; Baguet et al. 2012; Howard et al. 2013; Landenhed et al. 2015).

Previous epidemiological studies of AD have been hospital-based, have had incomplete ascertainment due to exclusion of out-of-hospital cases and predated widespread use of modern

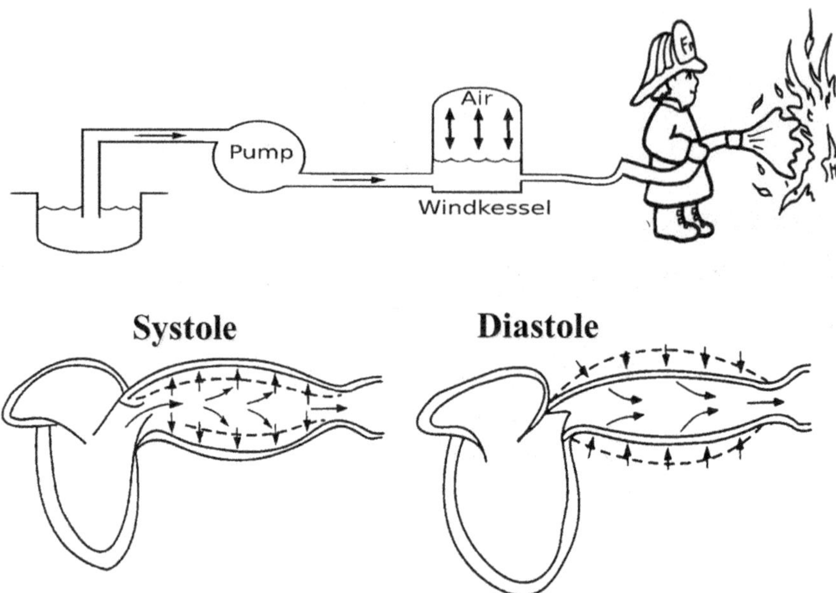

Fig. 2 Through the 'windkessel' effect, aorta acts as an elastic reservoir, converting the pulsatile ejection of blood into a steady stream of flow (see text for further explanations)

diagnostic technology, such as CT angiography. The first prospective study of acute aortic disease was conducted in a population of 92,728 in Oxfordshire, UK, during 2002–2012, as part of the Oxford Vascular Study (OXVASC) (Howard et al. 2013). The incidence of AD (6 per 100, 000 people per year) and of ruptured/symptomatic aortic aneurysms (11 per 100,000 people per year) in this study was higher than previously estimated (Howard et al. 2013), probably due to more complete inclusion of deaths prior to hospital admission. It is also possible that improvements in vascular imaging might have contributed and that the incidence of AD may have increased since previous studies. Even higher incidence rates of AD (15 per 100,000 patient-years) were recorded in the prospective cohort of 30,142 middle-aged individuals participating in the Malmö Diet and Cancer study, during up to 20 years of follow-up (Landenhed et al. 2015). In the same study hypertension was present in 86 % of individuals who subsequently developed AD. High blood pressure (BP) was strongly associated with incident AD (hazard ratio 2.64, 95 % CI 1.33–5.25), and conferred a population-attributable risk of 54 %

(Landenhed et al. 2015). Similarly, in the OXVASC study it has been observed that uncontrolled hypertension was the most significant treatable risk factor for AD. Premorbid control of BP was often poor, even though 67.3 % of patients were prescribed antihypertensive medications (Howard et al. 2013).

An abrupt, transient, severe increase in BP has been associated with acute AD through various mechanisms. Crack cocaine, which may cause transient hypertension due to catecholamine release, accounted for 37 % of dissections in a report of an inner city population (Manning and Black 2016). High-intensity weight lifting or other strenuous resistance training can also cause a transient elevation in blood pressure and has been reported as an antecedent (Manning and Black 2016). Hypertension is also the postulated mechanism when energy drinks or ergotism have been associated with aortic dissection (Manning and Black 2016).

Pathophysiology of dissection involves the separation of the tunica intima from the tunica media with subsequent penetration of blood. We have only limited understanding, however, of the mechanobiological processes that lead to this dreaded condition. Besides the link with poorly controlled hypertension, thoracic aortic aneurysms and dissections are associated with mutations in genes for extracellular matrix constituents, membrane receptors, contractile proteins, and associated signalling molecules (Humphrey et al. 2015). This grouping of factors suggests that these thoracic aorta diseases result, in part, from dysfunctional mechanosensing and mechanoregulation of the extracellular matrix by the intramural cells, which leads to a compromised structural integrity of the wall (Humphrey et al. 2015).

Some of the genetic mutations above mentioned are responsible for several syndromic and nonsyndromic genetic conditions that are associated with the development of thoracic aortic aneurysms and present with dissections at smaller diameters than usual. These conditions include Marfan syndrome, bicuspid aortic valve, Turner syndrome, Loeys-Dietz syndrome, and other less common diseases (Erbel et al. 2014; Baguet et al. 2012; Manning and Black 2016).

To prevent dissection of the aorta, timely operation on a patient with a known dilatation of the ascending aorta is advised, along with other supportive measures (Erbel et al. 2014; Baguet et al. 2012).

The wall tension, given by the product of the circumferential stress and wall thickness, is directly proportional to BP and vessel diameter, thus explaining why both hypertension and aortic dilatation are risk factors for aortic dissection (Erbel et al. 2014; Baguet et al. 2012). Indeed, an increased aortic root diameter (ARD) represents the main risk factor for thoracic aortic dissection and rupture and for aortic valve regurgitation (Erbel et al. 2014; Baguet et al. 2012).

It should be emphasized that thoracic aortic dimension alone seems not to be sufficient to detect subjects at high risk of aortic rupture and dissection. In fact, the aging process of the proximal elastic arteries, characterized by the progressive fracture of the elastic lamellae, account for both dilation (from the stretch after the fracture of a load-bearing material) and stiffening (through the transfer of stresses to more rigid collagenous components of the arterial wall) (Erbel et al. 2014; Baguet et al. 2012).

Although aortic surgery is usually recommended when the ascending aortic diameter reaches 5.5 cm in non-Marfan patients and 4.5 cm in Marfan patients (Erbel et al. 2014; Baguet et al. 2012), it has been recently shown that dissecting aortas are often sized well below the diameters defined by these surgical guidelines (Pape et al. 2007; Davies et al. 2006).

The International Registry of Acute Aortic Dissection study demonstrated that among patients with acute type A aortic dissection, aortic diameter at presentation was < 5.5 cm in most cases and < 5.0 cm in 40 % of the cases (Pape et al. 2007).

The usual underlying histopathologic changes in aortic tissue associated with aortic AD and often also with thoracic aneurysms are defined as "cystic medial degeneration or necrosis". These changes are known to occur to some extent with aging, but are accelerated by hypertension (Erbel et al. 2014; Baguet et al. 2012).

Although transthoracic echocardiography (TTE) is not the technique of choice for full assessment of the thoracic aorta, it is an excellent screening tool to evaluate aortic root morphology and dimensions, being widely available, cost effective, and safe. For these reasons, TTE is the most frequently used technique for measuring proximal aortic segments in clinical practice. It suffices to quantify maximum aortic root and proximal ascending aorta diameters when the acoustic window is adequate. Nevertheless, the technique is more limited for measuring the remaining aortic segments, for which transoesophageal echocardiography, computed tomography or magnetic resonance imaging are needed (Erbel et al. 2014; Baguet et al. 2012; Lang et al. 2015).

Measurements of aortic diameters are not always straightforward and some limitations inherent to all imaging techniques need to be acknowledged. No imaging modality has perfect resolution and reliable detection of aortic diameter at the same aortic segment over time requires standardized measurement; this includes similar determination of edges (inner-to-inner, or leading edge-to-leading edge, or outer-to-outer diameter measurement, according to the imaging modality). Whether the measurement should be done during systole or diastole has not yet been accurately assessed, but diastolic images give the best reproducibility (Erbel et al. 2014; Lang et al. 2015).

The available evidence regarding the prognostic role of aortic root size we will describe subsequently is mostly based on aortic root size measurements obtained by M-Mode echocardiography, under 2-dimensional control, at a single level (that is the widest point of Valsalva's sinuses). It is now recognized (Erbel et al. 2014; Lang et al. 2015) that this approach yields measurements that are 1–2 mm smaller than that recorded by 2-dimensional echocardiography and is biased by translational movement of the aortic root. Moreover, it has been observed that the correlates of aortic root may differ if its measurement is taken at different sites (i.e. annulus, supra-aortic ridge and ascending aorta) (Milan et al. 2013; Kim et al. 1996; Vriz et al. 2013; Campens et al. 2014).

3 Aortic Root and Hypertension

Intuitively, remodelling of the aortic root may be expected to occur in hypertensive subjects as a consequence of increased stress on the aortic wall due to the repeated hemodynamic overload.

For this reason arterial hypertension is commonly regarded as a predisposing condition for the development of thoracic aorta aneurysms (Erbel et al. 2014; Baguet et al. 2012). Even though linking dilatation of aortic root to high BP seems straightforward, the role of hypertension as determinant of aortic root enlargement remains controversial (Erbel et al. 2014; Baguet et al. 2012; Milan et al. 2013; Kim et al. 1996; Vriz et al. 2013; Campens et al. 2014; Vasan et al. 1995; Lam et al. 2010; O'Rourke and Nichols 2005; Mitchell et al. 2003; 2008; Ingelsson et al. 2008; Farasat et al. 2008; Roman et al. 1987; Tell et al. 1994; Palmieri et al. 2001; Bella et al. 2002; Agmon et al. 2003; Savage et al. 1979; Biaggi et al. 2009).

Vasan et al., using two-dimensionally guided M-mode measurement of the sinuses of Valsalva in the Framingham Heart Study, found a small direct relation between diastolic pressure and ARD, whereas both systolic and pulse pressures (PP) were inversely related to ARD after adjustment for age, height, and weight (Vasan et al. 1995). These results were confirmed in a longitudinal analysis of the same study, where each 10-mmHg increase in diastolic BP was associated with a larger predicted ARD in men (0.39 mm) than in women (0.19 mmHg), after adjustment for all other clinical covariates. Moreover, 10-mmHg increase in PP was related to a smaller predicted aortic root diameter in men (0.19 mm) and women (0.08 mm), after adjustment for age, BMI, and antihypertensive therapy (Lam et al. 2010).

These observations are in contrast with the classic notion that age-related Elastinc fragmentation, passive aortic dilatation, wall stiffening, and premature wave reflection lead directly to increasing PP with age (O'Rourke and Nichols 2005). In line with this traditional view, aortic root enlargement and increase in pulse pressure are two closely related phenomena, both linked to vascular aging (O'Rourke and Nichols 2005). On the contrary, these findings have led to the hypothesis that a smaller aortic root may play a key role in the pathogenesis of systolic hypertension by introducing a mismatch between ARD and blood flow so that forward wave amplitude is increased (Mitchell et al. 2003). Indeed, direct measurements of pulsatile hemodynamics in patients with systolic hypertension showed that although aortic root dilatation and stiffening occurred with increasing age, higher PP was associated with increased characteristic impedance and reduced rather than increased aortic root diameter (Mitchell et al. 2003). However, the only prospective analysis testing this hypothesis, performed in 3195 Framingham study participants with normal BP values at baseline, failed to show an association between incidence of hypertension and aortic root size (Ingelsson et al. 2008). The hypothesis that the association between aortic root size and BP may be related to specific subtypes of hypertension (isolated diastolic, isolated systolic, or systolic–diastolic hypertension) was not confirmed in a cross-sectional evaluation of 1256 Taiwanese patients (Farasat et al. 2008). In this study, after accounting for age and body surface area, ARD does not differ between normotensive and hypertensive individuals, even when the various patterns of hypertension are examined separately (Farasat et al. 2008), highlighting the importance of correctly matching cases and controls for those parameters which are known to be the main determinants of aortic size, namely sex, age and body size. Kim et al. (Kim et al. 1996) evaluated the size of ascending aorta in 110 normotensive individuals and 110 hypertensive patients matched for age and sex: after indexing aortic size for BSA, no significant difference was found between the two groups at the aortic annulus or at the SoV. In a study involving 102 patients with severe aortic regurgitation, Roman et al. found similar mean M-mode aortic diameters in normotensive and hypertensive groups (Roman et al. 1987).

Tell et al. in the Cardiovascular Health Study found a relation between diastolic but not systolic pressure and M-mode echocardiographic dimensions when the entire elderly cohort was analysed; however, when the "healthier" subgroup (no coronary heart disease or antihypertensive therapy) was examined, aortic diameter was not associated with blood pressure (Tell et al. 1994).

In a cross-sectional analysis of the 2096 hypertensive and 361 normotensive participants in the The Hypertension Genetic Epidemiology Network (HyperGEN) study (Palmieri et al. 2001), the prevalence of aortic root dilatation was similar between hypertensive and normotensive individuals and only a weak direct relation between ARD and office DBP was observed. In the Losartan Intervention for Endpoint reduction (LIFE) study (Bella et al. 2002) examining 947 hypertensive patients with electrocardiographic LVH no significant relationship between BP values and aortic dilatation was found. Other imaging evaluations (Vriz

et al. 2013; Campens et al. 2014; Bella et al. 2002; Agmon et al. 2003; Mitchell et al. 2008; Savage et al. 1979) and autopsy series (Sawabe et al. 2011; Virmani et al. 1991) examined this relation with mixed results. Nonetheless, recent data suggest a high prevalence of echocardiographic aortic root dilatation in the hypertensive population (Cipolli et al. 2009; Cuspidi et al. 2011; Covella et al. 2014).

In order to assess the prevalence of ARD dilatation in arterial hypertension, Covella and co-workers performed a meta-analysis including eight studies and a total of 10,791 hypertensive patients (Covella et al. 2014). Prevalence of ARD in the pooled population was 9.1 % with a marked difference between men and women (12.7 vs. 4.5 %). Hypertensive patients with ARD enlargement and those with normal aortic root size had similar office BP values (Covella et al. 2014).

On the contrary, in the PAMELA (Pressioni Arteriose Monitorate E Loro Associazioni) study (Cuspidi et al. 2014), conducted in 2051 individuals randomly selected from the population of Monza (Italy), and with a low global cardiovascular risk profile, office, home and 24-h ambulatory SBP and DBP showed a direct, significant correlation with ARD (Cuspidi et al. 2014).

Additionally, the Healthy Coronary Artery Risk Development in Young Adults (CARDIA) study provides longitudinal data on clinical correlates of aortic root size and dilatation through a 20-year period of early adulthood, in 3051 young adults aged 23–35 years (Teixido-Tura et al. 2015). Aortic root diameter measured by M-mode echocardiography at the end of the period of observation was positively correlated with the 20-year increase in diastolic, systolic, and mean arterial pressure and inversely related to pulse pressure (Teixido-Tura et al. 2015).

Very recently, in a large group of hypertensive individuals characterized by a high prevalence of chronic kidney disease (CKD), we found only a weak association, close to statistical significance (p = 0.08), between clinic diastolic BP and ARD either not indexed or normalized for height (Mulé et al. 2016).

Several reasons could explain the inconsistent findings of the studies above described: differences in study design, failure of cross-sectional studies to match hypertensive patients and normotensive individuals for all the potential confounding factors, definition of the aortic phenotype, and site and types of BP measurement. Whereas in the majority of studies only clinical BP measurements were available, out-of-office BP and central hemodynamics might be closer correlates of ARD enlargement (Kim et al. 1996; Cipolli et al. 2009; Cuspidi et al. 2014; Cuspidi et al. 2007).

Besides the aforementioned PAMELA study, that is the first one linking elevated out-of-office BP, as assessed either by home and ambulatory measurements, to aortic dilatation (Cuspidi et al. 2014), in a previous report of the same research group, average night-time diastolic BP, but not clinic or average 48 h BP, showed an independent association with ARD in 519 never-treated hypertensive patients (Cuspidi et al. 2007).

However, in the previously cited study of Kim et al. 24 h ambulatory BP readings were less strongly correlated to aortic diameters than casual blood pressure in the normotensive group, whereas ambulatory blood pressure was more correlated to aortic size in the hypertensive group (Kim et al. 1996). The physiological significance of this difference remains unclear.

A more accurate measurement of hemodynamic load may be achieved by non-invasive estimation of central arterial pressure and vascular compliance or by quantitative analysis of the arterial pressure waveform. Despite similar mean pressures, systolic and diastolic pressures may vary considerably with the degree of wave amplification, being maximal in the young, normotensive individual with a compliant vasculature (Erbel et al. 2014; Vasan et al. 1995).

Indeed, Milan and co-workers documented that, in a total of 190 untreated and treated essential hypertensive patients, central hemodynamic variables (aortic augmentation index and central pulse pressure) estimated by an applanation tonometry applied to the radial artery, were significantly associated with an increased ARD, whereas peripheral BP was not (Milan et al. 2011).

Moreover, assuming a relation between BP and aortic root diameter exists, the impact of the duration of high BP must be taken into account, as seem to suggest the relatively low prevalence of aortic root dilatation (3.7 %) among the untreated newly diagnosed hypertensive subjects examined by Cuspidi et al. (Cuspidi et al. 2007).

It is also possible that antihypertensive medications, taken by most of the patients enrolled in the investigations above reported, may have concealed the relation between BP and aortic root size. Last, but not least, the use of different methods for indexation of ARD may have in part contributed to the heterogeneous findings obtained in the investigations exploring the relationships between ARD and blood pressures.

Indeed, the best method for ARD indexation, as well as the normal values of aortic root size, are still a matter of debate (Table 1) (Erbel et al. 2014; Baguet et al. 2012; Pape et al. 2007; Davies et al. 2006; Lang et al. 2015; Vriz et al. 2013; Campens et al. 2014; Vasan et al. 1995; Palmieri et al. 2001; Bella et al. 2002; Cuspidi et al. 2007, 2011, 2014; Milan et al. 2011; Devereux et al. 2012). In the past years absolute measures were used to assess the size of aortic root, but the absolute aortic diameter is not a good enough marker of risk for aortic dissection (Erbel et al. 2014; Baguet et al. 2012; Pape et al. 2007; Davies et al. 2006; Lang et al. 2015). It is noteworthy that, as above reported, the majority of patients with acute type A aortic dissection had an aortic diameter less than 5.5 cm, a measure that is considered the cut-off value for suggesting aortic replacement by surgical guidelines (Pape et al. 2007).

For the great influence of BSA on aortic root dimensions, it has been proposed to normalize the absolute values of ARD for BSA (ARD/BSA) (Erbel et al. 2014; Baguet et al. 2012; Lang et al. 2015; Campens et al. 2014; Devereux et al. 2012; Hiratzka et al. 2010), considering also that such an indexation predicted the risk of rupture, dissection and death in patients with

Table 1 Cut-off values of aortic root size, measured by echocardiography at the sinuses of Valsalva, as suggested by different authors

Author, year	Not indexed (cm)	Indexed for BSA (cm/m^2)	Indexed for height (cm/m)
Roman et al., 1989	M: 4.0; F: 3.6	M: 2.1; F: 2.1	–
Vasan et al., 1995 (Framingham study)	–	95th percentiles that can be calculated by sex-specific regression equations	95th percentiles that can be calculated by sex-specific regression equations
Bella et al., 2002 (LIFE study)	–	>2SD above the regression line with BSA in a reference population	–
Palmieri et al., 2005 (HYPERGEN study)	–	97.5th percentiles that can be calculated by sex-specific regression equations	–
Cuspidi et al., 2006 (ETODH registry)	M: 4.0; F: 3.8	–	–
Cuspidi et al., 2007	M: 4.0; F: 3.7	–	–
Cipolli et al., 2009	M: 4.0; F: 3.7	–	–
Milan et al., 2011	–	2.0	–
Cuspidi et al., 2011	M: 3.9; F: 3.7	–	–
Baguet et al., 2012 (ESH newletter)		M: 2.1; F: 2.1	
Devereux et al., 2012	–	Nomograms based on age, sex and BSA	Nomograms based on age, sex and height
Milan et al., 2013	M: 3.9; F: 3.7	–	–
Cuspidi et al., 2014 (PAMELA study)	M: 3.8; F: 3.4	M: 2.1; F: 2.2	M: 2.3; F: 2.2
Campens et al., 2014	–	Gender-, age- and BSA- specific upper limits of normal and Z-score equations	–

thoracic aortic aneurysms, better than did unadjusted aortic root size (Erbel et al. 2014; Davies et al. 2006). Furthermore, ARD/BSA showed a significant association with mortality (Lai et al. 2010).

On the other hand, some authors have suggested that the use of body surface area as a means of adjustment for differences in body size is mathematically incorrect (Nidorf et al. 1992) and carries the potential risk of an under diagnosis in obese subjects, which are a substantial proportion of hypertensive patients, and of an over diagnosis in the individuals with lower BSA (e.g. women).

For these reasons, they advocate indexation of aortic diameter for height that is considered a more linear and mathematically sound way of comparing measurements. (Nidorf et al. 1992). Finally, some evidence suggests that ARD would have a better prognostic value when normalized to height (Cuspidi et al. 2014).

Regardless of the method used to measure BP, overall the contribution of it to aortic root dilatation has been shown to be substantially inferior than that of some non-hemodynamic factors.

4 Non-hemodynamic Determinants of Aortic Root Size

Besides BP, several factors influence aortic root dimension, including age, gender and anthropometric variables, such as height, weight and their derivatives body surface area and body mass index (BMI) (Erbel et al. 2014; Kim et al. 1996; Bella et al. 2002; Teixido-Tura et al. 2015; Devereux et al. 2012; Hiratzka et al. 2010; Lai et al. 2010; Nidorf et al. 1992; Reed et al. 1993; Roman et al. 1989). Of these factors, anthropometric variables have the greatest impact.

In some studies, height is the most important determinant of aortic root size compared with other anthropometric indexes, such as weight or body surface area (Lai et al. 2010; Nidorf et al. 1992; Reed et al. 1993). Original observations in Framingham study (Vasan et al. 1995) showed that height is the most important predictor, with every 10-cm increment in height associated with increment in aortic root size of 0.24 mm in men and 0.38 mm in women.

Weight also influences aortic dimensions with a 10-kg increase in weight associated with an increment in aortic root size of 0.87 in males and 0.68 mm in females (Vasan et al. 1995).

More recently, Campens et al. in a cohort of 849 children and adults (Campens et al. 2014) demonstrated that ARD measured by TTE at the sinuses of Valsalva correlated closely with height in the children, whereas in subjects > 15 years of age, height was less strongly correlated with aortic dimensions compared to BSA.

An association between age and aortic root size has been consistently reported in autopsy series and clinical studies (Milan et al. 2011, 2013; Kim et al. 1996; [12]; Vriz et al. 2013; Campens et al. 2014; Vasan et al. 1995; Lam et al. 2010; Agmon et al. 2003; Savage et al. 1979; Biaggi et al. 2009; Sawabe et al. 2011; Virmani et al. 1991; Cipolli et al. 2009; Cuspidi et al. 2007, 2011, 2014; Covella et al. 2014; Teixido-Tura et al. 2015; Mulé et al. 2016; Devereux et al. 2012; Hiratzka et al. 2010). In the most recent Framingham analysis (Lam et al. 2010) is reported a 0.9-mm increase of aortic dimension in men and 0.7 mm in women, for each successive decade of life, after adjustment for other determinants. The age-related increase of ARD is considered a consequence of fatigue and fracture of elastin fibers with subsequent remodelling (O'Rourke and Nichols 2005). This view applies the principles of material fatigue that relate fracture of non-living components with extent of pulsatile strain and the number of applied cycles of strain (i.e., heart beats). This theory explains both aortic dilation (from fracture of elastic components) and stiffening (from transfer of tension from elastin to collagenous fibers in the wall) (O'Rourke and Nichols 2005).

It is generally accepted that aortic dimensions are smaller in women than in men in adulthood, whereas aortic root size do not differ between the genders in infancy and childhood (Erbel et al. 2014; Lang et al. 2015; Vriz et al. 2013; Campens et al. 2014; Vasan et al. 1995). The physiologic basis for this difference has not been completely elucidated, but is likely related to the average smaller body size (and lean body mass) and the lesser absolute cardiac output, in women as compared to men (Erbel et al. 2014; Cuspidi et al. 2007; Hiratzka et al. 2010).

A greater propensity to outward aortic remodelling for men has been highlighted in a longitudinal analysis of more than 3000 Framingham patients (Lam et al. 2010), and this finding is consistent with the high male-to-female ratio seen in patients with thoracic aortic dissection (Pape et al. 2007). Sex steroids have been shown in vitro to regulate collagen and elastin deposition and gene expression of matrix metalloproteinases (MMPs) (Natoli et al. 2005).

Among the main cardiovascular risk factors, diabetes alone seems to be associated with reduced aortic diameters, at abdominal and thoracic level, as well as with a lower risk of aortic aneurysms and dissections (Shantikumar et al. 2010; Prakash et al. 2012).

The cause of the smaller aortic dimension in the diabetic population remains to be established.

It presumably arises from glycaemia-associated alterations in the vascular matrix, which protect against aortic enlargement. It is well known that the walls of aneurysmal aortas show increased proteolytic activity and accelerated matrix depletion (Freestone et al. 1995).

By contrast, diabetes is characterized by increased matrix deposition due to a combination of increased synthesis and reduced proteolysis

(Mauer 1994). It has been reported that wall stress in the aorta was reduced in diabetes, mainly due to an increased wall thickness (Astrand et al. 2007).

Continued excessive MMPs production and activation result in increased degradation of aortic wall elastin and collagen, with alteration in the mechanical properties of the aortic wall, leading to aneurysmal dilatation (Shantikumar et al. 2010; Prakash et al. 2012; Freestone et al. 1995; Karakaya et al. 2006). A down regulation of MMPs activity has been shown in arteries of diabetic patients, and high glucose levels accelerating synthesis of collagen might be the mechanism behind increased wall thickness, reduced aortic wall stress, decreased aneurysm prevalence and reduced frequency of aortic root dilatation (Shantikumar et al. 2010; Prakash et al. 2012; Singh et al. 2001; Portik-Dobos et al. 2002; Lam et al. 2003).

Indeed, it has been suggested that hyperglycaemia induced crosslinking of the collagen network in the aortic wall media, and this crosslinking resists proteolysis and inhibits secretion of the MMPs thought to mediate aortic aneurysm formation. Further, diabetes is also known to suppress plasmin, which activates the MMPs (Shantikumar et al. 2010; Prakash et al. 2012).

Hyperglycaemia is also associated with reduced adventitial neovascularization and decreased infiltration of inflammatory cells into the medial layer of the aorta (Shantikumar et al. 2010; Prakash et al. 2012). These processes could also reduce the expansion of aorta by reduction of vascular smooth muscle cell death and extracellular matrix degradation. Alternatively, it is possible that aortic dilatation may protect against the development of diabetes. Thoracic aorta disease is associated with increased circulating concentrations of insulin-like growth factor 1, an endocrine peptide endowed with antidiabetic effects (Shantikumar et al. 2010; Prakash et al. 2012).

Further evidence is required to determine the plausibility of these various pathophysiologic explanations for this seemingly paradoxical effect of diabetes on aortic size.

5 Aortic Root Dilatation and Subclinical Hypertensive Target Organ Damage

Current hypertension guidelines propose a risk stratification strategy based on BP levels as well as on the presence or not of concomitant cardiovascular risk factors, subclinical target organ damage (TOD) and associated clinical conditions (Mancia et al. 2013).

A great emphasis has been placed on the early detection of subclinical (or asymptomatic) cardiovascular and renal alterations, defined as hypertension related TOD (Mancia et al. 2013). This because the search for TOD in clinical practice allows a better cardiovascular risk profiling of patients with hypertension, being TOD unanimously regarded as a mediating step between risk factor exposure and CV events, that reflects the cumulative damaging effects from risk factors (Mancia et al. 2013).

Several alterations of hypertensive target organs have been described. Among these manifestations, most attention has been devoted to left ventricular hypertrophy (LVH), left ventricular dysfunction, left atrial enlargement, renal dysfunction, and abnormalities in small and medium-size arteries such as retinal and carotid vessels (Mancia et al. 2013).

An independent association between aortic root size, determined by X-ray scan, transthoracic or transoesophageal echocardiography, and LVH has been reported in different settings (Palmieri et al. 2001; Bella et al. 2002; Cipolli et al. 2009; Cuspidi et al. 2006, 2007, 2011, 2014; Covella et al. 2014; Mulé et al. 2016; Rayner et al. 2004; Iarussi et al. 2001). In the abovementioned meta-analysis of Covella et al. (Covella et al. 2014), left ventricular mass (LVM) was significantly greater in hypertensive patients with aortic root enlargement than in those with normal aortic root. Similarly, in our recent study we observed highly significant correlations between ARD and LVM either considered as absolute values or indexed for BSA or height (Mulé et al. 2016).

Interestingly, in a cross-sectional analysis of 438 hypertensive patients with LV hypertrophy

(266 women and 172 men) women with enlarged ARD had higher cardiac output, decreased peripheral vascular resistance, whereas men with ARD dilatation presented with a higher prevalence of concentric LV hypertrophy, suggesting that aortic root enlargement may be related to volume overload in women and to myocardial growth-related parameters in men (Cipolli et al. 2009).

Although the positive relationship between LVM and ARD could be simply mediated by hypertension itself, the dubious association of BP with ARD, does not support this hypothesis.

The most comprehensive assessment of the relation between aortic root size and TOD, at the cardiac and extra cardiac level, was performed in the large population of mostly treated essential hypertensive patients enrolled in the Evaluation of Target Organ Damage in Hypertension (ETODH) observational registry (Cuspidi et al. 2006). In this investigation the prevalence of LVH, carotid intima–media thickening (IMT), plaques and microalbuminuria was significantly higher in patients with aortic root dilatation (ARD > 40 mm in men and > 38 mm in men; n = 206; 6.1 %)) when compared to 3160 patients with normal aortic size (Cuspidi et al. 2006). Moreover, a lower E/A (early diastolic/late diastolic) mitral flow velocity ratio was found in patients with aortic root dilatation with respect to subjects with normal aortic root size (Cuspidi et al. 2006). In a multiple logistic regression analysis, in both untreated and treated hypertensive patients, the markers of TOD that remained independently associated with ARD dilatation were: LVH, E/A ratio and carotid IMT (Cuspidi et al. 2006).

Subsequently, the relationships between aortic root diameter and echocardiographic features of LV diastolic functions were investigated in 333 patients with preserved LV systolic function and at least one cardiovascular risk factor (hypertension, diabetes or dyslipidaemia) (Masugata et al. 2011). ARD was measured by M-mode echocardiography, and LV diastolic function was evaluated by measuring the peak velocity of early (E) and late (A) diastolic transmitral blood flow and peak early diastolic mitral annular velocity (E′) by Doppler echocardiography. Stepwise multiple regression analysis showed that E wave in women and E′ in men were independently associated with aortic root diameter. The authors concluded that aortic root dilatation might be a useful marker of subclinical LV diastolic dysfunction (Masugata et al. 2011).

6 Aortic Root Size and Renal Function

Even if the association of aortic stiffness with CKD, since its earlier stages, is largely demonstrated (Briet et al. 2006, 2012; Mulè et al. 2010; Geraci et al. 2015;), little attention has been paid to the relationships between renal function and aortic root size.

For this reason, we recently assessed the influence of estimated glomerular filtration rate (eGFR) on ARD in 611 hypertensive subjects with a high prevalence of CKD (Mulé et al. 2016).

We found that aortic root was significantly greater in hypertensive subjects with CKD when compared to their counterparts with normal renal function (Fig. 3). On the other hand, the hypertensive patients with elevated aortic root diameter, expressed either as absolute values or normalized for BSA or height, had significantly lower GFR, estimated using the Chronic Kidney Disease Epidemiology Collaboration (CKD-EPI) equation, than those with normal aortic root size (Fig. 4). Moreover, GFR was significantly and inversely associated with ARD, assessed by TTE (Fig. 5). This relation was detectable at univariate analyses, regardless of the method used to assess aortic root dimension, as absolute measure or indexed for height or BSA. However, in multivariate analyses, taking into account the effect of age, sex, duration of hypertension and other potentially confounding factors, only the association of eGFR with ARD/H and that between eGFR and ARD/BSA remained statistically significant (Fig 6) (Mulé et al. 2016).

Additionally, the receiver-operating characteristic curve analysis revealed that an estimated GFR value of about 50 ml/min/1.73 m^2

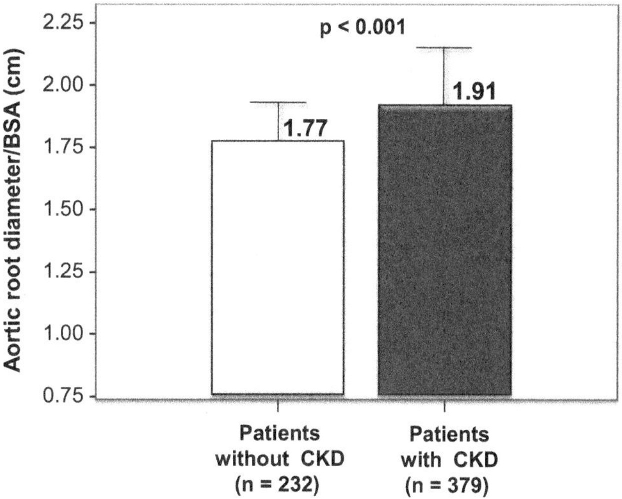

Fig. 3 Mean values (± SD) of aortic root diameter indexed for body surface area (BSA) in hypertensive patients with and without chronic kidney disease (CKD)

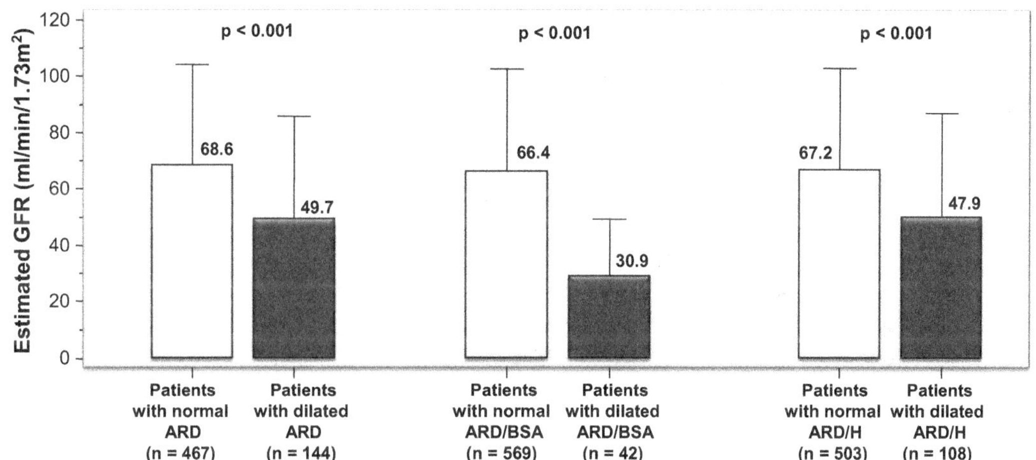

Fig. 4 Mean levels (± SD) of glomerular filtration rate (GFR) estimated with Chronic Kidney Disease Epidemiology Collaboration (CKD-EPI) equation in hypertensive patients with elevated aortic root diameter not indexed (>3.8 cm in men and > 3.4 cm in women), normalized for BSA (>2.1 cm/m^2 in men and > 2.2 cm/m^2 in women) and indexed for height (>2.3 cm/m in men and > 2.2 cm/m in women), as compared to subjects with normal aortic root size

represents the better threshold to distinguish hypertensive patients with dilated aortic root from those with a normal one, especially when aortic size is normalized for BSA. The practical implications of the very high negative predictive value (99 %) of this threshold, with respect to the detection of an enlarged ARD/BSA, are that patients with a GFR above this value, having clinical characteristics similar to those of our study population, have a very low probability

(1 %) to manifest a dilated ARD/BSA (Mulé et al. 2016) (Fig. 7).

Moreover, we observed a steeper age-related increase of ARD in CKD patients as compared to those with normal renal function. This seems to suggest that the inverse association between GFR and ARD that we found may be regarded as a manifestation of accelerated vascular aging, similar to that described in other arterial districts in the CKD patients (Briet et al. 2006).

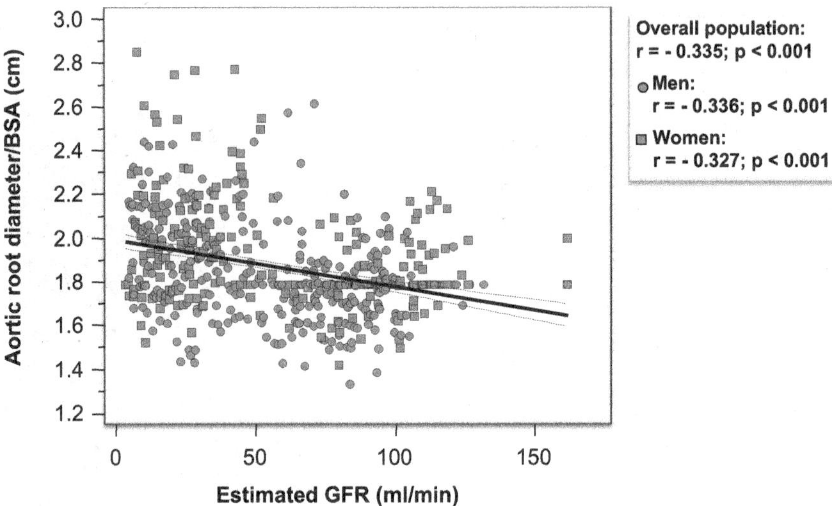

Fig. 5 The scatterplot describes in a population of hypertensive patients with a high prevalence of CKD, the inverse relationship between aortic root diameter indexed for body surface area (BSA) and glomerular filtration rate (GFR) estimated with Chronic Kidney Disease Epidemiology Collaboration (CKD-EPI) equation. The GFR was recalculated to adjust for BSA of each patient by multiplying by each individual's BSA and dividing by 1.73 m2, so that GFR was expressed in units of ml/min. The correlations did not differ in men (*grey squares*) and in women (*grey circles*)

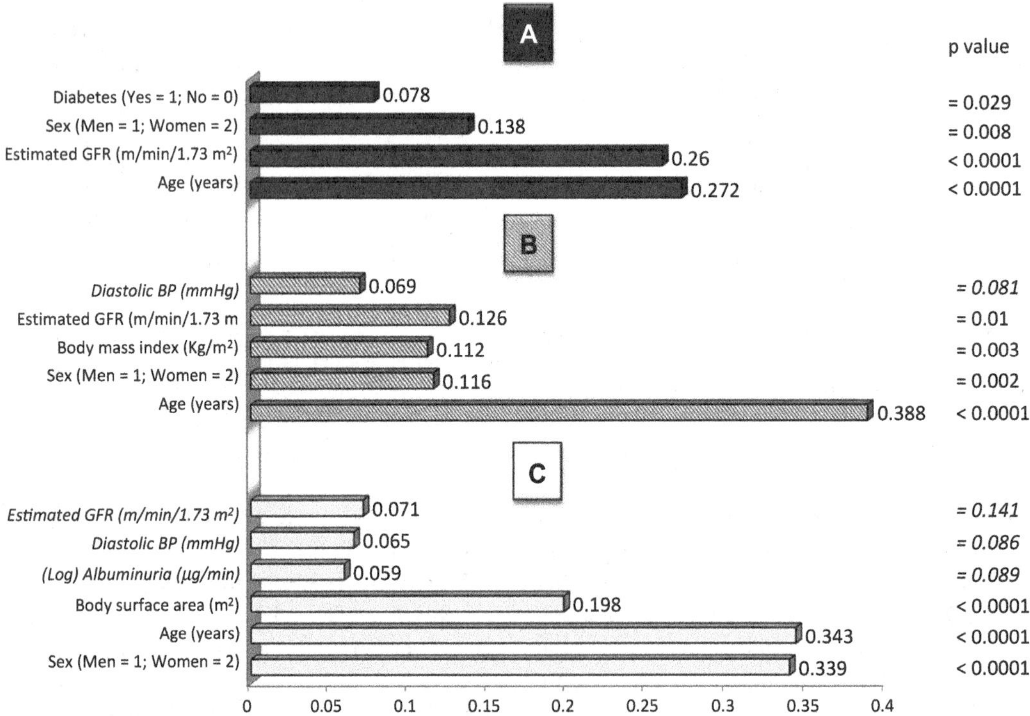

Fig. 6 Multivariate correlates of aortic root diameter indexed for BSA (**a**), normalized for height (**b**), and not indexed (**c**) in the study of Mulè et al. (Mulé et al. 2016). Each histogram represents the standardized regression coefficient. The variables showing an association not statistically significant, but with a p value ranging from 0.15 to 0.05, are presented in Italics

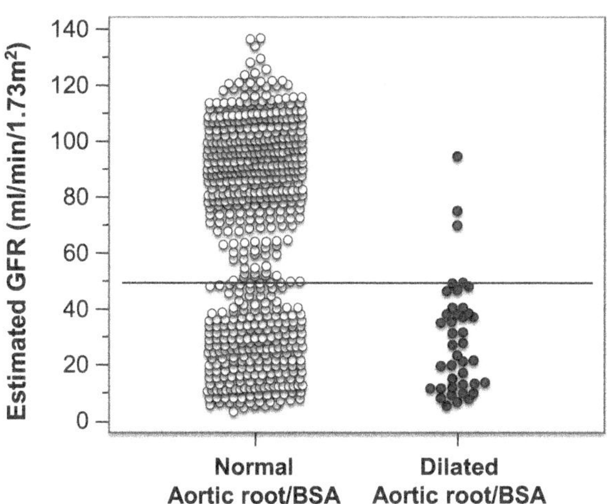

Fig. 7 Dot plot graph showing that in the study of Mulè et al. (Mulé et al. 2016) the value of estimated GFR able to better distinguish patients with enlarged ARD from those with normal aortic root size was 49.2 ml/min per 1.73 m2. The sensitivity and specificity of this value are also reported

The negative relationship between GFR and ARD/BSA in our study was attenuated, but remained significant in multivariate analyses, even taking into account the effect of LVM, either indexed for BSA or normalized for height$^{2.7}$ (Mulé et al. 2016). This probably because LVH and dilated ARD/BSA related to kidney dysfunction share only in part the same pathogenetic mechanisms.

It is conceivable that, at least in part, mechanisms similar to those responsible for the reduced large arteries elasticity may be the cause of aortic root enlargement in CKD patients: endothelial dysfunction, activation of the renin–angiotensin–aldosterone system and of the endothelins system, inflammation, oxidative stress and lipid peroxidation, increased homocysteine levels, abnormalities in tissue metalloproteinases, vascular smooth muscle cell hyperplasia, elastin fragmentation, reduced amount of elastic fibers and increased collagen content (Briet et al. 2006). On the other hand, it has been demonstrated that, in patients with mild-to-moderate CKD, arterial enlargement and increased arterial stiffness of the carotid artery occur in parallel with the decline in renal function (Briet et al. 2012).

Finally, it is noteworthy that some studies (Iribarren et al. 2007; Chun et al. 2014) reported an association between renal insufficiency and risk of developing abdominal aortic aneurysms. Even these evidences are not available to date for thoracic aorta, they seem to be in line with our findings and corroborate the notion that the unfavourable impact of an impaired renal function on the cardiovascular system may be extended also to the structure of the aorta.

7 Aortic Root Dilatation, In Absence of Aneurysmatic Alterasions, as Predictor of Cardiovascular Risk

Recent population-based studies showed that an enlarged ARD might predict an adverse prognosis, even in absence of aneurysmatic alterations (Cuspidi et al. 2014; Lai et al. 2010; Gardin et al. 2006; Lam et al. 2013).

In a bi-racial sample of the general population including 3993 elderly without overt cardiovascular disease at baseline, participating in the Cardiovascular Health Study, enlarged ARD was independently associated with an increased risk for stroke in men and women (hazard ratio 1.39 per cm, p = 0.015), CVD mortality in men and women (hazard ratio 1.48 per cm, p = 0.007), and total mortality in men and women taking antihypertensive medications (hazard ratio 1.46 per cm, p = 0.007), but not with incident myocardial infarction (hazard ratio 0.89, p = 0.39) (Gardin et al. 2006). Furthermore, the highest quintile of ARD was found to be a significant, but modest, predictor of incident congestive failure in men but not in women (Gardin et al. 2006).

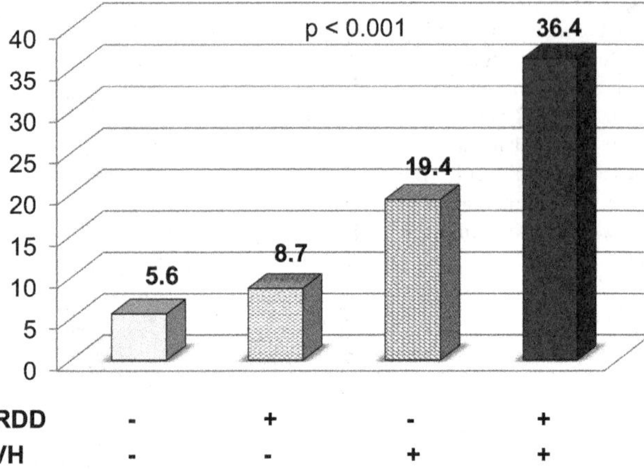

Fig. 8 Incidence (%) of cardiovascular events in the population of the PAMELA study (Cuspidi et al. 2014), divided in four groups according to the presence/absence of left ventricular hypertrophy (LVH) and aortic root diameter dilatation (ARDD)

The relationship between ARD and heart failure has been more recently examined in the Framingham Heart Study (Lam et al. 2013). The authors reported that among the 6483 middle-aged and older adults followed up over an 8-year period, the risk of incident heart failure increased with ARD values at baseline (Lam et al. 2013).

Furthermore, ARD indexed for BSA showed a significant association with all-cause death in the subjects aged < 65 years, enrolled in the Chin–Shan Community Cardiovascular Cohort (CCCC) study (Lai et al. 2010).

Moreover, in the PAMELA study, adjusting for several clinical covariates including demographics, BP and clinical risk factors, ARD indexed to height was a significant predictor of incident cardiovascular morbidity and mortality (hazard ratio 2.6) (Cuspidi et al. 2014).

It is important to note that the association between LVH and AR dilatation (as defined according to sex-specific criteria derived from the healthy fraction of the PAMELA population) was a stronger predictor of cardiovascular outcomes than that entailed by LVH alone (Fig. 8) (Cuspidi et al. 2014).

8 Conclusions

Although the relationship between BP and aortic root size is still a matter od debate, increasing evidence seems to support the notion that aortic root dilatation, even in absence of aneurysmatic alterations, may be regarded as an hypertensive organ damage paralleling other preclinical markers such as left ventricular hypertrophy (LVH) or microalbuminuria, whose unfavourable prognostic significance is firmly established. Future studies are needed to assess whether or not antihypertensive therapy is able to reduce aortic root dimension and the increased risk associated with its enlargement.

References

Agmon Y, Khandheria BK, Meissner I, Schwartz GL, Sicks JD, Fought AJ et al (2003) Is aortic dilatation an atherosclerosis-related process? Clinical, laboratory, and transesophageal echocardiographic correlates of thoracic aortic dimensions in the population with implications for thoracicaortic aneurysm formation. J Am Coll Cardiol 42:1076–1083. doi:10.1016/S0735-1097(03)00922-7

Astrand H, Rydén-Ahlgren A, Sundkvist G, Sandgren T, Länne T (2007) Reduced aortic wallstress in diabetes mellitus. Eur J Vasc Endovasc Surg 33: 592–598. doi: http://dx.doi.org/10.1016/j.ejvs.2006.11.011

Baguet JP, Chavanon O, Sessa C, Thony F, Lantelme P, Barone-Rochette G et al (2012) European Society of Hypertension scientific newsletter: hypertension and aortic diseases. J Hypertens 30:440–443. doi:10.1097/HJH.0b013e32834f867a

Bella JN, Wachtell K, Boman K, Palmieri V, Papademetriou V, Gerdts E et al (2002) Relation of left ventricular geometry and function to aortic root dilatation in patients with systemic hypertension and left ventricular hypertrophy (the LIFE study). Am J Cardiol 89:337–341

Biaggi P, Matthews F, Braun J, Rousson V, Kaufmann PA, Jenni R (2009) Gender, age, and body surface area are the major determinants of ascending aorta dimensions in subjects with apparently normal echocardiograms. J Am Soc Echocardiogr 22:720–725. doi:10.1016/j.echo.2009.03.012

Briet M, Bozec E, Laurent S, Fassot C, London GM, Jacquot C, Froissart M, Houillier P, Boutouyrie P (2006) Arterial stiffness and enlargement in mild-to-moderate chronic kidney disease. Kidney Int 69:350–357. doi:10.1038/sj.ki.5000047

Briet M, Boutouyrie P, Laurent S, London GM (2012) Arterial stiffness and pulse pressure in CKD and ESRD. Kidney Int 82:388–400. doi:10.1038/ki.2012.131

Campens L, Demulier L, De Groote K, Vandekerckhove K, De Wolf D, Roman MJ et al (2014) Reference values for echocardiographic assessment of the diameter of the aortic root and ascending aorta spanning all age categories. Am J Cardiol 114:914–920. doi:10.1016/j.amjcard.2014.06.024

Chun KC, Teng KY, Chavez LA, Van Spyk EN, Samadzadeh KM, Carson Teng KY et al (2014) Risk factors associated with the diagnosis of abdominal aortic aneurysm in patients screened at a regional veterans affairs health care system. Ann Vasc Surg 28:87–92. doi:10.1016/j.avsg.2013.06.016

Cipolli JAA, Souza FAS, Ferreira-Sae MCS, Magalhaes JAP, Figueiredo ES, Vidotti VG et al (2009) Sex-specific hemodynamic and nonhemodynamic determinants of aortic root size in hypertensive subjects with left ventricular hypertrophy. Hypertens Res 32:956–961. doi:10.1038/hr.2009.134

Covella M, Milan A, Totaro S, Cuspidi C, Re A, Rabbia F, Veglio F (2014) Echocardiographic aortic root dilatation in hypertensive patients: a systematic review and meta-analysis. J Hypertens 32:1928–1935. doi:10.1097/HJH.0000000000000286

Cuspidi C, Meani S, Fusi V, Valerio C, Sala C, Zanchetti A (2006) Prevalence and correlates of aortic root dilatation in patients with essential hypertension: relationship with cardiac and extra-cardiac organ damage. J Hypertens 24:573–580. doi:10.1097/01.hjh.0000209992.48928.1f

Cuspidi C, Meani S, Valerio C, Esposito A, Sala C, Masaidi M et al (2007) Ambulatory blood pressure, target organ damage and aortic root size in never treated essential hypertensives. J Hum Hypertens 21:531–538. doi:10.1038/sj.jhh.1002200

Cuspidi C, Negri F, Salvetti M, Lonati L, Sala C, Capra A et al (2011) Aortic root dilatation in hypertensive patients: a multicenter survey in echocardiographic practice. Blood Press 20:267–273. doi:10.3109/08037051.2011.565556

Cuspidi C, Facchetti R, Bombelli M, Re A, Cairoa M, Sala C et al (2014) Aortic root diameter and risk of cardiovascular events in a general population: data from the PAMELA study. J Hypertens 32:1879–1887. doi:10.1097/HJH.0000000000000264

Davies RR, Gallo A, Coady MA, Tellides G, Botta DM, Burke B et al (2006) Novel measurement of relative aortic size predicts rupture of thoracic aortic aneurysms. Ann Thorac Surg 81:169–177. doi:10.1016/S0003-4975(01)03236-2

Devereux RB, de Simone G, Arnett DK, Best LG, Boerwinkle E, Howard BV et al (2012) Normal limits in relation to age, body size and gender of two-dimensional echocardiographic aortic root dimensions in persons >/=15 years of age. Am J Cardiol 110:1189–1194. doi:10.1016/j.amjcard.2012.05.063

Erbel R, Aboyans V, Boileau C, Bossone E, Bartolomeo RD, Eggebrecht H et al (2014) 2014 ESC guidelines on the diagnosis and treatment of aortic diseases: document covering acute and chronic aortic diseases of the thoracic and abdominal aorta of the adult. The task force for the diagnosis and treatment of aortic diseases of the European Society of Cardiology. (ESC). Eur Heart J 35:2873–2926. doi:10.1093/eurheartj/ehu281

Farasat SM, Morrell CH, Scuteri A, Ting CT, Yin FCP, Spurgeon HA et al (2008) Do hypertensive individuals have enlarged aortic root diameters? Insights from studying the various subtypes of hypertension. Am J Hypertens 21:558–563. doi:10.1038/ajh.2008.10

Freestone T, Turner RJ, Coady A, Higman DJ, Greenhalgh RM, Powell JT (1995) Inflammation and matrix metalloproteinases in the enlarging abdominal aortic aneurysm. Arterioscler Thromb Vasc Biol 15:1145–1151. doi:10.1161/01.ATV.15.8.1145

Gardin JM, Arnold AM, Polak J, Jackson S, Smith V, Gottdiener J (2006) Usefulness of aortic root dimension in persons > 65 years of age in predicting heart failure, stroke, cardiovascular mortality, all-cause mortality and acute myocardial infarction (from the Cardiovascular Health Study). Am J Cardiol 97:270–275

Geraci G, Mulè G, Geraci C, Mogavero M, D'Ignoto F, Morreale M et al (2015) Association of renal resistive index with aortic pulse wave velocity in hypertensive patients. Eur J Prev Cardiol 22:415–422. doi:10.1177/2047487314524683

Hiratzka LF, Bakris GL, Beckman JA, Bersin RM, Carr VF, Casey DE Jr et al (2010) 2010 ACCF/AHA/AATS/ACR/ASA/SCA/SCAI/SIR/STS/SVM guidelines for the diagnosis and management of patients with Thoracic Aortic Disease: a report of the American College of Cardiology Foundation/American Heart Association Task Force on Practice Guidelines, American Association for Thoracic Surgery, American College of Radiology, American Stroke Association, Society of Cardiovascular Anesthesiologists, Society for Cardiovascular Angiography and Interventions, Society of Interventional Radiology, Society of Thoracic Surgeons, and Society for Vascular Medicine. Circulation 121:e266–e369. doi:10.1161/CIR.0b013e3181d4739e

Howard DP, Banerjee A, Fairhead JF, Perkins J, Silver LE, Rothwell PM, for the Oxford Vascular Study (2013) Population-based study of incidence and outcome of acute aortic dissection and premorbid risk factor control: 10-year results from the Oxford Vascular Study. Circulation 127: 2031–2037. doi: 10.1161/CIRCULATIONAHA.112.000483

Humphrey JD, Schwartz MA, Tellides G, Milewicz DM (2015) Role of mechanotransduction in vascular biology: focus on thoracic aortic aneurysms and dissections. Circ Res 116:1448–1461. doi:10.1161/CIRCRESAHA.114.304936

Iarussi D, Caruso A, Galderisi M, Covino FE, Dialetto G, Bossone E et al (2001) Association of left ventricular hypertrophy and aortic dilatation in patients with acute thoracic aortic dissection. Angiology 52:447–455

Ingelsson E, Pencina MJ, Levy D, Aragam J, Mitchell GF, Benjamin EJ, Vasan RS (2008) Aortic root diameter and longitudinal blood pressure tracking. Hypertension 52:473–477. doi:10.1161/HYPERTENSIONAHA.108.11415

Iribarren C, Darbinian JA, Go AS, Fireman BH, Lee CD, Grey DP (2007) Traditional and novel risk factors for clinically diagnosed abdominal aortic aneurysm: the Kaiser multiphasic health checkup cohort study. Ann Epidemiol 17:669–678. doi:10.1016/j.annepidem.2007.02.004

Karakaya O, Barutcu I, Esen AM, Dogan S, Saglam M, Karapinar H et al (2006) Relationship between circulating plasma matrix metalloproteinase-9 (gelatinase-B) concentration and aortic root dilatation. Am J Hypertens 19:361–365. doi:10.1016/j.amjhyper.2005.08.013

Kim M, Roman MJ, Cavallini C, Schwartz JE, Pickering TG, Devereux RB (1996) Effect of hypertension on aortic root size and prevalence of aortic regurgitation. Hypertension 28:47–52

Lai CL, Chien KL, Hsu HC, Su TC, Chen MF, Lee YT (2010) Aortic root dimension as an independent predictor for all-cause death in adults <65 years of age (from the Chin-Shan Community Cardiovascular Cohort Study). Echocardiography 27:487–495. doi:10.1111/j.1540-8175.2009.01072.x

Lam S, Verhagen NA, Strutz F, van der Pijl JW, Daha MR, van Kooten C (2003) Glucose-induced fibronectin and collagen type III expression in renal fibroblasts can occur independent of TGF-beta1. Kidney Int 63:878–888. doi:10.1046/j.1523-1755.2003.00824

Lam CS, Xanthakis V, Sullivan LM, Lieb W, Aragam J, Redfield MM et al (2010) Aortic root remodeling over the adult life course: longitudinal data from the Framingham Heart Study. Circulation 122:884–890. doi:10.1161/CIRCULATIONAHA.110.937839

Lam CSP, Gona P, Larson MG, Aragam J, Lee DS, Mitchell GF et al (2013) Aortic root remodeling and risk of heart failure in the Framingham Heart Study. J Am Coll Cardiol HF 1:79–83. doi:10.1016/j.jchf.2012.10.003

Landenhed M, Engström G, Gottsäter A, Caulfield MP, Hedblad B, Newton-Cheh C et al (2015) Risk profiles for aortic dissection and ruptured or surgically treated aneurysms: a prospective cohort study. J Am Heart Assoc 4, e001513. doi:10.1161/JAHA.114.001513

Lang RM, Badano LP, Mor-Avi V, Afilalo J, Armstrong A, Ernande L et al (2015) Recommendations for cardiac chamber quantification by echocardiography in adults: an update from the American Society of Echocardiography and the European Association of Cardiovascular Imaging. Eur Heart J Cardiovasc Imaging 16:233–271. doi:10.1093/ehjci/jev014

Mancia G, Fagard R, Narkiewicz K, Redon J, Zanchetti A, Böhm M, Task Force Members et al (2013) 2013 ESH/ESC Guidelines for the management of arterial hypertension. The Task Force for the management of arterial hypertension of the European Society of Hypertension (ESH) and of the European Society of Cardiology (ESC). J Hypertens 31:1281–1357. doi:10.1097/01.hjh.0000431740.32696.cc

Manning WJ, Black JH III. Clinical features and diagnosis of acute aortic dissection. In UpToDate. Retrieved from http://www.uptodate.com/home/index.html. Accessed 29 Mar 2016

Masugata H, Senda S, Murao K, Okuyama H, Inukai M, Hosomi N et al (2011) Aortic root dilatation as a marker of subclinical left ventricular diastolic dysfunction in patients with cardiovascular risk factors. J Int Med Res 39:64–70

Mauer SM (1994) Structural-functional correlations of diabetic nephropathy. Kidney Int 45:612–622. doi:10.1038/ki.1994.80

Milan A, Tosello F, Caserta M, Naso D, Puglisi E, Magnino C et al (2011) Aortic size index enlargement is associated with central hemodynamics in essential hypertension. Hypertens Res 34:126–132. doi:10.1038/hr.2010.185

Milan A, Tosello F, Naso D, Avenatti E, Leone D, Magnino C et al (2013) Ascending aortic dilatation, arterial stiffness and cardiac organ damage in essential hypertension. J Hypertens 31:109–116. doi:10.1097/HJH.0b013e32835aa588

Mitchell GF, Lacourciere Y, Ouellet J-P, Izzo JL Jr, Neutel J, Kerwin LJ et al (2003) Determinants of elevated pulse pressure in middle-aged and older subjects with uncomplicated systolic hypertension: the role of proximal aortic diameter and the aortic pressure-flow relationship. Circulation 108:1592–1598. doi:10.1161/01.CIR.0000093435.04334.1F

Mitchell GF, Conlin PR, Dunlap ME, Lacourciere Y, Arnold JMO, Ogilvie RI et al (2008) Aortic diameter, wall stiffness, and wave reflection in systolic hypertension. Hypertension 51:105–111. doi:10.1161/HYPERTENSIONAHA.107.099721

Mulè G, Cottone S, Cusimano P, Palermo A, Geraci C, Nardi E et al (2010) Unfavourable interaction of microalbuminuria and mildly reduced creatinine clearance on aortic stiffness in essential hypertension. Int J Cardiol 145:372–375. doi:10.1016/j.ijcard.2010.02.047

Mulé G, Nardi E, Morreale M, D'Amico S, Foraci AC, Nardi C et al (2016) Relationship between aortic root size and glomerular filtration rate in hypertensive patients. J Hypertens 34:495–505. doi:10.1097/HJH.0000000000000819

Natoli AK, Medley TL, Ahimastos AA, Drew BG, Thearle DJ, Dilley RJ et al (2005) Sex steroids modulate human aortic smooth muscle cell matrix protein deposition and matrix metalloproteinase expression. Hypertension 46:1129–1134. doi:10.1161/01.HYP.0000187016.06549.96

Nidorf SM, Picard MH, Triulzi MO, Thomas JD, Newee J, King ME et al (1992) New perspectives in the assessment of cardiac chamber dimensions during development and adulthood. J Am Coll Cardiol 19:983–988

O'Rourke MF, Nichols WW (2005) Aortic diameter, aortic stiffness, and wave reflection increase with age and isolated systolic hypertension. Hypertension 45:652–658. doi:10.1161/HYPERTENSIONAHA.107.099721

Palmieri V, Bella JN, Arnett DK, Roman MJ, Oberman A, Kitzman DW et al (2001) Aortic root dilatation at sinuses of valsalva and aortic regurgitation in hypertensive and normotensive subjects: the Hypertension Genetic Epidemiology Network Study. Hypertension 37:1229–1235. doi:10.1161/01.HYP.37.5.1229

Pape LA, Tsai TT, Isselbacher EM, Oh JK, O'gara PT, Evangelista A et al (2007) Aortic diameter > or = 5.5 cm is not a good predictor of type A aortic dissection: observations from the International Registry of Acute Aortic Dissection (IRAD). Circulation 116:1120–1127

Portik-Dobos V, Anstadt MP, Hutchinson J, Bannan M, Ergul A (2002) Evidence for a matrix metalloproteinase induction/activation system in arterial vasculature and decreased synthesis and activity in diabetes. Diabetes 51:3063–3068. doi:10.2337/diabetes.51.10.3063

Prakash SK, Pedroza C, Khalie YA, Milewicz DM (2012) Diabetes and reduced risk for thoracic aortic aneurysms and dissections: a nationwide case–control study. J Am Heart Assoc 1:jah3-e00032310.1161/JAHA.111.000323

Rayner BL, Goodman H, Opie LH (2004) The chest radiograph. A useful investigation in the evaluation of hypertensive patients. Am J Hypertens 17:507–510. doi:10.1016/j.amjhyper.2004.02.012

Reed CM, Richey PA, Pulliam DA, Somes GW, Alpert BS (1993) Aortic dimensions in tall men and women. Am J Cardiol 71:608–610

Roman MJ, Devereux RB, Niles NW, Hochreiter C, Kligfield P, Sato N et al (1987) Aortic root dilatation as a cause of isolated, severe aortic regurgitation. Ann Intern Med 106:800–807

Roman MJ, Devereux RB, Kramer-Fox R, O'Loughlin J (1989) Two-dimensional echocardiographic aortic root dimensions in normal children and adults. Am J Cardiol 64:507–512

Savage DD, Drayer JI, Henry WL, Mathews EC Jr, Ware JH, Gardin JM et al (1979) Echocardiographic assessment of cardiac anatomy and function in hypertensive subjects. Circulation 59:623–632. doi:10.1161/01.CIR.59.4.623

Sawabe M, Hamamatsu A, Chida K, Mieno MN, Ozawa T (2011) Age is a major pathobiological determinant of aortic dilatation: a large autopsy study of community deaths. J Atheroscler Thromb 18:157–165

Shantikumar S, Ajjan R, Porter KE, Scott DJA (2010) Diabetes and the abdominal aortic aneurysm. Eur J Vasc Endovasc Surg 39:200–207. doi:10.1016/j.ejvs.2009.10.014

Singh R, Song RH, Alavi N, Pegoraro AA, Singh AK, Leehey DJ (2001) High glucose decreases matrix metalloproteinase-2 activity in rat mesangial cells via transforming growth factor-beta1. Exp Nephrol 9:249–257, 52619

Teixido-Tura G, Almeida AL, Choi EY, Gjesdal O, Jacobs DR Jr, Dietz HC et al (2015) Determinants of aortic root dilatation and reference values among young adults over a 20-year period: coronary artery risk development in young adults study. Hypertension 66:23–29. doi:10.1161/HYPERTENSIONAHA.115.05156

Tell GS, Rutan GH, Kronmal RA, Bild DE, Polak JF, Wong ND et al (1994) Correlates of blood pressure in community-dwelling older adults. The Cardiovascular Health Study. Cardiovascular health study (CHS) Collaborative Research Group. Hypertension 23:59–67

Vasan RS, Larson MG, Levy D (1995) Determinants of echocardiographic aortic root size. The Framingham heart study. Circulation 91:734–740. doi:10.1161/01.CIR.91.3.734

Virmani R, Avolio AP, Mergner WJ, Robinowitz M, Herderick EE, Cornhill JF et al (1991) Effect of aging on aortic morphology in populations with high and low prevalence of hypertension and atherosclerosis. Comparison between occidental and Chinese communities. Am J Pathol 139:1119–1129

Vriz O, Driussi C, Bettio M, Ferrara F, D'Andrea A, Bossone E (2013) Aortic root dimensions and stiffness in healthy subjects. Am J Cardiol 112:1224–1229. doi:10.1016/j.amjcard.2013.05.068

Adv Exp Med Biol - Advances in Internal Medicine (2017) 2: 447–473
DOI 10.1007/5584_2016_98
© Springer International Publishing AG 2016
Published online: 19 October 2016

Treating Hypertension to Prevent Cognitive Decline and Dementia: Re-Opening the Debate

M. Florencia Iulita and Hélène Girouard

Abstract

Hypertension and dementia are two of the most prevalent and damaging diseases associated with aging. Chronic hypertension, particularly during mid-life, is a strong risk factor for late-life cognitive decline and impairment. Hypertension is also the number one risk factor for stroke and a major contributor to the pathogenesis of vascular dementia and Alzheimer's disease. Despite the vast epidemiologic and mechanistic evidence linking hypertension to cognitive impairment, and the positive effects of blood pressure lowering on reducing the risk of post-stroke dementia, uncertainty remains about the benefit of antihypertensive medication on other forms of dementia. This chapter reviews the link between hypertension and cognition, and discusses the evidence for and against the use of antihypertensive medication for dementia prevention.

Keywords

Hypertension • Cognitive dysfunction • Dementia • Stroke • Antihypertensive drugs • Vascular risk factors

Abbreviations

ABPM	ambulatory blood pressure monitoring
ACEI	angiotensin-converting enzyme inhibitor
AD	Alzheimer's disease
AngII	angiotensin II
ARB	angiotensin-II receptor blocker
ASCOT	Anglo-Scandinavian Cardiac Outcomes Trial
Aβ	amyloid-β
BBB	blood-brain barrier
BP	blood pressure

M.F. Iulita
Department of Neurosciences, Faculty of Medicine, Université de Montréal, 2900 Edouard-Montpetit, H3T 1J4 Montréal, QC, Canada
e-mail: florencia.iulita@umontreal.ca

H. Girouard (✉)
Department of Pharmacology, Faculty of Medicine, Université de Montréal, 2900 Edouard-Montpetit, H3T 1J4 Montréal, QC, Canada
e-mail: helene.girouard@umontreal.ca

CCB	calcium channel blocker
CI	confidence interval
DBP	diastolic blood pressure
DHP	dihydropyridine
DSM-IV	Diagnostic and Statistical Manual of Mental Disorders, 4th Edition
FDG-PET	Fludeoxyglucose (18^F)-Positron Emission Tomography
FINGER	Finnish Geriatric Intervention Study to Prevent Cognitive Impairment and Disability
HCTZ	hydrochlorothiazide
HOPE	Heart Outcomes Prevention Evaluation
HR	hazard ratio
HYVET	Hypertension in the Very Elderly Trial
ICD-10	International Classification of Diseases 10th Revision
JNC-8	Eighth Joint National Committee on the Prevention, Detection, Evaluation, and Treatment of High Blood Pressure
MCI	mild cognitive impairment
MMSE	mini mental state examination
MRC	Medical Research Council
MRI	magnetic resonance imaging
PiB-PET	Pittsburgh compound B-Positron Emission Tomography
PP	pulse pressure
PROGRESS	Perindopril Protection Against Recurrent Stroke Study
RRR	relative risk reduction
SBP	systolic blood pressure
SCOPE	Study on Cognition and Prognosis in the Elderly
SHEP	Systolic Hypertension in the Elderly
SPRINT	Systolic Blood Pressure Intervention Trial
SYST-EUR	Systolic Hypertension in Europe
VaD	vascular dementia

1 Introduction

Hypertension and dementia are two of the most prevalent and damaging diseases associated with aging, affecting millions of individuals worldwide (Global Health Observatory Data: World Health Organization). Together they represent a major public health concern given the increasing life expectancy of seniors in modern societies. Besides the heart and the kidneys, the brain is one of the major organs that suffer from the deleterious effects of hypertension, and such damage is strongly responsible for the mortality and morbidity associated with this disorder (Go et al. 2014).

Decades ago, hypertension was defined by an increase in diastolic blood pressure (DBP) above 90 mmHg. An increase in SBP was thought to be part of the normal aging process. Several studies later demonstrated that SBP was a stronger predictor of adverse cardiovascular events and mortality (Lewington et al. 2002; Kannel et al. 1971), what led afterwards to a change in the definition of hypertension to include both parameters (SBP $\geq$140 mmHg and/or DBP $\geq$90 mmHg).

Both DBP and SBP rise with increasing age; however the patterns of change are different. From age 20 to 60, both SBP and DBP increase in a linear fashion (Franklin et al. 1997); and this rise is mostly attributed to increased peripheral vascular resistance. With the onset of middle age (between age 50 and 60) DBP begins to plateau and declines thereafter, while SBP continues to increase progressively with advancing age, resulting in an increased pulse pressure (defined as the difference between SBP and DBP) (Franklin et al. 1997). With aging, the elastic properties of large conduit arteries such as the carotids and the aorta begin to degenerate; a phenomenon that results in increased arterial stiffness and explains the predominance of increased SBP over DBP in the elderly (Franklin 2006). As a result, isolated systolic hypertension is the most frequent subtype of hypertension in middle aged and elderly subjects (Franklin et al. 2001).

Several epidemiological studies have reported that chronic hypertension, particularly during mid-life, is a strong risk factor for late-life cognitive decline and impairment (Elias et al. 1993; Qiu et al. 2005; Abete et al. 2014). Cognitive impairment is a broad term that encompasses a group of symptoms that may be caused by different underlying pathologies. Thus, cognitive dysfunction may manifest in different ways, such as failure to remember recent events, forgetting words, difficulties in judgement and decision-making, getting lost in familiar surroundings, repetitive questioning; symptoms which are most often accompanied by drastic mood swings and personality changes (Trivedi 2006; Winblad et al. 2004). Cognitive impairment is one of the major causes of disability in the elderly and in many cases, a strong precursor to dementia (Bennett et al. 2002).

Hypertension is also the number one risk factor for stroke (Lawes et al. 2004) and a major contributor to the pathogenesis of vascular dementia (VaD) and Alzheimer's disease (AD) (Eftekhari et al. 2007), the most common causes of dementia in the elderly. Alzheimer's disease is a complex, multi-faceted neurodegenerative disorder leading to synaptic loss and neuronal dysfunction (Selkoe 2002). Its two major pathological substrates are extracellular aggregates of amyloid-β (Aβ) peptides and intracellular neurofibrillary tangles (Querfurth and LaFerla 2010; Blennow et al. 2006). Instead, vascular dementia refers to a heterogeneous group of brain disorders in which cognitive dysfunction is caused by cerebrovascular lesions (e.g. atherosclerosis, ischemic or haemorrhagic stroke, lacunes, microbleeds, carotid stenosis) (Iadecola 2013). Alzheimer's disease accounts for 60–80 % of all dementia cases, followed by vascular dementia (Alzheimer's Association 2015). Although traditionally the pathogenic hallmarks of these two types of dementia have been considered different, there is a growing recognition that mixed dementias with vascular and Alzheimer pathology are common, and that vascular factors are also major contributor to the pathogenesis of Alzheimer's disease (Iadecola 2010).

The negative effects of hypertension on cognitive function are best understood in terms of the brain's need for constant blood supply. The brain is a highly vascularized organ, and continued perfusion is vital to meet its high metabolic demand. Hypertension alters the structure and molecular composition of cerebral blood vessels and disrupts the homeostatic mechanisms that ensure an adequate blood supply to the brain at all times (Pires et al. 2013; Iadecola et al. 2009). Thus, damage to the cerebral vasculature compromises oxygen and glucose delivery for proper neuronal function, as well as the removal of metabolic waste and toxic proteins. These alterations render the brain more vulnerable to ischemic injury, white matter disease and to the development of neurodegenerative pathologies (Soros et al. 2013; Faraco and Iadecola 2013).

Although hypertension is regarded as a strong risk factor for stroke, cognitive dysfunction and dementia later in life, the evidence that antihypertensive therapy improves cognition and reduces dementia risk is less conclusive. While several studies report a strong effect of controlling blood pressure in reducing stroke risk by ~40 % and consequently, post-stroke dementia, the effects of antihypertensive medications on other forms of cognitive decline or dementia is less clear (Rouch et al. 2015).

In the present chapter we examine the pathophysiological link between hypertension and cognition, and discuss the evidence for and against the use of antihypertensive medications in preventing cognitive decline and dementia. We consider the limitations of observational studies and randomized controlled trials and offer a perspective on how this question could be re-examined in future clinical studies.

2 The Link Between Hypertension, Cognitive Decline and Dementia

It is well recognized that vascular risk factors, such as hypertension, diabetes, hypercholesterolemia, coronary heart disease and obesity are implicated in the pathogenesis of vascular dementia and Alzheimer's disease (de la Torre 2004; Barnes and Yaffe 2011). Hypertension is a leading risk factor for stroke, a condition which doubles the risk to develop dementia (Leys et al. 2005). Hypertension has been associated with impaired cognitive function, particularly affecting processing speed, attention, judgement and reasoning, and to a lesser extent episodic memory (Elias et al. 2012). For comprehensive reviews on the subject the reader is referred to (Qiu et al. 2005; Leys et al. 2005; Guo et al. 1997a; Kennelly et al. 2009; Hughes and Sink 2016; Duron and Hanon 2008; Birns and Kalra 2009; Gorelick et al. 2012).

Although the link between high blood pressure and cognitive dysfunction is well established, the onset and age at hypertension assessment are key factors that may influence an individual's risk to develop cognitive impairment and/or dementia in the future (Qiu et al. 2005).

2.1 Mid-Life Hypertension, Cognitive Decline and Dementia

Several large-scale observational studies including men and women have indicated that chronic hypertension, especially high SBP during midlife (~40–65 years), is associated with an increased risk of cognitive decline and dementia in late adulthood. A summary list of relevant studies is presented in Table 1.

The Framingham Study in the early 1990s was one of the first to show that blood pressure levels and chronicity of hypertension in individuals aged 55–88 years where inversely related to global cognitive performance and to specific measures of memory and attention, assessed 14 years after blood pressure examination (Elias et al. 1993). A similar adverse effect of midlife hypertension on late-life cognitive function was demonstrated by the Honolulu-Asia Aging Study (Launer et al. 1995). Although this program examined only men of Japanese-American origin, results demonstrated that the risk for poor cognitive function increased progressively with higher levels of SBP, which had been measured in the preceding two decades. In this report, there was not a significant association between midlife DBP and cognitive function. However, two additional Swedish studies with other large-scale men cohorts have found significant inverse correlations between DBP measured at age 50 and cognitive function 20 years later

(Kilander et al. 1998; Kilander et al. 2000). Extending these observations, the multiethnic Southall and Brent study showed a significant U shaped-association between mid-life DBP (at age 40–67) and cognitive impairment in the subsequent two decades (Taylor et al. 2013). In other words, both low and high DBP were found to have adverse effects on cognitive function later in life. The U-shaped relationship between DBP and cognition was more prominent in the older participants (50–67 years) than in the younger subjects (40–49 years), and surprisingly pulse pressure showed little evidence of association after covariate adjustment (Taylor et al. 2013).

If hypertension has a negative effect on cognitive function, when do cognitive deficits appear after the onset of high blood pressure? In a recent prospective cohort (a Dutch population including men and women), the Masstrich Aging Study examined the cognitive trajectories of individuals with prevalent and incident hypertension (age 25–84) over a period of 12 years (Kohler et al. 2014). Interestingly, it was found that subjects who developed hypertension during the study duration exhibited a slow, steady decline in memory and processing speed within 6–12 years after blood pressure assessment, suggesting that the onset of hypertension may offer a window for therapeutic brain protection.

With respect to dementia, epidemiologic studies have also shown a significant adverse effect of elevated mid-life blood pressure on the risk of developing vascular dementia and Alzheimer's disease in future years (Launer et al. 2000; Kivipelto et al. 2001; Wu et al. 2003; Yamada et al. 2003; Whitmer et al. 2005; Ninomiya et al. 2011). The Honolulu Heart Program, where a large cohort of Japanese-American men were followed over a period of 25 years, revealed that the risk of two of the most common subtypes of dementia (AD and VaD) was ~4 times higher (4.8 (95 % CI = 2.0–11.8)) for those individuals with untreated high SBP ($\geq$160 mmHg) and high DBP ($\geq$95 mmHg) (4.3 (95 % CI = 1.7–10.8) (Launer et al. 2000). Mid-life blood pressure (whether it was moderate or high) was not associated with dementia risk in men who received antihypertensive medication. This

Table 1 Summary of studies investigating the association between mid-life hypertension and late-life cognitive decline and dementia

Study	Participants[a]	Follow-up	Outcome	Main results
Kohler et al. (2014)	$n = 1805$, age 25–84 years	12 years	Verbal memory, executive function and processing speed (psychometric tests)	Baseline and incident HT ($\geq$140/ 90 mmHg) associated with a faster decline in memory and processing speed
Gottesman et al. (2014)	$n = 13{,}476$, age 45–64 years	20 years	Verbal learning, short-term memory and executive function (as a composite)	HT ($\geq$140/90 mmHg) at baseline was associated with a steeper cognitive decline later in life
Taylor et al. (2013)	$n = 1484$, age 40–67 years (multiethnic)	20 years	Global cognitive function, expressed as a composite	Low and high baseline DBP (quintiles) related to cognitive impairment
Ninomiya et al. (2011)	$n = 534$, age 65–79 years	32 years	AD and VaD (DSM-III and NINCDS-ADRDA	Greater mid-life BP (quartiles) associated with increased risk of VaD but not of AD
Whitmer et al. (2005)	$n = 8845$, mean age 42 years	30 years	Dementia (medical records)	Mid-life HT ($\geq$140/90 mmHg) associated with a 20–40 % increased risk of dementia
Wu et al. (2003)	$n = 301$, age >65 years	15 years	AD (DSM-IV)	Mid-life severe HT ($\geq$160/95 mmHg) was as a strong risk factor for AD later in life
Yamada et al. (2003)	$n = 1774$, age >65 years	25–30 years	AD and VaD (DSM-IV)	Higher SBP (continuous variable) associated with increased risk of VaD but not of AD
Kivipelto et al. (2001)	$n = 1449$ age 40–64 years	11–26 years	AD (DSM-IV and NINCDS-ADRDA)	High SBP ($\geq$160 mmHg) in mid-life was a significant risk factor for AD later in life
Kilander et al. (2000)	$n = 502$, age 50 years (men only)	20 years	Global cognitive function, measured with 13 psychometric tests	Low DBP ($\leq$70 mmHg) related to better performance in cognitive tests later in life
Launer et al. 2000	$n = 3703$, age 45–68 years (men only)	25–27 years	Dementia (DSM-III); AD (NINCDS-ADRDA)	Midlife severe HT ($\geq$160/95 mmHg) increased risk of late-life dementia in untreated subjects
Kilander et al. (1998)	$n = 999$, age 50 years (men only)	20 years	Global cognitive function, measured by the MMSE	Positive association between mid-life DBP and prospective cognitive decline
Launer et al. (1995)	$n = 3735$, mean age 53 (men only)	25 years	Cognitive function, measured by the CASI	Midlife SBP predictor of poor cognitive function. No association with DBP
Elias et al. (1993)	$n = 1702$, age 55–88 years	14–20 years	Global cognitive function, expressed as a composite score	Inverse relation between BP (continuous variable) and cognition

[a]Age refers to age at study inclusion. *AD* Alzheimer's disease, *BP* blood pressure, *CASI* cognitive abilities screening instrument, *DBP* diastolic blood pressure, *DSM-III/IV* Diagnostic and Statistical Manual for mental disorders 3rd and 4th edition, *HT* hypertension, *NINCDS-ADRDA* National Institute of Neurological and Communicative Disorders and Stroke – Alzheimer's Disease and Related Disorders Association, *MMSE* mini-mental state examination, *SBP* systolic blood pressure, *VaD* vascular dementia

study further reported a trend for an association between low DBP (<80 mmHg) and increased risk of both types of dementia, although it was not significant.

In line with the results of the Honolulu Heart Program, Kivipelto and colleagues later demonstrated in a Finnish population (including men and women) that individuals with mid-life isolated systolic hypertension (SBP $\geq$160 mmHg) exhibited a ~ 2 fold risk (CI = 1.0–5.5) of developing Alzheimer's disease over a follow-up period of 11–26 years (Kivipelto et al. 2001).

This risk was enhanced in people who also had high serum cholesterol levels ($\geq$6.5 mmol/L), and was not influenced by midlife DBP levels. The significant association between high SBP and dementia risk in the Honolulu Heart Program and in the Kivipelto cohort highlights the importance of monitoring and controlling isolated systolic hypertension. The lack of association between DBP and dementia in the study of Kivipelto and colleagues may be related to the fact that individuals with Alzheimer's disease were more likely to have received treatment for hypertension, which could have corrected DBP but not SBP levels, as discussed by the authors. Also, some individuals were followed for less than 20 years and the population was smaller compared to that from the Honolulu Heart Program. Despite these differences, both studies highlight the relevance of high mid-life SBP as a risk factor for dementia.

2.2 Late-Life Hypertension, Cognitive Dysfunction and Dementia

Even though the association between midlife hypertension, cognitive dysfunction and dementia is generally well supported, the relationship between high blood pressure in late life (65 + years) and cognition is less consistent. A summary list of relevant reports is depicted in Table 2.

Several cross-sectional and longitudinal studies have indicated a significant adverse effect of late-life hypertension (defined as BP $\geq$140–160/ 90–95 mmHg) on global cognition (Kilander et al. 1998; Cacciatore et al. 1997; Elias et al. 2003; Tzourio et al. 1999) as well as on specific cognitive domains like executive function (Kuo et al. 2004). However, such associations between high BP and cognitive decline could not be demonstrated in other elderly populations (Hebert et al. 2004; Tervo et al. 2004; Solfrizzi et al. 2004; Gottesman et al. 2014). In addition, evidence from other study cohorts suggest either the inverse relation; that low blood pressure in older adults is related

to poor global cognitive function, or even more complex U-shaped associations between late-life blood pressure and cognition (Launer et al. 1995; Guo et al. 1997b; Pandav et al. 2003; Waldstein et al. 2005). While high BP may be damaging to the brain by leading to atherosclerosis, white matter disease and altered neurovascular coupling (as reviewed later in this chapter), low BP may negatively affect cognition by leading to insufficient cerebral perfusion, rendering the brain more vulnerable to ischemic and neurodegenerative pathologies.

Similar discrepancies have been reported on the relationship between hypertension in old age and dementia (Qiu et al. 2005; Power et al. 2013). For example, a longitudinal study of 70 year-old residents of Gothenburg, Sweden, revealed a significant correlation between increased DBP ($\geq$100 mmHg) at age 70 and the risk of developing dementia 15 years later (Skoog et al. 1996). In a study with a shorter follow-up (6 years), SBP and DBP were found to confer opposing risks. While subjects with very high SBP were at higher risk of dementia, very low DBP ($\leq$65 mmHg), rather than high DBP, produced an adjusted relative risk of 1.7 (95 % CI = 1.1–2.4) for Alzheimer disease (Qiu et al. 2003). The association between low DBP on dementia risk was also found in other prospective cohorts (Verghese et al. 2003). The opposing trajectories of systolic and diastolic BP are in line with the concept that pulse pressure increases with older age, reflecting increased arterial stiffness; which could explain the positive associations between high SBP and low DBP with Alzheimer's disease.

In contrast, Morris and colleagues found no significant relation between Alzheimer's disease risk and high blood pressure measured 13 years before and 2 years after dementia diagnosis in subjects aged 65 or older (Morris et al. 2001). It should be noted that in this study only a small number of participants had high blood pressure at baseline, and that they tended to be older. Also, about 30 % of the population was receiving antihypertensive medication with diuretics or beta-blockers, although there was no association between antihypertensive use, Alzheimer's

Table 2 Summary of studies investigating the association between late-life hypertension and risk of cognitive decline and dementia

Study	Participants	Follow-up	Outcome	Main results
Ninomiya et al. (2011)	$n = 668$, age 65–79 years	17 years	AD and VaD (DSM-III and NINCDS-ADRDA)	Significant association between late-life BP level (defined by JNC-7) and VaD but not AD
Li et al. (2007)	$n = 2356$, age $\geq$65 years	8 years	Dementia (NINCDS-ADRDA)	High SBP ($\geq$160 mmHg) associated with increased risk of dementia (<70 years); risk declined with older age (70+)
Waldstein et al. (2005)	$n = 847$, age 39–96 years	11 years	Battery of six psychometric tests to assess attention, working and verbal memory, processing speed and executive function	At older ages, both high and low DBP were associated with poor performance on tests of executive function, confrontation naming and processing speed
Solfrizzi et al. (2004)	$n = 2963$, age 65–84 years	3.5 years	MCI (MMSE) and (DSM-III and NINCDS-ADRDA)	No significant effect of HT as a risk factor for MCI
Tervo et al. (2004)	$n = 747$, age 60–76 years	3 years	MCI (MMSE)	No effect of elevated blood pressure on conversion to MCI
Kuo et al. (2004)	$n = 70$, mean age 72 years	Cross-sectional study	Verbal and visual memory, visuo-spatial skills and executive function	Greater SBP (quartiles) associated to impairment in executive function
Hebert et al. (2004)	$n = 4284$, age $\geq$ 65 years	3–6 years	Global cognition (composite of four cognitive tests)	No significant association between SBP or DBP and cognitive change
Elias et al. (2003)	$n = 1423$, age 55–88 years	4–6 years	Learning, memory, executive function and abstract reasoning	Positive association between HT ($\geq$140/90 mmHg) and low cognitive performance only in men (not in women)
Qiu et al. (2003)	$n = 1270$, age 75–101 years	6 years	Dementia and AD (DSM-III)	Both high SBP (>180 mmHg) and low DBP ($\leq$65 mmHg) associated with an increased risk of dementia and AD
Verghese et al. (2003)	$n =$488, age $\geq$75 years	Median 6.7 years	Dementia (DSM-III)	High SBP (140–179 mmHg) and low DBP (<70 mmHg) influenced risk of developing AD
Morris et al. (2001)	$n = 378$, age $\geq$65 years	13 years	AD (NINCDS-ADRDA)	No association between high SBP ($\geq$160 mmHg) and risk of AD
Tzourio et al. (1999)	$n = 1172$, age 59–71 years	4 years	Global cognitive function, measured with the MMSE	High BP ($\geq$160/95 mmHg) associated with cognitive decline
Kilander et al. 1998	$n =$999, age 70 years (men only)	Cross-sectional study	Global cognitive function, measured with the MMSE	Greater DBP (quintiles) related to lower cognitive function
Cacciatore et al. (1997)	$n = 1106$, age 65–95 years	Cross-sectional study	Global cognitive function, measured with the MMSE	Greater DBP (but not SBP) associated with increased risk of cognitive impairment
Skoog et al. (1996)	$n = 382$, age 70 years	15 years	Dementia (DSM-III) and AD (NINCDS-ADRDA)	Subjects who developed dementia at age 79–85 had higher SBP and DBP at age 70 than people who remained dementia free

AD Alzheimer's disease, *BP* blood pressure, *CASI* cognitive abilities screening instrument, *DBP* diastolic blood pressure, *DSM-III/IV* Diagnostic and Statistical Manual for mental disorders 3rd and 4th edition, *HT* hypertension, *NINCDS-ADRDA* National Institute of Neurological and Communicative Disorders and Stroke – Alzheimer's Disease and Related Disorders Association, *MCI* mild cognitive impairment, *MMSE* mini-mental state examination, *SBP* systolic blood pressure, *VaD* vascular dementia disease and SBP measured between 4 and 13 years before diagnosis.

When examining the risk of high blood pressure on dementia across different age strata (65–74 years, 75–84 years and 85+), Li et al. found that only in the youngest age group there was a significant association between high SBP (>160 mmHg) and dementia (HR $= 1.6$, 95 % CI $= 1.01$–2.55) (Li et al. 2007). No such relationships were evident in the older participants, supporting the concept that the link between high blood pressure and dementia varies with age.

Since Alzheimer's disease has a long incubation phase that lasts decades, it is possible that late-life hypertension is not related to a disease that had begun decades before, or alternatively, if hypertension is indeed a risk factor, there may not be enough time for the clinical expression of dementia to manifest when hypertension occurs in late life.

Interestingly, prospective longitudinal studies with very long durations (between 32 and 37 years of follow-up) have revealed an inverted U-shaped trajectory of blood pressure in people who developed incident dementia. In the Honolulu-Asia Aging Study, the development of Alzheimer's disease or vascular dementia was related to a greater rise in SBP from midlife to late life followed by a decline in blood pressure in the years preceding the clinical diagnosis of dementia (Stewart et al. 2009).

Similar findings were presented by the Prospective Population Study of Women in Gothenburg, Sweden, a cohort that was followed for 37 years. In this study, the development of incident Alzheimer's disease (between ages 79 and 85) was related to higher midlife SBP and DBP and a steeper increase of SBP between age 46 and 70, followed by declines in blood pressure in the years before dementia onset (between ages 75 and 85) (Joas et al. 2012). This decline could be explained by a disturbed control of BP with neurodegeneration and/or by the fact that hypotension itself promotes degenerative processes. Interestingly, the same study showed that such variations in SBP were more pronounced in demented subjects treated for hypertension, suggesting that these treatments in women who became demented did not prevent well the increase in blood pressure.

2.3 Post-stroke Dementia

It is estimated that more than 70 % of patients with ischemic or haemorrhagic stroke have a history of high blood pressure (Miller et al. 2014). Dementia is a frequent cause of disability after stroke, occurring in approximately 25–30 % stroke survivors, although prevalence rates may vary among study populations (Henon et al. 2006; Barba et al. 2000). In fact, having a stroke increases the risk of developing dementia by 3–5 times, irrespective of its type (vascular, Alzheimer's or mixed), and this risk is highest within the first months after stroke (Leys et al. 2005).

Patients with post-stroke dementia have higher mortality rates and are often more impaired in functional daily activities (Henon et al. 2006). There is also a strong, linear association between stroke mortality and blood pressure (Palmer et al. 1992). Thus, it has been argued that among the modifiable risk factors, controlling blood pressure in patients with a prior stroke should result in a favourable reduction in the risk of developing dementia and cognitive impairment (Soros et al. 2013). Whether antihypertensive therapy is effective in preventing stroke-related cognitive decline and other forms of dementia will be discussed in Sect. 3 of this chapter.

2.4 How Does Hypertension Affect Cognitive Function?

Multiple mechanisms link hypertension to cognitive dysfunction and dementia (Fig. 1). High blood pressure affects the brain by altering the structure of the cerebral vasculature, by disrupting the mechanisms that regulate the cerebral circulation, as well as by contributing to the pathogenesis of Alzheimer's disease (Faraco and Iadecola 2013; Iadecola and Davisson 2008;

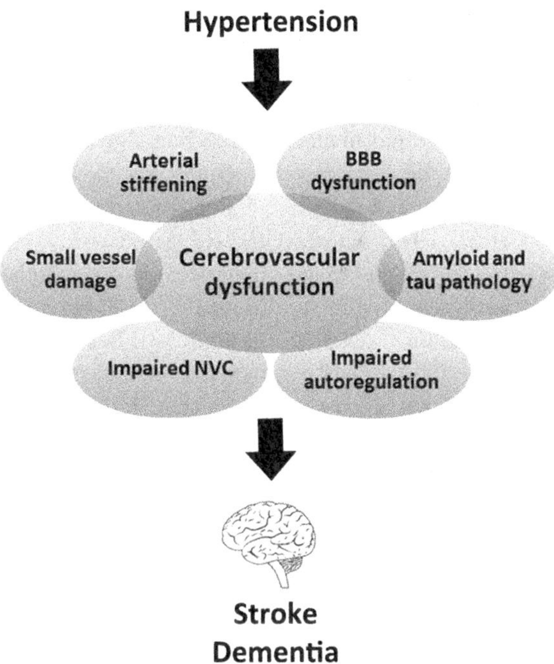

Fig. 1 The link between hypertension, cerebrovascular dysfunction and dementia. Persistent elevated blood pressure promotes the formation of atherosclerosis, leads to arterial smooth muscle hyperplasia and vascular remodelling, increasing arterial stiffening. The resulting increased pulsatility may promote reactive oxygen species production and inflammation in cerebral blood vessels and further lead to disruption in the blood brain barrier (*BBB*). Hypertension may also affect small cerebral arteries leading to microhemorrages and vessel wall necrosis, referred as lipohyalinosis. Besides affecting the structure of cerebral blood vessels, hypertension disrupts the mechanisms that regulate cerebral blood flow, such as neurovascular coupling (*NVC*) and cerebral autoregulation. These changes compromise the clearance of brain metabolites, such as amyloid-β and tau, favouring their accumulation. Taken together, the structural and functional alterations induced by hypertension lead to cerebrovascular dysfunction and render the brain more vulnerable to degenerative and ischemic disease

Girouard and Iadecola 2006; Skoog and Gustafson 2006). These effects will be briefly reviewed.

2.4.1 Structural Alterations in Cerebral Blood Vessels

Hypertension promotes the formation of atherosclerosis in large extracranial and intracranial arteries, leading to a reduced vascular lumen and hypoperfusion followed by vascular occlusion and ischemic injury, and consequently, to increased stroke risk (Hollander et al. 1993). Studies in rodents suggest that a moderate reduction in cerebral blood flow affects brain homeostasis. At declining flow rates, protein synthesis is inhibited first, at blood flow values approximately 80 % of the normal flow rate (Xie et al. 1989; Jacewicz et al. 1986), followed by alterations in glucose utilization and energy metabolism, the release of neurotransmitters (particularly of the inhibitory type), and finally by anoxic depolarization (at <20 % of normal flow rate) (Hossmann 1994). Chronic hypoperfusion has also been proposed as an early factor driving the neurodegenerative process of Alzheimer's disease (Zlokovic 2011; de la Torre 2002).

Elevated blood pressure also induces occluding lesions in small cerebral arteries and arterioles supplying the white matter, known as lipohyalinosis. This refers to thickening of the vessel wall or in severe cases to vessel wall necrosis, which may lead to rupture (Lammie

2002). Thus, such morphological alterations facilitate the appearance of lacunes (infarcts of <20 mm in diameter) and microinfarcts (<1 mm in diameter), as well as microbleeds and large cerebral haemorrhages, leading to white matter damage, (Havlik et al. 2002). Notably, these vascular lesions have been associated to reduced cognitive function (Skoog et al. 1996; Kapasi and Schneider 2016; Wolf et al. 2000) and to an accelerated progression from mild cognitive impairment (MCI) to dementia (Clerici et al. 2012).

Sustained elevations in blood pressure may also lead to adaptive changes in cerebral blood vessels (i.e. vascular remodelling) to counteract the adverse effects of increased pulsatile stress induced by hypertension (Intengan and Schiffrin 2001). Vascular smooth muscle cells may grow in size or undergo a rearrangement that leads to reduced vessel lumen and capacity to dilate; and accumulation of extracellular matrix proteins may further lead to greater vessel wall thickness (Intengan and Schiffrin 2001; Baumbach and Heistad 1989; Heistad et al. 1990). Accumulation of collagen deposits and elastin fragmentation may also occur in large arteries, leading to reduced distensibility and vascular stiffening (Kaess et al. 2012). Arterial stiffness is often a neglected aspect of hypertension, which deserves further attention as it has been related to stroke, cognitive impairment and dementia (Pase et al. 2012; Hanon et al. 2005), although the pathogenic mechanisms involved continue to be elucidated (Sadekova et al. 2013).

2.4.2 Alterations in Cerebrovascular Function

Besides affecting the mechanical properties of cerebral blood vessels, hypertension interferes with the homeostatic mechanisms that control the regulation of cerebral blood flow. In experimental models, hypertension (induced by the infusion of angiotensin-II) impaired the endothelium-dependent relaxation of cerebral blood vessels as well as functional hyperemia, which is the increase in cerebral blood flow in response to neuronal activity (Kazama et al. 2004; Girouard et al. 2006). Alterations in

neurovascular coupling are also supported by human studies. Patients with untreated hypertension have reduced evoked cerebral blood flow responses in the posterior parietal cortex when engaged in a memory task (Jennings et al. 2005).

Given that the integrity of endothelial cells is vital for the regulation of blood-brain barrier (BBB) permeability, the negative effects of hypertension on endothelial function inevitably impact on BBB maintenance (Abbott et al. 2010). Several lines of evidence point at oxidative stress, matrix metallo-protease activation and inflammation as the underlying mechanisms linking hypertension to BBB breakdown (Kahles et al. 2007; Yang and Rosenberg 2011).

In addition, hypertension alters cerebral autoregulation (Immink et al. 2004), which is the mechanism by which cerebral blood flow remains constant within a certain range of arterial pressures (60–150 mmHg). Taken together, the changes induced by hypertension compromise cerebral perfusion and render the brain more vulnerable to stroke and to neurodegenerative lesions. Interestingly, endothelium-dependent relaxation and functional hyperemia are altered in experimental models of Alzheimer's disease (Niwa et al. 2000a, b; Park et al. 2004) as well as in humans suffering from this disorder (Hock et al. 1997; Rosengarten et al. 2006; Janik et al. 2016).

2.4.3 Alzheimer's Disease Pathology

It is known that cerebrovascular lesions, such as those caused by hypertension, worsen cognitive performance and increase the likelihood of dementia development in individuals who also exhibit Alzheimer's neuropathology (Snowdon et al. 1997; Esiri et al. 1999; Chi et al. 2013). Interestingly, histopathological analyses from the Honolulu-Asia Aging Study have demonstrated that people with elevated midlife blood pressure exhibited greater number of cortical and hippocampal amyloid plaques and neurofibrillary tangles, as well as reduced brain weight later in life (Petrovitch et al. 2000).

Likewise, Shah and colleagues recently reported that the risk of Alzheimer's disease was higher in individuals with declining levels of plasma Aβ; an interaction which was enhanced by midlife blood pressure (Shah et al. 2012). In this study, reduced plasma Aβ was related to an increased likelihood of cerebral amyloid angiopathy (deposition of amyloid within the walls of cerebral blood vessels); suggesting that hypertension may interfere with the vascular clearance of Aβ leading to amyloid accumulation. As a case in point, experimental models of chronic and acute hypertension reproduce the enhanced deposition of Aβ in cerebral blood vessels and in the brain parenchyma, and also exhibit an altered permeability of the blood-brain barrier (Carnevale et al. 2012; Gentile et al. 2009; Faraco et al. 2016).

3 Treating Hypertension to Prevent Cognitive Decline and Dementia

Given the ample epidemiological and mechanistic evidence linking hypertension with lower cognitive abilities, a logical question emerges: does blood pressure control slow down cognitive decline and prevent dementia? A beneficial effect of antihypertensive medication on cognitive decline and dementia incidence is suggested by several observational studies with short/medium-term follow-ups (i.e. between 412 years) (Kohler et al. 2014; Tzourio et al. 1999; Qiu et al. 2003; Joas et al. 2012; Gelber et al. 2013; Khachaturian et al. 2006; Guo et al. 1999, 2001). Interestingly, Peila and colleagues suggested that the protective effect of antihypertensive therapy (after adjusting for age, education, *APOE* ε4 status, midlife and late-life BP) is proportional to its use: the longer the duration of treatment, the lower the risk of incident dementia and its subtypes (AD and VaD) (Peila et al. 2006). Despite these encouraging observations, the true effect of blood pressure lowering drugs on cognition can only be assessed by randomized placebo-controlled clinical trials. These are summarized in Table 3.

The **Systolic Hypertension in Europe (SYST-EUR)** trial was one of the first double-blind studies to show a significant reduction in the incidence of dementia (AD and VaD) due to antihypertensive treatment (Forette et al. 1998). This trial enrolled dementia-free subjects (with no prior history of stroke) who were 60+ years and had high SBP (160–219 mmHg). Active treatment consisted of nitrendipine, a calcium channel blocker (CCB), which could be combined with a diuretic (hydrochlorothiazide: HCTZ) and/or with enalapril, an angiotensin-converting enzyme (ACE) inhibitor. The goal of the study was to reach a threshold of SBP reduction of at least 150 mmHg. The SYST-EUR trial was stopped early after 2 years due to a significant reduction in stroke-related events (by ~40 % $P < 0.001$) in the treatment group. At this time point, nitrendipine also reduced the incidence of all cause dementia by 50 % ($P = 0.05$), including Alzheimer's, vascular and mixed dementia cases. These findings were based on a total of 32 incident dementia cases (all forms). After the trial stopped, all participants (those previously treated and those in the placebo group) were invited to continue or begin treatment with the same BP-lowering regimen for another 2 years (Forette et al. 2002). Interestingly, this second phase showed that immediate antihypertensive therapy was more effective at reducing dementia risk compared to delayed treatment, supporting the observation from Peila et al. discussed above (Peila et al. 2006).

Despite comparable subject demographics to the SYST-EUR trial (participants aged 60+, SBP ranging from 160 to 219 mmHg) and a similarly reduced stroke risk (by 36 %), the **Systolic Hypertension in the Elderly Program (SHEP)** study did not find a significant protective effect of blood pressure lowering on dementia incidence, after a follow-up of 4.5 years (relative risk reduction; RRR: 14 %; 95 % CI: −26 to 54 %; $P = 0.44$) (SHEP Cooperative Research Group 1991). No distinction between AD and VaD dementia was made. It should be also noted that the antihypertensive regimen was different, consisting primarily of chlorthalidone (a diuretic). Thus, it is possible that for dementia prevention it may not be just about lowering blood pressure but also about the choice of

Table 3 Randomized controlled trials assessing the effect of antihypertensive drugs on cognitive decline and dementia

Trial	Participants	Follow-up	Intervention	Outcome	Main results
SYST-EUR	$n = 2902$ with ISH, mean age 70 years	4 years	CCB (nitrendipine) and/or ACEI (enalapril) and/or diuretic (HCTZ) vs. placebo	Dementia (AD, VaD and mixed) by DSM-III and MMSE	Significant dementia (AD and VaD) risk reduction by 55 % (95 % CI: 24–73 %) in treated group
SHEP	$n = 4376$ with ISH, age >60 years	4.5 years	Diuretic (chlorthalidone) with BB (atenolol) or reserpine vs. placebo	Dementia (Short-CARE test)	14 % (95 % CI: −26 to 54 %) reduction in dementia (non significant) in treated group
SCOPE	$n = 4964$ with ESH, age 70–89 years	3.7 years	ARB (candesartan) with possible addition of diuretic (HCTZ) and/or open-label AH	Dementia and cognitive function (ICD-10 and MMSE)	Comparable incidence of dementia (all cause) and rate of cognitive decline between placebo and active treatment groups
MRC	$n = 2584$ with ESH, age 65–74 years	4.5 years	Diuretic (HCTZ) or BB (atenolol) vs. placebo	Change in cognitive function (measured by the PAL and TMT tests)	No significant effect of active treatment on change in cognitive function
PROGRESS	$n = 6105$ with prior stroke or TIA, mean age 64 years	3.9 years	ACEI (perindopril) with possible addition of diuretic (indapamide) vs. placebo	Dementia and cognitive decline (DSM-IV and MMSE)	Significant reduction in the risk of dementia with recurrent stroke by 34 % (95 % CI: 3–55 %) and of cognitive decline with recurrent stroke by 45% (95% CI: 21-61%)
HOPE	$n = 9297$ with vascular risk factors, age ≥ 55 years	4.5 years	ACEI (ramirpil) vs. placebo	Stroke, TIA and cognitive function	Significant reduction in stroke-related cognitive decline by 41 % (95 % CI: 6–63 %)
HYVET-COG	$n = 3336$ with ESH, age ≥ 55 years	2.2 years	Diuretic (indapamide) with possible addition of ACEI (perindropil) vs. placebo	Cognitive decline and dementia (assessed by MMSE)	No significant difference in incident dementia rates between active treatment and placebo

AD Alzheimer's disease, *ACEI* angiotensin-converting enzyme inhibitors, *AH* antihypertensive, *ARB* angiotensin receptor blocker, *BB* beta-blocker, *CCB* calcium channel blocker, *CI* confidence interval, *DSM-III/IV* Diagnostic and Statistical Manual for mental disorders 3rd and 4th edition, *ESH* essential hypertension, *HCTZ* hydrochlorothiazide, *HOPE* heart outcomes prevention evaluation, *HYVET-COG* hypertension in thevery elderly trial cognitive function assessment, *ICD-10* International Statistical Classification of Diseases and Related Health Problems 10th edition, *ISH* isolated systolic hypertension, *MMSE* mini-mental state examination, *MRC* Medical Research Council, *PAL* paired-associates learning, *PROGRESS* The Perindopril Protection Against Recurrent Stroke Study, *SCOPE* Study on Cognition and Prognosis in the Elderly, *SHEP* Systolic Hypertension in the Elderly Program, *Short-CARE* short-comprehensive assessment and referral evaluation, *SYST-EUR* systolic hypertension in Europe, *TIA* transient ischemic attack, *TM* trail making, *VaD* vascular dementia

antihypertensive drug. In particular CCBs of the dihydropyridine (DHP) type, as used in the SYST-EUR trial, could be beneficial in the context of Alzheimer's disease given that sustained intracellular calcium elevations may promote Aβ production and tau phosphorylation (Paris et al. 2011; Green and LaFerla 2008; Yu et al. 2009). This suggests that DHP-CCBs may have additional protective effects on the brain other than decreasing BP.

In a subsequent report about the SHEP trial, it was observed that the non-significant cognitive and functional effects of the treatment might have been due to differential dropout between the groups; i.e. participants who missed the annual cognitive assessments tended to be older, to be in the placebo group and to have a higher occurrence of cardiovascular events. In other words, selective attrition may have biased the lack of significant differences between active treatment and placebo (Di Bari et al. 2001). Another important consideration is that due to ethical reasons, participants with high blood pressure in the placebo group also received open-label antihypertensive medication. These limitations put into question the observation that BP lowering does not affect dementia.

The **Study on Cognition and Prognosis in the Elderly (SCOPE)** was a prospective, double-blind trial designed to assess whether antihypertensive treatment with candesartan, an angiotensin-II type I (AT1) receptor blocker (ARB), was effective in reducing cardiovascular events, cognitive decline and dementia in elderly patients (70–89 years) with moderate high blood pressure (SBP 160–179 mmHg) (Lithell et al. 2003). Additional open-label antihypertensive drugs (i.e. HCTZ, diuretic, CCBs), were included as needed in both groups.

After 3.7 years of follow-up and after achieving considerable reductions in blood pressure and non-fatal stroke risk (by 27.8 %), no difference was noted in global cognition scores or dementia incidence between the two groups, assessed with the mini-mental state examination (MMSE) and ICD-10 criteria. Considering that by the end of the trial both candesartan and placebo groups had received additional AH medication and that both obtained significant BP reductions (from 166.0/90.3 to 145.2/79.9 in candesartan arm and 166.6/90/4 to 148.5/81.6 in placebo arm), it is possible that this could be masking any treatment benefit. The fact that a significant stroke risk reduction was seen with candesartan treatment (compared to placebo) could further highlight a protective cerebrovascular effect mediated through AT1 receptor antagonism. In addition, as the authors acknowledged, the rates of dementia incidence in

the study cohort were lower (approximately 6.5 cases per 1000 patient years) compared to what would be expected for the age range (70–89 years) of the subjects, thus limiting the study's power to detect a significant difference on the treatment. Notably, in a later report, SCOPE participants were segregated based on baseline cognitive function into high and low. This new analysis revealed that the incidence of dementia was higher in subjects with initially lower cognitive function, and importantly, that MMSE scores in the active treatment subgroup declined less than in the placebo group (Skoog et al. 2005).

Similarly, in a first report of the **Medical Research Council (MRC)** study, a subgroup of hypertensive subjects ($n = 2584$; age 65–74; SBP 160–209 mmHg, DBP < 115 mmHg) who received treatment with a diuretic (HCTZ + amiloride) or a beta-blocker (atenolol) were examined longitudinally with a neuropsychological testing battery, that included the paired associate learning and trail making tests, over a period of 4.5 years. These tests evaluate episodic memory and new learning as well as executive functions. The trial reported no difference in the rate of change of semantic memory and attention scores between the treated and placebo groups (Prince et al. 1996). When a subset of these patients ($n = 387$) were followed for an extended period of 9–12 years, it was found that poorer global cognition at follow-up was significantly associated to a smaller decline in SBP during the study period (Cervilla et al. 2000), suggesting that more extensive trial durations may be needed to detect significant differences in cognition.

The **Perindopril Protection Against Recurrent Stroke Study (PROGRESS)** trial evaluated the efficacy of monotherapy with perindopril (an ACE inhibitor), or in combination with indapamide (a thiazide-like diuretic), compared to other antihypertensive therapies in reducing the risk of cognitive decline and dementia in subjects with pre-existing stroke or transient ischemic attack (mean age 64 years). Contrary to the other studies discussed before, cognitive decline and dementia incidence (assessed by the MMSE and DSM-IV criteria) were primary outcomes in the PROGRESS trial analysis. After a mean follow-up of 3.9 years, the study showed a clear benefit of combination therapy in reducing the risk of post-stroke dementia and cognitive decline by 34 % (95 % CI: 3–55 %) and 45 % (95 % CI: 21–61 %) respectively, in individuals with recurrent stroke. Despite this positive observation, the effect was not significant in patients with dementia in the absence of repeated stroke events (Tzourio et al. 2003). In line with the PROGRESS study, the Heart Outcomes Prevention Evaluation (HOPE) trial revealed a significant 41 % reduction in stroke-related functional impairment (cognition, motor weakness, speech and swallowing) in patients with cardiovascular risk factors treated with an ACE inhibitor (ramipril) (Bosch et al. 2002). In the HOPE trial, an effect on dementia incidence was not evaluated.

A commonality of all previous studies was the testing of antihypertensive medication for cognitive protection in 'young' older adults (60–75 years). The double-blind, placebo-controlled **Hypertension in the Very Elderly Trial (HYVET)** included a cognitive assessment sub-study (HYVET-COG) to examine the benefit of treating very old hypertensive subjects (80+, SBP 160–200 mmHg; DBP < 110 mmHg), with no dementia at baseline (Peters et al. 2008). Participants received indapamide (a diuretic) with the possible addition of perindropil (ACE inhibitor) to reach a target blood pressure of <150/80 mmHg. The study had a short follow-up (mean 2.2 years) due to positive effects on stroke and total mortality reduction. At this time, although there was a risk reduction of 14 % in dementia incidence between active treatment and placebo, these differences were not statistically significant, likely due to the short follow-up and the low number of patients who had developed dementia.

In brief, several observational studies and some, but not all, randomized controlled trials support the use of antihypertensive medication for dementia prevention. While the protective effect of blood pressure control on cognition is consistent for stroke-related cognitive decline,

the beneficial effect of antihypertensive drugs on other forms of dementia has not been supported by some trials and further questioned in several meta-analyses (Power et al. 2011; McGuinness et al. 2009). The reasons for such conflicting results will be discussed in the next section.

4 Antihypertensive Treatment and Dementia Prevention: Assessing the Evidence

The conflicting results of some randomized controlled trials and meta-analyses put into question the efficacy of antihypertensive drugs for preventing cognitive decline and dementia. However, certain methodological considerations, as briefly discussed above, may have negatively biased these outcomes. These are further reviewed below along with possible recommendations for future trial design and data analysis.

4.1 Patient Heterogeneity

Several trials have tested the efficacy of antihypertensive therapies for dementia prevention in heterogeneous patient populations, and such analyses may have negatively biased the results of these studies. Instead, looking at the effect of blood pressure lowering on subgroup of patients, rather than globally, may reveal positive effects of such drugs on cognition. An example of this is the outcome of the PROGRESS and HOPE trials, which revealed significant reductions in cognitive decline and dementia in patients with recurrent stroke but not in patients who developed dementia without a new stroke (Tzourio et al. 2003; Bosch et al. 2002).

Patients could also be segregated by genetic polymorphisms that have an impact on cognition. The best studied genetic risk factor for Alzheimer's disease is the E4 allele of apolipoprotein E (ApoE4) (Poirier et al. 1993). This variant favours Aβ aggregation and impairs its clearance (Verghese et al. 2013). ApoE4 carriers exhibit a greater decline in cerebral blood flow in brain regions typically affected by Alzheimer's pathology (temporal, frontal and parietal cortices) (Thambisetty et al. 2010). In individuals with hypertension, the presence of an E4 allele synergistically accelerates cognitive decline (Yasuno et al. 2012). Notably, none of the randomised trials discussed in this chapter have evaluated the effect of antihypertensives on cognition in individuals with E4 alleles. The PROGRESS trial reported a comparable number of E4 carriers between the treatment and placebo group but did not conduct sub analyses on E4 carriers. This could be something to take into consideration in the design of future trials.

Age at hypertension onset is another key factor to consider, as it is well established that the negative effects of hypertension on cognitive function are more important in middle age. Therefore, timely control of blood pressure in patients in their 50s–60s may confer greater cognitive protection than in very elderly patients (80+).

Sex and ethnicity are also important criteria. There is evidence from human and animal studies that males and females are affected differently by hypertension. The incidence of hypertension and ischemic stroke is lower in premenopausal women, and such protection has been attributed to reproductive hormones, particularly estrogen (Sandberg and Ji 2012). In experimental models of hypertension, male and ovariectomized female mice exhibit attenuated cerebrovascular responses to whisker stimulation or acetylcholine, while young female mice are relatively spared (Girouard et al. 2008). Interestingly, after women enter menopause the incidence of hypertension is even higher than in men (Ong et al. 2008). Besides hypertension, the prevalence of Alzheimer's disease is higher in women older than 80 years than in men, with faster rates of cognitive decline after dementia diagnosis (Mielke et al. 2014). Therefore, a better understanding of the mechanisms underlying sex differences in the impact of high blood pressure and dementia will allow for a better choice of therapies for each particular group. For such analyses, it will be important to consider men and women separately but also to segregate them into

age categories that take into account pre- and post-menopause.

In a similar manner, ethnicity may also account for differences in blood pressure responses to antihypertensive therapy. In the Anglo-Scandinavian Cardiac Outcomes Trial (ASCOT), the blood pressure lowering effect of atenolol (a beta blocker) and amlodipine (a CCB) differed among different ethnic groups: black patients were significantly less responsive to atenolol compared to Caucasians, while amlodipine was equally effective in both groups (Gupta et al. 2010). In combination therapy (amlodipine + perindopril), South-Asians exhibited a greater blood pressure lowering response compared to white and black patients (Gupta et al. 2010). These findings should be taken into consideration for the future design of trials as well as for guidelines on blood pressure management.

Overall, the factors mentioned above suggest that the classification of patient populations is essential, and that analyses in subgroups of subjects may unmask previously unrecognized differences in the protective effect of antihypertensives.

4.2 Choice of Antihypertensive Drug

The fact that different classes of antihypertensive drugs were used across different trials makes it difficult to conclude whether lack of benefit is due to the drug itself, or simply to blood pressure lowering. In other words, some antihypertensive therapies might be beneficial to protect cognition beyond their blood pressure lowering properties.

The potential benefit of treatment with CCB for Alzheimer's disease and vascular dementia have been suggested by a Cochrane meta-analysis (Lopez-Arrieta and Birks 2002) and also demonstrated by the SYST-EUR trial. The latter also revealed a significant benefit of nitrendipine on reducing stroke risk. In a meta-analysis of 13 studies, Angeli and colleagues further concluded that the effect on stroke is more significant for dihydropyridine CCBs and that it appears to be independent from the degree of blood pressure lowering, hinting at potential neuroprotective effects of CCB (Angeli et al. 2004). CCB work by reducing the number of open calcium channels in cell membranes, thereby restricting the influx of calcium into cells. This mechanism of action is relevant in the context of amyloid pathologies given that Aβ is known to disrupt calcium homeostasis by inducing the formation of calcium-permeable pores on the cell membrane, leading to neurodegeneration (Yu et al. 2009).

In the first report of the SCOPE trial a protective effect of candesartan (an ARB) on dementia incidence was not demonstrated (Lithell et al. 2003), although a sub-study with a longer follow-up revealed a lower reduction in MMSE scores in patients with active treatment (Skoog et al. 2005). In agreement, the OSCAR study (Observational Study on Cognitive function And SBP Reduction) supported the use of ARBs for the protection of cognitive function (Hanon et al. 2008). OSCAR was a large ($n = 25{,}745$), multi-ethnic longitudinal open-label trial to assess the benefit of 6-month eprosartan treatment (a highly selective AT1 receptor antagonist) on cognitive decline and BP reduction in individuals with isolated systolic hypertension, aged 50+ years (Pathak et al. 2007). The MMSE was used to assess global cognitive function. In its primary report, it was observed that even after a short follow-up, treatment with eprosartan (as monotherapy or in combination with other AH drugs) led to an improvement in MMSE scores from baseline (+0.8 points; $P < 0.0001$) (Hanon et al. 2008). There was a strong correlation between the degree of SBP reduction and MMSEs score improvement at completion. In a subsequent publication, it was shown that, besides BP reduction, eprosartan treatment also diminished pulse pressure (Radaideh et al. 2011), suggesting that the protective effects of AT1 receptor antagonism could also include a reduction of arterial stiffness, which could further lead to a cognitive benefit.

The PROGRESS and HYVET-COG trials supported the efficacy of ACE inhibitors in preventing stroke-related cognitive decline and

dementia. ACE inhibitors lower blood pressure by inhibiting the production of angiotensin II (AngII), a potent vasoconstrictor (Brown and Vaughan 1998). AngII has deleterious effects on cognitive (Duchemin et al. 2013) and cerebrovascular functions (Kazama et al. 2004; Girouard et al. 2006), which could also explain the benefit of inhibiting its production, particularly in ischemic diseases. ACE inhibitors have been linked with other mechanisms relevant to dementia, such as their capacity to antagonize the effects of AngII on the inhibition of acetylcholine release (Barnes et al. 1992; Savaskan 2005), as well as by their effect on the modulation of inflammation, which is another hallmark of neurodegenerative diseases (Montecucco et al. 2009). To date, the clinical benefit of ACE inhibitors for non-stroke related dementias remains to be demonstrated.

In summary, even if all antihypertensive drugs lower blood pressure, the choice of a particular class of drug may be important for preventing (or delaying) different causes of cognitive decline and dementia. From the evidence available, it appears that dihydropyridine CCBs and AT1 receptor antagonists could have an additional beneficial effect on cognition in sporadic dementias, while AT1 receptor antagonists and ACE inhibitors have better efficacy in preventing cognitive decline and dementia associated with stroke compared to drugs that similarly lower blood pressure.

4.3 Study Duration and Sensitivity of Neuropsychological Tests

In contrast to longitudinal observational studies with follow-up periods of 20–30 years, most randomized clinical trials have run for shorter periods (maximum 4–5 years). A limited follow-up duration, especially when enrolling patients in their 60–70s who are dementia-free may not be sufficient time to detect significant changes in incidence dementia rates.

There is a growing recognition that Alzheimer's disease has a decades-long asymptomatic or 'incubation' phase, where the pathological changes that lead to dementia are present despite the absence of cognitive or functional deficits (Sperling et al. 2011; Dubois et al. 2010). It is known that this preclinical phase, in which biomarkers are abnormal, is also characterized by very subtle deficits in cognition while functional activities are spared (Sperling et al. 2013). In that sense, longer follow-ups with cognitive decline and dementia as a primary outcome are needed as well as more sensitive cognitive tests. The MMSE test, which has been widely used in many randomized trials and is still a hallmark in the clinic, is not particularly sensitive for detecting subtle changes in cognition (Pendlebury et al. 2012). An alternative test that could be considered is the Montreal Cognitive Assessment (MoCA) (Nasreddine et al. 2005), with the advantage that besides assessing multiple cognitive domains it also evaluates several aspects of executive functions, that are particularly affected in vascular cognitive disorders. This test is recommended in the Vascular Cognitive Impairment Harmonization Standards from the National Institute of Neurological Disorders and Stroke–Canadian Stroke Network (Hachinski et al. 2006).

A further advantage of the MoCA test is the possibility of screening for cognitive deficits in specific domains, separating memory from executive function scores. This is an important consideration for future trials, which could help detect more subtle deficits in specific domains that may appear masked by a normal global cognitive performance. As a case in point, the Canadian Study of Health and Aging found that in individuals with cognitive impairment (mean age 83.06 years) there was no association between dementia incidence and hypertension during a follow-up of 5 years. The same was true for subjects who only had a memory deficit. However, in individuals with executive dysfunction, 57.7 % subjects with hypertension progressed to dementia, whereas the rate of progression was 28 % for normotensives (Oveisgharan and Hachinski 2010).

In addition, self-to-self comparisons should be encouraged, as this analysis would reveal true cognitive change or decline, as opposed to comparing a single test value at a single time point. It should be noted that, except for the PROGRESS study, cognition was a secondary outcome in all the other randomized controlled studies.

Considering the long asymptomatic phase of Alzheimer's disease and the short duration of most antihypertensive drug trials, the inclusion of fluid (CSF, plasma) or imaging biomarkers (e.g. PiB-PET; MRI, FDG-PET) should be encouraged in future trials. An intervention that may appear to be ineffective on preventing dementia (using cognitive or functional outcomes as endpoints) may demonstrate efficacy on reducing pathological biomarkers, thus providing the grounds for re-evaluating such therapy with a different study design.

4.4 Blood Pressure Lowering Regimen: Standard vs. Intensive

Many randomized trials were conducted in subjects with very high blood pressure (SBP 160–219 mmHg) and aimed to reach a reduction of at least 150 mmHg. Is it possible that blood pressure should be reduced beyond what current guidelines recommend (140 mmHg) to observe a positive effect on cognitive function and dementia prevention?

The Systolic Blood Pressure Intervention Trial (SPRINT) is the first study to compare the efficacy of standard (SBP <150–140 mmHg) versus intensive (SBP < 120 mmHg) blood pressure lowering therapy on reducing cardiovascular risk, dementia incidence and the rate of cognitive decline, as primary endpoints. The study has been conducted in hypertensive patients (SBP >130 mmHg or higher) with cardiovascular risk factors, except for diabetes or a previous stroke (those patients were excluded). Rather than focusing on specific drug classes, SPRINT focused on comparing two different blood pressure lowering endpoints.

In a first communication, the SPRINT Research Group reported that after 3 years of follow-up, intensive blood pressure lowering significantly reduced cardiovascular events and mortality rates by ~30 %. It should be noted that patients in the intensive group also exhibited a higher frequency of adverse events compared to the standard-treatment group, including hypotension, syncope, electrolyte abnormalities, and acute kidney injury or failure (Perkovic and Rodgers 2015). The subset study focusing on cognition and dementia (SPRINT-MIND) is not currently completed. Based on the positive results of the first analysis, the field awaits with excitement whether intensive treatment will also have a positive effect on dementia.

In line with the SPRINT principles, results from an ongoing clinical study comparing the cognitive performance of untreated normotensive subjects to that of individuals with controlled hypertension (age range 65–85 years) revealed a strong correlation between the % of daily BP over 135 mmHg and poor performance on tests of executive function (Noriega-de-la-Colina et al. 2016). Likewise, the OSCAR study showed that individuals with a tighter control of SBP (<140 mmHg) had a greater improvement of MMSE scores compared to subjects whose SBP ranged between 140 and 160 mmHg following treatment (Hanon et al. 2008). Taken together, the results of these studies reinforce the SPRINT hypothesis that a more intensive BP reduction (lower threshold) should have positive effects on cognition in people with hypertension.

4.5 Neglecting the Contribution of Other Parameters Associated to Hypertension

4.5.1 Arterial Stiffness

It is well accepted that stiffening of large elastic arteries occurs with aging, and that such process can be accelerated by hypertension (Franklin et al. 1997; Benetos et al. 2002). Similarly, in young adult hypertensive subjects, the pulsatile stress induced by increased blood pressure may lead to vascular remodelling and elastin fragmentation and result in arterial stiffening. Interestingly, arterial stiffness has been demonstrated as an antecedent factor to hypertension in young normotensive adults, suggesting a bidirectional interaction between the two processes (Dernellis and Panaretou 2005).

The significance of arterial stiffness is best highlighted by epidemiological studies revealing its role as a strong risk factor for cognitive decline, dementia and amyloid accumulation (Pase et al. 2012; Hughes et al. 2015). Therefore, if antihypertensive drugs are efficient at lowering blood pressure but not at correcting arterial stiffness it is expected that reducing blood pressure may not have an impact on preventing cognitive decline and dementia. As a case in point, Mackenzie and colleagues reported that while four different kinds of antihypertensive drugs were capable of reducing peripheral systolic pressure as well as pulse pressure, most of them were not efficient at reducing central arterial stiffness (Mackenzie et al. 2009).

Future trials should therefore consider the contribution of arterial stiffness to cognitive decline and incorporate other measures, such as pulse wave velocity (a surrogate of arterial stiffness), besides brachial blood pressure to assess the influence of hypertension and arterial stiffness on cognition. In addition, given that arterial stiffness is a significant link between hypertension and dementia, future trials should focus on interventions that correct these two parameters. Evidence suggests that DHP-CCBs and ACE inhibitors are superior to other antihypertensive drugs in reducing central arterial stiffening (Janic et al. 2014; Dudenbostel and Glasser 2012).

4.5.2 Circadian Variations in Blood Pressure

It is physiologically normal that blood pressure levels vary during a 24 h period. Blood pressure typically falls during the first hours of sleep (around 10–20 % drop) and rises in the morning during wakefulness (<15 mmHg) (Pickering et al. 2006). This marked increase in blood pressure is known as morning surge. Besides having high blood pressure, individuals with hypertension may exhibit a distorted pattern of blood pressure variations, such as an exacerbated morning surge or a diminished (<10 %) nocturnal blood pressure drop (Neutel et al. 2008). The latter is referred as non-dipping pattern.

The current standard assessment of blood pressure in clinical practise provides a static BP value that is not informative of such diurnal variations. These parameters are important for several reasons. Firstly, exacerbated morning surge is a common phenomenon in hypertensive subjects, even in those with mild hypertension (Neutel et al. 2008). Prospective studies have demonstrated significant associations between increased morning surge and stroke risk as well as cardiovascular events and cardiac mortality, independent of the 24 h blood pressure level (Kario et al. 2003; Gosse et al. 2004). Second, there is a strong relation between the non-dipping pattern and low cognitive function, vascular dementia and cerebrovascular lesions (Kilander et al. 1998; Yamamoto et al. 2005).

Morning surge and the nocturnal drop in BP can be assessed through ambulatory blood pressure monitoring (ABPM), which involves the use of a blood pressure monitor that takes several readings during the day and night. This information could be highly beneficial in clinical trials of antihypertensive drugs to better understand the link between the different BP parameters and cognitive decline. It could also help evaluate whether a certain drug (or drug class) maintains its effect throughout the 24 h cycle and thus help select the most adequate drug with the proper pharmacodynamic profile to target a particular group of patients.

In brief, this discussion reinforces the concept that hypertension, just like dementia, is a complex disorder which needs to be studied in light of the many factors presented above, before ruling out that blood pressure management will not have an impact on preventing cognitive decline and dementia.

5 Conclusion: How Can We Treat Hypertension to Protect the Brain?

Hypertension is one of the most common diseases associated with aging and it is well established that timely blood pressure control is the gold standard for stroke prevention. Despite the solid mechanistic and epidemiological evidence linking hypertension (particularly in middle age) to cognitive impairment, uncertainty remains regarding the benefit of blood pressure control on dementia prevention, particularly for patients without a prior history of stroke. Future randomized controlled trials are needed to answer this question -which remains open- taking into account the complexity of hypertension and the contribution of factors such as age, gender, ethnicity, genetic polymorphisms, the mechanism of action of blood pressure lowering drugs and the need for more sensitive cognitive tests and longer follow-ups.

With the evidence available, current guidelines from the American Heart Association recommend antihypertensive treatment for cognitive protection and dementia prevention in patients with a history of stroke or at risk for vascular cognitive impairment. For other individuals, it is mentioned that blood pressure lowering could be useful in preventing dementia if treatment occurs during middle-age, whereas for patients aged 80+ it is recognized that such benefit is not well established (Gorelick et al. 2011).

To what extent should blood pressure be reduced across different age groups? According to the most recent report from the Eighth Joint National Committee on the Prevention, Detection, Evaluation, and Treatment of High Blood Pressure (JNC-8) the target blood pressure for most individuals should be <140/90 mmHg and lower (130/80 mmHg) for people with albuminuria and chronic kidney disease or diabetes mellitus (James et al. 2014). In terms of age, a blood pressure target of 130/80 mmHg or lower is recommended for young adults, while a less tight control is preferred for persons older than 60 years (<150/90 mmHg) (James et al. 2014). The guidelines from the Canadian Hypertension Education Program concur (Daskalopoulou et al. 2015).

In terms of medication initiation, for people over 80 years the JNC-8 recommends antihypertensive treatment to be initiated if BP is >150/90 mmHg, while the threshold for starting antihypertensive medication in younger adults is

>140/90 mmHg (James et al. 2014). Given the recent results of the SPRINT study that an intensive reduction in BP (<120 mmHg) resulted in a 25 % risk reduction of major cardiovascular events (including stroke), it could be expected that current guidelines for hypertension management may be modified in the near future.

What is less clear is how to treat -or whether it is safe to treat- older people with already established dementia, cognitive impairment and hypertension. No specific recommendations exist from the JNC-8 or the European Society of Hypertension. A growing body of evidence from epidemiological studies indicates that excessive blood pressure reduction may be harmful in older patients with pre-existing cognitive and physical disability (Poortvliet et al. 2013; Sabayan et al. 2012). Recently, Mossello and colleagues examined the association between blood pressure (measured by ABPM), cognitive score change (assessed by the MMSE) in a population of elderly patients (mean age 79 years) with MCI (32 %) and Alzheimer's disease (68 %). They found that individuals with dementia or MCI who were being treated with antihypertensives and whose daytime SBP was in the lowest tertile ($\leq$128 mmHg) exhibited greater cognitive decline over a period of 9 months, compared with subjects in the intermediate and highest tertiles (Mossello et al. 2015). Although the population studied was small (172 subjects) and the follow-up was short, their findings are consistent with the concept that aggressive blood pressure lowering may not be beneficial for elderly individuals with pre-existing cognitive impairment. Considering that large artery stiffness, reduced microvascular density and impaired cerebrovascular regulation increase with age, the elevated blood pressure may serve as a compensatory mechanism to ensure proper perfusion to the brain, and thus be critical for cognitive function. Meanwhile, the neurodegenerative process in individuals with dementia may affect blood pressure regulation leading to a decline in blood pressure that further compromises cerebral perfusion. Therefore, as eloquently stated by Sabayan and Westerdorp, a 'one size fits all' approach in hypertension management needs to be revisited, and the concept of 'the lower the better' may not apply to all patient subgroups (Sabayan and Westendorp 2015).

Is antihypertensive therapy the only route for cognitive protection? The Finnish Geriatric Intervention Study to Prevent Cognitive Impairment and Disability (FINGER) is a randomised controlled trial that tested the effect of a multi-domain intervention to prevent cognitive decline in the elderly at risk of dementia. FINGER enrolled subjects aged 60–77 years who were assigned to an 'active intervention' (diet, exercise, cognitive training, monitoring and management of vascular risk factors and social activity) or to 'placebo' (general medical advice). After 2 years, people in the active intervention group exhibited significantly higher scores in tests of memory, executive function and processing speed (Ngandu et al. 2015).

The initial results of the FINGER study are consistent with the concept that the detection and control of vascular risk factors, such as blood pressure, could have a significant impact on the prevention of cognitive impairment and dementia. In agreement, Barnes and Yaffe reported several years ago that about 5 % (1.7 million) of Alzheimer's disease cases are potentially attributable to hypertension (during mid-life), and, importantly, if the prevalence of hypertension were reduced by only by 10 % (for instance by primary prevention with lifestyle modification), that would result in 160 000 less Alzheimer cases worldwide (Barnes and Yaffe 2011).

At present, the vast evidence for the contribution of vascular factors such as hypertension to the pathogenesis of dementia calls for new randomized controlled trials to further investigate the potential of blood pressure management on promoting healthy cognitive aging.

Acknowledgements MFI would like to acknowledge support from the Herbert H. Jasper Postdoctoral Research Fellowship in Neurosciences from the Groupe de Recherche sur le Système Nerveux Central (GRSNC), Université de Montréal, and from a Bourse Postdoctorale from the Fonds de recherche du Québec – Santé (FRQS). HG would like to acknowledge support from the Heart and Stroke Foundation of Canada, the Canadian Institutes of Health Research and the Canadian Foundation for Innovation. HG is the holder of an investigator award from the FRQS.

References

Abbott NJ, Patabendige AA, Dolman DE, Yusof SR, Begley DJ (2010) Structure and function of the blood-brain barrier. Neurobiol Dis 37(1):13–25

Abete P, Della-Morte D, Gargiulo G, Basile C, Langellotto A, Galizia G et al (2014) Cognitive impairment and cardiovascular diseases in the elderly. A heart-brain continuum hypothesis. Ageing Res Rev 18:41–52

Alzheimer's Association (2015) 2015 Alzheimer's disease facts and figures. [updated Mar; cited 11 3]. 332–384. Available from: http://www.ncbi.nlm.nih.gov/pubmed/25984581

Angeli F, Verdecchia P, Reboldi GP, Gattobigio R, Bentivoglio M, Staessen JA et al (2004) Calcium channel blockade to prevent stroke in hypertension: a meta-analysis of 13 studies with 103,793 subjects. Am J Hypertens 17(9):817–822

Barba R, Martinez-Espinosa S, Rodriguez-Garcia E, Pondal M, Vivancos J, Del Ser T (2000) Poststroke dementia : clinical features and risk factors. Stroke 31 (7):1494–1501

Barnes DE, Yaffe K (2011) The projected effect of risk factor reduction on Alzheimer's disease prevalence. Lancet Neurol 10(9):819–828

Barnes JM, Barnes NM, Costall B, Coughlan J, Kelly ME, Naylor RJ et al (1992) Angiotensin-converting enzyme inhibition, angiotensin, and cognition. J Cardiovasc Pharmacol 19(Suppl 6):S63–S71

Baumbach GL, Heistad DD (1989) Remodeling of cerebral arterioles in chronic hypertension. Hypertension 13(6 Pt 2):968–972

Benetos A, Adamopoulos C, Bureau JM, Temmar M, Labat C, Bean K et al (2002) Determinants of accelerated progression of arterial stiffness in normotensive subjects and in treated hypertensive subjects over a 6-year period. Circulation 105(10):1202–1207

Bennett DA, Wilson RS, Schneider JA, Evans DA, Beckett LA, Aggarwal NT et al (2002) Natural history of mild cognitive impairment in older persons. Neurology 59(2):198–205

Birns J, Kalra L (2009) Cognitive function and hypertension. J Hum Hypertens 23(2):86–96

Blennow K, de Leon MJ, Zetterberg H (2006) Alzheimer's disease. Lancet 368(9533):387–403

Bosch J, Yusuf S, Pogue J, Sleight P, Lonn E, Rangoonwala B et al (2002) Use of ramipril in preventing stroke: double blind randomised trial. BMJ 324(7339):699–702

Brown NJ, Vaughan DE (1998) Angiotensin-converting enzyme inhibitors. Circulation 97(14):1411–1420

Cacciatore F, Abete P, Ferrara N, Paolisso G, Amato L, Canonico S et al (1997) The role of blood pressure in cognitive impairment in an elderly population. Osservatorio Geriatrico Campano Group. J Hypertens 15(2):135–142

Carnevale D, Mascio G, D'Andrea I, Fardella V, Bell RD, Branchi I et al (2012) Hypertension induces brain beta-amyloid accumulation, cognitive impairment, and memory deterioration through activation of receptor for advanced glycation end products in brain vasculature. Hypertension 60(1):188–197

Cervilla JA, Prince M, Joels S, Lovestone S, Mann A (2000) Long-term predictors of cognitive outcome in a cohort of older people with hypertension. Br J Psychiatry 177:66–71

Chi NF, Chien LN, Ku HL, Hu CJ, Chiou HY (2013) Alzheimer disease and risk of stroke: a population-based cohort study. Neurology 80(8):705–711

Clerici F, Caracciolo B, Cova I, Fusari IS, Maggiore L, Galimberti D et al (2012) Does vascular burden contribute to the progression of mild cognitive impairment to dementia? Dement Geriatr Cogn Disord 34(3–4):235–243

Daskalopoulou SS, Rabi DM, Zarnke KB, Dasgupta K, Nerenberg K, Cloutier L et al (2015) The 2015 Canadian Hypertension Education Program recommendations for blood pressure measurement, diagnosis, assessment of risk, prevention, and treatment of hypertension. Can J Cardiol 31(5):549–568

de la Torre JC (2002) Alzheimer disease as a vascular disorder: nosological evidence. Stroke 33 (4):1152–1162

de la Torre JC (2004) Is Alzheimer's disease a neurodegenerative or a vascular disorder? Data, dogma, and dialectics. Lancet Neurol 3(3):184–190

Dernellis J, Panaretou M (2005) Aortic stiffness is an independent predictor of progression to hypertension in nonhypertensive subjects. Hypertension 45 (3):426–431

Di Bari M, Pahor M, Franse LV, Shorr RI, Wan JY, Ferrucci L et al (2001) Dementia and disability outcomes in large hypertension trials: lessons learned from the systolic hypertension in the elderly program (SHEP) trial. Am J Epidemiol 153(1):72–78

Dubois B, Feldman HH, Jacova C, Cummings JL, Dekosky ST, Barberger-Gateau P et al (2010) Revising the definition of Alzheimer's disease: a new lexicon. Lancet Neurol 9(11):1118–1127

Duchemin S, Belanger E, Wu R, Ferland G, Girouard H (2013) Chronic perfusion of angiotensin II causes cognitive dysfunctions and anxiety in mice. Physiol Behav 109:63–68

Dudenbostel T, Glasser SP (2012) Effects of antihypertensive drugs on arterial stiffness. Cardiol Rev 20 (5):259–263

Duron E, Hanon O (2008) Hypertension, cognitive decline and dementia. Arch Cardiovasc Dis 101 (3):181–189

Eftekhari H, Uretsky S, Messerli FH (2007) Blood pressure, cognitive dysfunction, and dementia. J Am Soc Hypertens 1(2):135–144

Elias MF, Wolf PA, D'Agostino RB, Cobb J, White LR (1993) Untreated blood pressure level is inversely related to cognitive functioning: the Framingham Study. Am J Epidemiol 138(6):353–364

Elias MF, Elias PK, Sullivan LM, Wolf PA, D'Agostino RB (2003) Lower cognitive function in the presence of obesity and hypertension: the Framingham heart study. Int J Obes Relat Metab Disord 27(2):260–268

Elias MF, Goodell AL, Dore GA (2012) Hypertension and cognitive functioning: a perspective in historical context. Hypertension 60(2):260–268

Esiri MM, Nagy Z, Smith MZ, Barnetson L, Smith AD (1999) Cerebrovascular disease and threshold for dementia in the early stages of Alzheimer's disease. Lancet 354(9182):919–920

Faraco G, Iadecola C (2013) Hypertension: a harbinger of stroke and dementia. Hypertension 62(5):810–817

Faraco G, Park L, Zhou P, Luo W, Paul SM, Anrather J et al (2016) Hypertension enhances Abeta-induced neurovascular dysfunction, promotes beta-secretase activity, and leads to amyloidogenic processing of APP. J Cereb Blood Flow Metab 36(1):241–252

Forette F, Seux ML, Staessen JA, Thijs L, Birkenhager WH, Babarskiene MR et al (1998) Prevention of dementia in randomised double-blind placebo-controlled Systolic Hypertension in Europe (Syst-Eur) trial. Lancet 352(9137):1347–1351

Forette F, Seux ML, Staessen JA, Thijs L, Babarskiene MR, Babeanu S et al (2002) The prevention of dementia with antihypertensive treatment: new evidence from the Systolic Hypertension in Europe (Syst-Eur) study. Arch Intern Med 162(18):2046–2052

Franklin SS (2006) Hypertension in older people: part 1. J Clin Hypertens (Greenwich) 8(6):444–449

Franklin SS, Gustin W 4th, Wong ND, Larson MG, Weber MA, Kannel WB et al (1997) Hemodynamic patterns of age-related changes in blood pressure. The Framingham Heart Study. Circulation 96(1):308–315

Franklin SS, Jacobs MJ, Wong ND, L'Italien GJ, Lapuerta P (2001) Predominance of isolated systolic hypertension among middle-aged and elderly US hypertensives: analysis based on National Health and Nutrition Examination Survey (NHANES) III. Hypertension 37(3):869–874

Gelber RP, Ross GW, Petrovitch H, Masaki KH, Launer LJ, White LR (2013) Antihypertensive medication use and risk of cognitive impairment: the Honolulu-Asia aging study. Neurology 81(10):888–895

Gentile MT, Poulet R, Di Pardo A, Cifelli G, Maffei A, Vecchione C et al (2009) Beta-amyloid deposition in brain is enhanced in mouse models of arterial hypertension. Neurobiol Aging 30(2):222–228

Girouard H, Iadecola C (2006) Neurovascular coupling in the normal brain and in hypertension, stroke, and Alzheimer disease. J Appl Physiol (1985) 100 (1):328–335

Girouard H, Park L, Anrather J, Zhou P, Iadecola C (2006) Angiotensin II attenuates endothelium-dependent responses in the cerebral microcirculation through nox-2-derived radicals. Arterioscler Thromb Vasc Biol 26(4):826–832

Girouard H, Lessard A, Capone C, Milner TA, Iadecola C (2008) The neurovascular dysfunction induced by angiotensin II in the mouse neocortex is sexually dimorphic. Am J Physiol Heart Circ Physiol 294(1): H156–H163

Global Health Observatory Data: World Health Organization. Available from: http://www.who.int/gho/ncd/ risk_factors/blood_pressure_prevalence_text/en/

Go AS, Mozaffarian D, Roger VL, Benjamin EJ, Berry JD, Blaha MJ et al (2014) Heart disease and stroke statistics--2014 update: a report from the American Heart Association. Circulation 129(3):e28–e292

Gorelick PB, Scuteri A, Black SE, Decarli C, Greenberg SM, Iadecola C et al (2011) Vascular contributions to cognitive impairment and dementia: a statement for healthcare professionals from the American Heart Association/American Stroke Association. Stroke 42 (9):2672–2713

Gorelick PB, Nyenhuis D, American Society of Hypertension Writing Group, Materson BJ, Calhoun DA, Elliott WJ et al (2012) Blood pressure and treatment of persons with hypertension as it relates to cognitive outcomes including executive function. J Am Soc Hypertens 6(5):309–315

Gosse P, Lasserre R, Minifie C, Lemetayer P, Clementy J (2004) Blood pressure surge on rising. J Hypertens 22 (6):1113–1118

Gottesman RF, Schneider AL, Albert M, Alonso A, Bandeen-Roche K, Coker L et al (2014) Midlife hypertension and 20-year cognitive change: the atherosclerosis risk in communities neurocognitive study. JAMA Neurol 71(10):1218–1227

Green KN, LaFerla FM (2008) Linking calcium to Abeta and Alzheimer's disease. Neuron 59(2):190–194

Guo Z, Viitanen M, Fratiglioni L, Winblad B (1997a) Blood pressure and dementia in the elderly: epidemiologic perspectives. Biomed Pharmacother 51 (2):68–73

Guo Z, Fratiglioni L, Winblad B, Viitanen M (1997b) Blood pressure and performance on the mini-mental state examination in the very old. Cross-sectional and longitudinal data from the Kungsholmen project. Am J Epidemiol 145(12):1106–1113

Guo Z, Fratiglioni L, Zhu L, Fastbom J, Winblad B, Viitanen M (1999) Occurrence and progression of dementia in a community population aged 75 years and older: relationship of antihypertensive medication use. Arch Neurol 56(8):991–996

Guo Z, Fratiglioni L, Viitanen M, Lannfelt L, Basun H, Fastbom J et al (2001) Apolipoprotein E genotypes and the incidence of Alzheimer's disease among persons aged 75 years and older: variation by use of antihypertensive medication? Am J Epidemiol 153 (3):225–231

Gupta AK, Poulter NR, Dobson J, Eldridge S, Cappuccio FP, Caulfield M et al (2010) Ethnic differences in blood pressure response to first and second-line antihypertensive therapies in patients randomized in the ASCOT Trial. Am J Hypertens 23(9):1023–1030

Hachinski V, Iadecola C, Petersen RC, Breteler MM, Nyenhuis DL, Black SE et al (2006) National Institute of Neurological Disorders and Stroke-Canadian Stroke Network vascular cognitive impairment harmonization standards. Stroke 37(9):2220–2241

Hanon O, Haulon S, Lenoir H, Seux ML, Rigaud AS, Safar M et al (2005) Relationship between arterial stiffness and cognitive function in elderly subjects with complaints of memory loss. Stroke 36 (10):2193–2197

Hanon O, Berrou JP, Negre-Pages L, Goch JH, Nadhazi Z, Petrella R et al (2008) Effects of hypertension therapy based on eprosartan on systolic arterial blood pressure and cognitive function: primary results of the observational study on cognitive function and systolic blood pressure reduction open-label study. J Hypertens 26(8):1642–1650

Havlik RJ, Foley DJ, Sayer B, Masaki K, White L, Launer LJ (2002) Variability in midlife systolic blood pressure is related to late-life brain white matter lesions: the Honolulu-Asia aging study. Stroke 33(1):26–30

Hebert LE, Scherr PA, Bennett DA, Bienias JL, Wilson RS, Morris MC et al (2004) Blood pressure and late-life cognitive function change: a biracial longitudinal population study. Neurology 62(11):2021–2024

Heistad DD, Mayhan WG, Coyle P, Baumbach GL (1990) Impaired dilatation of cerebral arterioles in chronic hypertension. Blood Vessels 27(2–5):258–262

Henon H, Pasquier F, Leys D (2006) Poststroke dementia. Cerebrovasc Dis 22(1):61–70

Hock C, Villringer K, Muller-Spahn F, Wenzel R, Heekeren H, Schuh-Hofer S et al (1997) Decrease in parietal cerebral hemoglobin oxygenation during performance of a verbal fluency task in patients with Alzheimer's disease monitored by means of near-infrared spectroscopy (NIRS)–correlation with simultaneous rCBF-PET measurements. Brain Res 755 (2):293–303

Hollander W, Prusty S, Kemper T, Rosene DL, Moss MB (1993) The effects of hypertension on cerebral atherosclerosis in the cynomolgus monkey. Stroke 24 (8):1218–1226; discussion 26–7

Hossmann KA (1994) Viability thresholds and the penumbra of focal ischemia. Ann Neurol 36(4):557–565

Hughes TM, Sink KM (2016) Hypertension and its role in cognitive function: current evidence and challenges for the future. Am J Hypertens 29(2):149–157

Hughes TM, Craft S, Lopez OL (2015) Review of 'the potential role of arterial stiffness in the pathogenesis of Alzheimer's disease'. Neurodegener Dis Manag 5 (2):121–135

Iadecola C (2010) The overlap between neurodegenerative and vascular factors in the pathogenesis of dementia. Acta Neuropathol 120(3):287–296

Iadecola C (2013) The pathobiology of vascular dementia. Neuron 80(4):844–866

Iadecola C, Davisson RL (2008) Hypertension and cerebrovascular dysfunction. Cell Metab 7(6):476–484

Iadecola C, Park L, Capone C (2009) Threats to the mind: aging, amyloid, and hypertension. Stroke 40(3 Suppl): S40–S44

Immink RV, van den Born BJ, van Montfrans GA, Koopmans RP, Karemaker JM, van Lieshout JJ (2004) Impaired cerebral autoregulation in patients with malignant hypertension. Circulation 110 (15):2241–2245

Intengan HD, Schiffrin EL (2001) Vascular remodeling in hypertension: roles of apoptosis, inflammation, and fibrosis. Hypertension 38(3 Pt 2):581–587

Jacewicz M, Kiessling M, Pulsinelli WA (1986) Selective gene expression in focal cerebral ischemia. J Cereb Blood Flow Metab 6(3):263–272

James PA, Oparil S, Carter BL, Cushman WC, Dennison-Himmelfarb C, Handler J et al (2014) 2014 evidence-based guideline for the management of high blood pressure in adults: report from the panel members appointed to the Eighth Joint National Committee (JNC 8). JAMA 311(5):507–520

Janic M, Lunder M, Sabovic M (2014) Arterial stiffness and cardiovascular therapy. Biomed Res Int 2014:621437

Janik R, Thomason LA, Chaudhary S, Dorr A, Scouten A, Schwindt G et al (2016) Attenuation of functional hyperemia to visual stimulation in mild Alzheimer's disease and its sensitivity to cholinesterase inhibition. Biochim Biophys Acta 1862(5):957–965

Jennings JR, Muldoon MF, Ryan C, Price JC, Greer P, Sutton-Tyrrell K et al (2005) Reduced cerebral blood flow response and compensation among patients with untreated hypertension. Neurology 64(8):1358–1365

Joas E, Backman K, Gustafson D, Ostling S, Waern M, Guo X et al (2012) Blood pressure trajectories from midlife to late life in relation to dementia in women followed for 37 years. Hypertension 59(4):796–801

Kaess BM, Rong J, Larson MG, Hamburg NM, Vita JA, Levy D et al (2012) Aortic stiffness, blood pressure progression, and incident hypertension. JAMA 308 (9):875–881

Kahles T, Luedike P, Endres M, Galla HJ, Steinmetz H, Busse R et al (2007) NADPH oxidase plays a central role in blood-brain barrier damage in experimental stroke. Stroke 38(11):3000–3006

Kannel WB, Gordon T, Schwartz MJ (1971) Systolic versus diastolic blood pressure and risk of coronary heart disease. The Framingham study. Am J Cardiol 27(4):335–346

Kapasi A, Schneider JA (2016) Vascular contributions to cognitive impairment, clinical Alzheimer's disease, and dementia in older persons. Biochim Biophys Acta 1862(5):878–886

Kario K, Pickering TG, Umeda Y, Hoshide S, Hoshide Y, Morinari M et al (2003) Morning surge in blood pressure as a predictor of silent and clinical cerebrovascular disease in elderly hypertensives: a prospective study. Circulation 107(10):1401–1406

Kazama K, Anrather J, Zhou P, Girouard H, Frys K, Milner TA et al (2004) Angiotensin II impairs neurovascular coupling in neocortex through NADPH oxidase-derived radicals. Circ Res 95(10):1019–1026

Kennelly SP, Lawlor BA, Kenny RA (2009) Blood pressure and the risk for dementia: a double edged sword. Ageing Res Rev 8(2):61–70

Khachaturian AS, Zandi PP, Lyketsos CG, Hayden KM, Skoog I, Norton MC et al (2006) Antihypertensive medication use and incident Alzheimer disease: the Cache County study. Arch Neurol 63(5):686–692

Kilander L, Nyman H, Boberg M, Hansson L, Lithell H (1998) Hypertension is related to cognitive impairment: a 20-year follow-up of 999 men. Hypertension 31(3):780–786

Kilander L, Nyman H, Boberg M, Lithell H (2000) The association between low diastolic blood pressure in middle age and cognitive function in old age. A population-based study. Age Ageing 29(3):243–248

Kivipelto M, Helkala EL, Laakso MP, Hanninen T, Hallikainen M, Alhainen K et al (2001) Midlife vascular risk factors and Alzheimer's disease in later life: longitudinal, population based study. BMJ 322 (7300):1447–1451

Kohler S, Baars MA, Spauwen P, Schievink S, Verhey FR, van Boxtel MJ (2014) Temporal evolution of cognitive changes in incident hypertension: prospective cohort study across the adult age span. Hypertension 63(2):245–251

Kuo HK, Sorond F, Iloputaife I, Gagnon M, Milberg W, Lipsitz LA (2004) Effect of blood pressure on cognitive functions in elderly persons. J Gerontol A Biol Sci Med Sci 59(11):1191–1194

Lammie GA (2002) Hypertensive cerebral small vessel disease and stroke. Brain Pathol 12(3):358–370

Launer LJ, Masaki K, Petrovitch H, Foley D, Havlik RJ (1995) The association between midlife blood pressure levels and late-life cognitive function. The Honolulu-Asia Aging Study. JAMA 274 (23):1846–1851

Launer LJ, Ross GW, Petrovitch H, Masaki K, Foley D, White LR et al (2000) Midlife blood pressure and dementia: the Honolulu-Asia aging study. Neurobiol Aging 21(1):49–55

Lawes CM, Bennett DA, Feigin VL, Rodgers A (2004) Blood pressure and stroke: an overview of published reviews. Stroke 35(4):1024

Lewington S, Clarke R, Qizilbash N, Peto R, Collins R, Prospective Studies Collaboration (2002) Age-specific relevance of usual blood pressure to vascular mortality: a meta-analysis of individual data for one million adults in 61 prospective studies. Lancet 360 (9349):1903–1913

Leys D, Henon H, Mackowiak-Cordoliani MA, Pasquier F (2005) Poststroke dementia. Lancet Neurol 4 (11):752–759

Li G, Rhew IC, Shofer JB, Kukull WA, Breitner JC, Peskind E et al (2007) Age-varying association between blood pressure and risk of dementia in those aged 65 and older: a community-based prospective cohort study. J Am Geriatr Soc 55(8):1161–1167

Lithell H, Hansson L, Skoog I, Elmfeldt D, Hofman A, Olofsson B et al (2003) The Study on Cognition and Prognosis in the Elderly (SCOPE): principal results of a randomized double-blind intervention trial. J Hypertens 21(5):875–886

Lopez-Arrieta JM, Birks J (2002) Nimodipine for primary degenerative, mixed and vascular dementia. Cochrane Database Syst Rev 3:CD000147

Mackenzie IS, McEniery CM, Dhakam Z, Brown MJ, Cockcroft JR, Wilkinson IB (2009) Comparison of the effects of antihypertensive agents on central blood pressure and arterial stiffness in isolated systolic hypertension. Hypertension 54(2):409–413

McGuinness B, Todd S, Passmore P, Bullock R (2009) Blood pressure lowering in patients without prior cerebrovascular disease for prevention of cognitive impairment and dementia. Cochrane Database Syst Rev 4:CD004034

Mielke MM, Vemuri P, Rocca WA (2014) Clinical epidemiology of Alzheimer's disease: assessing sex and gender differences. Clin Epidemiol 6:37–48

Miller J, Kinni H, Lewandowski C, Nowak R, Levy P (2014) Management of hypertension in stroke. Ann Emerg Med 64(3):248–255

Montecucco F, Pende A, Mach F (2009) The renin-angiotensin system modulates inflammatory processes in atherosclerosis: evidence from basic research and clinical studies. Mediators Inflamm 2009:752406

Morris MC, Scherr PA, Hebert LE, Glynn RJ, Bennett DA, Evans DA (2001) Association of incident Alzheimer disease and blood pressure measured from 13 years before to 2 years after diagnosis in a large community study. Arch Neurol 58(10):1640–1646

Mossello E, Pieraccioli M, Nesti N, Bulgaresi M, Lorenzi C, Caleri V et al (2015) Effects of low blood pressure in cognitively impaired elderly patients treated with antihypertensive drugs. JAMA Intern Med 175(4):578–585

Nasreddine ZS, Phillips NA, Bedirian V, Charbonneau S, Whitehead V, Collin I et al (2005) The Montreal Cognitive Assessment, MoCA: a brief screening tool for mild cognitive impairment. J Am Geriatr Soc 53 (4):695–699

Neutel JM, Schumacher H, Gosse P, Lacourciere Y, Williams B (2008) Magnitude of the early morning blood pressure surge in untreated hypertensive patients: a pooled analysis. Int J Clin Pract 62 (11):1654–1663

Ngandu T, Lehtisalo J, Solomon A, Levalahti E, Ahtiluoto S, Antikainen R et al (2015) A 2 year multidomain intervention of diet, exercise, cognitive training, and vascular risk monitoring versus control to prevent cognitive decline in at-risk elderly people (FINGER): a randomised controlled trial. Lancet 385 (9984):2255–2263

Ninomiya T, Ohara T, Hirakawa Y, Yoshida D, Doi Y, Hata J et al (2011) Midlife and late-life blood pressure and dementia in Japanese elderly: the Hisayama study. Hypertension 58(1):22–28

Niwa K, Younkin L, Ebeling C, Turner SK, Westaway D, Younkin S et al (2000a) Abeta 1-40-related reduction in functional hyperemia in mouse neocortex during somatosensory activation. Proc Natl Acad Sci U S A 97(17):9735–9740

Niwa K, Carlson GA, Iadecola C (2000b) Exogenous A beta1-40 reproduces cerebrovascular alterations resulting from amyloid precursor protein overexpression in mice. J Cereb Blood Flow Metab 20(12):1659–1668

Noriega-de-la-Colina A, Wu R, Desjardins-Crépeau L, Lamarre-Cliche M, Larochelle P, Bherer L, Girouard H (eds) (2016) Correlation between cognitive decline and blood pressure in elderly patients with controlled hypertension. In: 10th annual meeting of the Canadian Association for Neuroscience, 29 May–1 June, 2016, Toronto, Canada

Ong KL, Tso AW, Lam KS, Cheung BM (2008) Gender difference in blood pressure control and cardiovascular risk factors in Americans with diagnosed hypertension. Hypertension 51(4):1142–1148

Oveisgharan S, Hachinski V (2010) Hypertension, executive dysfunction, and progression to dementia: the canadian study of health and aging. Arch Neurol 67 (2):187–192

Palmer AJ, Bulpitt CJ, Fletcher AE, Beevers DG, Coles EC, Ledingham JG et al (1992) Relation between blood pressure and stroke mortality. Hypertension 20 (5):601–605

Pandav R, Dodge HH, DeKosky ST, Ganguli M (2003) Blood pressure and cognitive impairment in India and the United States: a cross-national epidemiological study. Arch Neurol 60(8):1123–1128

Paris D, Bachmeier C, Patel N, Quadros A, Volmar CH, Laporte V et al (2011) Selective antihypertensive dihydropyridines lower Abeta accumulation by targeting both the production and the clearance of Abeta across the blood-brain barrier. Mol Med 17 (3–4):149–162

Park L, Anrather J, Forster C, Kazama K, Carlson GA, Iadecola C (2004) Abeta-induced vascular oxidative stress and attenuation of functional hyperemia in mouse somatosensory cortex. J Cereb Blood Flow Metab 24(3):334–342

Pase MP, Herbert A, Grima NA, Pipingas A, O'Rourke MF (2012) Arterial stiffness as a cause of cognitive decline and dementia: a systematic review and meta-analysis. Intern Med J 42(7):808–815

Pathak A, Hanon O, Negre-Pages L, Sevenier F, Oscar Investigators (2007) Rationale, design and methods of the OSCAR study: observational study on cognitive function and systolic blood pressure reduction in hypertensive patients. Fundam Clin Pharmacol 21 (2):199–205

Peila R, White LR, Masaki K, Petrovitch H, Launer LJ (2006) Reducing the risk of dementia: efficacy of long-term treatment of hypertension. Stroke 37 (5):1165–1170

Pendlebury ST, Mariz J, Bull L, Mehta Z, Rothwell PM (2012) MoCA, ACE-R, and MMSE versus the National Institute of Neurological Disorders and Stroke-Canadian Stroke Network Vascular Cognitive Impairment Harmonization Standards Neuropsychological Battery after TIA and stroke. Stroke 43 (2):464–469

Perkovic V, Rodgers A (2015) Redefining blood-pressure targets–SPRINT starts the marathon. N Engl J Med 373(22):2175–2178

Peters R, Beckett N, Forette F, Tuomilehto J, Clarke R, Ritchie C et al (2008) Incident dementia and blood pressure lowering in the Hypertension in the Very Elderly Trial cognitive function assessment (HYVET-COG): a double-blind, placebo controlled trial. Lancet Neurol 7(8):683–689

Petrovitch H, White LR, Izmirilian G, Ross GW, Havlik RJ, Markesbery W et al (2000) Midlife blood pressure and neuritic plaques, neurofibrillary tangles, and brain weight at death: the HAAS. Honolulu-Asia aging Study. Neurobiol Aging 21(1):57–62

Pickering TG, Shimbo D, Haas D (2006) Ambulatory blood-pressure monitoring. N Engl J Med 354 (22):2368–2374

Pires PW, Dams Ramos CM, Matin N, Dorrance AM (2013) The effects of hypertension on the cerebral circulation. Am J Physiol Heart Circ Physiol 304 (12):H1598–H1614

Poirier J, Davignon J, Bouthillier D, Kogan S, Bertrand P, Gauthier S (1993) Apolipoprotein E polymorphism and Alzheimer's disease. Lancet 342(8873):697–699

Poortvliet RK, Blom JW, de Craen AJ, Mooijaart SP, Westendorp RG, Assendelft WJ et al (2013) Low blood pressure predicts increased mortality in very old age even without heart failure: the Leiden 85-plus study. Eur J Heart Fail 15(5):528–533

Power MC, Weuve J, Gagne JJ, McQueen MB, Viswanathan A, Blacker D (2011) The association between blood pressure and incident Alzheimer disease: a systematic review and meta-analysis. Epidemiology 22(5):646–659

Power MC, Tchetgen EJ, Sparrow D, Schwartz J, Weisskopf MG (2013) Blood pressure and cognition: factors that may account for their inconsistent association. Epidemiology 24(6):886–893

Prince MJ, Bird AS, Blizard RA, Mann AH (1996) Is the cognitive function of older patients affected by anti-hypertensive treatment? Results from 54 months of the Medical Research Council's trial of hypertension in older adults. BMJ 312(7034):801–805

Qiu C, von Strauss E, Fastbom J, Winblad B, Fratiglioni L (2003) Low blood pressure and risk of dementia in the Kungsholmen project: a 6-year follow-up study. Arch Neurol 60(2):223–228

Qiu C, Winblad B, Fratiglioni L (2005) The age-dependent relation of blood pressure to cognitive function and dementia. Lancet Neurol 4(8):487–499

Querfurth HW, LaFerla FM (2010) Alzheimer's disease. N Engl J Med 362(4):329–344

Radaideh GA, Choueiry P, Ismail A, Eid E, Berrou JP, Sedefdjian A et al (2011) Eprosartan-based hypertension therapy, systolic arterial blood pressure and cognitive function: analysis of Middle East data from the OSCAR study. Vasc Health Risk Manag 7:491–495

Rosengarten B, Paulsen S, Molnar S, Kaschel R, Gallhofer B, Kaps M (2006) Acetylcholine esterase inhibitor donepezil improves dynamic cerebrovascular regulation in Alzheimer patients. J Neurol 253 (1):58–64

Rouch L, Cestac P, Hanon O, Cool C, Helmer C, Bouhanick B et al (2015) Antihypertensive drugs, prevention of cognitive decline and dementia: a systematic review of observational studies, randomized controlled trials and meta-analyses, with discussion of potential mechanisms. CNS Drugs 29(2):113–130

Sabayan B, Westendorp RG (2015) Blood pressure control and cognitive impairment–why low is not always better. JAMA Intern Med 175(4):586–587

Sabayan B, Oleksik AM, Maier AB, van Buchem MA, Poortvliet RK, de Ruijter W et al (2012) High blood pressure and resilience to physical and cognitive decline in the oldest old: the Leiden 85-plus study. J Am Geriatr Soc 60(11):2014–2019

Sadekova N, Vallerand D, Guevara E, Lesage F, Girouard H (2013) Carotid calcification in mice: a new model to study the effects of arterial stiffness on the brain. J Am Heart Assoc 2(3):e000224

Sandberg K, Ji H (2012) Sex differences in primary hypertension. Biol Sex Differ 3(1):7

Savaskan E (2005) The role of the brain renin angiotensin system in neurodegenerative disorders. Curr Alzheimer Res 2(1):29–35

Selkoe DJ (2002) Alzheimer's disease is a synaptic failure. Science 298(5594):789–791

Shah NS, Vidal JS, Masaki K, Petrovitch H, Ross GW, Tilley C et al (2012) Midlife blood pressure, plasma beta-amyloid, and the risk for Alzheimer disease: the Honolulu Asia aging study. Hypertension 59 (4):780–786

SHEP Cooperative Research Group (1991) Prevention of stroke by antihypertensive drug treatment in older persons with isolated systolic hypertension. Final results of the Systolic Hypertension in the Elderly Program (SHEP). SHEP Cooperative Research Group. JAMA 265(24):3255–3264

Skoog I, Gustafson D (2006) Update on hypertension and Alzheimer's disease. Neurol Res 28(6):605–611

Skoog I, Lernfelt B, Landahl S, Palmertz B, Andreasson LA, Nilsson L et al (1996) 15-year longitudinal study of blood pressure and dementia. Lancet 347 (9009):1141–1145

Skoog I, Lithell H, Hansson L, Elmfeldt D, Hofman A, Olofsson B et al (2005) Effect of baseline cognitive function and antihypertensive treatment on cognitive and cardiovascular outcomes: Study on Cognition and Prognosis in the Elderly (SCOPE). Am J Hypertens 18 (8):1052–1059

Snowdon DA, Greiner LH, Mortimer JA, Riley KP, Greiner PA, Markesbery WR (1997) Brain infarction and the clinical expression of Alzheimer disease. The Nun Study. JAMA 277(10):813–817

Solfrizzi V, Panza F, Colacicco AM, D'Introno A, Capurso C, Torres F et al (2004) Vascular risk factors, incidence of MCI, and rates of progression to dementia. Neurology 63(10):1882–1891

Soros P, Whitehead S, Spence JD, Hachinski V (2013) Antihypertensive treatment can prevent stroke and cognitive decline. Nat Rev Neurol 9(3):174–178

Sperling RA, Aisen PS, Beckett LA, Bennett DA, Craft S, Fagan AM et al (2011) Toward defining the preclinical stages of Alzheimer's disease: recommendations from the National Institute on Aging-Alzheimer's Association workgroups on diagnostic guidelines for Alzheimer's disease. Alzheimers Dement 7 (3):280–292

Sperling RA, Johnson KA, Doraiswamy PM, Reiman EM, Fleisher AS, Sabbagh MN et al (2013) Amyloid deposition detected with florbetapir F 18 ((18)F-AV-45) is related to lower episodic memory performance in clinically normal older individuals. Neurobiol Aging 34(3):822–831

Stewart R, Xue QL, Masaki K, Petrovitch H, Ross GW, White LR et al (2009) Change in blood pressure and incident dementia: a 32-year prospective study. Hypertension 54(2):233–240

Taylor C, Tillin T, Chaturvedi N, Dewey M, Ferri CP, Hughes A et al (2013) Midlife hypertensive status and cognitive function 20 years later: the Southall and Brent revisited study. J Am Geriatr Soc 61 (9):1489–1498

Tervo S, Kivipelto M, Hanninen T, Vanhanen M, Hallikainen M, Mannermaa A et al (2004) Incidence and risk factors for mild cognitive impairment: a population-based three-year follow-up study of cognitively healthy elderly subjects. Dement Geriatr Cogn Disord 17(3):196–203

Thambisetty M, Beason-Held L, An Y, Kraut MA, Resnick SM (2010) APOE epsilon4 genotype and longitudinal changes in cerebral blood flow in normal aging. Arch Neurol 67(1):93–98

Trivedi JK (2006) Cognitive deficits in psychiatric disorders: current status. Indian J Psychiatry 48 (1):10–20

Tzourio C, Dufouil C, Ducimetiere P, Alperovitch A (1999) Cognitive decline in individuals with high blood pressure: a longitudinal study in the elderly. EVA study group. Epidemiology of vascular aging. Neurology 53(9):1948–1952

Tzourio C, Anderson C, Chapman N, Woodward M, Neal B, MacMahon S et al (2003) Effects of blood pressure lowering with perindopril and indapamide therapy on dementia and cognitive decline in patients with cerebrovascular disease. Arch Intern Med 163 (9):1069–1075

Verghese J, Lipton RB, Hall CB, Kuslansky G, Katz MJ (2003) Low blood pressure and the risk of dementia in very old individuals. Neurology 61(12):1667–1672

Verghese PB, Castellano JM, Garai K, Wang Y, Jiang H, Shah A et al (2013) ApoE influences amyloid-beta (Abeta) clearance despite minimal apoE/Abeta association in physiological conditions. Proc Natl Acad Sci U S A 110(19):E1807–E1816

Waldstein SR, Giggey PP, Thayer JF, Zonderman AB (2005) Nonlinear relations of blood pressure to cognitive function: the Baltimore longitudinal study of aging. Hypertension 45(3):374–379

Whitmer RA, Sidney S, Selby J, Johnston SC, Yaffe K (2005) Midlife cardiovascular risk factors and risk of dementia in late life. Neurology 64(2):277–281

Winblad B, Palmer K, Kivipelto M, Jelic V, Fratiglioni L, Wahlund LO et al (2004) Mild cognitive impairment–beyond controversies, towards a consensus: report of the International Working Group on Mild Cognitive Impairment. J Intern Med 256(3):240–246

Wolf H, Ecke GM, Bettin S, Dietrich J, Gertz HJ (2000) Do white matter changes contribute to the subsequent development of dementia in patients with mild cognitive impairment? A longitudinal study. Int J Geriatr Psychiatry 15(9):803–812

Wu C, Zhou D, Wen C, Zhang L, Como P, Qiao Y (2003) Relationship between blood pressure and Alzheimer's disease in Linxian County, China. Life Sci 72 (10):1125–1133

Xie Y, Mies G, Hossmann KA (1989) Ischemic threshold of brain protein synthesis after unilateral carotid artery occlusion in gerbils. Stroke 20(5):620–626

Yamada M, Kasagi F, Sasaki H, Masunari N, Mimori Y, Suzuki G (2003) Association between dementia and midlife risk factors: the Radiation Effects Research Foundation adult health study. J Am Geriatr Soc 51 (3):410–414

Yamamoto Y, Akiguchi I, Oiwa K, Hayashi M, Ohara T, Ozasa K (2005) The relationship between 24-hour blood pressure readings, subcortical ischemic lesions and vascular dementia. Cerebrovasc Dis 19 (5):302–308

Yang Y, Rosenberg GA (2011) Blood-brain barrier breakdown in acute and chronic cerebrovascular disease. Stroke 42(11):3323–3328

Yasuno F, Tanimukai S, Sasaki M, Ikejima C, Yamashita F, Kodama C et al (2012) Effect of plasma lipids, hypertension and APOE genotype on cognitive decline. Neurobiol Aging 33(11):2633–2640

Yu JT, Chang RC, Tan L (2009) Calcium dysregulation in Alzheimer's disease: from mechanisms to therapeutic opportunities. Prog Neurobiol 89(3):240–255

Zlokovic BV (2011) Neurovascular pathways to neurodegeneration in Alzheimer's disease and other disorders. Nat Rev Neurosci 12(12):723–738

Adv Exp Med Biol - Advances in Internal Medicine (2017) 2: 475–488
DOI 10.1007/5584_2016_78
© Springer International Publishing AG 2016
Published online: 9 October 2016

Measurement of Arterial Stiffness: A Novel Tool of Risk Stratification in Hypertension

János Nemcsik, Orsolya Cseprekál, and András Tislér

Abstract

Cardiovascular diseases are the leading causes of morbidity and mortality in industrialized countries worldwide, despite highly effective preventive treatments available. As a difference continues to exist between the estimated and true number of events, further improvement of risk stratification is an essential part of cardiovascular research.

Among hypertensive patients measurement of arterial stiffness parameters, like carotid-femoral pulse wave velocity (cfPWV) or brachial-ankle pulse wave velocity (baPWV) can contribute to the identification of high-risk subpopulation of patients. This is a hot topic of vascular research including the possibility of the non-invasive measurement of central hemodynamics, wave reflections and recently, 24-h arterial stiffness monitoring as well. This chapter discusses the past and the present of this area including the scientific achievements with cfPWV, baPWV and other measures, provides a short overview of methodologies and the representation of arterial stiffness parameters in guidelines.

Keywords

Hypertension • Arterial stiffness • Pulse wave velocity • Guidelines

1   Introduction

Hypertension has many aspects and a wild range of medical professions are involved in its research and treatment, like cardiology, angiology, endocrinology, nephrology, neurology or psychiatry. In this chapter we focus on the arteries, especially their mechanical

J. Nemcsik (✉)
Department of Family Medicine, Semmelweis University, 1023 Mecset utca 17. II/25A, Budapest, Hungary

Health Service of Zugló (ZESZ), Budapest, Hungary
e-mail: janos.nemcsik@gmail.com

O. Cseprekál
Department of Transplantation and Surgery, Semmelweis University, Budapest, Hungary

A. Tislér
Ist Department of Medicine, Semmelweis University, Budapest, Hungary

properties, that can be non-invasively measured with the identification and analysis of pulse wave curves leading to the evaluation of arterial stiffness, wave reflection and central hemodynamic parameters. The spread of this research area and its implantation into clinical practice might lead to the development of a new profession, which could be called "arteriology".

The palpation of the pulse is a fundamental part of physical examination since the early ages of the Greek and Chinese medicine (Kuriyama 1999). The first European milestone of vascular research is dated back to 1628, when William Harvey described the basics of circulation in his classical text "de Motu Cordis…" (Harvey 1628; O'Rourke et al. 2001). Pulse wave analysis is rooted in the nineteenth century, when after the theoretical basis of Marey (Marey 1860), Frederick Akbar Mahomed developed sphygmograph, described normal radial pressure waveform and demonstrated differences from carotid wave (Mahomed 1872). In the middle of the twentieth century McDonald enlightened that this difference is based on wave reflection (McDonald 1960) and Womersley introduced transfer functions to characterize vascular beds in the frequency domain, an invention, that led to the development of the modern pulse wave analysis (O'Rourke et al. 2001; Womersley 1957). The history of arterial stiffness measurement begins in 1985, when Levy, Targett and their co-workers described in two articles the first device and computer program to automatically record and calculate pulse wave velocity (PWV) (Levy et al. 1985; Targett et al. 1985).

The shape of pulse wave curves is changing with age-associated arterial stiffening due to increased wave reflections, as it is demonstrated in Fig. 1. The pathopysiological background of this phenomenon is complex. It is thought, that with ageing, the chronic cyclical stress on the wall of large arteries leads to elastin fracturing and thinning, which is accelerated in the presence of hypertension (Nichols and O'Rourke 2005). Since in adulthood the production of elastin is not possible, this process leads to the irreversible change of the elastin/collagen ratio, which causes the stiffening of the large arteries

(Powell et al. 1992). Among the autocrine, paracrine and neuroendocrine effects leading to an increase in arterial stiffening, the role of the renin-angiotensin-aldosterone system have been extensively studied. Its activation stimulate multiple inflammatory pathways, such as tissue growth factor-β and NF-kB, promoting reactive oxygen species production with reduction in nitric oxide bioavailability (Usui et al. 2000; Gibbons et al. 1992; Fok and Cruickshank 2015). In hypertension, systemic arterial compliance was strongly and negatively correlated with plasma aldosterone level (Blacher et al. 1997). Other deleterious effects of inflammatory processes are the impair of the balance between the production of proteases and their inhibitors and the promotion of the synthesis of advanced glycation end-products (AGEs). Matrix metalloproteases are proteases that are responsible for the accelerated breakdown of elastin and destruction of the molecular folding of collagen. AGEs promote the irreversible cross-linking of collagen, which together with overexpression of MMPs, eventuate in a stiff extracellular matrix (Fok and Cruickshank 2015). Sodium is also an important player in the process of arterial stiffening. High sodium concentration itself leads to the hypertrophy of vascular smooth muscle cells (Gu et al. 1998). In sodium-sensitive, borderline-hypertensive patients large artery compliance was found reduced compared to age-matched sodium-resistant subjects which suggests alterations in the viscoelastic properties of arterial wall characteristics in sodium-sensitive patients (Draaijer et al. 1993).

It remains a conundrum, whether arterial stiffening is a cause or a consequence of hypertension? It was a widely accepted belief, that increased arterial stiffness is a consequence of hypertension. But in contrast to this dogma, in treated hypertensive patients baseline arterial stiffness measures were found to be associated with longitudinal increases of systolic blood pressure, mean arterial pressure and pulse pressure (Coutinho et al. 2014). Moreover, in an analysis of the Framingham Heart Study higher arterial stiffness was associated with blood pressure progression and incident hypertension

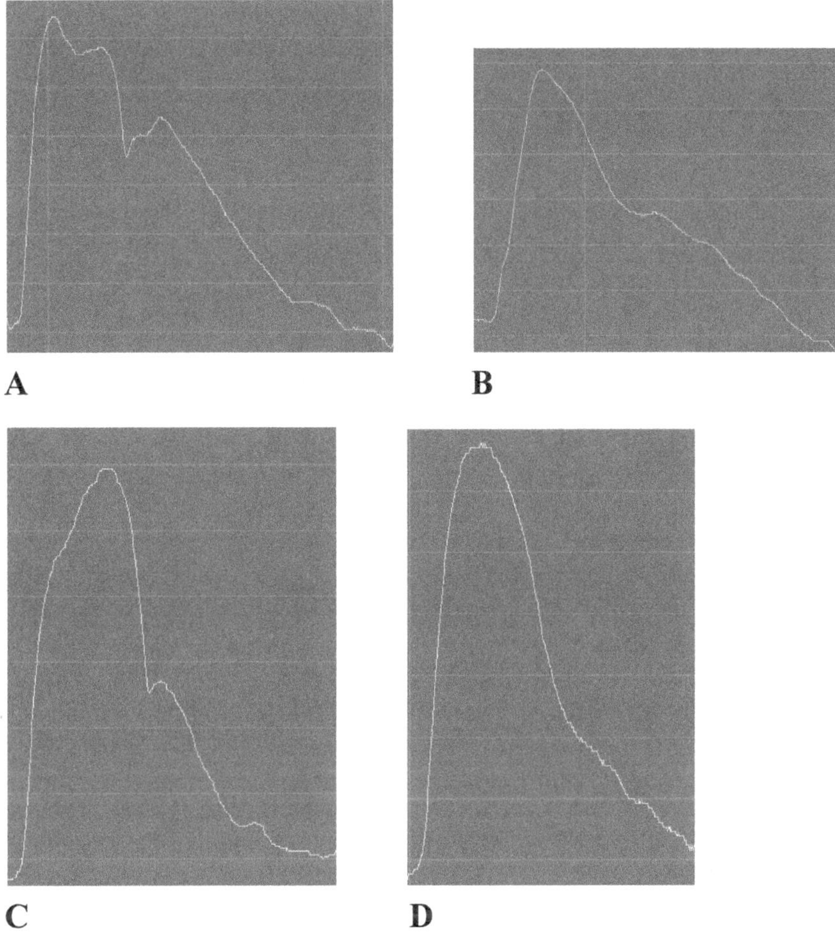

Fig. 1 Changes of pulse wave curves with ageing. (**a**) carotid wave of a young patient (26 years); (**b**) femoral wave of a young patient (26 years); (**c**) carotid wave of an aged patient (78 years); (**d**) femoral wave of an aged patient (78 years). Evaluated with the tonometric PulsePen device

7 years later, but higher blood pressure at the initial examination was not associated with progressive arterial stiffening (Kaess et al. 2012).

What is might mostly approaching the truth is, that arterial stiffening is both a cause and a consequence of hypertension in a sort of vicious circle. Elastic and muscular type arteries adapt differently to hemodynamic changes caused by the left ventricule construction. The ability of large and elastic arteries to accommodate for the nonlinear pressure-volume changes caused by stroke volume (conduit and Windkessel function) can be characterized by several functional and structural parameters, especially compliance, distensibility, that provides information about the extrinsic features of the arteries, meanwhile i.e. elastic modulus (Young's) describe the intrinsic elastic properties of the vessel walls. The conduit and Windkessel functions of the aorta balance the effect of pressure-volume overload that generate central pulse pressure. It transfers toward the peripheral muscular vessels those of smaller inner diameter, thinner and stiffer vessel wall (London and Pannier 2010). The altered geometry and structure of muscular type arteries protect small vessels against higher pulse pressure from the central arteries that is called phenomenon of impedance mismatch. During aging the elasticity of the arterial wall decreases and become stiffer. Thus after a prime age small vessels can not be protected against the pressure load, that lead to increased shear stress and endothelial damage in the periphery. Physiologically, the transfer of pulse pressure is displayed as pulse wave that is reflected back from the points of vessel junctions and reach the heart at the diastolic phase. Stiffer arteries – transition from elastic to muscular type arteries and that of resistance arteries – can reflect the pulse wave earlier, thus the augmented pressure approach the heart cycle during the systolic phase causing pressure burden on the left ventricle.

Structural damage and functional deterioration of arteries reinforce the hemodynamic vicious circle of stiffness and high blood pressure, while highlighting the chicken and the egg debate of the possible origin of hypertension *per se*. These findings also underscore the importance of the better understanding of the pathophysiology of arterial stiffening, with the hope of providing a new potential targets for the prevention of hypertension.

2 Aortic and Carotid-Femoral Pulse Wave Velocity

The most accepted and wildly used arterial stiffness parameter is pulse wave velocity (PWV), derived from less flow velocity, but rather diameter and pressure waveforms recorded at different points of the arterial tree. PWV, as the Bramwell-Hill equation demonstrates, is a functional measurement of distensibility, which is defined by a volume change in proportion to a change in pressure relative to the initial volume (Bramwell and Hill 1922):

$$PWV = \sqrt{\frac{V \times \Delta P}{\rho \times \Delta V}}$$

where PWV is the pulse wave velocity, V is the volume, P is the pressure and ρ is the blood density. Consequently, PWV is closely related to changes in volume and arterial pressure as well. Arterial wall properties are also important in determining PWV, and these are described by

the Moens-Kroteweg equation (Nichols and O'Rourke 2005):

$$PWV = \sqrt{E_{inc} \times \frac{h}{\rho} \times D}$$

where PWV is the pulse wave velocity, E_{inc} is the Young's elastic modulus of arterial wall (a measure of the arterial wall mechanical properties), h is the arterial wall thickness, ρ is the blood density and D is the vessel diameter. An increase in wall stiffness (E_{inc}) and/or in wall thickness is accompanied with an increase in PWV and arterial calibre is inversely proportional to PWV. Taken together, arterial stiffness can be modulated directly by the changes in vascular tone, arterial wall mechanical properties and thickness and also indirectly, by changes in blood pressure (Fok and Cruickshank 2015).

As the thoracic and abdominal aorta gives the largest contribution to the arterial buffering function (Isnard et al. 1989), aortic PWV (aPWV) is an arterial stiffness parameter of high priority. As the exact evaluation of aPWV requires invasive intervention or MRI, methodologies with limited possibility of involvement into epidemiological studies, surrogate methodologies are used for approximations of aPWV. Among them, carotid-femoral PWV (cfPWV), the velocity of pulse as it travels from the heart to the carotid and to the femoral artery, is the most commonly applied non-invasive method and considered as the "gold standard" measurement of arterial stiffness (Laurent et al. 2006). cfPWV is usually evaluated using the "foot-to-foot" velocity method from a number of waveforms. Surface tonometry probes are usually applied at the right common carotid artery and the right femoral artery. cfPWV is calculated using the following formula:

$$cfPWV = D/Dt$$

where $cfPWV$ is carotid-femoral pulse wave velocity, D is the distance between the two recording sites and Dt is the time delay between the "foot" of the carotid and the femoral waveforms. The "foot" of the wave is defined at the end of diastole, when the steep rise of the waveform begins (Vlachopoulos et al. 2015). The unit of cfPWV is meter/second (m/s).

From this formula it is clear, that a crucial point of cfPWV evaluation is the correct measurement of the travelled distance. Different measurement methodologies can lead to different PWV values which can also have different prognostic significances (Nemeth et al. 2011). For a long time there has been no agreement in this field until 2012, when consensus document was published recommending the use of the 80 % of the direct carotid to femoral distance as it provides only 0.4 % difference with MRI-calculated value (Van Bortel et al. 2012). Another important point of view in respect of methodological considerations is the accuracy of distance measurement between the carotid and femoral sites. In women the breast contour and in both sexes obesity can limit the use of tape measure, so it is recommended to apply sliding caliper instead of tape (Bossuyt et al. 2013).

Several devices are commercially available to measure directly cfPWV. The first was the Complior System (Alam Medical, Vincennes, France), which is based on the simultaneous recording of arterial pulse waves at carotid and femoral sites, through mechanotransducer probes (Asmar et al. 1995). The next was the SphygmoCor system (AtCor, Sydney, Australia), which uses a large-band piezoelectronic probe (applanation tonometer) and records consecutively carotid and femoral arterial pulse waves, with both signals being synchronized to the same ECG R wave (Wilkinson et al. 1998). The PulsePen (Diatecne, Milano, Italy) is based also on applanation tonometry and uses successive carotid and femoral pulse waves synchronized with ECG (Salvi et al. 2004). The Vicorder (Skidmore Medical Limited, Bristol, United Kingdom) is based on oscillometric technique to measure cfPWV through the inflation of a neck pad and a cuff around the thigh (van Leeuwen-Segarceanu et al. 2010). Moreover, cfPWV can also be measured by pulsed Doppler ultrasound with a Linear Array, with ECG gating, as it was demonstrated by Calabia et al. (2011). However, among these devices Complior and SpygmoCor are the most frequently used ones, also in epidemiologic studies.

Before implementation of a novel biomarker into clinical practice the applicant must fulfill different criteria, as Table 1. demonstrates. From this point of view cfPWV fulfill almost all requirements.

A number of studies have proven, that cfPWV is associated with different cardiovascular pathophysiological conditions and has strong prognostic value. Apart from the dominant effect of ageing (McEniery et al. 2005), hypertension was found to be another main contributor to enhanced arterial stiffening (Simon et al. 1985). In uncomplicated essential hypertension the

Table 1 Criteria for vascular biomarkers to qualify as clinical surrogate endpoints

1. Proof of concept	Do novel biomarker levels differ between subjects with and without outcome?
2. Prospective validation	Does the novel biomarker predict development of future outcomes in a prospective cohort or nested case-cohort study?
3. Incremental value	Does it add predictive information over and above established, standard risk markers?
4. Clinical utility	Does it change predicted risk sufficiently to change recommended therapy?
5. Clinical outcomes	Does the use of the novel biomarker improve clinical outcomes, especially when tested in a randomized clinical trial?
6. Cost-effectiveness	Does the use of the biomarker improve clinical outcomes sufficiently to justify the additional costs?
7. Ease of use	Is it easy to use, allowing widespread application?
8. Methodological consensus	Is the biomarker measured uniformly in different laboratories? Are study results directly comparable?
9. Reference values (or cut-off values)	Are there published reference values, or, at least, cut-off values?

Adapted from Vlachopoulos et al. (2015)

independent predictive value of cfPWV from classic cardiovascular risk factors was clearly demonstrated (Boutouyrie et al. 2002; Laurent et al. 2001, 2003). Moreover, its predictive value was also confirmed in end-stage renal disease (Blacher et al. 1999), in patients after ischemic stroke (Gasecki et al. 2012), in elderly subjects (Meaume et al. 2001; Sutton-Tyrrell et al. 2005) and in the general population (Mattace-Raso et al. 2006). The independent predictive value of cfPWV was even confirmed by a recent meta-analysis, in which Ben-Shlomo et al. nicely demonstrated that after the adjustment of additional risk factors an increase in 1 SD change in log cfPWV is related to 30 %, 28 % and 17 % increase in cardiovascular (CV) events, CV mortality and all-cause mortality, respectively (Ben-Shlomo et al. 2014). In the practical interpretation of the results, for a 60-year-old man who is a non-smoker, non-diabetic, normotensive and normolipemic, a 1 m/s increase in cfPWV leads to a 7 % increase of the hazard for CV events (Ben-Shlomo et al. 2014; Vlachopoulos et al. 2014). The independent association with all-cause mortality suggests that the impact of arterial stiffening extends beyond the diseases of CV system.

The clinical utility of cfPWV measurement was confirmed by two studies and a meta-analysis demonstrating that patients at intermediate risk could be reclassified into a higher or lower CV risk category when cfPWV is measured (Mattace-Raso et al. 2006; Sehestedt et al. 2009; Mitchell et al. 2010). In the Framingham study for individuals at intermediate CV risk, addition of cfPWV resulted in upward reclassification of 14.3 % of participants who experienced a CV event and downward reclassification of 1.4 % of participants who did not experience a CV event, yielding a net reclassification of 15.7 % (Mitchell et al. 2010). Based on the above-mentioned results it is obvious, the cfPWV fulfills the requirements of the 1–4 points of Table 1.

According to point 5., the influence of cfPWV modification for clinical outcome, there is only one study available so far, in which in patients with end-stage renal disease the lack of the decrease of cfPWV in response to blood pressure medication was a predictor of all-cause and cardiovascular mortality (Guerin et al. 2001). A randomized clinical trial called Statégie de Prévention Cardiovasculaire Basée sur la Rigidité Arterielle Study (SPARTE) was started in 2012 in 40 French clinical centres with the planned involvement of 3000 hypertensive patients and with the follow-up period of 4 years, aiming to test the hypothesis that a therapeutic strategy that targets the normalization of arterial stiffness is more effective in preventing CV events than usual care. In the control group, the target is blood pressure, while in the active group the target is aortic stiffness with the aim of normalizing it to <10 m/s (Laurent et al. 2012). Without the result of this and other future trials with similar setups, there is a lack of evidence on broader patient population that the normalization of cfPWV or any other arterial stiffness parameter has positive impact on CV outcome above that of reaching the blood pressure target values.

No data are currently available about the cost-effectiveness of cfPWV measurement. Potentially, the spread of the technology could reduce device prices, however no marked reduction was observed in the latest years. The main expense is the salary of the examiner, which geographically can differ markedly. Considering the high reclassification rate of patients and the comparison of cost with other powerful, but costly biomarkers, like coronary calcium score, cfPWV is probably a cost-effective risk stratification methodology.

The accurate and reproducible measurement of cfPWV requires moderate expertise. It is easy in most of the cases, but obesity and picnic stature may render measurements challenging. A true disadvantage of cfPWV measurement is the manipulation in the inguinal region which can be uncomfortable for some patients.

An expert consensus document on the measurement of aortic stiffness on the daily practice using cfPWV is available involving such scientific communities, like the Artery Society, the European Society of Hypertension and the European Network for Noninvasive Investigation of Large Arteries (Van Bortel et al. 2012).

Reference values of cfPWV have been established in 2010 involving 1455 healthy

Table 2 Distribution of carotid-femoral pulse wave velocity (m/s) according to the age category in healthy population (1455 subjects)

Age category (years)	Mean ($\pm$2 SD)	Median (10–90 pc)
<30	6.2 (4.7–7.6)	6.1 (5.3–7.1)
30–39	6.5 (3.8–9.2)	6.4 (5.2–8.0)
40–49	7.2 (4.6–9.8)	6.9 (5.9–8.6)
50–59	8.3 (4.5–12.1)	8.1 (6.3–10.0)
60–69	10.3 (5.5–15.0)	9.7 (7.9–13.1)
$\geq$70	10.9 (5.5–16.3)	10.6 (8.0–14.6)

Adapted from Arterial Stiffness' Collaboration (2010)
SD standard deviation, *10 pc* the upper limit of the 10th percentile, *90 pc* the lower limit of the 90th percentile

subjects together with 11,092 patients with different CV risk factors (Arterial Stiffness' Collaboration 2010). However, this paper was published before the consensus document on distance measurement (Van Bortel et al. 2012), but cfPWV values were calculated according to the later accepted 80 % of the direct carotid-femoral distance. Table 2. demonstrates the distribution of cfPWV according to the age category in apparently healthy population.

As a consequence that cfPWV fulfills almost all the nine requirements of Table 1 to be an accepted biomarker, it has already been involved into some guidelines. It was first recommended as a marker of subclinical organ damage with the value >12 m/s in 2007, in the guideline of the European Society of Hypertension (ESH) and the European Society of Cardiology (ESC), for the management of arterial hypertension (Mancia et al. 2007). In the next ESH-ESC hypertension guideline in 2013 cfPWV is recommended to be evaluated as a measure of asymptomatic organ damage with the strength of class **IIa**, level of evidence **B** (Mancia et al. 2013). In the recent ESC- Artery Society position paper, the evaluation of cfPWV as a vascular biomarker is recommended as a class **IIa**, level of evidence **A** method (Vlachopoulos et al. 2015). Pulse wave velocity measurement is also recommended in the recent ESC- European Association for the Study of Diabetes guideline, as a useful cardiovascular marker, adding predictive value to the usual risk estimate (Ryden et al. 2013). In 2010, in the American College of Cardiology Foundation (ACCF)/American Heart Association (AHA) task force document

the measurement of cfPWV was not recommended to be used in asymptomatic adults, outside of research settings (Greenland et al. 2010) and cfPWV measurement was even not mentioned in the next ACC/AHA guideline for the assessment of cardiovascular risk (Goff et al. 2014). However, in a recently published AHA scientific statement it is declared that it is reasonable to measure arterial stiffness to provide incremental information beyond standard CV disease risk factors in the prediction of future CV disease events (class: **IIa**, level of evidence: **A**) (Townsend et al. 2015). With this statement document the position of cfPWV measurement in the cardiovascular risk stratification has become similar both in Europe and in America.

3 Oscillometric Approximations of Aortic Pulse Wave Velocity

As cfPWV measurement is partly operator-dependent and the manipulation in the inguinal region can cause discomfort for the subject, oscillometric approximations of aortic PWV through a brachial cuff can have perspectives in the future. Mobil-o-Graph (Wassertheurer et al. 2010), Arteriograph (Horvath et al. 2010) and Vasotens (Ageenkova and Purygina 2011) are such devices, and all of them are able per se or have versions developed for 24-h blood pressure and arterial stiffness monitoring as well (Laszlo et al. 2015). So far none of these new techniques is involved in the recommendations as an alternative of cfPWV (Vlachopoulos et al. 2015; Mancia et al. 2013; Townsend et al. 2015). As in case of these new methodologies in validation studies the determination coefficients (R^2) in comparison with gold-standard methods are mostly between 0.4 and 0.7, which reflect very imperfect agreement, experts do not recommend their involvement into prospective studies (Boutouyrie et al. 2014a). This fact can lead to a catch-22, as a manufacturer company per se rarely have enough funds to perform large population-based investigations. A solution for this discrepancy were the use of gold-standard and oscillometric methods parallel in prospective studies, which could provide both answers for clinical questions and validations of these alternative methodologies.

4 Brachial-Ankle Pulse Wave Velocity and Other Promising Parameters

In this paragraph we would like to provide an overview of an arterial stiffness parameter which is widely accepted and used in Japan and China and the cumulating data with this methodology also enabled its involvement into guidelines. Brachial-ankle pulse wave velocity (baPWV) is a simple-to-assess stiffness marker of the large and middle-size arteries. It is measured with a volume-plethysmographic device (eg VP1000, VP2000, OMRON Health Care Co. Ltd., Kyota, Japan) using four cuffs placed on both arms (brachial) and ankles, connected to plethysmographic and oscillometric sensors, recording the brachial and posterior tibial pressure waveforms (Vlachopoulos et al. 2015; Tomiyama et al. 2006). Travel distance is calculated using the path lengths from the suprasternal notch to the brachium (Lb) and from the suprasternal notch to the ankle (La) with a correction for the height of the individual using validated equations. baPWV is calculated with the following equation:

$$baPWV = {}^{(La-Lb)}\!/_{\Delta Tba},$$

where ΔTba is the time interval between the wavefront of the brachial waveform and that of the ankle waveform (Vlachopoulos et al. 2015; Tomiyama et al. 2006).

It has been demonstrated, that baPWV is closely correlated with cfPWV and invasively assessed aortic PWV and the presence of CV risk factors is linked with its elevated value (Yamashina et al. 2002, 2003; Tomiyama and Yamashina 2010). Prospective studies have confirmed that baPWV is a useful predictor of future CV events not only in essential hypertension (Munakata et al. 2012), but also in general population (Ninomiya et al. 2013), in end-stage renal disease (Kitahara et al. 2005), in diabetes (Maeda et al. 2014), in patients with acute coronary syndrome (Tomiyama et al. 2005) and heart failure (Meguro et al. 2009). In a meta-analysis it was demonstrated that a 1 m/s increase in baPWV corresponds with an increase of 12 %, 13 % and 6 % in total cardiovascular events, cardiovascular mortality and all-cause mortality, respectively (Vlachopoulos et al. 2012). It seems, that an optimal cutoff value of baPWV is 18 m/s in the assessment of high risk for CV disease (Ninomiya et al. 2013; Tomiyama et al. 2005). Moreover, as baPWV can predict the development of hypertension or stage III chronic kidney disease (Yambe et al. 2007; Takase et al. 2011; Chen et al. 2011; Tomiyama et al. 2010), in healthy subjects under the age of 60, and baPWV values between 14 and 18 m/s lifestyle modifications are recommended by some experts of this field (Yamashina et al. 2003; Tomiyama et al. 2016).

Although lots of achievements have been succeeded in respect of baPWV to be an accepted CV biomarker, but there are still some incomplete requirements. No consensus document is available on the measurement methodology, only the manufacturer's instructions. Reference values have been published only in Chinese populations (Ai et al. 2011; Wang et al. 2009), data are missing in Caucasian or other races. So far, the potential clinical advantage of baPWV over traditional risk scores have not been proven. Although it has been demonstrated that baPWV improves for the treatment of hypertension, dyslipidemia, diabetes or lifestyle modifications (Toyama et al. 2012, 2016), only one study reported so far, that improvement of baPWV obtained after 6 months of conventional therapy was a reliable marker of a better prognosis in patients with coronary artery disease (Orlova et al. 2010).

Based on these findings, in the recent ESC position paper on vascular biomarkers baPWV is recommended for primary and secondary CV disease prevention with the class of **IIb**, level of evidence **B** (Vlachopoulos et al. 2015). The recent AHA recommendation states that baPWV is useful in cardiovascular outcome predictions in Asian populations, but longitudinal studies in the United States and Europe by these methods are lacking (Class **I**; Level of Evidence **B**) (Townsend et al. 2015).

Unfortunately the limited extent of this book chapter does not permit the detailed description of other parameters that also can have future perspectives. Parameters of pulse wave analysis and central hemodynamics can be estimated alone or connected with cfPWV measurement. Other parameters can be evaluated with specific devices. Some of these measures are already mentioned in the recommendations. The recent ESC/ESH hypertension guideline states that augmentation index and central blood pressure can be helpful risk stratification tools in young patients with isolated systolic hypertension, however, more data are needed before central hemodynamic indices are recommended for routine use in hypertensive patients in general (Mancia et al. 2013). In the recent ESC biomarker position paper the usefulness of the measurement of central hemodynamics/wave reflections for primary and secondary CV disease prevention is judged as **IIb/B** (recommendation/level of evidence) (Vlachopoulos et al. 2015). The AHA scientific statement declares that the use of wave separation analysis is recommended when investigations are focused specifically on the role of wave reflection as either an exposure for CV outcome or a target for intervention (class **I**, level of evidence **B**). The same document states that similarly to baPWV, the measurement of cardiac ankle vascular stiffness index is useful in CV outcome prediction in Asian populations, but longitudinal studies in the United States and Europe are lacking (class **I**, level of evidence

B) (Townsend et al. 2015). The measurement of carotid stiffness parameters is also promising. A recent meta-analysis demonstrated that greater carotid stiffness is associated with a higher incidence of stroke independently of cfPWV and modestly improved risk prediction of stroke beyond Framingham stroke risk score factors and cfPWV (van Sloten et al. 2015). In summary, this research area is far not limited only for cfPWV or baPWV, the complexity is growing with new candidates with further potential in helping risk stratification and individual therapy adjustment.

5 How Can We Improve the Arterial Stiffness of Our Patients?

Many non-pharmacological interventions can improve arterial stiffness and/or wave reflection, like dietary changing including weight loss and salt reduction (Pase et al. 2011; Dengo et al. 2010), aerobic exercise training (Edwards et al. 2004; Edwards and Lang 2005), passive vibration (Sanchez-Gonzalez et al. 2012) and enhanced external counterpulsation treatment (Nichols et al. 2006). For maximal cardiovascular benefits, these interventions must be initially introduced immediately and continued over an extended period of time (Townsend et al. 2015).

In respect of pharmaceutical interventions, it is demonstrated, that different kind of blood pressure medications have beneficial effect for arterial stiffening (Fok and Cruickshank 2015). The reduction of aortic PWV was confirmed with the administration of renin inhibitor (Virdis et al. 2012), angiotensin converting enzyme (ACE) inhibitors/angiotensin AT1 receptor blockers (ARBs) (Mitchell et al. 2002, 2005; Karalliedde et al. 2008; Boutouyrie et al. 2014b), an endothelin-A receptor antagonist (Dhaun et al. 2009), with spironolactone and hydrochlorotiazide monotherapy in elderly (Kithas and Supiano 2010), or with ACE inhibitor/ARBs in combination with spironolactone (Edwards et al. 2009). The problem with these interventions, that the destiffening effect of a blood pressure medication can hardly be divided from the effect of blood pressure reduction per se, however, some authors state that the observed destiffening effect is at least partly independent of blood pressure reduction (Karalliedde et al. 2008; Boutouyrie et al. 2014b; Edwards et al. 2009). One compound with a direct destiffening effect was tested so far, but the advanced glycation end-products crosslink breaker alagebrium after promising initial results (Kass et al. 2001; Zieman et al. 2007) unfortunately did not get through all the clinical pharmacological phases, probably due to the financial problems of the developing company.

Numerous nutritional supplements have been found to improve arterial stiffening like flavonoids (Lilamand et al. 2014), omega-3 and soy isoflavone (Pase et al. 2011) or tetrahydrobiopterin (Moreau et al. 2012; Pierce et al. 2012). As these interventions are also often accompanied with blood pressure reduction, their blood-pressure independent destiffening effect is not unambiguous as well. So the clinical importance of blood pressure-independent destiffening is still a pending question and such studies like the above-mentioned SPARTE (Laurent et al. 2012) are needed to give us answers.

6 Conclusions, Future Directions

In hypertensive patients the measurement of arterial stiffening, especially cfPWV is already a recommended method to detect target organ damage both in Europe and in America. Its role in risk stratification seems to be clarified, but the potential benefit in cardiovascular outcome from treating hypertensive patients until a certain cfPWV goal value is not confirmed yet. Besides cfPWV, other measures of arterial stiffness are getting closer to be recommended in clinical use, like baPWV, or different wave reflection parameters. Recently devices measuring 24-h ambulatory arterial stiffness have become available on the market, opening a new field of research interest. These findings confirm that the study of large artery structure and function is becoming an essential part of hypertension care.

References

Ageenkova OA, Purygina MA (2011) Central aortic blood pressure, augmentation index, and reflected wave transit time: reproducibility and repeatability of data obtained by oscillometry. Vasc Health Risk Manag 7:649–656, Pubmed Central PMCID: PMC3225346, Epub 2011/12/06. eng

Ai ZS, Li J, Liu ZM, Fan HM, Zhang DF, Zhu Y et al (2011) Reference value of brachial-ankle pulse wave velocity for the eastern Chinese population and potential influencing factors. Braz J Med Biol Res = Revista brasileira de pesquisas medicas e biologicas/ Sociedade Brasileira de Biofisica [et al] 44 (10):1000–1005, Epub 2011/08/31. eng

Arterial Stiffness' Collaboration (2010) Determinants of pulse wave velocity in healthy people and in the presence of cardiovascular risk factors: 'establishing normal and reference values'. Eur Heart J 31 (19):2338–2350, Pubmed Central PMCID: PMC2948201. Epub 2010/06/10. eng

Asmar R, Benetos A, Topouchian J, Laurent P, Pannier B, Brisac AM et al (1995) Assessment of arterial distensibility by automatic pulse wave velocity measurement. Validation and clinical application studies. Hypertension 26(3):485–490, Epub 1995/09/01. eng

Ben-Shlomo Y, Spears M, Boustred C, May M, Anderson SG, Benjamin EJ et al (2014) Aortic pulse wave velocity improves cardiovascular event prediction: an individual participant meta-analysis of prospective observational data from 17,635 subjects. J Am Coll Cardiol 63(7):636–646, Epub 2013/11/19. eng

Blacher J, Amah G, Girerd X, Kheder A, Ben Mais H, London GM et al (1997) Association between increased plasma levels of aldosterone and decreased systemic arterial compliance in subjects with essential hypertension. Am J Hypertens 10(12 Pt 1):1326–1334, Epub 1998/01/27. eng

Blacher J, Guerin AP, Pannier B, Marchais SJ, Safar ME, London GM (1999) Impact of aortic stiffness on survival in end-stage renal disease. Circulation 99 (18):2434–2439, Epub 1999/05/11. eng

Bossuyt J, Van De Velde S, Azermai M, Vermeersch SJ, De Backer TL, Devos DG et al (2013) Noninvasive assessment of carotid-femoral pulse wave velocity: the influence of body side and body contours. J Hypertens 31(5):946–951, Epub 2013/03/21. eng

Boutouyrie P, Tropeano AI, Asmar R, Gautier I, Benetos A, Lacolley P et al (2002) Aortic stiffness is an independent predictor of primary coronary events in hypertensive patients: a longitudinal study. Hypertension 39(1):10–15, Epub 2002/01/19. eng

Boutouyrie P, Fliser D, Goldsmith D, Covic A, Wiecek A, Ortiz A et al (2014a) Assessment of arterial stiffness for clinical and epidemiological studies: methodological considerations for validation and entry into the European Renal and Cardiovascular Medicine registry. Nephrol Dial Transpl 29(2):232–239, Epub 2013/10/03. eng

Boutouyrie P, Beaussier H, Achouba A, Laurent S (2014b) Destiffening effect of valsartan and atenolol: influence of heart rate and blood pressure. J Hypertens 32(1):108–114, Epub 2013/11/28. eng

Bramwell JCH, Hill AV (1922) Velocity of transmission of the pulse wave. Lancet 199(5149):891–892

Calabia J, Torguet P, Garcia M, Garcia I, Martin N, Guasch B et al (2011) Doppler ultrasound in the measurement of pulse wave velocity: agreement with the Complior method. Cardiovasc Ultrasound 9:13, Pubmed Central PMCID: PMC3098145, Epub 2011/04/19. eng

Chen SC, Chang JM, Liu WC, Tsai YC, Tsai JC, Hsu PC et al (2011) Brachial-ankle pulse wave velocity and rate of renal function decline and mortality in chronic kidney disease. Clin J Am Soc Nephrol 6(4):724–732, Pubmed Central PMCID: PMC3069362, Epub 2011/04/02. eng

Coutinho T, Bailey KR, Turner ST, Kullo IJ (2014) Arterial stiffness is associated with increase in blood pressure over time in treated hypertensives. J Am Soc Hypertens 8(6):414–421, Pubmed Central PMCID: PMC4103613, Epub 2014/06/24. eng

Dengo AL, Dennis EA, Orr JS, Marinik EL, Ehrlich E, Davy BM et al (2010) Arterial destiffening with weight loss in overweight and obese middle-aged and older adults. Hypertension 55(4):855–861, Pubmed Central PMCID: PMC2859827, Epub 2010/03/10. eng

Dhaun N, Macintyre IM, Melville V, Lilitkarntakul P, Johnston NR, Goddard J et al (2009) Blood pressure-independent reduction in proteinuria and arterial stiffness after acute endothelin-a receptor antagonism in chronic kidney disease. Hypertension 54(1):113–119, Epub 2009/06/10. eng

Draaijer P, Kool MJ, Maessen JM, van Bortel LM, de Leeuw PW, van Hooff JP et al (1993) Vascular distensibility and compliance in salt-sensitive and salt-resistant borderline hypertension. J Hypertens 11(11):1199–1207, Epub 1993/11/01. eng

Edwards DG, Lang JT (2005) Augmentation index and systolic load are lower in competitive endurance athletes. Am J Hypertens 18(5 Pt 1):679–683, Epub 2005/05/11. eng

Edwards DG, Schofield RS, Magyari PM, Nichols WW, Braith RW (2004) Effect of exercise training on central aortic pressure wave reflection in coronary artery disease. Am J Hypertens 17(6):540–543, Epub 2004/06/05. eng

Edwards NC, Steeds RP, Stewart PM, Ferro CJ, Townend JN (2009) Effect of spironolactone on left ventricular mass and aortic stiffness in early-stage chronic kidney disease: a randomized controlled trial. J Am Coll Cardiol 54(6):505–512, Epub 2009/08/01. eng

Fok H, Cruickshank JK (2015) Future treatment of hypertension: shifting the focus from blood pressure lowering to arterial stiffness modulation? Curr Hypertens Rep 17(8):67, Epub 2015/07/15. eng

Gasecki D, Rojek A, Kwarciany M, Kubach M, Boutouyrie P, Nyka W et al (2012) Aortic stiffness predicts functional outcome in patients after ischemic stroke. Stroke J Cereb Circ 43(2):543–544, Epub 2011/11/15. eng

Gibbons GH, Pratt RE, Dzau VJ (1992) Vascular smooth muscle cell hypertrophy vs. hyperplasia. Autocrine transforming growth factor-beta 1 expression determines growth response to angiotensin II. J Clin Invest 90(2):456–461, Pubmed Central PMCID: PMC443121, Epub 1992/08/01. eng

Goff DC Jr, Lloyd-Jones DM, Bennett G, Coady S, D'Agostino RB, Gibbons R et al (2014) 2013 ACC/AHA guideline on the assessment of cardiovascular risk: a report of the American College of Cardiology/American Heart Association Task Force on Practice Guidelines. Circulation 129(25 Suppl 2): S49–S73, Epub 2013/11/14. eng

Greenland P, Alpert JS, Beller GA, Benjamin EJ, Budoff MJ, Fayad ZA et al (2010) 2010 ACCF/AHA guideline for assessment of cardiovascular risk in asymptomatic adults: a report of the American College of Cardiology Foundation/American Heart Association Task Force on Practice Guidelines. Circulation 122(25):e584–e636, Epub 2010/11/26. eng

Gu JW, Anand V, Shek EW, Moore MC, Brady AL, Kelly WC et al (1998) Sodium induces hypertrophy of cultured myocardial myoblasts and vascular smooth muscle cells. Hypertension 31(5):1083–1087, Epub 1998/05/12. eng

Guerin AP, Blacher J, Pannier B, Marchais SJ, Safar ME, London GM (2001) Impact of aortic stiffness attenuation on survival of patients in end-stage renal failure. Circulation 103(7):987–992, Epub 2001/02/22. eng

Harvey W (1628) de Motu Cordis et Sanguinis Animalibus. William Fitzer Frankfurt

Horvath IG, Nemeth A, Lenkey Z, Alessandri N, Tufano F, Kis P et al (2010) Invasive validation of a new oscillometric device (Arteriograph) for measuring augmentation index, central blood pressure and aortic pulse wave velocity. J Hypertens 28(10):2068–2075, Epub 2010/07/24. eng

Isnard RN, Pannier BM, Laurent S, London GM, Diebold B, Safar ME (1989) Pulsatile diameter and elastic modulus of the aortic arch in essential hypertension: a noninvasive study. J Am Coll Cardiol 13(2):399–405, Epub 1989/02/01. eng

Kaess BM, Rong J, Larson MG, Hamburg NM, Vita JA, Levy D et al (2012) Aortic stiffness, blood pressure progression, and incident hypertension. Jama 308(9):875–881, Pubmed Central PMCID: PMC3594687, Epub 2012/09/06. eng

Karalliedde J, Smith A, DeAngelis L, Mirenda V, Kandra A, Botha J et al (2008) Valsartan improves arterial stiffness in type 2 diabetes independently of blood pressure lowering. Hypertension 51 (6):1617–1623, Epub 2008/04/23. eng

Kass DA, Shapiro EP, Kawaguchi M, Capriotti AR, Scuteri A, de Groof RC et al (2001) Improved arterial compliance by a novel advanced glycation end-product crosslink breaker. Circulation 104 (13):1464–1470, Epub 2001/09/26. eng

Kitahara T, Ono K, Tsuchida A, Kawai H, Shinohara M, Ishii Y et al (2005) Impact of brachial-ankle pulse wave velocity and ankle-brachial blood pressure index on mortality in hemodialysis patients. Am J Kidney Dis 46(4):688–696, Epub 2005/09/27. eng

Kithas PA, Supiano MA (2010) Spironolactone and hydrochlorothiazide decrease vascular stiffness and blood pressure in geriatric hypertension. J Am Geriatr Soc 58(7):1327–1332, Pubmed Central PMCID: PMC3064882, Epub 2010/06/11. eng

Kuriyama S (1999) The expressiveness of the body and the divergence of Greek and Chinese medicine. Zone Books, New York

Laszlo A, Reusz G, Nemcsik J (2015) Ambulatory arterial stiffness in chronic kidney disease: a methodological review. Hypertens Res 3, Epub 2015/12/04. Eng

Laurent S, Boutouyrie P, Asmar R, Gautier I, Laloux B, Guize L et al (2001) Aortic stiffness is an independent predictor of all-cause and cardiovascular mortality in hypertensive patients. Hypertension 37 (5):1236–1241, Epub 2001/05/23. eng

Laurent S, Katsahian S, Fassot C, Tropeano AI, Gautier I, Laloux B et al (2003) Aortic stiffness is an independent predictor of fatal stroke in essential hypertension. Stroke J Cereb Circ 34(5):1203–1206, Epub 2003/04/05. eng

Laurent S, Cockcroft J, Van Bortel L, Boutouyrie P, Giannattasio C, Hayoz D et al (2006) Expert consensus document on arterial stiffness: methodological issues and clinical applications. Eur Heart J 27 (21):2588–2605, Epub 2006/09/27. eng

Laurent S, Briet M, Boutouyrie P (2012) Arterial stiffness as surrogate end point: needed clinical trials. Hypertension 60(2):518–522, Epub 2012/06/27. eng

Levy B, Targett RC, Bardou A, McIlroy MB (1985) Quantitative ascending aortic Doppler blood velocity in normal human subjects. Cardiovasc Res 19 (7):383–393, Epub 1985/07/01. eng

Lilamand M, Kelaiditi E, Guyonnet S, Antonelli Incalzi R, Raynaud-Simon A, Vellas B et al (2014) Flavonoids and arterial stiffness: promising perspectives. Nutr Metab Cardiovasc Dis 24 (7):698–704, Epub 2014/03/25. eng

London GM, Pannier B (2010) Arterial functions: how to interpret the complex physiology. Nephrol Dial Transpl 25(12):3815–3823, Epub 2010/10/16. eng

Maeda Y, Inoguchi T, Etoh E, Kodama Y, Sasaki S, Sonoda N et al (2014) Brachial-ankle pulse wave velocity predicts all-cause mortality and cardiovascular events in patients with diabetes: the Kyushu Prevention Study of Atherosclerosis. Diabetes Care 37 (8):2383–2390, Epub 2014/06/06. eng

Mahomed F (1872) The physiology and clinical use of the sphygmograph. Med Times Gazette 1:62

Mancia G, De Backer G, Dominiczak A, Cifkova R, Fagard R, Germano G et al (2007) 2007 Guidelines for the management of arterial hypertension: the Task Force for the Management of Arterial Hypertension of the European Society of Hypertension (ESH) and of the European Society of Cardiology (ESC). Eur Heart J 28(12):1462–1536, Epub 2007/06/15. eng

Mancia G, Fagard R, Narkiewicz K, Redon J, Zanchetti A, Bohm M et al (2013) 2013 ESH/ESC guidelines for the management of arterial hypertension: the Task Force for the Management of Arterial Hypertension of the European Society of Hypertension (ESH) and of the European Society of Cardiology (ESC). Eur Heart J 34(28):2159–2219, Epub 2013/06/19. eng

Marey E (1860) Recherches sur le pouls an moyen d'un nouvel appareil enregisteur: le sphygmographe. E Thunot et Cie, Paris

Mattace-Raso FU, van der Cammen TJ, Hofman A, van Popele NM, Bos ML, Schalekamp MA et al (2006) Arterial stiffness and risk of coronary heart disease and stroke: the Rotterdam Study. Circulation 113 (5):657–663, Epub 2006/02/08. eng

McDonald D (1960) Blood flow in arteries. Edward Arnold, London

McEniery CM, Yasmin, Hall IR, Qasem A, Wilkinson IB, Cockcroft JR (2005) Normal vascular aging: differential effects on wave reflection and aortic pulse wave velocity: the Anglo-Cardiff Collaborative Trial (ACCT). J Am Coll Cardiol 46(9):1753–1760, Epub 2005/11/01. eng

Meaume S, Benetos A, Henry OF, Rudnichi A, Safar ME (2001) Aortic pulse wave velocity predicts cardiovascular mortality in subjects >70 years of age. Arterioscler Thromb Vasc Biol 21(12):2046–2050, Epub 2001/12/18. eng

Meguro T, Nagatomo Y, Nagae A, Seki C, Kondou N, Shibata M et al (2009) Elevated arterial stiffness evaluated by brachial-ankle pulse wave velocity is deleterious for the prognosis of patients with heart failure. Circ J 73(4):673–680, Epub 2009/02/28. eng

Mitchell GF, Izzo JL Jr, Lacourciere Y, Ouellet JP, Neutel J, Qian C et al (2002) Omapatrilat reduces pulse pressure and proximal aortic stiffness in patients with systolic hypertension: results of the conduit hemodynamics of omapatrilat international research study. Circulation 105(25):2955–2961, Epub 2002/06/26. eng

Mitchell GF, Lacourciere Y, Arnold JM, Dunlap ME, Conlin PR, Izzo JL Jr (2005) Changes in aortic stiffness and augmentation index after acute converting enzyme or vasopeptidase inhibition. Hypertension 46 (5):1111–1117, Epub 2005/10/19. eng

Mitchell GF, Hwang SJ, Vasan RS, Larson MG, Pencina MJ, Hamburg NM et al (2010) Arterial stiffness and cardiovascular events: the Framingham Heart Study. Circulation 121(4):505–511, Pubmed Central PMCID: PMC2836717, Epub 2010/01/20. eng

Moreau KL, Meditz A, Deane KD, Kohrt WM (2012) Tetrahydrobiopterin improves endothelial function and decreases arterial stiffness in estrogen-deficient postmenopausal women. Am J Phys Heart Circ Phys 302(5):H1211–H1218, Pubmed Central PMCID: PMC3311456, Epub 2012/01/17. eng

Munakata M, Konno S, Miura Y, Yoshinaga K (2012) Prognostic significance of the brachial-ankle pulse wave velocity in patients with essential hypertension: final results of the J-TOPP study. Hypertens Res 35 (8):839–842, Epub 2012/04/27. eng

Nemeth ZK, Studinger P, Kiss I, Othmane Tel H, Nemcsik J, Fekete BC et al (2011) The method of distance measurement and torso length influences the relationship of pulse wave velocity to cardiovascular mortality. Am J Hypertens 24(2):155–161, Epub 2010/11/06. eng

Nichols WW, O'Rourke MF (2005) McDonald's blood flow in arteries: theoretical, experimental and clinical applications, 5th edn. Hodder Arnold, London

Nichols WW, Estrada JC, Braith RW, Owens K, Conti CR (2006) Enhanced external counterpulsation treatment improves arterial wall properties and wave reflection characteristics in patients with refractory angina. J Am Coll Cardiol 48(6):1208–1214, Epub 2006/09/19. eng

Ninomiya T, Kojima I, Doi Y, Fukuhara M, Hirakawa Y, Hata J et al (2013) Brachial-ankle pulse wave velocity predicts the development of cardiovascular disease in a general Japanese population: the Hisayama Study. J Hypertens 31(3):477–483, discussion 83. Epub 2013/ 04/26. eng

O'Rourke MF, Pauca A, Jiang XJ (2001) Pulse wave analysis. Br J Clin Pharmacol 51(6):507–522, Pubmed Central PMCID: PMC2014492, Epub 2001/06/26. eng

Orlova IA, Nuraliev EY, Yarovaya EB, Ageev FT (2010) Prognostic value of changes in arterial stiffness in men with coronary artery disease. Vasc Health Risk Manag 6:1015–1021, Pubmed Central PMCID: PMC2988619, Epub 2010/12/04. eng

Pase MP, Grima NA, Sarris J (2011) The effects of dietary and nutrient interventions on arterial stiffness: a systematic review. Am J Clin Nutr 93(2):446–454, Epub 2010/12/15. eng

Pierce GL, Jablonski KL, Walker AE, Seibert SM, DeVan AE, Black SM et al (2012) Tetrahydrobiopterin supplementation enhances carotid artery compliance in healthy older men: a pilot study. Am J Hypertens 25 (10):1050–1054, Pubmed Central PMCID: PMC3482981, Epub 2012/06/08. eng

Powell JT, Vine N, Crossman M (1992) On the accumulation of D-aspartate in elastin and other proteins of the ageing aorta. Atherosclerosis 97(2–3):201–208, Epub 1992/12/01. eng

Ryden L, Grant PJ, Anker SD, Berne C, Cosentino F, Danchin N et al (2013) ESC Guidelines on diabetes, pre-diabetes, and cardiovascular diseases developed in collaboration with the EASD: the Task Force on diabetes, pre-diabetes, and cardiovascular diseases of the European Society of Cardiology (ESC) and developed in collaboration with the European Association for the Study of Diabetes (EASD). Eur Heart J 34 (39):3035–3087, Epub 2013/09/03. eng

Salvi P, Lio G, Labat C, Ricci E, Pannier B, Benetos A (2004) Validation of a new non-invasive portable tonometer for determining arterial pressure wave and pulse wave velocity: the PulsePen device. J Hypertens 22(12):2285–2293, Epub 2004/12/23. eng

Sanchez-Gonzalez MA, Wong A, Vicil F, Gil R, Park SY, Figueroa A (2012) Impact of passive vibration on pressure pulse wave characteristics. J Hum Hypertens 26(10):610–615, Epub 2011/06/24. eng

Sehestedt T, Jeppesen J, Hansen TW, Rasmussen S, Wachtell K, Ibsen H et al (2009) Risk stratification with the risk chart from the European Society of Hypertension compared with SCORE in the general population. J Hypertens 27(12):2351–2357, Epub 2009/11/17. eng

Simon AC, Levenson J, Bouthier J, Safar ME, Avolio AP (1985) Evidence of early degenerative changes in large arteries in human essential hypertension. Hypertension 7(5):675–680, Epub 1985/09/01. eng

Sutton-Tyrrell K, Najjar SS, Boudreau RM, Venkitachalam L, Kupelian V, Simonsick EM et al (2005) Elevated aortic pulse wave velocity, a marker of arterial stiffness, predicts cardiovascular events in well-functioning older adults. Circulation 111(25):3384–3390, Epub 2005/06/22. eng

Takase H, Dohi Y, Toriyama T, Okado T, Tanaka S, Sonoda H et al (2011) Brachial-ankle pulse wave velocity predicts increase in blood pressure and onset of hypertension. Am J Hypertens 24(6):667–673, Epub 2011/02/19. eng

Targett RC, Levy B, Bardou A, McIlroy MB (1985) Simultaneous Doppler blood velocity measurements from aorta and radial artery in normal human subjects. Cardiovasc Res 19(7):394–399, Epub 1985/07/01. eng

Tomiyama H, Yamashina A (2010) Non-invasive vascular function tests: their pathophysiological background and clinical application. Circ J 74(1):24–33, Epub 2009/11/19. eng

Tomiyama H, Koji Y, Yambe M, Shiina K, Motobe K, Yamada J et al (2005) Brachial – ankle pulse wave velocity is a simple and independent predictor of prognosis in patients with acute coronary syndrome. Circ J 69(7):815–822, Epub 2005/07/01. eng

Tomiyama H, Hashimoto H, Hirayama Y, Yambe M, Yamada J, Koji Y et al (2006) Synergistic acceleration of arterial stiffening in the presence of raised blood pressure and raised plasma glucose. Hypertension 47 (2):180–188, Epub 2005/12/29. eng

Tomiyama H, Tanaka H, Hashimoto H, Matsumoto C, Odaira M, Yamada J et al (2010) Arterial stiffness and declines in individuals with normal renal function/ early chronic kidney disease. Atherosclerosis 212 (1):345–350, Epub 2010/07/03. eng

Tomiyama H, Matsumoto C, Shiina K, Brachial-Ankle YA, PWV (2016) Current status and future directions as a useful marker in the management of cardiovascular disease and/or cardiovascular risk factors. J Atheroscler Thromb 23(2):128–146, Epub 2015/11/13. eng

Townsend RR, Wilkinson IB, Schiffrin EL, Avolio AP, Chirinos JA, Cockcroft JR et al (2015) Recommendations for improving and standardizing vascular research on arterial stiffness: a scientific statement from the American Heart Association. Hypertension 66(3):698–722, Pubmed Central PMCID: PMC4587661, Epub 2015/07/15. eng

Toyama K, Sugiyama S, Oka H, Iwasaki Y, Sumida H, Tanaka T et al (2012) Combination treatment of rosuvastatin or atorvastatin, with regular exercise improves arterial wall stiffness in patients with coronary artery disease. PLoS ONE 7(7):e41369, Pubmed Central PMCID: PMC3400658, Epub 2012/07/26. eng

Usui M, Egashira K, Tomita H, Koyanagi M, Katoh M, Shimokawa H et al (2000) Important role of local angiotensin II activity mediated via type 1 receptor in the pathogenesis of cardiovascular inflammatory changes induced by chronic blockade of nitric oxide synthesis in rats. Circulation 101(3):305–310, Epub 2000/01/25. eng

Van Bortel LM, Laurent S, Boutouyrie P, Chowienczyk P, Cruickshank JK, De Backer T et al (2012) Expert consensus document on the measurement of aortic stiffness in daily practice using carotid-femoral pulse wave velocity. J Hypertens 30(3):445–448, Epub 2012/01/27. eng

van Leeuwen-Segarceanu EM, Tromp WF, Bos WJ, Vogels OJ, Groothoff JW, van der Lee JH (2010) Comparison of two instruments measuring carotid-femoral pulse wave velocity: Vicorder versus SphygmoCor. J Hypertens 28(8):1687–1691, Epub 2010/05/26. eng

van Sloten TT, Sedaghat S, Laurent S, London GM, Pannier B, Ikram MA et al (2015) Carotid stiffness is associated with incident stroke: a systematic review and individual participant data meta-analysis. J Am Coll Cardiol 66(19):2116–2125, Epub 2015/11/07. eng

Virdis A, Ghiadoni L, Qasem AA, Lorenzini G, Duranti E, Cartoni G et al (2012) Effect of aliskiren treatment on endothelium-dependent vasodilation and aortic stiffness in essential hypertensive patients. Eur Heart J 33(12):1530–1538, Epub 2012/03/28. eng

Vlachopoulos C, Aznaouridis K, Terentes-Printzios D, Ioakeimidis N, Stefanadis C (2012) Prediction of cardiovascular events and all-cause mortality with brachial-ankle elasticity index: a systematic review and meta-analysis. Hypertension 60(2):556–562, Epub 2012/06/27. eng

Vlachopoulos C, Aznaouridis K, Stefanadis C (2014) Aortic stiffness for cardiovascular risk prediction: just measure it, just do it! J Am Coll Cardiol 63 (7):647–649, Epub 2013/11/19. eng

Vlachopoulos C, Xaplanteris P, Aboyans V, Brodmann M, Cifkova R, Cosentino F et al (2015) The role of vascular biomarkers for primary and secondary prevention. A position paper from the European Society of Cardiology Working Group on peripheral circulation: Endorsed by the Association for Research into Arterial Structure and Physiology (ARTERY) Society. Atherosclerosis 241(2):507–532, Epub 2015/06/29. eng

Wang X, Xie J, Zhang LJ, Hu DY, Luo YL, Wang JW (2009) Reference values of brachial-ankle pulse wave velocity for Northern Chinese. Chin Med J 122 (18):2103–2106, Epub 2009/09/29. eng

Wassertheurer S, Kropf J, Weber T, van der Giet M, Baulmann J, Ammer M et al (2010) A new oscillometric method for pulse wave analysis: comparison with a common tonometric method. J Hum Hypertens 24(8):498–504, Pubmed Central PMCID: PMC2907506, Epub 2010/03/20. eng

Wilkinson IB, Fuchs SA, Jansen IM, Spratt JC, Murray GD, Cockcroft JR et al (1998) Reproducibility of pulse wave velocity and augmentation index measured by pulse wave analysis. J Hypertens 16(12 Pt 2):2079–2084, Epub 1999/01/14. eng

Womersley J (1957) The mathematical analysis of the arterial circulation in a state of oscillatory motion. Dayton, Ohio: Wright Air Development Center, Technical Report Wade-TR 56–614

Yamashina A, Tomiyama H, Takeda K, Tsuda H, Arai T, Hirose K et al (2002) Validity, reproducibility, and clinical significance of noninvasive brachial-ankle pulse wave velocity measurement. Hypertens Res 25 (3):359–364, Epub 2002/07/24. eng

Yamashina A, Tomiyama H, Arai T, Hirose K, Koji Y, Hirayama Y et al (2003) Brachial-ankle pulse wave velocity as a marker of atherosclerotic vascular damage and cardiovascular risk. Hypertens Res 26 (8):615–622, Epub 2003/10/22. eng

Yambe M, Tomiyama H, Yamada J, Koji Y, Motobe K, Shiina K et al (2007) Arterial stiffness and progression to hypertension in Japanese male subjects with high normal blood pressure. J Hypertens 25(1):87–93, Epub 2006/12/05. eng

Zieman SJ, Melenovsky V, Clattenburg L, Corretti MC, Capriotti A, Gerstenblith G et al (2007) Advanced glycation endproduct crosslink breaker (alagebrium) improves endothelial function in patients with isolated systolic hypertension. J Hypertens 25(3):577–583, Epub 2007/02/07. eng

Adv Exp Med Biol - Advances in Internal Medicine (2017) 2: 489–496
DOI 10.1007/5584_2016_172
© Springer International Publishing AG 2016
Published online: 19 November 2016

Primordial Prevention of Cardiometabolic Risk in Childhood

Meryem A. Tanrikulu, Mehmet Agirbasli, and Gerald Berenson

Abstract

Fetal life and childhood are important in the development of cardiometabolic risk and later clinical disease of atherosclerosis, hypertension and diabetes mellitus. Molecular and environmental conditions leading to cardiometabolic risk in early life bring us a challenge to develop effective prevention and intervention strategies to reduce cardiovascular (CV) risk in children and later disease. It is important that prevention strategies begin at an early age to reduce future CV morbidity and mortality. Pioneering work from longitudinal studies such as Bogalusa Heart Study (BHS), the Finnish Youth Study and other programs provide an awareness of the need for public and health services to begin primordial prevention. The impending CV risk beginning in childhood has a significant socioeconomic burden. Directions to achieve primordial prevention of cardiometabolic risk in children have been developed by prior longitudinal studies. Based on those studies that show risk factors in childhood as precursors of adult CV risk, implementation of primordial prevention will have effects at broad levels. Considering the epidemic of obesity, the high prevalence of hypertension and cardiometabolic risk, prevention early in life is valuable. Comprehensive health education, such as 'Health Ahead/Heart Smart', for all elementary school age children is one approach to begin primordial prevention and

M.A. Tanrikulu (✉)
İstanbul Maltepe State Hospital, Zumrutevler Mah.
Mevlana Halid Caddesi No: 21, Nishadalar Sitesi, 12.
Blok Daire: 41, Maltepe, 34852 Istanbul, Turkey
e-mail: matanrikulu@yahoo.com

M. Agirbasli
Department of Cardiology Istanbul, Medeniyet University
Medical School, Istanbul, Turkey

G. Berenson
Department of Internal Medicine-Section of Cardiology,
New Orleans, LA 70112, USA

can be included in public education beginning in kindergarten along with the traditional education subject matter.

Keywords

Childhood cardiometabolic risk • Childhood and adolescence metabolic syndrome • Primordial prevention

Abbreviations

AAP   American Academy of Pediatrics
AHA   American Heart Association
BHS   Bogalusa Heart Study
BMI   Body mass index
CV   Cardiovascular
PEP   Prevention Education Program
SHPPS   School Health Policies and Programs Study
T2DM   Type 2 Diabetes Mellitus

1   Introduction

Cardiometabolic risk factors tend to cluster and directly increase the risk for cardiovascular (CV) diseases and type 2 diabetes mellitus (T2DM). The burden from CV disease impacts general health and has an important socioeconomic burden on global health (Ford 2004). Cardiometabolic risk factors are known to start early in childhood (Webber et al. 1995; Weiss et al. 2004) and therefore, being prevalent in the pediatric population needs to be structured into a correct stratification of future CV risk. In fact, longitudinal studies indicate that findings of arterial high blood pressure and metabolic syndrome in childhood translate into high CV and heart disease risk in adulthood. The aim of intervention in children with cardiometabolic risk is to achieve an optimal reduction of such risk. Lifestyle modifications and public awareness attempt to counteract the effects of the underlying risk factors (abdominal obesity, physical inactivity and atherogenic diet) (Misra et al. 2010). Moreover, starting from childhood physicians should screen for metabolic disturbances and associated metabolic risk factors (high blood pressure, dyslipidemia, insulin resistance and prothrombotic and proinflammatory states).

Childhood and adolescence are particularly vulnerable periods of life to the effects of cardiometabolic risk and later development of atherosclerosis, hypertension and diabetes mellitus. Even fetal life influences adult CV disease, through low birth weight (Lopez-Lopez et al. 2015; Sipola-Leppänen and Kajantie 2015). A better understanding of mechanisms leading to cardiometabolic risk in early life will lead to more effective prevention and intervention strategies to reduce metabolic stress in children, underlying silent CV disease and later manifest disease (Berenson et al. 2005). Therefore, early prevention strategies beginning in childhood are the most logical steps to reduce future CV morbidity and mortality. Primordial preventive efforts for cardiometabolic risk in children have been recognized as necessary steps to improve the future health of children loading into adulthood.

Lifestyle interventions are the first step in achieving cardiometabolic risk reduction in children and adolescents. The promotions of exercise and energy expenditure are key lifestyle interventions. Other lifestyle changes also have a beneficial effect on specific cardiometabolic risk populations and must be encouraged in specific children.

Maintenance of lifestyle changes in children requires counseling the parents and frequently confounded by socioeconomic conditions. These, remain to be difficult in the long term. The School Breakfast Program is one such example (Williams 2014). This program provides breakfast to public and nonprofit private schools and residential childcare institutions to provide free and reduced-price breakfasts to eligible children. The aim is to target children who do not eat a healthy breakfast at home. Children who eat healthy school breakfast will less likely to be overweight and will have improved nutrition, eat more fruits, vegetables, protein. The emphasis in nutrition has to be stressed through education.

In this review, we will concisely consider the efforts to stratify and primordially prevent cardiometabolic risk in children.

2 Childhood Obesity and Endemic Proneness to Develop Metabolic Syndrome

Undoubtedly, the prevalence of cardiometabolic risk increases several fold among obese children and adolescents. An alarming global epidemic of childhood obesity, hypertension and T2DM (Hannon et al. 2005) fueled the consideration and worldwide recognition of cardiometabolic risk in children and adolescents as a global public health concern (Cook et al. 2003; de Ferranti et al. 2004). Yet, there is a tendency to overlook cardiometabolic risk factors in children. For instance, high blood pressure (hypertension) in children is blood pressure that is same or above than 95 % of children who are the same sex, age and height. Given the fact that, a simple target blood pressure level does not indicate high blood pressure in all age and gender groups for children since changes occur as they grow, physicians tend to underestimate the consequences of high blood pressure in children. Fortunately, there are now non-invasive measures of silent changes of the CV system. Several companies invest in non-invasive instruments for precise measurement of blood pressure and endothelial function. Surely, lifestyle changes, such as improving eating habits and exercising more, can help reduce high blood pressure in children, for some children, medications can still be necessary to prevent

end-organ damage (Simonetti et al. 2011; Tu et al. 2011; Pacifico et al. 2011).

Prevention and treatment strategies for cardiometabolic risk in children focus on weight management, prevention of obesity and insulin resistance. Environmental and social factors such as diet and physical activity influence high blood pressure, dyslipidemia and obesity in children. Cigarette smoking and tobacco use are also common among adolescents, yet, these as well as other risk factors are all controllable. Lifestyle and behavioral influence on CV risk begin early in life and preventive measures should meet this challenge. Healthy lifestyle should be adopted in childhood, to modulate CV risk effectively later in life. Surely, we need long-term data related to the CV disease and T2DM risk from pediatric cardiometabolic risk. Concerns exist about the safety of forceful strategies in children who are still growing and developing. Moreover, chronic alterations in sex hormone secretion in children may affect the timing of puberty, final stature, and body composition, as well as cause of early-onset obesity, cardiometabolic risk and T2DM.

Furthermore differences exist in the criteria, definition and prevalence of cardiometabolic risk in children and adolescents between populations (Deboer 2010). Environmental factors, physical activity and eating habits not only differ among populations but also change during the transition of puberty and adolescence (Lazarou et al. 2009). Therefore, conclusive guidelines for global assessment of cardiometabolic risk in children are unlikely to be imminent.

3 Primordial Prevention

For over 30 years, Bogalusa Heart Study (BHS), the Finnish Youth Study, the Muscatine Study and other population studies provided further understanding of the early origin of CV disease beginning in childhood (Berenson et al. 1998). Environment and lifestyle related problems such as poor eating behavior, use of tobacco, alcohol and addicting drugs begin early in life and contribute to development of adult heart disease (Berenson et al. 1995).

Prevention strategies can diverge as: (1) population or public health strategy and (2) a high risk model. But in these strategies, need to include addressing special problems in children that affect health of children, such as drop-out rate in schools and violent behavior.

3.1 Population or Public Health Strategy

Primary care physicians, pediatricians and cardiologists can play a major leadership role in the prevention of adult heart diseases beginning in childhood. Physicians are encouraged to obtain and understand risk factor profiles in children, along with a family history of heart disease.

It is important to incorporate health education into the public school system starting in the kindergarten. A public health approach to prevention of CV disease can be introduced early through health education and health promotion programs (Berenson and Pickoff 1995). 'Health Ahead/Heart Smart' program is an example of a public health model focusing on school children and individuals at a young age (Downey et al. 1987; Berenson 1998). This program addresses the broad problem of CV risk and obesity and incorporates primordial prevention. Students have achieved weight reduction and improved physical activity in schools implementing the program aggressively (Berenson 2012). This program has been introduced into a geographic area of a Parish (County) of Louisiana State in United States to involve all elementary age students (approximately 5000 children). The program succeeded in controlling obesity with the involvement of parents and community resources.

3.2 High Risk Offspring Model

This model is for parents and children who have already developed risk factors or clinical heart disease (Berenson et al. 1993; Johnson and

Table 1 Universal criteria to identify children at high risk

Waist circumference ≥90th percentile
Waist/height ratio >0.5
Body mass index >90th percentile
Fasting plasma glucose ≥86 mg/dL
Triglycerides >75th percentile
High-density lipoprotein cholesterol <25th percentile
Systolic or diastolic blood pressure >75th percentile
Positive family history for diabetes mellitus or metabolic syndrome

Agirbasli et al. (2016)

Nicklas 1995). Table 1 briefly summarizes universally accepted criteria identifying children at high risk (Agirbasli et al. 2016). It is especially important to identify children of parents who have had established vascular disease by age 60 or have hypertension, diabetes, or other risk factors (Berenson and Pickoff 1995). The 'Heart Smart Family Health Promotion' program is a unique approach to education and skills development aimed at improving the CV health of entire family. A multidisciplinary team, consisting of a cardiologist, physician and nurse specialist interested in CV prevention, a nutritionist, an exercise person and a psychologist, teaches families, including children, on a weekly basis. Enhanced social support and self-confidence are needed to succeed (Johnson and Nicklas 1995) and are integrated into the program. This program has been shown to be successful in risk factor reduction (Berenson 2012).

Prevention Education Program (PEP) Family Health Study is an observational study to assess the effects of 1 year of sustained general lifestyle advice in school-children and their parents (Schwandt et al. 2011). PEP is an intergenerational lifestyle habits that affect CV risk factors within biological families. As lifestyle habits are predictable, they may be used for implementation of family-based CV disease prevention strategies which are models for high-risk families (Schwandt et al. 2010). PEP reveals that improvement in CV risk factors is possible by lifestyle enhancement. Decreases in insulin resistance and dyslipidemia following weight reduction have also been accomplished (Grulich-Henn et al. 2011).

The development of life skills necessary for maintaining optimal wellness, including social issues, such as prevention of smoking, alcohol and drug use, violent behavior, teenage pregnancy and dropping out of school are emphasized (Berenson 2010). Early evaluations of this program indicated favorable changes in health knowledge, eating habits, physical activity and clinical CV risk factors of the children (Johnson and Nicklas 1995).

The primordial strategies (Berenson 2009) include healthy diet and physical exercise to obtain CV fitness and prevent obesity, hypertension and hypercholesterolemia together with prevention of smoking, alcohol and other drug usage starting from kindergarten.

4 Tobacco Use and Parental Smoking

Substantial scientific evidence documents the association between CV risk factors and tobacco use of adolescents and parental smoking (Juonala et al. 2012). Thus, preventive measures will have the greatest impact when applied at an early age (Wynder 1995). Young children can be protected from tobacco smoke exposure only if their parents quit smoking. Moreover, recently maternal smoking is shown to be a risk factor for higher BMI and obesity index particularly in children whose mothers had smoked during pregnancy (Ino et al. 2012). Educational programs should focus on social support and family based approach. Skill- training programs in smoking prevention in adolescents are also essential components (Weintraub et al. 2011).

5 Health Education for Public Schools

Increasing childhood obesity is linked to increasing cardiometabolic risk consequences, including CV disease and T2DM. American Heart Association (AHA) and American Academy of Pediatrics (AAP) have reported recommendations for CV health and risk reduction in children and adolescents including screening programs, dietary and physical activity recommendations (Weintraub et al. 2011; Gidding et al. 2012). At each well-child visit, heart disease-related health behaviors should be assessed and monitored. CV risk factor screening with school-based (and preschool) health assessments would also assist in early identification of children at risk (Roger et al. 2012).

Adequate intake of micronutrients and physical activity appropriate for the maintenance of a normal weight for height; are encouraged (Gidding et al. 2005).

The School Health Policies and Programs Study (SHPPS) focused on health-promoting physical school environment policies and programs (Jones et al. 2007). Concerted public health efforts to coordinate culturally-appropriate parental and caregiver education, home lifestyle changes, dietary and exercise modifications may reverse the current trajectory of obesity epidemic.

6 Future Directives

According to 2011–2012 data from National Health and Nutrition Examination Survey (National Center for Health Statistics), in United States, among children 2–19 years of age, 31.7 % are overweight or obese and 16.9 % are obese. Mexican American boys or girls and African American girls are disproportionately affected (Roger et al. 2012). Approximately 30 % of overweight children have three cardiometabolic risk factors and 9 out of 10 have at least one risk factor (Cruz and Goran 2004).

Perhaps the most effective method to reach a total population under risk is to incorporate a comprehensive health education program like 'Health Ahead/Heart Smart' into public education starting in kindergarten.

Family history should be updated for obesity, hypertension, dyslipidemia, diabetes, and smoking before age 55 for men and age 65 for women in order to identify children and adolescents who are at high risk for CV disease (Weintraub et al. 2011).

The epidemic of childhood obesity, which resulted in increased cardiometabolic risk prevalence, has become a major health problem due to its future consequences. Programs should become a component of national health-care reform (Wynder 1995). Future research priority should also be given to testing new models delivering risk prevention and treatment in the health systems and primary care practices. Evidence-based therapies should be disseminated to primary care practices.

7 Conclusion

The coexistence of multiple risk factors starts an early form of atherosclerosis in childhood (Newman et al. 1986). Cardiometabolic risk in children and its many consequences including T2DM and silent CV disease present serious threats to the current and future health of youth. Screening and identifying children and adolescents for CV risk and encouraging them and their families through healthy lifestyle changes should be implemented as a global strategy. Health education and health promotion of children require cooperation as a community and family effort. Health care providers together with primary care providers should develop and test the primordial prevention strategies in large cohort studies. Pioneering work from longitudinal studies such as BHS need to incorporate into improved educational efforts. The awareness of the public and health services improved concerning the impending CV risk. It is likely primordial prevention can have an effect at a broad level, considering the high prevalence of obesity, cardiometabolic risk, and their consequences of heart disease, atherosclerosis, hypertension and T2DM. We recommend comprehensive health education such as 'Health Ahead/Heart Smart' to be included in public education beginning in kindergarten equal to the traditional education subject matter.

References

Agirbasli M, Tanrikulu AM, Berenson GS (2016) Metabolic syndrome: bridging the gap from childhood to adulthood. Cardiovasc Ther 34(1):30–36. doi:10.1111/1755-5922.12165

Berenson GS (ed) (1998) Introduction of comprehensive health promotion for elementary schools: the health ahead/heart smart program. Vintage Press Inc, New York

Berenson GS (2009) Cardiovascular risk begins in childhood: a time for action. Am J Prev Med 37(1 Suppl): S1–S2. doi:10.1016/j.amepre.2009.04.018

Berenson GS (2010) Cardiovascularhealth promotion for children: a model for a Parish (County)-wide program (implementation and preliminary results). Prev Cardio 13(1):23–28. doi:10.1111/j.1751-7141.2009.00049.x

Berenson GS (2012) Bogalusa Heart Study group. Health consequences of obesity. Pediatr Blood Cancer 58 (1):117–121. doi:10.1002/pbc.23373

Berenson GS, Pickoff AS (1995) Preventive cardiology and its potential influence on the early natural history of adult heart diseases: the Bogalusa Heart Study and the Heart Smart Program. Am J Med Sci 310(Suppl 1): S133–S138

Berenson GS, Harsha DW, Johnson CC (1993) Teach families to be heart smart. Patient Care 6:134–135

Berenson GS, Wattigney WA, Bao W, Srinivasan SR, Radhakrishnamurthy B (1995) Rationale to study the early natural history of heart disease: the Bogalusa Heart Study. Am J Med Sci 310(Suppl 1):S22–S28

Berenson GS, Srinivasan SR, Bao W, Newman WP 3rd, Tracy RE, Wattigney WA (1998) Association between multiple cardiovascular risk factors and the early development of atherosclerosis. Bogalusa Heart Study. N Engl J Med 338(23):1650–1656

Berenson GS, Srnivasan RS, Bogalusa Heart Study Group (2005) Cardiovascular risk factors in youth with implications for aging: the Bogalusa Heart Study. Neurobiol Aging 26(3):303–307

Cook S, Weitzman M, Auinger P, Nguyen M, Dietz WH (2003) Prevalence of a metabolic syndrome phenotype in adolescents: findings from NHANES-III, 1988–1994. Arch Pediatr Adolesc Med 157 (8):821–827

Cruz ML, Goran MI (2004) The metabolicsyndrome in children and adolescents. Curr Diab Rep 4(1):53–62

de Ferranti SD, Gauvreau K, Ludwig DS, Neufeld EJ, Newburger JW, Rifai N (2004) Prevalence of the metabolic syndrome in American adolescents. Circulation 110(16):2494–2497

Deboer MD (2010) Underdiagnosis of metabolic syndrome in non-hispanic black adolescents: a call for ethnic-specific criteria. Curr Cardiovasc Risk Rep 4 (4):302–310

Downey AM, Frank GC, Webber LS, Harsha DW, Virgilio SJ, Franklin FA et al (1987) Implementation of "Heart Smart:" a cardiovascular school health promotion program. J Sch Health 57(3):98–104

Ford ES (2004) The metabolic syndrome and mortality from cardiovascular disease and all-causes: findings from the National Health and Nutrition Examination Survey II Mortality study. Atherosclerosis 173 (2):309–314

Gidding SS, Dennison BA, Birch LL, Daniels SR, Gillman MW, Lichtenstein AH, et al.; American Heart Association; American Academy of Pediatrics (2005) Dietary recommendations for children and adolescents: a guide for practitioners: consensus statement from the American Heart Association. Circulation 112(13):2061–2075

Gidding SS, Daniels SR, Kavey RE; for the Expert Panel on Cardiovascular Health and Risk Reduction in Youth (2012) Developing the 2011 integrated pediatric guidelines for cardiovascular risk reduction. Pediatrics. 129(5):e1311–e1319. doi: 10.1542/peds.2011-2903

Grulich-Henn J, Lichtenstein S, Hörster F, Hoffmann GF, Nawroth PP, Hamann A (2011) Moderate weight reduction in an outpatient obesity intervention program significantly reduces insulin resistance and risk factors for cardiovascular disease in severely obese adolescents. Int J Endocrinol 2011:541021. doi:10.1155/2011/541021

Hannon TS, Rao G, Arslanian SA (2005) Childhood obesity and type 2 diabetes mellitus. Pediatrics 116 (2):473–480

Ino T, Shibuya T, Saito K, Inaba Y (2012) Relationship between body mass index of offspring and maternal smoking during pregnancy. Int J Obes (London) 36 (4):554–558. doi:10.1038/ijo.2011.255

Johnson CC, Nicklas TA (1995) Health ahead-heart smart family approach to prevention of cardiovascular disease. Am J Med Sci 310(Suppl 1):S127–S132

Jones SE, Axelrad R, Wattigney WA (2007) Healthy and safe school environment, Part II, Physical school environment: results from the School Health Policies and Programs Study 2006. J Sch Health 77(8):544–556

Juonala M, Magnussen CG, Venn A, Gall S, Kähönen M, Laitinen T et al (2012) Parental smoking in childhood and brachial artery flow-mediated dilatation in young adults: the cardiovascular risk in young Finns study and the childhood determinants of adult health study. Arterioscler Thromb Vasc Biol 32(4):1024–1031. doi:10.1161/ATVBAHA.111.243261

Lazarou C, Panagiotakos DB, Matalas AL (2009) Lifestyle factors are determinants of children's blood pressure levels: the CYKIDS study. J Hum Hypertens 23 (7):456–463. doi:10.1038/jhh.2008.151

Lopez-Lopez J, Lopez-Jaramillo P, Camacho PA, Gomez-Arbelaez D, Cohen DD (2015) The link between fetal programming, inflammation, muscular strength, and blood pressure. Mediators Inflamm 2015:710613. doi:10.1155/2015/710613, Epub 2015 Sep 27

Misra A, Singhal N, Khurana L (2010) Obesity, the metabolic syndrome, and type 2 diabetes in developing countries: role of dietary fats and oils. J Am Coll Nutr 29(3 Suppl):289S–301S

Newman WP 3rd, Freedman DS, Voors AW, Gard PD, Srinivasan SR, Cresanta JL et al (1986) Relation of serum lipoprotein levels and systolic blood pressure to early atherosclerosis. The Bogalusa Heart Study. N Engl J Med 314(3):138–144

Pacifico L, Anania C, Osborn JF, Ferraro F, Bonci E, Olivero E et al (2011) Low 25(OH)D3 levels are associated with total adiposity, metabolic syndrome, and hypertension in Caucasian children and adolescents. Eur J Endocrinol 165(4):603–611. doi:10.1530/EJE-11-0545

Roger VL, Go AS, Lloyd-Jones DM, Benjamin EJ, Berry JD, Borden WB, et al.; American Heart Association Statistics Committee and Stroke Statistics Subcommittee (2012) Heart disease and stroke statistics–2012 update: a report from the American Heart Association. Circulation. 125(1):e2–e220. doi: 10.1161/CIR.0b013e31823ac046

Schwandt P, Haas GM, Liepold E (2010) Lifestyle and cardiovascular risk factors in 2001 child-parent pairs: the PEP Family Heart Study. Atherosclerosis 213 (2):642–648. doi:10.1016/j.atherosclerosis.2010.09.032

Schwandt P, Bertsch T, Haas GM (2011) Sustained lifestyle advice and cardiovascular risk factors in 687 biological child-parent pairs: the PEP Family Heart Study. Atherosclerosis 219(2):937–945. doi:10.1016/j.atherosclerosis.2011.09.032

Simonetti GD, Schwertz R, Klett M, Hoffmann GF, Schaefer F, Wühl E (2011) Determinants of blood pressure in preschool children: the role of parental smoking. Circulation 123(3):292–298. doi:10.1161/CIRCULATIONAHA.110.958769

Sipola-Leppänen M, Kajantie E (2015) Should we assess cardiovascular risk in young adults born preterm? Curr Opin Lipidol 26(4):282–287. doi:10.1097/MOL.0000000000000190

Tu W, Eckert GJ, DiMeglio LA, Yu Z, Jung J, Pratt JH (2011) Intensified effect of adiposity on blood pressure in overweight and obese children. Hypertension 58(5):818–824. doi:10.1161/HYPERTENSIONAHA.111.175695

Webber LS, Osganian V, Luepker RV, Feldman HA, Stone EJ, Elder JP et al (1995) Cardiovascular risk factors among third grade children in four regions of the United States. The CATCH study: Child and Adolescent Trial for Cardiovascular Health. Am J Epidemiol 141(5):428–439

Weintraub WS, Daniels SR, Burke LE, Franklin BA, Goff DC Jr, Hayman LL, et al.; American Heart Association Advocacy Coordinating Committee; Council on Cardiovascular Disease in the Young; Council on the Kidney in Cardiovascular Disease; Council on Epidemiology and Prevention; Council on CardiovascularNursing; Council on Arteriosclerosis; Thrombosis and Vascular Biology; Council on Clinical Cardiology, and Stroke Council (2011) Value of primordial and primary prevention for cardiovascular disease: a policy statement from the American Heart Association. Circulation 124(8):967–990. doi: 10.1161/CIR.0b013e3182285a81

Weiss R, Dziura J, Burgert TS, Tamborlane WV, Taksali SE, Yeckel CW et al (2004) Obesity and the metabolic syndrome in children and adolescents. N Engl J Med 350(23):2362–2374

Williams PG (2014) The benefits of breakfast cereal consumption: a systematic review of the evidence base. Adv Nutr 5(5):636S–673S. doi:10.3945/an.114. 006247

Wynder EL (1995) From the discovery of risk factors for coronary artery disease to the application of preventive measures. Am J Med Sci 310(Suppl 1): S119–S122

Adv Exp Med Biol - Advances in Internal Medicine (2017) 2: 497–510
DOI 10.1007/5584_2016_37
© Springer International Publishing AG 2016
Published online: 16 July 2016

Emotional Stress as a Risk for Hypertension in Sub-Saharan Africans: Are We Ignoring the Odds?

Leoné Malan and Nico T. Malan

Abstract

Globally most interventions focus on improving lifestyle habits and treatment regimens to combat hypertension as a non-communicable disease (NCD). However, despite these interventions and improved medical treatments, blood pressure (BP) values are still on the rise and poorly controlled in sub-Saharan Africa (SSA). Other factors contributing to hypertension prevalence, such as chronic emotional stress, might provide some insight for future health policy approaches.

Currently, Hypertension Society guidelines do not mention emotional stress as a probable cause for hypertension. Recently the 2014 World Global Health reports, suggested that African governments should consider using World Health Organization hypertension data as a proxy indicator for social well-being. However, the possibility that a stressful life and taxing environmental factors might disturb central neural control of BP regulation has largely been ignored in SSA.

Linking emotional stress to vascular dysregulation is therefore one way to investigate increased cardiometabolic challenges, neurotransmitter depletion and disturbed hemodynamics. Disruption of stress response pathways and subsequent changes in lifestyle habits as ways of coping with a stressful life, and as probable cause for hypertension prevalence in SSA, may be included in future preventive measures. We will provide an overview on emotional stress and central neural control of BP and will include also implications thereof for clinical practice in SSA cohorts.

1   Hypertension Prevalence in Sub-Saharan Africa (SSA)

As a non-communicable disease (NCD), hypertension is responsible for an estimated 45 % of deaths due to heart disease and 51 % of deaths due to stroke globally (World Health

L. Malan (✉) and N.T. Malan
Hypertension in Africa Research Team (HART),
North-West University, Hoffman street, Private Bag
X6001, Potchefstroom 2520, South Africa
e-mail: leone.malan@nwu.ac.za

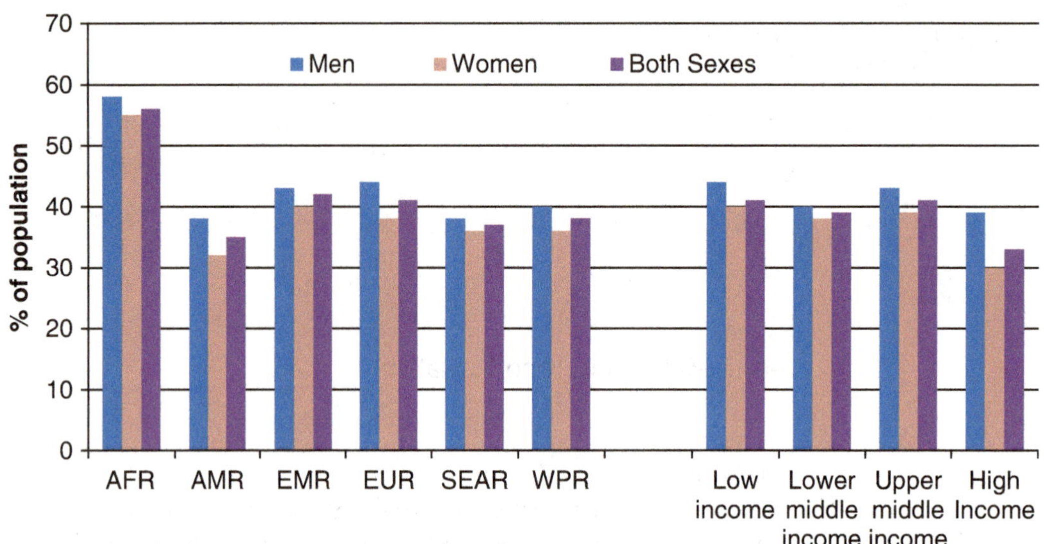

Fig. 1 Hypertension prevalence in six World Health Organization regions. Where: *AFR* WHO African Region, *AMR* WHO Region of the Americas, *EMR* WHO Eastern Mediterranean Region, *EUR* WHO European Region, *SEAR* WHO South-East Asia Region, *WPR* WHO Western Pacific Region (World Health Organisation 2014). Where: % raised blood pressure (SBP 140+ and/or DBP 90+ or on meds), ages 25+, age standardized

Organisation 2014). Of the WHO's six regions, the African region has the highest prevalence of hypertension with an estimate of 46 % in adults aged 25 and above, according to WHO's Global status report on NCD's (World Health Organisation 2014) (Fig. 1). The prevalence of elevated BP was consistently increased, with low, lower middle and upper middle income countries all having rates in the region of 40 %.

However, more recent findings provide a far more disturbing picture. A prospectively followed teachers' cohort from South Africa [173 black (aged 47.5 ± 7.8 years; 186 white (aged 49.6 ± 9.9 years)] showed that Blacks had a substantially higher 24 h hypertension prevalence (66 %) as opposed to Whites (42 %) (Hamer et al. 2015; Malan et al. 2016). Furthermore, the composite cardiovascular disease (CVD) burden in this Black cohort over 3 years (defined as history of physician diagnosed heart disease, use of anti-hypertensives, anti-diabetic, or statin medications at either time point) was higher compared to Whites (49.1 vs. 32.0 %, p = 0.012) (Hamer et al. 2015). In another South African cohort study including 1,994 Blacks older than 30 years, hypertension prevalence was 48 % (Schutte et al. 2012) whereas it ranged from 19 to 48 % in cohorts from Ghana (Bosu 2010).

The large variation in separate studies' data raises concern about the real situation. One possibility may be the lack of hypothesis driven prospective findings on hypertension prevalence in SSA. Another more controversial matter is that hypertension research did not receive enough attention over the last decade, with funding bodies mostly supporting infectious disease research in SSA (Peck et al. 2013; Tagoe and Dake 2011; World Health Organisation 2014) Fortunately enough, at present the attention seems to be shifting and Nigeria, one of many developing countries, recently reported that NCD's have become a growing problem (Peck et al. 2013; World Health Organisation 2014). At a Tanzanian hospital this was also the case since NCDs accounted for half of all deaths. Here, hypertension was the second most common cause of death overall and the leading cause of death in patients >50 years old (Peck et al. 2013). Due to overwhelming evidence of hypertension as a causative factor for deaths in SSA (World Health Organisation 2014), it is of the utmost importance, therefore, to progress with hypothesis driven research on hypertension prevalence and secondary outcomes in prospective cohort studies.

The examination as to whether emotional stress is a causative factor for hypertension or other NCDs has largely been understudied in SSA. Currently, the Sympathetic activity and Ambulatory Blood Pressure in Africans (SABPA) study is the only prospective cohort study in SSA where the study design (central neural control) was based on findings from studies over the previous 20 years (Malan et al. 2015). Cross-sectional data revealed that coping disability, cognitive emotional distress and a lack of social support were factors involved in NCDs development and progression in teachers from an urban environment (Malan et al. 2008, 2012, 2015; Venter et al. 2014). In this cohort, sympathetic hyperactivity was associated with cardiometabolic risk, namely hypertension prevalence, sympathovagal imbalance and depressed heart rate variability, all which contribute to vulnerability for cardiovascular risk (Lambert et al. 1994; Malan et al. 2013; Pal et al. 2014; Van Lill et al. 2011). It was also shown that factors leading to sympathetic hyperactivity included a stressful life and coping with continuous and taxing emotional demands (McEwen and Gianaros 2010). As a consequence, cardiometabolic demands will increase so to induce continuous adjustments by the brain to control sensitivity levels of organ systems in maintaining homeostasis (Gross 1998).

2 Central Neural Control of BP

As early as 1878 Claude Bernard postulated that maintenance of a stable internal environment is a prerequisite for the development of a complex functional nervous system (Gross 1998). Metabolic balance is maintained as neurons store glycogen as endogenous neuronal glycogen, which protects neuronal tolerance to hypoxic stress (Saez et al. 2014). Therefore, the brain maintains homeostasis by adjusting the sensitivity of target organs to neural and metabolic inputs (Gross

1998; McDougall et al. 2015; Saez et al. 2014) For example, the regular and continuous contractions of a normally functioning heart muscle must be able to respond to the changing requirements of the body's tissues.

It is also important to note that BP is centrally controlled, whereby no set-point for BP exists in the central nervous system (Nishida et al. 2012). If a set point existed, the BP control system would become a completely closed, self-contained system always causing BP to return to the set level independent of demands in organs and tissues. This implies that organs and tissues will not be protected even though the circulatory system itself may be. Therefore, neural BP regulation seems to be dynamic and acts as a phasic control in the circulatory system essential for maintaining life (Gross 1998; Nishida et al. 2012) When cardiometabolic demands increase, it is essential that the cardiovascular system, an open system, is able to respond with compensatory increases in BP to maintain homeostasis. Whether hypertension is the result of a compensatory elevation of BP to maintain organ function has been questioned (Mancia et al. 2013). Surely, fluctuations in BP are deemed physiologically necessary when cardiometabolic demands increase in an attempt to maintain homeostasis. Hypertension, however, represents a permanent shift in normal values, necessary for optimal organ function, but leading to end-organ damage. The "safety" or threshold levels for BP still needs in-depth investigations as hypertension prevalence is increasing despite medical interventions or treatment regimens to lower BP.

Despite these views, a neurophysiological approach showed that increased cardiometabolic demands in a hypertensive individual will be taxing to neuronal health because depletion or attenuated neurotransmitter secretion may induce neural and adrenal fatigue and/or depression (Cabib 1996; De Kock et al. 2012, 2015; Dobrunz and Stevens 1997). Long-term changes in a neuron or synapse will result in a permanent change in a neuron's excitatory properties and can cause synaptic fatigue (Cabib 1996). This may occur from much more or less activation that could potentially lead to synaptic depression. Indeed, short-term depression as well as habituation have been located in the sensory part of the defence response pathway, as well as at the axon terminals of sensory afferents in the brain stem (caudal pontine reticular nucleus) (Kvetnansky et al. 2009). In support, higher metabolic demands revealed reduced cerebral respiratory quotient in depressed subjects (Lambert et al. 1994). Neural fatigue or depression may thus impair metabolism in subcortical areas which regulate emotions such as the dorsolateral prefrontal cortex and the amygdala (Barton et al. 2007; LeDoux 2012; Taylor et al. 2013). A threat to homeostasis is thus sensed where the response has a degree of specificity depending, among other things, on the particular challenge to homeostasis, the organism's perception of the stressor and its ability to cope with it (LeDoux 2012). An important feature of successful coping with stress is that physiological systems are not only turned-on efficiently by a particular stressor but are also turned-off again after cessation of the stressor to conserve resources. However, coping with chronic stress, will have a turned-off reaction when cardiometabolic demands increase in hypertensive individuals as cognitive or memory performance was related to blunted parietal cerebral cortex blood flow responses (Jennings et al. 2005). Whereas turned-on reactions in hypertensives resulted in compensatory regional cerebral blood flow in the mesencephalon (or midbrain) which correlated with prefrontal cerebral blood flow (Jennings et al. 2005). Once again, a set-point for BP can be questioned.

In support of this notion, central neural control of subcortical areas regulating emotion, such as the dorsolateral prefrontal cortex and the amygdala, was associated with impaired metabolism and depression (Barton et al. 2007; LeDoux 2012; Taylor et al. 2013). Linking emotional distress to vascular dysregulation is therefore one way to investigate increased cardiometabolic challenges (Akinroye 2013; Kadirvelu et al. 2012; Lambert et al. 2000; Malan et al. 1992, 1996). Defensive coping responses included increased cardiometabolic challenges, depletion of neurotransmitters and

disturbed hemodynamics in urban-dwelling Blacks from the North-West region of South Africa (De Kock et al. 2012, 2015; Malan et al. 2008, 2012, 2013, 2015, 2016; Scheepers et al. 2016).

Central neural control is thus actively involved with emotional stress upon activation of stress response pathways. These pathways include the sympatho-adrenal medullary (SAM) and hypothalamic-pituitary-adrenal cortical axis (HPAA), both facilitating inflammatory, glycolysis and adrenergic responses (Taylor et al. 2013). Indeed, sympathetic hyperactivity is present in about 30 % of depressed patients, independent of hypertensive status (Barton et al. 2007). Other findings support the notion of sympathetic hyperactivity and neural fatigue, as attenuated acute stress pathway responses (De Kock et al. 2012; Taylor et al. 2013) and chronic defensiveness were shown in a SSA Black cohort. (Malan et al. 2015) Indeed, in this cohort, chronic depression in conjunction with hypertension prevalence was more prevalent in Blacks than in Whites (28.67 % vs. 5.29 · %; P ≤ 0.001) (Malan et al. 2016). Therefore, chronic emotional distress seems to facilitate higher metabolic demands and may even further contribute to increased risk of stroke (Taylor et al. 2013). In agreement, Biccard (Biccard 2008) also showed that Blacks from SSA are more likely to be diagnosed with symptomatic occlusive vascular disease or vascular dysregulation indicating increased stroke risk.

Additionally, recent studies support the notion that the cardiovascular system is regulated by cortical modulation (Mazzeo et al. 2014; Nagai et al. 2010; Stahrenberg et al. 2013). Insular cortex damage is suggested to be associated with cardiovascular system dysregulation such as ECG, cardiac stress (Tropinin T) and sympathovagal disturbances (Mazzeo et al. 2014; Nagai et al. 2010; Stahrenberg et al. 2013). Increased sympathetic nervous system activity therefore may serve as a pathophysiological event affecting the relationship between the insular cortex and cardiovascular dysregulation (Nagai et al. 2010). The insular cortex, amygdala and anterior cingulate gyrus are involved in processing the information related to emotional significance, such as the defence response to external stressors. Therefore, the insular cortex is implicated in BP control in cooperation with subcortical autonomic centres.

3 Factors Burdening Central Neural Control of BP

Important background factors are to be considered as possible obstacles for BP control in SSA. Social supportive systems are not in place (Kadirvelu et al. 2012) and Mayosi et al. (2012) urged the launch of an integrated model of health care at all levels in South Africa, which has to be supported by a robust surveillance system. However, upstream determinants of ill health, such as a lack of resources, poverty and insufficient quality education, may lie beyond the reach of the health sector in Africa (Seedat 2015). Therefore, if social support systems are not in place, self-management of NCDs in SSA will remain poor.

Another factor which may seriously compromise mental well-being is the level of violence in South Africa. According to a non-governmental organisation, registered as a non-profit company with the aim of protecting the rights of minorities, 17,805 persons were murdered in South Africa in 1 year (2014–2015) (National Development Plan 2016). That is an average of 48.8 murders per day. The country's homicide figure has subsequently increased with 4.6 % since 2013/2014. Attempted murder showed an increase of 3.2 %, while robbery with aggravating circumstances increased drastically by 8.5 %. These figures are an example of the high levels of aggression currently prevailing in South Africa and unfortunately are also spreading to the youth. The impact of this threat on emotional health is documented in WHO reports on mental well-being (Lund et al. 2011; Reed et al. 2012; World Health Organisation 2008, 2010). Threats to well-being or survival, actual or potential may increase a vicious cycle of fear, not feeling safe and anxiety (Reed et al. 2012). Subsequent autonomic, cardiovascular and neuroendocrine activation and specific behaviour

patterns have been associated with a hypervigilant state in an attempt to cope with these adverse or unexpected situations (World Health Organisation 2010). Vulnerability and an elevated risk of psychological distress will thus enforce increases in poor lifestyle habits and NCDs in an attempt to cope with these situations.

3.1 Stress Appraisal – The Defence Response

In more than 400 studies, little consensus could be found about how to conceptualize or classify how people cope with or appraise stress situations (Skinner et al. 2003). Coping functions at a number of levels and involves a plethora of behaviours, cognitions, and perceptions. At the highest level are sets of basic adaptive processes which intervene between stress and its psychological, social, and physiological outcomes. Coping inventories of Carver et al. (1989) and Amirkhan (1990) primarily focussed on problem-solving (defence) vs. emotional avoidance (defeat), and social support seeking behaviours. The above described defence response in two separate bi–ethnic gender group studies, performed 10 years apart, was related to similar outcomes, i.e. disturbed cardiometabolic responses (Malan et al. 2006, 2012, 2014). Given the focus of our review, our approach will be from a neurophysiological angle, as sensory perception and a hypervigilant state burden central neural control, thereby overloading an individual's resources, so to induce neural and adrenal fatigue (De Kock et al. 2012, 2015; Malan et al. 2008, 2012, 2013, 2015; Scheepers et al. 2015, 2016). This concurs (Fig. 2) with most recent neuroscience research findings (LeDoux 2012).

A defensive state is triggered by activity in survival circuits that detect threats and generate automatic defence and a general arousal state due to widespread release of aminergic neuromodulators (Moscarello and LeDoux 2013). Memory processing or thoughts are implicated in this process with emotions resulting from the cognitive processing of actual situations. Coping has been defined as "cognitive

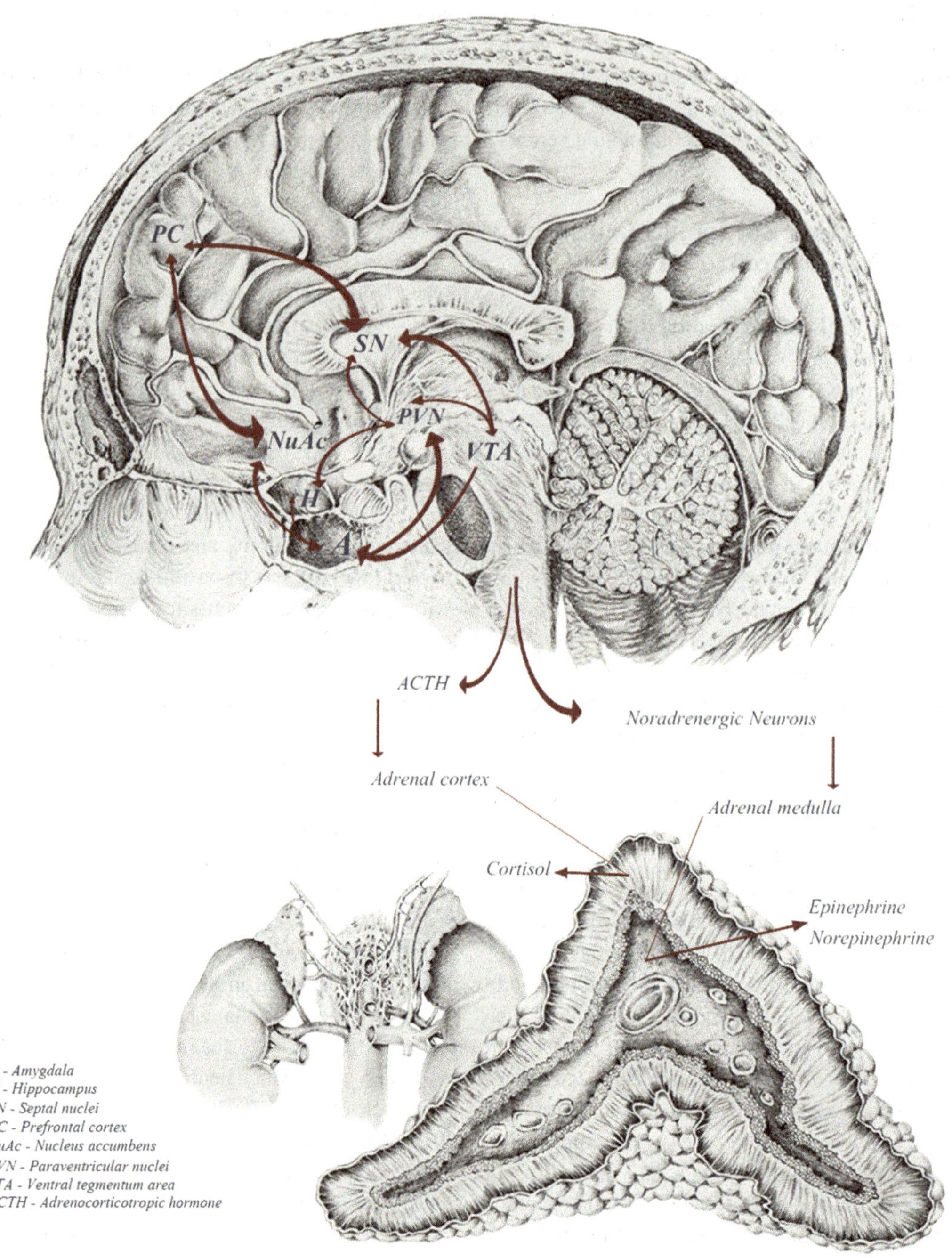

Fig. 2 Proposed sensory-motor integrative defensive responses involve sensory perception and a state of consciousness of environmental changes (internal and external) in the thalamus. Memory processing or thoughts are implicated in the process. Downstream signalling in the insula region will activate emotional responses in the amygdala whereas the importance of the stimuli as a threat or a challenge is weighted in the hippocampus. The nucleus accumbens will regulate motivation for recognition of stimuli in the prefrontal cortex. The paraventricular nucleus in the hypothalamus will respond and activate the autonomic nervous system motor output pathway; considering the integrated emotional response in the ventral tegmentum area. Output signals will be conducted via the brain stem to the heart (Permission to use diagram granted by the artists: A de Kock and AJG du Plessis, April, 2016)

and behavioural efforts to manage specific external or internal demands (and conflicts between them) that are appraised as taxing to the resources of a person" (Amirkhan 1990). Coping resources can be divided into internal psychological resources (e.g. personality characteristics) and external environmental resources (e.g. social support). Coping also has behavioural facets (activities to deal with stress) as well as physiological implications (neuro-endocrine activity and cardiovascular reactivity) (Moscarello and LeDoux 2013).

Chronic stress experience, such as the psychosocial stress of an urban-dwelling lifestyle, and ultimately acculturation (Malan et al. 1992, 1996) may however exacerbate cardiovascular reactivity to acute stressors (Malan et al. 2006, 2012, 2013), and predispose to hypertension (Malan et al. 2006, 2012). When coping is successful, the vagal system is typically activated to decrease secretion of stress mediators and to normalise autonomic activity, whilst α_2-adrenergic receptor binding activates a negative feedback loop to decrease norepinephrine levels (Huang et al. 2012). However, chronic stress, sleep deprivation or apnoea, sedentary lifestyles, stimulant abuse, abdominal obesity, insulin resistance, hypertension, and depression, can all cause chronic sympathetic hyperactivity with disruption of autonomic homeostasis (Curtis and O'Keefe 2002; Malan et al. 2013). Overwhelming or sustained stress may therefore interfere with coping ability, causing distress and hyperactivity of the SAM system, as the body tries to cope with increasing demands. As such neither the vagal system nor the negative feedback mechanism of the α_2-adrenergic receptors will be able to reduce the amounts of norepinephrine released (Curtis et al. 2002; Huang et al. 2012; Malan et al. 2012). Concentrations will increase even further and may culminate in norepinephrine overload, enforcing a hypervigilant defensive coping state. Indeed, findings have revealed that prolonged SAM activation and/or norepinephrine overload can further increase vasoconstriction, alter cardiovascular stress responses, and facilitate hypertension, endothelial dysfunction as well as atherosclerosis risk

(De Kock et al. 2012, 2015; Malan et al. 2008, 2012, 2013, 2015, 2016; Scheepers et al. 2016).

Cross-cultural differences in coping have been related to perspectives on the Self in a western context. The Self is the basis of what the individual thinks, feels and does and reflects the relative importance of the individual-self versus social-self (Chang 1996) The Self-construct, as social construct, is a cultural construct that shows cross-cultural variance. In collectivistic groups, the Self is defined as part of the inner group. Independency in collectivistic groups (in the Black African culture) means that the individual does not want to be a burden to his/her inner group (Van der Wateren 1997). Independency in individualistic cultures (in the White Western culture) indicates a need in the individual to act his/her own way (Triandis et al. 1990). In an urban environment, Black individuals may find it difficult to maintain their traditional way of life and in order to survive, may feel the need to abandon their traditional beliefs. The social support they experienced in a traditional setting will disappear (Malan et al. 1992, 1996, 2008; Vorster et al. 2005). Thus Whites might be able to find solutions for their own problems whereas Blacks depending on support and approval from their inner group might be more Indeed, they sought more social support, as coping strategy, to adapt in an urban environment (Malan et al. 2008, 2013, 2015).

In the African Black, it could imply that if defence coping on a long-term basis becomes untenable because the situation is judged as "no way out", a shift towards defeat, neural fatigue or depression is a conceivable outcome (De Kock et al. 2012, 2015; Malan et al. 2006, 2008). This implies a physiological neural fatigue or reaction with enhanced sympathetic activity, especially vascular reactivity (Malan et al. 2006, 2012, 2013). On behavioural level, the urban Black individuals still reported a defence coping reaction style, but with a physiological reaction resembling emotional distress or neural fatigue (De Kock et al. 2012). The "normal" physiological reaction pattern changes where defence coping (in-control) is dissociated from the normal physiological reaction and is exhibited as a

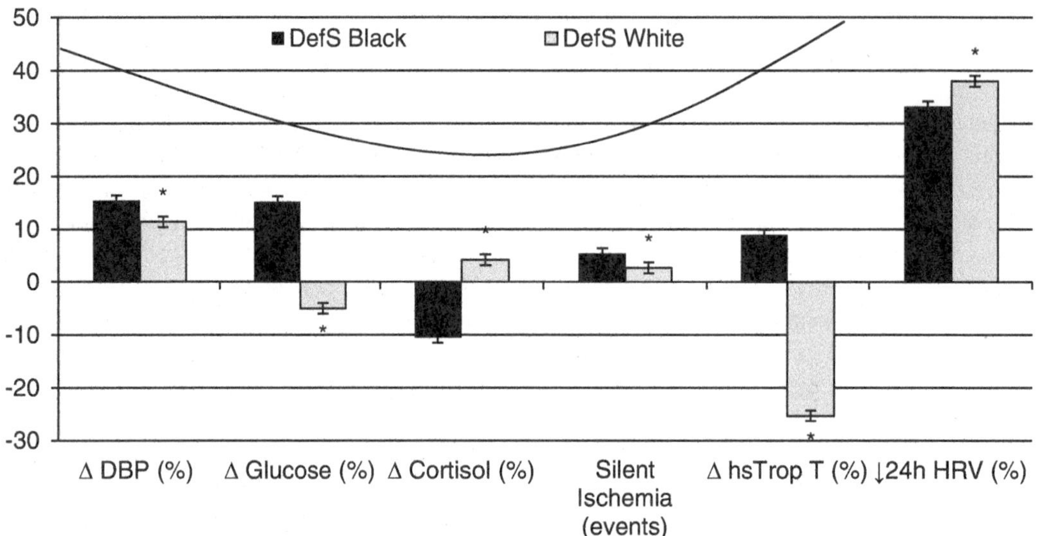

Fig. 3 Adjusted central control (BP-glucose) and coronary artery risk markers including changes (Δ) during exposure to a 1 min mental stressor test in an ethnic cohort utilising defence coping, independent of *concomitant* confounders. *, P ≤ 0.05

physiological neural fatigue or loss-of-control reaction. This pattern could indicate a physiological adaptation process where African Blacks with an inherent collectivistic cultural context are living in an individualistic cultural environment and, if anticipated support is not forthcoming, stress will be exacerbated (Ryff and Singer 2002). Adaptive learned behaviours of defensive coping Africans might therefore reflect life choices of smoking and alcohol consumption, which appears to be ineffective in handling normal challenges of daily life (Malan et al. 2014). Their enhanced vascular reactivity due to alpha-adrenergic stimulation and / or beta-adrenergic hyporesponsiveness (Malan et al. 2012, 2013) will have permissive effects on cortisol (De Kock et al. 2012, 2015), and may further impact on depression or distress via the HPAA (Björntorp 2001; Folkow 2000). Therefore, it appears that coping styles, as possible risk factors for cardiometabolic disturbance, may be contributing to the development of hypertension in an urban-dwelling environment.

Unpublished data in defensive coping African Black vs. Whites reinforce the notion of disruption in central neural control of BP. Defence coping increases activation of HPAA pathways during exposure to an acute mental stressor (Stroop 1935), similar to everyday life stress (Kidd et al. 2014). Responses to an acute mental stressor indicative of emotional distress are presented in Fig. 3. Vasoconstrictive responses (DBP) and lower cortisol responses are accompanied by increased insular region activation, high sensitive Troponin T release and 24 h silent ischemic events. Central neural control activation occurs via acutely increased metabolic changes, i.e. glucose responses which support the defence response. The pattern is maladaptive in urban-dwelling Blacks and emotional distress seems to disrupt homeostatic control. Hence, SAM activation will induce a depression in heart rate variability (HRV) to maintain central neural control.

3.2 Emotional Stress and an Urban-Dwelling Lifestyle

As early as 1929, Donnison (1929) screened approximately 1,000 male Kenyans, aged 15–80 years, living in primitive conditions in a native reserve. He showed that BP was similar or slightly lower in aged compared to younger

Kenyans. Sobngwi et al. (2004) supported these findings, showing that lifetime exposure to urbanization was associated with increases in obesity, BP, and diabetes but not with age. Similarly Danaei et al. (2011) reported increases in systolic blood pressure (SBP) in 5.4 million participants from low to middle income countries when moving from a traditional rural area to an urbanized area. In Ghana West Africa, the odds ratios for being hypertensive were 1.9 (1.3–2.9; P < 0.01) for urban men and 1.9 (1.3–2.8; P < 0.0001) for urban women, independent of age (Agyemang 2006).

Since 1989, transition from an rural to an urban-dwelling environment in approximately 4,000 Black Africans from the Venda, Botswana and the North-West regions in South Africa, was related to cultural disruption, increases in emotional distress, hypertension prevalence (Malan L, et al. 2006, 2008, 2012; Malan NT, et al. 1992, 1996; Vorster et al. 2005) as well as vascular changes such as angiogenesis (Venter et al. 2014). Apart from cultural disruption, other aggravating factors, like crime, come into play emphasizing why an urban-dwelling lifestyle has been recognized as a potent psychosocial stressor for CVD risk (Björntorp 2001; Malan et al. 2006). Official crime statistics of 2016 in SSA recorded that in only one of the urban-dwelling areas in SSA about 78 % car hijackings, 74 % of car thefts, and 57 % of house robberies occurred compared to other urban-dwelling areas (South African Cities Urban Safety Reference Group (USRG) 2016). In agreement, BeLue et al., showed increased CVD risk in urban environments (BeLue et al. 2009).

Apart from cultural disruption, these statistics additionally emphasize the burden of an urban-dwelling lifestyle in SSA (BeLue et al. 2009). Overall, psychosocial stress has been associated with the more negative spectrum of health effects i.e., increases in perceived stress, hypocortisolism, vascular responsiveness, central obesity, hypertension prevalence and other risk factors for NCDs (Danaei et al. 2011; Malan et al. 1992; Malan et al. 2015, 2016; Rosmond 2005; Sobngwi et al. 2004). These findings are supported by the synergistic effect of cardiometabolic risk markers and defensiveness in African men (De Kock et al. 2015; Malan et al. 2008, 2015; Scheepers et al. 2015, 2016). An urban over-demanding and unsafe environment seemingly increase demands on central neural control systems and coping with these demands may be taxing on the cardiovascular system (Malan et al. 2006, 2008), if endured chronically (Malan et al. 2015, 2016). Subsequently, higher demands on central neural control centres, if chronically challenged, will increase NCDs morbidity, as has just been shown by Hamer et al. (2015), von Känel et al. (2016) and Malan et al. (2016) From these findings, it is apparent that acculturated communities are even more vulnerable to NCDs than even those having lived their entire lives in an urban environment (Malan et al. 1996; Sobngwi et al. 2004). Neurobiological pathway regulation and behavioural or lifestyle factors are thus instrumental to cope with a taxing environment.

3.3 Behavioural Risk Factors – Neurobiological Pathways

Psychological distress and coping disability have been associated with dysregulated neurobiological pathways and changes in behavioural risk factors such as a poor diet, physical inactivity, increases in smoking and alcohol consumption (Alberts et al. 2005; Cois and Ehrlich 2014; Deasy et al. 2014; Layte and Whelan 2009; Parrott 1999; Sinha and Jastreboff 2013; WHO 2014).

3.3.1 Obesity

Chronic and high levels of repeated and uncontrollable stress result in dysregulation of the HPAA, with changes in glucocorticoid gene expression affecting energy homeostasis and feeding behaviour (Könner 2011; Sinha and Jastreboff 2013). Chronic stress persistently increases glucocorticoids, and promotes central obesity which, in the presence of insulin will decrease HPAA activity (Björntorp 2001). With chronic stress, corticotrophin, glucocorticoids and catecholamine activities are altered to increase sensitization of reward pathways (including the ventral tegmental area, nucleus accumbens, dorsal striatum and the prefrontal cortex areas) (Könner 2011). These pathways influence preference for addictive substances, highly palatable foods and increases drug/food craving and intake (Tyrka et al. 2012). The extra-hypothalamic projections of corticotrophin are involved in subjective and behavioural responses to stress, while release of neuropeptide Y (NPY) during stress and increased NPY mRNA in the arcuate nucleus of the hypothalamus, amygdala and hippocampus, increase feeding, but also decrease anxiety and stress (Maniam and Morris 2012). This motivational circuit overlaps with limbic regions controlling emotions (e.g. the amygdala, hippocampus, and insula) that play a role in experiencing emotions and stress, and in learning and memory processes involved in negotiating behavioural and cognitive responses critical for adaptation and homeostasis (Maniam and Morris 2012). The coping or self-medicating functions of these habitual behaviours make the costs of giving them up particularly difficult and limit the ability to adopt healthy but challenging behaviours (Lutfey and Freese 2005).

3.3.2 Physical Inactivity

Hallgren et al. (2016) demonstrated that exercise interventions reduced depression and moderated sensitivity to stress. However, they stated that longitudinal studies are still needed to confirm long term outcomes. Indeed, both smoking and physical inactivity alleviated stress in the short term, but it was shown to increase stress levels in the long term (Sinha and Jastreboff 2013). In SSA, behavioural risk markers were also related to increases in NCDs (Groenewald et al. 2007; Hamer et al. 2011; World Health Organisation 2014). South Africans additionally demonstrated high rates of physical inactivity prevalence rates, with 46.4 % of men and 55.7 % of women, not meeting the recommended guidelines (McGuire et al. 2009; World Health Organisation 2014). However, we could not replicate findings that physical activity of different intensity was directly associated with markers of

chronic stress or telomere length in an African teachers' cohort (von Känel et al. 2016).

3.3.3 Smoking and Alcohol Habits

In South Africa, the prevalence of tobacco use varies by population group and gender and the use of tobacco in women is at very high levels (Groenewald et al. 2007). Alcohol consumption however, remains the most serious concern in SSA (Malan et al. 2016; Zatu et al. 2016), mostly so in men (Bosu 2010). In a meta-analysis involving under-developed and middle-income countries, South Africa was rated as one of the countries with the highest hypertension prevalence rates, with alcohol abuse, in individuals younger than 50 years, being one of the most significant predictors for hypertension in Blacks (Lloyd-Sherlock et al. 2014).

Alcohol abuse was independently associated with BP, transient 24 h ischemic events, autonomic dysfunction and structural vascular disease in Ghana (Agyemang 2006), Uganda (Bosu 2010; Kotwani et al. 2013) and South Africa (Malan et al. 2013, Malan et al. 2014; Oosthuizen et al. in press). Gamma glutamyl transferase, a marker of alcohol consumption (Hastedt et al. 2013), predicted cardiovascular [HR = 2.76 (1.49–5.12)] and all-cause mortality [HR = 2.47 (1.75–3.47)] and hypertension development [(HR = 1.31 (1.06–1.62)] in 1,471 black South Africans over 5 years (Zatu et al. 2016).

Alcohol consumption of more than 58 g/day predicted subcortical silent brain infarction and was recognised as a risk factor for stroke [OR, 2.58 (95 % CI, 1.50 to 4.45)] (Kobayashi et al. 1997). The impact of alcohol abuse in Blacks may thus be detrimental to subcortical and vascular health in Blacks. Alcohol is a central nervous system depressant, which can induce higher metabolic demands and vascular depression (Hastedt et al. 2013; Kobayashi et al. 1997; Van Deventer and Lindeque 2015). Therefore, statistical adjustment for alcohol abuse in data analyses fails to provide a clear answer when considering the effect of ethanol on the brain, vasculature and metabolism. Alcohol abuse as defence mechanism to cope with a taxing environment (Malan et al. 2014, 2015, 2016) might thus induce depression. Whether depression *per se* truly reflects emotional distress or alternatively, whether alcohol abuse induces subcortical depression and ischemia in Blacks, however, remains to be investigated.

4 From Basic Research to Clinical Practice

In comparison with data from other countries, South Africa has lower rates of depression, than the USA but higher rates than Nigeria, where general practioners fail to detect 33–50 % of depressive disorders in patients (Ngcobo and Pillay 2008; Tomlinson et al. 2009). However, depression has recently been acknowledged as a risk factor for cardiac remodelling and poor prognosis in patients with coronary heart disease (Lichtman et al. 2014). Presently, we underscore the importance of emotional distress when utilizing chronic defence coping as it was associated with left ventricular hypertrophy, neural and adrenal fatigue in a Black cohort from SSA (De Kock et al. 2012, 2015; Malan et al. 2016; Mashele et al. 2014). We have observed that emotional distress increased cardiometabolic demands and disrupted central neural control of BP in a Black cohort from SSA (Malan et al. 2016). We cautiously suggest that more hypotheses-driven longitudinal studies are needed to inform the medical community on emotional stress as an important cause of a high prevalence of hypertension. If not investigated, implementation of interventions for preventive health care programs will be slowed down.

Africans behaviourally might thus be masking the truth by reporting emotional well-being, which contrasts with physiological loss of control with disturbed central neural control increasing blood pressure and thus hypertension prevalence. Currently, recommendations are for (1) longitudinal studies focussing on emotional stress; (2) screening of BP, ECGs (depressed HRV), central obesity as well as for signs of depression to detect disturbed central neural control; and lastly, we recommend (3) appointment of school counsellors to support the acquirement of healthy coping strategies at a tender age which may prove to be more effective compared to changing the lifestyle habits of adults (Vedanthan et al. 2016).

Acknowledgements The SABPA study and findings on emotional stress and hypertension would not have been possible without the volunteering participant sample, the dedicated input of the Hypertension in Africa Research Team (HART), GJ Motlhasedi (Fieldworker), C Lessing (Research Nurse), S Péter (MD) and in-kind analyses of the national and international expert team.

Conflicts of Interest No conflicts of interest declared.

References

Agyemang C (2006) Rural and urban differences in blood pressure and hypertension in Ghana. West Afr Public Health 120(6):525–533

Akinroye K (2013) Nigerians wake up to high blood pressure. Bull World Health Organ 91:242–243

Alberts M, Urdal P, Steyn K, Stensvold I, Tverdal A, Nel JH et al (2005) Prevalence of cardiovascular diseases and associated risk factors in a rural black population of South Africa. Eur J Cardiovasc Prev Rehab 12 (4):347–354

Amirkhan JH (1990) A factor analytically derived measure of coping: the coping strategy indicator. J Pers Soc Psych 59:1066–1074

Barton DA, Dawood T, Lambert EA, Esler MD, Haikerwal D, Brenchley C, Socratous F, Kaye DM, Schlaich MP, Hickie I, Lambert GW (2007) Sympathetic activity in major depressive disorder: identifying those at increased cardiac risk? J Hypertens 25(10):2117–2124

BeLue R, Okoror TA, Iwelunmor J, Taylor KD, Degboe AN, Agyemang C, Ogedegbe G (2009) An overview of cardiovascular risk factor burden in sub-Saharan African countries: a socio-cultural perspective. Glob Health 5:1

Biccard BM (2008) Anaesthesia for vascular procedures: how do South African patients differ? SAJAA 14:109e115

Björntorp P (2001) Do stress reactions cause abdominal obesity and comorbidities? Obes Rev 2:73–86

Bosu WK (2010) Epidemic of hypertension in Ghana: a systematic review. BMC Public Health 10:418

Cabib SS (1996) Stress, depression and the mesolimbic dopamine system. Psycho-Pharmacol (Berl) 128 (4):331–342

Carver CS, Scheier MF, Weintraub JK (1989) Assessing coping strategies: a theoretically base approach. J Pers Soc Psych 57(2):267–283

Chang EC (1996) Cultural differences in optimism, pessimism, and coping: predictors of subsequent adjustment in Asian American and Caucasian American college students. J Couns Psych 43(1):113–123

Cois A, Ehrlich R (2014) Analysing the socioeconomic determinants of hypertension in South Africa: a structural equation modelling approach. BMC Public Health 14(1):414

Curtis BM, O'Keefe JH (2002) Autonomic tone as a cardiovascular risk factor: the dangers of chronic fight or flight. Mayo Clin Proc 77:45–54

Danaei G, Finucane MM, Lu Y, Singh GM, Cowan MJ, Paciorek CJ et al (2011) National, regional, and global trends in fasting plasma glucose and diabetes prevalence since 1980: systematic analysis of health examination surveys and epidemiological studies with 370 country-years and 2 · 7 million participants. Lancet 378(9785):31–40

De Kock A, Malan L, Potgieter JC, Steenekamp W, Van der Merwe M-T (2012) Metabolic syndrome indicators and target organ damage in urban active coping African and Caucasian men: the SABPA Study. Exp Clin Endocrin Diab 120(5):282–287

De Kock A, Malan L, Hamer M, Cockeran M, Malan NT (2015) Defensive coping and renovascular disease risk – adrenal fatigue in a cohort of Africans and Caucasians: the SABPA study. Phys Behav 147(8):213–219

Deasy C, Coughlan B, Pironom J, Jourdan D, Mcnamara PM (2014) Psychological distress and lifestyle of students: implications for health promotion. Health Prom Int. doi:10.1093/heapro/dau086

Dobrunz LE, Stevens CF (1997) Heterogeneity of release probability, facilitation, and depletion at central synapses. Neuron 18:995–1008

Donnison CP (1929) Blood pressure in the African native: its bearing upon the aetiology of hyperpiesa and arteriosclerosis. Lancet 223:6–7

Folkow B (2000) Perspectives on the integrative functions of the 'sympatho-adreno-medullary system'. Auton Neurosci 83:101–115

Groenewald P, Vos T, Norman R, Laubscher R, Van Walbeek C, Saloojee U et al (2007) Estimating the burden of disease attributable to smoking in South Africa in 2000. S Afr Med J 97(8):674–681

Gross CG (1998) Claude Bernard and the constancy of the internal environment. Neuroscientist 4(5):380–385

Hallgren M, Herring MP, Owen N, Dunstan D, Ekblom Ö, Helgadottir B, Nakitanda OA, Forsell Y (2016) Exercise, physical activity, and sedentary behavior in the treatment of depression: broadening the scientific perspectives and clinical opportunities. Front Psychiatr 7:36. doi:10.3389/fpsyt.2016.00036

Hamer M, Von Känel R, Reimann MNT, Schutte AE, Huisman HW, Malan L (2015) Progression of cardiovascular risk factors in Black Africans: 3 year follow up of the SABPA cohort study. Atherosclerosis 238:52e54

Hamer M, Malan L, Malan NT, Schutte AE, Huisman HW, van Rooyen JM, Schutte R, Fourie CMT, Seedat YK (2011) Objectively assessed health behaviors and sub-clinical atherosclerosis in black and white Africans: the SABPA study. Atherosclerosis 215:237–242

Hastedt M, Büchner M, Rothe M, Gapert R, Herre S, Krumbiegel F et al (2013) Detecting alcohol abuse: traditional blood alcohol markers compared to ethyl glucuronide (EtG) and fatty acid ethyl esters (FAEEs) measurement in hair. Foren Sci Med Pathol 9(4):471–477

Huang HP, Zhu FP, Chen XW, Xu ZQ, Zhang CX, Zhou Z (2012) Physiology of quantal norepinephrine release from somatodendritic sites of neurons in locus coeruleus. Front Mol Neurosci 5(29):1–5

Jennings JR, Muldoon MF, Ryan C, Price JC, Greer P, Sutton-Tyrrell K, van der Veen FM, Meltzer CC (2005) Reduced cerebral blood flow response and compensation among patients with untreated hypertension. Neurology 64(8):1358–1365

Kadirvelu A, Sadasivan S, Ng SH (2012) Social support in type II diabetes care: a case of too little, too late. Diabetes Metab Synd Obes Targets Ther 5:407–417

Kidd T, Livia A, Steptoe A (2014) The relationship between cortisol responses to laboratory stress and cortisol profiles in daily life. Biol Psych 99:34–40

Kobayashi S, Okada K, Koide H, Bokura H, Yamaguchi S (1997) Subcortical silent brain infarction as a risk factor for clinical stroke. Stroke 28:1932–1939

Könner AC (2011) Role for insulin signaling in catecholaminergic neurons in control of energy homeostasis. Cell Metab 13:720–728

Kotwani P, Kwarisiima D, Clark TD, Kabami J, Geng EH, Jain V et al (2013) Epidemiology and awareness of hypertension in a rural Ugandan community: a cross-sectional study. BMC Public Health 13:1151

Kvetnansky R, Sabban EL, Palkovits M (2009) Catecholaminergic systems in stress: structural and molecular genetic approaches. Phys Rev 89(2):535–606

Lambert GW, Ferrier C, Kaye D, Kalff V, Kelly MJ, Cox HS et al (1994) Monoaminergic neuronal activity in subcortical brain regions in essential hypertension. Blood Press 3:55–66

Lambert G, Johansson M, Agren H, Friberg P (2000) Evidence of reduced central nervous system norepinephrine and dopamine turnover in patients with depressive illness. Arch Gen Psychiatry 57:787–793

LeDoux J (2012) Rethinking the emotional brain. Neuron 73(4):653–676

Lichtman J, Froelicher FS, Blumenthal JA, Carney RM, Doering LV, Frasure-Smith N et al (2014) Depression as a risk factor for poor prognosis among patients with acute coronary syndrome: systematic review and recommendations. A scientific statement from the American Heart Association. Circulation 129:1350–1369

Lloyd-Sherlock P, Beard J, Minicuci N, Ebrahim S, Chatterjii S (2014) Hypertension among older adults in low- and middle-income countries: prevalence, awareness and control. Int J Epidem 43(1):116–128

Lund C, De Silva M, Plagerson S, Cooper S, Crisholm D, Das J et al (2011) Poverty and mental disorders: breaking the cycle in low-income and middle-income countries. Lancet 378:1502–1514

Lutfey K, Freese J (2005) Toward some fundamentals of fundamental causality: socioeconomic status and health in the routine clinic visit for diabetes. Am J Sociol 110:1326–1372

Malan NT, Van der Merwe JS, Eloff FC, Huisman HW, Kruger A, Eloff FC et al (1992) A comparison of cardiovascular reactivity of rural Blacks, Urban Blacks and Whites. Stress Med 8:214–246

Malan NT, Brits JS, Eloff FC, Huisman HW, Kruger A, Laubscher PJ et al (1996) The influence of acculturation on endocrine reactivity during acute stress in urban black males. Stress Med 12:55–63

Malan L, Schutte AE, Malan NT, Wissing MP, Vorster HH, Steyn HS et al (2006) Specific coping strategies of Africans during urbanization: comparing cardiovascular responses and perception of health data. Biol Psych 72(3):305–310

Malan L, Malan NT, Wissing MP, Seedat YK (2008) Coping with urbanization: a cardiometabolic risk? Biol Psych 79:323–328

Malan L, Hamer M, Schlaich MP, Lambert GW, Harvey BH, Reimann M et al (2012) Facilitated defensive coping, silent ischaemia and ECG left-ventricular hypertrophy: the SABPA study. J Hypertens 30:543–550

Malan L, Hamer M, Schlaich MP, Lambert GW, Ziemssen T, Reimann M et al (2013) Defensive coping facilitates higher blood pressure and early sub-clinical structural vascular disease via alterations in heart rate variability: the SABPA study. Atherosclerosis 227:391–397

Malan L, Oosthuizen W, Scheepers JD, Möller-Wolmarans M, Malan NT (2014) Coping and autonomic dysfunction act in tandem with alcohol-related sub-clinical atherosclerosis: the SABPA Study. In: Raines J (ed) Substance abuse: prevalence, genetic and environmental risk factors and prevention. Nova Science Publishers, New York, pp 107–128

Malan L, Hamer M, Frasure-Smith N, Steyn HS, Malan NT (2015) COHORT PROFILE: sympathetic activity and ambulatory blood pressure in Africans (SABPA) prospective cohort study. Int J Epidem 6:1814–1822

Malan L, Hamer M, von Känel R, Schlaich MP, Reimann M, Frasure-Smith N et al (2016) Chronic depression symptoms and salivary NOx associated with retinal vascular dysregulation: the SABPA study. Nitric Oxide 55–56:10–17

Mancia G, Fagard R, Narkiewicz K, Redo J, Zanchetti A, Böhm M et al (2013) 2013 ESH/ESC guidelines for the management of arterial hypertension. The Task Force for the management of arterial hypertension of the European Society of Hypertension (ESH) and of the European Society of Cardiology. J Hypertens 31:1281–1357

Maniam J, Morris MJ (2012) The link between stress and feeding behaviour. Neuropharmacology 63:97–110

Mashele N, Malan L, Van Rooyen JM, Harvey BH, Potgieter JC, Hamer M (2014) Blunted neuroendocrine responses linking depressive symptoms and ECG left ventricular hypertrophy in black Africans: the SABPA study. Cardiovasc Endocrin 3:59–65

Mayosi BM, Flisher AJ, Lalloo UG, Sitas F, Tollman SM, Bradshaw D (2012) The burden of non-communicable diseases in South Africa. Lancet 374(9693):934–947

Mazzeo AT, Micalizzi A, Mascia L, Scicolone A, Siracusano L (2014) Brain–heart crosstalk: the many faces of stress-related cardiomyopathy syndromes in anaesthesia and intensive care. Br J Anaesth 112(5):803–815

McDougall SJ, Münzberg H, Derbenev AV, Zsombok A (2015) Central control of autonomic functions in health and disease. Front Neurosci 8:440. doi:10.3389/fnins.2014.00440

McEwen BS, Gianaros PJ (2010) Central role of the brain in stress and adaptation: links to socioeconomic status, health, and disease. Ann NY Acad Sci 1186:190–222

McGuire KA, Janssen I, Ross R (2009) Ability of physical activity to predict cardiovascular disease beyond commonly evaluated cardiometabolic risk factors. Am J Cardiol 104:1522–1526

Moscarello JM, LeDoux JE (2013) Active avoidance learning requires prefrontal suppression of amygdala-mediated defensive reactions. J Neurosci 33(9):3815–3823

Nagai M, Hoshide S, Kario K (2010) The insular cortex and cardiovascular system: a new insight into the brain-heart axis. J Am Soc Hypertens 4(4):174–182

National Development Plan(2016) South Africa, Vision 2030. The State of Urban Safety in South Africa Report

Ngcobo M, Pillay PJ (2008) Depression in African women presenting for psychological services at a general hospital. Afr J Psychiatr 11:133–137

Nishida Y, Tandal-Hiruma M, Kemuriyama T, Hagisawa K (2012) Long-term blood pressure control: is there a set-point in the brain? J Physiol Sci 62:147–161

Oosthuizen W, Malan L, Scheepers JD, Cockeran M, Malan NT (in press) The defence response and alcohol intake: a coronary artery disease risk? J Clin Exp Hypertens

Pal GK, Adithan C, Dutta TK, Pal P, Nanda N, Lalitha V et al (2014) Association of hypertension status and cardiovascular risks with sympathovagal imbalance in first degree relatives of type 2 diabetics. J Diab Invest 5(4):449–455

Parrott AC (1999) Does cigarette smoking cause stress? Am Psychol 54(10):817–820

Peck RN, Green E, Mtabaji J, Majinge C, Smart LR, Downs JA et al (2013) Hypertension-related diseases as a common cause of hospital mortality in Tanzania: a 3-year prospective study. J Hypertens 31(9):1806–1811

Reed RV, Fazel M, Jones L, Panter-Brick C, Stein A (2012) Mental health of displaced and refugee children resettled in low-income and middle-income countries: risk and protective factors. Lancet 379:250–265

Rosmond R (2005) Role of stress in the pathogenesis of the metabolic syndrome. Psychoneuroendocrinology 30:1–10

Ryff CD, Singer B (2002) From social structure to biology. In: Snyder CR, Lopez SJ (eds) Handbook of positive psychology. Oxford University Press, Oxford, pp 541–555

Saez I, Duran J, Sinadinos C, Beltran A, Yanes O, Tevy MF et al (2014) Neurons have an active glycogen metabolism that contributes to tolerance to hypoxia. J Cerebral Blood Flow Met 34:945–955

Scheepers JD, Malan L, De Kock A, Malan NT, Cockeran M, von Känel R (2015) Ethnic disparity in defensive coping endothelial responses: the SABPA study. Phys Behav 147(8):306–312

Scheepers JD, Malan L, von Ka¨nel R, De Kock A, Cockeran M, Malan NT (2016) Hypercoagulation and hyperkinetic blood pressure indicative of physiological loss-of-control despite behavioural control in Africans: the SABPA study. Blood Pressure, 1–9 [Epub ahead of print]. PMID: 26806201

Schutte AE, Schutte R, Huisman HW, van Rooyen JM, Fourie CM, Malan NT et al (2012) Are behavioural risk factors to be blamed for the conversion from optimal blood pressure to hypertensive status in Black South Africans? A 5-year prospective study. Int J Epidemiol 41(4):1114–1123

Seedat YK (2015) Why is control of hypertension in sub-Saharan Africa poor? Cardiovasc J Afr 26 (4):193–195

Sinha R, Jastreboff AM (2013) Stress as a common risk factor for obesity and addiction. Biol Psychiatry 73 (9):827–835

Skinner EA, Edge K, Altman J, Sherwood H (2003) Searching for the structure of coping: a review and critique of category systems for classifying ways of coping. Psych Bull 129(2):216–269

Sobngwi E, Mbanya J-C, Unwin N, Porcher R, Kengne A-P, Fezeu L et al (2004) Exposure over the life course to an urban environment and its relation with obesity, diabetes, and hypertension in rural and urban Cameroon. Int J Epidemiol 33:769–776

South African Cities Urban Safety Reference Group (USRG) (2016) The state of urban safety in South Africa report 2016. South African Cities Network: http://www.saferspaces.org.za/uploads/files/State-of-Urban-Safety-Brochure-web.pdf

Stahrenberg R, Niehaus C-F, Edelmann F, Mende M, Wohlfahrt J, Wasser K et al (2013) High-sensitivity troponin assay improves prediction of cardiovascular risk in patients with cerebral ischaemia. J Neurol Neurosurg Pscyhiatr 84(5):479–487

Stroop JR (1935) Studies of interference in serial verbal reactions. J Exp Psych 18:643–662

Tagoe HA, Dake FAA (2011) Healthy lifestyle behaviour among Ghanaian adults in the phase of a health policy change. Glob Health 7:7

Taylor WD, Aizenstein HJ, Alexopoulos GS (2013) The vascular depression hypothesis: mechanisms linking vascular disease with depression. Mol Psych 18 (9):963–974

Tomlinson M, Grimsrud AT, Stein DJ, Williams DR, Myer L (2009) The epidemiology of major depression in South Africa: results from the South African Stress and Health study. SA Med J 99(5, 2):367–373

Triandis HC, McCusker C, Hui CH (1990) Multimethod probes of individualism and collectivism. J Pers Soc Psych 59:1006–1020

Tyrka AR, Walters OC, Price LH, Anderson GM, Carpenter LL (2012) Altered response to neuroendocrine challenge linked to indices of the metabolic syndrome in healthy adults. Horm Metab Res 44:543–549

Van der Wateren E (1997) Dynamics of values, coping styles and psychological health in a young group. MA dissertation, Potchefstroom University for Christian Higher Education, Potchefstroom, 189 p

Van Deventer CA, Lindeque JZ, Jansen van Rensburg PJ, Malan L, Van der Westhuizen FH, Louw R (2015) Use of metabolomics to elucidate the metabolic perturbation associated with hypertension in a black South African male cohort: the SABPA study. J Am Soc Hypertens 9(2):104–14

Van Lill AS, Malan L, van Rooyen JM, Ziemssen T, Reimann M (2011) Baroreceptor sensitivity and left ventricular hypertrophy in urban South African men: the SABPA Study. Blood Pressure 20:355–361

Vedanthan R, Bansilal S, Soto AV, Kovacic JC, Latina J, Jaslow R et al (2016) Family-based approaches to cardiovascular health promotion. J Am Coll Cardiol 67(14):1725–1737

Venter PC, Malan L, Schutte AE (2014) Psychosocial stress but not hypertensive status associated with angiogenesis in Africans. Blood Press 23(5):307–314

von Känel R, Bruwer EJ, De Ridder JH, Swanepoel M, Hamer M, Cockeran M, Malan L (2016) Association between objectively measured physical activity, chronic stress and leukocyte telomere length. J Sport Med Phys Fitness [Epub ahead of print]. PMID: 27074439

Vorster HH, Venter CS, Wissing MP, Margetts BM (2005) The nutrition and health transition in the North West Province of South Africa: a review of the THUSA (Transition and Health during Urbanisation of South Africans) study. Public Health Nutr 8(5):480–490

World Health Organisation (2008) Closing the gap in a generation: health equity through action on the social determinants of health. World Health Organization, Geneva. Accessed Mar 2016.

World Health Organisation (2010) Mental health and development: targeting people with mental health conditions as a vulnerable group. World Health Organization, Geneva. Accessed Mar 2016.

World Health Organisation. (2014)The World health report: Non-communicable diseases country profiles 2014. Report, 1-207. World Health Organisation, Geneva. Accessed Mar 2016

Zatu MC, Van Rooyen JM, Kruger A, Schutte AE (2016) Alcohol intake, hypertension development and mortality in black South Africans. Eur J Prev Cardiol 23 (3):308–315

Adv Exp Med Biol - Advances in Internal Medicine (2017) 2: 511–540
DOI 10.1007/5584_2016_90
© Springer International Publishing AG 2016
Published online: 30 December 2016

Endothelial Dysfunction and Hypertension

Dildar Konukoglu and Hafize Uzun

Abstract

In the past, endothelium was thought to be only a mechanical barrier. Today, endothelium is known to be a tissue regulating vascular tone, cell growth and the interaction between the leukocytes, thrombocytes and the vessel wall. It also synthesizes growth factors and thrombo-regulatory molecules and responds to physical and chemical signals. Even though the term "endothelial dysfunction" is generally used for deterioration of endothelium-dependent vasodilatation; the term also includes the abnormalities between endothelium and leukocytes, thrombocytes and regulatory molecules and conditions resulting in aberrant endothelium activation. Healthy endothelium is essential for cardiovascular control. Thus, it plays an important role in pathogenesis of many diseases and cardiovascular problems such as atherosclerosis, systemic and pulmonary hypertension, cardiomyopathies and vasculitides. The aim of this chapter is to explain endothelial dysfunction and the circulating molecules of endothelial cells as they become potential targets of therapeutic approach for hypertension. This chapter reviews the roles of endothelial dysfunction in hypertension by addressing (1) the nature of endothelial function, (2) mechanisms of endothelial dysfunction and its relationship with the diseases (3) also endothelial function testing (4) the role of endothelial dysfunction and hypertension and (4) the effects of antihypertensive therapeutic options on the endothelial dysfunction. In addition to these, the role of endothelial dysfunction in white coat hypertension has been discussed. The key connections between hypertension and endothelial dysfunction are vitally important for future studies to permit new interventions to be designed and released.

D. Konukoglu and H. Uzun (✉)
Cerrahpasa Medical Faculty, Department of
Biochemistry, Istanbul University, Istanbul, Turkey
e-mail: huzun59@hotmail.com

Keywords

Endothelial dysfunction • Atherosclerosis • Hypertension • White coat hypertension • Coagulation • Fibrinolysis • Inflammatory mediators • Endothelium-derived relaxing factors • Endothelium-derived contracting factors: angiogenesis

1 Introduction

The term endothelial dysfunction is used to describe the altered metabolism of available nitric oxide (NO) or imbalance of several endothelium-derived relaxing and constrictor factors. Between the blood and the vascular wall, the endothelium forms both mechanical and biological barrier (Vanhoutte et al. 2009). Interactions between platelets and leukocytes with the vessel wall, impairment of vascular tone, inflammation, free radical formation and oxidation of lipids and vascular smooth muscle cell proliferation can be activate endothelial cells (ECs) (Lerman and Burnett Jr 1992). ECs function by secreting relaxing and/or contracting molecules. ECs are exposed to the shear stress resulting from blood flow and can convert mechanical stimuli into intracellular or biochemical signals (e.g., proliferation, apoptosis, migration, permeability, remodeling and gene expression) (Li et al. 2005a). As a result, endothelial dysfunction is related to several diseases including atherosclerosis, cancer metastasis, inflammatory diseases and hypertension (Rajendran et al. 2013).

Hypertension is defined as the presence of chronically elevated systemic arterial or diastolic blood pressure (BP) above a certain threshold whereas sustained hypertension is defined as systolic BP >140 mm Hg in medical environment and daytime ambulatory systolic BP >135 mm Hg, and/or medical environment diastolic BP >90 mm Hg and daytime ambulatory diastolic BP >85 mm Hg (Weber et al. 2014). Thus, the patients with sustained hypertension have increased BP levels in the medical environment (in clinics or office) and out of the medical environment (at home). Sustained high blood pressure is also an indicator of the age, diet, stress, sedentary lifestyle, all or the combination of these factors. It has been suggested that sustained hypertension is closely related to both target organ damage and organ function failure including heart, kidneys, and brain. Pathophysiology of hypertension is related to several factors, including genetics, activation of the sympathetic nervous system, the rennin- angiotensin (AT)- aldosterone system, endothelial dysfunction, impaired capillary blood flow and inflammatory mediators (Dawes et al. 2008; Oparil et al. 2003).

2 The Nature of Endothelial Function

Three layers of the artery wall from outside to inside comprise; tunica adventitia, tunica media and tunica intima. The layer of tunica adventitia; contains nerve endings, perivascular adipose tissue and connective elements, such as fibroblasts and collagen. It plays important roles in the vascular development and remodeling. The second layer, vascular smooth muscle, regulates the response of constriction and dilatation of the blood vessels. The mechanical stimuli, such as shear stress and pressure, or pharmacological stimuli activate the contraction of the vascular smooth muscle cells by increasing the intracellular calcium concentration. Tunica intima, the innermost layer of the vascular arterial wall, consists of monolayer ECs and connective tissues lie beneath the ECs. Substances can pass through the connection between ECs or are absorbed by the cells. As the vascular vessel sizes are about 60–80 nm in diameter, endothelium provides restriction for larger particles and

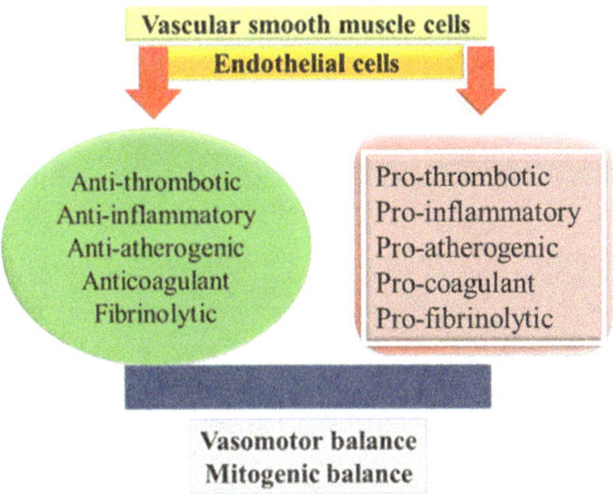

Fig. 1 Activities of endothelial cells. Vasomotor and mitogenic balance is provided by molecules secreted by endothelial cells and vascular smooth muscle cell. These cells have several paracrine functions by producing and secreting several molecules including vasoactive, inflammatory, vasculoprotective, angiogenic, thrombotic and antithrombotic

prevents the interaction between the blood cells and the vessel wall (Wilson and Lerman 2001; Vestweber 2012).

Multiprotein complexes containing transmembrane proteins (such as claudins, occludins, and junction adhesion molecules) and cytosol proteins that connect membrane proteins to the intracellular cytoskeleton form intercellular junctions between ECs (Chistiakov et al. 2015). The endothelium is also considered as an endocrine organ, while it demonstrates several paracrine functions by producing and secreting vasoactive, inflammatory, vasculoprotective, angiogenic, thrombotic and antithrombotic molecules (Fig. 1). Like the other endocrine organs, endothelium possesses receptors that display various cellular and hormonal events (Table 1).

2.1 Regulation of Vascular Tonicity

Vascular tonicity is regulated by atrial natriuretic peptide, eicosanoids, adrenal steroids, sodium, and water excretion and by the control of neurologic, kallikrein- kinin, reno-medullary endothelial systems. Molecules such as endothelin-1 (ET-1), angiotensin II (AT-II),

Table 1 Molecules which are produced and secreted by endothelial cells

Regulation of vascular tonicity	
Vasodilatation	Nitric oxide
	Prostacyclin
	Endothelium-derived hyperpolarizing factors
	Adenosine
Vasoconstriction	Endothelin-1
	Angiotensin II
	Thromboxane A_2
	Reactive oxygen species
Balancing of blood fluidity and thrombosis	
Coagulation	Heparin cofactor 2
	Factor V
	Protein S
	Protein C
	Thrombomodulin
	Tissue factor
	von Willebrand factor
Fibrinolysis	Tissue plasminogen activator
	Prostaglandins
	Plasminogen activator inhibitor type 1
	Urokinase
Vascular inflammatory and immunological process control	
Cytokines	Interleukin -1
	Interleukin-6
	Interleukin-8
	Monocyte chemoattractant protein-1
Adhesion molecules	Transforming growth factor
	Tumor necrosis factor
	Vascular cell adhesion protein 1
	Intercellular adhesion molecule 1
	Selectins
Growth factors	Basic fibroblast growth factor
	Insulin like growth factor
	Platelet derived growth factor
	Transforming growth factor

thromboxane A_2 (TXA$_2$), and reactive oxygen species (ROS) are known as endothelium-derived relaxing factors, whereas NO and prostacyclin are known as endothelium-derived hyperpolarizing factors (EDHFs) (Dawes et al. 2008). In healthy endothelial tissues, a

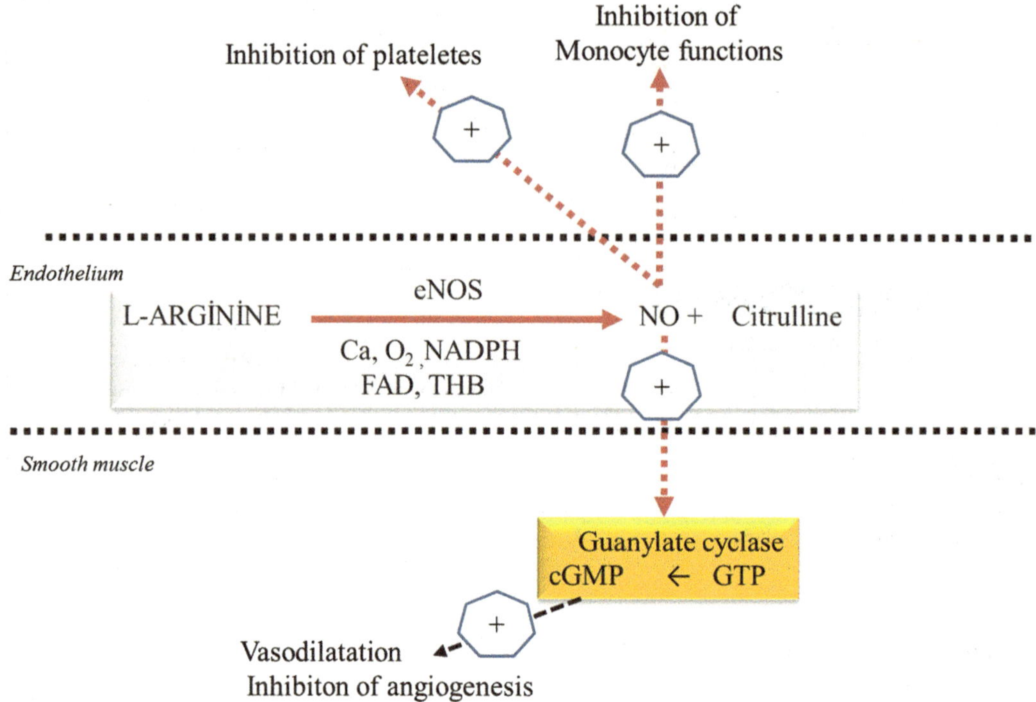

Fig. 2 Nitric oxide (NO) is synthesized by endothelial nitric oxidase synthase (eNOS) can activate soluble guanylate cyclase. cGMP is produced. Vasodilatation occurs, and angiogenesis is inhibited. NO inhibits both platelet and monocyte functions (Şekil Türkçe)

balance between endothelium-derived relaxing factors (EDRFs) and endothelium-derived contracting factors (EDCFs) is maintained. Disturbance of this balance causes endothelial dysfunction (Cahill and Redmond 2016).

Nitric Oxide (NO) Vascular smooth muscle cells release: Endothelium-derived NO, the known most powerful vasodilator which activates the soluble guanylate cyclase. Soluble Guanylate cyclase (sGS) enzyme converts GTP to cyclic GMP (cGMP) which activates protein kinase G that leads decreases in the cytosolic calcium concentrations. NO can also affect cellular activity, independently of sGC activation, by the stimulation of the endoplasmic reticulum calcium ATPase, reducing the intracellular calcium concentration and cause relaxation of the smooth muscle. The release of inflammation, vascular cell proliferation, platelet adhesion, and tissue factor are inhibited by NO (Laher 2014).

NO is synthesized from an L-arginine by the enzyme nitric oxide synthases (NOS) as a free radical (Fig. 2). There are three distinct genes encoding NOS isozymes; neuronal NOS (nNOS or NOS-1), cytokine-inducible NOS (iNOS or NOS-2) and endothelial NOS (eNOS or NOS-3) (Melikian et al. 2009) (Table 2). The production of NO from L-arginine by NOS requires the presence of various co-factors including tetrahydrobiopterin, flavin adenine dinucleotide, flavin mononucleotide, calmodulin (calcium binding protein) and iron protoporphyrin (Palmer et al. 1988). nNOS is expressed in the central and peripheral nervous systems, in cardiac and skeletal myocytes, smooth muscles and ECs. NO produced in the nervous systems by nNOS is associated with the regulation of neuronal excitability and synaptic plasticity, memory and learning processes. It has been suggested that the expression of vascular nNOS is also upregulated by stimulation with

Table 2 The forms of NO synthase

	Gene	Main Localization (s)	Functions	Stimulation
Neuronal NOS (nNOS;NOS-1) (calcium-dependent)	Chromosome 12	Central and peripheral nervous systems	Regulation of neuronal excitability and synaptic plasticity,	Angiotensin II
				Platelet-derived growth factor
		Cardiac and skeletal myocytes Smooth muscle and endothelial cells	Memory and learning processes	
Inducible NOS (iNOS;NOS-2) (calcium-independent)	Chromosome 17	Immune system	Participation in anti-microbial and anti-tumor activities (e.g.oxidative burst of macrophages)	Proinflammatory cytokines (Interleukin-1, Tumor necrosis factor α, Interferon γ)
		Cardiovascular system		
		Smooth muscle cells		
Endothelial NOS (eNOS; NOS-3) (calcium–dependent)	Chromosome 7	Endothelium	Regulating vascular function	Shear stress
				Acetylcholine
				Bradykinin
				Histamine

AT-II and platelet-derived growth factor (Dawson et al. 1991). iNOS is minimal under physiological conditions and is calcium insensitive. When iNOS is stimulated, it continuously produces NO. Induction of iNOS occurs mainly during infection and chronic inflammation. iNOS is expressed in vascular smooth muscle cells following exposure to pro-inflammatory cytokines. It is reported that inflammation-induced iNOS production in the endothelium is related to the vascular dysfunction by limiting the availability of BH_4 for e NOS (Lowenstein and Padalko 2004; Gunnett et al. 2005). eNOS is the major isoform for the regulation of vascular function. The activity of eNOS and the production of NO can be stimulated by shear stress, acetylcholine, bradykinin and histamine by both calcium-dependent and independent ways (Laher 2014). Acetylcholine, bradykinin and histamine bind to specific receptors on the endothelial cell membrane and increase the intracellular concentration of calcium. In a calcium-independent manner, the activation of eNOS is due to the post-translational modification of the enzyme including phosphorylation by NOS kinase and dephosphorylation by phosphatases

(Kellogg et al. 2005; Bae et al. 2003). Phosphorylation alters the activity of eNOS, and different sites of phosphorylation can have an opposing effect.The endogenous competitive inhibitor for eNOS is called asymmetric dimethyl arginine (ADMA) (Arora et al. 2013; Zhao et al. 2014). The inhibition of eNOS is correlated with plasma ADMA levels, and plasma ADMA levels are inversely related to endothelium-dependent vasodilation (Vestweber 2012). The acute and chronic rise in the shear stress of blood up-regulates the expression and the activity of eNOS, and thus the release of EDRF/NO (Kolluru et al. 2010; Michel and Vanhoutte 2010). AT-II by binding to its receptor produces bradykinins which stimulate eNOS consequently increases the formation of NO (Yayama et al. 2006).

Additionally, the products of the metabolism of NO are nitrite and nitrate which act as a reservoir of NO. Under certain conditions, several enzymes, such as xanthine oxidoreductase, mitochondrial cytochrome oxidase, aldehyde dehydrogenase 2 and cytochrome P450 reductase, catalyze the reduction of nitrite or nitrate to NO (Weitzberg et al. 2010).

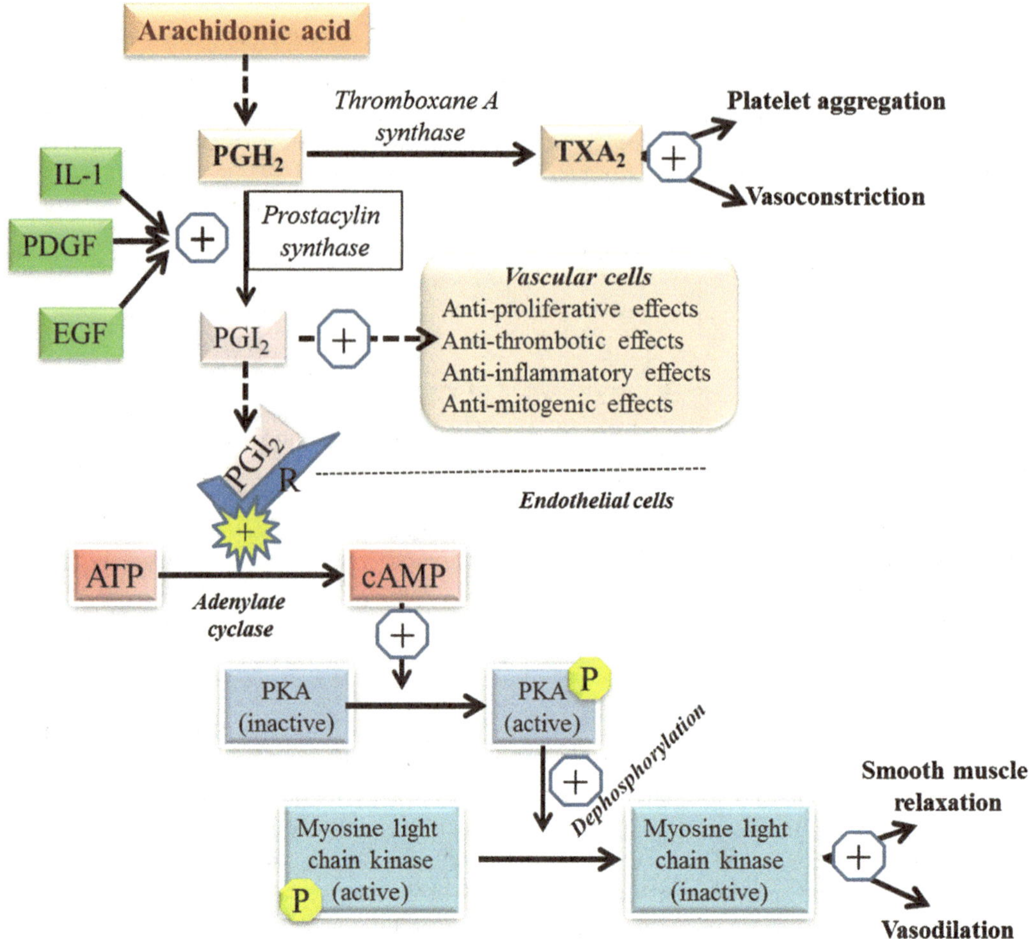

Fig. 3 The synthesis of the prostacyclin from prostaglandin (*PG*) G2 and thromboxane (*TX*) A2. TXA$_2$ shows interactions in contrast to PGI$_2$. *IL-1* Interleukin-1, *PDGF* Platelet derived growth factor, *EGF* Epidermal growth factor, *R* PGI$_2$ receptor

Prostacyclin Another vasodilator molecule is prostacyclin (also called prostaglandin I$_2$ or PGI$_2$) which is a prostaglandin that belongs to the eicosanoid family of lipid molecules. Prostacyclin is produced in ECs in response to inflammatory mediators, including interleukin (IL)-1 and platelet-derived and epidermal growth factors from prostaglandin H$_2$ (PGH$_2$) by the action of the enzyme prostacyclin synthase (Fig. 3). Like NO, it inhibits platelet activation and act as an effective vasodilator (Cahill and Redmond 2016; Siti et al. 2015). PGI$_2$ is released by healthy ECs and performs its function via paracrine signaling that involves G protein-coupled receptors on both ECs and platelets.

PGI$_2$ binds to endothelial prostacyclin receptors and raise cAMP levels in the cytosol. cAMP activates protein kinase A (PKA) which promotes the dephosphorylation of the myosin light chain kinase. Dephosphorylation of the enzyme results in the inhibition of myosinlight-chainkinase. This leads relaxation of the smooth muscle relaxation and vasodilation (Francis et al. 2010). Prostacyclin has also antiproliferative, antithrombotic, anti-inflammatory and antimitogenic effects on vascular cells. On the other hand, prostanoids, such as PGD$_2$ and PGF$_{2,}$ produced in vascular endothelium modulating intracellular Ca^{2+} concentration produce vasoconstriction (Siti et al. 2015).

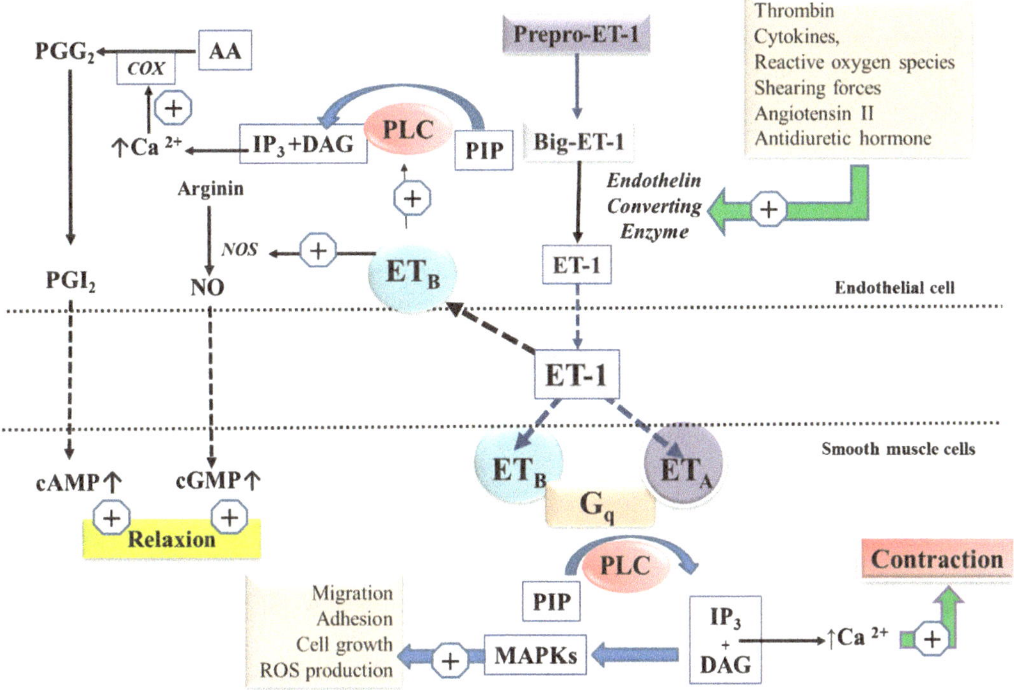

Fig. 4 Endothelin (ET); receptors (ET$_A$ and ET$_B$), mechanisms and effects. *PLC* Phospholipase C, *PIP* Phosphatidyl inositol diphosphate, *IP$_3$* Inositol triphosphate, *DAG* Diacylglycerol, *MAPK* Mitogen activated kinase, *AA* Arachidonic acid, *PGG$_2$* Prostaglandin G$_2$, *PGI$_2$* Prostaglandin I$_2$

Endothelium-Derived Hyperpolarizing Factor The term of EDHF represents a mechanism rather than a specific factor (Luksha et al. 2009). Prostacyclin and NO can be considered as an endothelium-derived hyperpolarizing substance. Because most of the available inhibitors of cyclooxygenase abolish the production of prostaglandins in vascular tissues, any endothelium-dependent hyperpolarization observed in the presence of one of these inhibitors is unlikely to involve prostacyclin. NO can also hyperpolarize, or repolarize, vascular smooth muscle cells by activating, in either a c-GMP dependent or –independent pathways through potassium channels such as K-ATP. NO interacts with other ionic channels of the smooth muscle, including chloride and cationic channels and also influences the membrane potential of the smooth muscle cells indirectly in an autocrine fashion (Félétou and Vanhoutte 2006). Members of a class of arachidonic acid derivatives, the epoxyeicosatrienoic acid, hydrogen peroxide, C-type natriuretic peptide, have been suggested to function as an EDHF in some vascular beds. These molecules are accepted as non-NO–non-PGI$_2$– EDHFs. EDHF is proposed to be a substance and/or electrical signal that is generated or synthesized in and released from the endothelium. Its function is to hyperpolarize vascular smooth muscle cells, causing these cells to relax. EDHFs are able to activate ion channels, and initiate smooth muscle hyperpolarization and relaxation (Luksha et al. 2009). Calcium-activated K+ channels are opened by EDHFs in vascular smooth muscle cells. The effects of EDHF's are highest on the small arteries, and are very significant for the regulation of organ blood flow, peripheral vascular resistance and blood pressure, particularly when production of NO is depressed (Michel and Vanhoutte 2010; Luksha et al. 2009; Félétou and Vanhoutte 2006; Khazaei et al. 2008).

Endothelins Endothelins (ETs) are potent vasoconstrictor molecules having a key role in vascular homeostasis (Fig. 4). Although there are three types of ET, vascular ECs produce only ET-1 which has prominent roles (Wang and Zhao 2010). ET-1 is a 21 amino acid peptide that is synthesized from a 39 amino acid precursor named pre-pro endothelin. Active endothelin molecule is generated by the actions of an endothelin converting enzyme (ECE) found on the endothelial cell membranes. There are two basic types of ET-1 receptors: ET_A and ET_B. Both of these receptors are coupled to a G-protein and to the formation of IP_3 (Barton 2011; Kedzierski and Yanagisawa 2001). In blood vessels, the ET_A receptor is dominant under normal conditions. ET-1 produces vasoconstriction through activation of L-type Ca^{+2} channels by binding to ET-A receptors on vascular smooth muscle cells. In addition to the presence of both ET_A and ET_B receptors on the smooth muscle, ET_B receptors are also found on the endothelium, and under the control of vascular tone, considerable cross-talk between ET, NO and prostacyclin occur (Vanhoutte et al. 2009). When ET-1 binds to endothelial ET_B receptors, the formation of NO is stimulated but in the absence of smooth muscle endothelin receptor stimulation, NO causes vasodilation. The other effects of ETs include cell growth, embryonic development, renal functions, neurophysiological functions (such as pain signaling), cardiovascular homeostasis, cancer cell growth, endocrine function, inflammation, pulmonary functions (such as bronchoconstriction) and reproductive system functions (Khazaei et al. 2008). ET-1 production and release are stimulated by AT-II, antidiuretic hormone (ADH), thrombin, cytokines, reactive oxygen species, and shearing forces acting on the vascular endothelium. The ET-1 release is inhibited by prostacyclin, atrial natriuretic peptide and NO (Davenport et al. 2016).

Angiotensin I and II Angiotensin II (AT-II) cause structural changes and vasoconstriction in the arterial wall by affecting many cellular and intracellular events in smooth muscle. Two types of AT-II receptors on ECs are determined. AT-II type-1 receptor is particularly involved in the contraction of vascular smooth muscle cells.

AT-II-type-1 receptor blockers increase the release of NO and prostaglandins whereas AT II- type-2 receptors provide the activation of the endothelial relaxation (Masuyer et al. 2014; Jiang et al. 2014).

Thromboxane Thromboxane (TX) A_2 is a member of the eicosanoid lipid family. TXA_2 is generated from prostaglandin H_2 by thromboxane-A synthase. TXA_2 acts by binding to the G-protein-coupled thromboxane receptors. Thromboxane is a vasoconstrictor, and it facilitates platelet aggregation (Fig. 3). Therefore, TXA_2 shows interactions in contrast to prostacyclin (Bauer et al. 2014; Korbecki et al. 2014).

Adenosine The vascular ECs releases adenosine to produce vaso-relaxation through activation of purinergic (P_2) receptors. Adenosine release is related to local oxygen tension. Also, adenosine metabolites play roles in local vasoregulation and in the physiological control of blood pressure (Ralevic and Dunn 2015).

2.2　Inflammatory and Immune Response of ECs

Many stimuli associated with inflammatory and immune vascular diseases have been reported to induce endothelial cell apoptosis (Winn and Harlan 2005a). Endothelial cells produce and react to a variety of cytokines (these include chemokines, colony-stimulating factors (CSF), Interleukins (IL), growth factors, and interferons (IFN) and other mediators). Therefore, ECs have important roles in defense and inflammation. The chemokines from ECs affect leukocytes (neutrophils, eosinophils), T lymphocytes, natural killer cells and monocytes. Since ECs are located at the tissue-blood interface, they present several chemokines to circulating leukocytes. When production of chemokines is elevated, Tumor Necrosis Factor (TNF)-α and IL-1 for the receptor (so called as decoy receptor) are released into the circulation (Vanhoutte et al. 2009). IL-1 and TNF-α are synergistically effective on the expression of pro-inflammatory genes in various cells. Endothelial cells also produce granulocyte macrophage CSF (GM-CSF), granulocyte CSF (G-CSF), macrophage CSF (M-CSF), the stem cell factors, IL-1 and IL-6 and TNF receptors. ECs by themselves are targets of the inflammatory response. TNF-α and TNF-β are produced by activated macrophages and activated T cells, respectively. These activate ECs and neutrophil aggregation, as well as NO synthesis. Inflammatory disease progression depends on the balance between pro-inflammatory and anti-inflammatory cytokines. ECs involve the systemic anti-inflammatory response by producing anti-inflammatory cytokines such as an IL-1 receptor, IL-10, IL-13, and Transforming Growth Factor (TGF)-β. Anti-inflammatory cytokines can either block the process initiated by pro-inflammatory cytokines or suppress the inflammatory cascade. While cytokines such as IL-4, IL-10, IL-13, and TGF-β suppress the production of IL-1, TNF-α, other pro-inflammatory cytokines block the production of these cytokines (Mai et al. 2013). TGF-β is also produced by macrophages, T cells, and endothelium and generally works as a growth inhibitor of ECs. Additionally, IL-8 stimulates proliferation and migration of ECs and have angiogenic properties (Medzhitov 2008; Levesque et al. 1990).

ECs facilitate leukocyte movement into tissues through adhesion molecules such as E-selectin, P-selectin, intercellular adhesion molecule-1 (ICAM-1) and vascular cell adhesion molecule (VCAM). Resting ECs are considered not to be adhesive to circulating leukocytes. ICAM-2 is expressed on resting ECs, whereas ICAM-1 and VCAM are minimal on resting state and their expression can be increased by cytokines and endotoxin activation. Lymphocytes, platelets, and other leukocytes can interact with ECs under basal conditions via the L-selectin receptor. When lymphocytes are activated, they express integrins, which interact with ICAM and VCAM. L-selectin, as an adhesion molecule, and β2 integrin are involved in the adherence of leukocytes to ECs. Activated ECs also secrete platelet activating factor (PAF) and stimulate the expression of P-selectin and E-selectin. PAF upregulates integrins on leukocytes. Activated platelets binds to CD40 on ECs (Vanhoutte et al. 2009; Tuttolomondo et al. 2012; Tummala et al. 1999; Szmitko et al. 2003).

The endothelium is also capable of expressing various growth factors including G-CSF, M-CSF, GM-CSF, platelet-derived growth factor (PDGF), vascular endothelial growth factor (VEGF), and fibroblast growth factors (FGF). CSFs and growth factors produced by the endothelium are also important for hematopoiesis which increases the number of immune cells in the circulation during inflammation (Croft et al. 2009).

The immune system has important roles in the defense mechanism against infections or in response to tissue injury. Dendritic cells (DC), macrophages, natural killer (NK) T cells, and Toll-like receptors (TLRs) are components of the immune system. ECs actively participate in both innate and adaptive immune responses through producing cytokines and chemokines which recruit phagocytes to the site of infection. Endothelial permeability is also increased, allowing for additional trafficking of immune cells during inflammation. Although ECs at rest do not interact with leukocytes, activated ECs increase the expression of adhesion molecules and chemokines and interact with immune cells during the inflammatory process. ECs also can serve as antigen presenting cells by expressing both MHC I and II molecules and presenting endothelial antigens to T cells during inflammation. Both TLRs (TLR2 and TLR4) and NLRs are expressed in inflamed endothelium. When inflammation is dominated by TH1 cells, ECs express chemokine ligand 10 (CXCL10) and E-selectin, which favors the recruitment of TH1 cells. EC surface molecules such as lymphocyte function-associated antigen (LFA)-3 and ICAM-1 increase the production of IL-2 and IL-4 by T cells. ECs with activated T cells enhance IFN-γ production via OX40 (CD134) signaling (OX40 is a member of the TNFR/TNF superfamily and are expressed on the activated CD4 and CD8 T cells). An anti-angiogenic cytokine derived from ECs, vascular endothelial growth inhibitor functions to suppress ECs proliferation in a cell cycle-dependent manner lipopolysaccharide, which induce ECs to produce IL-1, IL-8, and monocyte chemotactic protein-1 (MCP-1). Like LPS, tumor necrosis factor-α (TNF-α), and interferon-γ (IFN-γ) can induce TLR2 expression via an NF-kB-dependent pathway. ECs also express CD14, a known receptor for LPS and IFN-α, which is an important cytokine in regulating innate immune responses against viruses (Mai et al. 2013; Croft et al. 2009; Rodriguez-Iturbe et al. 2014).

Under healthy conditions, ECs express the lectin-like oxidized low-density lipoprotein (oxLDL) receptor (LOX-1) at low levels. Expression of LOX-1 in ECs is elevated in response to stimulation by oxLDL, pro-inflammatory cytokines, and pro-atherogenic factors such as AT-II. OxLDL also induces cell surface adhesion molecule expression and impair NO production in ECs by increasing superoxide generation. LOX-1 has a role in the mediation of endothelial phagocytosis of aged red blood cells and apoptotic cells. LOX-1-mediated phagocytotic activity can be inhibited by oxLDL. Thus, LOX-1 is important in endothelial-mediated vascular homeostasis and coagulation prevention under physiological conditions (Pirillo et al. 2013; Dunn et al. 2008).

ECs can also induce suppressive immune function in T cells. Mechanistically, after contact with ECs, regulatory T cells upregulate the expression of programmed death-1 receptor and increase the production of anti-inflammatory cytokines IL-10 and TGF-β (Tselios et al. 2014; Pastrana et al. 2012).

Recently, it has been shown that ECs also induce cellular signaling by endothelial microparticles (EMPs). EMPs are small plasma membrane-derived vesicles (0.1–1.5 μm in diameter), are released by various cell types during cell activation or apoptosis (a type of programmed cell death). Microparticle formation induced by various factors, including TNF-α, IL-1β, thrombin, calcium ionophore, and reactive oxygen species. Microparticles express surface antigens from their cells of origin which allow for the identification of their sources. Circulating EMPs are biomarkers of inflammation and contribute to the pathological state. Depending on the nature of the stimulus, EMPs contain endothelial proteins such as ICAM-1, integrin, and cadherin. EMPs also have endothelial nuclear materials such as microRNA, RNA, and DNA, which can induce intracellular signaling via the transfer of these nuclear materials and proteins to target cells. EMPs also have pro-coagulant and pro-adhesive properties, which promote coagulation and vascular inflammation. EMPs were also found to induce the maturation of plasmacytoid dendritic cells. Plasmacytoid dendritic cells matured by EMPs secrete pro-inflammatory cytokines IL-6 and IL-8 (Yuana et al. 2013; Bernal-Mizrachi et al. 2003; Helbing et al. 2014a).

2.3 The Link Between Hemostasis and Coagulation and ECs

The endothelium plays a pivotal role in the regulation of the hemostatic balance, and endothelial and smooth muscle cells express several proteins participating in hemostasis. Hemostasis is a complex event. Multiple interactions between blood cells and the damaged vessel wall, the coagulation proteins, and blood cells and the cell-cell interactions are required in the hemostatic process (Fig. 5). In physiological state, healthy ECs express antiplatelet and anticoagulant molecules that prevent platelet aggregation and fibrin formation, respectively. Injury to endothelium leads to loss of protective molecules and the appearance of adhesive and pro-coagulant activities. When coagulation proteins are activated by their specific receptors on the vascular cell surface, in turn, these cells lead to the expression of genes involved in coagulation, angiogenesis, leukocyte adhesion and regulation of the vascular wall tone (Stenina 2003; Yau et al. 2015).

Tissue factor (TF) is the receptor for factor VII and is a pro-coagulant. It is inhibited by tissue factor pathway inhibitor (TFPI), which is synthesized by ECs and is one of the most important endothelium-derived inhibitors of the blood

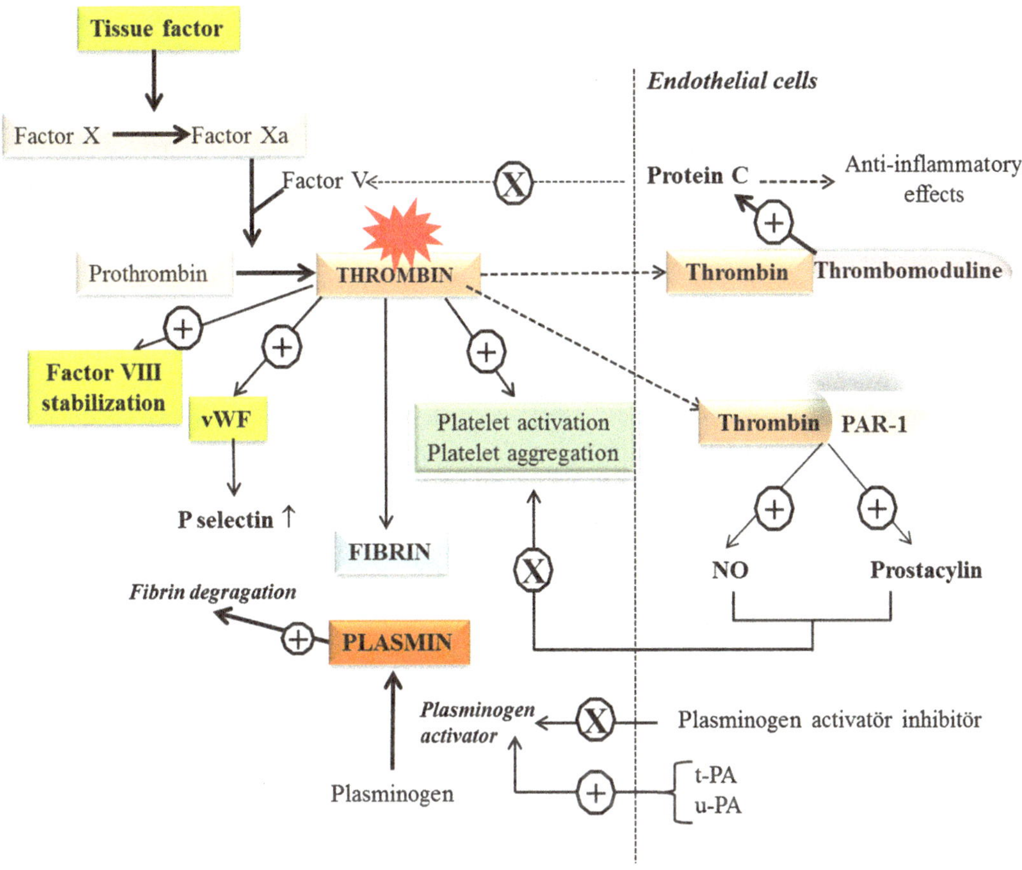

Fig. 5 Endothelium has both anticoagulant and coagulant activities (*see text*); *PAR-1* Protease-activated receptor-1, *t-PA* Tissue type plasminogen activator, *u-PA* urokinase type plasminogen activator, *vWF* von Willebrand factor (Şekilde Türkçe Karakterler mevcut)

coagulation cascade. TF activates factor X, which then combines with factor Va to convert prothrombin to thrombin. Thrombin has pro-coagulant activity. It binds to thrombomodulin which is expressed on the ECs surface. Thrombomodulin requires for the pro-coagulant effects of thrombin as a cofactor in normal vessels. The thrombin-thrombomodulin complex activates protein C. This process is forced by the endothelial protein C receptor (EPCR). Activated protein C (APC) is an effective anticoagulant through the inactivation of factor Va. Thrombin is also chemotactic for polymorphonuclear leukocytes and is a potent inducer of platelet activating factor (PAF) expression in ECs. Thrombin is also involved in the process of inflammation and can up-regulate endothelial cell P-selectin expression

through von Willebrand factor (vWF). Endothelium also produces and secretes vWF, mediating platelet adhesion and shear stress-induced aggregation. vWF, which is also synthesized within megakaryocytes and the α-granules of platelets, is a multimeric adhesion glycoprotein. vWF is essential for platelet adhesion to collagen via the platelet receptor glycoprotein Ib-FV-FIX at sites of vascular injury. The vWF binds and stabilizes factor VIII and is a cofactor for platelet binding to exposed extracellular matrix in injured vessel walls (Vanhoutte et al. 2009; Stenina 2003; Yau et al. 2015; Steffel et al. 2006; Esmon 2006).

Under physiological conditions, the endothelium prevents thrombosis. Endothelial protease-activated receptors (PARs) serve as sensors for proteases and initiate a cascade of cell signals upon activation by thrombin, APC, FXa, the

TF/FVIIa/FXa complex, high concentrations of plasmin, and matrix metalloproteases. Thrombin-mediated activation of PAR-1 is responsible for the production of NO and prosta-cyclin, which limits platelet activation, induces the activation of Weibel-Palade bodies, releasing VWF and t-PA, and mediates the surface expo-sure of TF. Thus, PARs (especially PAR-2) play an important role in the pro-coagulant response upon stimulation, and this induces pro-inflammatory responses (Lacave et al. 1989; Lijnen and Collen 1997).

Platelets play a fundamental role in preventing blood loss by forming the platelet hemostatic plug and to serve as a platform for coagulation factors. Platelet-endothelium interactions play an impor-tant role in the activation and regulation of platelets. While an intact endothelium inhibits the adhesion of platelets, through the release of NO and PGI_2, activated ECs express a variety of molecules and receptors that increase platelet adhesion to the site of injury. In ECs, Weibel-Palade bodies store, vWF, P-selectin, angiopoietin-2, t-PA, and ET-1, which are active participants of platelet adhesion, leukocyte recruit-ment, inflammation modulation, fibrinolysis, and vasoconstriction, respectively. Following vascular insult or in the presence of vasoactive agents such as histamine, bradykinin, and thrombin, endothe-lial Weibel-Palade bodies fuse with the plasma membrane and release these products into the space wherein they perform their specific functions (Francis et al. 2010). Normal ECs also produce enzymes called ectonucleotidases, which dephosphorylates ADP to AMP and then to aden-osine and inhibit platelet aggregation, and release matrix metalloproteases (MMPs) to cleave platelet aggregates. TXA_2 produced by activated platelets, has prothrombotic properties, stimulating activa-tion of new platelets as well as increasing platelet aggregation. Platelet aggregation is achieved by mediating expression of the glycoprotein complex GP IIb/IIIa in the cell membrane of platelets. Circulating fibrinogen binds to these receptors on adjacent platelets, further strengthening the clot (Yau et al. 2015; Steffel et al. 2006; Esmon 2006; Perutelli et al. 1992; Lacave et al. 1989; Lijnen and Collen 1997).

ECs synthesize and secrete plasminogen activator (PA) to degrade the clot and plasminogen activator inhibitor (PAI), and thus provide anticoagulant and pro-coagulant regu-latory mechanisms, respectively. Additionally, MMPs are released from ECs to cleave platelet aggregates. Fibrin degradation is trigged by some fibrinolytic molecules, such as tissue –type PA (t-PA) and urokinase-type PA (u-PA). t-PA is pre-dominantly found in ECs while u-PA is expressed in ECs, macrophages, renal epithelial cells and some tumor cells. T-PA convert plasminogen to plasmin. Both plasminogen and plasminogen activators (t-PA and u-PA) bind to specific cellular receptors; assembly of components of the fibrino-lytic system at the endothelial cell surface results in stimulation of fibrinolytic activity. Thus, t-PA provides an essential method for removal of blood clots (Salame et al. 2000; Shih and Hajjar 1993; Barnathan et al. 1990).

2.4   Hemodynamic Factors and Endothelial Cell

Flow rate and pressure in the blood vessels also affect the smooth muscle tone. The increase in flow velocity (shear stress), via ion channels (cal-cium, potassium and sodium) stimulates eNOS activity and the synthesis of NO from ECs. The increase in pressure reduces both the stress and release of endothelin from NO; vascular shear stress can also influence the coagulant potential of ECs. Arterial shear stress can induce the tran-scription factors. Likewise, reduced venous shear stress can induce hypoxia and stimulate the release of P-selectin and von Willebrand factor from ECs. The nature of the shear stress also has a significant influence on the type of thrombi that forms. Arte-rial clots form under high shear stress after athero-sclerotic plaque rupture and are rich in platelets (called as white clot). In contrast, venous thrombi develop under low shear stress and are rich in fibrin and red blood cells (called as red clot). It has been indicated that plasma viscosity is a major determi-nant of capillary blood flow, and alteration in plasma viscosity contributes to impaired blood flow and to increased cardiovascular risk

(Reneman et al. 2006; Ballermann et al. 1998; Li et al. 2005b; Ercan et al. 2003).

2.5 Angiogenesis

Since ECs are an important component of blood vessels, they can be triggered to induce angiogenesis upon stimulation (Francis et al. 2010). VEGF is an angiogenic factor produced by ECs, with specific receptors on the endothelium. The formation of new blood vessels from pre-existing endothelium is mediated by VEGF. VEGF also contributes to the inflammatory response through stimulation of the release of adhesion molecules, MMPs and NO, via the transcription factor activator protein-1 (AP-1) (Kim and Byzova 2014; Jaipersad et al. 2014).

The coagulation system plays a major role in the development of angiogenesis. Activated protein C stimulates angiogenesis in brain endothelium, and cross-linked fibrin serves as a scaffold for ECs to synthesize new blood vessels. Platelets contain a rich source of vasoactive agents and chemokines, such as serotonin, TA_2, PAF and pro-angiogenic growth factors, such as vascular VEGF. VEGF can stimulate/upregulate eNOS and has physiological role for the normal endothelial control of vasomotor tone (Jaipersad et al. 2014).

An anti-angiogenic cytokine derived from ECs, vascular endothelial growth inhibitor functions to suppress EC proliferation in a cell cycle-dependent manner. These compounds stimulate ECs proliferation and promote the growth of new blood vessels. The expression of TF has been shown to induce tumor angiogenesis through TF-FVIIa-dependent PAR-2 activation which induces the expression of VEGF, IL-8, and MMP-7. It has been suggested that TF isoform may play a prominent role in promoting the angiogenesis (Mai et al. 2013; Yau et al. 2015).

Laminar shear stress is also a potent antiapoptotic stimulus in ECs. Some postulated mechanisms of protection include up-regulation of NOS, as well (Ercan et al. 2014).

3 Endothelial Dysfunction

Healthy endothelium has some athero-protective role including promotion of vasodilation, antioxidant and anti-inflammatory effects, inhibition of both leukocyte adhesion and migration and smooth muscle cell proliferation and migration. Healthy endothelium has anticoagulant and profibrinolytic effects, as well as the inhibitory effects on platelet aggregation and adhesion. Impaired endothelium-dependent vasodilation is also associated with the state of endothelial activation which is characterized by elevated pro-inflammatory and pro-coagulatory events (Fig. 6). The major factors for endothelial dysfunction are a reduction of the NO bioavailability, impairment in the response of vascular smooth muscle to the vasodilators, the elevated sensitivity of ECs against

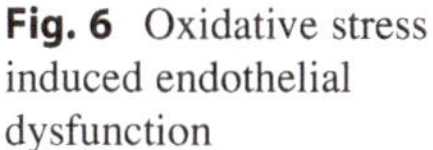

Fig. 6 Oxidative stress induced endothelial dysfunction

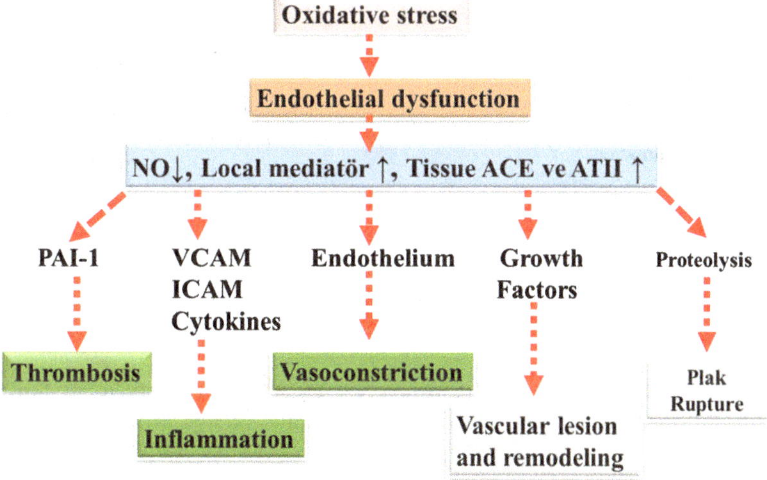

vasoconstrictors, increased production of the vasoconstrictor substances, or elevated shear stress (Fig. 7). Traditional and nontraditional risk factors for cardiovascular events, diabetes mellitus, atherosclerosis and hypertension are associated with enhanced ROS or increased oxidative stress. Increased oxidative stress is considered as a major mechanism involved in the pathogenesis of endothelial dysfunction. Disturbance of NO metabolism (elevated degradation of NO, inactivation of NO, or presence of NO inhibitors; Fig. 8) may be due to the elevation in oxidative stress (González et al. 2014; Bonetti et al. 2003).

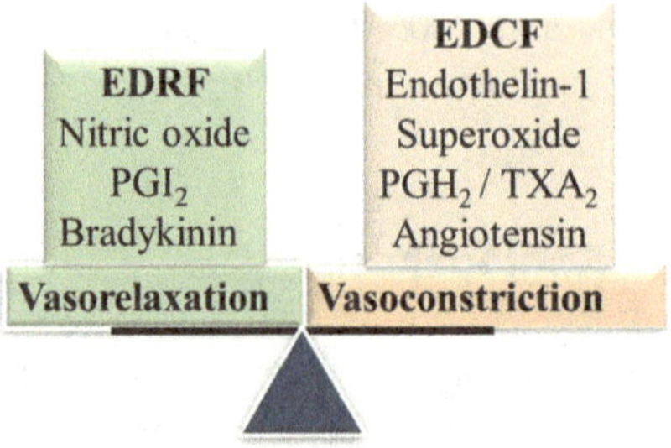

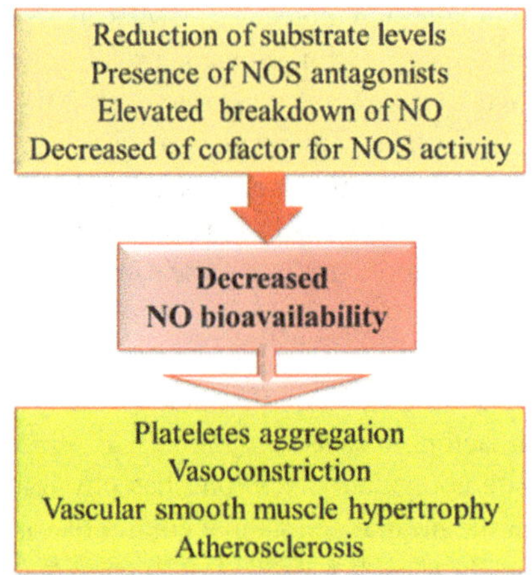

Fig. 7 A balance between endothelium-derived relaxing factors (EDRFs) and endothelium-derived contracting factors (EDCFs)

3.1   NO and Endothelial Dysfunction: The Link with Oxidative Stress

Oxidative stress has been implicated in the pathophysiology of many cardiovascular conditions, including hypertension. ROS significantly increase the influence of stimulants such as inflammation, radiation, high partial oxygen pressure, advanced age, obesity, and chemical substances. Oxidative stress that increases on a cellular level results in oxidative damage by altering the structure of molecules such as deoxyribonucleic acid, amino acid, protein, lipid, and carbohydrate (Fig. 9). A particularly important radical for

Fig. 8 Nitric oxide (NO) bioavailability

Fig. 9 Oxidative stress has been implicated in the pathophysiology of many cardiovascular conditions, including hypertension. ROS significantly increase the influence of stimulants such as inflammation, insulin resistance, dyslipidemia, advanced age and obesity which are related to decreased nitric oxide bioavailability

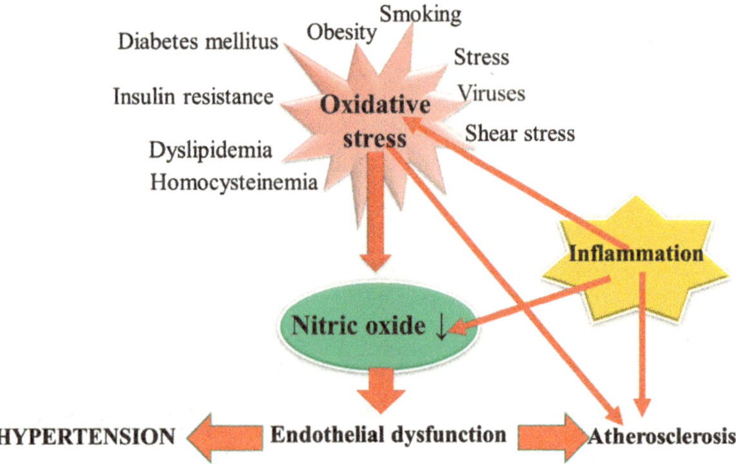

cardiovascular biology is superoxide, which is formed by the one-electron reduction of oxygen. Superoxide can serve as both an oxidant and as a reductant and is a progenitor for other ROS. Other radicals include the hydroxyl radical, lipid peroxyl radical, and alkoxyl radicals. Other molecules, including peroxynitrite, hypochlorous acid, and hydrogen peroxide are not radicals but have strong oxidant properties and are, therefore, included as ROS. Another a group of molecules is the reactive nitrogen species (RNS) including NO, the nitrogen dioxide radical, and the nitro sodium cation. The main sources for oxidative excess in the vasculature are adenine dinucleotide phosphate (NADPH) oxidase (NOX), xanthine oxidase, the mitochondrial and uncoupled NOS (Zhao et al. 2014; Bonetti et al. 2003; Ferroni et al. 2006).

NOX catalyzes the reduction of molecular oxygen by NADPH as an electron donor, thus generating superoxide. Superoxide anion is a major determinant of NO synthesis and availability, and can act as a vasoconstrictor. Superoxide combines with NO, which is synthesized by eNOS, to form peroxynitrite, in turn, peroxynitrite oxidizes and destabilizes eNOS to produce more superoxide. Superoxide also leads to BH4 oxidation, which is a cofactor for NO synthesis. Vascular superoxide is derived primarily from NOX when stimulated by hormones such as AT-II and ET-1. Xanthine oxidase is also an important source for oxygen free radical present in the vascular endothelium. It involves purine metabolism. During this process oxygen is reduced to superoxide (González et al. 2014).

eNOS is an important source of superoxide and peroxynitrite. In addition AT-II, acting through the AT1 receptor stimulates NOX causing the accumulation of superoxide, hydrogen peroxide, and peroxynitrite. Peroxynitrite is generated from NO in the increased oxidative stress conditions. It plays proatherogenic roles by leading to oxidation of LDL and degradation of the eNOS cofactor. ROS upregulate VCAM-1, ICAM-1 and MCP-1. Oxidative excess is also linked to a pro-inflammatory state of the vessel wall. Inflammation decreases NO bioavailability. On the other hand, under pathological conditions,

EDHF can compensate for the loss of NO in arteries. The effects of EDHF are greatest at the level of small arteries. The changes in the EDHF action are of critical importance for the regulation of organ blood flow, peripheral vascular resistance, and blood pressure (Luksha et al. 2009; Ceriello 2008).

3.2 Asymmetric Dimethylarginine and Endothelial Dysfunction

Asymmetric dimethylarginine (ADMA) is endogenous competitive inhibitor of eNOS. It is created in protein methylation, a common mechanism of post-translational protein modification, which is catalyzed by N-methyltransferases. ADMA is eliminated by excretion through the kidneys or metabolism to citrulline by the enzyme dimethylarginine dimethylaminohydrolase (DDAH). ADMA is one of the molecules associated with oxidative stress. Oxidative stress increases the plasma ADMA levels by increasing the activity of enzymes that take part in the production of ADMA and by decreasing the activity of enzymes that take part in metabolizing ADMA. The increased ADMA levels decrease the release of NO by inhibiting NOS. As NO decreases, hemodynamic changes and endothelial dysfunction occurs. Overexpression of DDAH also decreases ADMA levels and increase eNOS activity. Protein arginine methyltransferases, which produce methylated arginines, were shown to be upregulated by shear stress, and this upregulation was associated with enhanced ADMA generation (Endemann and Schiffrin 2004; Papageorgiou et al. 2015; Siervo et al. 2011).

3.3 LDL Oxidation and Endothelial Dysfunction

Oxidation plays a role in the pathogenesis of atherosclerosis. The oxidation of LDL triggers the uptake of the uptake of oxLDL by macrophages and the formation of foam cell. Also, oxidation processes may result in oxidized

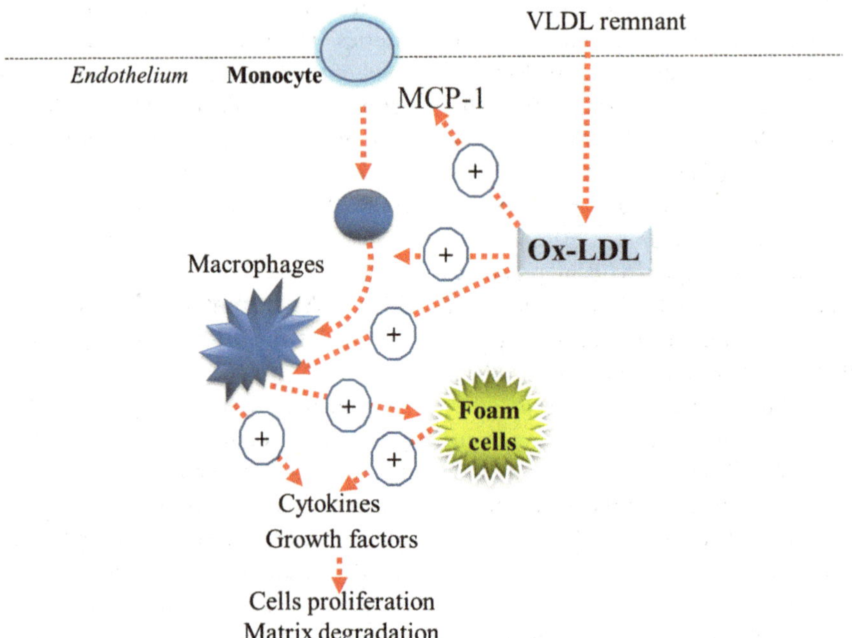

Fig. 10 oxLDL activates macrophages and generation of foam cells. Foam cells trigger the both production and secretion of growth factors and cytokines which stimulate cells proliferation and matrix degradation. *MCP-1* Monocytechemotactic factor-1

lipids with pro-inflammatory effect (Fig. 10). The other lipids which present in the blood vessel wall lead to inflammation and atherosclerosis (Stancel et al. 2016; Ouweneel and Van Eck 2016).

oxidative stress initiators. Also, Hcy mediates LDL-autoxidation and changes the redox thiol status in mitochondrial gene expression. Homocysteine and/or adenosine exposure of ECs cause apoptosis (McCully 2015; Pushpakumar et al. 2014).

3.4 Homocysteinemia and Endothelial Dysfunction

Homocysteine (Hcy) is a sulfhydryl-containing amino acid. It is synthesized from the demethylation of methionine. The presentation of either methyl tetrahydrofolate or betaine, Hcy may be converted into methionine by methylation reaction or may be metabolized to cysteine by the sulfuration reaction. It has been shown that hyperhomocysteinemia is a major and independent risk factor for cardiovascular disease. Hcy cause arteriosclerosis by damaging the endothelium either directly or by altering oxidative status. In presence of hyperhomocysteinemia, Hcy autoxidation occurs, which may stimulate the production of hydroxyl radicals, as known as

3.5 Coagulation and Inflammation Pathways and Endothelial Dysfunction

Endothelial dysfunction is responsible for inflammation and blood coagulation. During endothelial dysfunction, ECs become activated and contribute to the pathogenesis of thrombosis. Hypoxic conditions often lead to endothelial dysfunction and promote the release of VWF from ECs. Inflammation can be accompanied by thrombosis. Proinflammatory cytokines, such as TNF-α and IL-1, upregulate the production of TF and VWF, while attenuating the expression of thrombomodulin, NO and prostacyclin. Patients with systemic inflammation show an impaired protein C system due to impaired protein C synthesis and impaired protein C activation. While protein C is synthesized by hepatocytes, ECs can regulate protein C activation through the expression of thrombomodulin. As such, thrombomodulin levels are significantly downregulated by the presence of pro-inflammatory cytokines, such as TNF-α and IL-1, resulting in diminished protein C activation. These events result in a shift from anti-thrombotic to pro-thrombotic conditions (Yau et al. 2015; Goldenberg and Kuebler 2015; Kleinegris et al. 2012).

3.6 Shear Stress and Endothelial Dysfunction

Normally high shear stress is beneficial as it promotes adaptive dilatation or structural remodeling of the artery wall through endothelium-mediated mechanisms In addition, growth status of ECs can be regulated by shear stress. It has been shown that shear stress suppresses the EC apoptosis, and can be attenuated by the inhibition of NO production. Anti-apoptotic effect of shear stress is mediated by the up-regulation of eNOS. Although the inter-normal endothelium does not allow the passage of macromolecules such as oxLDL, shear stress, by a variety of mechano-sensors effects, activate intracellular signaling pathways, thus modulating gene expression and cellular functions such as proliferation, apoptosis, migration, permeability, and alignment (Li et al. 2005a). It has been demonstrated that the rheological impairment of dyslipidemic patients was related with endothelial dysfunction and this was a possible cause of both micro and macrovascular complications. Plasma viscosity, ADMA and oxLDL values were significantly higher in subjects with dyslipidemia. Plasma NO concentration was decreased in dyslipidemic subjects compared to the normo-lipidemic subjects (Ercan et al. 2014). Additionally, plasma viscosity, an early atherosclerotic risk factor, might be helpful in the assessment of cardiovascular risk in obese subjects along with classical cardiovascular risk factors such as plasma cholesterol and atherogenic index (Konukoglu et al. 2009).

3.7 Insulin Resistance and Endothelial Dysfunction

Endothelial dysfunction may also favor insulin resistance. It has been reported that the insulin resistance syndrome can be involved as the diverse consequences of endothelial dysfunction in different vascular beds. Insulin resistance is frequently associated with other abnormalities that can affect endothelial function, such as hyperglycemia, hypertension, dyslipidemia, and altered coagulation/fibrinolysis. Insulin resistance leads to endothelial dysfunction and may contribute to obesity (Fig. 11). Obesity leads to insulin resistance and endothelial dysfunction, mainly through fat-derived metabolic products, hormones, and adipocytokines. Obesity, insulin resistance, and endothelial dysfunction closely coexist in type 2 diabetes. The mechanisms are numerous and complex. Non-pharmacological and pharmacological interventions targeting obesity and/or insulin resistance demonstrate an amelioration of endothelial dysfunction and low-grade inflammation (Muniyappa and Sowers 2013; Rao et al. 2015; Prieto et al. 2014).

4 The Links Between Endothelial Dysfunction and Sustained Hypertension

Endothelial dysfunction was initially identified as impaired vasodilation to specific stimulus of acetylcholine or bradykinin. Endothelium dysfunction leads to functional changes in the microvasculature with a predominant and deleterious constrictive tone. Endothelial dysfunction, as a risk factor involves several pathological conditions. Hypertension is also an important risk factor for atherosclerosis and endothelial dysfunction. In hypertension, sustained elevation of systemic pressure in the microvasculature leads to premature aging and increased turnover

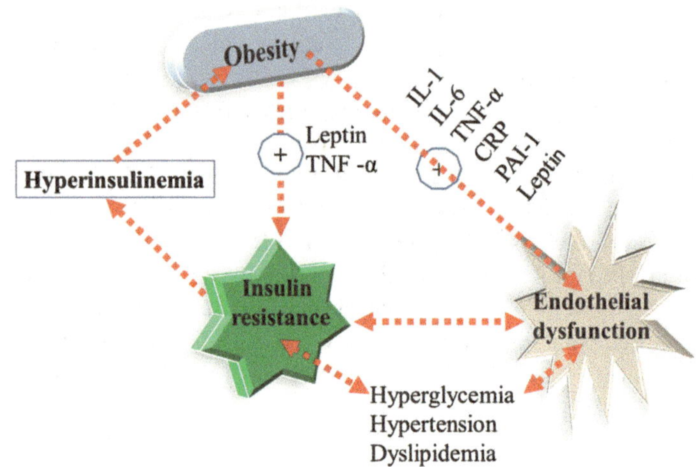

Fig. 11 Insulin resistance and endothelial dysfunction. *IL* Interleukin, *TNF* Tumor necrosis factor, *CRP* C-reactive protein, *PAI-I* Plasminogen activator inhibitor –I

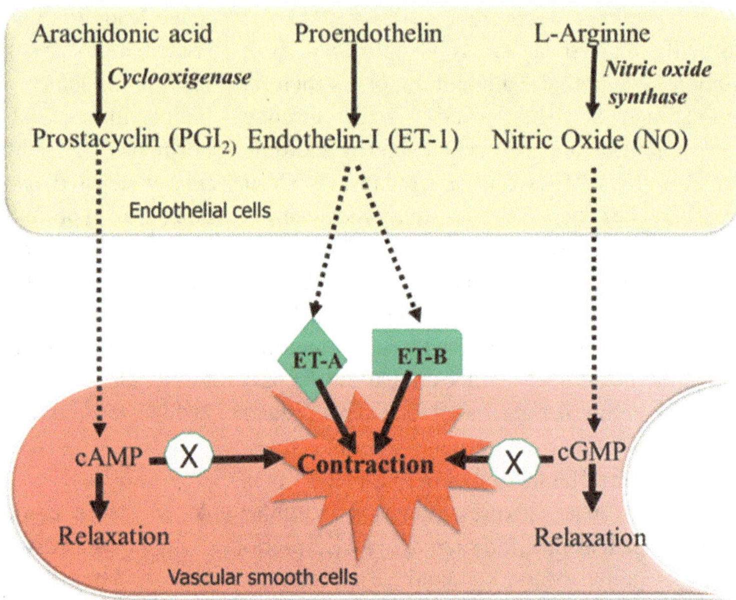

Fig. 12 Impaired response of endothelium to vasoconstriction in hypertension

of ECs. The endothelium has an impaired ability to release EDRFs, resulting in vasoconstriction (Fig. 12). Hypertension has been linked to deficient levels of NO and increased vascular production of ROS. There are some structural changes in the vascular wall in hypertension. Hypertension results in structural alterations in microcirculatory beds such as remodeling and rarefaction. It is remodeling that is responsible for the majority of the chronic elevation in systemic vascular resistance seen in hypertension (Kiowski 1999; McIntyre et al. 1999; Jacobsen et al. 2011)

Reduction in NO synthesis leads to arterial vasoconstriction and hypertension. Chronic administration of NOS inhibitors causes sustained hypertension. NO plays a role in facilitating sodium excretion so that systemic inhibition of NOS promotes salt and water retention (Melikian et al. 2009). Together these findings suggest that a reduction in NO-mediated dilatation will increase arterial resistance and enhance the susceptibility of the cardiovascular system to pressor stimuli. The role of the endothelium and NO in systemic hypertension is very controversial. Although an impaired release of relaxing factors may partly be associated with the pathogenesis of hypertension (Michel and Vanhoutte 2010; Lüscher et al. 1989), it now appears that endothelium-dependent relaxation is heterogeneously affected in this condition. In some vascular beds of hypertensive rats such as the aorta, mesenteric, carotid and cerebral vessels, endothelium-dependent relaxation is impaired (Calver et al. 1993; Luscher and Vanhoutte 1986; Dohi et al. 1990). In contrast, in coronary and renal arteries of spontaneously hypertensive rats, endothelial function does not seem to be affected by high blood pressure (Luscher 1991; Tschudi et al. 1991).

Despite the fact that mechanisms underlying hypertension are not yet fully elucidated, the evidence shows that oxidative stress plays a central role in its pathophysiology. In general, oxidative stress is defined as excess formation and/or insufficient removal of highly reactive molecules such as ROS and reactive nitrogen species (RNS). ROS promote vasoconstriction and vascular remodeling, increasing systemic vascular resistance, a common finding in most cases of human hypertension. ROS promote vasoconstriction and vascular hypertrophy. NOX is up-regulated by humoral and mechanical signals in hypertension. In hypertension, both endothelial xanthine oxidase and ROS are increased, which is associated with increased arteriolar tone. Xanthine oxidase may play a role in end-organ damage in hypertension (Gimenez et al. 2016; Santilli et al. 2015; Montezano et al. 2015a; Virdis et al. 2011).

Hypertension is associated with lipid peroxidation due to an impaired oxidant/antioxidant status (Armas-Padilla et al. 2007). Increased lipid peroxidation and decreased antioxidants with aging indicate that per oxidative damage further increases with higher blood pressure and the aging process. It has been shown that, there was a significant relationship between acetylcholine-dependent vasodilation

and plasma levels of selectins, MCP-1 and thiobarbituric acid-reactive substances (TBARS; as a marker of lipid peroxidation) (Lee et al. 2012; Ahmad et al. 2013; Rodrigo et al. 2013). Previously reported study was to evaluate the influence of aging on the levels of TBARS, lipid hydroperoxide (LOOH), and 8-iso-prostaglandin F2α (8-iso-PGF2α) in elderly hypertensives (Yavuzer et al. 2016a). The results of this study demonstrated that serum TBARS, LOOH and 8-iso-PGF2α levels were significantly high in the elderly hypertensive patients. The relationship between miRNA, NO and eNOS with subclinical atherosclerosis in patients with hypertension has been evaluated (Cengiz et al. 2015). Decreased levels of NO and eNOS and increased miRNA expression were found in this study. This report suggests that miRNA might be involved in the early stages of atherosclerotic process in hypertensive patients. Population-based observational studies have reported an inverse relationship between various plasma antioxidants and blood pressure. Decreased antioxidant activity (SOD, catalase) and reduced levels of ROS scavengers (vitamin E, glutathione) might contribute to oxidative stress in human hypertension (Rodrigo et al. 2007; Loukogeorgakis et al. 2010). Plasma vitamin C levels are inversely related to blood pressure in normotensive and hypertensive cohorts (Block et al. 2008). Amelioration of impaired endothelial function and protection against vascular damage by reducing oxidative stress through exercise, healthy diet, and smoking cessation, but not through antioxidant supplementation, should provide additional therapeutic benefit in the management of patients with hypertension. Until more is known about the molecular mechanisms, whereby ROS cause vascular damage and hypertension in humans, therapies targeting oxidative stress should focus on promoting vascular health through lifestyle and healthy behavioral modifications, such as exercise, nutrition, and smoking cessation (Michalsen and Li 2013).

On the other hand, oxidative stress and endothelial dysfunction are known to be associated with inflammation and can contribute to hypertension; however, whether inflammation is a cause or effect of hypertension is not clear. Inflammation is a protective response to injury or infection. The acute phase protein, C-reactive protein (CRP), is considered as inflammatory marker showing the strongest association with hypertension. It has been demonstrated that hypertensive patients commonly have higher plasma CRP levels. Hypertensive patients have been reported to have higher plasma concentrations of pro-inflammatory cytokines. Inflammation has been shown to down regulate NOS activity. Chronic inflammation can also trigger oxidative stress, which has been associated with hypertension (Crowley 2014; Yasunari et al. 2002).

There is also evidence for involvement of immune cells in human hypertension. Hypertensive patients with nephrosclerosis have higher renal infiltration of CD4+ and CD8+ T cells than normotensives (Youn et al. 2013). Circulating levels of CXC chemokine receptor type 3 (CXCR3), which is well-known tissue-homing chemokine for T cells, have been reported to be elevated in hypertensive patients (Youn et al. 2013). On the other hand, HT induces vascular wall injury and remodeling. The immune system is a sensitive sensor of tissue injury and is involved in the repair (Winn and Harlan 2005b). Hypertensive factors such as AT II, salt, or aldosterone directly activate the innate immune system (De Ciuceis et al. 2014; De Miguel et al. 2015). This process also leads complement activation and toll-like receptors (TLR) as well as ROS production. Autoimmunity can also be directed against vascular wall antigen. Due to the autoantibodies against AT receptor develop in some hypertensives, it is considered that innate immunity can be a secondary cause of hypertension and adaptive immunity can cause or aggravate hypertension. Therefore immunity may be a potential therapeutic target in hypertension in the future (Wenzel et al. 2016; Anders et al. 2015; Idris-Khodja et al. 2014).

Hypertensive individuals are also at increased risk for type 2 diabetes. They are often overweight, insulin resistant, and have endothelial dysfunction. Interestingly, it has been reported that even non-obese hypertensive individuals have abnormalities in endothelial function and findings that suggest that hypertension might impair endothelial function independently from the effects of weight (Ferri et al. 1998). Insulin has both pro- and anti-atherogenic actions, and endothelin-1-dependent vasoconstrictor actions on the vasculature. Endothelin is secreted by ECs, causes vasoconstriction and elevates blood pressure. Endothelin receptor antagonists reduce blood pressure and peripheral vascular resistance in both normotensive controls and patients with mild to moderate essential hypertension, supporting the interpretation that endothelin plays a role in the pathogenesis of hypertension (Lin et al. 2015; Kobayashi et al. 2008). Leptin is a hormone which is secreted by adipocytes and related with obesity. Leptin regulates energy balance and has also sympathetic, vascular and renal actions that can influence blood pressure (Vaněčková et al. 2014). Recent evidence suggests that hyperleptinemia may induce the systemic oxidative stress and decrease the amount of bioactive NO levels possibly due to its degradation by reactive oxygen species. This may be one of the most important mechanisms in the generation of hypertension in obesity (Bełtowski 2012). It has been reported that that plasma leptin and TBARS levels were increased in obesity, and obese hypertensives have significantly higher plasma leptin levels, TBARS levels and lower NO levels than obese normotensives (Konukoglu et al. 2006). Therefore, hyperleptinemia may be an important contributor to the generation of hypertension in obesity.

Hypertension may be associated with impaired fibrinolysis. Fibrinolytic markers such as PAI-1, tPA, and tPA/PAI-1 complex are independently associated with the development of hypertension (Tabak et al. 2009). In a previous study, it has been suggested that, plasma Hcy, which have thrombotic effects, does not have predictive values for indication of cardiovascular disease. However, in the presence of other risk factors (e.g. hyperlipidemia, hypertension, obesity, and/or hyperinsulinemia), Hcy may have a permissive role on the endothelium damage even in the normohomocysteinemic range. The effects of Hcy seemed to be related with free radical generating systems in hypertensives (Konukoglu et al. 2003).

Microparticles (MPs) consist of the EMPs, leukocyte microparticles (LMs) and platelet microparticles (PMPs). MPs are assayed by flow cytometry. Recent data indicate that altered, activated ECs release EMPs into circulation. MPs are furthermore involved in the progression of impaired endothelial function as well as in angiogenesis (Helbing et al. 2014b). There are only few study to show the relationship between MPs and arterial hypertension (Preston et al. 2003; Marques et al. 2013). It has been found that both EMPs and PMPs were significantly increased in hypertensives and that EMPs were correlated with the level of blood pressures. EMPs can be found in several conditions which are associated with arterial hypertension, such as preeclampsia (Marques et al. 2013). It has been found that, EMPs reduce NO in patients with myocardial infarction [135] (Burada EMPler MI'lı hastalarda NO seviyelerini azaltır demek mi istedik?). At the present time, it is considered that circulating MPs might be novel therapeutic targets in microparticle mediated diseases (Helbing et al. 2014b).

5 Antihypertensive Therapy and Endothelial Dysfunction

Current therapies for human hypertension include AT-II type 1 receptor blockers (ARB), Angiotensin-converting enzyme inhibitors (ACEIs), diuretics, calcium channel antagonists, and β-blockers. Treatment with commonly used antihypertensive drugs reduce the risk of total major cardiovascular events, and more importantly, it appears that the higher the reduction in blood pressure, the larger the reduction in cardiovascular risk (James et al. 2014). It has been well documented that endothelium dysfunction can be improved by the use of a statin drug and aspirin, Mediterranean diet, aerobic exercise and weight loss (Montezano et al. 2015b).

Hypertension management guidelines categorize ACEIs and ARB interchangeably as first-line treatments in uncomplicated hypertension (Hirata et al. 2010). These medications have different mechanisms of action and quite different evidence bases (Sindone et al. 2016). The AT-IR leads to vasoconstriction, cell growth, and cell proliferation; the AT-IIR has the opposite effect. The AT-IR is antinatriuretic; the AT-IIR is natriuretic. The AT-IR stimulation results in free radicals; AT-II R stimulation produces *NO* which can neutralize free radicals. The AT-IR induces plasminogen activator inhibitor-1 (*PAI-1*) and other growth family pathways; the AT-II R does not. The ARB binds to and blocks selectively at the AT-IR, promoting stimulation of the receptor by AT-II (Chappell 2016; Matavelli and Siragy 2015). ACEIs prevent the breakdown of bradykinin, a mediator that stimulates the endothelium to generate NO. ACEIs increase NO bioavailability by decreasing the synthesis of AT-II and by enhancing serum levels of NO-releasing bradykinin via inhibition of its degradation. Moreover, ACEIs may also enhance the activity of endothelium-derived hyperpolarizing factor under certain conditions (Mendoza-Torres et al. 2015; Su 2015). On the other hand, it has been reported that treated hypertensive patients with ACEIs had lower plasma sPLA and oxLDL levels and higher Paraoxonase-1 activities than hypertensive patients without therapy (Rao et al. 2015). Therefore, ACEI treatment may also help reduce inflammation and oxidative stress in hypertensives. Short and long-term ACEI administration may be lead an improvement in both coronary and peripheral endothelial function in patients with CAD and/or its risk factors, but the magnitude of this effect may vary depending on the compound used, the presence of risk factors, and genetic variables (Ferroni et al. 2006; Mullen et al. 1998). Additionally, in contrast to ACEIs, controversial results have been reported regarding the effect of AT receptor antagonists on endothelial function (Chappell 2016; Prasad et al. 2001; Li et al. 2014). Recently published data results have been shown that ARBs improve peripheral endothelial function, however, the effect couldn't be maintained for a long time (Prasad et al. 2000).

Some β-blockers have endothelial protective effects. It can improve the endothelium-dependent vasodilator responses by increasing NO release and reducing prothrombotic blood levels of fibrinogen, homocysteine and plasminogen activator inhibitor-1 (e.g. nebivolol, as a β_1-antagonist) (Tzemos et al. 2001), or by its antioxidant capacity (e.g.carvedilol, a non-selective β_1- and β_2 antagonist with α-antagonist property) in patients with essential hypertension (Zepeda et al. 2012). It has been also suggested that the combination of a beta blocker with an ACE inhibitor have more beneficial effect on endothelial function than monotherapy in hypertensive patients with obesity (Vyssoulis et al. 2004). Therefore this combination can be used for the treatment of endothelial dysfunction associated with hypertension, as well as diabetes or atherosclerosis.

Dihydropyridine calcium channel blockers protect against ROS-induced endothelial cell death They have an endothelial protective effect against oxLDL induced ROS, antioxidant activity related to reduction in lipid peroxidation and associated ROS generation (Kelly et al. 2012) or an anti-inflammatory effect as indicated by decreased CRP and IL-6 levels as well as leukocyte activation (Napoli et al. 1999). Combination of calcium channel blockers (e.g. amlodipine) with a renin inhibitor improves endothelial dysfunction in hypertensive patients linked to its NO-releasing action and anti-inflammatory effect (Yasu et al. 2013; Celık et al. 2015).

Angiotensin-(1-7) is a metabolite of AT-I under the action of various enzymes. It can also be generated from AT-II (He et al. 2014). In ECs, AT-(1-7) activates eNOS and inhibits AT II-induced NAD (P) H oxidase activation (Trask and Ferrario 2007). Chronic treatment with AT-(1-7) improves renal endothelial dysfunction by increasing NO release (Arora et al. 2013) and eNOS expression (Costa et al. 2010). Otherwise, AT-(1-7) restores NO/cGMP by production and migration, decreases NOX activity, and enhances survival and proliferation of endothelial progenitor cells isolated from the blood of diabetics (Jarajapu et al. 2013).

ETB receptor on both ECs and vascular smooth muscle cells mediates vasodilatation and constriction, respectively. Although it has been demonstrated that the long term treatment with mixed ETA-receptor and ETB-receptor antagonists (as endothelin receptor antagonist, ERA, bosentan) decreases blood pressure in the patients with mild-to-moderate essential hypertension, suggesting that endothelin may be used in such patients (Krum et al. 1998), development of endothelin drug class for the indication of systemic hypertension has been discontinued because of toxicity (teratogenicity, testicular atrophy, and hepatotoxicity) (Spence et al. 1999; Thaete et al. 2001). Nowadays, ERAs were only used for the treatment of pulmonary arterial hypertension (Chaumais et al. 2015).

It has been indicated that aggressive treatment of dyslipidemia and hypertension was very important by decreasing the development of the atherosclerosis (Hsueh and Quiñones 2003). The thiazolidinediones which are peroxisome proliferator-activated receptor–γ agonists improve glucose and lipid metabolism. These drugs have recently been shown to improve endothelial function in the early stages of insulin resistance (Salomone and Drago 2012).

As a result of this, it is currently difficult to precisely define the possible links between endothelial dysfunction and hypertension or its effects on target organs such as the heart, brain or kidneys. Despite the difficulty of distinguishing the possible direct effects of antihypertensive drugs on endothelial function from indirect protection secondary to the decreased blood pressure, the effects of various antihypertensive drugs on endothelial dysfunction have been tested (Mancia et al. 2013).

6 The Links Between Endothelial Dysfunction and White Coat Hypertension

White coat hypertension (WCH) is a term used for people not receiving antihypertensive medication who have a persistently high office blood pressure ($\geq$ 140/90 mmHg) together with a normal; ambulatory blood pressure ($<$135/85 mmHg) or home blood pressure (Soma et al. 1996). Subjects with WCH are characterized by elevated arterial pressure in the physician's office, but "normal" pressure at other times. Many studies reported that white coat effect can be seen mostly in women, children and elderly. In order not to cause possible risks of inaccurate treatment in these patients, ambulatory blood pressure measurements should be done regularly and treatment decision should be given accordingly.

The prognosis in the patients with WCH remains uncertain. Several studies indicate a good prognosis of this condition by demonstrating a low-degree of end organ damage (Pickering et al. 1988; White et al. 1989). Other authors report WCH exhibits end-organ damage (Cardillo et al. 1993; Hoegholm et al. 1994) and metabolic abnormalities such as hyperlipidemia, impaired insulin sensitivity, elevated blood glucose, and increased serum insulin levels (Bjorklund et al. 2002; Julius et al. 1990; Weber et al. 1994). Sustained hypertension causes atherosclerotic changes and it is one of the main risk factors of coronary artery disease. It is not clear, if WCH also causes atherosclerosis as it is associated with other target organ changes similar to those associated with sustained hypertension. Clinical surveys on endothelial dysfunction in WCH are controversial (Hlubocka et al. 2002; Vaindirlis et al. 2000a; Gomez-Cerezo et al. 2002). In meta-analyses, the patients with WCH were not significantly different from true normotensive individuals when adjusted for age, gender and other covariates (Fagard and Cornelissen 2007; Pierdomenico and Cuccurullo 2011; Franklin et al. 2012). On the other hand, other meta-analyses state that common carotid intima-media thickness is greater in WCH patients than in true normotensive individuals and is not different from sustained hypertensive patients (Cuspidi et al. 2015a). In few meta-analyses indicate that WCH is not an entirely benign condition (Briasoulis et al. 2016; Cuspidi et al. 2015b;

Stergiou et al. 2014). WCH might not be considered as an innocent trait. It seems to be an important clinical situation requiring a close follow-up.

Various studies also observed the presence of endothelial dysfunction and abnormal angiogenesis with increased values of ET-1, homocysteine and vascular VEGF accompanying with a decrease in NO in WCH (Tabak et al. 2009; Uzun et al. 2004; Karter et al. 2004; Curgunlu et al. 2005a; Curgunlu et al. 2005b; Caner et al. 2006; Marchi-Alves and Carnio 2009; Lengyel et al. 2012; Yavuzer et al. 2015). The relationship of oxidative stress and NO is well known. Increased NO levels in WCH patients may be the result of enhanced oxidative stress. It indicates the increased oxidative stress which was probably the leading cause of endothelial dysfunction. The elevated oxidative status is a strong risk factor for coronary artery disease. Procalcitonin (PCT) levels in WCH patients are significantly and consistently higher than normotensives (Yavuzer et al. 2016b). Systemic inflammation moderately occurs in the WCH. PCT monitoring may be a useful biomarker in inflammation related to atherosclerosis and early stage hypertension.

Even though several studies described WCH as a benign entity and showed no difference in cardiovascular events and deaths between WCH and normotensive patients, other studies have indicated similar or at least close rates of death or cardiovascular events in patients with WCH and clinical hypertensive patients (Verdecchia et al. 1996; Strandherg and Salomaa 2000). The early detection of these patients by ambulatory blood pressure monitorization might prevent future mortality and morbidity. To sum up, white coat effect is not an innocent phenomenon like normal blood pressure nor as hazardous as clinical hypertension. WCH may thus be a transition state between normotension and hypertension. It may be concluded that vascular changes in WCH were not structural but functional. Further studies are needed to assess the increased cardiovascular risk in WCH conferred by endothelial dysfunction.

Conclusion Endothelial dysfunction is a common mechanism involved in many cardiovascular diseases, and plays a critical role in the development of diseases or contributes to the development and progression of organ damages. Multiple mechanisms such as inflammation, increased ROS and RNS, cellular apoptosis, increased vasoconstrictor production, decreased vasodilator production and vascular remodeling are involved in endothelial dysfunction. In endothelial dysfunction, NO bioavailability seems to play a central role in the development and progress of hypertension, as well as diabetes or atherosclerosis. It appears that a drug with endothelium-protective property may yield therapeutic benefits. Endothelial dysfunction is more prevalent in WCH than in true normotensive individuals, but it is either equal or better in WCH as compared to sustained hypertension. Therefore, the evaluation of endothelium-improving action may be helpful for the hypertension related cardiovascular events.

References

Ahmad A, Singhal U, Hossain MM, Islam N, Rizvi I (2013) The role of the endogenous antioxidant enzymes and malondialdehyde in essential hypertension. J Clin Diagn Res 7:987–990

Anders HJ, Baumann M, Tripepi G, Mallamaci F (2015) Immunity in arterial hypertension: associations or causalities. Nephrol Dial Transplant 30:1959–1964

Armas-Padilla MC, Armas-Hernández MJ, Sosa-Canache B, Cammarata R, Pacheco B, Guerrero J, Carvajal AR, Hernández-Hernández R, Israili ZH, Valasco M (2007) Nitric oxide and malondialdehyde in human hypertension. Am J Ther 14:172–176

Arora P, Arora A, Sharma S (2013) Vascular endothelium dysfunction and hypertension: insight on molecular basics. Innov Pharm Pharmacother 1:199–219

Bae SW, Kim HS, Cha YN, Park YS, Jo SA, Jo I (2003) Rapid increase in endothelial nitric oxide production by bradykinin is mediated by protein kinase A signaling pathway. Biochem Biophys Res Commun 306:981–987

Ballermann BJ, Dardik A, Eng E, Liu A (1998) Shear stress and the endothelium. Kidney Int Suppl 67: S100–S108

Barnathan ES, Kuo A, Karikó K, Rosenfeld L, Murray SC, Behrendt N, Rønne E, Weiner D, Henkin J, Cines DB (1990) Characterization of human endothelial cell urokinase-type plasminogen activator receptor protein and mRNA. Blood 76:1795–1806

Barton M (2011) The discovery of endothelium-dependent contraction: the legacy of Paul M. Vanhoutte Pharmacol Res 63:455–462

Bauer J, Ripperger A, Frantz S, Ergün S, Schwedhelm E, Benndorf RA (2014) Pathophysiology of isoprostanes in the cardiovascular system: implications of isoprostane-mediated thromboxane A2 receptor activation. Br J Pharmacol 171:3115–3131

Bełtowski J (2012) Leptin and the regulation of endothelial function in physiological and pathological conditions. Clin Exp Pharmacol Physiol 39:168–178

Bernal-Mizrachi L, Jy W, Jimenez JJ, Pastor J, Mauro LM, Horstman LL, de Marchena E, Ahn YS (2003) High levels of circulating endothelial microparticles in patients with acute coronary syndromes. Am Heart J 145:962–970

Bjorklund K, Lind L, Vessby B, Andren B, Lithell H (2002) Different metobolic predictors of white-coat and sustained hypertension over a 20-year follow up. Circulation 106:63–68

Block G, Jensen CD, Norkus EP, Hudes M, Crawford PB (2008) Vitamin C in plasma is inversely related to blood pressure and change in blood pressure during the previous year in young Black and White women. Nutr J 7:35.1–9

Bonetti PO, Lerman LO, Lerman A (2003) Endothelial dysfunction: a marker of atherosclerotic risk. Arterioscler Thromb Vasc Biol 23:168–175

Boulanger CM, Scoazec A, Ebrahimian T, Henry P, Mathieu E, Tedgui A, Mallat Z (2001) Circulating microparticles from patients with myocardial infarction cause endothelial dysfunction. Circulation 104:2649–2652

Briasoulis A, Androulakis E, Palla M, Papageorgiou N, Tousoulis D (2016) White-coat hypertension and cardiovascular events: a meta-analysis. J Hypertens 34:593–599

Cahill PA, Redmond EM (2016) Vascular endothelium – gatekeeper of vessel health. Atherosclerosis 248:97–109

Calver A, Collier J, Vallance P (1993) Nitric oxide and cardiovascular control. Exp Physiol l78:303–326

Caner M, Karter Y, Uzun H, Curgunlu A, Vehid S, Balci H, Yucel R, Güner I, Kutlu A, Yaldiran A, Oztürk E (2006) Oxidative stress in human in sustained and white coat hypertension. Int J Clin Pract 60:1565–1571

Cardillo C, Felice FD, Campia U, Folli G (1993) Psychological reactivity and cardiac end organ changes in white coat hypertension. Hypertension 21:836–844

Celık T, Balta S, Karaman M, Ahmet Ay S, Demırkol S, Ozturk C, Dınc M, Unal HU, Yılmaz MI, Kılıc S, Kurt G, Tas A, Iyısoy A, Quartı-Trevano F, Fıcı F, Grassı G (2015) Endocan, a novel marker of endothelial dysfunction in patients with essential hypertension: comparative effects of amlodipine and valsartan. Blood Press 24:55–60

Cengiz M, Yavuzer S, Kılıçkıran Avcı B, Yürüyen M, Yavuzer H, Dikici SA, Karataş ÖF, Özen M, Uzun H, Öngen Z (2015) Circulating miR-21 and eNOS in subclinical atherosclerosis in patients with hypertension. Clin Exp Hypertens 37:643–649

Ceriello A (2008) Possible role of oxidative stress in the pathogenesis of hypertension. Diabetes Care Am Diabetes Assoc 31(Supl 2):S181–S184

Chappell MC (2016) Biochemical evaluation of the renin-angiotensin system: the good, bad, and absolute? Am J Physiol Heart Circ Physiol 310:H137–H152

Chaumais MC, Guignabert C, Savale L, Jaïs X, Boucly A, Montani D, Simonneau G, Humbert M, Sitbon O (2015) Clinical pharmacology of endothelin receptor antagonists used in the treatment of pulmonary arterial hypertension. Am J Cardiovasc Drug 15:13–26

Chistiakov DA, Orekhov AN, Bobryshev YV (2015) Endothelial barrier and its abnormalities in cardiovascular disease. Front Physiol 6:1–11

Coban E, Ozdoğan M, Ermiş C (2004) Plasma levels of homocysteine in patients with white-coat hypertension. Int J Clin Pract 58:997–999

Costa MA, Lopez Verrilli MA, Gomez KA, Nakagawa P, Peña C, Arranz C, Gironacci MM (2010) Angiotensin-(1-7) upregulates cardiac nitric oxide synthase in spontaneously hypertensive rats. Am J Physiol Heart Circ Physiol 299:H1205–H1211

Croft M, So T, Duan W, Soroosh P (2009) The significance of OX40 and OX40L to T cell biology and immune disease. Immunol Rev 229:173–191

Crowley SD (2014) The cooperative roles of inflammation and oxidative stress in the pathogenesis of hypertension. Antioxid Redox Signal 20:102–120

Curgunlu A, Uzun H, Bavunoğlu I, Karter Y, Genç H, Vehid S (2005a) Increased circulating concentrations of asymmetric dimethylarginine (ADMA) in white coat hypertension. J Hum Hypertens 19:629–633

Curgunlu A, Karter Y, Uzun H, Aydin S, Ertürk N, Vehid S, Simsek G, Kutlu A, Oztürk E, Erdine S (2005b) Hyperhomocysteinemia: an additional risk factor in white coat hypertension. Int Heart J 46:245–254

Cuspidi C, Sala C, Tadic M, Rescaldani M, Grassi G, Mancia G (2015a) Is white-coat hypertension a risk factor for carotid atherosclerosis? A review and meta-analysis. Blood Press Monit 20:57–63

Cuspidi C, Rescaldani M, Tadic M, Sala C, Grassi G, Mancia G (2015b) White-coat hypertension, as defined by ambulatory blood pressure monitoring, and subclinical cardiac organ damage: a meta-analysis. J Hypertens 33:24–32

Davenport AP, Hyndman KA, Dhaun N, Southan C, Kohan DE, Pollock JS, Pollock DM, Webb DJ, Maguire JJ (2016) Endothelin. Pharmacol Rev 68:357–418

Dawes MG, Bartlett G, Coats AJ, Juszczak E (2008) Comparing the effects of white coat hypertension and sustained hypertension on mortality in a UK primary care setting. Ann Fam Med 6:390–396

Dawson TM, Bredt DS, Fotuhi M, Hwang PM, Snyder SH (1991) Nitric oxide synthase and neuronal NADPH diaphorase are identical in brain and peripheral tissues. Proc Natl Acad Sci 88:7797–7801

De Ciuceis C, Rossini C, La Boria E, Porteri E, Petroboni B, Gavazzi A, Sarkar A, Rosei EA, Rizzoni D (2014) Immune mechanisms in hypertension. High Blood Press Cardiovasc Prev 21:227–234

De Miguel C, Rudemiller NP, Abais JM, Mattson DL (2015) Inflammation and hypertension: new understandings and potential therapeutic targets. Curr Hypertens Rep 17:507

Dohi Y, Thiel MA, Buhler FR, Luscher TF (1990) Activation of the endothelial L-arginine pathway in pressurized mesenteric resistance arteries: effect of age and hypertension. Hypertension 15:170–179

Dunn S, Vohra RS, Murphy JE, Homer-Vanniasinkam S, Walker JH, Ponnambalam S (2008) The lectin-like oxidized low-density-lipoprotein receptor: a pro-inflammatory factor in vascular disease. Biochem J 409:349–355

Endemann DH, Schiffrin EL (2004) Endothelial dysfunction. J Am Soc Nephrol 15:1983–1992

Ercan M, Konukoglu D, Onen S (2003) Plasma viscosity as a cardiovascular risk marker in patients with proteinuria. Clin Hemorheol Microcirc 29:111–116

Ercan M, Firtina S, Konukoglu D (2014) Comparison of plasma viscosity as a marker of endothelial dysfunction with nitric oxide and asymmetric dimethylarginine in subjects with dyslipidemia. Clin Hemorheol Microcirc 57:315–323

Esmon CT (2006) Inflammation and the activated protein C anticoagulant pathway. Semin Thromb Hemost 32 (Suppl 1):49–60

Fagard RH, Cornelissen VA (2007) Incidence of cardiovascular events in white-coat, masked and sustained hypertension vs. true normotension: a meta-analysis. J Hypertens 25:2193–2198

Félétou M, Vanhoutte PM (2006) Endothelium-derived hyperpolarizing factor: where are we now? Arterioscler Thromb Vasc Biol 26:1215–1225

Ferri C, Desideri G, Baldoncini R, Bellini C, De Angelis C, Mazzocchi C, Santucci A (1998) Early activation of vascular endothelium in nonobese, non-diabetic essential hypertensive patients with multiple metabolic abnormalities. Diabetes 47:660–667

Ferroni P, Basili S, Paoletti V, Davì G, Psaty BM (2006) Endothelial dysfunction and oxidative stress in arterial hypertension. Nutr Metab Cardiovasc Dis 16:222–233

Francis SH, Busch JL, Corbin JD, Sibley D (2010) cGMP-dependent protein kinases and cGMP phosphodiesterases in nitric oxide and cGMP action. Pharmacol Rev 62:525–563

Franklin SS, Thijs L, Hansen TW, Li Y, Boggia J, Kikuya M, Björklund-Bodegård K, Ohkubo T, Jeppesen J, Torp-Pedersen C, Dolan E, Kuznetsova T, Stolarz-Skrzypek K, Tikhonoff V, Malyutina S, Casiglia E, Nikitin Y, Lind L, Sandoya E, Kawecka-Jaszcz K, Imai Y, Wang J,

Ibsen H, O'Brien E, Staessen JA, International Database on Ambulatory Blood Pressure in Relation to Cardiovascular Outcomes Investigators (2012) Significance of white-coat hypertension in older persons with isolated systolic hypertension: a meta-analysis using the International Database on Ambulatory Blood Pressure Monitoring in Relation to Cardiovascular Outcomes population. Hypertension 59:564–571

Gimenez M, Schickling BM, Lopes LR, Miller FJ Jr (2016) Nox1 in cardiovascular diseases: regulation and pathophysiology. Clin Sci 130:151–165

Goldenberg NM, Kuebler WM (2015) Endothelial cell regulation of pulmonary vascular tone, inflammation, and coagulation. Comp Physiol 5:531–559

Gomez-Cerezo J, Ríos Blanco JJ, Suárez García I, Moreno Anaya P, García Raya P, Vázquez-Muñoz E, Barbado Hernández FJ (2002) Noninvasive study of endothelial function in white coat hypertension. Hypertension 40:304–309

González J, Valls N, Brito R, Rodrigo R (2014) Essential hypertension and oxidative stress: new insights. World J Cardiol 6:353–366

Gunnett C, Lund D, McDowell A, Faraci F, Heistad D (2005) Mechanisms of inducible nitric oxide synthaseemediated vascular dysfunction. Arterioscler Thromb Vasc Biol 25:1617–1622

He Y, Si D, Yang C, Ni L, Li B, Ding M, Yang P (2014) The effects of amlodipine and S(-)-amlodipine on vascular endothelial function in patients with hypertension. Am J Hypertens 27:27–31

Helbing T, Olivier C, Bode C, Moser M, Diehl P (2014) Role of microparticles in endothelial dysfunction and arterial hypertension. World J Cardiol 6:1135–1139

Hirata Y, Nagata D, Suzuki E, Nishimatsu H, Suzuki J, Nagai R (2010) Diagnosis and treatment of endothelial dysfunction in cardiovascular disease. Int Heart J 51:1–6

Hlubocka Z, Umnevora V, Heller S et al (2002) Circulating intercellular cell adhesion molecule-1, endothelin-1and von willebrand factor-markers of endothelial dysfunction in uncomplicated essensial hypertension: the effect of treatment with ACE inhibitors. J Hum Hypertens 16:557–562

Hoegholm A, Bang LE, Kristensen KS, Nielsen JW, Holm J (1994) Microalbuminuria in 411 untreated individuals with established hypertension, white coat hypertension and normotension. Hypertension 24:101–105

Hsueh WA, Quiñones MJ (2003) Role of endothelial dysfunction in insulin resistance. Am J Cardiol 92:10J–17J

Idris-Khodja N, Mian MO, Paradis P, Schiffrin EL (2014) Dual opposing roles of adaptive immunity in hypertension. Eur Heart J 35:1238–1244

Jacobsen JC, Hornbech MS, Holstein-Rathlou NH (2011) Significance of microvascular remodelling for the vascular flow reserve in hypertension. Interface Focus 1:117–131

Jaipersad AS, Lip GY, Silverman S, Shantsila E (2014) The role of monocytes in angiogenesis and atherosclerosis. J Am Coll Cardiol 63:1–11

James PA, Oparil S, Carter BL, Cushman WC, Dennison-Himmelfarb C, Handler J, Lackland DT, LeFevre ML, MacKenzie TD, Ogedegbe O, Smith SC Jr, Svetkey LP, Taler SJ, Townsend RR, Wright JT Jr, Narva AS, Ortiz E (2014) 2014 evidence-based guideline for the management of high blood pressure in adults: report from the panel members appointed to the Eighth Joint National Committee (JNC 8). JAMA 311:507–520

Jarajapu YP, Bhatwadekar AD, Caballero S, Hazra S, Shenoy V, Medina R, Kent D, Stitt AW, Thut C, Finney EM, Raizada MK, Grant MB (2013) Activation of the ACE2/angiotensin-(1-7)/Mas receptor axis enhances the reparative function of dysfunctional diabetic endothelial progenitors. Diabetes 62:1258–1269

Jiang F, Yang J, Zhang Y, Dong M, Wang S, Zhang Q, Liu FF, Zhang K, Zhang C (2014) Angiotensin-converting enzyme 2 and angiotensin 1-7: novel therapeutic targets. Nat Rev Cardiol 11:413–426

Julius S, Mejia A, Jones K et al (1990) 'White coat' versus 'sustained' borderline hypertension in Tecimseh, Michigan. Hypertension 16:617–623

Karter Y, Ertürk NT, Aydín S, Curgunlu A, Uzun H, Vehid S, Kutlu AO, Yaldiran A, Oztürk E, Erdine S, Sipahioğlu F (2003) Endothelial dysfunction in sustaincd and white coat hypertension. Am J Hypertens 16:892

Karter Y, Aydin S, Curgunlu A, Uzun H, Ertürk N, Vehid S, Kutlu A, Simsek G, Yücel R, Arat A, Ozturk E, Erdine S (2004) Endothelium and angiogenesis in white coat hypertension. J Hum Hypertens 18:809–814

Kedzierski RM, Yanagisawa M (2001) Endothelin system: the double-edged sword in health and disease. Annu Rev Pharmacol Toxicol 41:851–876

Kellogg D, Zhao J, Coey U, Green J (2005) Acetylcholine-induced vasodilation is mediated by nitric oxide and prostaglandins in human skin. J Appl Physiol 98:629–632

Kelly AS, Gonzalez-Campoy JM, Rudser KD, Katz H, Metzig AM, Thalin M, Bank AJ (2012) Carvedilol-lisinopril combination therapy and endothelial function in obese individuals with hypertension. J Clin Hypertens 14:85–91

Khazaei M, Moien-afshari F, Laher I (2008) Vascular endothelial function in health and diseases. Pathophysiology 15:49–67

Kim YW, Byzova TV (2014) Oxidative stress in angiogenesis and vascular disease. Blood 123:625–631

Kiowski W (1999) Endothelial dysfunction in hypertension. Clin Exp Hypertens 21:635–646

Kleinegris MC, Ten Cate-Hoek AJ, Ten Cate H (2012) Coagulation and the vessel wall in thrombosis and atherosclerosis. Pol Arch Med Wewn 122:557–566

Kobayashi T, Nogami T, Taguchi K, Matsumoto T, Kamata K (2008) Diabetic state, high plasma insulin and angiotensin II combine to augment endothelin-1-induced vasoconstriction via ETA receptors and ERK. Br J Pharmacol 155:974–983

Kolluru GK, Sinha S, Majumder S, Muley A, Siamwala JH, Gupta R, Chatterjee S (2010) Shear stress promotes nitric oxide production in endothelial cells by sub-cellular delocalization of eNOS: a basis for shear stress mediated angiogenesis. Nitric Oxide 22:304–315

Konukoglu D, Serin O, Ercan M, Turhan M (2003) Plasma homocysteine levels in obese and non-obese subjects with or without hypertension; its relationship with oxidative stress and copper. Clin Biochem 36:405–408

Konukoglu D, Serin O, Turhan MS (2006) Plasma leptin and its relationship with lipid peroxidation and nitric oxide in obese female patients with or without hypertension. Arch Med Res 37:602–606

Konukoglu D, Firtina S, Serin O, Cavusoglu C (2009) Relationship among plasma secretory phospholipase A2, oxidized low density lipoprotein & paraoxonase activities in hypertensive subjects treated with angiotensin converting enzyme inhibitors. Indian J Med Res 129:390–394

Korbecki J, Baranowska-Bosiacka I, Gutowska I, Chlubek D (2014) Cyclooxygenase pathways. Acta Biochim Pol 61:639–649

Krum H, Viskoper RJ, Lacourciere Y, Budde M, Charlon V (1998) The effect of an endothelin-receptor antagonist, bosentan, on blood pressure in patients with essential hypertension. Bosentan Hypertension Investigators. N Engl J Med 338:784–790

Lacave R, Rondeau E, Ochi S, Delarue F, Schleuning WD, Sraer JD (1989) Characterization of a plasminogen activator and its inhibitor in human mesangial cells. Kidney Int 35:806–811

Laher I (ed) (2014) Systems biology of free radicals and antioxidants book. Springer, Berlin/Heidelberg

Lee R, Margaritis M, Channon KM, Antoniades C (2012) Evaluating oxidative stress in human cardiovascular disease: methodological aspects and considerations. Curr Med Chem 19:2504–2520

Lengyel S, Katona E, Zatik J, Molnár C, Paragh G, Fülesdi B, Páll D (2012) The impact of serum homocysteine on intima-media thickness in normotensive, white-coat and sustained hypertensive adolescents. Blood Press 21:39–44

Lerman A, Burnett JC Jr (1992) Intact and altered endothelium in regulation of vasomotion. Circulation 86 (suppl III):III-12–II-19

Levesque MJ, Nerem RM, Sprague EA (1990) Vascular endothelial cell proliferation in culture and the influence of flow. Biomaterials 11:702–707

Li Y, Haga C, Chien S (2005) Molecular basis of the effects of shear stress on vascular endothelial cells. J Biomech 38:1949–1971

Li S, Wu Y, Yu G, Xia Q, Xu Y (2014) Angiotensin II receptor blockers improve peripheral endothelial function: a meta-analysis of randomized controlled trials. PLoS One 9, e90217

Lijnen HR, Collen D (1997) Endothelium in hemostasis and thrombosis. Prog Cardiovasc Dis 39:343–350

Lin YJ, Juan CC, Kwok CF, Hsu YP, Shih KC, Chen CC, Ho LT (2015) Endothelin-1 exacerbates development of hypertension and atherosclerosis in modest insulin resistant syndrome. Biochem Biophys Res Commun 460:497–503

Loukogeorgakis SP, van den Berg MJ, Sofat R, Nitsch D, Charakida M, Haiyee B, de Groot E, MacAllister RJ, Kuijpers TW, Deanfield JE (2010) Role of NADPH oxidase in endothelial ischemia/reperfusion injury in humans. Circulation 121:2310–2316

Lowenstein CJ, Padalko E (2004) iNOS (NOS2) at a glance. J Cell Sci 117:2865–2867

Luksha L, Agewall S, Kublickiene K (2009) Endothelium-derived hyperpolarizing factor in vascular physiology and cardiovascular disease. Atherosclerosis 202:330–344

Luscher TF (1991) Endothelium-derived nitric oxide: the endogenous nitrovasodilator in the human cardiovascular system. Eur Heart J 12(Suppl E):2–11

Luscher TF, Vanhoutte PM (1986) Endothelium-dependent contractions to acetylcholine in the aorta of the spontaneously hypertensive rat. Hypertension 8:344–348

Lüscher TF, Yang ZH, Diederich D, Bühler FR (1989) Endothelium-derived vasoactive substances: potential role in hypertension, atherosclerosis, and vascular occlusion. J Cardiovasc Pharmacol 14(Suppl 6):S63–S69

Mai J, Virtue A, Shen J, Wang H, Yang X-F (2013) An evolving new paradigm: endothelial cells–conditional innate immune cells. J Hematol Oncol 6:61

Mancia G, Fagard R, Narkiewicz K et al (2013) ESH/ESC guidelines for the management of arterial hypertension: the Task Force for the Management of Arterial Hypertension of the European Society of Hypertension (ESH) and of the European Society of Cardiology (ESC). Eur Heart J 34:2159–2219

Marchi-Alves LM, Carnio EC (2009) Is there any correlation between insulin resistance and nitrate plasma concentration in white coat hypertensive patients? Cardiol Res Pract 2009:376735

Marques FK, Campos FM, Sousa LP, Teixeira-Carvalho-A, Dusse LM, Gomes KB (2013) Association of microparticles and preeclampsia. Mol Biol Rep 40:4553–4559

Masuyer G, Yates CJ, Sturrock ED, Acharya KR (2014) Angiotensin-I converting enzyme (ACE): structure, biological roles, and molecular basis for chloride ion dependence. Biol Chem 395:1135–1149

Matavelli LC, Siragy HM (2015) AT2 receptor activities and pathophysiological implications. J Cardiovasc Pharmacol 65:226–232

McCully KS (2015) Homocysteine and the pathogenesis of atherosclerosis. Expert Rev Clin Pharmacol 8:211–219

McIntyre M, Bohr DF, Dominiczak AF (1999) Endothelial function in hypertension: the role of superoxide anion. Hypertension 34:539–545

Medzhitov R (2008) Origin and physiological roles of inflammation. Nature 454:428–435

Melikian N, Seddon MD, Casadei B, Chowienczyk PJ, Shah AM (2009) Neuronal nitric oxide synthase and human vascular regulation. Trends Cardiovasc Med 19:256–262

Mendoza-Torres E, Oyarzún A, Mondaca-Ruff D, Azocar A, Castro PF, Jalil JE, Chiong M, Lavandero S, Ocaranza MP (2015) ACE2 and vasoactive peptides: novel players in cardiovascular/renal remodeling and hypertension. Ther Adv Cardiovasc Dis 9:217–237

Michalsen A, Li C (2013) Fasting therapy for treating and preventing disease – current state of evidence. Forsch Komplementmed 20:444–453

Michel T, Vanhoutte PM (2010) Cellular signaling and NO production. Pflugers Arch - Eur J Physiol 459:807–816

Montezano AC, Tsiropoulou S, Dulak-Lis M, Harvey A, Camargo Lde L, Touyz RM (2015a) Redox signaling, Nox5 and vascular remodeling in hypertension. Curr Opin Nephrol Hypertens 24:425–433

Montezano AC, Dulak-Lis M, Tsiropoulou S, Harvey A, Briones AM, Touyz RM (2015b) Oxidative stress and human hypertension: vascular mechanisms, biomarkers, and novel therapies. Can J Cardiol 31:631–641

Mullen MJ, Clarkson P, Donald AE, Thomson H, Thorne SA, Powe AJ, Furuno T, Bull T, Deanfield JE (1998) Effect of enalapril on endothelial function in young insulin-dependent diabetic patients: a randomized, double-blind study. J Am Coll Cardiol 31:1330–1335

Muniyappa R, Sowers JR (2013) Role of insulin resistance in endothelial dysfunction. Rev Endocr Metab Disord 14:5–12

Napoli C, Salomone S, Godfraind T, Palinski W, Capuzzi DM, Palumbo G, D'Armiento FP, Donzelli R, de Nigris F, Capizzi RL, Mancini M, Gonnella JS, Bianchi A (1999) 1,4-Dihydropyridin ealcium channel blockers inhibit plasma and LDL oxidation and formation of oxidation-specific epitopes in the arterial wall and prolong survival in stroke-prone spontaneously hypertensive rats. Stroke 30:1907–1915

Oparil S, Zaman MA, Calhoun DA (2003) Pathogenesis of hypertension. Ann Intern Med 139:761–776

Ouweneel AB, Van Eck M (2016) Lipoproteins as modulators of atherothrombosis: from endothelial function to primary and secondary coagulation. Vascul Pharmacol 82:1–10

Palmer RM, Ashton D, Moncada S (1988) Vascular endothelial cells synthesize nitric oxide from L-arginine. Nature 333:664–666

Papageorgiou N, Androulakis E, Papaioannou S, Antoniades C, Tousoulis D (2015) Homoarginine in the shadow of asymmetric dimethylarginine: from nitric oxide to cardiovascular disease. Amino Acids 47:1741–1750

Pastrana JL, Sha X, Virtue A, Mai J, Cueto R, Lee IA, Wang H, Yang XF (2012) Regulatory T cells and Atherosclerosis. J Clin Exp Cardiol 2012(Suppl 12):002–019

Perutelli P, Marchese P, Mori PG (1992) The glycoprotein IIb/IIIa complex of the platelets. An activation-dependent integrin. Recenti Prog Med 83:100–104

Pickering TG, James GD, Boddie C, Harshfield GA, Blank S, Laragh JH (1988) How common is white coat hypertension. JAMA 259:225–228

Pierdomenico SD, Cuccurullo F (2011) Prognostic value of white-coat and masked hypertension diagnosed by ambulatory monitoring in initially untreated subjects: an updated meta-analysis. Am J Hypertens 24:52–58

Pierdomenico SD, Bucci A, Lapenna D, Lattanzio FM, Talone L, Cuccurullo F, Mezzetti A (2003) Circulating homocysteine levels in sustained and white coat hypertension. J Hum Hypertens 17:165–170

Pirillo A, Norata GD, Catapano AL (2013) LOX-1, OxLDL, and atherosclerosis. Mediators Inflamm 2013:1–13

Prasad A, Tupas-Habib T, Schenke WH, Mincemoyer R, Panza JA, Waclawiw MA, Ellahham S, Quyyumi AA (2000) Acute and chronic angiotensin-1 receptor antagonism reverses endothelial dysfunction in atherosclerosis. Circulation 101:2349–2354

Prasad A, Halcox JPJ, Waclawiw MA, Quyyumi AA (2001) Angiotensin type 1 receptor antagonism reverses abnormal coronary vasomotion in atherosclerosis. J Am Coll Cardiol 38:1089–1095

Preston RA, Jy W, Jimenez JJ, Mauro LM, Horstman LL, Valle M, Aime G, Ahn YS (2003) Effects of severe hypertension on endothelial and platelet microparticles. Hypertension 41:211–217

Prieto D, Contreras C, Sánchez A (2014) Endothelial dysfunction, obesity and insulin resistance. Curr Vasc Pharmacol 12:412–426

Pushpakumar S, Kundu S, Sen U (2014) Endothelial dysfunction: the link between homocysteine and hydrogen sulfide. Curr Med Chem 21:3662–3672

Rajendran P, Rengarajan T, Thangavel J, Nishigaki Y, Sakthisekaran D, Sethi G, Nishigaki I (2013) The vascular endothelium and human diseases. Int J Biol Sci 9:1057–1069

Ralevic V, Dunn WR (2015) Purinergic transmission in blood vessels. Auton Neurosci 191:48–66

Rao A, Pandya V, Whaley-Connell A (2015) Obesity and insulin resistance in resistant hypertension: implications for the kidney. Adv Chronic Kidney Dis 22:211–217

Reneman RS, Arts T, Hoeks AP (2006) Wall shear stress—an important determinant of endothelial cell function and structure in the arterial system in vivo. Discrepancies with theory. J Vasc Res 43:251–269

Rodrigo R, Prat H, Passalacqua W, Araya J, Guichard C, Bächler JP (2007) Relationship between oxidative stress and essential hypertension. Hypertens Res 30:1159–1167

Rodrigo R, Libuy M, Feliú F, Hasson D (2013) Oxidative stress-related biomarkers in essential hypertension and ischemia-reperfusion myocardial damage. Dis Markers 35:773–790

Rodriguez-Iturbe B, Pons H, Quiroz Y, Lanaspa M, Johnson RJ (2014) Autoimmunity in the pathogenesis of hypertension. Nat Rev Nephrol 10:56–62

Salame MY, Samani NJ, Masood I, deBono DP (2000) Expression of the plasminogen activator system in the human vascular wall. Atherosclerosis 152:19–28

Salomone S, Drago F (2012) Effects of PPARγ ligands on vascular tone. Curr Mol Pharmacol 5:282–291

Santilli F, D'Ardes D, Davì G (2015) Oxidative stress in chronic vascular disease: from prediction to prevention. Vasc Pharmacol 74:23–37

Shih GC, Hajjar KA (1993) Plasminogen and plasminogen activator assembly on the human endothelial cell. Proc Soc Exp Biol Med 202:258–264

Siervo M, Corander M, Stranges S, Bluck L (2011) Post-challenge hyperglycaemia, nitric oxide production and endothelial dysfunction: the putative role of asymmetric dimethylarginine (ADMA). Nutr Metab Cardiovasc Dis 21:1–10

Sindone A, Erlich J, Lee C, Newman H, Suranyi M, Roger SD (2016) Cardiovascular risk reduction in hypertension: angiotensin-converting enzyme inhibitors, angiotensin receptor blockers. Where are we up to? Intern Med J 46:364–372

Siti HN, Kamisah Y, Kamsiah J (2015) The role of oxidative stress, antioxidants and vascular inflammation in cardiovascular disease. Vasc Pharmacol 71:40–56

Soma J, Aakhus S, Dahl K, Slørdahl S, Wiseth R, Widerøe TE, Skjaerpe T (1996) Hemodynamics in white coat hypertension compared to ambulatory hypertension and normotension. Am J Hypertens 9:1090–1098

Spence S, Anderson C, Cukierski M, Patrick D (1999) Teratogenic effects of the endothelin receptor antagonist L-753,037 in the rat. Reprod Toxicol 13:15–29

Stancel N, Chen CC, Ke LY, Chu CS, Lu J, Sawamura T, Chen CH (2016) Interplay between crp, atherogenic ldl, and lox-1 and its potential role in the pathogenesis of atherosclerosis. Clin Chem 62:320–327

Steffel J, Lüscher TF, Tanner FC (2006) Tissue factor in cardiovascular diseases: molecular mechanisms and clinical implications. Circulation 113:722–731

Stenina OI (2003) Regulation of gene expression in vascular cells by coagulation proteins. Curr Drug Targets 4:143–158

Stergiou GS, Asayama K, Thijs L, Kollias A, Niiranen TJ, Hozawa A, Boggia J, Johansson JK, Ohkubo T, Tsuji I, Jula AM, Imai Y, Staessen JA, International Database on HOme blood pressure in relation to Cardiovascular Outcome (IDHOCO) Investigators (2014) Prognosis of white-coat and masked hypertension: International Database of HOme blood pressure in relation to Cardiovascular Outcome. Hypertension 63:675–682

Strandherg TE, Salomaa V (2000) White coat effect, blood pressure and mortality in men: prospective cohort study. Eur Heart J 21:1714–1718

Su JB (2015) Vascular endothelial dysfunction and pharmacological treatment. World J Cardiol 7:719–741

Szmitko PE, Wang CH, Weisel RD, de Almeida JR, Anderson TJ, Verma S (2003) New markers of inflammation and endothelial cell activation: part I. Circulation 108:1917–1923

Tabak O, Gelisgen R, Uzun H, Kalender B, Balci H, Curgunlu A, Simsek G, Karter Y (2009) Hypertension and hemostatic/fibrinolytic balance disorders. Clin Invest Med 32:E285–E290

Thaete LG, Neerhof MG, Silver RK (2001) Differential effects of endothelin A and B receptor antagonism on fetal growth in normal and nitric oxide-deficient rats. J Soc Gynecol Investig 8:18–23

Trask AJ, Ferrario CM (2007) Angiotensin-(1-7): pharmacology and new perspectives in cardiovascular treatments. Cardiovasc Drug Rev 25:162–174

Tschudi MR, Criscione L, Luscher TF (1991) Effect of aging and hypertension on endothelial function of rat coronary arteries. J Hypertens 9:164–165

Tselios K, Sarantopoulos A, Gkougkourelas I, Boura P (2014) T regulatory cells: a promising new target in atherosclerosis. Crit Rev Immunol 34:389–397

Tummala PE, Chen XL, Sundell CL, Laursen JB, Hammes CP, Alexander RW, Harrison DG, Medford RM (1999) Angiotensin II induces vascular cell adhesion molecule-1 expression in rat vasculature: potential link between the renin-angiotensin system and atherosclerosis. Circulation 100:1223–1229

Tuttolomondo A, Di Raimondo D, Pecoraro R, Arnao V, Pinto A, Licata G (2012) Atherosclerosis as an inflammatory disease. Curr Pharm Des 18:4266–4288

Tzemos N, Lim PO, MacDonald TM (2001) Nebivolol reverses endothelial dysfunction in essential hypertension: a randomized, double-blind, crossover study. Circulation 104:511–514

Uzun H, Karter Y, Aydin S, Curgunlu A, Simşek G, Yücel R, Vehiyd S, Ertürk N, Kutlu A, Benian A, Yaldiran A, Oztürk E, Erdine S (2004) Oxidative stress in white coat hypertension; role of paraoxonase. J Hum Hypertens 18:523–528

Vaindirlis I, Peppa-Patrikiou M, Dracopoulou M, Manoli I, Voutetakis A, Dacou-Voutetakis C (2000) 'White coat hypertension' in adolescents: increased values of urinary cortisol and endothelin. J Pediatr 136:359–364

Vaněčková I, Maletínská L, Behuliak M, Nagelová V, Zicha J, Kuneš J (2014) Obesity-related hypertension: possible pathophysiological mechanisms. J Endocrinol 223:R63–R78

Vanhoutte PM, Shimokawa H, Tang EH, Feletou M (2009) Endothelial dysfunction and vascular disease. Acta Physiol 196:193–222

Verdecchia P, Schillaci G, Boldrini P, Ciucci A, Porcellati C (1996) White coat hypertension. Lancet 348:1444–1445

Vestweber D (2012) Relevance of endothelial junctions in leukocyte xtravasation and vascular permeability. Ann N Y Acad Sci 1257:184–192

Virdis A, Duranti E, Taddei S (2011) Oxidative stress and vascular damage in hypertension: role of angiotensin II. Int J Hypertens 2011, 916310

Vyssoulis GP, Marinakis AG, Aznaouridis KA, Karpanou EA, Arapogianni AN, Cokkinos DV, Stefanadis CI (2004) The impact of thirdgeneration beta-blocker antihypertensive treatment on endothelial function and the prothrombotic state: effects of smoking. Am J Hypertens 17:582–589

Wang Y, Zhao S (2010) Vasoactivators and placental vasoactivity. Morgan & Claypool Life Sciences, San Rafael

Weber MA, Neutel JM, Smith DH, Graettinger WF (1994) Diagnosis of mild hypertension by ambulatory blood pressure monitoring. Circulation 90:2291–2298

Weber MA, Schiffrin EL, White WB, Mann S, Lindholm LH, Kenerson JG, Flack JM, Carter BL, Materson BJ, Ram CV, Cohen DL, Cadet JC, Jean-Charles RR, Taler S, Kountz D, Townsend R, Chalmers J, Ramirez AJ, Bakris GL, Wang J, Schutte AE, Bisognano JD, Touyz RM, Sica D, Harrap SB (2014) Clinical practice guidelines for the management of hypertension in the community a statement by the American Society of Hypertension and the International Society of Hypertension. J Hypertens 32:3–15

Weitzberg E, Hezel M, Lundberg JO (2010) Nitrate-nitrite-nitric oxide pathway: implications for anesthesiology and intensive care. Anesthesiology 113:1460–1475

Wenzel U, Turner JE, Krebs C, Kurts C, Harrison DG, Ehmke H (2016) Immune mechanisms in arterial hypertension. J Am Soc Nephrol 27:677–686

White WB, Schulman P, McCabe EJ, Dey HM (1989) Average daily blood pressure, not office blood pressure, determines cardiac function in patients with hypertension. JAMA 261:873–877

Wilson SH, Lerman A (2001) Function of vascular endothelium. In: Heart physiology and pathophysiology, vol 27. Elsevier Inc., New York

Winn RK, Harlan JM (2005) The role of endothelial cell apoptosis in inflammatory and immune diseases. J Thromb Haemost 3:1815–1824

Yasu T, Kobayashi M, Mutoh A, Yamakawa K, Momomura S, Ueda S (2013) Dihydropyridine calcium channel blockers inhibit non-esterified-fatty-acid-induced endothelial and rheological dysfunction. Clin Sci 125:247–255

Yasunari K, Maeda K, Nakamura M, Yoshikawa J (2002) Oxidative stress in leukocytes is a possible link between blood pressure, blood glucose, and C-reacting protein. Hypertension 39:777–780

Yau JW, Teoh H, Verma S (2015) Endothelial cell control of thrombosis. BMC Cardiovasc Disord 15:130

Yavuzer S, Yavuzer H, Cengiz M, Erman H, Altıparmak MR, Korkmazer B, Balci H, Simsek G, Yaldıran AL, Karter Y, Uzun H (2015) Endothelial damage in white coat hypertension: role of lectin-like oxidized low-density lipoprotein-1. J Hum Hypertens 29:92–98

Yavuzer H, Yavuzer S, Cengiz M, Erman H, Doventas A, Balci H, Erdincler DS, Uzun H (2016a) Biomarkers of lipid peroxidation related to hypertension in aging. Hypertens Res 39:342–348

Yavuzer H, Cengiz M, Yavuzer S, Rıza Altıparmak M, Korkmazer B, Balci H, Yaldıran AL, Uzun H (2016b) Procalcitonin and Pentraxin-3: current biomarkers in inflammation in white coat hypertension. J Hum Hypertens 30:424–429

Yayama K, Hiyoshi H, Imazu D, Okamoto H (2006) Angiotensin II stimulates endothelial NO synthase phosphorylation in thoracic aorta of mice with abdominal aortic banding via type 2 receptor. Hypertension 48:958–964

Youn JC, Yu HT, Lim BJ, Koh MJ, Lee J, Chang DY, Choi YS, Lee SH, Kang SM, Jang Y, Yoo OJ, Shin EC, Park S (2013) Immunosenescent CD8+ T clls and C-X-C cemokine receptor type 3 chemokines are increased in human hypertension. Hypertension 62:126–133

Yuana Y, Sturk A, Nieuwland R (2013) Extracellular vesicles in physiological and pathological conditions. Blood Rev 27:31–39

Zepeda RJ, Castillo R, Rodrigo R, Prieto JC, Aramburu I, Brugere S, Galdames K, Noriega V, Miranda HF (2012) Effect of carvedilol and nebivolol on oxidative stress-related parameters and endothelial function in patients with essential hypertension. Basic Clin Pharmacol Toxicol 111:309–316

Zhao Y, Vanhoutte PM, Leung SWS (2014) Vascular nitric oxide: beyond eNOS. J Pharmacol Sci 129:83–94

Adv Exp Med Biol - Advances in Internal Medicine (2017) 2: 541–560
DOI 10.1007/5584_2016_48
© Springer International Publishing AG 2016
Published online: 11 September 2016

Cerebellar Adrenomedullinergic System. Role in Cardiovascular Regulation

Leticia Figueira and Anita Israel

Abstract

Adrenomedullin (AM) is a multifunctional peptide which exerts numerous biological activities through the activation of AM1 (CRLR + RAMP2) and AM2 (CRLR + RAMP3) receptors. AM immunoreactivity, AM binding sites and CRLR, RAMP1, RAMP2 and RAMP3 are expressed in rat cerebellar vermis. AM binding sites are discretely and differentially distributed in the rat cerebellar cortex with higher levels detected in SHR when compared with WKY rats. In addition, there is an up-regulation of cerebellar CGRP1 (CRLR + RAMP1) and AM2 (CRLR + RAMP3) receptors and a down-regulation of AM1 (CRLR + RAMP2) receptor during hypertension associated with a decreased AM expression. These changes may constitute a mechanism which contributes to the development of hypertension, and supports the notion that cerebellar AM is involved in the regulation of blood pressure. Cerebellar AM activates ERK, increases cAMP, cGMP and nitric oxide, and decreases antioxidant enzyme activity. These effects are mediated through AM_1 receptor since they are blunted by AM(22-52). AM-stimulated cAMP production is mediated through AM2 and CGRP receptors. *In vivo* administration of AM into the cerebellar vermis caused a profound, specific and dose-dependent hypotensive effect in SHR, but not in normotensive WKY rats. This effect was mediated through AM1 receptor since it was abolished by AM(22-52). In addition, AM injected into the cerebellar vermis reduced vasopressor response to footshock stress. These findings demonstrate dysregulation of cerebellar AM system during hypertension, and suggest that cerebellar AM plays an important role in the regulation of blood pressure. Likewise, they constitute a novel mechanism of blood pressure control which has not been described so far.

L. Figueira
Laboratory of Neuropeptides, School of Pharmacy,
Universidad Central de Venezuela, Caracas, Venezuela

School of Bioanalysis, Department of Health Sciences,
Universidad de Carabobo, Carabobo, Venezuela

A. Israel (✉)
Laboratory of Neuropeptides, School of Pharmacy,
Universidad Central de Venezuela, Caracas, Venezuela
e-mail: astern88@gmail.com

Keywords
Adrenomedullin • CRLR • RAMPs • Cerebellum • Vermis • AM(22-52) • Hypertension

1   Introduction

Adrenomedullin (AM) is a multifunctional peptide with 52-(human (h)) or 50-(rat (r)) amino acid residues (Fig. 1), which is a member of the calcitonin/calcitonin gene-related peptide (CGRP) superfamily [4, 5]. It was first isolated from human pheochromocytoma extracts by Kitamura et al. [51], whom found that AM was able to elevate 3',5' cyclic adenosine monophosphate (cAMP) production in human platelets and to exert a potent and long-lasting hypotensive effect in rats. Adrenomedullin is synthesized as part of a larger precursor molecule, termed preproadrenomedullin. In both rat and human this precursor consists of 185 amino acids [51, 82], while the porcine precursor has 188 residues [52]. Preproadrenomedullin contains a 21-amino acid N-terminal signal peptide that immediately precedes a 20-amino acid amidated peptide, designated proadrenomedullin N-terminal 20 peptide or PAMP [51].

AM immunoreactivity, AM mRNA and the peptide itself are found in the circulation and in lung, spleen, kidney, heart, adrenal gland and brain. AM has also been found to be secreted from endothelial and vascular smooth muscle cells [5, 42, 44, 104, 105]. AM is involved in the regulation of blood pressure and body fluid balance. In effect, systemic AM administration elicits potent, dose-dependent vasodilatatory effects, reduces blood pressure, increases urine output and urinary sodium excretion. On the other hand, AM is an antioxidant substance, since AM attenuates reactive oxygen species (ROS) production mediated by the stimulation of nicotinamide adenine dinucleotide phosphate-oxidase (NAD(P)H oxidase) [49, 50, 76, 92, 112, 113]. Additionally, AM may directly inhibit NAD(P)H oxidase activity eliciting protective effects [76]. Thus, it is clear that AM is capable to reduce free radicals and ROS production mediated by NAD(P)H oxidase stimulation, through inhibition of enzyme activity [76].

AM exerts multiples biological activities through the activation of two specific receptors, the AM type 1 (AM1) and type 2 (AM2) receptors, formed from the obligate co-expression of a class-B, G protein coupled receptor (GPCR), the calcitonin receptor-like receptor (CRLR) and receptor activity-modifying proteins (RAMPs) 2 or 3, respectively [4, 61, 74]. The calcitonin gene-related peptide 1 (CGRP1) receptor is formed of a complex between CRLR and RAMP1 [61]. Thus, the CRLR/RAMP1 heterodimer defines the CGRP1 receptor and the association between RAMP2 or RAMP3/CRLR forms a functional AM1 and AM2 receptor, respectively [54] (Fig. 2). AM1 receptors are highly selective for AM over CGRP and other peptides, while AM2 receptor binds both AM and AM2 (intermedin) with high affinities [43]. AM also has appreciable affinity for the CGRP1 receptor [36]. Thus, RAMPs regulates the ligand selectivity of CRLR [5]. CGRP1 receptor is effectively antagonized by CGRP(8-37); meanwhile AM1 receptor is more effectively blocked by a selective AM receptor antagonist, h-AM(22-52) or r-AM (20-50) than by CGRP(8-37). Unlike the pharmacological features of the AM1 receptor, AM2 receptor differs among species. In h-AM2 receptors, AM is more effectively blocked by a selective AM-receptor antagonist, but in r-AM2, the CGRP1 receptor antagonist are more potent than AM-blockers [54].

AM receptors and binding sites for AM are found in several body regions [21]. The CRLR mRNA and peptide are predominantly expressed in the lung, blood vessels, liver, midgut, rectum, urethra, adrenal cortex, uterus, coronary artery endothelial and smooth muscle cells [37, 54,

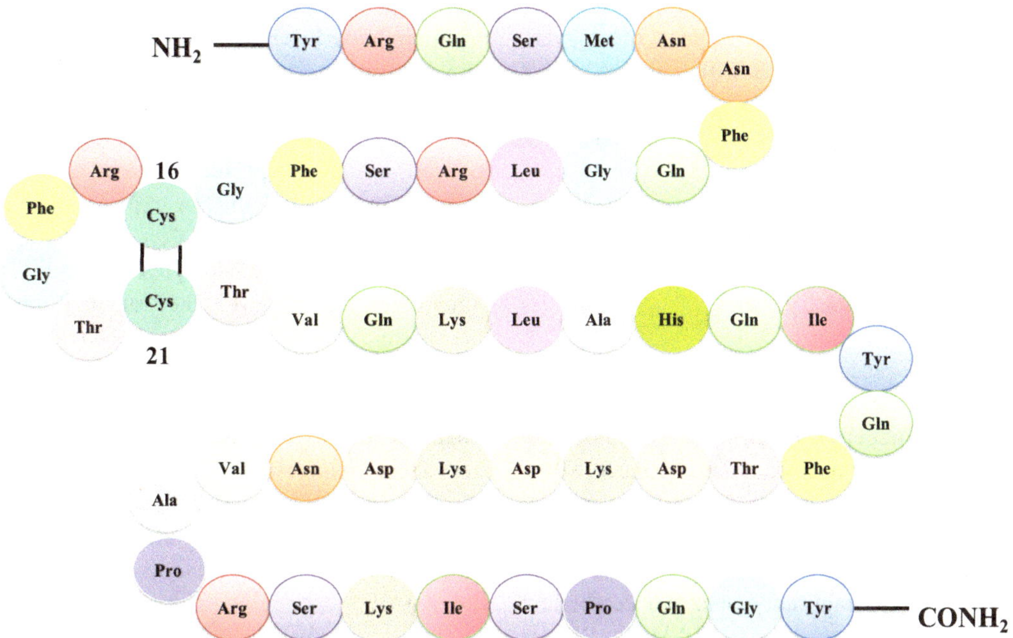

Fig. 1 Structure of adrenomedullin. h-AM is formed by a ring structure of 52 amino acid residues held by a disulfide bond between Cys-16 and Cys-21; with a Tyr residue amidated in the C-terminal portion. These structural features are necessary for its biological activity

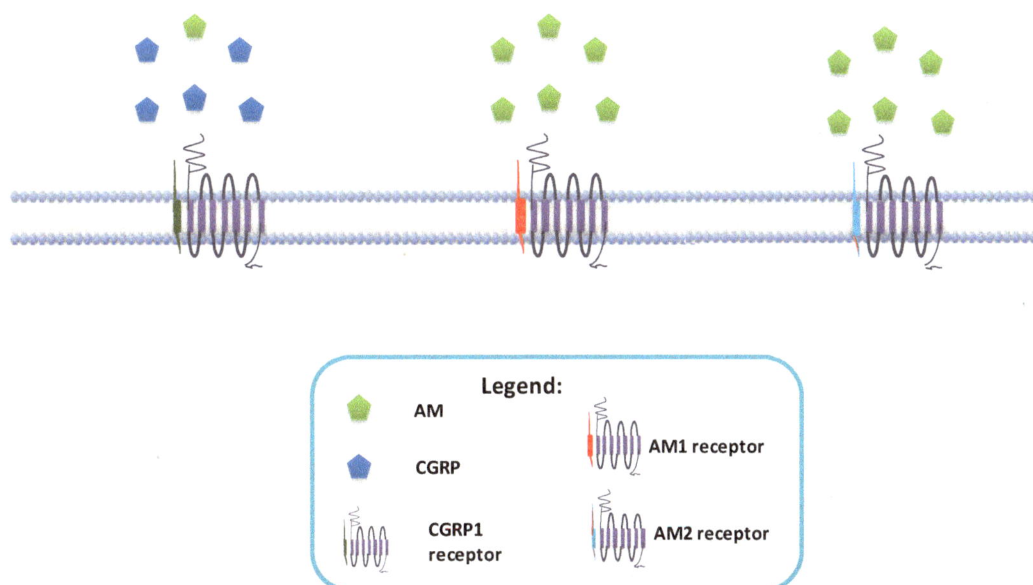

Fig. 2 Adrenomedullin type 1 (AM1) and type2 (AM2) receptors, formed from the obligate co-expression of the calcitonin receptor-like receptor (CRLR) and receptor activity-modifying proteins (RAMPs) 2 or 3, respectively. Thus, CRLR/RAMP2 heterodimer (*red* and *purple*) or CRLR/RAMP3 (*blue* and *purple*) preferentially bind AM. While the calcitonin gene-related peptide 1 (CGRP1) receptor is formed of a complex between CRLR and RAMP1 (*green* and *purple*) and preferentially bind CGRP [61]

72]. The distribution of RAMP1 expression have been reported in fat, thymus, spleen, uterus, pancreas and bladder; while RAMP2 and RAMP3 is expressed in the lung, kidney, heart, liver, spleen, uterus, ovary and placenta [21, 36, 54, 61, 67].

2 Adrenomedullin Receptor Subtypes in the Central Nervous System

AM and its receptors are locally produced and expressed in the central nervous system (CNS) and are particularly localized to the autonomic nuclei, including nucleus tractus solitarii (NTS), lateral parabrachial nucleus and rostral ventrolateral medulla, cerebral cortex, pituitary gland, thalamus, hypothalamus, brainstem, medulla oblongata, midbrain, amygdala and cerebellum [5, 42, 47, 58, 73, 86, 88, 107]. RAMP1 mRNA is found in the hippocampus, nucleus accumbens, caudate–putamen, cerebral cortex and cerebellum; RAMP2 mRNA is expressed in numerous brain areas, including autonomic nuclei such as the paraventricular nucleus, supraoptic nucleus, arcuate and ventromedial nuclei, as well as in the NTS, area postrema and dorsal motor nucleus of the vagus, hippocampus, olfactory bulb, choroid plexus and cerebellum; and RAMP3 mRNA is expressed in the cerebral cortex, thalamus and cerebellum [95, 100]. These findings suggest the existence of a central adrenomedullinergic system of physiological relevance.

Several studies support that hypertension may influence AM and its receptor component expression both in the periphery and in the CNS. In fact, AM concentration is increased in the plasma and tissues during hypertension [36, 74]. In addition, the expression pattern of RAMPs isoforms in a given cell may change in physiological and pathological conditions determining the responsiveness to AM and CGRP [5]. Hypertension induced by restraint stress reduced prepro-AM mRNA level in the hypothalamic paraventricular nucleus, supraoptic nucleus, NTS, dorsal motor nucleus of the vagus, area postrema and subfornical organ [88]. It has been reported changes in brain mRNA RAMP2 expression in response to blood pressure manipulations. In effect, decreased blood pressure induced by nitroprusside infusion elicited an increase in RAMP2 mRNA expression in the NTS, while increased blood pressure induced by phenylephrine infusion elicited a decrease in RAMP-2 mRNA expression in the paraventricular nucleus and NTS. This data provide anatomical and physiological evidence for a homeostatic role for AM in the brain and suggest that central AM may participate in the regulation of sympathetic activity [95]. Effectively, it has been shown that chronic stress induced by immobilization for seven consecutive days produced an enhanced expression of AM in the cerebrospinal fluid-contacting nucleus [106] and chronic footshock and noise stress for fifteen consecutive days produced an up-regulation of prepro-AM and RAMP3 expression in hypothalamus and pituitary gland [56]. Also, chronic stress caused an increase in CRLR expression in medulla oblongata and decrease in the midbrain and hypothalamus. While RAMP2 expression was increased in medulla oblongata and hypothalamus, suggesting that increased hypothalamic prepro-AM, RAMP2 and RAMP3 may be a protection mechanism for resetting hypertension induced by chronic stress and suggests that AM may be related to the development of the stress-induced hypertension [56].

3 Adrenomedullinergic System in Cerebellum Vermis

The emphasis for a role of the systemic circulating AM in the regulation of fluid and electrolyte balance, arterial pressure and the pathophysiology of cardiovascular disease have recently shift, and now is focused on the local tissue AM. Studies have demonstrated the importance of a tissue AM system. As essential requirement for a tissue AM system is that all of the components necessary for the biosynthesis of the active peptide reside within the tissue. This requires a demonstration that peptides mRNAs, its receptor components and biosynthetic enzymes are in detectable quantities, and that the peptide synthesis actually occurs locally. Although some of the components may be taken up into the tissue from the circulation, even in the presence of a local system, the *de novo* tissue generation of AM and its interaction with AM receptors on the same (autocrine) or adjacent (paracrine) cells defines the local system. In addition, it should be demonstrated that the biologically active product is regulated within the tissue independently of the systemic circulation, and the reduction or elimination of the action of the product results in a physiological response [9]. In regard to brain and specifically in the cerebellum, there is sufficient evidence indicating the existence of a local functional cerebellar adrenomedullinergic system.

In this respect, it has been demonstrated the presence of AM, AM receptors and their receptor components in cerebellum vermis [24, 30, 75]. AM immunoreactivity, AM binding sites and CRLR, RAMP1, RAMP2 and RAMP3 expression are detected in rat cerebellum [10, 86, 94, 102]. In fact, it has been demonstrated by light and electron microscopy AM-like immunoreactivity in cerebellar Purkinje cells and mossy terminal nerve fibers as well as neurons of the cerebellar nuclei [66, 86, 87]. In addition, the presence of RAMP1 and RAMP2 mRNA in Purkinje cells and RAMP3 mRNA in cerebellar granular cells has been shown [100]. Likewise, CRLR and RAMP1 were detected on the surface of the Purkinje cell bodies and in their processes [19, 65]. This evidence indicates that AM could participate in cerebellar functions as an autocrine/paracrine factor.

Moreover, the evidence suggests that the expression and function of adrenomedullinergic system components could be altered during growth. In fact, RAMP1, RAMP3 and CRLR expression in rat cerebellar vermis increased with age, without changes for AM and RAMP2 expression [24, 30]. Similar findings have been shown for CGRP1 receptor (CRLR/RAMP1) expressed in cerebellar cortical neuron and glial, which suffer of marked changes during cerebellum development. Indeed, autoradiographic and immunofluorescence studies followed by con-focal analysis in rat cerebellum demonstrated a lower CGRP1 receptor density in Purkinje cells and molecular cells during development and their increase during maturity, suggesting that CGRP1 and its receptor may promote a coordinated development of cerebellar glial cells, an effect driven mainly by the CGRP released by climbing fibers [64].

Likewise, AM activates several signaling pathways and regulates ROS metabolism centrally [91, 101, 103]. In cerebellum AM activates extracellular signal-regulated kinases (ERK), increases cAMP production probably through the activation of protein kinase A (PKA); increases cyclic guanosine monophosphate (cGMP) production and nitric oxide (NO) accumulation. These effects are mediated through the activation of AM_1 receptor, since AM specific receptor blocker, AM(22-52), blunted AM action, meanwhile AM-induced increase of cAMP production is mediated through stimulation of AM2 and CGRP receptors [26–30] (Fig. 3). In this sense, Endo and Launey [20] found that NO-cGMP-protein kinase G (PKG) pathway plays an important role in the activation of ERK1/2 in Purkinje cells of rat cerebellum. This high levels in the cerebellar NO/cGMP [63], the enzyme guanylil cyclase (GC) [68], cGMP [22] and cGMP-dependent protein kinase in cerebellar Purkinje cells [57] suggest that the NO/cGMP signaling pathway could act as a neurotransmitter in the cerebellum. Futhermore, nitric oxide synthase (NOS) and soluble GC are colocalized and activated in various regions of the cerebellum [16]. In contrast to cAMP, which is homogeneously distributed in different brain areas, cGMP is 10 to 50 times more concentrated in the cerebellum than in other brain areas. cGMP is believed to exert its effects through cGMP-dependent protein kinase (cGPK), the activity and expression is specifically detected in the cerebellum, mainly concentrated in the Purkinje cells [57].

AM has been described as an endogenous antioxidant substance as it is cytoprotective against organ damage [69, 92]. In fact, AM regulate cerebellar metabolism of ROS, since AM decreased thiobarbituric acid reactive substances (TBARS) production, and catalase (CAT),

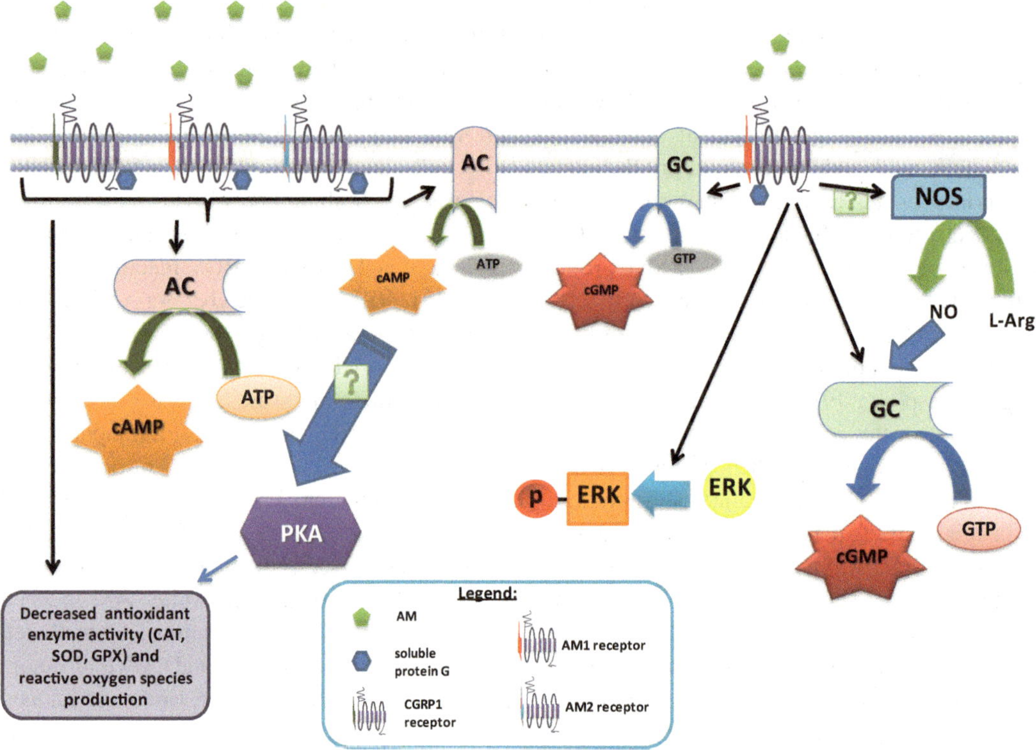

Fig. 3 Adrenomedullin receptor signaling pathways in rat cerebellar vermis. AM reduces SOD, CAT and GPx enzyme activity mediated by PKA, via activation of CGRP and AM receptor subtypes. Meanwhile, AM increases ERK activity, NO and cGMP production via activation of AM1 receptor; and increases cAMP production through CGRP1 and AM receptor subtypes (*AC* adenylil cyclase, *AM* adrenomedullin, *ATP* adenosine triphosphate, *CAT* catalase, *cAMP* cyclic adenosine monophosphate, *cGMP* cyclic guanosine monophosphate, *ERK* extracellular signal-regulated kinases, *GC* guanylil cyclase, *GPx* glutathione peroxidase, *Gs* soluble protein G, *GTP* guanosine triphosphate, *NO* nitric oxide, *NOS* nitric oxide synthase, *p-ERK* phospho-extracellular signal-regulated kinases, *PKA* protein kinase A, *SOD* superoxide dismutase)

glutathione peroxidase (GPx) and superoxide dismutase (SOD) basal activity in cerebellar vermis of male *Sprague Dawley* rats [23, 31] as it was also reported in other organs such as kidney and liver [14, 114]. This decrease in enzyme activity in cerebellar vermis suggests that AM is capable of reducing ROS production, because the reduction of antioxidant enzymes activity was accompanied by a decrease in lipid peroxidation. Likewise, this effect is mediated by PKA, since pretreatment with PKI-(6-22) amide, a PKA inhibitor, was able to reverse the inhibitory effect of AM on the basal activity of antioxidant enzymes (Fig. 3), as has been reported by other studies in several tissues [92, 112]. Moreover, AM(22-50) and CGRP(8-37) blunted AM-induced decrease of antioxidant enzymes activity indicating that this effect is mediated through stimulation of both AM and CGRP$_1$, receptors. These data support the role of AM in the regulation of cerebellar antioxidant enzyme activity and suggests the existence of a functional local cerebellar adrenomedullinergic system of physiological relevance.

4   Cerebellar Adrenomedullinergic System During Hypertension

There is evidence that cerebellum participates in blood pressure regulation and of changes of AM and its receptor components expression in

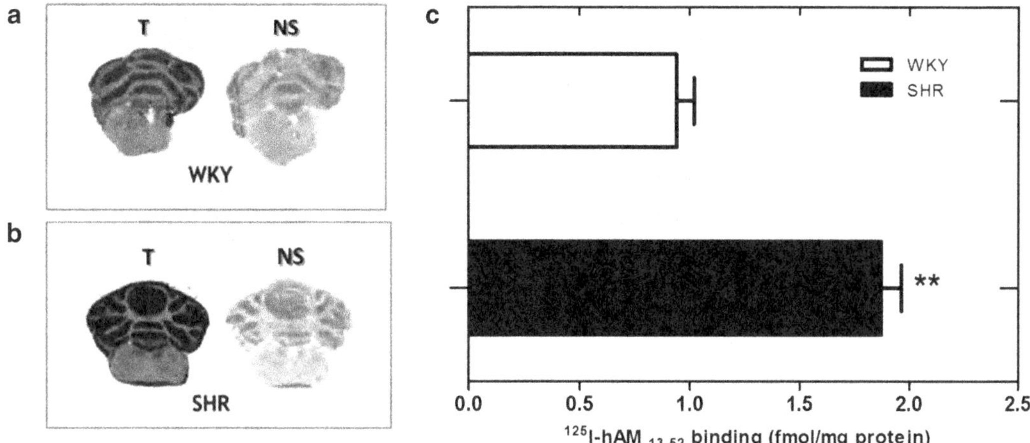

Fig. 4 Autoradiographic localization of ^{125}**h-AM (13-52) binding in coronal sections of rat cerebellum.** Sections of WKY (Panel A) and SHR (Panel B) rat cerebellum. Quantification of ^{125}h-AM(13-52) binding (Panel C). *T* Total binding, *NS* Non-specific binding (Modified and reprinted with permission from Pastorello et al. [75])

several regions of CNS during hypertension. In support for that, in the pioneer work of Pastorello et al. [75] who reported the distribution and levels of AM receptor binding sites in the brain of 16-week-old normotensive Wistar Kyoto (WKY) and spontaneously hypertensive (SHR) rats, using ^{125}I-hAM(13-52) as radioligand. As previously reported by Juaneda et al. [48], it was demonstrated that AM receptors are discretely and differentially distributed in the rat cerebellum cortex. However, higher levels of AM binding sites were detected in the granular cell layer of the cerebellum of SHR when compared with WKY rats [75] (Fig. 4). The increase in cerebellar AM receptors during hypertension could be interpreted as an up-regulation mechanism of cerebellar binding sites to compensate the increase in blood pressure in SHR rats; or they could represent a primary alteration which would result in a secondary alteration in the autonomic regulatory mechanisms in cerebellum with the consequent increase in blood pressure.

Figueira and Israel [30] showed the notion of a dysregulation of AM cerebellar system during hypertension in 16-week-old WKY and SHR rats in the cerebellar vermis. Quantification of AM, CRLR, RAMP1, RAMP2 and RAMP3 expression using western blot analysis, demonstrated an up-regulation of cerebellar vermis CGRP1 (CRLR + RAMP1) and AM2 (CRLR + RAMP3) receptors and a down-regulation of AM1 (CRLR + RAMP2) receptor during hypertension associated with a decreased AM expression (Fig. 5). The reduction in AM expression in vermis of SHR rats could be responsible for the up-regulation of AM2 receptors and binding sites observed by autoradiography [24, 30].

It is known that CRLR/RAMP2 complex constitutes the pathway for AM biological activity, and it is believed that altered expression of RAMPs is associated with alterations of AM response [36]. Therefore, RAMP2 is mainly expressed in the basal state while expression levels of RAMP3 remain relatively low [36]. In pathological conditions like hypertension, there are phenotype changes of RAMPs expression, from a high response (high expression of RAMP2) to a low response to AM (high expression of RAMP3) [30, 36]. Therefore, the decreased expression of RAMP2 and AM suggest that these changes may constitute a mechanism which contributes to the development of hypertension, and supports the notion that this peptide is involved in the regulation of blood pressure in cerebellum. Furthermore, up-regulation of CRLR, RAMP1 and RAMP3 expression would

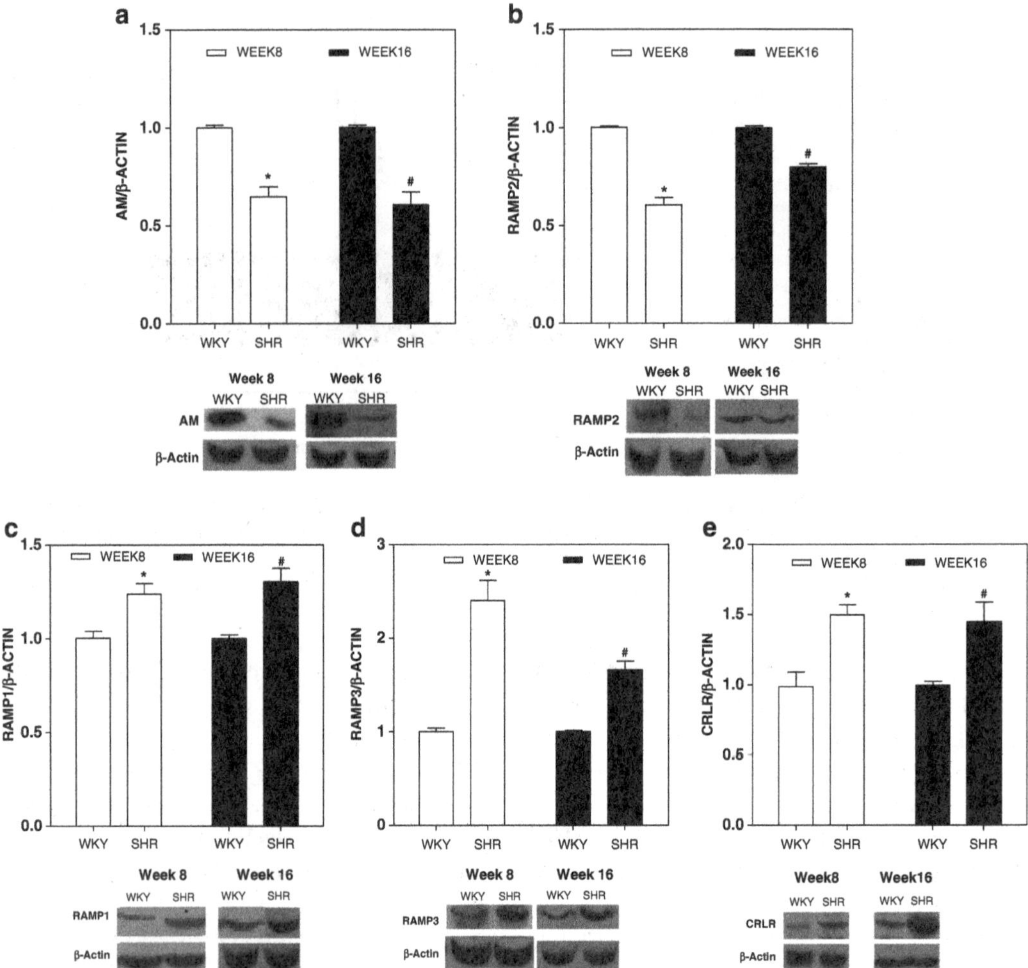

Fig. 5 Effect of hypertension on adrenomedullin and its receptor components in cerebellar vermis. AM expression and of its receptor components CRLR, RAMP1, RAMP2 and RAMP3 are altered in SHR rats when compared with WKY rats. In SHR rats AM and RAMP2 expression are reduced while CRLR, RAMP1 and RAMP3 expression are increased. Cerebellar vermis expression of AM (Panel A), RAMP2 (Panel B), RAMP1 (Panel C), RAMP3 (Panel D) and CRLR (Panel E) in 8 and 16 week-old WKY and SHR rats. Results are expressed as mean ± S.E.M. AM, RAMP1, RAMP2, RAMP3 and CRLR expression was normalized with that of β-actin (N = 10). *p < 0.0001 vs. WKY 8 week old. #p < 0.0001 vs. WKY 16 week old (Modified and reprinted with permission from Figueira and Israel [30])

promote the interaction of AM with CGRP1 and AM2 receptors, rather than AM1 receptors, thereby favoring the compensatory mechanism to increased blood pressure. Alternatively, these changes could be the initial disturbance that would result in dysregulation of the mechanisms controlling blood pressure, since these changes are present from the early stages of life (8 weeks) of hypertensive rats [30]. In fact, lowering blood pressure with an oral antihypertensive treatment during eleven days, reversed AM and its receptor components expression to those levels found in normotensive rats [33], suggesting that hypertension induces adaptive changes to compensate a rise of blood pressure (Fig. 6). Meanwhile, the antihypertensive treatment, to restore AM and RAMP2 expression would increase AM1 receptor expression and

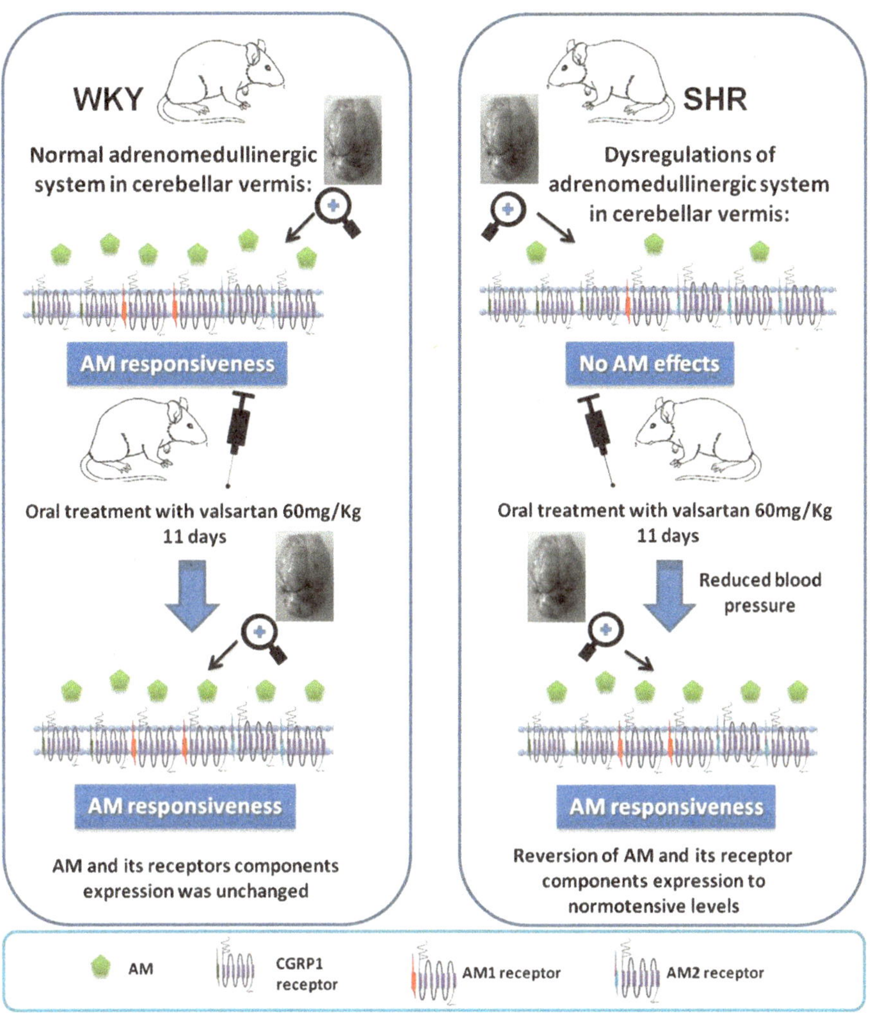

Fig. 6 **Effect of lowering blood pressure on AM and its receptor components expression in cerebellar vermis of WKY and SHR rats**. AM expression and of its receptor components CRLR, RAMP1, RAMP2 and RAMP3 are altered in SHR rats when compared with WKY rats. In SHR rats, AM and RAMP2 expression are reduced while CRLR, RAMP1 and RAMP3 expression are increased. Oral antihypertensive treatment with valsartan during eleven days, reversed AM and its receptor components expression to those levels found in normotensive rats and reestablished the AM responsiveness (*AM* adrenomedullin, *SHR* spontaneously hypertensive rats, *WKY* Wistar Kyoto rats)

would promote AM responsiveness via AM1 receptor. Therefore, reversion with peripheral administration of an antihypertensive may represent a strategy to compensate the primary abnormality in the control of blood pressure and opens the possibility of a novel mechanism in antihypertensive therapy suggesting that cerebellum may play a role in the regulation of arterial blood pressure.

5 Role of Brain Adrenomedullin in Blood Pressure Control

AM is a peptide which exerts important roles in the regulation of cardiovascular function. At peripheral level, AM administration reduces blood pressure due to a decrease in peripheral vascular resistance [5, 38, 40]. It has been demonstrated that AM exerts its vasodilator action by an endothelium-dependent and independent mechanism. In this regard, most studies have indicated that AM induces endothelium-independent vasodilation by activating CGRP receptors with subsequent activation of cAMP production in vascular smooth muscle cells. Also, AM can activate potassium channels in smooth muscle cells causing hyperpolarization [81]. Additionally, AM through their specific receptors on endothelial cells induces endothelium-dependent vasodilation [39], since AM activates endothelial NOS (eNOS) by at least two mechanisms. First, AM increases intracellular calcium levels, which stimulates eNOS activity [91], and secondly, AM activates phosphatidylinositide 3-kinase/Akt (PIK3/Akt) pathway, which phosphorylates eNOS and increases the enzyme activity even at low calcium concentrations [70]. In fact, Hayakawa et al. [39] found that AM relaxed rat aorta, pre-contracted with phenylephrine, in a dose-dependent manner, observing that endothelium denudation attenuated vasodilator response, suggesting that NO-cGMP signaling pathway is involved in the mechanism of AM-induced vasorelaxation in aorta. Furthermore, AM is capable of inhibiting the production of vasoconstrictors such as endothelin-1 [5].

AM effects at the CNS cannot be predicted based on the effects induced by this peptide peripherally [38]. Indeed, AM exerts several effects in the CNS. Central AM administration results in various neuroendocrine responses such as the inhibition of arginine vasopressin secretion induced by hypovolemic and osmotic stimuli, and an increase of oxytocin secretion by activating hypothalamic oxytocin-producing cells [85, 111]; likewise intracerebroventricular (*icv*) administration of AM elevated plasma adrenocorticotropic hormone (ACTH) levels [89]. In addition, central administration of AM inhibits water drinking and salt appetite [99] and increases urinary water, sodium and potassium excretion, in a dose-dependent manner in conscious hydrated rats [17, 45]. Central administration of AM increases atrial natriuretic peptide release [12, 98]. Furthermore, microinjection of AM into the area postrema and the rostral ventrolateral medulla causes a hypertensive effect; while in the paraventricular nucleus of the hypothalamus produces hypotension [1, 46, 108]. This evidence indicates that central AM may play an important role in body fluid homeostasis and central regulation of the cardiovascular system.

In this regard, administration of AM into the area postrema [1, 110] or *icv* caused an increase in blood pressure in a dose-dependent manner [45, 83, 84], an effect mediated through CGRP receptor [80, 96]. While, Samson [84] suggested that the central AM pressor action is mediated through specific AM receptors, since administration of AM in the lateral and fourth ventricles elevates blood pressure in conscious rats, and this effect was not blocked by the antagonist of CGRP receptor. Furthermore, Xu and Krukoff [107] showed that AM administration into the rostral ventrolateral medulla increased blood pressure and heart rate in dose-dependent manner, through AM specific receptors and mediated by glutamate involving N-methyl-D-aspartate (NMDA) and non-NMDA receptors; additionally NO synthetized from neuronal NOS (nNOS) contributes with the vasopressor effect induced by AM through a signaling pathway associated with soluble GC. This data indicate that AM in the rostral ventrolateral medulla causes a hypertensive effect potentiating glutamatergic and nitrergic neurotransmission, since both glutamatergic and nitrergic inhibition blunted AM induced effects in the rostral ventrolateral medulla [107].

On the other hand, AM administration in the paraventricular nucleus has been shown to cause a decrease in blood pressure [93] which is mediated by NO and gamma-aminobutyric acid (GABA), since blockade of $GABA_A$ receptor and inhibition of NO production attenuated the decrease in blood pressure induced by AM. These results suggest that AM in the paraventricular nucleus activates cells producing NO, increasing GABAergic neurotransmission and lowering blood pressure [107]. Furthermore, it has been shown that *icv* administration of AM stimulates NO production in the hypothalamus and activates neurons which produce NO in the paraventricular nucleus

[89]. Likewise, microinjection of sodium nitroprusside, a NO donor, in the paraventricular nucleus lowers blood pressure and heart rate [116], suggesting that NO in this nucleus is one of the candidates mediating the hypertensive effect of AM. In addition, GABA exerts a tonic inhibitory effect on sympathetic nervous system in paraventricular nucleus [13, 59]; in fact, the selective antagonist of $GABA_A$ receptor, bicuculline, blocked AM-induced hyperpolarization of paraventricular nucleus magnocellular neurons, suggesting that GABA can contribute to AM hypotensive effect within the paraventricular nucleus [34].

Currently there are few reports on the possible effect on blood pressure exerted by AM administration into cerebellum, however the anatomical evidence and our *in vitro* results [23–31] point to a functional role in the regulation of blood pressure.

6 The Cerebellum as a Cardiovascular Regulator

The physiological mechanisms involved in AM actions in cerebellum are elusive and not yet clarified and could be multiple and complex. Moreover, there is little information about the role of the cerebellum in cardiovascular regulation.

There is anatomical evidence of a possible role for cerebellum in the regulation of cardiovascular function obtained from animal models and humans which show that vestibular cerebellar system and their cerebellar connections contribute to cardiovascular control during movement and posture alteration [15]. Various brain regions involved in cardiovascular control receive nerve signals from the cerebellum specifically from the fastigial nucleus and posterior cerebellar cortex [6–8, 18]. Furthermore, anatomical evidence supports the role of fastigial nucleus in cardiovascular function. Indeed, it has been identified various cardiovascular modules, such as fastigial nucleus, anterior vermis, posterior vermis, uvula (lobe IX), nodulus (lobe X); because stimulation of these structures involves changes in blood pressure, respiratory rate and vascular resistance [71]. In effect, after integrating the current research in the role of cardiovascular regulation of the cerebellum, Nisimaru [71] proposed the existence of five cardiovascular modules in the cerebellum dedicated to cardiovascular control. The first, a discrete rostral portion of the fastigial nucleus and the overlying medial portion of the anterior vermis (lobules I, II and III), this module controls the baroreflex. The second is formed by the anterior vermis which constitutes a microcomplex with parabrachial nucleus. The third is formed by caudal fastigial nucleus and posterior portion of vermis (lobes VII and VIII), controlling the vestibule sympathetic reflex. The fourth is integrated by the medial portion of the uvula with the NTS and parabrachial nucleus. The fifth module includes the lateral edge of the nodulus, and the uvula together with parabrachial nucleus and vestibular nuclei, which constitutes a cardiovascular microcomplex that controls the magnitude and/or timing of sympathetic nerve responses and stability of the mean arterial blood pressure during changes of head position and body posture. The lateral nodulus-uvula appears to be an integrative cardiovascular control center involving both the baroreflex and the vestibule-sympathetic reflex (Fig. 7) [71].

The major functions of these multiple microcomplexes are considered to be adaptive controls of the vestibule-sympathetic reflex and the baroreflex. This system combines feedback and feedforward control systems. The feedforward pathway from vestibular labyrinth to the vestibular nucleus (VN) and the feedback pathway from baroreceptors to the NTS and parabrachial nucleus converge on the common controller part in the rostral ventrolateral medulla. This combined control system maintains the mean arterial blood pressure against head movements and any perturbation of blood pressure under adaptative control by the five cardiovascular microcomplexes [71].

The functional evidence suggests that cerebellum may play a role in the regulation of arterial blood pressure. In fact, it has been shown that stimulation of several regions of the cerebellum

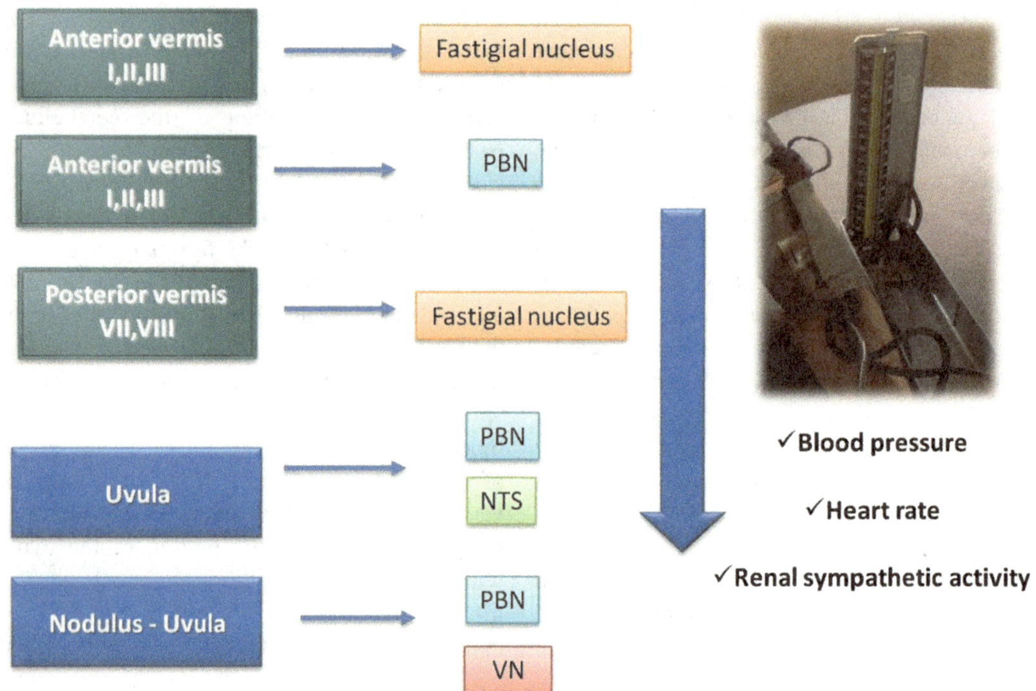

Fig. 7 Cerebellar cardiovascular modules. *PBN* Parabraquial nucleus, *NTS* Nucleus of tratus solitarii, *VN* Vestibular nucleus [71]. Studies in different animal species have shown that electrical stimulation of fastigial nucleus produces a pronounced pressor response, which may be due to connections of this nuclei with other important and recognized cardiovascular modules [7, 8, 71]. Meanwhile, electric stimulation of anterior vermis, the medial cortical regions of lobules I, II and III, posterior vermis (lobules VII and VII) and uvula (lobule IX) induces bradycardia, blood pressure fall and transient inhibition of sympathetic renal activity [3, 7, 71, 79]

produces changes in arterial blood pressure and heart rate [71, 78, 97]. It has been reported in anesthetized rabbits that electric stimulation of anterior vermis, the medial cortical regions of lobules I, II and III, posterior vermis (lobules VII and VII) and uvula (lobule IX) induces bradycardia, blood pressure fall and transient inhibition of sympathetic renal activity (Fig. 7) [3, 7, 71, 79], and in cats evoked a depressor response [77]. Also, Rocha et al. [79] found that stimulation of the posterior vermis caused a cardiovascular response characterized by hypotension and bradycardia. These findings provide clear evidence of the role of cerebellar vermis in regulating blood pressure.

It is well established that the posterior vermis projects to the caudal region of fastigial nucleus, and anterior vermis projects to the rostral portion of the fastigial nucleus [7]. In this regard, evidence show that electrical stimulation of the rostral region of fastigial nucleus in anaesthetized cats and rabbits caused a pressor response [8]; and this effect was abolished with alpha-adrenergic blocker or with sympathectomy, indicating that this action is mediated by sympathetic nervous system activity [71].

Several studies in different animal species have shown that electrical stimulation of fastigial nucleus produces a pronounced pressor response, which may be due to the connections of this nucleus with other important and recognized cardiovascular modules; since it has been established that neurons in the rostral portion of the fastigial nucleus project to the NTS, parabrachial nucleus, in a way that through these projections the rostral portion of the fastigial nucleus can participate in the cardiovascular control and the baroreceptor reflex [7, 8,

71]. Other cerebellar areas such interpositus and lateral nuclei fail to induce significant changes in blood pressure and heart rate [71].

7 Cerebellar Adrenomedullin in Cardiovascular Regulation

As there is an anatomical substrate, AM receptors and signaling pathways responding to AM in the cerebellum [23–27], it is plausible to expect that AM administered *in vivo* into the cerebellum may cause actions in cardiovascular regulation. Our results point to this possibility since we demonstrated that microinjection of AM into the cerebellar vermis of hypertensive rats causes a powerful and significant hypotensive response, which is specific and dose-dependent (0.02–200 pmol/5 μL) [30]. In effect, in SHR rats, administration of AM (200 pmol/ 5 μL) into cerebellar vermis produced a marked and significant hypotensive action when compared with vehicle (reduction of -20 to -40 mmHg). This hypotensive effect is manifested only during hypertension since in

WKY rats, administration of vehicle or AM (200 pmol/5 μL) into cerebellar vermis increased mean arterial pressure (MAP) in similar magnitude. The specificity of the hypotensive action of AM administered into the cerebellar vermis of SHR rats is based on the fact that microinjection of the peptide outside the vermis did not cause the hypotensive effects, and *in situ* administration of a pressor peptide such as angiotensin II (ANG II) or vehicle into cerebellar vermis increased MAP in similar magnitude in both WKY and SHR rats. AM's actions in the cerebellar vermis in SHR rats are mediated through AM1 receptor, as AM receptor specific antagonist, AM(22-52) (200 pmol/5 μL), co-injected with AM (200 pmol/5 μL) blunted AM's hypotensive effect, while CGRP(8-37) (200 pmol/ 5 μL) had no effect on AM actions (Fig. 8) [30]. These results provide the first functional evidence *in vivo* of a role for AM in the cerebellar vermis in the control of blood pressure.

The cause of the differences in the AM action among normotensive and hypertensive rats may be variable and has been described for other brain structures, since the intravenous infusion of AM reduces blood pressure in both

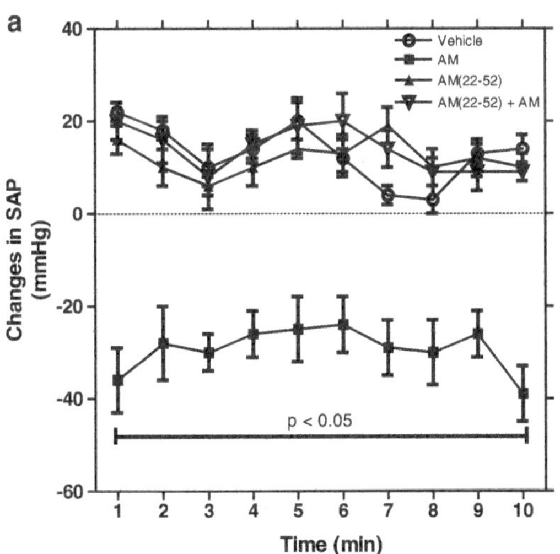
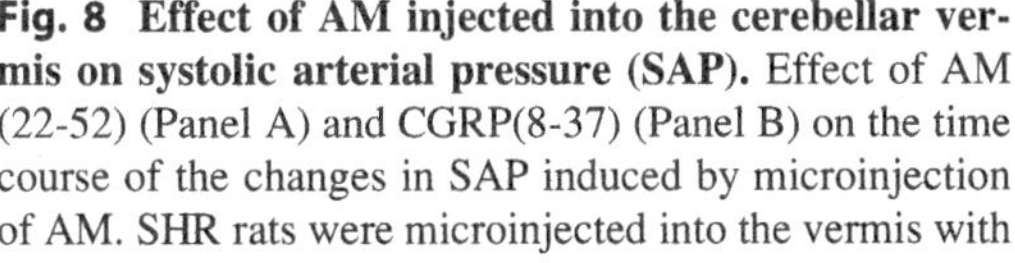

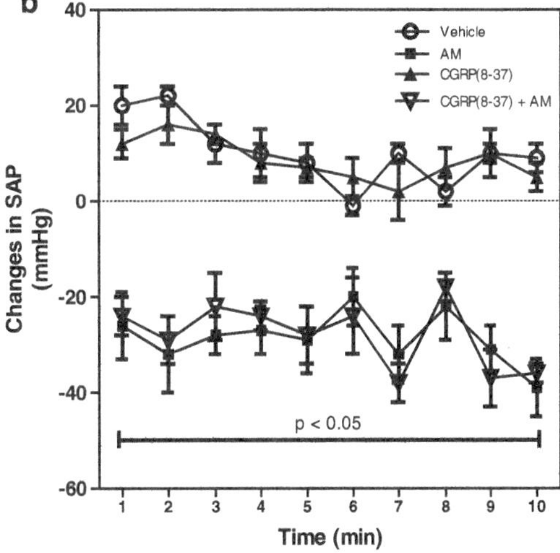

Fig. 8 Effect of AM injected into the cerebellar vermis on systolic arterial pressure (SAP). Effect of AM (22-52) (Panel A) and CGRP(8-37) (Panel B) on the time course of the changes in SAP induced by microinjection of AM. SHR rats were microinjected into the vermis with vehicle (5 μL), AM (200 pmol/5 μL), AM(22-52) (200 pmol/5 μL), AM + AM(22-52), CGRP(8-37) (200 pmol/5 μL) and AM + CGRP(8-37). Results are expressed as mean ± S.E.M. (N = 8). *p < 0.05 *vs.* its own control

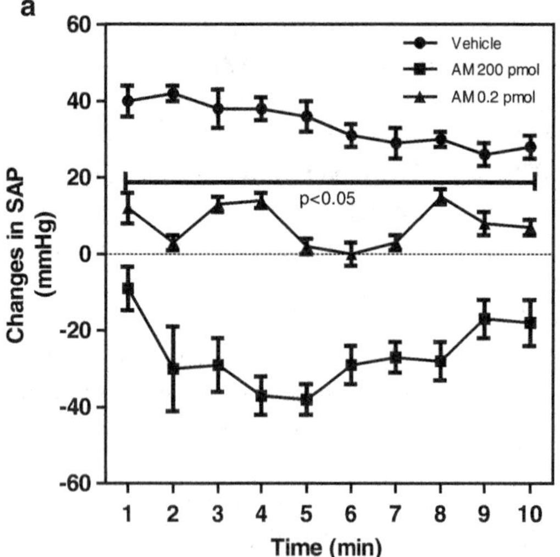

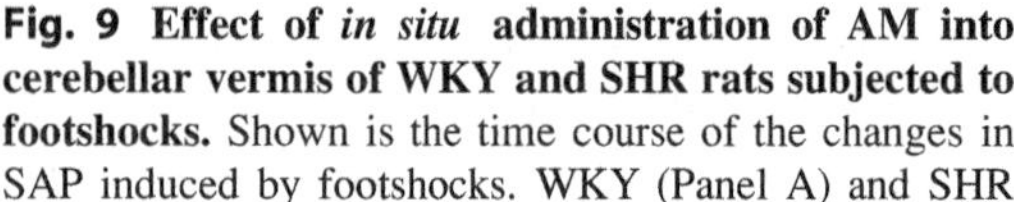

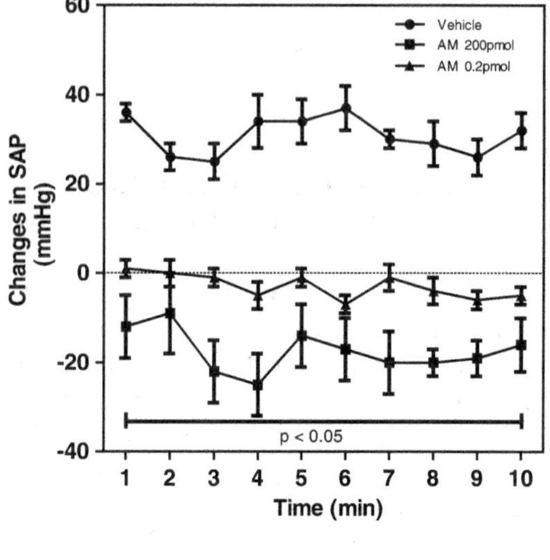

Fig. 9 Effect of *in situ* administration of AM into cerebellar vermis of WKY and SHR rats subjected to footshocks. Shown is the time course of the changes in SAP induced by footshocks. WKY (Panel A) and SHR (Panel B) rats were microinjected into the vermis with vehicle (5 μL) or AM (0.2 or 200 pmol/5 μL). Results are expressed as mean ± S.E.M. (N = 8). *p < 0.05 vs. vehicle

normotensive and hypertensive rats in a dose dependent manner; however the fall in blood pressure was higher in hypertensive rats compared to the normotensive [41]. Similarly, it was reported that rostral ventrolateral medulla neurons of SHR rats are more sensitive and have an increased response to ANG II with respect to WKY rats [11]. Therefore, the hypotensive effect induced by the intracerebellar administration of AM in SHR could be due to an increase in sensitivity and response in SHR compared with WKY rats. Alternatively, this differential response may be the manifestation of the cerebellar dysregulation of signaling pathways, or AM and AM1 receptor expression which are reduced during hypertension [25, 30].

The possible mechanism of the hypotensive action of AM when injected into the cerebellar vermis of SHR rats has not been established so far, but could be associated with the regulation of sympathetic efflux and seems to require a stimulated system. If so, AM administration into the cerebellar vermis should counteract the pressor response produced by acute stress. In this regard, Figueira and Israel [32] demonstrated that microinjection of AM into the cerebellar vermis was able to decrease the pressor response

induced by footshocks in WKY and SHR rats (Fig. 9), an experimental model of stress which increases sympathetic – adrenal system activity, catecholamine release to circulation, heart rate and blood pressure [55, 60].

AM inhibitory effect on sympathoadrenal response observed in this work is difficult to explain currently, but we might speculate that the cerebellum through its neuroanatomical connections from the fastigial nucleus and mediated through the NO/cGMP signaling pathway could represent a powerful counteregulator for the excitatory effects of brain nuclei involved in blood pressure regulation during stress. It is known that fastigial nucleus plays an important role in regulating the autonomic nervous system, since this nucleus projects to brainstem structures such as rostral ventrolateral medulla, which in turn receives innervations from the hypothalamic paraventricular and supraoptic nucleus [71]. In addition, NO producing neurons are located in autonomic nuclei such as hypothalamic paraventricular and supraoptic nucleus, nucleus tractus solitarii, ventrolateral and intermediolateral column of the spinal cord [53]. In paraventricular nucleus, NO inhibits sympathetic activity through the stimulation of

GABAergic interneurons [2, 115]. Meanwhile, in the nucleus tractus solitarii and ventrolateral medulla, NO has both sympatho-excitatory as sympatho-inhibitory effects suggesting that in brainstem NO regulates the sympathetic efflux through a balance of the outputs of these autonomic centers [53]. Furthermore, intracerebral administration of AM stimulates NO production in the hypothalamus and activates NO producing neurons in the paraventricular nucleus [98]. Stimulation of sympathetic outflow by AM *icv* administration together with inhibition of sympathetic outflow induced by NO in the paraventricular nucleus, suggests that AM-induced stimulation of the nitrergic system in the hypothalamus, could be part of a feedback mechanism, which acts to restore the homeostatic balance [90]. In support of this, it has been reported that *icv* administration of low doses of AM causes inhibition of renal sympathetic activity [62]. In addition, Fujita et al. [35] found that endogenous AM in the brain inhibits sympathetic activation through its antioxidant action. Meanwhile, Xu and Krukoff [109] indicated that in the rostral ventrolateral medulla AM exerts an inhibitory effect on baroreflex activity through an AM specific receptor mechanism in which activation of PKA is involved.

Altogether, this data points for a role of sympathetic system in cerebellar AM-mediated regulation of blood pressure and opens a new avenue for the involvement of cerebellar AM during stress.

8   Conclusions and Perspectives

During hypertension exists a dysregulation of cerebellar vermis AM, its receptor components and AM signaling pathways. Reduction of peripheral blood pressure after oral administration of valsartan is able to reverse changes in cerebellar expression of AM and its receptor components of hypertensive rats; indicating that these alterations represent the primary abnormality leading to hypertension; therefore reversion with peripheral administration of an antihypertensive drug, may represent a strategy to compensate the primary abnormality in the control of blood pressure and opens the possibility of a novel strategy in antihypertensive therapy. In addition, under hypertensive conditions AM administered into cerebellar vermis exerts a profound, dose-dependent hypotensive effect. These actions are mediated through AM1 receptor since there were blocked by AM(22-52), but not by CGRP(8-37). In addition, cerebellar AM is able to antagonize the pressor response induced by footshocks, suggesting that cerebellar AM may be involved in stress control. Our data demonstrates the existence of a cerebellar adrenomedullinergic system of physiological relevance during stress and hypertension. Likewise, they constitute a novel mechanism of blood pressure control which has not been described so far.

Abbreviations List

ACTH	Adrenocorticotropic hormone
AM	Adrenomedullin
AM1 receptor	AM type 1 receptor
AM2 receptor	AM type 2 receptor
ANG II	Angiotensin II
ATP	Adenosine triphosphate
cAMP	3',5' cyclic adenosine monophosphate
CAT	Catalase
cGMP	Cyclic guanosine monophosphate
cGPK	cGMP-dependent protein kinases
CGRP	Calcitonin gene-related peptide
CNS	Central nervous system
CRLR	Calcitonin receptor-like receptor
eNOS	Endothelial nitric oxide synthase
ERK	Extracellular signal-regulated kinases
GABA	Gamma-aminobutyric acid
GC	Guanylil cyclase
GPCR	G protein coupled receptor
GPx	Glutathione peroxidase
Gs	Soluble protein G
GTP	Guanosine triphosphate

h	Human
icv	Intracerebroventricular
MAP	Mean arterial pressure
NAD(P)H oxidase	Nicotinamide adenine dinucleotide phosphate-oxidase
NMDA	N-methyl-D-aspartate
nNOS	neuronal nitric oxide synthase
NO	Nitric oxide
NOS	Nitric oxide synthase
NTS	Nucleus tractus solitarii
p-ERK	phospho- extracellular signal-regulated kinases
PIK3/Akt	Phosphatidylinositide 3-kinases/Akt
PKA	Protein kinase A
PKG	Protein kinase G
r	Rat
RAMPs	Receptor activity-modifying proteins
ROS	Reactive oxygen species
SAP	Systolic arterial pressure
SHR	Spontaneously hypertensive rat
SOD	Superoxide dismutase
TBARS	Thiobarbituric acid reactive substances
VN	Vestibular nucleus
WKY	Wistar Kyoto rat

Acknowledgements This study was supported by Grants from People's Ministry of Science, Technology and Industry, Science Mission Project, Subproject 7, ECCV No. 2007001585, PEII-20122000760, CDCH-UCV AIA-06.8402.2012 and PG-06-06-8669-2013.

References

1. Allen M, Smith P, Ferguson A (1997) Adrenomedullin microinjection into the area postrema increases blood pressure. Am J Physiol 272:R1698–R1703
2. Bains J, Ferguson A (1997) Nitric oxide regulates NMDA- driven GABAergic inputs to type I neurons of the rat paraventricular nucleus. J Physiol 499:733–746
3. Baumel Y, Jacobson GA, Cohen D (2009) Implications of functional anatomy on information processing in the deep cerebellar nuclei. Front Cell Neurosci 3:1–8
4. Bell D, Zhao Y, Kelso E, McHenry E, Rush L, Lamont V, Nicholls P, McDermott B (2006) Upregulation of adrenomedullin and its receptor components during cardiomyocyte hypertrophy induced by chronic inhibition of nitric oxide synthesis in rats. Am J Physiol Heart Circ Physiol 290:H904–H914
5. Beltowski J, Jamroz A (2004) Adrenomedullin – what do we know 10 years since its discovery? Pol J Pharmacol 56:5–27
6. Bradley D, Ghelarducci B, Spyer K (1991) The role of the posterior cerebellar vermis in cardiovascular control. Neurosci Res 12(1):45–56
7. Bradley D, Ghelarducci B, Paton J, Spyer K (1987) The cardiovascular response elicited from the posterior cerebellar cortex in the anaesthetized and decerebrated rabbit. J Physiol 383:537–550
8. Bradley D, Paton J, Spyer K (1987) Cardiovascular responses evoked from the fastigial region of the cerebellum in anaesthetized and decerebrated rabbits. J Physiol 392:475–491
9. Carey R, Siragy H (2003) Newly recognized components of the renin-angiotensin system: potential roles in cardiovascular and renal regulation. Endocrine Rev 24(3):261–271
10. Chakravarty P, Suthar T, Coppock H, Nicholl C, Bloom S, Legon S, Smith D (2000) CGRP and adrenomedullin binding correlates with transcript levels for calcitonin receptor – like receptor (CRLR) and receptor activity modifying proteins (RAMPs) in rat tissues. Br J Pharmacol 130:189–195
11. Chan R, Chan Y, Wong T (1991) Responses of cardiovascular neurons in the rostral ventrolateral medulla of the normotensive Wistar Kyoto and spontaneously hypertensive rats to iontophoretic application of angiotensin II. Brain Res 556:145–150
12. Charles CJ, Rademaker MT, Richards AM, Cooper GJS, Coy DH, Nicholls MG (1998) Hemodynamic, hormonal, and renal effects on intracerebroventricular adrenomedullin in conscious sheep. Endocrinology 139:1746–1751
13. Chen QH, Haywood JR, Toney GM (2003) Sympathoexcitation by PVN injected bicuculline requires activation of excitatory amino acid receptors. Hypertension 42:725–731
14. Cikcikoglu N, Yurekli M, Yildirim N (2010) Investigation of some antioxidant enzymes activities depending on adrenomedullin treatment and cold stress in rat liver tissue. Turk J Biochem 35 (2):140–144
15. Cui J, Mukai C, Iwase S, Sawasaki N, Kitazawa H, Mano T, Sugiyama Y, Wada Y (1997) Response to vestibular stimulation of sympathetic outflow to muscle in humans. J Autonom Nerv Syst 66:154–162
16. de Vente J, Hopkins D, Markerink-van M, Emson P, Schmidt H, Steinbusch H (1998) Distribution of nitric oxide synthase and nitric oxide-receptive, cyclic GMP producing structures in the rat brain. Neuroscience 87(1):207–241

17. Díaz E, Israel A (2001) Effect of adrenomedullin receptor and calcitonin gene – related peptide receptor antagonists on centrally mediated adrenomedullin renal action. Brain Res Bull 55(1):29–35

18. Dormer K (1984) Modulation of cardiovascular response to dynamic exercise by fastigial nucleus. J Appl Physiol 56:1369–1377

19. Edvinsson L, Eftekhari S, Salvatore C, Warfvinge K (2010) Cerebellar distribution of calcitonin gene-related peptide (CGRP) and its receptor components calcitonin receptor-like receptor (CLR) and receptor activity modifying protein 1 (RAMP1) in rat. Mol Cell Neurosci 5:1–7

20. Endo S, Launey T (2003) Nitric oxide activates extracellular signal – regulated kinase 1/2 and enhances declustering of ionotropic glutamate receptor subunit 2/3 in rat cerebellar Purkinje cells. Neurosc Lett 350:122–126

21. Eto T (2001) A review of the biological properties and clinical implications of adrenomedullin and proadrenomedullin N terminal 20 peptide (PAMP), hypotensive and vasodilating peptides. Peptides 22:1693–1711

22. Ferrendelli JA (1978) Distribution and regulation of cyclic GMP in the central nervous system. Adv Cyclic Nucleotide Res 9:453–464

23. Figueira L, Israel A (2013) Efecto de la adrenomedulina sobre la actividad de las enzimas antioxidantes cerebelosas. Rev Fac Far 76(1–2):40–49

24. Figueira L, Israel A (2013) Desregulación del sistema adrenomedulinérgico cerebeloso en la hipertensión arterial. Rev Latin Hipert 8(1):9–15

25. Figueira L, Israel A (2013) Efecto hipotensor de la adrenomedulina cerebelosa. Rev Latin Hipert 8 (3):62–67

26. Figueira L, Israel A (2014) Efecto de la adrenomedulina cerebelosa sobre las quinasas reguladas por señales extracelulares en la hipertensión. Rev Fac Far 77(1–2):46–53

27. Figueira L, Israel A (2014) Señalización de la adrenomedulina en el vermis del cerebelo de la rata. Arch Vene Farmacol Terap 33(3):92–97

28. Figueira L, Israel A (2015) Efecto de la adrenomedulina sobre la producción de GMPc/óxido nítrico en el vermis de cerebelo durante la hipertensión. Rev Fac Far 78(1–2):77–83

29. Figueira L, Israel A (2015) Efecto de la hipertensión sobre la acción antioxidante de la adrenomedulina cerebelosa. Rev Fac Far 78(1–2):43–50

30. Figueira F, Israel A (2015) Role of cerebellar adrenomedullin in blood pressure regulation. Neuropeptides 52:59–66

31. Figueira L, Israel A (2015) Cerebellar adrenomedullin: new target for blood pressure regulation. Ther Targets Neurolog Dis 2:e1039. doi: 10.14800/ttnd.1039

32. Figueira L, Israel A (2016a) Papel de la adrenomedulina cerebelosa durante el estrés. Invest Clínica 57(3):280–292

33. Figueira L, Israel A (2016b) Effect of valsartan on cerebellar adrenomedullin system dysregulation during hypertension. The Cerebellum. doi: 10.1007/s12311-016-0780-2

34. Follwell MJ, Ferguson AV (2002) Adrenomedullin influences magnocellular and parvocellular neurons of paraventricular nucleus via separate mechanisms. Am J Physiol Regul Integr Comp Physiol 283: R1293–R1302

35. Fujita M, Kuwaki T, Ando K, Fujita T (2005) Sympatho – inhibitory action of endogenous adrenomedullin through inhibition of oxidative stress in the brain. Hypertension 45:1165–1172

36. Gibbons C, Dackor R, Dunworth W, Fritz-Six K, Caron K (2007) Receptor Activity – modifying proteins: RAMPing up adrenomedullin signaling. Mol Endocrinol 21(4):783–796

37. Han ZQ, Coppock HA, Smith DM, Van-Noorden S, Makgoba MW, Nichols CG, Legon S (1997) The interaction of CGRP and adrenomedullin with a receptor expressed in the rat pulmonary vascular endothelium. J Mol Endocrinol 18:267–72

38. Hanna F, Buchanan K (1996) Adrenomedullin: a novel cardiovascular regulatory peptide. Q J Med 89:881–884

39. Hayakawa H, Hirata Y, Kakoki M, Suzuki Y, Nishimatsu H, Nagata D, Suzuki E, Kikuchi K, Nagano T, Kangawa K, Matsuo H, Sugimoto T, Omata M (1999) Role of nitric oxide-cGMP pathway in adrenomedullin-induced vasodilation in the rat. Hypertension 33:689–693

40. Haynes J, Cooper M (1995) Adrenomedullin and calcitonin gene – related peptide in the rat isolated kidney and in the anaesthetized rat: in vitro and in vivo effects. Eur J Pharmacol 280:91–94

41. He H, Bessho H, Fujisawa Y, Horiuchi K, Tomohiro A, Kita T, Aki Y, Kimura S, Tamaki T, Abe Y (1995) Effects of a synthetic rat adrenomedullin on regional hemodynamics in rats. Eur J Pharmacol 273:209–214

42. Hinson J, Kapas S, Smith D (2000) Adrenomedullin, a multifunctional regulatory peptide. Endocr Rev 21(2):138–167

43. Hong Y, Hay D, Quirion R, Poyner D (2012) The pharmacology of adrenomedullin 2/intermedin. Br J Pharmacol 166(1):110–120

44. Ichiki Y, Kitamura K, Kangawa K, Kawamoto M, Matsuo H, Eto T (1994) Distribution and characterization of inmunoreactive adrenomedullin in human tissue and plasma. FEBS Lett 338:6–10

45. Israel A, Diaz E (2000) Diuretic and natriuretic action of adrenomedullin administered intracerebroventricularly in conscious rats. Regul Pept 89:13–18

46. Ji S, He R (2002) Microinjection of adrenomedullin in rostral ventrolateral medulla increases blood pressure, heart rate and renal sympathetic nerve activity in rats. Acta Phys Sin 54(6):460–466

47. Juaneda C, Dumont Y, Chabot J, Fournier A, Quirion R (2003) Adrenomedullin receptor binding sites in rat brain and peripheral tissues. Eur J Pharmacol 474:165–174

48. Juaneda C, Dumont Y, Chabot JG, Quirion R (2001) Autoradiographic distribution of adrenomedullin receptors in the rat brain. Eur J Pharmacol 421:R1–R2

49. Kato K, Yin H, Agata J, Yoshida H, Chao L, Chao J (2003) Adrenomedullin gene delivery attenuates myocardial infarction and apoptosis after ischemia and reperfusion. Am J Physiol Heart Circ Physiol 285:H1506–H1514

50. Kawai J, Ando K, Tojo A, Shimosawa T, Takahashi K, Onozato M, Yamasaki M, Ogita T, Nakaota T, Fujita T (2004) Endogenous adrenomedullin protects against vascular response to injury in mice. Circulation 109:1147–1153

51. Kitamura K, Kangawa K, Kawamoto M, Ichiki Y, Nakamura S, Matsuo H, Eto T (1993) Adrenomedullin: a novel hypotensive peptide isolated from human pheochromocytoma. Biochem Biophys Res Commun 192:553–560

52. Kitamura K, Kangawa K, Kojima M, Ichiki Y, Matsuo H, Eto T (1994) Complete amino acid sequence of porcine adrenomedullin and cloning of cDNA encoding its precursor [published erratum appears in FEBS Lett 1994 Jul 11;348(2):220]. FEBS Lett 338:306–310

53. Krukoff TL (1999) Central actions of nitric oxide in regulation of autonomic functions. Brain Res Rev 30:52–65

54. Kuwasako K, Cao YN, Nagoshi Y, Kitamura K, Eto T (2004) Adrenomedullin receptors: pharmacological features and possible pathophysiological roles. Peptides 25:2003–2012

55. Kvetnansky R, Sun C, Lake C, Thoa N, Torda T, Kopin I (1978) Effect of handling and forced immobilization on rat plasma levels of epinephrine, norepinephrine, and dopamine-beta-hydroxylase. Endocrinology 103:1868–1874

56. Li X, Li L, Shen L, Qian Y, Cao Y, Zhu D (2004) Changes of adrenomedullin and its receptor components mRNAs expression in the brain stem and hypothalamus- pitutitary – adrenal axis of stress – induced hypertensive rats. Acta Physiol Sin 56 (6):723–729

57. Lohmann S, Walter U, Miller P, Greengard P, De Camilli P (1981) Immunohistochemical localization of cyclic GMP-dependent protein kinase in mammalian brain. Proc Natl Acad Sci USA 78(1):653–657

58. Macchi V, Porzionato A, Belloni A, Stecco C, Parenti A, De Caro R (2006) Immunohistochemical mapping of adrenomedullin in the human medulla oblongata. Peptides 27:1397–1404

59. Martin DS, Segura T, Haywood JR (1991) Cardiovascular responses to bicuculline in the paraventricular nucleus of the rat. Hypertension 18:48–55

60. McCarty R, Gold P (1996) Catecholamine, stress, and disease: a psychobiological perspective. Psychosom Med 58:590–597

61. McLatchie L, Fraser N, Main M, Wise A, Brown J, Thompson N, Solari R, Lee M, Foord S (1998) RAMPs regulate the transport and ligand specificity of the calcitonin-receptor-like receptor. Nature 393 (6683):333–339

62. Mitsuhiko S, Shimokawa A, Kunitake T, Kato K, Hanamori T, Kitamura K, Eto T, Kannnan H (1998) Central actions of adrenomedullin on cardiovascular parameters and sympathetic outflow in conscious rats. Am J Physiol (Regulatory Integrative Comp Physiol) 274:R979–R984

63. Moncada S, Higgs A (1993) The L-arginine-nitric oxide pathway. N Engl J Med 329(27):2002–2012

64. Morara S, Rosina A, Provini L, Forloni G, Caretti A, Wimalawansa S (2000) Calcitonin gene-related peptide receptor expression in the neurons and glia of developing rat cerebellum: an autoradiographic and immunohistochemical analysis. Neurosci 100 (2):381–391

65. Morara S, Wimalawansa S, Rosina A (1998) Monoclonal antibodies reveal expression of the CGRP receptor in Purkinje cells, interneurons and astrocytes of rat cerebellar cortex. NeuroReport 9:3755–3759

66. Muñoz M, Martínez A, Cuttitta F, González A (2001) Distribution of adrenomedullin-like immunoreactivity in the central nervous system of the frog. J Chem Neuroanat 21:105–123

67. Nagae T, Mukoyama M, Sugawara A, Mori K, Yahata K, Kasahara M, Suganami T, Makino H, Fujinaga Y, Yoshioka T, Tanaka I, Nakao K (2000) Rat receptor-activity-modifying proteins (RAMPs) for adrenomedullin/CGRP receptor: cloning and up-regulation in obstructive nephropathy. Biochem Biophys Res Commun 270:89–93

68. Nakane M, Ichikawa M, Deguchi T (1983) Light and electron microscopic demonstration of guanylate cyclase in rat brain. Brain Res 273(1):9–15

69. Nishimatsu H, Shindo T, Takeuchi T, Moriyama N, Hirata Y, Kitamura T (2002) Role of endogenous adrenomedullin in the regulation of ischemic renal injury – studies on transgenic and knockout mice of adrenomedullin gene. J Urol 167:97–97

70. Nishimatsu H, Suzuki E, Nagata D, Moriyama N, Satonaka H, Walsh K, Sata M, Kangawa K, Matsuo H, Goto A, Kitamura T, Hirata Y (2001) Adrenomedullin induces endothelium-dependent vasorelaxation via the phosphatidylinositol 3-kinase/Akt-dependent pathway in rat aorta. Circ Res 89:63–70

71. Nisimaru N (2004) Cardiovascular modules in the cerebellum. Jpn J Physiol 54:431–448

72. Njuki F, Nicholl CG, Howard A, Mak JC, Barnes PJ, Girgi SI, Legon S (1993) A new calcitonin-receptor like sequence in rat pulmonary blood vessels. Clin Sci 85:385–388

73. Owji A, Gardiner J, Upton P, Mahmoodi M, Ghatei M, Bloom S, Smith D (1996) Characterization and molecular identification of adrenomedullin binding sites in the rat spinal cord: a comparison with calcitonin gene – related peptide receptors. J Neurochem 67:2172–2179

74. Pan C, Jaing W, Zhong G, Zhao J, Pang Y, Tang C, Qi Y (2005) Hypertension induced by nitric oxide synthase inhibitor increases responsiveness of ventricular myocardium and aorta of rat tissue to adrenomedullin stimulation *in vitro*. Life Science 78:398–405

75. Pastorello M, Díaz E, Csibi A, Garrido MR, Chabot J-G, Quirion R, Israel A (2007) Papel de la adrenomedulina cerebelosa en la hipertensión arterial. Arch Vene Farmacol Terap 26(2):98–104

76. Rahman M, Nishiyama A, Guo P, Nagai Y, Xing G, Fujisawa Y, Yan Y, Kimura S, Hosomi N, Omori K, Abe Y, Kohno M (2006) Effects of adrenomedullin on cardiac oxidative stress and collagen accumulation in aldosterone – dependent malignant hypertensive rats. J Phamacol Exp Ther 318:1323–1329

77. Rasheed B, Manchada S, Anand B (1970) Effects of stimulation of paleo cerebellum on certain vegetative functions in the cat. Brain Res 20:293–308

78. Rector D, Richard C, Harper R (2006) Cerebellar fastigial nuclei activity during blood pressure challenges. J Appl Physiol 101:549–555

79. Rocha I, Goncalves V, Bettencourt M, Silva L (2008) Effect of stimulation of sub-lobule IX-b of the cerebellar vermis on cardiac function. Physiol Res 57:701–707

80. Saita M, Shimokawa A, Kunitake T, Kato K, Hanamori T, Kitamura K, Eto T, Kannan H (1998) Central actions of adrenomedullin on cardiovascular parameters and sympathetic outflow in conscious rats. Am J Physiol 274:R979–R984

81. Sakai K, Saito K, Ishizuka N (1998) Adrenomedullin synergistically interacts with endogenous vasodilators in rats: a possible role of K(ATP) channels. Eur J Pharmacol 359:151–159

82. Sakata J, Shimokubo T, Kitamura K, Nakamura S, Kangawa K, Matsuo H, Eto T (1993) Molecular cloning and biological activities of rat adrenomedullin, a hypotensive peptide. Biochem Biophys Res Commun 195:921–992

83. Samson W, Murphy T, Resch Z (1998) Central mechanisms for the hypertensive effects of preproadrenomedullin – derived peptides in conscious rats. Am J Physiol 274:R1505–R1509

84. Samson W (1999) Adrenomedullin and the control of fluid and electrolyte homeostasis. Annu Rev Physiol 61:363–389

85. Serino R, Ueta Y, Hara Y, Nomura M, Yamamoto Y, Shibuya I, Hattori Y, Kitamura K, Kangawa K, Russell J, Yamashita H (1999) Centrally administered adrenomedullin increases plasma oxytocin level with induction of c-fos messenger ribonucleic acid in the paraventricular and supraoptic nuclei of the rat. Endocrinology 140:2334–2342

86. Serrano J, Uttenthal O, Martínez A, Fernández P, Martínez J, Alonso D, Bentura M, Santacana M, Gallardo J, Martínez R, Cutitta F, Rodrigo J (2000) Distribution of adrenomedullin – like inmunoreactivity in the rat central nervous system by light and electron microscopy. Brain Res 853:245–268

87. Serrano J, Encinas J, Fernández A, Castro S, Alonso D, Fernández P, Richart A, Bentura M, Santacana M, Cuttitta F, Martínez A, Rodrigo J (2003) Distribution of immunoreactivity for the adrenomedullin binding protein, complement factor H, in the rat brain. Neuroscience 116:947–962

88. Shan J, Krukoff T (2001) Distribution of preproadrenomedullin mRNA in the rat central nervous system and its modulation by physiological stressors. J Comp Neurol 432:88–100

89. Shan J, Krukoff T (2001) Intracerebroventricular adrenomedullin stimulates the hypothalamic-pituitary-adrenal axis, the sympathetic nervous system and production of hypothalamic nitric oxide. J Neuroendocrinol 13(11):975–984

90. Shan J, Stachniak T, Jhamandas J, Krukoff T (2003) Autonomic and neuroendcrine actions of adrenomedullin in the brain: mechanisms for homeostasis. Reg Pept 112:33–40

91. Shimekake Y, Nagata K, Ohta S, Kambayashi Y, Teraoka H, Kitamura K, Eto T, Kangawa K, Matsuo H (1995) Adrenomedullin stimulates two signal transduction pathways, cAMP accumulation and Ca (2+) mobilization, in bovine aortic endothelial cells. J Biol Chem 270:4412–4417

92. Shimosawa T, Shibagaki Y, Ishibashi K, Kitamura K, Kangawa K, Kato S, Ando K, Fujita T (2002) Adrenomedullin, an endogenous peptide, counteracts cardiovascular damage. Circulation 105:106–111

93. Smith PM, Ferguson AV (2001) Adrenomedullin acts in the rat paraventricular nucleus to decrease blood pressure. J Neuroendocrinol 13:467–471

94. Sone M, Takahashi K, Satoh F, Murakami O, Totsune K, Ohneda M, Sasano H, Ito H, Mouri T (1997) Specific adrenomedullin binding sites in the human brain. Peptides 18(8):1125–1129

95. Stachniak T, Krukoff T (2003) Receptor activity modifying protein 2 distribution in the rat central nervous system and regulation by changes in blood pressure. J Neuroendocrinol 15(9):840–850

96. Takahashi H, Watanabe T, Nishimura M, Nakanishi T, Sakamoto M, Yoshimura Y, Masuda M, Murakani T (1994) Centrally induced vasopressor and sympathetic responses to a novel endogenous peptide, adrenomedullin, in anesthetized rats. Am J Hypertens 7:478–482

97. Tandon O, Malhotra V, Bhaskar V, Shankar P (2006) Cerebellar control of visceral response – possible mechanisms involved. Indian J Exp Biol 44:429–435

98. Taylor M, Samson WA (2004) Possible mechanism for the action of adrenomedullin in brain to stimulate stress hormone secretion. Endocrinology 145:4890–4896

99. Taylor M, Samson W (2001) Adrenomedullin and central cardiovascular regulation. Peptides 22:1803–1207

100. Ueda T, Ugawa S, Saishin Y, Shimada S (2001) Expression of receptor – activity modifying protein (RAMP) mRNAs in the mouse brain. Mol Brain Res 93:36–45

101. Uezono Y, Shibuya I, Ueda Y, Tanaka K, Oishi Y, Yanagihara N, Ueno S, Toyohira Y, Nakamura T, Yamashita H, Izumi F (1998) Adrenomedullin increases intracellular Ca^{+2} and inositol 1,4,5 – triphosphate in human oligodendroglial cell line KG-1C. Brain Res 786:230–234

102. Uezono Y, Nakamura E, Ueda Y, Shibuya I, Ueta Y, Yokoo H, Yanagita T, Oyohira Y, Kobayashi H, Yanagihara N, Wada A (2001) Production of cAMP by adrenomedullin in human oligodendroglial cell line KG1C: comparison with calcitonin gene – related peptide and amylin. Brain Res Mol Brain Res 97:59–69

103. Vanhoose A, Emery M, Jimenez L, Winder D (2002) ERK Activation by G-protein-coupled receptors in mouse brain is receptor identity-specific. J Biol Chem 277(11):9049–9053

104. Wang Z, Martorell B, Wälchli T, Vogel O, Fischer J, Born W, Vogel J (2015) Calcitonin gene-related peptide (CGRP) receptors are important to maintain cerebrovascular reactivity in chronic hypertension. PLoS One 10(4):e0123697. http://dx.doi.org/10.1371/journal.pone.0123697 (eCollection 2015)

105. Wei Y, Cao Y, Zhu Y, Chang J, Tang J (1998) Immunohistochemistry and reverse transcription-PCR for detecting adrenomedullin in the central nervous system. Chin Med J 111:793–796

106. Wu H, Song S, Liu H, Xing D, Wang X, Fei Y, Li G, Zhang C, Li Y, Zhang L (2015) Role of adrenomedullin in the cerebrospinal fluid-contacting nucleus in the modulation of immobilization stress. Neuropeptides 51:43–54

107. Xu Y, Krukoff T (2004) Adrenomedullin in the rostral ventrolateral medulla increases arterial pressure and heart rate: roles of glutamate and nitric oxide. Am J Physiol 287:R729–R734

108. Xu Y, Krukoff T (2004) Decrease in arterial pressure induced by adrenomedullin in the hypothalamic paraventricular nucleus is mediated by nitric oxide and GABA. Regul Pept 119(1–2):21–30

109. Xu Y, Krukoff TL (2006) Adrenomedullin in the rostral ventrolateral medulla inhibits baroreflex control of heart rate: a role for protein kinase A. Br J Pharmacol 148:70–77

110. Yang B, Ferguson A (2003) Adrenomedullin influences dissociated rat area postrema neurons. Regul Pept 112:9–17

111. Yokoi H, Arima H, Murase T, Kondo K, Iwasaki Y, Oiso Y (1996) Intracerebroventricular injection of adrenomedullin inhibits vasopressin release in conscious rats. Neurosci Lett 216:65–67

112. Yoshimoto T, Fukai N, Sato R, Sugiyama T, Ozawa N, Shichiri M, Hirata Y (2004) Antioxidant effect of adrenomedullin on angiotensin II-induced reactive oxygen species generation in vascular smooth muscle cells. Endocrinology 145(7):3331–3337

113. Yoshimoto T, Gochou N, Fukai N, Sugiyama T, Shichiri M, Hirata Y (2005) Adrenomedullin inhibits angiotensin II-induced oxidative stress and gene expression in rat endothelial cells. Hypertens Res 28(2):165–172

114. Yurekli M, Esrefoglu M, Dogru M, Dogru A, Gul M, Whidden M (2009) Adrenomedullin reduces antioxidant defense system and enhances kidney tissue damage in cadmium and lead exposed rats. Environ Toxicol 24:279–286

115. Zhang J, Patel K (1998) Effect of nitric oxide within the paraventricular nucleus on renal sympathetic nerve discharge: role of GABA. Am J Physiol 275:R728–R734

116. Zhang K, Mayhan WG, Patel KP (1997) Nitric oxide within the paraventricular nucleus mediates changes in renal sympathetic nerve activity. Am J Physiol 273:R864–R872

Adv Exp Med Biol - Advances in Internal Medicine (2017) 2: 561–581
DOI 10.1007/5584_2016_75
© Springer International Publishing AG 2016
Published online: 13 December 2016

Recent Advances in the Genetics of Hypertension

Loo Keat Wei, Anthony Au, Lai Kuan Teh, and Huey Shi Lye

Abstract

Hypertension is a silent killer worldwide, caused by both genetic and environmental factors. Until now, genetic and genomic association studies of hypertension are reporting different degree of association on hypertension. Hence, it is essential to gather all the available information on the reported genetic loci and to determine if any biomarker(s) is/are significantly associated with hypertension. Current review concluded the potential biomarkers for hypertension, with regards to electrolyte and fluid transports, as well as sodium/potassium ions homeostasis, which are supported by the results of case-controls and meta-analyses.

Keywords

Hypertension • Genetic • GWAS • Polymorphism • Meta-analysis

List of Abbreviations

BP	Blood pressure
SBP	Systolic blood pressure
DBP	Diastolic blood pressure
SNP	Single nucleotide polymorphism
RAS	Renin-angiotensin-aldosterone system
REN	Renin
AGT	Angiotensinogen
Ang II	Angiotensin II
ACE	Angiotensin-converting enzyme
AGTR1	Angiotensin II type I receptor
AGTR2	Angiotensin II type 2 receptor

L.K. Wei (✉)
Department of Biological Science, Faculty of Science, Universiti Tunku Abdul Rahman, Bandar Barat, 31900 Kampar, Perak, Malaysia
e-mail: wynnelkw@gmail.com

A. Au
Institute of Bioproduct Development and Department of Bioprocess Engineering, Faculty of Chemical Engineering, Universiti Teknologi Malaysia, 81300, Skudai, Malaysia

L.K. Teh
Department of Biomedical Science, Faculty of Science, Universiti Tunku Abdul Rahman, Jalan Universiti, Bandar Barat, 31900 Kampar, Perak, Malaysia

H.S. Lye
Department of Agricultural and Food Science, Faculty of Science, Universiti Tunku Abdul Rahman, Jalan Universiti, Bandar Barat, 31900 Kampar, Perak, Malaysia

CYP11B2	Aldosterone synthase
ECE-1/ECE-2	Endothelin converting enzyme 1/2
EDN1/EDN2	Endothelin 1/2
EDNRA/ ENDRBB	Endothelin receptor A/B
eNOS	Endothelial nitric oxide synthase
ApoB/ApoC/ ApoE	Apolipoprotein B/C/E
LPL	Lipoprotein lipase
VLDL	Very low density lipoprotein
ENaC	Epithelial sodium channel
SCNN1A/ SCNN1B/ SCNN1G	Sodium channel non voltage gated 1 alpha subunit/beta subunit/gamma subunit
TSC	Thiazide sensitive Na^+Cl^- cotransporter
ATP1A2	ATPase, Na^+/K^+ transporting, alpha 2 polypeptide
ATP1B1	ATPase, Ca^{++} transporting, plasma membrane 1
ADD	Alpha-adducin
NEDD4L	Neural precursor cell expressed developmentally downregulated gene 4-like
SNS	Sympathetic nervous system
ADRB1	β1-adrenergic receptor
ADRB2	β2-adrenergic receptor
cAMP	Cyclic adenosine monophosphate
IGF-1	Insulin-like growth factor 1
IGF-1R	Insulin-like growth factor 1 receptor
GWAS	Genome-wide association studies
WTCCC	Wellcome Trust Case control consortium
RYR2	Ryanodine receptor 2
WNK1	WNK lysine Deficient Protein Kinase 1
UMOD	Uromodulin
PMS1	Post-meiotic segregation increased 1
SLC24A4	Solute carrier family 24 member 4
YWHAZ	Tyrosine 3-monooxygenasel-trytophan 5-monooxygenase activation protein, zeta polypeptide
IPO7	Importin 7
P4HA2	Prolyl 4-hydroxylase, alpha polypeptide II
CHARGE	Cohorts for Heart and Aging Research in Genome Epidemiology
ICBP	International Consortium for Blood pressure
NPR3-C5orf23	Natriuretic peptide receptor 3-chromosome 5 open reading frame 23
HFE	Human hemochromatosis protein
BAT2-BAT5	HLA-B associated transcript 2-HLA-B associated transcript 5
PLCE1	Phospholipase C epsilon 1
FLJ32810-TMEM133	rho-type guanosine triphosphate activating protein-transmembrane gene 133
GNAS-EDN3	Guanine nucleotide-binding protein alpha stimulating activity polypeptide 1-endothelin 3
MTHFR-NPPB	Methylenetetrahydrofolate reductase-natriuretic peptide B
CACNB2	Calcium channel voltage dependent beta 2 subunit
C10orf107	Chromosome 10 open reading frame 107
CYP1A1-ULK3	Cytochrome P450 family 1 subfamily A polypeptide-unc 51 like kinase 3
ANP	Natriuretic peptides encompass atrial natriuretic peptide
BNP	Brain-natriuretic peptide
CNP	C-type natriuretic peptide
INVEST-GENES	International Verapamil SR-Trandolapril Study Genetic Substudy

1 Introduction

Hypertension or high blood pressure (BP), the "silent killer", is the most common disorder worldwide. It is a condition in which abnormal high BP is found in the arteries. There are two types of hypertension, namely, essential and secondary hypertension. Essential hypertension that deals with unknown cause of this disorder accounts for 95 % of hypertension cases. Meanwhile, secondary hypertension often associated with endocrine diseases, cancer, renal diseases, pregnancy, drug induced and others. Untreated and uncontrolled hypertension can lead to several complications, including coronary artery disease, cerebrovascular disease, renal disease and peripheral arterial disease.

In general, the diagnosis of hypertension is based on the measurement of systolic blood pressure (SBP) and diastolic blood pressure (DBP). Multiple BP measurements obtained from separate occasions over a period of time is taken into account when diagnosing hypertension. The BP measurement can be done at the outpatient clinic or in a nonclinical setting (Shimamoto et al. 2014). Methods and criterion used to diagnose hypertension and BP measurement are shown in Table 1. Whereas, detailed classification of hypertension based on DBP and SBP were summarized in Fig. 1. According to American Heart Association, 32.6 % of United State adults ($\geq$20 years of age) are diagnosed with high BP from the year of 2009 to 2012. Among the diagnosed individuals, 54.1 % still able to control their BP, 76.5 % on anti-hypertensive medicine, 82.7 % aware of their hypertension condition, however 17.3 % of them did not seek for medical care (Mozaffarian et al. 2016).

Moreover, it is clear that hypertension may arise from a complex interplay between environmental and genetic factors. Due to different genetic profiles, male and African-Americans tend to have higher risk of hypertension as compared to female and in other ethnicities (Mozaffarian et al. 2016). Hence, it is pertinent to determine which candidate genes are mediating the susceptibility risk of hypertension, especially in regards to (i) renin-angiotensin-aldosterone system; (ii) vasomotor system; (iii) lipid metabolism; (iv) sodium regulating system; and (v) sympathetic nervous system.

2 Candidate Genes in Hypertension

2.1 Renin-Angiotensin-Aldosterone System

Renin-angiotensin-aldosterone system (RAS) pathway involves several genes such as *renin (REN)*, *angiotensinogen (AGT)*, *angiotensin-converting enzyme (ACE)*, *angiotensin II type 1 receptor (AGTR1)*, *angiotensin II type 2 receptor (AGTR2)* and *aldosterone synthase (CYP11B2)*, which regulating the homeostasis of arterial pressure, tissue perfusion and extracellular volume (Atlas 2007; Cat et al. 2013). Within the RAS, juxtaglomerular cells release REN in response to the reduction of circulated

Table 1 Blood pressure measurement modified from JSH guideline (2014)

Type	Method	Criterion for hypertension measurement (mm Hg)
Clinical	Auscultation	$\geq$140/90
	Automatic sphygmomanometer	
Nonclinical	Home blood pressure measurement	$\geq$135/85
	Ambulatory blood pressure monitoring	$\geq$130/80 for 24 h
		$\geq$135/85 for daytime
		$\geq$120/70 for nighttime

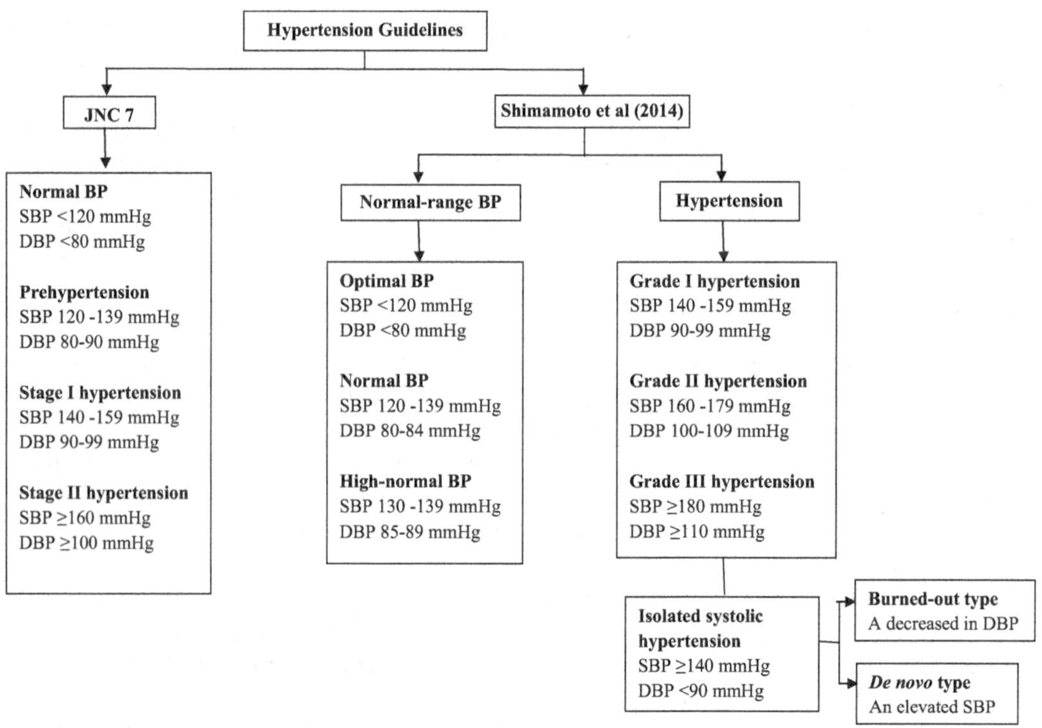

Fig. 1 Hypertension guidelines in JNC 7 and JSH 2014 (Chobanian 2003)

blood volume, renal perfusion pressure and sodium chloride concentration in the tubular fluid. REN cleaves the circulating AGT to form biologically inert decapeptide Ang I (angiotensin I), further converted to Ang II (angiotensin II) by ACE. Ang II is mediated by AGTR1 and AGTR2 to produce aldosterone. As a feedback inhibition, both Ang II and aldosterone restore renal perfusion, regulate sodium and fluid reabsorption, and inhibit subsequent release of REN, in order to restore circulating homeostasis and mediate BP (Atlas 2007; Cat et al. 2013). As shown in Table 2, it has been hypothesized that single nucleotide polymorphisms (SNPs) of *REN*, *AGT*, *AGTR1*, *AGTR2*, *ACE* and *CYP11B2* genes can dysregulate RAS and thus influence the pathophysiology of hypertension (Atlas 2007; Cat et al. 2013). SNPs of *REN rs*12750854, *ACE* rs4646994, *AGT rs*699, *rs*4762 and *rs*5050 are associated with DBP (Sethi et al. 2003; Fang et al. 2010; Penesova et al. 2006; Vangjeli et al. 2010; Fayyad and Aziz 2015).

In fact, aortic stiffness and left ventricular mass are the predictors for hypertension progression (Kim et al. 2014). Of which, elderly with aortic stiffness and carrying *AGTR1* rs5186 and rs275653 polymorphisms may prone to hypertension (Lajemi et al. 2001; Lacolley et al. 2009). *AGTR2* rs5194, rs12710567 and rs1403543 polymorphisms may cause hypertension by mediating left ventricular mass (Alfakih et al. 2004; Carstens et al. 2010; Huber et al. 2010). The accumulated plasma ACE disturbs homeostasis control of endothelial function by mediating aortic stiffness (Ljungberg et al. 2011). Moreover, high BP can become severe if an individual is carrying *CYP11B2* rs1799998 polymorphism (Matsubara et al. 2004). This SNP increases the aldosterone-to-renin ratio, while reducing the aldosterone production (Matsubara et al. 2004). Low levels of aldosterone induces extra sodium and fluid accumulation, in turn dysregulates BP and causes hypertension (Harrison-Bernard 2009; Mishra et al. 2012).

2.2 Vasomotor System

Vasomotor system consists of endothelin and endothelial nitric oxide that maintain vasoconstriction and vasodilation activities respectively (Table 2). *Endothelin converting enzyme 1 (ECE-1)* and *endothelin converting enzyme 2 (ECE-2)* are expressed in vascular endothelium and neuronal tissues, respectively. Among their isoforms, ECE-1b serves as the main player for BP regulation (Valdenaire et al. 1999). *ECE1b* rs213045 and rs213046 polymorphisms may increase *ECE* gene and protein expressions (Annapareddy et al. 2016), that subsequently promote ECE bind to vasoconstrictive receptors such as G-protein couple receptors, endothelin receptor A (EDNRA) and endothelin receptor B (EDNRB), to exert its vasoconstrictive effect (Ling et al. 2013). The receptor polymorphisms of *EDNRA* rs5335 and rs5343 alter *EDNRA* gene expression and endothelin binding (Rahman et al. 2008) as well as increase DBP and SBP in response to different salt sensitivity i.e. either salt depletion or repletion. On the other hand, a decrease in BP is observed among salt-sensitive individuals who carry *EDRNB* rs5351 polymorphism (Caprioli et al. 2008). Nonetheless, *endothelin 1 (EDN1)* rs5370 and *endothelin 2 (EDN2)* rs5800 polymorphisms increase the production of endothelin, enhance the calcium sensitivity on arteries, and subsequently mediate the progression of hypertension (Iglarz et al. 2002; Panoulas et al. 2008; Dhawan et al. 2014). The endothelial nitric oxide synthase (eNOS) produces nitric oxide and vasodilates the blood vessels to lower BP levels. Dysregulated eNOS may reduce about 50 % of the nitric oxide levels at the basal blood flow, and subsequently restrict endothelial diastolic function (Förstermann and Münzel 2006). This dysregulation is mainly related to *eNOS* rs1799983 and variable tandem repeat 4a/4b polymorphisms, which also associated with

hypertension risk (Tang et al. 2008a; Patkar et al. 2009; Yan-yan 2011).

2.3 Lipid Metabolism

Genetic polymorphisms of *apolipoprotein B (ApoB)*, *apolipoprotein C (ApoC)*, *apolipoprotein E (ApoE)* and *lipoprotein lipase (LPL)* genes within the lipid metabolism pathways have been associated with the variations in BP and the propensity of hypertension (Table 2). ApoB and ApoE are the major constituents for chylomicrons that catabolize triglyceride-rich lipoprotein particles. *ApoB* rs693 and *ApoE* E4E4 polymorphisms may impair the clearance of chylomicrons and VLDL remnants, which lead to the higher levels of triglycerides and cholesterol (Tang et al. 2008b; Das et al. 2009; Wei et al. 2015a, 2015b). This phenomenon promotes intimal-medial carotid artery thickening and susceptibility risk to hypertension (Paternoster et al. 2008; Rossi et al. 2001). Meanwhile, ApoC3 is a VLDL protein that inhibits LPL activity while destroying triglyceride-rich remnants catabolism. In particular, *ApoC3* rs5128 and rs4225 as well as *LPL* rs320 and rs328 polymorphisms induce high levels of triglycerides, high BP and thus increase the susceptibility risk of hypertension (Salah et al. 2009; Muñoz-Barrios et al. 2012; Ghattas et al. 2013).

2.4 Sodium Regulating System

BP is influenced by the efficiency of sodium reabsorption. Increase in sodium channel activity promotes sodium reabsorption and sodium retention, thereby elevating BP (Sun et al. 2011). Gene polymorphisms encoded for renal ion channels and sodium reabsorption transporters were summarized in Table 2.

Being the pertinent component in sodium reabsorption, epithelial sodium channel (ENaC) is involved in the first step of active sodium reabsorption in urinary bladder and renal collecting duct, which maintains the water and electrolyte homeostasis. ENaC consists of α-, β-

Table 2 Candidate genes for hypertension

System involved	Gene/protein and function	[a]Chromosomal location	Polymorphism	References
RAS	REN activates RAS	1q32	Insertion/deletion	Ying et al. (2010)
			7828A>T (rs6693954)	Sun et al. (2011)
			−5312C>T (rs12750854)	Vangjeli et al. (2010)
			10631A>G (rs2368564)	Ahmad et al. (2005)
			−4021C>T	Zhu et al. (2003)
			10795 T>G (rs5707)	Mansego et al. (2008)
	AGT is the substrate for angiotensin I	1q42-43	235M>T (rs669)	Sethi et al. (2003)
			174T>M (rs4762)	Fang et al. (2010)
			−20A>C (rs5050)	Fayyad et al. (2015)
	ACE degrades angiotensin I to form angiotensin II	17q23	Insertion/deletion (rs4646994)	Ramu et al. (2011)
	AGTR1 regulates aldosterone secretion	3q24	+1166A>C (rs5186)	Bonnardeaux et al. (1994)
			32611C>T (rs12695895)	Nie et al. (2010)
			+573 C>T (rs5182)	Martínez-Rodríguez et al. (2012)
	AGTR2 is a receptor for angiotensin II	X-chromosome	−1332A>G (rs5194)	Alfakih et al. (2004)
			+1675G>A (rs1403543)	Huber et al. (2010)
			1334T>C (rs12710567)	Zhang et al. (2003)
	CYP11B2 for cholesterol and steroids biosynthesis	8q22	−344C>T (rs1799998);	Matsubara et al. (2004)
Vasomotor system	EDN1 modulates vasomotor tone, and stimulates cell proliferation and remodeling	6p24.1	5665G>T (rs5370)	Iglarz et al. (2002)
	EDN2 regulates cell growth and vasoconstriction	1p34.2	985A>G (rs5800)	Hu et al. (2010)
	EDNRA mediates vasoconstriction and cell proliferation	EDNRA: 4q31.22	1363C>T (rs5343)	Benjafield et al. (2003)
			70C>G (rs5335)	Rahman et al. (2008)
	EDNRB clears ET-1 and releases vasodilator	13q22	1065G>A (rs5351)	Caprioli et al. (2008)
	ECE-1 involves in endothelin biosynthesis	1p36.1	839T>G (rs213046)	Funke-Kaiser et al. (2003)
			338C>A (rs213045)	
	eNOS is a vasodilator that inhibits smooth muscle cell proliferation and regulates BP	7q36	894G>T (rs 1799983)	Tang et al. (2008)
			Intron 4a/b or 27-bp-VNTR	Patkar et al. (2009)
			[a]*(the a-deletion has 4 tandem 27 bp repeats; b-insertion has 5 repeats)*	

Category	Gene and function	Chromosomal location[a]	Polymorphism	Reference
Lipid metabolism	*APOB* carries fats and fat-like substances (such as cholesterol) in the bloodstream	2p24-p23	3'VNTR	Frossard et al. 1(999)
			7673C>T (rs693)	Tang et al. (2008)
	APOC3 inhibits LPL and hepatic lipase to hydrolyze TG-rich particles, and regulates TG homeostasis	11q23.3	3206G>T (rs4225)	Tang et al. (2008)
			3,238 C>G (rs5128)	Ghattas et al. (2013)
	APOE packs cholesterols and other fats to the bloodstream	19q13.2 (coded by ε2, ε3, ε4 allele)	ε4allele, E3E4 and E4E4 genotypes, 388 T>C (rs rs429358), 526C>T (rs7412)	Li et al. (2003) and de Leeuw et al. (2004)
	LPL hydrolyzes TG and releases monoglycerides and free fatty acids as well as regulates HDL concentration	8p22	447S>X (rs328)	Sallah et al. (2009)
			27496 T>G (rs320)	Mu˜noz-Barrios et al. (2012)
Sodium regulating system	*SCNN1A* controls sodium ions and water transport into cells	12p13	2139G>A (rs4149623)	Iwai et al. (2002)
	SCNN1B controls sodium ions and water transport into cells	16p12.2-p12.1	594T>M (rs1799979)	Baker et al. (1998) and Yang et al. (2014)
	SCNN1G controls sodium ions and water transport into cells	16p12	−173G>A (rs5718)	Iwai et al. (2001)
	TSC regulates sodium chloride reabsorption by moving the charged sodium and chlorine ions across cell membrane	16q13	1420C>T	Melander et al. (2000)
			2736G>A	
			48591A>G (rs7204044)	Chang et al. (2011)
			56900931C>T (rs13306673)	
	NEDD4L regulates *ENaC* expression via ubiquitination	18q21	−326G>A (rs4149601)	Fava et al. (2006)
			276721 T>C (rs2288774)	
			55874441C>T (rs513563)	Russo et al. (2005)
			297555 T>C (rs3865418)	
	ATP1A2 maintains electrochemical gradients of sodium and potassium ions across the plasma membrane	1q23.2	–	Faruque et al. (2011)
	ATP1B1 maintains electrochemical gradients of sodium and potassium ions across the plasma membrane	1q24	29223G>A (rs2901029)	Faruque et al. (2011)
			14173C>T (rs3766031)	
			15513A>G (rs3766032)	
			30114G>A (rs12079745)	
			30989C>T (rs1138486)	
			20025T>A (rs2982468)	
Sympathetic nervous system	*GNB3* translates signals from cell surface into cell, and mediates hormones and peptides signaling	12p13	825C>T (rs5443)	Tozawa (2001)
	GCG-R regulates blood glucose levels and glucose homeostasis	17q25	118G>A (rs1801483)	Brand et al. (1999)
	IGF-1R exerts multiple physiologic effects on vasculature	15q26.3	−328C>T (rs8034564)	Horio et al. (2010)
			275124A>C (rs1464430)	

[a]chromosomal location based on genetic home reference (https://ghr.nlm.nih.gov/gene/)

and γ-subunits that encodes *sodium channel non voltage gated 1 alpha subunit (SCNN1A)*, *sodium channel non voltage gated 1 beta subunit (SCNN1B)* and *sodium channel non voltage gated 1 gamma subunit (SCNN1G)* genes, respectively (Sun et al. 2011). It has been reported that *SCNN1A* rs4149623 may decrease *SCNN1A* gene expression and subsequently reduce sodium reabsorption efficiency in the kidney (Iwai et al. 2002). *SCNN1A* rs4149623 may prevent individuals from the risk of hypertension, however, this SNP is a risk marker for hypertension among Japanese population (Iwai et al. 2002). *SCNN1B* rs1799979 alters β-ENaC protein structure and causes protein kinase C phosphorylation, which inhibits sodium channel activity and thus increases sodium retention and elevates BP (Yang et al. 2014). *SCNN1G* rs5718 reduces pulse pressure and SBP, in which dropping of pulse pressure (8 mmHg) and SBP (11 mmHg) have been observed among hypertensive patients (Iwai et al. 2001). Sodium reabsorption efficiency may also be regulated by *thiazide sensitive Na$^+$ Cl$^-$ cotransporter (TSC)* 2736G > A and 1420C > T polymorphisms. These SNPs up-regulate *TSC* gene expression and promote sodium reabsorption in thick ascending limb and distal convoluted tubule, which induce BP before and during the early phase of hypertension development (Manning et al. 2002; Keszei et al. 2007).

The absorbed sodium ions are transported across cell membrane to maintain electrolytes homeostasis (Sun et al. 2011). Several lines of evidence suggested that rs2901029, rs3766031, rs12079745, rs1138486, rs3766032 and rs2982468 polymorphisms in both *ATPase, Na$^+$/K$^+$ transporting, alpha 2 polypeptide (ATP1A2)* and *ATPase, Ca^{++} transporting, plasma membrane 1 (ATP1B1)* genes are deviating the electrochemical gradients of sodium and potassium ions across plasma membrane, and lead to higher BP (Chang et al. 2007; Xiao et al. 2009; Faruque et al. 2011). In addition, *alpha-adducin (ADD)* gene polymorphisms, such as *ADD1* rs4961, *ADD2* rs4984 and *ADD3* rs3731566 may dysregulate TSC and enhance constitutive tubular sodium reabsorption, which

lead to higher salt-sensitivity (Tikhonoff et al. 2003; Zafarmand et al. 2008; Seidlerová et al. 2009; Dimke et al., 2011). Increased salt sensitivity is also associated with *neural precursor cell expressed developmentally down-regulated 4-like E3 ubiquitin protein ligase (NEDD4L)* rs4149601 polymorphism through ENaC regulation. All in all, dysregulation of genes associated with sodium regulating system are contributed to the susceptibility risk of hypertension (Russo et al. 2005; Fava et al. 2006; Luo et al. 2009).

2.5 Sympathetic Nervous System

Sympathetic nervous system (SNS) is controlled by α- and β-adrenergic receptors that actively interact with G-proteins (Table 2). Among the available adrenergic receptors, the associations between β1-adrenergic receptor *(ADRB1)* and β2-adrenergic receptor *(ADRB2)* with hypertension risk are discussed. Both subunits that control BP by mediating cardiac output and peripheral resistance are believed to play a major role in hypertension (Soualmia 2012). ADRB1 belong to G-coupled receptor superfamily that located at the intracellular cytoplasmic tail. *ADRB1* rs1801253 polymorphism decreases it's receptor activity, affects the binding of ADRB1 on G-proteins, and is associated with lower mean values of SBP and DBP as well as the risk of hypertension (Johnson et al. 2011b). The ADRB2 regulates the vasodilation of smooth muscle cells via activation of cyclic adenosine monophosphate (cAMP) signalling pathway (Snyder et al. 2008). The risk of hypertension is multiplied among *ADRB2* rs1042713 carriers in an elderly population (Soudani et al. 2014).

In addition, the health status of vasculature also mediated by insulin-like growth factor 1 (IGF-1), a strong promoter for the growth of cardiomyocyte. Genetic polymorphisms of *IGF-1 receptor (IGF-1R)* have been associated with atherosclerosis, hypertension, angiogenesis, and diabetes (Higashi et al. 2012). Specifically, *IGF-1R* rs8034564 polymorphism contributes to abnormal left ventricular hypertrophy geometry changes that deteriorates the hypertension progression (Horio et al. 2010).

3 GWAS and Hypertension

Thus far, 26 candidate genes have been discussed, yet none of the single SNPs can protrude their significant role in affecting the risk of hypertension, which possibly due to the low modest effect of these SNPs. This phenomenon urges a drastic shift to genome-wide association studies (GWAS) that allow an unbiased investigation of genetic causes of hypertension, and providing a more convincing result as compared to the candidate genes approach. GWAS uses a dense panel of SNPs to determine the association between multiple genetic biomarkers and complex disorders such as hypertension and diabetes, have received a great attention since 2006. GWAS idea is based on 'common disease common variant' hypothesis, which emphasizes that common disease is related to small effect size of genetic variations with an allelic frequency higher than 5 % in the population (Gibson 2012). The GWAS with different degree of associations on hypertension were summarized in Table 3.

The Wellcome Trust Case Control Consortium, WTCCC (Burton et al. 2007) was pioneering GWAS-hypertension project. WTCCC investigated 2000 cases each for seven common diseases and 3000 shared controls (Table 3). Seven common diseases were hypertension, coronary artery disease, rheumatoid arthritis, bipolar disorder, Crohn's disease, type 1 and type 2 diabetes. Two thousand hypertension cases were recruited from British Genetics of Hypertension (BRIGHT) study. Among the 3000 shared controls, 1500 of them were recruited from the 1958 British Birth Cohort and the rests of the samples were the blood donors who participated in GWAS-hypertension project. Twenty-one SNPs with p values lower than 5×10^{-8} were discovered across the entire genome. Of which, nine SNPs for Crohn's disease, five for type 1 diabetes, three for type

2 diabetes, two for rheumatoid arthritis, and one for both coronary artery disease and bipolar disorder.

Even though the strongest polymorphism has been identified for hypertension, rs2820037 gained statistical significance at 7.7×10^{-7}; yet, it failed to achieve genome-wide significance threshold of 5×10^{-8} (Burton et al. 2007). This SNP is located on chromosome 1q43 and is mapped to the nearest *ryanodine receptor 2* (*RYR2*) gene. RYR2 is abundantly found in cardiac muscle and modulates calcium ion flow rate from sarcoplasmic reticulum. RYR2 is also exerting a direct effect on cardiac depolarisation and myocardial contractile dysfunction (Galati et al. 2016). It has been reported that genetic variation of *RYR2* increases the risk of malignant ventricular arrhythmias, but the severity of arrhythmias can be further deteriorated among hypertensive individuals (Galati et al. 2016). Hence, rs2820037 polymorphism causes arrhythmias, which is secondary to hypertension. Moreover, no direct relationship between the genetic variations within *RYR2* and hypertension was observed so far. The possible explanation is that this SNP was unable to achieve the genome-wide significance threshold of 5×10^{-8} in WTCCC (Burton et al. 2007).

In addition, rs146888326 polymorphism that has been identified to be associated with the severity of hypertension, was not associated with hypertension in WTCCC (Burton et al. 2007). Supposedly, rs1468326 polymorphism that situated at 3 kb upstream of *WNK lysine deficient protein kinase 1* (*WNK1*) gene promoter region can modify WNK1 expression, regulate sodium homeostasis, increase BP and hypertension risk (Newhouse et al. 2005). The non-significant association observed between rs1468326 polymorphism and hypertension in GWAS could be due to the poorly tagged of this SNP on the Affymetrix chips. Also, other nearby SNPs may exhibit larger effect size than rs1468326 (Burton et al. 2007). Nonetheless, misclassification bias is the main concern of WTCCC as this study was not purposely designed for hypertension. Misclassification bias may dilute the detecting power of the

Table 3 GWAS of hypertension

Study (cohort)	Ethnicity	Sample size	Number of SNP covered	Key finding highlighted in GWAS			Summary of the translated protein/ enzyme for the mapped gene
				rs number	P value	Mapped gene	
Burton et al. (2007)	Caucasians	5000	469,557	rs2820037	7.7×10^{-7}	RYR2	Calcium channel that modulates flow rate of calcium ion from sarcoplasmic reticulum and supplies calcium ion for cardiac muscle.
Kato et al. (2008)	Asians	940	80,795	rs3755351	1.7×10^{-5}	ADD2	Membrane-cytoskeleton-associated protein that predominantly expressed in the brain to enhance the assembly of spectrin-actin network. It binds to calmodulin in regulating BP.
Adeyemo et al. (2009) (HUFS)	African American	1017	808,465	rs9791170	5.1×10^{-7}	P4HA2	Prolyl 4-hydroxylase for collagen synthesis.
Org et al. (2009) (KORA S3)	Caucasians	1644	395,912	rs11646213	5.3×10^{-8}	CDH13	Calcium-dependent cell adhesion protein that protects vascular endothelial cells from apoptosis.
Wang et al. (2009)	Caucasians	542	79,447	rs6749447	1.6×10^{-7}	STK39	Serine threonine kinase that acts as an intermediate for cellular stress response pathway and phosphorylates cation-chloride-coupled co-transporters.
Padmanabhan et al. (2010)	Caucasians	3320	551,629	rs13333226	3.6×10^{-11}	UMOD	Constitutive inhibitor of calcium crystallization in renal fluids that protects against urinary tract infection.
Johnson et al. (2011)	Caucasians	86,588	49,452	rs2004776	6.7×10^{-14}	AGT	Pre-angiotensinogen degrades by renin in decreasing the BP level.
		33,638	55,692	rs11105354	1.1×10^{-10}	ATP2B1	As described before.

phenotypes, especially if the hypertensive control samples may be misclassified as cases (Burton et al. 2007). This is an extremely serious problem in GWAS where each SNP carried relatively small effect sizes, and in fact, misclassifying as low as 5 % of controls as cases can reduce the power of study by 10 % (Burton et al. 2007).

Subsequent GWAS suggested that rs13333226 polymorphism decreases the risk of hypertension (Padmanabhan et al. 2010). Rs13333226 polymorphism that located at 1617 base pairs upstream to the transcription start site, is mapped to 5′ end of *uromodulin* (*UMOD*) gene. *UMOD* encodes for uromodulin, the most abundant extracellular glycosylphosphatidy-linositol anchored glycoprotein expressed in the ascending limb of Henley (Padmanabhan et al. 2010). Rs13333226 polymorphism is involved in sodium homeostasis, by decreasing urinary uromodulin excretion and promoting sodium reabsorption at proximal tubular (Padmanabhan et al. 2010). Since excessive sodium reabsorption and its accumulation has resulted in water reten-tion and high BP, it is suggested that dysregulation of sodium homeostasis may causes hypertension via WNK-sodium chloride cotransporter pathway (Fujita 2014).

The first GWAS-hypertension study among African American has been reported by Adeyemo et al. (2009). Despite from the 30 SNPs discov-ered, only five SNPs attained genome-wide signif-icance threshold of 5×10^{-8} and were associated with SBP. These five SNPs were respectively mapped to *post-meiotic segregation increased 1* (*PMS1*), intergenic AL365265.23, *solute carrier family 24 member 4* (*SLC24A4*), *tyrosine 3-monooxygenase/tryptophan 5-monooxygenase activation protein, zeta polypeptide* (*YWHAZ*) and *importin 7* (*IPO7*) genes. Unfortunately, none of them were associated with hypertension. The strongest marker for hypertension, rs9791170 was failed to attain genome-wide sig-nificance threshold of 5×10^{-8} among West Africans (Adeyemo et al. 2009). Rs9791170 polymorphism which located at 6 kb upstream of *prolyl 4-hydroxylase, alpha polypeptide II* (*P4HA2*), is believed to exert distal anti-stress effects among hypertensive individuals. P4HA2 catalyzes the post-translational formation of 4-hydroxyproline, while the latter is an indicator for *de novo* proline synthesis. Even though pro-line has been reported to modulate anti-oxidation activity in human fibroblasts and immortalized cell lines (Kuo et al. 2016), there is no direct relationship between 4-hydroxyproline and

hypertension. Hence, this could be a possible reason for the non-significant association between rs9791170 polymorphism and hyperten-sion. Moreover, in the subsequent replication studies by Fox et al. (2011), Jin et al. (2011) and Kidambi et al. (2012), none of these SNPs achieved genome-wide significance threshold of 5×10^{-8} (Table 3).

4 GWAS Meta-Analysis and Hypertension

Currently, several meta-analysis of GWAS have been performed to identify the genetic variations of hypertension with very small effect sizes. Meta-analysis allows the synthesized results from all eligible studies to attain higher level of conclusion, by refining significance p value and estimating the effect size (Bush and Moore 2012; Au et al. 2015). Normally, GWAS-BP studies tend to report a huge number of participants which is believed to provide sufficient statistical power to decrease BP variations from various next generation sequencing platforms and BP measurement techniques. However, we only focused on hypertensive subjects than combining the results with BP, diastolic and systolic phenotypes. This is to avoid false positive findings because continuous traits such as BP always exhibit greater statistical power as com-pared to dichotomous traits i.e. hypertension, which the latter is unlikely to report a genome-wide significance p value of 5×10^{-8} (Ehret 2010). As shown in Table 4, meta-analysis of GWAS resulted in eight SNPs (rs17367504, rs11191548, rs12946454, rs16998073, rs1530440, rs653178, rs1378942 and rs16948048), which were significantly associated with hypertension (Newton-Cheh et al. 2009). Among these SNPs, only rs17367504, rs16998073 and rs1378942 polymorphisms achieved genome-wide significance threshold of 5×10^{-8} (Newton-Cheh et al. 2009).

Similarly, Cohorts for Heart and Aging Research in Genome Epidemiology (CHARGE) suggested that 20, 13 and 10 SNPs discovered by GWAS were associated with DBP, SBP and

Table 4 Meta-analysis of GWAS on hypertension

Study (cohort)	Ethnicity	Sample size	Key finding highlighted in GWAS			Summary of the translated protein/enzyme for the mapped gene
			rs number	P value	Mapped gene	
Levy et al. (2009)	Caucasians	29,136	rs2681472	1.7×10^{-8}	*ATP2B1*	Magnesium-dependent enzyme that maintain intracellular calcium homeostasis.
			rs11105354	1.8×10^{-8}		
			rs11105364	2.1×10^{-8}		
			rs17249754	2.2×10^{-8}		
			rs11105368	2.2×10^{-8}		
			rs12579302	2.2×10^{-8}		
			rs11105378	2.8×10^{-8}		
			rs12230074	2.8×10^{-8}		
			rs2681492	8.4×10^{-8}		
			rs4842666	3.4×10^{-7}		
			rs7640747	4.8×10^{-7}	*ITGA9*	Alpha Integrin that mediate cell-cell and cell-matrix adhesion.
			rs11105328	7.1×10^{-7}		
			rs743395	7.5×10^{-7}		
			rs11014166	7.8×10^{-7}	*CACNB2*	Subunit of voltage-dependent calcium channel that increases peak calcium current.
Levy et al. (2009) (joint meta-analysis)	Caucasians	63,569	rs2681472	1.8×10^{-11}	*ATP2B1*	As described before.
Newton-Cheh et al. (2009)	Caucasians	34,433	rs17367504	2×10^{-9}	*MTHFR*	Reductase in one carbon metabolism pathway that reduces 5,10-methylenetetrahydrofolate to 5-methyltetrahydrofolate.
			rs11191548	3×10^{-13}	*NT5C2*	Hydrolyze purine nucleotides and involves in purine metabolism.
			rs12946454	2×10^{-5}	*PLCD3*	Phospholipase that hydrolyze phospholipids to second messengers, and increases cystolic calcium ion concentration for subsequent cellular response.
			rs16998073	7×10^{-10}	*FGF5*	Oncogene for mitogenic and cell survival activities.
			rs1530440	2×10^{-3}	*C10orfl07*	No significant function.
			rs653178	8×10^{-7}	*ATXN2*	Predominately located at Golgi apparatus for epidermal growth factor receptor trafficking.
			rs1378942	2×10^{-14}	*CSK*	Non-receptor tyrosine kinase that mediates immune response, and cell growth.

			rs16948048	1×10^{-4}	ZNF652	Transcriptional repressor.
International Consortium for Blood Pressure Genome-Wide Association Studies 2011	Caucasians	200,000	rs2932538	2.9×10^{-7}	MOV10	RNA helicase for RNA-dependent gene silencing.
			rs13082711	3.6×10^{-4}	SLC4A7	Sodium bicarbonate cotransporter that mediates intracellular pH for visual sensory transmission.
			rs419076	3.1×10^{-4}	MECOM	Oncoprotein and transcription regulator for apoptosis and hematopoiesis.
			rs13107325	4.9×10^{-7}	SLC39A8	Solute-carrier that responsible for zinc influx during inflammation.
			rs13139571	2.5×10^{-5}	GUCY1A3-GUCY1B3	GUCY1A3: soluble guanylate cyclases that converts GTP to GMP and pyrophosphate. GUCY1B3: converts GTP cGMP for nitric oxide binding.
			rs1173771	3.2×10^{-10}	NRP3-C5orf23	Natriuretic peptide receptor clears the circulating and extracellular natriuretic peptides via endocytosis.
			rs11953630	1.7×10^{-7}	EBF1	Transcriptional activator that recognizes palindromic sequence.
			rs1799945	1.8×10^{-10}	HFE	Membrane protein that mediates iron absorption.
			rs805303	1.1×10^{-10}	BAT2-BAT5	A locus that encompasses BAT2, BAT3, BAT4, BAT5, BAG6, CSNK2B, LY6G5B, LY6G5C.
			rs4373814	8.5×10^{-8}	CACNB2 (5')	As described before.
			rs932764	9.4×10^{-9}	PLCE1	Phospholipase that hydrolyze phosphatidylinositol 4,5-bisphosphate to second messengers for subsequent cell differentiation activity.
			rs7129220	1.1×10^{-3}	ADM	Preprohormone that enhances angiogenesis for malignant hypertension.
			rs633185	5.4×10^{-11}	FLJ32810-TMEM133	FLJ32810: GTPase activating protein that may affect blood pressure. TMEM133: Unknown gene function.
			rs2521501	7.0×10^{-7}	FURIN-FES	FURIN: Subtilisin-like proprotein convertase for tumor progression. FES: Tyrosine-specific protein kinase that maintains cellular transformation.
			rs1327235	4.6×10^{-4}	JAG1	Ligand for notch 1 receptor that involves in hematopoiesis.
			rs6015450	4.2×10^{-14}	GNAS-EDN3	GNAS: A locus for maternally, paternally and biallelically imprinting regulations. EDN3: Endothelins for neural crest-derived cell lineages.

(continued)

Table 4 (continued)

Study (cohort)	Ethnicity	Sample size	Key finding highlighted in GWAS			
			rs number	P value	Mapped gene	Summary of the translated protein/enzyme for the mapped gene
			rs17367504	2.3×10^{-10}	*MTHFR-NPPB*	MTHFR: Reductase in one carbon metabolism pathway that reduces 5,10-methylenetetrahydrofolate to 5-methyltetrahydrofolate. NPPB: Cardiac hormone that inhibits renin and aldosterone secretion for cardiovascular homeostasis.
			rs1458038	1.9×10^{-7}	*FGF5*	As described before.
			rs1813353	6.2×10^{-10}	*CACNB2 (3′)*	As described before.
			rs4590817	9.8×10^{-9}	*C10orf107*	As described before.
			rs11191548	1.4×10^{-5}	*CYP17A1-NT5C2*	CYP17A1: Monooxygenase for steroidogenic pathway that generates glucocorticoids and androgens. NT5C2: As described before.
			rs381815	3.4×10^{-6}	*PLEKHA7*	Responsible for zonula adherens, biogenesis and maintenance.
			rs17249754	1.1×10^{-14}	*ATP2B1*	Magnesium-dependent enzyme that maintain intracellular calcium homeostasis.
			rs3184504	2.6×10^{-6}	*SH2B3*	Negative regulator for cytokine signalling.
			rs10850411	5.2×10^{-6}	*TBX5-TBX3*	TBX5: Transcription factor for heart development. TBX3: Transcriptional repressor for tetrapod development.
			rs1378942	1.0×10^{-8}	*CYP1A1-ULK3*	CYP1A1: Monooxygenase that hydrolyze polycyclic aromatic hydrocarbons. ULK3: Serine tyrosine kinase that mediates Sonic hedgehog signalling and autophagy.
			rs12940887	1.2×10^{-7}	*ZNF652*	As described before.
Johnson et al. (2011)	Caucasians	86,588	rs1801253	3.3×10^{-4}	*ADRB1*	Adrenergic receptor that modulates physiological effects of hormone epinephrine and neurotransmitter norepinephrine for ocular hypotension.
			rs2004776	3.7×10^{-7}	*AGT*	Pre-angiotensinogen degrades by renin in decreasing the blood pressure level.
			rs4305	3.0×10^{-5}	*ACE*	Peptidase that converts angiotensin I into angiotensin II to maintain blood pressure and fluid-electrolyte balance.

Kato et al. (2011)	Asians	19,608	rs17030613	2.1×10^{-7}	*CAPZA1*	Actin binding protein that mediates the growth of actin filament.
			rs16849225	3.5×10^{-6}	*FIGN*	ATP-dependent microtubule severing protein that suppresses the growth of microtubule.
			rs1173766	4.8×10^{-9}	*NPR3*	Natriuretic peptide receptor that cleans circulating and extracellular natriuretic peptides via endocytosis.
			rs11066280	4.0×10^{-8}	*PTPN11*	Protein tyrosine phosphatase that involves in signalling pathway of mitotic cycle.
			rs35444	6.2×10^{-5}	*TBX3*	Transcriptional repressor for tetrapod development.

hypertension, respectively (p < 4×10^{-7}) (Levy et al. 2009). A subsequent joint meta-analysis between CHARGE and Global Blood Pressure Genetics (Global BPgen) consortia concluded that only single SNP of rs2681472 attained genome-wide significance for hypertension (p < 5×10^{-8}) (Levy et al. 2009). This SNP is mapped to plasma membrane *ATP2B1*. ATP2B1 is an ion-transport ATPase that predominately expressed in the vascular endothelium. ATP2B1 functions as a pertinent modulator for intracellular calcium homeostasis that is involved in the vascular smooth muscles dilations and contractions (Brini and Carafoli 2011). Three Japanese teams i.e. Tabara et al. (2010), Takeuchi et al. (2010) and Miyaki et al. (2012) have extended the *ATP2B1* SNPs analysis on 14,105, 1526 and 735 Japanese subjects, respectively. Tabara et al. (2010) concluded that *ATP2B1* rs11105378 polymorphism exhibits stronger association towards hypertension followed by *ATP2B1* rs2681472 polymorphism. Although Takeuchi et al. (2010) reported that rs2681472 polymorphism was significantly associated with hypertension, this SNP failed to attain genome wide significance threshold (p = 0.002). However, subsequent meta-analyses by Xi et al. (2012) and Xi et al. (2014) confirmed a significant association between rs2681472 polymorphism and hypertension. In the subsequent replication study, Miyaki et al. (2012) confirmed that another SNP (rs17249754) significantly increased the risk towards hypertension by two-folds. And their result also found to be consistent with International Consortium for Blood Pressure (ICBP) GWAS (2011). ICBP GWAS has identified 11 indexed SNPs that associated with hypertension risk at genome wide threshold of 5×10^{-8}. The indexed SNPs were rs1173771, rs1799945, rs805303, rs932764, rs633185, rs6015450, rs17367504, rs1813353, rs4590817, rs17249754 and rs1378942. These SNPs were mapped to *natriuretic peptide receptor 3-chromosome 5 open reading frame 23 (NPR3-C5orf23), human hemochromatosis protein (HFE), HLA-B associated transcript 2-HLA-B associated transcript 5 (BAT2-BAT5), phospholipase C epsilon 1 (PLCE1), rho-type guanosine triphosphate activating protein-transmembrane gene 133 (FLJ32810-TMEM133), guanine nucleotide-binding protein alpha stimulating activity polypeptide 1-endothelin 3 (GNAS-EDN3), methylenetetrahydrofolate reductase-natriuretic peptide B (MTHFR-NPPB), calcium channel voltage dependent beta 2 subunit (CACNB2), chromosome 10 open reading frame 107 (C10orf107), cytochrome P450 family 1 subfamily A polypeptide-unc 51 like kinase 3 (CYP1A1-ULK3)* and *ATP2B1*, respectively (Table 4). Of which, several genes of interest will be discussed in the subsequent paragraphs.

Natriuretic peptides encompass atrial natriuretic peptide (ANP), brain-natriuretic peptide (BNP) and C-type natriuretic peptide (CNP), which are associated with hypertension risk. CNP mediates intracellular electrolyte volume via RAS and sodium homeostasis, is removed by NPR3 via sequential internalization and degradation processes (Pereira et al. 2013). The rate of CNP removal is decreased in the presence of *NPR3* rs1173771 polymorphism, that has been revealed as the protective factor in Algerian patients with hypertension (Lardjam-Hetraf et al. 2015) as well as associated with orthostatic hypotension (Fedorowski et al. 2012). Meanwhile, the production of ANP and BNP are stimulated by mechanical stretching on atrial wall, and further enhanced in the presence of rs17367504 polymorphism (Song et al. 2015). The rs17367504 polymorphism that mapped to *MTHFR-NPPB* locus has been associated with 24 h DBP and SBP (Tomaszewski et al. 2010), and increased risk of orthostatic hypertension by 1.13-folds (95 % CI 1.02–1.24, p = 0.02) (Fedorowski et al. 2012).

Furthermore, a link between ANP, BNP, innate immune response and rs805303 polymorphism has been proposed to be associated with the risk of hypertension (Hong et al. 2013). Likewise, the excessive consumption of deoxycorticosterone acetate and salt as well as the progressive iron overloading may cause hepatic antioxidant-oxidant imbalance that subsequently lead to oxidative stress (Kremastinos and Farmakis 2011; Trott and Harrison 2014). In fact, *HFE* rs1799945 polymorphism is one of the culprit for the intracellular iron accumulation and oxidative stress event (Ludwiczek et al. 2007; Kremastinos and Farmakis 2011). The oxidative stress event is deteriorated with the accumulation of inositol 1,4,5-triphosphate and particularly in the presence of *PLCE1* rs932764 polymorphism (Zhang and Huang 2012). Additionally, this polymorphism promotes the hydrolysis of phosphatidylinositol-4,5-bisphosphate to diacylglycerol and inositol 1,4,5-triphosphate (Zhang and Huang 2012). Mass production of vascular inositol 1,4,5-triphosphate stimulates the release of calcium ions and leads to vascular resistance towards blood flow and thus contributes to hypertension risk (Abou-Saleh et al. 2013).

Released calcium ions are modulated by calcium channels, during the transportation of calcium ions into cells (Nie et al. 2010). Calcium channel families encompass α_1, α_2, β, δ and γ subunits. For instance, *CACNB2* that encodes an $\beta2$-regulatory subunit is targeting on $\alpha1$ cell surface expression in the regulation of calcium channels activities (Nie et al. 2010). During anti-hypertensive treatment, calcium channel blockers (antihypertensive drugs) bound on α_1 subunits to block calcium ion from flowing through the channel, by which *CACNB2* genetic polymorphisms may exert different antihypertensive effects (Nie et al. 2010). INternational VErapamil SR-Trandolapril STudy GENEtic Substudy (INVEST-GENES) suggested that hypertensive individuals with *CACNB2* rs2357928 GG genotype may predict a better response to β-blocker compared, as compared with calcium channel blocker (Nie et al. 2010).

Moreover, among ICBP GWAS identified SNPs, it has been confirmed that *zinc finger protein 831 (ZNF831)* rs6015450 was significantly increased the risk of hypertension by 1.29-folds (95 % confident interval (CI) 1.09–1.53, p = 0.003), even though this SNP did not attained genome wide association threshold of 5×10^{-8} (Juhola et al. 2012). It is hypothesized that rs6015450 would be more precise if it is mapped to 5′ end upstream of *ZNF831* gene, as Juhola et al. (2012) also agreed that rs6015450 is mapped to *ZNF831* instead of GNAS-*EDN3*.

5 Conclusion

In overall, we concluded that candidate gene polymorphisms involved in renin-angiotensin-aldosterone system, vasomotor system, lipid metabolism, sodium regulating system; and sympathetic nervous system may play a role in the development of hypertension. Furthermore, SNPs discovered in GWAS that mapped on *ATP2B1*, *NPR3* and *PLCE1* genes may influence the susceptibility risk of hypertension. Therefore, it is pertinent to highlight that SNPs in the genes related to dysregulation of calcium/sodium homeostasis and calcium/sodium transport as well as activation of immune response and oxidative stress are associated with the pathophysiological process of hypertension.

Acknowledgement We acknowledge the financial support from a Fundamental Research Grant Scheme (FRGS/1/2015/SKK08/UTAR/02/3).

References

Abou-Saleh H, Pathan AR, Daalis A, Hubrack S, Abou-Jassoum H, Al-Naeimi H et al (2013) Inositol 1, 4, 5-trisphosphate (IP3) receptor up-regulation in hypertension is associated with sensitization of Ca^{2+} release and vascular smooth muscle contractility. J Biol Chem 288(46):32941–32951

Adeyemo A, Gerry N, Chen G, Herbert A, Doumatey A, Huang H et al (2009) A genome-wide association study of hypertension and blood pressure in African Americans. PLoS Genet 5(7):e1000564–e1000575

Alfakih K, Maqbool A, Sivananthan M, Walters K, Bainbridge G, Ridgway J et al (2004) Left ventricle mass index and the common, functional, X-linked angiotensin II type-2 receptor gene polymorphism (−1332 G/A) in patients with systemic hypertension. Hypertension 43(6):1189–1194

Annapareddy SNR, Kumbakonam VS, Elumalai R, Ramanathan G, Periyasamy S, Lakkakula BVKS (2016) ECE1 gene variant shows tendency toward chronic kidney disease advancement among autosomal polycystic kidney disease patients. Hong Kong J Nephrol 18:20–25

Atlas SA (2007) The renin-angiotensin aldosterone system: pathophysiological role and pharmacologic inhibition. J Manag Care Pharm 13(8 Supp B):9–20

Au A, Griffiths LR, Cheng K-K, Kooi CW, Irene L, Wei LK (2015) The influence of OLR1 and PCSK9 gene polymorphisms on ischemic stroke: evidence from a meta-analysis. Sci Rep 5:18224. doi:10.1038/srep18224

Brini M, Carafoli E (2011) The plasma membrane Ca^{2+} ATPase and the plasma membrane sodium calcium exchanger cooperate in the regulation of cell calcium. Cold Spring Harb Perspect Biol 3(2):a004168–a004185

Burton PR, Clayton DG, Cardon LR, Craddock N, Deloukas P, Duncanson A et al (2007) Genome-wide association study of 14,000 cases of seven common diseases and 3,000 shared controls. Nature 447 (7145):661–678

Bush WS, Moore JH (2012) Genome-wide association studies. PLoS Comput Biol 8(12):e1002822–e1002833

Caprioli J, Mele C, Mossali C, Gallizioli L, Giacchetti G, Noris M et al (2008) Polymorphisms of EDNRB, ATG, and ACE genes in salt-sensitive hypertension. Can J Physiol Pharmacol 86(8):505–510

Carstens N, van der Merwe L, Revera M, Heradien M, Goosen A, Brink PA et al (2010) Genetic variation in angiotensin II type 2 receptor gene influences extent of left ventricular hypertrophy in hypertrophic cardiomyopathy independent of blood pressure. J Renin Angiotensin Aldosterone Syst 12(3):274–280

Cat AND, Montezano AC, Touyz RM (2013) Renin–angiotensin–aldosterone system: new concepts. Hypertension 84–100

Chang Y-PC, Liu X, Kim JDO, Ikeda MA, Layton MR, Weder AB et al (2007) Multiple genes for essential-hypertension susceptibility on chromosome 1q. Am J Hum Genet 80(2):253–264

Chobanian AV, Bakris GL, Black HR, Cushman WC, Green LA, Izzo JL et al. (2003) The seventh report of the Joint National Committee on Prevention, Detection, Evaluation, and Treatment of High Blood Pressure (JNC 7). JAMA 289(19):2560–2571.

Das B, Pawar N, Saini D, Seshadri M (2009) Genetic association study of selected candidate genes (ApoB, LPL, Leptin) and telomere length in obese and hypertensive individuals. BMC Med Genet 10(1):99–112

Dhawan V, Sharma I, Mahajan N, Sangwan SM, Jain S (2014) Implication of endothelin-2 and oxidative stress biomarkers in essential hypertension. J Hypertens 3(170):1095–2167

Dimke H, San-Cristobal P, de Graaf M, Lenders JW, Deinum J, Hoenderop JGJ et al (2011) γ-Adducin stimulates the thiazide-sensitive NaCl cotransporter. J Am Soc Nephrol 22(3):508–517

Ehret GB (2010) Genome-wide association studies: contribution of genomics to understanding blood pressure and essential hypertension. Curr Hypertens Rep 12 (1):17–25

Fang YJ, Deng HB, Thomas GN, Tzang CH, Li CX, Xu ZL et al (2010) Linkage of angiotensinogen gene polymorphisms with hypertension in a sibling study of Hong Kong Chinese. J Hypertens 28(6):1203–1209

Faruque MU, Chen G, Doumatey A, Huang H, Zhou J, Dunston GM et al (2011) Association of ATP1B1, RGS5 and SELE polymorphisms with hypertension and blood pressure in African-Americans. J Hypertens 29(10):1906–1912

Fava C, Von Wowern F, Berglund G, Carlson J, Hedblad B, Rosberg L et al (2006) 24-h ambulatory blood pressure is linked to chromosome 18q21-22 and genetic variation of NEDD4L associates with cross-sectional and longitudinal blood pressure in Swedes. Kidney Int 70(3):562–569

Fayyad HAR, Aziz IH (2015) Genetic polymorphism of angiotensinogen gene in high blood pressure. World J Pharm Pharm Sci 4(10):1910–1917

Fedorowski A, Franceschini N, Brody J, Liu C, Verwoert GC, Boerwinkle E et al (2012) Orthostatic hypotension and novel blood pressure-associated gene variants: genetics of Postural Hemodynamics (GPH) Consortium. Eur Heart J 33(18):2331–2341

Förstermann U, Münzel T (2006) Endothelial nitric oxide synthase in vascular disease: from marvel to menace. Circulation 113(13):1708–1714

Fox ER, Young JH, Li Y, Dreisbach AW, Keating BJ, Musani SK et al (2011) Association of genetic variation with systolic and diastolic blood pressure among African Americans: the Candidate Gene Association Resource study. Hum Mol Genet 20(11):2273–2284

Fujita T (2014) Mechanism of salt-sensitive hypertension: focus on adrenal and sympathetic nervous systems. J Am Soc Nephrol 25(6):1148–1155

Galati F, Galati A, Massari S (2016) RyR2 QQ2958 genotype and risk of malignant ventricular arrhythmias. Cardiol Res Pract 2016, Available from: http://dx.doi.org/10.1155/2016/2868604

Ghattas M, Badawy H, Mesbah N, Abo-Elmatty D (2013) Apolipoprotein CIII3238C/G gene polymorphism influences oxidized low-density lipoprotein with a risk of essential hypertension. J Biochem Pharmacol Res 1(3):143–147

Gibson G (2012) Rare and common variants: twenty arguments. Nat Rev Genet 13(2):135–145

Harrison-Bernard LM (2009) The renal renin-angiotensin system. Adv Physiol Educ 33(4):270–274

Higashi Y, Sukhanov S, Anwar A, Shai S-Y, Delafontaine P (2012) Aging, atherosclerosis, and IGF-1. J Gerontol A Biol Sci Med Sci 67(6):626–639

Hong GL, Chen XZ, Liu Y, Liu YH, Fu X, Lin SB et al (2013) Genetic variations in MOV10 and CACNB2 are associated with hypertension in a Chinese Han population. Genet Mol Res 12(4):6220–6227

Horio T, Kamide K, Takiuchi S, Yoshii M, Miwa Y, Matayoshi T et al (2010) Association of insulin-like growth factor-1 receptor gene polymorphisms with left ventricular mass and geometry in essential hypertension. J Hum Hypertens 24(5):320–326

Huber M, Völler H, Jakob S, Reibis R, Do V, Bolbrinker J et al (2010) Role of the angiotensin II type 2 receptor gene (+1675G/A) polymorphism on left ventricular hypertrophy and geometry in treated hypertensive patients. J Hypertens 28(6):1221–1229

Iglarz M, Benessiano J, Philip I, Vuillaumier-Barrot S, Lasocki S, Hvass U et al (2002) Preproendothelin-1 gene polymorphism is related to a change in vascular reactivity in the human mammary artery in vitro. Hypertension 39(2):209–213

International Consortium for Blood Pressure Genome-Wide Association Studies (2011) Genetic variants in novel pathways influence blood pressure and cardiovascular disease risk. Nature 478(7367):103–109

Iwai N, Baba S, Mannami T, Katsuya T, Higaki J, Ogihara T et al (2001) Association of sodium channel γ-subunit promoter variant with blood pressure. Hypertension 38(1):86–89

Iwai N, Baba S, Mannami T, Ogihara T, Ogata J (2002) Association of a sodium channel α subunit promoter variant with blood pressure. J Am Soc Nephrol 13 (1):80–85

Jin HS, Hong KW, Lim JE, Oh B (2011) Replication of an African-American GWAS on blood pressure and hypertension in the Korean population. Genes Genomics 33(2):127–132

Johnson T, Gaunt TR, Newhouse SJ, Padmanabhan S, Tomaszewski M, Kumari M et al (2011a) Blood pressure loci identified with a gene-centric array. Am J Hum Genet 89(6):688–700

Johnson AD, Newton-Cheh C, Chasman DI, Ehret GB, Johnson T, Rose L et al (2011b) Association of hypertension drug target genes with blood pressure and hypertension in 86588 individuals. Hypertension 57 (5):903–910

Juhola J, Oikonen M, Magnussen CG, Mikkilä V, Siitonen N, Jokinen E et al (2012) Childhood physical, environmental and genetic predictors of adult hypertension: the cardiovascular risk in young Finns study. Circulation 126(4):402–409

Kato N, Miyata T, Tabara Y, Katsuya T, Yanai K, Hanada H et al (2008) High-density association study and nomination of susceptibility genes for hypertension in the Japanese National Project. Hum Mol Genet 17 (4):617–627

Kato N, Takeuchi F, Tabara Y, Kelly TN, Go MJ, Sim X et al (2011) Meta-analysis of genome-wide association studies identifies common variants associated with blood pressure variation in east Asians. Nat Genet 43(6):531–538

Keszei AP, Tisler A, Backx PH, Andrulis IL, Bull SB, Logan AG (2007) Molecular variants of the thiazide-sensitive Na+−Cl- cotransporter in hypertensive families. J Hypertens 25(10):2074–2081

Kidambi S, Ghosh S, Kotchen JM, Grim CE, Krishnaswami S, Kaldunski ML et al (2012) Non-replication study of a genome-wide association study for hypertension and blood pressure in African Americans. BMC Med Genet 13(1):27–35

Kim JY, Park JB, Kim DS, Kim KS, Jeong JW, Park JC et al (2014) Gender difference in arterial stiffness in a multicenter cross-sectional study: the Korean Arterial Aging Study (KAAS). Pulse 2(1-4):11–17

Kremastinos DT, Farmakis D (2011) Iron overload cardiomyopathy in clinical practice. Circulation 124 (20):2253–2263

Kuo M-L, Lee MB-E, Tang M, den Besten W, Hu S, Sweredoski MJ et al (2016) PYCR1 and PYCR2 interact and collaborate with RRM2B to protect cells from overt oxidative stress. Sci Rep 6:18846. doi:10.1038/srep18846

Lacolley P, Challande P, Osborne-Pellegrin M, Regnault V (2009) Genetics and pathophysiology of arterial stiffness. Cardiovasc Res 81(4):637–648

Lajemi M, Labat C, Gautier S, Lacolley P, Safar M, Asmar R et al (2001) Angiotensin II type 1 receptor − 153A/G and 1166A/C gene polymorphisms and increase in aortic stiffness with age in hypertensive subjects. J Hypertens 19(3):407–413

Lardjam-Hetraf SA, Mediene-Benchekor S, Ouhaibi-Djellouli H, Meroufel DN, Boulenouar H, Hermant X et al (2015) Effects of established blood pressure loci on blood pressure values and hypertension risk in an Algerian population sample. J Hum Hypertens 29 (5):296–302

Levy D, Ehret GB, Rice K, Verwoert GC, Launer LJ, Dehghan A et al (2009) Genome-wide association study of blood pressure and hypertension. Nat Genet 41(6):677–687

Ling L, Maguire JJ, Davenport AP (2013) Endothelin-2, the forgotten isoform: emerging role in the cardiovascular system, ovarian development, immunology and cancer. Br J Pharmacol 168(2):283–295

Ljungberg LU, De Basso R, Alehagen U, Björck HM, Persson K, Dahlström U et al (2011) Impaired abdominal aortic wall integrity in elderly men carrying the angiotensin-converting enzyme D allele. Eur J Vasc Endovasc Surg 42(3):309–316

Ludwiczek S, Theurl I, Muckenthaler MU, Jakab M, Mair SM, Theurl M et al (2007) Ca^{2+} channel blockers reverse iron overload by a new mechanism via divalent metal transporter-1. Nat Med 13(4):448–454

Luo F, Wang Y, Wang X, Sun K, Zhou X, Hui R (2009) A functional variant of NEDD4L is associated with hypertension, antihypertensive response, and orthostatic hypotension. Hypertension 54(4):796–801

Manning J, Beutler K, Knepper MA, Vehaskari VM (2002) Upregulation of renal BSC1 and TSC in prenatally programmed hypertension. Am J Physiol Renal Physiol 283(1):F202–F206

Matsubara M, Sato T, Nishimura T, Suzuki M, Kikuya M, Metoki H et al (2004) CYP11B2 polymorphisms and home blood pressure in a population-based cohort in Japanese: the Ohasama study. Hypertens Res 27 (1):1–6

Mishra A, Srivastava A, Mittal T, Garg N, Mittal B (2012) Impact of renin-angiotensin-aldosterone system gene polymorphisms on left ventricular dysfunction in coronary artery disease patients. Dis Markers 32(1):33–41.

Miyaki K, Htun NC, Song Y, Ikeda S, Muramatsu M, Shimbo T (2012) The combined impact of 12 common variants on hypertension in Japanese men, considering GWAS results. J Hum Hypertens 26(7):430–436

Mozaffarian D, Benjamin EJ, Go AS, Arnett DK, Blaha MJ, Cushman M et al (2016) Heart disease and stroke statistics-2016 update a report from the American Heart Association. Circulation 133:e38–e360

Muñoz-Barrios S, Guzmán-Guzmán IP, Muñoz-Valle JF, Salgado-Bernabé AB, Salgado-Goytia L, Parra-Rojas I (2012) Association of the HindIII and S447X polymorphisms in LPL gene with hypertension and type 2 diabetes in Mexican families. Dis Markers 33 (6):313–320

Newhouse SJ, Wallace C, Dobson R, Mein C, Pembroke J, Farrall M et al (2005) Haplotypes of the WNK1 gene associate with blood pressure variation in a severely hypertensive population from the British Genetics of Hypertension study. Hum Mol Genet 14 (13):1805–1814

Newton-Cheh C, Johnson T, Gateva V, Tobin MD, Bochud M, Coin L et al (2009) Genome-wide association study identifies eight loci associated with blood pressure. Nat Genet 41(6):666–676

Nie SJ, Wen-Ru T, Bi-Feng C, Jin L, Wen Z, Sheng-Jun L et al (2010) Haplotype-based case-control study of the human AGTR1 gene and essential hypertension in Han Chinese subjects. Clin Biochem 43(3):253–258

Org E, Eyheramendy S, Juhanson P, Gieger C, Lichtner P, Klopp N et al (2009) Genome-wide scan identifies CDH13 as a novel susceptibility locus contributing to blood pressure determination in two European populations. Hum Mol Genet 18(12):2288–2296

Padmanabhan S, Melander O, Johnson T, Di Blasio AM, Lee WK, Gentilini D et al (2010) Genome-wide association study of blood pressure extremes identifies variant near UMOD associated with hypertension. PLoS Genet 6(10):e1001177–e1001188

Panoulas VF, Douglas KMJ, Smith JP, Taffé P, Stavropoulos-Kalinoglou A, Toms TE et al (2008) Polymorphisms of the endothelin-1 gene associate with hypertension in patients with rheumatoid arthritis. Endothelium 15(4):203–212

Paternoster L, González NAM, Lewis S, Sudlow C (2008) Association between apolipoprotein E genotype and carotid intima-media thickness may suggest a specific effect on large artery atherothrombotic stroke. Stroke 39(1):48–54

Patkar S, Charita BH, Ramesh C, Padma T (2009) High risk of essential hypertension in males with intron 4 VNTR polymorphism of eNOS gene. Indian J Hum Genet 15(2):49–53

Penesova A, Cizmarova E, Kvetnansky R, Koska J, Sedlakova B, Krizanova O (2006) Insertion/deletion polymorphism on ACE gene is associated with endothelial dysfunction in young patients with hypertension. Horm Metab Res 38(9):592–597.

Pereira NL, Lin D, Pelleymounter L, Moon I, Stilling G, Eckloff BW et al (2013) Natriuretic peptide receptor-3 gene (NPR3) nonsynonymous polymorphism results in significant reduction in protein expression because

of accelerated degradation. Circ Cardiovasc Genet 6 (2):201–210

Rahman T, Baker M, Hall DH, Avery PJ, Keavney B (2008) Common genetic variation in the type A endothelin-1 receptor is associated with ambulatory blood pressure: a family study. J Hum Hypertens 22 (4):282–288

Rossi A, Baldo-Enzi G, Ganzaroli C, Coscetti G, Calabrò A, Baiocchi MR et al (2001) Relationship of early carotid artery disease with lipoprotein (a), apolipoprotein B, and fibrinogen in asymptomatic essential hypertensive patients and normotensive subjects. J Investig Med 49(6):505–513

Russo CJ, Melista E, Cui J, DeStefano AL, Bakris GL, Manolis AJ et al (2005) Association of NEDD4L ubiquitin ligase with essential hypertension. Hypertension 46(3):488–491

Salah A, Khan M, Esmail N, Habibullah S, Al LY (2009) Genetic polymorphism of S447X lipoprotein lipase (LPL) and the susceptibility to hypertension. J Crit Care 24(3):e11–e14

Seidlerová J, Staessen JA, Bochud M, Nawrot T, Casamassima N, Citterio L et al (2009) Arterial properties in relation to genetic variations in the adducin subunits in a white population. Am J Hypertens 22(1):21–26

Sethi AA, Nordestgaard BG, Tybjærg-Hansen A (2003) Angiotensinogen gene polymorphism, plasma angiotensinogen, and risk of hypertension and ischemic heart disease a meta-analysis. Arterioscler Thromb Vasc Biol 23(7):1269–1275

Shimamoto K, Ando K, Fujita T, Hasebe N, Higaki J, Horiuchi M et al (2014) The Japanese Society of Hypertension guidelines for the management of hypertension. Hypertens Res 37:253–392

Snyder EM, Johnson BD, Joyner MJ (2008) Genetics of β2-adrenergic receptors and the cardiopulmonary response to exercise. Exerc Sport Sci Rev 36 (2):98–105

Song W, Wang H, Wu Q (2015) Atrial natriuretic peptide in cardiovascular biology and disease (NPPA). Gene 569(1):1–6

Soualmia H (2012) Candidate genes in hypertension. In: Khullar M (ed) Genetics and pathophysiology of essential hypertension, 1st edn. InTech, Rijeka, pp 139–168

Soudani NY, Fakhoury RM, Kaissi SS, Zgheib NK (2014) The role of genetic polymorphisms in endothelial nitric oxide synthase and beta2-adrenergic receptors with risk of hypertension in a sample of Lebanese people. Saudi Med J 35(3):255–260

Sun B, Williams JS, Pojoga L, Chamarthi B, Lasky-Su J, Raby BA et al (2011) Renin gene polymorphism: its relationship to hypertension, renin levels and vascular responses. J Renin Angiotensin Aldosterone Syst 12 (4):564–571

Tabara Y, Kohara K, Kita Y, Hirawa N, Katsuya T, Ohkubo T et al (2010) Common Variants in the ATP2B1 Gene Are Associated With Susceptibility to

Hypertension The Japanese Millennium Genome Project. Hypertension 56(5):973–980

Takeuchi F, Isono M, Katsuya T, Yamamoto K, Yokota M, Sugiyama T et al (2010) Blood pressure and hypertension are associated with 7 loci in the Japanese population. Circulation 121(21):2302–2309

Tang W, Yang Y, Wang B, Xiao C (2008a) Association between a G894T polymorphism of eNOS gene and essential hypertension in Hani and Yi minority groups of China. Arch Med Res 39(2):222–225

Tang M, Dai Y, Huang Y, Cai X, Tian X, Tu Z (2008b) The univariation and multiple linear regression analyses for seventeen SNPs in thirteen cardiovascular disease-predisposing genes and blood pressure in Chinese Han males. Clin Exp Hypertens 30(7):648–661

Tikhonoff V, Kuznetsova T, Stolarz K, Bianchi G, Casiglia E, Kawecka-Jaszcz K et al (2003) Blood pressure phenotypes in relation to the β-adducin C1797T polymorphism in the European Project on Genes in Hypertension (EPOGH). Blood Press Monit 8(4):151–154

Tomaszewski M, Debiec R, Braund PS, Nelson CP, Hardwick R, Christofidou P et al (2010) Genetic architecture of ambulatory blood pressure in the general population insights from cardiovascular gene-centric array. Hypertension 56(6):1069–1076

Trott DW, Harrison DG (2014) The immune system in hypertension. Adv Physiol Educ 38(1):20–24

Valdenaire O, Lepailleur-Enouf D, Egidy G, Thouard A, Barret A, Vranckx R et al (1999) A fourth isoform of endothelin-converting enzyme (ECE-1) is generated from an additional promoter. Eur J Biochem 264 (2):341–349

Vangjeli C, Clarke N, Quinn U, Dicker P, Tighe O, Ho C et al (2010) Confirmation that the renin gene distal enhancer polymorphism REN-5312C/T is associated with increased blood pressure. Circ Cardiovasc Genet 3(1):53–59

Wang Y, O'Connell JR, McArdle PF, Wade JB, Dorff SE, Shah SJ et al (2009) Whole-genome association study identifies STK39 as a hypertension susceptibility gene. Proc Natl Acad Sci 106(1):226–231

Wei LK, Menon S, Griffiths LR, Gan SH (2015a) Signaling pathway genes for blood pressure, folate and cholesterol levels among hypertensives: an epistasis analysis. J Hum Hypertens 29(2):99–104

Wei LK, Au A, Menon S, Gan SH, Griffiths LR (2015b) Clinical Relevance of MTHFR, eNOS, ACE, and ApoE Gene Polymorphisms and Serum Vitamin Profile among Malay Patients with Ischemic Stroke. J Stroke Cerebrovasc 9:2017–2025

Xi B, Tang W, Wang Q (2012) Polymorphism near the ATP2B1 gene is associated with hypertension risk in East Asians: a meta-analysis involving 15909 cases and 18529 controls. Blood Press 21(2):134–138

Xi B, Shen Y, Zhao X, Chandak GR, Cheng H, Hou D et al (2014) Association of common variants in/near six genes (ATP2B1, CSK, MTHFR, CYP17A1, STK39 and FGF5) with blood pressure/hypertension risk in Chinese children. J Hun Hypertens 28(1):32–36

Xiao B, Zhang Y, Niu W, Gao P, Zhu D (2009) Association of ATP1B1 single-nucleotide polymorphisms with blood pressure and hypertension in a Chinese population. Clin Chim Acta 407(1):47–50

Yang H-C, Liang Y-J, Wu Y-L, Chung C-M, Chiang K-M, Ho H-Y et al (2009) Genome-wide association study of young-onset hypertension in the Han Chinese population of Taiwan. PLoS ONE 4(5):e5459–e5470

Yang X, He J, Gu D, Hixson JE, Huang J, Rao DC et al (2014) Associations of epithelial sodium channel genes with blood pressure changes and hypertension incidence: the GenSalt study. Am J Hypertens 27 (11):1370–1376

Yan-yan L (2011) Endothelial nitric oxide synthase G894T gene polymorphism and essential hypertension in the Chinese population: a meta-analysis involving 11,248 subjects. Intern Med 50(19):2099–2106

Zafarmand MH, van der Schouw YT, Grobbee DE, de Leeuw PW, Bots ML (2008) α-adducin Gly460Trp variant increases the risk of stroke in hypertensive Dutch women. Hypertension 51(6):1665–1670

Zhang A, Huang S (2012) Progress in pathogenesis of proteinuria. Int J Nephrol 2012, Available from: http://dx.doi.org/10.1155/2012/314251

Adv Exp Med Biol - Advances in Internal Medicine (2017) 2: 583–598
DOI 10.1007/5584_2016_80
© Springer International Publishing AG 2016
Published online: 26 November 2016

The Role of DNA Methylation in Hypertension

Masashi Demura and Kiyofumi Saijoh

Abstract

DNA methylation is the covalent modification of DNA that affects its function, without altering DNA sequences. Three important roles of DNA methylation include intrauterine programming, acquired predisposition, and transgenerational inheritance. A wide variety of factors can affect DNA methylation. Intrauterine programming involves drastic changes in DNA methylation patterns during cellular development and differentiation, which have a long-lasting effect on the predisposition of offspring. Influences from the mother, including maternal nutritional status, modify intrauterine epigenetic programming. In contrast to the rapid and drastic changes in utero, postnatal factors in daily life can also continue to slowly and dynamically change DNA methylation patterns in both somatic and germ cells. Epigenetic changes occurring in germ cell DNA exert a transgenerational impact on the phenotype of future generations, thus providing a means for ancestral transmission of environmental experiences. Despite adaptive ability, mismatch effect of transgenerational inheritance could be potentially harmful to health if environment has changed, and the acquired acclimatization is no longer beneficial. Increasing evidence from both human and animal studies indicates that DNA methylation exerts a causal impact on the development of hypertension. Therefore, an adverse outcome of maternal malnutrition could be the development of hypertension in offspring, whereby nutritional factors or disease conditions could induce phenotypes susceptible to hypertension through alteration of DNA methylation patterns. These factors are likely to alter DNA methylation patterns in all tissues including germ cells, and despite no direct evidence of an association

M. Demura (✉) and K. Saijoh
Department of Hygiene, Graduate School of Medical
Science, Kanazawa University, Kanazawa 920-8640,
Japan
e-mail: m-demura@med.kanazawa-u.ac.jp

between transgenerational epigenetic inheritance and hypertension, it is likely to play a role.

Keywords

Intrauterine programming • Epigenetics • Gene transcription • Epigenetic inheritence • Epigenetic biomarkers • Histone acetylation

1 Introduction

Hypertension is a chronic disease condition, of which approximately 90 % of cases are classified as essential hypertension without a definitive cause. Multifactorial mechanisms are involved in the development of hypertension. Dynamic interaction between genetic and environmental factors is thought to cause an increase in blood pressure (Beilin 1990). The underlying pathogenetic basis of hypertension development is of crucial importance for the development of preventive and therapeutic strategies. Family history of essential hypertension is a well-known major risk factor for hypertension development and, implies possible underlying genetic mechanisms for blood pressure regulation.

While several studies have successfully identified hypertension susceptibility genes (Adeyemo et al. 2009; Levy et al. 2009; Newton-Cheh et al. 2009; Hong et al. 2010; Padmanabhan et al. 2010; International Consortium for Blood Pressure Genome-Wide Association et al. 2011; Kato et al. 2011, 2015; Wain et al. 2011; Franceschini et al. 2013; Ganesh et al. 2013), such studies have clearly shown that gene polymorphism only partially contributes to the pathogenesis of hypertension. More surprisingly, whole-genome sequencing has revealed that many people carry disease-causing genetic mutations without disease symptoms (MacArthur and Tyler-Smith 2010; MacArthur et al. 2012; Dewey et al. 2014). This indicates that unidentified heritable factors, rather than genetic factors, play a role in the expression of the disease state. These observations can be explained by epigenetic mechanisms that, despite their heritability, are

potentially modifiable through environmental factors. Epigenetics refers to phenomena that are involved in regulating gene expression without changing the DNA sequence. Epigenetic modifications include DNA methylation, histone modification, and non-coding RNA (ncRNA). There is a growing body of evidence showing the role of several epigenetic mechanisms in a wide variety of human diseases (Marchal and Miotto 2015; Bohacek and Mansuy 2015; Szyf 2015).

It has been hypothesized that once established, DNA methylation patterns are stably maintained. However, a growing body of evidence has revealed that DNA methylation patterns dynamically responded to various environmental stimuli. Environmental factors influencing DNA methylation patterns include chemicals (Arai et al. 2011), infection (Nakajima et al. 2009; Maekita et al. 2006; Li et al. 2004), smoking (Oka et al. 2009; Zhang et al. 2014), exercise (Ronn et al. 2013; Denham et al. 2015), learning (Miller and Sweatt 2007; Miller et al. 2010) and climate (Bind et al. 2014). Other conditions, diseased and non-diseased induce changes in DNA methylation patterns in adult human tissues (Wang et al. 2014a; Nilsson et al. 2015; Liu et al. 2015; Ronn et al. 2015). Although epigenetic alterations in blood DNA do not clearly explain the pathogenesis of hypertension, there are a number of studies showing an association between DNA methylation in blood and hypertension. Global DNA methylation is low in blood DNA from hypertensive patients and its level depends on the progression of hypertension (Smolarek et al. 2010). Candidate gene approaches have successfully identified differentially methylated sites in blood DNA (Friso et al. 2008; Zhang et al. 2013; Pizzolo et al. 2015). Hypertension-related changes of DNA methylation in the blood have been found in a genome-wide approach (Kato et al. 2015; Wang et al. 2013). The combination of both genetic and epigenetic factors will exert a profoundly important impact on the hypertensive phenotype.

This chapter focuses on the current evidence, in mammals, that environment and disease-associated factors can influence blood pressure in association with epigenetic modifications, especially DNA methylation. We discuss the nature of the underlying DNA methylation, including how and when DNA methylation can be induced, as well as the molecular mechanisms of DNA methylation induction and maintenance. In addition, we refer limitations in the current understanding of DNA methylation as causal factors for the development of hypertension, and discuss future perspectives for the use of epigenetic knowledge in preventative and therapeutic medicine.

2 DNA Methylation Maintenance

DNA methylation occurs at cytosine residues and is a major epigenetic modification. TET family proteins catalyze the conversion of methylcytosine (5mC) to hydroxymethylcytosine (5hmC). In addition, TET proteins can generate 5-formylcytosine (5fC) from 5hmC, followed by conversion of 5fC to 5-carboxylcytosine (5caC) through oxidation. 5fC and 5caC are specifically recognized and excised by thymine-DNA glycosylase (TDG). Oxidation of 5mC by TET proteins, followed by TDG-mediated base excision repair (TDG/BER) constitutes a pathway for active DNA demethylation (Fig. 1a).

Subsequent induction of methyl group modification by DNA methyltransferases 1, 3A and 3B (DNMT1, DNMT3A and DNMT3B) maintains DNA methylation patterns. DNMT3A and DNMT3B induce de novo DNA methylation whereas DNMT1 primarily methylates the opposite strand of 5mC, maintaining DNA

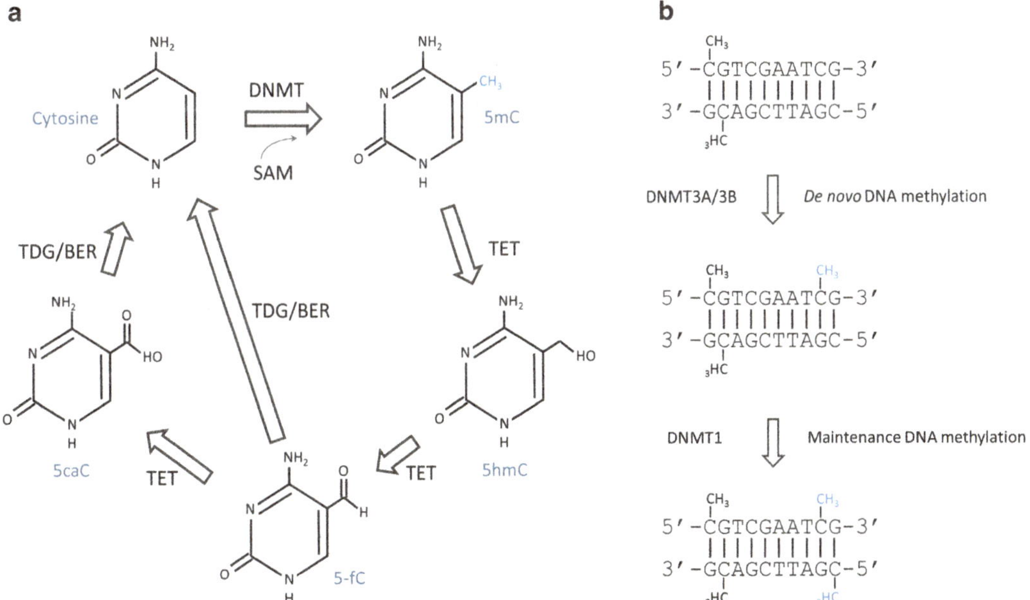

Fig. 1 (a) Dynamic cycle of DNA demethylation and remethylation (*DNMT* DNA methyltransferase, *SAM* S-adenosyl methionine, *5mC* methylcytosine, *5hmC* hydroxymethylcytosine, *5fC* 5-formylcytosine, *5caC* carboxylcytosine, *TET* ten-eleven translocation enzyme, *TDG* thymine-DNA glycosylase, *TDG/BER* TDG-mediated base excision repair) (**b**) DNA methylation by DNMTs

methylation patterns (Fig. 1b). This model of DNA demethylation and remethylation is the most widely accepted, although several other mechanisms of active DNA demethylation and remethylation have been proposed (Chen et al. 2013; Wang et al. 2014b; Thillainadesan et al. 2012a).

3 DNA Methylation and Gene Transcription

DNA methylation at gene promoter sequences is generally associated with transcriptional silencing or decreased gene expression. DNA methylation physically disturbs the locus by preventing transcriptional proteins binding to the promoter, and by interacting with proteins known as methyl-CpG-binding domain proteins (MBDs). MBD proteins attract additional proteins to the locus, including histone deacetylases and other chromatin remodeling proteins. This forms compact, inactive chromatin, termed heterochromatin.

DNA methylation has been shown to play a role in the transcriptional activity of a number of genes involved in blood pressure regulation. The renin-angiotensin-aldosterone system (RAAS) plays a major role in efficient fluid retention, and as such is involved in maintaining blood pressure, and in the pathogenesis of essential hypertension. Components of RAAS including human *AGT* (Wang et al. 2014a), human *ACE* (Riviere et al. 2011), rat *Agtr1b* (Bogdarina et al. 2007) and human *CYP11B2* (Demura et al. 2010) have been shown to be negatively regulated by DNA methylation. Similarly, when CpG island sequences of the human *AGTR1* promoter were cloned into a reporter plasmid its transcriptional activity was dependent upon DNA methylation (unpublished observation). DNA methylation has been demonstrated to decrease the transcriptional activity of *HSD11B2* whose loss of function mutation causes the syndrome of apparent mineralocorticoid excess and hypertension (Alikhani-Koopaei et al. 2004). In spontaneous hypertensive rats, increased expression with low promoter DNA

methylation is observed in *Slc12a2* that maintains ionic balance, thereby regulating blood pressure (Lee et al. 2010).

4 DNA Methylation Dynamics During Intrauterine Programming

After fertilization, the erasure of epigenetic factors (called genomic initialization) progresses until embryo implantation (preimplantation programming). The initialized cells attain the totipotent ability to change into any cell type. In humans, DNA methylation patterns are largely erased in the paternal genome, except in paternally imprinted regions and transposable elements. In contrast, the maternal genome methylation patterns are almost entirely maintained and demethylation occurs to a much lesser extent (Okae et al. 2014). Global DNA demethylation of the mouse maternal genome, however, takes place by passive dilution through DNA replication during initialization (passive DNA demethylation) (Lee et al. 2014).

DNA remethylation on both paternal and maternal genome occurs during human embryonic development, with global DNA methylation level reaching at almost 80 % in the early post-implantation embryos (Guo et al. 2014, 2015). Cell lineage-specific DNA methylation patterns are established through the course of differentiation. Primordial germ cells (PGCs), which can give rise to sperm and oocytes, show a drastic decrease in global DNA methylation to less than 10 % at approximately 10–11 weeks of gestation (Guo et al. 2015). In human somatic tissues a tissue-specific signature exists at 9 weeks gestation, however, further gain or loss of DNA methylation occurs in a substantial number of genomic regions during the first and second trimester, and the DNA methylation patterns in fetal somatic tissues become comparable to those of the corresponding adult tissues. *De novo* DNA methylation is associated with cessation of developmental processes, while DNA demethylation is observed, thereby activating tissue-specific functions (Slieker et al. 2015). DNA sequence-specific-transcription factors regulate both active DNA demethylation and *de novo* DNA methylation during embryonic (Feldmann et al. 2013; Lienert et al. 2011) and fetal (Slieker et al. 2015) development. In contrast to DNA methylation patterns during adulthood, which remain relatively stable, DNA methylation dynamics during intrauterine life are much more dramatic.

Although DNA methylation is extensively erased in human preimplantation embryos and PGCs, the erasure is incomplete (Tang et al. 2015). In addition to changes in DNA methylation related to development and differentiation, DNA can also become hypermethylated or hypomethylated by maternal factors at various genomic loci in human fetal cells during intrauterine life (Drake et al. 2015; Chhabra et al. 2014; Chang et al. 2011; Chen et al. 2014). If changes in DNA methylation patterns occurring by maternal factors are not erased or diluted during intrauterine life, they tend to postnatally persist in somatic and germ cells. Maintained methylation patterns in somatic cells affect phenotype associated with DNA methylation patterns. In other words, the factor influences postnatal constitution. The epigenetic changes in germ cells are maintained and carried forward to the offspring, even in the absence of the initial trigger in a phenomenon known as transgenerational inheritance. The regions that evade global DNA demethylation in the preimplantation embryos and PGCs would potentially represent hotspots of transgenerational epigenetic inheritance (Tang et al. 2015).

5 Postnatal DNA Methylation Dynamics

Various environmental and health factors can induce changes in DNA methylation in both somatic and germ cells throughout postnatal life. Cytosines of CpG dinucleotides are either methylated or unmethylated at the cellular level. DNA methylation patterns in regulatory regions, including promoters and cis-acting elements, exert a profound impact on transcriptional

activity. The number of cells with an unmethylated promoter determines the expression level of the corresponding gene in a given tissue. It therefore follows that tissue DNA methylation patterns are of physiological importance to constitution. Dynamic changes in DNA methylation patterns influence two crucial aspects of constitution (acquired predisposition) and non-Mendelian inheritance (transgenerational epigenetic inheritance) (Fig. 2).

It is important to understand the signals that influence the dynamics of DNA methylation patterns. *In vitro* and *in vivo* studies have shown that active and gradual DNA demethylation (Miller and Sweatt 2007; Miller et al. 2010; Wang et al. 2014a, b; Thomassin et al. 2001; Demura et al. 2015) (Fig. 3a) or *de novo* methylation (Wang et al. 2014b; Ishikawa et al. 2015; Thillainadesan et al. 2012b; Wajapeyee et al. 2013; Serra et al. 2014) (Fig. 3b) following long-term stimulation or suppression occurs around a transcription factor-binding site (TFBS) and a transcription start site (TSS), respectively. Stimulatory signals switch the gene expression phenotype from an inactive to an active state within a tissue, whereas suppressive signals switch the gene expression phenotype from an active to an inactive state (Fig. 4). Therefore, although changes in DNA methylation patterns almost always causes changes in transcriptional activity, they are a consequence rather than a cause.

There are examples of what happens to DNA methylation patterns when transcriptional signals (activation or repression) are removed. *In vitro* studies using cultured hepatocytes showed that glucocorticoid-induced DNA demethylation at a distal enhancer element of the rat *Tat* gene is maintained for at least 3 months following glucocorticoid withdrawal (sustained type of active DNA demethylation) (Thomassin et al. 2001). Conversely, DNA demethylation within the promoters of both *AGT* (Wang et al. 2014a) and *CYP11B2* (Demura et al. 2010) upon stimulation is reversed when the stimuli (interleukin 6 for *AGT*, potassium for *CYP11B2*) are removed (reversed type of active DNA demethylation) (Demura et al. 2015).

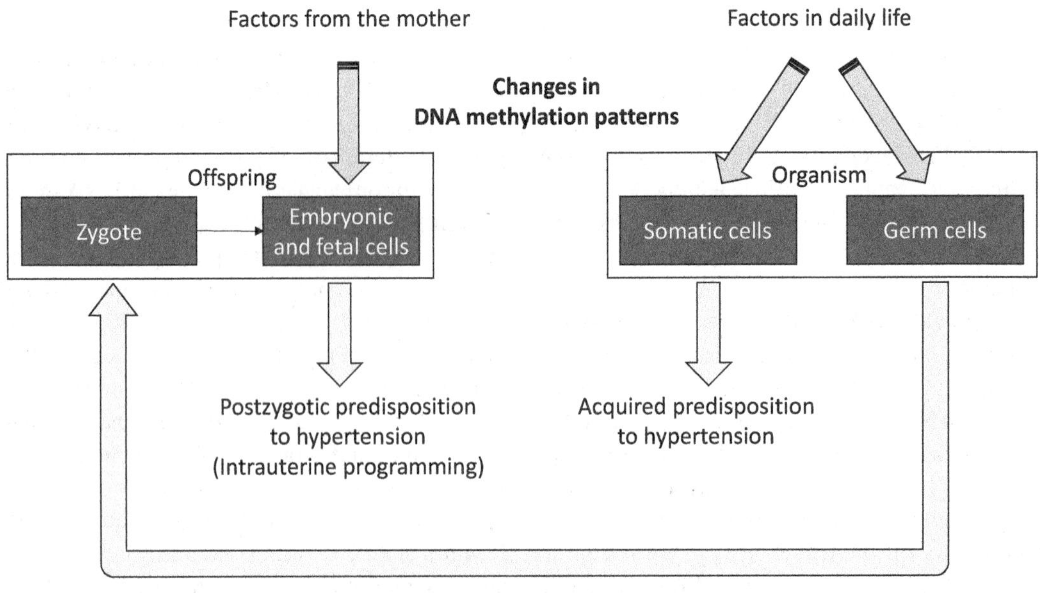

Fig. 2 Proposed model: "DNA methylation changes susceptibility to hypertension"

Miller et al. have elegantly offered valuable insight into the dynamics of DNA methylation patterns and memory formation. Fear conditioning transiently induces low DNA methylation at the *Reln* locus (that promotes memory), and high DNA methylation at the *Ppp1cc* locus (that suppresses memory) in the hippocampus where short memory is formed. These hippocampal changes are reversed 1 day following fear-conditioning removal (Miller and Sweatt 2007). By contrast, fear conditioning induces high DNA methylation, and associated decreased gene expression, in the memory suppressor *Ppp3ca* in the dorsomedial prefrontal cortex where remote memory is stored. This cortical change lasts at least 1 month following fear-conditioning removal (Miller et al. 2010). These examples demonstrate that some factor can evoke gene-targeted and bidirectional changes when and where needed, upregulating some genes with active DNA demethylation, and downregulating others with *de novo* DNA methylation.

Dynamic changes in DNA methylation patterns are typically divided into 4 types* reversed DNA demethylation (Miller and Sweatt

2007; Wang et al. 2014a; Demura et al. 2015) (Fig. 5a), sustained DNA demethylation (Thomassin et al. 2001) (Fig. 5b), reversed DNA methylation (Miller and Sweatt 2007) (Fig. 5c) and sustained DNA methylation patterns (Miller et al. 2010) (Fig. 5d). Sustained patterns of DNA demethylation (Fig. 5b) and methylation (Fig. 5d) are more likely to exert an impact on phenotype through epigenetic phenomena including acquired predisposition, transgenerational epigenetic inheritance and intrauterine programming.

6 Molecular Mechanisms Underlying DNA Methylation Dynamics

Two independent research groups have described that transcriptional activation by estrogen induces cyclical DNA demethylation and remethylation of the promoters and first exons of several estrogen-responsive genes (Metivier et al. 2008; Kangaspeska et al. 2008). During estrogen stimulation, the TDG/BER system demethylates DNA by replacing a methylated cytosine with an unmethylated cytosine. The DNA is then remethylated by DNMTs. The periodic time interval of DNA demethylation and remethylation is approximately 20–40 min. However, long-term stimulation or suppression result in gradual DNA demethylation (Fig. 3a) or *de novo* methylation (Fig. 3b) around a TFBS and a TSS over days or years. The degree of changes in DNA methylation depends on distance from a TFBS or a TSS (Fig. 3). Therefore, the tendency to maintain DNA methylation patterns appear to be due to the competition between TDG/BER system and DNMT enzymes. Additional factors are required to induce gradual changes in DNA methylation patterns in the face of this competition.

A balance between DNA methylation and demethylation activities in the nucleus has a role in the gradual changes in DNA methylation patterns. More importantly, protein complexes responsible for DNA methylation and demethylation activities need to be locally recruited and formed. Recent evidence shows that ncRNAs play a key role in regulating DNA methylation patterns in a locus-specific fashion. Antisense long ncRNA upregulates TCF21 gene expression with low DNA methylation of the promoter. The long ncRNA sequence is complementary to that of the TCF21 promoter, and interacts with both the TCF21 promoter and GADD45A that recruits TET and TDG for base excision and repair (Arab et al. 2014). Another example is that of the DNMT1-interacting long ncRNAs. These

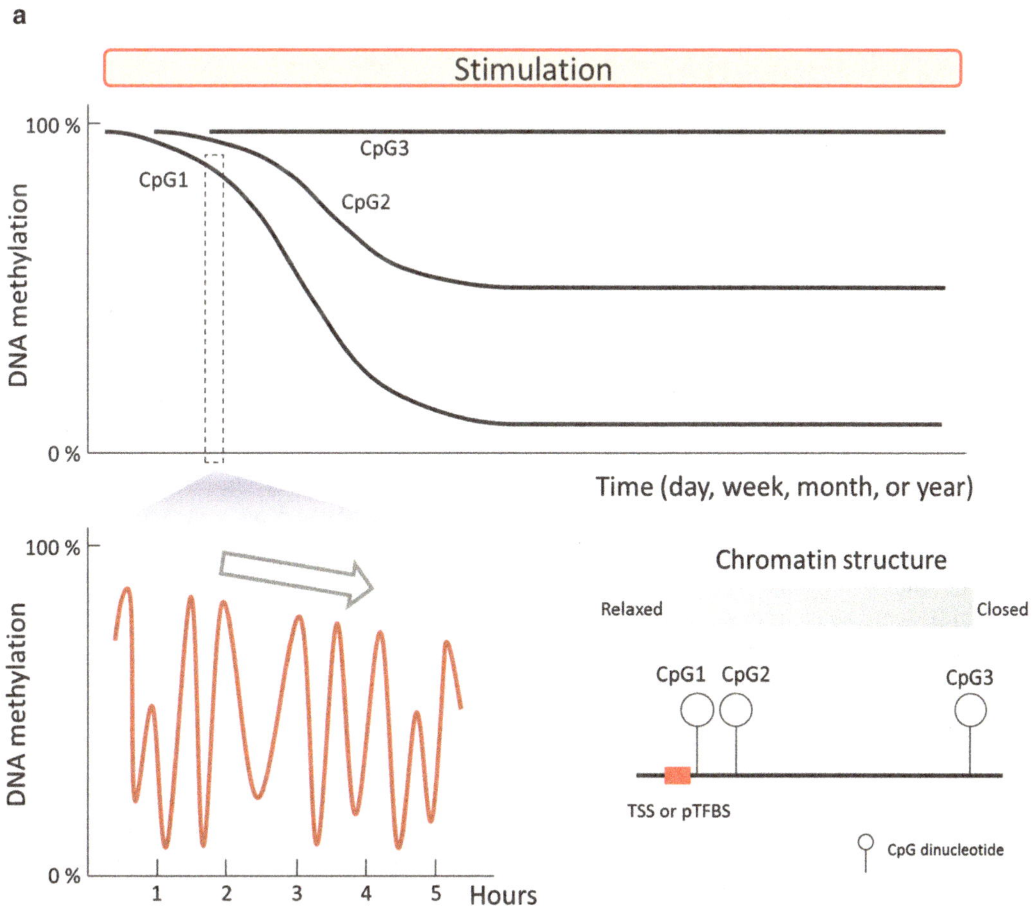

Fig. 3 Schematic representation of dynamic changes in DNA methylation patterns by either stimulation (**a**) or suppression(**b**) (*TSS* transcription start site, *pTFBS* positive transcription factor-binding site, *nTFBS* negative transcription factor-binding site)

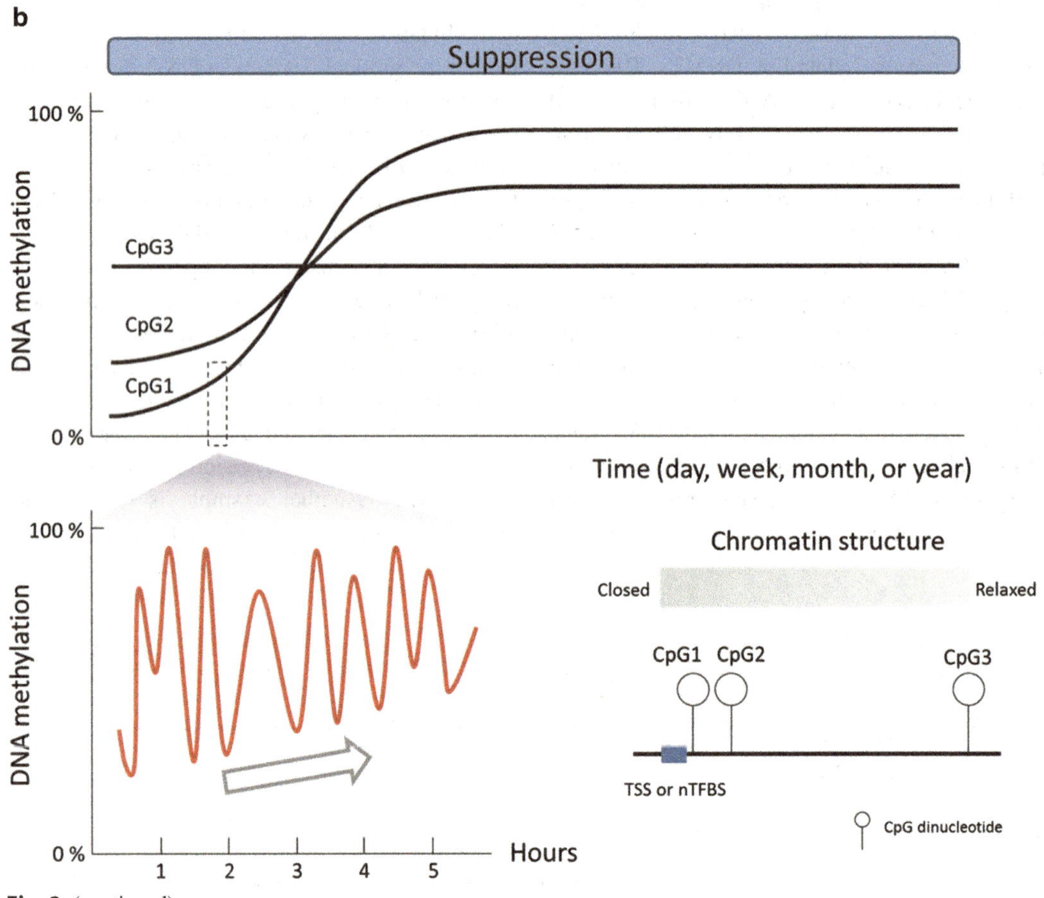

Fig. 3 (continued)

ncRNAs arise from corresponding gene-specific loci and act as a shield, halting DNMT1 and thus preventing DNA methylation at their site of transcription (Di Ruscio et al. 2013).

DNMT1 maintains DNA methylation patterns by methylating the opposite DNA strand of *de novo* hemi-methylated CpG dinucleotides (Fig. 1b). Once double-stranded DNA methylation has been achieved, double-stranded demethylation would be resistant to erasure (James et al. 2003). Blocking gene-specific DNA methylation by DNMT1-interacting long ncRNAs may be required to establish and maintain low DNA methylation after stimulation removal (sustained DNA demethylation, Fig. 5b). Conversely, genomic loci lacking expression of DNMT1-interacting long ncRNAs may maintain high DNA methylation after suppression removal (sustained DNA methylation, Fig. 5d). The presence or absence of DNMT1-interacting long ncRNAs expression may explain four types of gene-specific changes in DNA methylation patterns upon stimulation or suppression.

7 Intrauterine Programming and Hypertension

A maternal diet low in protein increases the susceptibility of offspring to hypertension. The Dutch famine cohort shows that children from mothers with insufficient protein intake, in relation to carbohydrate intake, during the third trimester of pregnancy had higher blood pressure in adulthood (Roseboom et al. 1999, 2001a). In addition, the famine is associated with glucose

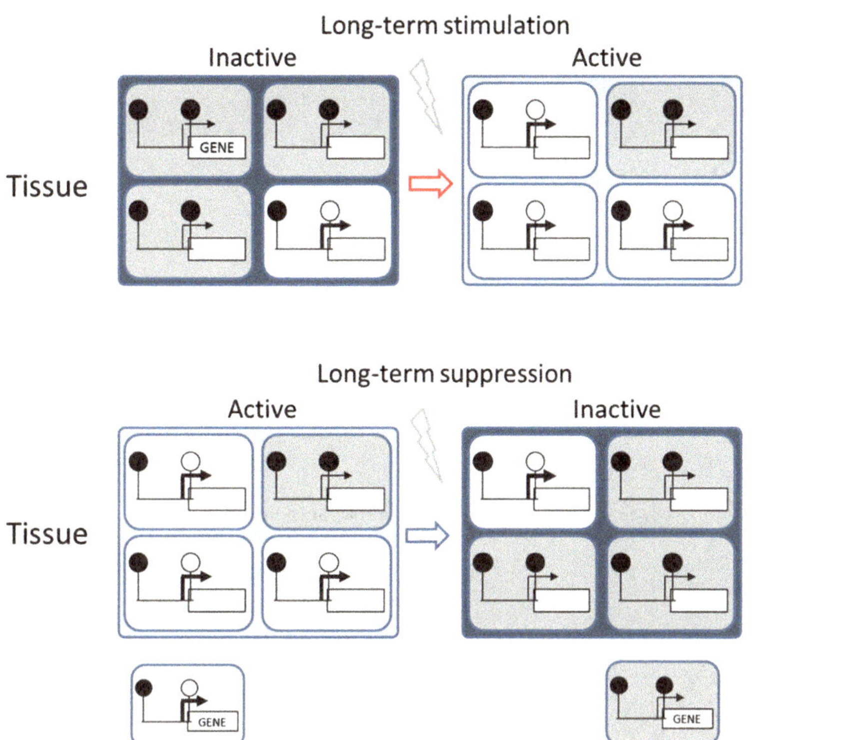

Fig. 4 Gene expression phenotype conversion

intolerance, obesity, and elevated serum cholesterol in later life (Roseboom et al. 2001b). Reduced representation bisulfite sequencing (RRBS) analysis, that covers only 5–10 % of all genomic CpG dinucleotides, was used to identify the Dutch famine-associated changes in DNA methylation in genes that could be responsible for the adverse metabolic profile (Heijmans et al. 2008; Tobi et al. 2014). More comprehensive analyses, such as whole genome bisulfite sequencing (WGBS) (that covers >70 % of human genomic CpG dinucleotides), is likely to identify changes in the methylation of genes involved in the development of hypertension.

Maternal low protein diets in rat (Kwong et al. 2000) and mouse (Watkins et al. 2008) programs offspring to develop hypertension. In rats, offspring of mothers fed a low protein diet develop hypertension with decreased DNA methylation and subsequent increased expression of the type 1b angiotensin II receptor gene (*Agtr1b*) in the adrenal gland (Bogdarina et al. 2007). These changes, involved in developing hypertension, are seen very early in life and last until at least 12 weeks of age, suggestive of a sustained type of DNA demethylation. In contrast, angiotensinogen in the liver shows increased expression at 1 week of age, and is normalized by 12 weeks. Despite lacking data on DNA methylation, it is predicted that *Agt* will show a returned type of DNA demethylation. Similar findings of increased *Agtr1* expression have been reported in sheep following a maternal undernutrition diet (Whorwood et al. 2001).

When maternal glucocorticoid synthesis is pharmacologically blocked during the first two weeks of pregnancy, the maternal low protein diet-associated hypertension in the offspring is ameliorated. This is associated with a concomitant normalization of gene expression and DNA methylation of *Agtr1b* in the rat adrenal gland (Bogdarina et al. 2010), suggesting that the

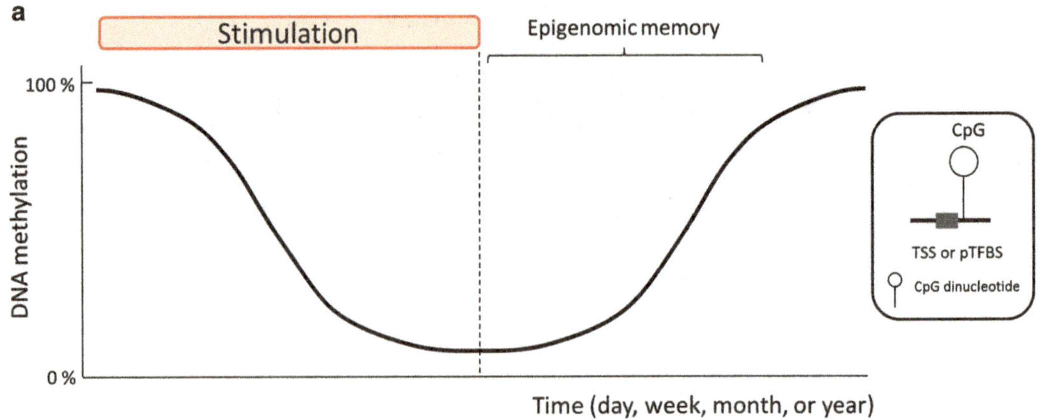

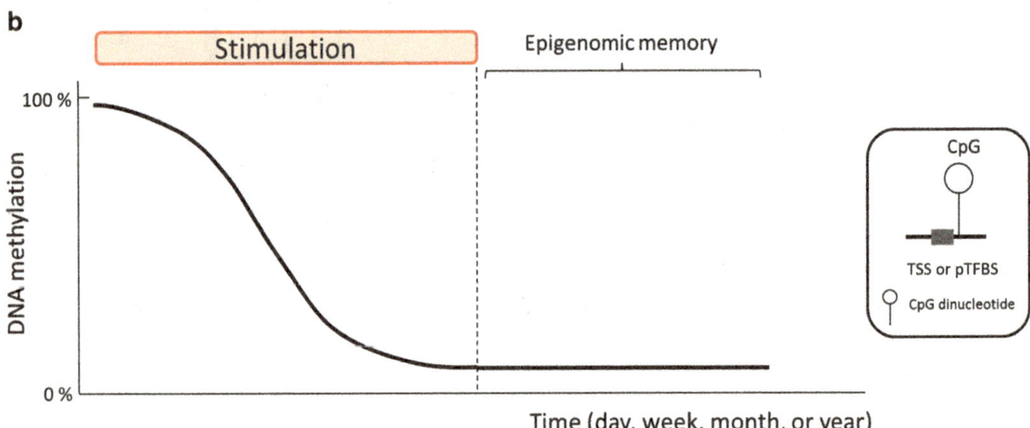

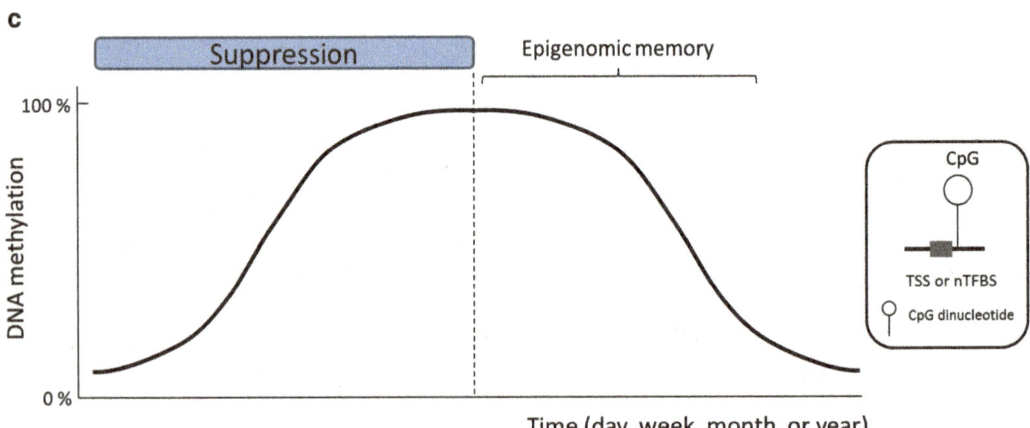

Fig. 5 Schematic representation of dynamic changes in DNA methylation patterns upon some signal and its cessation. (**a**) Reversed DNA demethylation. (**b**) Sustained DNA demethylation. (**c**) Reversed DNA methylation. (**d**) Sustained DNA methylation (*TSS* transcription start site, *pTFBS* positive transcription factor-binding site, *nTFBS* negative transcription factor-binding site)

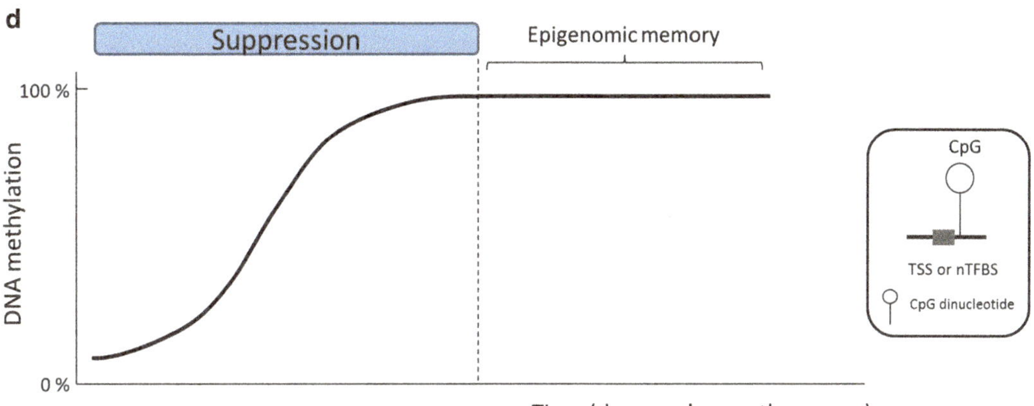

Fig. 5 (continued)

maternal hypothalamic-pituitary-adrenal axis plays a central role in the development of hypertension associated with prenatal exposure to a maternal low protein diet.

8 Acquired Predisposition and Hypertension

Tissue DNA methylation patterns are of physiological importance to constitution. One human study evaluated the association between DNA methylation and acquired predisposition for hypertension (Wang et al. 2014a). Visceral adipose tissue (VAT) surrounding cortisol-producing adenoma (Cushing's syndrome, CS), aldosterone-producing adenoma (APA), and non-functioning adenoma (NFA) were examined. Both cortisol and aldosterone were found to have the ability to stimulate VAT *AGT* transcription, with accompanying *AGT* promoter DNA demethylation. Cortisol and aldosterone exert differential effects through binding and activation of a subfamily of NR3C glucocorticoid receptors (GRs) (NR3C1) and mineralocorticoid receptors (MRs) (NR3C2), respectively. The sites of DNA demethylation at the *AGT* locus appear to be associated with GR or MR binding sites (Wang et al. 2014a; Demura et al. 2015). This study demonstrates that disease conditions such as CS and APA cause acquired predisposition to susceptibility to hypertension through DNA demethylation of VAT *AGT*.

Surgical removal of the tumor does not always restore blood pressure to normal levels in CS and APA, suggesting that the DNA methylation patterns induced by excess circulating cortisol and aldosterone are not fully reversed. A genome-wide analysis of DNA methylation is necessary to elucidate whether changes in DNA methylation patterns are reversed or sustained in a locus-specific fashion following surgical treatment for CS and APA. Such analysis is likely to have a large impact on our understanding of the role of DNA methylation in hypertension.

High DNA methylation around a TSS is associated with the absence of RNA polymerase II. Conversely, low DNA methylation around a TSS is associated with the presence of either active (high transcription levels) or stalled (low transcription levels) RNA polymerase II (Takeshima et al. 2009). The combination of high promoter DNA methylation and intermediate DNA methylation around the TSS of VAT *AGT* in NFA reflects suppression of VAT *AGT* transcription (Wang et al. 2014a; Demura et al. 2015). Excessive salt in contemporary diets reduces circulating RAAS levels (Oliver et al. 1975). Collectively, although VAT would be a major site of AGT production, high promoter DNA methylation of VAT *AGT* in NFA is considered to be adaptive response against an overabundance of salt in contemporary society.

Salt is a well-recognized risk factor for the development of hypertension. In rats, high-salt diets suppresses the level of circulating RAAS, yet VAT *Agt* expression is increased and accompanied by low *Agt* promoter methylation (Wang et al. 2014a; Demura et al. 2015). Using RRBS analysis, exposure to a high-salt diet for just 7 days induces significant changes in DNA methylation and hydroxymethylation patterns in the renal outer medulla (Liu et al. 2014).

As described, concrete, although limited, examples are available that demonstrate that disease conditions and dietary factors can induce an acquired predisposition to hypertension. Further insights into the relationship between DNA methylation and hypertension will be gleaned from additional studies in this area.

9 Transgenerational Epigenetic Inheritance and Hypertension

Whilst several animal studies have illustrated transgenerational inheritance, there is currently no direct and definitive evidence showing transgenerational epigenetic inheritance in hypertension. In addition to their target organs, environmental factors and disease conditions can cause changes in DNA methylation patterns in all tissues including germ cells. Changes in germ cells are less apparent than those that occur in target tissues (Dias and Ressler 2014). From an evolutionary perspective, this system would provide the ability to adapt to environmental circumstances and aid in preservation of the species.

In rats, fetal alcohol exposure increases DNA methylation at the *Pomc* promoter in sperm and these changes persists across at least three generations (Govorko et al. 2012). In rats, fetal alcohol exposure increases DNA methylation at the *Pomc* promoter in sperm and these changes persists across at least three generations (Anway et al. 2005). In mice, odor fear conditioning induces targeted changes in gene expression and DNA methylation in sperm as well as the olfactory nerve, which persists across at least two generations. More importantly, in this study *in vitro* fertilization using sperm from an odor-conditioned mouse reproduced the same changes in behavior, gene expression, and DNA

methylation (Dias and Ressler 2014), indicating that sperm contains a certain signal to mediate transgenerational inheritance and DNA methylation patterns are a likely candidate for the mediator.

Postnatal experiences also alter the DNA methylation patterns of several genes in sperm. In mice, postnatal traumatic stress induces gene-targeted and bidirectional changes in sperm as well as the brain, thereby upregulating some genes with low DNA methylation and downregulating others with high DNA methylation (Franklin et al. 2010). Similar changes in DNA methylation patterns are observed in the sperm of both parent and offspring, and in the relevant somatic tissues of the offspring, which is strongly indicative of transgenerational inheritance.

Although data supporting transgenerational inheritance of epigenetic changes, including DNA methylation, is lacking there are a number of supportive examples are in humans. Firstly, the offspring of prenatally undernourished fathers during the Dutch-famine become obese (Vccncndaal et al. 2013). Nutrition intake of grandparents appears to influence the mortality of grandchildren (Kaati et al. 2002; Pembrey et al. 2006; Bygren et al. 2014), suggesting transgenerational responses in humans. Another study analyzed four generations of a family showed that the allelic asymmetry of DNA methylation observed in somatic cells was also present in germ cells (Tang et al. 2016). Additionally, exercise induces changes in the DNA methylation patterns of many genes in human sperm (Denham et al. 2015). Despite indirect, these observations indicate that transgenerational epigenetic inheritance, in association with DNA methylation, occurs in humans. Taken together, transgenerational epigenetic inheritance related to hypertension is likely to exist in humans.

The molecular mechanism by which transgenerational inheritance takes place remains largely unknown. *De novo* DNA methylation and DNA demethylation are targeted to particular regulatory elements in both somatic and germ cells. Extracellular vesicles containing proteins and ncRNAs can mediate intercellular communication between somatic and germ cells (Cossetti et al. 2014; Devanapally et al. 2015). Therefore, DNA-binding transcription factors and ncRNAs emerge as a strong candidate contributing directly to transgenerational inheritance.

10 Conclusion and Emerging Concept

DNA methylation patterns have been thought to be stably maintained. However, life experiences, environmental factors, and disease conditions can dynamically alter DNA methylation patterns. More importantly, it is becoming increasingly clear that these various factors can change DNA methylation patterns in germ cells as well as in somatic tissues, leading to heritable changes in traits and behaviors.

Previous studies have revealed that genetic factors have a limited capacity for coping with the question of the development and inheritance of hypertension. Epigenetic mechanisms have led to an enormous paradigm shift in our understanding of phenotypes and heritability. Environmental changes during intrauterine and early postnatal life can lead to changes in DNA methylation patterns with altered gene expression. Such changes could result in increased susceptibility to hypertension in adulthood. In addition, although gradual, changes in DNA methylation patterns in adulthood may also affect a susceptibility to hypertension.

DNA methylation patterns vary from tissue to tissue, and even within tissues, thus conferring on DNA a particular cellular identity. Meanwhile, it is undeniably true that experiences, environmental factors, and disease conditions make their own epigenetic mark on DNA. Mapping changes in the patterns of DNA demethylation and *de novo* DNA methylation in response to various factors will open new avenues for diagnostics, health promotion, and disease prevention.

Acknowledgements This chapter was supported by the Japan Society for Takeda Science Foundation (to M Demura).

References

Adeyemo A, Gerry N, Chen G, Herbert A, Doumatey A, Huang H et al (2009) A genome-wide association study of hypertension and blood pressure in African Americans. PLoS Genet 5(7):e1000564

Alikhani-Koopaei R, Fouladkou F, Frey FJ, Frey BM (2004) Epigenetic regulation of 11 beta-hydroxysteroid dehydrogenase type 2 expression. J Clin Invest 114(8):1146–1157

Anway MD, Cupp AS, Uzumcu M, Skinner MK (2005) Epigenetic transgenerational actions of endocrine disruptors and male fertility. Science 308 (5727):1466–1469

Arab K, Park YJ, Lindroth AM, Schafer A, Oakes C, Weichenhan D et al (2014) Long noncoding RNA TARID directs demethylation and activation of the tumor suppressor TCF21 via GADD45A. Mol Cell 55(4):604–614

Arai Y, Ohgane J, Yagi S, Ito R, Iwasaki Y, Saito K et al (2011) Epigenetic assessment of environmental chemicals detected in maternal peripheral and cord blood samples. J Reprod Dev 57(4):507–517

Beilin LJ (1990) Diet and lifestyle in hypertension: changing perspectives. J Cardiovasc Pharmacol 16 (Suppl 7):S62–S66

Bind MA, Zanobetti A, Gasparrini A, Peters A, Coull B, Baccarelli A et al (2014) Effects of temperature and relative humidity on DNA methylation. Epidemiology 25(4):561–569

Bogdarina I, Welham S, King PJ, Burns SP, Clark AJ (2007) Epigenetic modification of the renin-angiotensin system in the fetal programming of hypertension. Circ Res 100(4):520–526

Bogdarina I, Haase A, Langley-Evans S, Clark AJ (2010) Glucocorticoid effects on the programming of AT1b angiotensin receptor gene methylation and expression in the rat. PLoS ONE 5(2):e9237

Bohacek J, Mansuy IM (2015) Molecular insights into transgenerational non-genetic inheritance of acquired behaviours. Nat Rev Genet 16(11):641–652

Bygren LO, Tinghog P, Carstensen J, Edvinsson S, Kaati G, Pembrey ME et al (2014) Change in paternal grandmothers' early food supply influenced cardiovascular mortality of the female grandchildren. BMC Genet 15:12

Chang H, Zhang T, Zhang Z, Bao R, Fu C, Wang Z et al (2011) Tissue-specific distribution of aberrant DNA methylation associated with maternal low-folate status in human neural tube defects. J Nutr Biochem 22(12):1172–1177

Chen CC, Wang KY, Shen CK (2013) DNA 5-methylcytosine demethylation activities of the mammalian DNA methyltransferases. J Biol Chem 288(13):9084–9091

Chen D, Zhang A, Fang M, Fang R, Ge J, Jiang Y et al (2014) Increased methylation at differentially methylated region of GNAS in infants born to gestational diabetes. BMC Med Genet 15:108

Chhabra D, Sharma S, Kho AT, Gaedigk R, Vyhlidal CA, Leeder JS et al (2014) Fetal lung and placental methylation is associated with in utero nicotine exposure. Epigenetics 9(11):1473–1484

Cossetti C, Lugini L, Astrologo L, Saggio I, Fais S, Spadafora C (2014) Soma-to-germline transmission of RNA in mice xenografted with human tumour cells: possible transport by exosomes. PLoS ONE 9 (7):e101629

Demura M, Wang F, Yoneda T, Karashima S, Cheng Y, Yamagishi M et al (2010) Epigenetic transcriptional repression of the human CYP11B2 gene. Endocr J 57: S339

Demura M, Demura Y, Takeda Y, Saijoh K (2015) Dynamic regulation of the angiotensinogen gene by DNA methylation, which is influenced by various stimuli experienced in daily life. Hypertens Res 38 (8):519–527

Denham J, O'Brien BJ, Harvey JT, Charchar FJ (2015) Genome-wide sperm DNA methylation changes after 3 months of exercise training in humans. Epigenomics 7(5):717–731

Devanapally S, Ravikumar S, Double-stranded JAM, RNA (2015) made in C. elegans neurons can enter the germline and cause transgenerational gene silencing. Proc Natl Acad Sci U S A 112(7):2133–2138

Dewey FE, Grove ME, Pan C, Goldstein BA, Bernstein JA, Chaib H et al (2014) Clinical interpretation and implications of whole-genome sequencing. JAMA 311(10):1035–1045

Di Ruscio A, Ebralidze AK, Benoukraf T, Amabile G, Goff LA, Terragni J et al (2013) DNMT1-interacting RNAs block gene-specific DNA methylation. Nature 503(7476):371–376

Dias BG, Ressler KJ (2014) Parental olfactory experience influences behavior and neural structure in subsequent generations. Nat Neurosci 17(1):89–96

Drake AJ, O'Shaughnessy PJ, Bhattacharya S, Monteiro A, Kerrigan D, Goetz S et al (2015) In utero exposure to cigarette chemicals induces sex-specific disruption of one-carbon metabolism and DNA methylation in the human fetal liver. BMC Med 13:18

Feldmann A, Ivanek R, Murr R, Gaidatzis D, Burger L, Schubeler D (2013) Transcription factor occupancy can mediate active turnover of DNA methylation at regulatory regions. PLoS Genet 9(12):e1003994

Franceschini N, Fox E, Zhang Z, Edwards TL, Nalls MA, Sung YJ et al (2013) Genome-wide association analysis of blood-pressure traits in African-ancestry individuals reveals common associated genes in African and non-African populations. Am J Hum Genet 93 (3):545–554

Franklin TB, Russig H, Weiss IC, Graff J, Linder N, Michalon A et al (2010) Epigenetic transmission of the impact of early stress across generations. Biol Psychiatry 68(5):408–415

Friso S, Pizzolo F, Choi SW, Guarini P, Castagna A, Ravagnani V et al (2008) Epigenetic control of 11 beta-hydroxysteroid dehydrogenase 2 gene promoter is related to human hypertension. Atherosclerosis 199(2):323–327

Ganesh SK, Tragante V, Guo W, Guo Y, Lanktree MB, Smith EN et al (2013) Loci influencing blood pressure identified using a cardiovascular gene-centric array. Hum Mol Genet 22(8):1663–1678

Govorko D, Bekdash RA, Zhang C, Sarkar DK (2012) Male germline transmits fetal alcohol adverse effect on hypothalamic proopiomelanocortin gene across generations. Biol Psychiatry 72(5):378–388

Guo H, Zhu P, Yan L, Li R, Hu B, Lian Y et al (2014) The DNA methylation landscape of human early embryos. Nature 511(7511):606–610

Guo F, Yan L, Guo H, Li L, Hu B, Zhao Y et al (2015) The transcriptome and DNA methylome landscapes of human primordial germ cells. Cell 161(6):1437–1452

Heijmans BT, Tobi EW, Stein AD, Putter H, Blauw GJ, Susser ES et al (2008) Persistent epigenetic differences associated with prenatal exposure to famine in humans. Proc Natl Acad Sci U S A 105 (44):17046–17049

Hong KW, Go MJ, Jin HS, Lim JE, Lee JY, Han BG et al (2010) Genetic variations in ATP2B1, CSK, ARSG and CSMD1 loci are related to blood pressure and/or hypertension in two Korean cohorts. J Hum Hypertens 24(6):367–372

International Consortium for Blood Pressure Genome-Wide Association, Ehret GB, Munroe PB, Rice KM, Bochud M, Johnson AD et al (2011) Genetic variants in novel pathways influence blood pressure and cardiovascular disease risk. Nature 478(7367):103–109

Ishikawa K, Tsunekawa S, Ikeniwa M, Izumoto T, Iida A, Ogata H et al (2015) Long-term pancreatic beta cell exposure to high levels of glucose but not palmitate induces DNA methylation within the insulin gene promoter and represses transcriptional activity. PLoS ONE 10(2):e0115350

James SJ, Pogribny IP, Pogribna M, Miller BJ, Jernigan S, Melnyk S (2003) Mechanisms of DNA damage, DNA hypomethylation, and tumor progression in the folate/methyl-deficient rat model of hepatocarcinogenesis. J Nutr 133(11 Suppl 1):3740S–3747S

Kaati G, Bygren LO, Edvinsson S (2002) Cardiovascular and diabetes mortality determined by nutrition during parents' and grandparents' slow growth period. Eur J Hum Genet 10(11):682–688

Kangaspeska S, Stride B, Metivier R, Polycarpou-Schwarz M, Ibberson D, Carmouche RP et al (2008) Transient cyclical methylation of promoter DNA. Nature 452(7183):112–115

Kato N, Takeuchi F, Tabara Y, Kelly TN, Go MJ, Sim X et al (2011) Meta-analysis of genome-wide association studies identifies common variants associated with blood pressure variation in east Asians. Nat Genet 43(6):531–538

Kato N, Loh M, Takeuchi F, Verweij N, Wang X, Zhang W et al (2015) Trans-ancestry genome-wide association study identifies 12 genetic loci influencing blood pressure and implicates a role for DNA methylation. Nat Genet

Kwong WY, Wild AE, Roberts P, Willis AC, Fleming TP (2000) Maternal undernutrition during the preimplantation period of rat development causes blastocyst abnormalities and programming of postnatal hypertension. Development 127(19):4195–4202

Lee HA, Baek I, Seok YM, Yang E, Cho HM, Lee DY et al (2010) Promoter hypomethylation upregulates Na+-K+-2Cl- cotransporter 1 in spontaneously hypertensive rats. Biochem Biophys Res Commun 396 (2):252–257

Lee HJ, Hore TA, Reik W (2014) Reprogramming the methylome: erasing memory and creating diversity. Cell Stem Cell 14(6):710–719

Levy D, Ehret GB, Rice K, Verwoert GC, Launer LJ, Dehghan A et al (2009) Genome-wide association study of blood pressure and hypertension. Nat Genet 41(6):677–687

Li X, Hui AM, Sun L, Hasegawa K, Torzilli G, Minagawa M et al (2004) p16INK4A hypermethylation is associated with hepatitis virus infection, age, and gender in hepatocellular carcinoma. Clin Cancer Res 10 (22):7484–7489

Lienert F, Wirbelauer C, Som I, Dean A, Mohn F, Schubeler D (2011) Identification of genetic elements that autonomously determine DNA methylation states. Nat Genet 43(11):1091–1097

Liu Y, Liu P, Yang C, Cowley AW Jr, Liang M (2014) Base-resolution maps of 5-methylcytosine and 5-hydroxymethylcytosine in Dahl S rats: effect of salt and genomic sequence. Hypertension 63 (4):827–838

Liu F, Sun Q, Wang L, Nie S, Li J (2015) Bioinformatics analysis of abnormal DNA methylation in muscle samples from monozygotic twins discordant for type 2 diabetes. Mol Med Rep 12(1):351–356

MacArthur DG, Tyler-Smith C (2010) Loss-of-function variants in the genomes of healthy humans. Hum Mol Genet 19(R2):R125–R130

MacArthur DG, Balasubramanian S, Frankish A, Huang N, Morris J, Walter K et al (2012) A systematic survey of loss-of-function variants in human protein-coding genes. Science 335(6070):823–828

Maekita T, Nakazawa K, Mihara M, Nakajima T, Yanaoka K, Iguchi M et al (2006) High levels of aberrant DNA methylation in Helicobacter pylori-infected gastric mucosae and its possible association with gastric cancer risk. Clin Cancer Res 12(3 Pt 1):989–995

Marchal C, Miotto B (2015) Emerging concept in DNA methylation: role of transcription factors in shaping DNA methylation patterns. J Cell Physiol 230 (4):743–751

Metivier R, Gallais R, Tiffoche C, Le Peron C, Jurkowska RZ, Carmouche RP et al (2008) Cyclical DNA methylation of a transcriptionally active promoter. Nature 452(7183):45–50

Miller CA, Sweatt JD (2007) Covalent modification of DNA regulates memory formation. Neuron 53 (6):857–869

Miller CA, Gavin CF, White JA, Parrish RR, Honasoge A, Yancey CR et al (2010) Cortical DNA methylation maintains remote memory. Nat Neurosci 13 (6):664–666

Nakajima T, Yamashita S, Maekita T, Niwa T, Nakazawa K, Ushijima T (2009) The presence of a methylation fingerprint of Helicobacter pylori infection in human gastric mucosae. Int J Cancer 124 (4):905–910

Newton-Cheh C, Johnson T, Gateva V, Tobin MD, Bochud M, Coin L et al (2009) Genome-wide association study identifies eight loci associated with blood pressure. Nat Genet 41(6):666–676

Nilsson E, Matte A, Perfilyev A, de Mello VD, Kakela P, Pihlajamaki J et al (2015) Epigenetic alterations in human liver from subjects with type 2 diabetes in parallel with reduced folate levels. J Clin Endocrinol Metab 100(11):E1491–E1501

Oka D, Yamashita S, Tomioka T, Nakanishi Y, Kato H, Kaminishi M et al (2009) The presence of aberrant DNA methylation in noncancerous esophageal mucosae in association with smoking history: a target for risk diagnosis and prevention of esophageal cancers. Cancer 115(15):3412–3426

Okae H, Chiba H, Hiura H, Hamada H, Sato A, Utsunomiya T et al (2014) Genome-wide analysis of DNA methylation dynamics during early human development. PLoS Genet 10(12):e1004868

Oliver WJ, Cohen EL, Neel JV (1975) Blood pressure, sodium intake, and sodium related hormones in the Yanomamo Indians, a "no-salt" culture. Circulation 52(1):146–151

Padmanabhan S, Melander O, Johnson T, Di Blasio AM, Lee WK, Gentilini D et al (2010) Genome-wide association study of blood pressure extremes identifies variant near UMOD associated with hypertension. PLoS Genet 6(10):e1001177

Pembrey ME, Bygren LO, Kaati G, Edvinsson S, Northstone K, Sjostrom M et al (2006) Sex-specific, male-line transgenerational responses in humans. Eur J Hum Genet 14(2):159–166

Pizzolo F, Friso S, Morandini F, Antoniazzi F, Zaltron C, Udali S et al (2015) Apparent mineralocorticoid excess by a novel mutation and epigenetic modulation by HSD11B2 promoter methylation. J Clin Endocrinol Metab 100(9):E1234–E1241

Riviere G, Lienhard D, Andrieu T, Vieau D, Frey BM, Frey FJ (2011) Epigenetic regulation of somatic angiotensin-converting enzyme by DNA methylation and histone acetylation. Epigenetics 6(4):478–489

Ronn T, Volkov P, Davegardh C, Dayeh T, Hall E, Olsson AH et al (2013) A six months exercise intervention influences the genome-wide DNA methylation pattern in human adipose tissue. PLoS Genet 9(6):e1003572

Ronn T, Volkov P, Gillberg L, Kokosar M, Perfilyev A, Jacobsen AL et al (2015) Impact of age, BMI and HbA1c levels on the genome-wide DNA methylation and mRNA expression patterns in human adipose tissue and identification of epigenetic biomarkers in blood. Hum Mol Genet 24(13):3792–3813

Roseboom TJ, van der Meulen JH, Ravelli AC, van Montfrans GA, Osmond C, Barker DJ et al (1999) Blood pressure in adults after prenatal exposure to famine. J Hypertens 17(3):325–330

Roseboom TJ, van der Meulen JH, Ravelli AC, Osmond C, Barker DJ, Bleker OP (2001a) Effects of prenatal exposure to the Dutch famine on adult disease in later life: an overview. Mol Cell Endocrinol 185 (1-2):93–98

Roseboom TJ, van der Meulen JH, Ravelli AC, Osmond C, Barker DJ, Bleker OP (2001b) Effects of prenatal exposure to the Dutch famine on adult disease in later life: an overview. Twin Res 4(5):293–298

Serra RW, Fang M, Park SM, Hutchinson L, Green MR (2014) A KRAS-directed transcriptional silencing pathway that mediates the CpG island methylator phenotype. Elife 3:e02313

Slieker RC, Roost MS, van Iperen L, Suchiman HE, Tobi EW, Carlotti F et al (2015) DNA methylation landscapes of human fetal development. PLoS Genet 11(10):e1005583

Smolarek I, Wyszko E, Barciszewska AM, Nowak S, Gawronska I, Jablecka A et al (2010) Global DNA methylation changes in blood of patients with essential hypertension. Med Sci Monit 16(3):CR149–CR155

Szyf M (2015) Nongenetic inheritance and transgenerational epigenetics. Trends Mol Med 21 (2):134–144

Takeshima H, Yamashita S, Shimazu T, Niwa T, Ushijima T (2009) The presence of RNA polymerase II, active or stalled, predicts epigenetic fate of promoter CpG islands. Genome Res 19(11):1974–1982

Tang WW, Dietmann S, Irie N, Leitch HG, Floros VI, Bradshaw CR et al (2015) A unique gene regulatory network resets the human germline epigenome for development. Cell 161(6):1453–1467

Tang A, Huang Y, Li Z, Wan S, Mou L, Yin G et al (2016) Analysis of a four generation family reveals the widespread sequence-dependent maintenance of allelic DNA methylation in somatic and germ cells. Sci Rep 6:19260

Thillainadesan G, Chitilian JM, Isovic M, Ablack JN, Mymryk JS, Tini M et al (2012) TGF-beta-dependent active demethylation and expression of the p15ink4b tumor suppressor are impaired by the ZNF217/CoREST complex. Mol Cell 46(5):636–649

Thomassin H, Flavin M, Espinas ML, Grange T (2001) Glucocorticoid-induced DNA demethylation and gene memory during development. EMBO J 20 (8):1974–1983

Tobi EW, Goeman JJ, Monajemi R, Gu H, Putter H, Zhang Y et al (2014) DNA methylation signatures link prenatal famine exposure to growth and metabolism. Nat Commun 5:5592

Veenendaal MV, Painter RC, de Rooij SR, Bossuyt PM, van der Post JA, Gluckman PD et al (2013) Transgenerational effects of prenatal exposure to the 1944-45 Dutch famine. BJOG 120(5):548–553

Wain LV, Verwoert GC, O'Reilly PF, Shi G, Johnson T, Johnson AD et al (2011) Genome-wide association study identifies six new loci influencing pulse pressure and mean arterial pressure. Nat Genet 43 (10):1005–1011

Wajapeyee N, Malonia SK, Palakurthy RK, Green MR (2013) Oncogenic RAS directs silencing of tumor suppressor genes through ordered recruitment of transcriptional repressors. Genes Dev 27(20):2221–2226

Wang X, Falkner B, Zhu H, Shi H, Su S, Xu X et al (2013) A genome-wide methylation study on essential hypertension in young African American males. PLoS ONE 8(1):e53938

Wang F, Demura M, Cheng Y, Zhu A, Karashima S, Yoneda T et al (2014a) Dynamic CCAAT/enhancer binding protein-associated changes of DNA methylation in the angiotensinogen gene. Hypertension 63 (2):281–288

Wang KY, Chen CC, Shen CK (2014b) Active DNA demethylation of the vertebrate genomes by DNA methyltransferases: deaminase, dehydroxymethylase or demethylase? Epigenomics 6(3):353–363

Watkins AJ, Ursell E, Panton R, Papenbrock T, Hollis L, Cunningham C et al (2008) Adaptive responses by mouse early embryos to maternal diet protect fetal growth but predispose to adult onset disease. Biol Reprod 78(2):299–306

Whorwood CB, Firth KM, Budge H, Symonds ME (2001) Maternal undernutrition during early to midgestation programs tissue-specific alterations in the expression of the glucocorticoid receptor, 11beta-hydroxysteroid dehydrogenase isoforms, and type 1 angiotensin ii receptor in neonatal sheep. Endocrinology 142 (7):2854–2864

Zhang LN, Liu PP, Wang L, Yuan F, Xu L, Xin Y et al (2013) Lower ADD1 gene promoter DNA methylation increases the risk of essential hypertension. PLoS ONE 8(5):e63455

Zhang Y, Yang R, Burwinkel B, Breitling LP, Brenner H (2014) F2RL3 methylation as a biomarker of current and lifetime smoking exposures. Environ Health Perspect 122(2):131–137

Adv Exp Med Biol - Advances in Internal Medicine (2017) 2: 599–613
DOI 10.1007/5584_2016_79
© Springer International Publishing AG 2016
Published online: 9 October 2016

Metabolomics, Lipidomics and Pharmacometabolomics of Human Hypertension

Anthony Au, Kian-Kai Cheng, and Loo Keat Wei

Abstract

Hypertension is a common but complex human disease, which can lead to a heart attack, stroke, kidney disease or other complications. Since the pathogenesis of hypertension is heterogeneous and multifactorial, it is crucial to establish a comprehensive metabolomic approach to elucidate the molecular mechanism of hypertension. Although there have been limited metabolomic, lipidomic and pharmacometabolomic studies investigating this disease to date, metabolomic studies on hypertension have provided greater insights into the identification of disease-specific biomarkers, predicting treatment outcome and monitor drug safety and efficacy. Therefore, we discuss recent updates on the applications of metabolomics technology in human hypertension with a focus on metabolic biomarker discovery.

Keywords

Metabolomics • Lipidomics • Pharmacometabolomics • Hypertension

1 Introduction

Hypertension is a symptomless disease which can lead to serious complications, including metabolic syndrome, blurred vision, memory loss, kidney failure, stroke and damage to the heart and coronary arteries (Messerli et al. 2007).

A. Au (✉)
Institute of Bioproduct Development and Department of Bioprocess Engineering, Faculty of Chemical Engineering, Universiti Teknologi Malaysia, 81300 Johor, Malaysia
e-mail: auzlanthony@gmail.com

K.-K. Cheng
Institute of Bioproduct Development and Department of Bioprocess Engineering, Faculty of Chemical Engineering, Universiti Teknologi Malaysia, 81300 Johor, Malaysia

Innovation Centre in Agritechnology, Universiti Teknologi Malaysia, 81300 Johor, Malaysia

L.K. Wei
Centre for Biodiversity Research, Universiti Tunku Abdul Rahman, Bandar Barat, 31900 Kampar, Perak, Malaysia

Department of Biological Science, Faculty of Science, Universiti Tunku Abdul Rahman, Bandar Barat, 31900 Kampar, Perak, Malaysia

Hypertension can be classified into primary (essential or idiopathic), secondary (non essential), and to a lesser extent, isolated systolic hypertension, malignant hypertension, white coat hypertension, and resistant hypertension. Around 90–95 % of hypertensive patients are primary hypertension, as a result of interaction between genetic and lifestyle factors; whereas the remaining 5–10 % are categorized as secondary hypertension, due to renal diseases, endocrine disorders, or side effect of medications (Poulter et al. 2015).

Diagnosis of hypertension is based on sphygmomanometer to measure the pressures exerted during the heart beats (systolic) and resting between beats (diastolic). Normal blood pressure reading is under 120/80 mm Hg (systolic over diastolic), while 140/90 mm Hg and above are considered high blood pressure. Hypertension can be managed with several anti-hypertensive drugs, such as beta-blockers (e.g. atenolol), thiazide diuretics (e.g. hydrochlorothiazide), angiotensin converting enzyme inhibitors (e.g. captopril), calcium channel blockers (e.g. amlodipine) and alpha-1 antagonist (e.g. terazosin) (Chobanian et al. 2003). Other treatments may include lipid-lowering drugs (e.g. statins and fibrates) that can prevent dyslipidemia, diabetes mellitus, cardiovascular and cerebrovascular diseases in hypertensive patients (Jacobson and Zimmerman 2006).

Since pathogenesis and pathophysiology of hypertension may changes during the course of hypertension, it is important to establish a new 'omics' approach for early prediction and elucidate the molecular mechanism of hypertension (Thongboonkerd 2005; Nikolic et al. 2014). Consequently, this would be beneficial for the prevention and management of hypertension as well as promote the development of new therapeutic strategies and improved diagnostic methods to meet future demands.

2 Metabolomics, Lipidomics and Pharmacometabolomics

'Omics' approaches, including genomics (DNA), transcriptomics (RNA), proteomics (proteins), and metabolomics (metabolites), play a pivotal role in our understanding of human biology and diseases such as hypertension (Fig. 1). Metabolomics is one of the 'omics' approaches that study the global metabolic profile in biological samples (e.g. cells, tissues and body fluids), by using analytical techniques with the combination of cheminformatics, bioinformatics and statistics analyses (Madsen et al. 2010).

Fig. 1 Omics' approaches

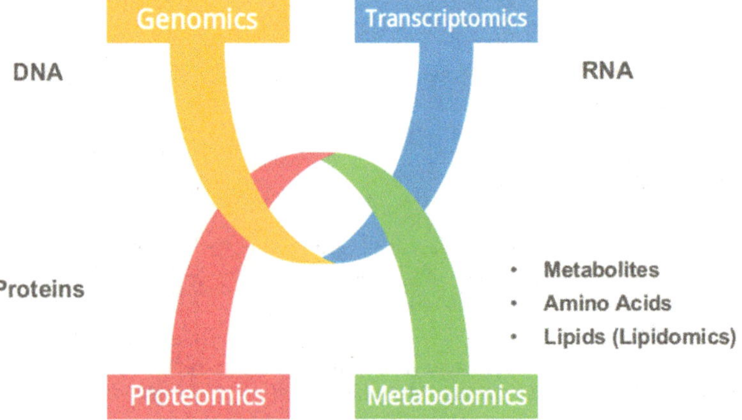

Lipidomics is a subfield of metabolomics, which focuses on the identification and quantitation of the complete set of lipids on a metabolic basis and further associated with diseases or treatments. Pharmacometabolomics is an emerging field that positively contributes to personalized medicine, involves the identification of metabolic patterns that can predict the response of drug treatment in human diseases. Pharmacometabolomics also helps to investigate the effects of drugs on metabolism and identify the metabolic pathways that correspond to drug-response phenotype and metabolic adverse effects (Kaddurah-Daouk et al. 2014).

Human metabolome consisted of approximately 4229 endogenous metabolites in serum sample (Psychogios et al. 2011). Metabolites represent the intermediate and end products of metabolic reactions and cellular processes, and may have diverse functions in different organisms. Metabolites usually have low molecular weight of less than 1500 Dalton, and biological molecules including carbohydrates, fatty acids, and amino acids can be considered as metabolites. Metabolites also vary depending on their polarity, solubility and volatility. For instance, amino acids are hydrophilic polar metabolites, while lipids are hydrophobic non-polar metabolites.

3 Targeted and Untargeted Metabolomics

An appropriate experimental design is required to ensure that the metabolomic data is able to answer the questions of interest (Fig. 2). Two distinct metabolomic strategies, namely targeted and untargeted approaches have been applied to the analysis of metabolites. Targeted metabolomic approach is on the basis of hypothesis-driven manner and also used for biomarkers validation (Griffiths et al. 2010; Wei et al. 2010). Targeted metabolomics is the measurement of a select group of metabolites, typically focusing on one

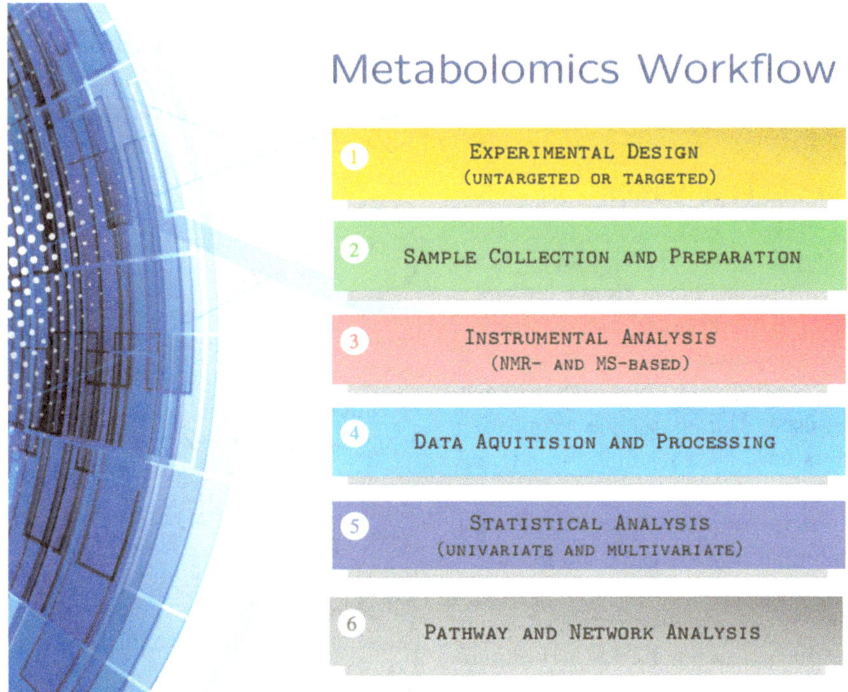

Fig. 2 Metabolomics workflow

or more related pathways of interest (Dudley et al. 2010). It is normally performed using mass spectrometry (MS) based approach. By taking this approach, a novel association between metabolites and diseases may be revealed and enables a more comprehensive understanding on metabolic functions and pathways (Roberts et al. 2012).

In contrast to targeted metabolomics, untargeted approaches allow the unbiased detection of full set of metabolites in the biological samples. This approach offers the opportunity for the discovery of novel metabolites and metabolic pathways without prior knowledge of the identified metabolites (Patti et al. 2012). Therefore, untargeted metabolomics is classified as discovery-phase or hypothesis-generating research. Untargeted metabolomics can be performed by nuclear magnetic resonance (NMR) and MS approaches, in order to measure and quantify as many metabolites as possible (Alonso et al. 2015). However, the challenging part of this approach is build upon the complexity and pleiotropic nature of metabolomic data as well as the protocol and time required to analyze the massive data sets (Patti et al. 2012; Roberts et al. 2012).

4 Sample Preparation

The initial step in a metabolic profiling is the extraction of metabolites from biological samples. Metabolite extraction varies profoundly depending on study objectives, sample availability (cell, tissue or body fluid) and analytical platform to be used. During sample acquisition, several factors have been identified to interfere with metabolomic outcomes. For instance, gender, age, diurnal variations, diet, exercise and drug consumption may influence the metabolic profile of an individual (Yin et al. 2015). In addition, type of blood-collection tubes (such as lithium heparin, potassium EDTA and citrate), duration between sample collection and processing, transportation, storage and repeating freeze-thaw cycles of samples may also affect the

analytical results (Yin and Xu 2014; Yin et al. 2015).

In the consideration of complex, heterogeneous and dynamic nature of metabolome, metabolite extraction can be performed in order to separate and maximize the total number of metabolites detected. The procedure of metabolite extraction is specific to samples types and metabolites of interest (Patti 2011). Liquid-liquid extraction and solid phase extraction are the most commonly used methods for metabolites extraction (Yin and Xu 2014). Metabolites should be quenched immediately to stop metabolism for example by perchloric acid treatment or freezing at $-80\ ^\circ$C or liquid nitrogen prior to extraction. During extraction process, different solvents such as methanol, isopropanol, chloroform, acetonitrile or their combinations are used, thus allow the separation of polar and non-polar metabolites and also protein depletion (Bruce et al. 2008; Sellick et al. 2011; Sapcariu et al. 2014). Lipids are usually extracted with chloroform–methanol aqueous mixtures (Jung et al. 2011). As a result, the upper aqueous soluble phase is consisted of polar metabolites, while non-polar metabolites are remained in the lower organic phase. However, it has been suggested that minimal sample preparation may lead to the production of accurate, reliable, and unbiased data (Dunn et al. 2011).

5 Analytical Instrumentation

High-throughput analytical platforms allow the simultaneous separation and comprehensive detection of metabolites present in biological samples, mainly based on either NMR spectroscopy or MS technologies. These including, but are not limited to ^{1}H-NMR spectroscopy, ^{13}C-NMR spectroscopy, ^{15}N-NMR spectroscopy, ^{31}P-NMR spectroscopy, gas chromatography-MS (GC-MS), gas chromatography-flame ionization detection (GC-FID), capillary electrophoresis-MS (CE-MS), direct infusion-MS (DI-MS) and liquid chromatography-MS (LC-MS). High-resolution magic-angle spinning NMR spectroscopy can be used for metabolic profiling of intact tissues without any pretreatment of samples (Beckonert et al. 2010).

6 Nuclear Magnetic Resonance Based Method

NMR spectroscopy is a rapid and effective technique for untargeted metabolomics, as it can identify and quantify a wide range of metabolites in biological samples. This technique is a non-destructive method and requires only minimal sample preparation. ^{1}H-NMR spectroscopy is the one of most common used methods for metabolomic analysis, and to a lesser extent ^{13}C-, ^{15}N- and ^{31}P-NMR (Keun and Athersuch 2011). The principle of NMR involved the absorption of radiant energy by atomic nuclei (^{1}H) in the presence of a magnetic field (Lane 2012). At the same field, different atomic nuclei within a molecule will generate different resonance frequencies. These signals will provide the chemical and structural information on the detected molecule.

However, NMR has relatively low analytical sensitivity that detects only high-abundance metabolites, thus leads to a requirement for greater initial sample volume (Bothwell and Griffin 2011). Moreover, complex datasets may result in peaks overlapping or similar coupling constants in one-dimensional NMR. This can be overcome by applying two- and three-dimensional NMR spectroscopy methods such as J-resolved spectroscopy, spin-echo correlated spectroscopy, diffusion ordered spectroscopy and ultrafast J-Resolved correlation spectroscopy (Ludwig and Viant 2010; Dunn et al. 2011; Larive et al. 2014). Furthermore, high-resolution magic angle spinning (HRMAS) NMR spectroscopy can be performed on intact tissues without sample preparation (Bothwell and Griffin 2011; Larive et al. 2014). During the process, sample is spun at magic angle (54°44') to the magnetic field with high speed (2000–6000 Hz), in order to reduce or remove the chemical shift anisotropy and dipole-dipole couplings (Salek et al. 2011).

7 Mass Spectrometry Based Method

MS coupled with liquid chromatography (LC) or gas chromatography (GC), enables the ionization and subsequent separation of the ions and fragment ions according to their mass-to-charge (m/z) ratio (Pitt 2009). In LC-MS, several types of atmospheric pressure ionization methods are used for the ionization of different categories of metabolites. Of which, the most commonly used electrospray ionization is used for the initial screening of unknown metabolites (Xiao et al. 2012). Atmospheric-pressure chemical ionization and atmospheric-pressure photoionization are suitable for the detection of non-polar metabolites and have been widely applied in lipidomic studies (Xiao et al. 2012). There are different types of MS analyzers, including ion trap, time-of-flight, orbitrap, and quadrupole MS (Fuhrer and Zamboni 2015).

The high resolution of GC combined with the MS detection, and more recently GC × GC-MS, provides an excellent system for performing global metabolic profiling, with the help of metabolome databases in the identification of unknown compounds (Patti et al. 2012). However for GC-MS based method, sample derivatization is required prior to data acquisition. For aqueous metabolites, the common practice is to use a two-step derivatization processes (methoximation followed by silylation) prior to GC-MS analysis to reduce polarity and increase thermal stability and volatility (Cheng et al. 2014). The benefits of GC-MS based strategies may include very high resolution, good sensitivity and robustness; these are further enhanced by a two dimensional GC × GC-MS. The metabolites elute from the first column are separated based on volatility and followed by polarity in the second column (Lenz and Wilson 2007).

Compared to NMR and GC-MS, LC-MS based method is able to detect a larger numbers (200–500) of metabolites, and therefore has been recommended for global metabolite profiling (Patti et al. 2012). In many ways, LC-MS analysis can be performed using reversed-phase gradient chromatography, electrospray ionization probe and Z-spray ion source in order to obtain the most comprehensive metabolic profile (Cheng et al. 2014). LC-MS may reduce the interference between analytes and background by improving gaps (ion suppression) or peaks (ion enhancement) signals (Lenz and Wilson 2007). However, it is suggested that identified metabolites have to be confirmed and validated with authentic metabolic standards.

The sensitivity of MS is determined by metabolite's pK, hydrophobicity and ionization potential (Want et al. 2007). Therefore, quenching and metabolite extraction method as well as sample handling and storage may affect the amount of variability in the sample results. Another limitation of MS is the lower reproducibility as compared with NMR method. Despite these limitations, MS platform still outperforms NMR-based method for the detection of low-abundance and large quantity of metabolites (Theodoridis et al. 2011). MS possesses a greater sensitivity than NMR spectroscopy that capable to detect very low-abundance metabolites at picogram level (Dunn et al. 2011). By showing their respective pros and cons, the combination strategy of MS with NMR spectroscopy has proven to be effective and becomes increasingly popular in metabolomic studies.

In addition, advancement of new technology has been made in utilizing triple quadrupole (QqQ) MS for the quantitatively measurement of metabolites with higher sensitivity and specificity (Patti et al. 2012). QqQ MS consists of precursor ion scan, neutral loss scan, product ion scan, and selected reaction monitoring to filter and detect the metabolites with more sensitive and specific to their molecular weight and structure (Pitt 2009). QqQ MS is coupled with other separation techniques (LC, GC, and CE) and multiple reaction monitoring, in order to enhances its selectivity and sensitivity. Hence, QqQ MS technology provides excellent depth and breadth of metabolome coverage, and is well-suited for targeted metabolome analysis and quantification of metabolites.

8 Data Acquisition and Analysis

Data acquisition and analysis are conducted to identify the particular metabolites that could potentially serve as biomarkers for diseases. Putative identification of metabolites is initially carried out by matching the actual m/z values and theoretical m/z values in various databases such as Human Metabolome Database (http://www.hmdb.ca/), HumanCyc (http://humancyc.org/), LipidMaps (http://www.lipidmaps.org/), MassBank (http://www.massbank.jp/?lang=en) and Metlin (https://metlin.scripps.edu/index.php) (Johnson et al. 2014). Metabolomic data acquisition and processing can be performed by metabolomic softwares such as AMDIS, CODA, HighChem MassFrontier, LECO ChromaTOF, MathDAMP, MetAlign, MZMine, SpectralWorks AnalyzerPro, TargetSearch, WMSM and XCMS (Shulaev 2006; Kind and Fiehn 2010; Patti et al. 2012).

Metabolomics data has been analyzed with a wide range of statistical analyses, in order to reduce the number of variables and examine the difference between groups (Bartel et al. 2013). These analyses can be classified into either univariate analysis of t-test and ANOVA (analysis of variance) or multivariate analysis such as the widely used PCA (principal components analysis), PLS (Partial least squares) regression, and PLS-DA (PLS-discriminant analysis). In addition, metabolomics data have also been analysed using MANOVA (multivariate analysis of variance), ASCA (ANOVA-simultaneous component analysis), OPLS (orthogonal-PLS), OPLS-DA (OPLS-discriminant analysis), SIMCA (Soft independent modelling of class analogies), HCA (hierarchical cluster analysis), SOMs (self-organizing maps), SVM (Support vector machines) and Random Forest (Sugimoto et al. 2012; Bartel et al. 2013). Differential metabolic profiles between two groups can be compared using parametric Student t-tests and Wilcoxon rank sum nonparametric tests, while ANOVA test is applied for multiple groups (Bartel et al. 2013). In contrast, multivariate methods analyzed and compared between different metabolic features and interactions between them (Bartel et al. 2013; Alonso et al. 2015). These multivariate analyses can be classified into unsupervised (PCA, ASCA, HCA and SOMs) and supervised (PLS regression, OPLS, SIMCA and SVM) methods (Sugimoto et al. 2012; Bartel et al. 2013). Unsupervised methods analyze data irrespective to the type of study samples; whereas supervised methods categorize the study samples according to the phenotypes prior to analysis and more appropriate for constructing risk prediction models (Alonso et al. 2015).

Bioinformatic tools have contributed to metabolomics field by transforming the metabolomic raw data obtained into biologically meaningful information (Johnson et al. 2014). A number of bioinformatic databases are currently publicly available for metabolomic data analysis and visualization tools, including KEGG (http://www.genome.ad.jp/kegg/), BioCyc (http://biocyc.org/), DOME (http://medicago.vbi.vt.edu), MapMan (http://gabi.rzpd.de/projects/MapMan/), MetaCyc (http://metacyc.org/), MetNet (http://metnet.vrac.iastate.edu/) and KaPPA-View (http://kpv.kazusa.or.jp/kappa-view/) (Shulaev 2006; Johnson et al. 2014; Sas et al. 2015). Other bioinformatics tools for pathway mapping and network visualization include Paintomics, VANTED (Visualization and Analysis of Networks containing Experimental Data), and MetaboAnalyst. In order to build a network of genes-metabolites pathways interaction, several network tool such as MetScape, MBRole (Metabolites Biological Role), MSEA (Metabolite Set Enrichment Analysis), MetaMapp, 3Omics, ProMeTra and *mummichog* attempted to extend this approach to metabolite biomarkers discovery (Shulaev 2006; Johnson et al. 2014; Sas et al. 2015).

9 Metabolomic Biomarkers

As indicated in Table 1, a number of metabolites have been discovered in metabolomics studies associated with incident hypertension (Holmes et al. 2008; Liu et al. 2011; Zheng et al. 2013a, b;

Zhong et al. 2014; Nikolic et al. 2015; van Deventer et al. 2013; Wang et al. 2015). These metabolites may serve as biomarkers for early diagnosis, prevention and treatment of this disease.

Carbohydrate metabolism alterations were found to be associated with hypertension, and patients with essential hypertension demonstrated impaired glucose tolerance, insulin resistance and abnormal glucose metabolism (García-Puig et al. 2006). In conjunction with the elevated level of glucose, altered levels of other monosaccharides, disaccharides and polysaccharides were observed in hypertensive patients. Of which, the levels of lactate, galactose, glucosamine, glycerol, 4-hydroxyphenyllactate, 2-hydroxyvaleric acid, 2-ketoglutaric acid, oxalic acid, sorbose, sucrose, sorbitol, inosose and myo-inositol were increased, whereas fructose, cellobiose, methyluric acid, lactobionic acid, indole carboxylic acid, tricarballylic acid formate and glucuronide were decreased (Liu et al. 2011; Zhong et al. 2014; van Deventer et al. 2013; Wang et al. 2015). These results suggest that carbohydrate metabolism dysregulation may play an important role in hypertension, through sodium retention, renal tubular sodium reabsorption, sympathetic nervous system and adverse effects of anti-hypertensive drugs (Gambardella et al. 1993; Sechi et al. 1997; Savica et al. 2010).

Several lines of evidence also indicated that free fatty acids were significantly associated with the development of hypertension (Fagot-Campagna et al. 1998; Wang et al. 2008), possibly by regulating vascular tone and microvascular function, inhibiting endothelium-dependent vasodilatation and increasing blood pressure (de Jongh et al. 2004; Spijkers et al. 2011). Furthermore, increased levels of free fatty acids may contributed to hypertension through the alteration of membrane microviscosity and lipid metabolism, by modulating ion transport, pH regulation, intracellular Ca2+ handling and signaling pathway (Zicha et al. 1999). Interestingly, findings from metabolomic studies indicated that the levels of very low-density lipoprotein, low-density lipoprotein, acetone,

Table 1 Association of metabolic changes with incident hypertension

Metabolomic markers		Techniques employed	Statistical analysis	References
Increased concentrations	Decreased concentrations			
Alanine	Formate, hippurate and N-methylnicotinate	^{1}H-NMR	OPLS-DA	Holmes et al. (2008)
Choline	Urea, α-1 Acid glycoprotein	^{1}H-NMR	OPLS and PLS-DA	De Meyer et al. (2008)
D-glucose, D-galactose, glucosamine, L-sorbose, sucrose, D-sorbitol, inosose, myo-inositol, heptanoic acid, 1-stearoylglycerol, oleic acid, 1-palmitoylglycerol, nonanoic acid, eicosanoic acid, hexanoic acid, pipecolic acid, L-ornithine, L-lysine, pyroglutamic acid, L-histidine, L-alanine, glutamine, L-isoleucine, α-aminoadipic acid, N-acetylglycine, L-tyrosine, homocysteine, L-aspartic acid, glutamic acid, L-tryptophan, allantoin, 3-amino-2-piperidone, urea and 2-ketoglutaric acid	D-Fructose, D-cellobiose, lactobionic acid, glycerol 3-phosphate	GC-TOF-MS	PCA, PLS and OPLS	Liu et al. (2011)
4-Hydroxyhippurate, 5α-androstan-3β,17β-diol disulfate, androsterone sulfate and epiandrosterone sulfate	–	GC-MS and LC-MS	PCA	Zheng et al. (2013a, b)
Very low density lipoprotein, low density lipoprotein, lactic acid, acetone and acetylformic acid	Valine, alanine, glucose, inose, p-hydroxyphenylalanine and methylhistidine	^{1}H-NMR	PLS-DA, OPLS-DA and *t*-test	Zhong et al. (2014)
Oxalic acid, fumaric acid, glycerol, adenine, pyrophosphate and uric acid	L-Valine, L-isoleucine, glycine, L-threonine, L-methionine, ornithine, L-asparagine, L-glutamine, citrulline, L-lysine, L-tyrosine, L-tryptophan, L-cystine and capric acid	GC-MS	PCA, Mann-Whitney-Wilcoxon	Wang et al. (2015)
3-OH-Sebacic acid, 2-OH-isovalerate, 4-OH-phenyl-lactate, tricarballylic acid and lactic acid	Hesperetin, hexenoylcarnitine, fumaric acid, methylguanosine, N-acetylarylamine, kynurenic acid, phenylglyoxylate, indole carboxylate glucuronide, methyluric acid, dimethyluracil and trimethyl-L-lysine	GC-MS and LC-MS	PCA	van Deventer et al. (2013)
Talose, lyxose, glucose-1-phosphate, methylmalonic acid, malonic acid, shikimic acid	Threonine, nicotinoyl glycine, phenylalanine, aspartic acid, Gly-Pro, galactose, thymol, noradrenaline, methyl-beta-D-galactopyranoside, 2-methoxyestrone, alpha-tocopherol	GC-MS	t-test/ Wilcoxon rank sum test	Hao et al. (2016)

^{1}H-NMR Proton nuclear magnetic resonance
GC-TOF-MS Gas chromatography time-of-flight mass spectrometry
GC-MS Gas chromatography mass spectrometry
LC-MS Liquid chromatography mass spectrometry
OPLS Orthogonal partial least square
PLS-DA Partial least square discriminant analysis
OPLS-DA Orthogonal partial least square discriminant analysis
PCA Principal component analysis
PLS Partial least square

1-stearoylglycerol, 1-palmitoylglycerol, and free fatty acids such as oleic acid, nonanoic acid, ecosanoic acid, hexanoic acid, and heptanoic acid were significantly higher among hypertensive patients compared to normotensive controls (Liu et al. 2011; Zhong et al. 2014).

Another metabolic pathway that is repeatedly found to be perturbed in hypertensive patients is amino acid metabolism. Amino acids, including alanine, histidine, isoleucine, lysine, homocysteine, ornithine, tyrosine, p-hydroxyphenylalanine, methylhistidine, aspartic acid, glutamine, glutamic acid and pyroglutamic acid were observed at higher concentrations in blood samples of patients with hypertension (Liu et al. 2011; Zhong et al. 2014). However, isoleucine, glycine, threonine, phynylalanine, methionine, ornithine, asparagine, glutamine, citrulline, lysine, tyrosine, tryptophan, cystin, hexenoylcarnitine and trimethyl-L-lysine were found to have lower concentrations in other metabolomic studies (van Deventer et al. 2013; Wang et al. 2015). Alanine is found in dietary sources of proteins, but is particularly concentrated in meats. Alanine was positively associated with high blood pressure, which in agreement with several metabolomic studies (Holmes et al. 2008; Liu et al. 2011; Zhong et al. 2014). In addition, other amino acids, branched chain amino acids and sex steroid metabolites such as 5α-androstan-3β,17β-diol sulfate, androsterone sulfate and epiandrosterone sulfate, were independently associated with increased risk of hypertension (Zheng et al. 2013a, b).

Urea, the main metabolite of protein metabolism, has become an independent predictor of hypertension (De Meyer et al. 2008; Liu et al. 2011). Likewise, uric acid and allantoin were observed at higher levels in hypertensive patients, in contrast to dimethyluracil and methyluric acid (Liu et al. 2011; van Deventer et al. 2013; Wang et al. 2015). The underlying mechanism could be explained by the regulation of urinary sodium (Na) homeostasis via an effect of diuresis and natriuresis (Cirillo et al. 2002). In hypertensive patients, urinary urea was inversely associated with blood pressure, as the higher urea level may reduce glomerular filtration rate and impaired renal function (Cirillo et al. 2002; Martin et al. 2005).

Researchers also highlighted changes in metabolites originated from gut microorganism, indicating a possible link between gut microflora activities with hypertension. Notably, microbial metabolites (such as formate, hippurate, 4-hydroxyhippurate and lyxose) detectable blood and urine in humans were found significantly changed and can be associated with to the development of hypertension (Hao et al. 2016; Holmes et al. 2008; Zheng et al. 2013a, b). Together, these finding shows a promising future research direction for hypertension.

10 Lipidomic Biomarkers

The number of lipidomic studies related to hypertension is limited (Graessler et al. 2009; Hu et al. 2011; Kulkarni et al. 2013). As shown in Table 2, the identified lipid metabolites were ether phosphatidylcholine, ether phosphatidylethanolamine, lysophosphatidylcholine, phosphatidylcholine, sphingomyelin, cholesteryl ester, triacylglycerol, monohexosylceramide, phosphatidylinositol and diacylglycerol, which mainly involved in lipid signaling pathway. Dysregulation of this signaling pathway may contribute to the pathogenesis of human diseases such as inflammation, cancer and metabolic disease (Wymann and Schneiter 2008). For instance, sphingomyelins consisted of phosphocholine or phosphoethanolamine as their phospholipid polar head group and served as substrates for the hydrolysis of ceramides through action of sphingomyelinases (Hannun and Obeid 2008). Sphingomyelinases enzymes further break down sphingomyelin to generate ceramide and phosphocholine, which may, in turn, accelerate the formation of diacylglycerol from phosphocholine (Hannun and Obeid 2008). Therefore, diacylglycerol (final product of lipid signaling pathway), together with the second messenger inositol-1,4,5-triphosphate, play important roles in regulating protein kinase C activity and calcium release (Hannun and Obeid 2008). Moreover, it has been reported that the

Table 2 Association of lipid metabolites with incident hypertension

Lipidomic markers	Techniques employed	Statistical analysis	References
Ether phosphatidylcholine(36:4, 36:5, 38:4, 38:5, 34:2, 36:3, 34:1, 40:5) and ether phosphatidylethanolamine(38:5, 38:6, 40:5)	LC-ESI-MS/MS	SOLAR software	Graessler et al. (2009)
Lysophosphatidylcholine(22:6), phosphatidylcholine(40:6), sphingomyelin(16:1, 24.2), cholesteryl ester(20:4, 22:6) and triacylglycerol(48:0, 48:1, 48:2, 48:3, 50:0, 50:1, 50:2, 50:3, 50:4, 50:5, 52:1, 52:2, 52:3, 52:4, 52:5, 52:6, 54:2, 54:3, 54:4, 54:5, 54:6, 56:5, 56:6, 56:7, 56:8, 56:9)	LC-IT-TOF-MS	PCA, ANOVA	Hu et al. (2011)
Monohexosylceramide(22:0, 24:0, 24:1), phosphatidylcholine(34:4, 34:1, 36:2, 40:6), phosphatidylinositol(34:1, 36:2, 40:6) and diacylglycerol(16:0/18:0, 16:0/20:3, 16:0/22:5, 16:0/22:6, 16:1/18:1, 18:0/18:1, 18:0/24:0)	LTQ Orbitrap hybrid MS	PCA, MANCOVA, ANOVA	Kulkarni et al. (2013)

LC-ESI-MS/MS Liquid chromatography-electrospray ionization-tandem mass spectrometry
LC-IT-TOF-MS Liquid chromatography ion trap time-of-flight mass spectrometry
LTQ Orbitrap hybrid MS LTQ Orbitrap hybrid mass spectrometry
PCA Principal component analysis
ANOVA Analysis of variance
MANCOVA Multivariate analysis of variance

accumulation of triacylglycerol lipid species may induce lipotoxicity in hypertension (Hu et al. 2010). Therefore, there is a strong biological plausibility for the role of lipid signaling molecules in pathophysiology of hypertension (Kulkarni et al. 2013).

11 Pharmacometabolomic Biomarkers

Recently, the promise of pharmacometabolomics for hypertensive patients has been delivered in several studies (Wikoff et al. 2013; Altmaier et al. 2014; Rotroff et al. 2015). These studies investigated the effects of the five major classes of anti-hypertensive drugs on human metabolism and identified the metabolic pathways response to drug treatment. The potential pharmacometabolomic markers associated with these outcomes were further highlighted in Table 3.

Beta blockers, or known as beta-adrenergic blocking agents, may lower the blood pressure by blocking the effects of epinephrine (adrenaline) and norepinephrine (noradrenaline) hormones on b-adrenergic receptors (Frishman 1988). Free fatty acids such as oleic acid, linoleic acid, palmitoleic acid, palmitic acid, 3-hydroxybutanoic acid, arachidonic acid,

3-hydroxybutyrate methyl-hexadecanoic acid, dihomolinoleate, 10-nonadecenoate, stearic acid, myristic acid and heptadecanoic acid were significantly decreased in patients treated with beta-blockers. Meanwhile, elevated levels of sugar alcohol (including threitol, arabitol, allo-inositol) and amino acids (including pyroglutamine, homocitrulline, salicylate, hydroxyisovaleroyl-carnitine, 2-methylbutyroyl-carnitine) were observed. Beta-blockers (both propanolol and atenolol) may attenuate lipolysis by lowering the plasma free fatty acid levels (Deacon 1978). Lipolysis is stimulated by catecholamine hormones, including adrenaline and noradrenaline, and is regulated by the beta-adrenergic receptors (Millet et al. 1998). Therefore, it seems that beta-blockers may cause metabolic changes in fatty acid biosynthesis and glycerolipid metabolism pathways. Moreover, these metabolic perturbations are greatly influenced by ethnicity (e.g. Causcasians and African Americans) (Wikoff et al. 2013; Rotroff et al. 2015).

Thiazide diuretic (hydrochlorothiazide) is used to treat high blood pressure, by inhibiting sodium reabsorption within the kidney's distal tubule, which leads to increased excretion of sodium and water in urine (Duarte and Cooper-DeHoff 2010). Decreased levels of dipeptide and

Table 3 Association of metabolic changes with anti-hypertensive drugs

Anti-hypertensive drugs	Pharmacometabolomic markers		Techniques employed	Statistical analysis	References
	Increased concentrations	Decreased concentrations			
Beta-blockers	Alpha ketoglutaric acid, threitol, arabitol, dihydroabietic acid, conduritol-beta-epoxide and allo-inositol	Oleic acid, linoleic acid, palmitoleic acid, palmitic acid, 3-hydroxy-butanoic acid, arachidonic acid, methyl-hexadecanoic acid, myristic acid, threonine, stearic acid, glycerol-alpha-phosphate	GC-TOF-MS	Wilcoxon signed rank	Wikoff et al. (2013)
	Pyroglutamine, homocitrulline, salicylate, hydroxyisovaleroyl-carnitine and 2-methylbutyroyl-carnitine	Serotonin, dihomolinoleate, 3-hydroxybutyrate, 10-nonadecenoate, margarate, and eicosenoate	UHPLC-MS-MS and GC-MS	Linear regression test	Altmaier et al. (2014)
	6-deoxyglucitol, threitol, uracil, talose, 1-monoolein, hydroxycarbamate, allo-inositol and 2,3,5-trihydroxypyrazine	Linoleic acid, oleic acid, palmitic acid, palmitoleic acid, 3-hydroxy-butanoic acid, arachidonic acid, methyl-hexadecanoic acid, heptadecanoic acid and threonine	GC-TOF-MS	Wilcoxon signed-rank test	Rotroff et al. (2015)
Thiazide diuretics	Pseudouridine, c-glycosyl-tryptophan, glutarylcarnitine, homocitrulline and urate	Phenylalanyl-phenylalanine	UHPLC-MS-MS and GC-MS	Linear regression test	Altmaier et al. (2014)
	Uric acid, ribonic acid, 1-hexadecanol, erythritol, kynurenine, glycero-gulo-heptose, dihydroabietic acid, 2-ketoisocaproic acid, aconitic acid, behenic acid, glucose 1-phosphate and glycine	Threonine, aminomalonic acid, glutamine, serine, phytol, phosphoethanolamine and methoxytryosine	GC-TOF-MS	Wilcoxon signed-rank test	Rotroff et al. (2015)
ACE inhibitors	Des-Arg9-bradykinin	Phenylalanyl-phenylalanine and aspartyl-phenylalanine	UHPLC-MS-MS and GC-MS	Linear regression test	Altmaier et al. (2014)
Statins	1-Arachidonoyl-glycerophosphocholine, 1-arachidonoylglycerol-phosphoethanolamine, isobutyrylcarnitine, 1-docosahexaenoyl-glycerophosphocholine, alpha-tocopherol and uridine	7-alpha-hydroxy-3-oxo-4-cholestenoate, 1-palmitoyl-glycero-phosphoinositol, lathosterol and glycochenodeoxycholate			
Fibrates	2-Hydroxyisobutyrate, 3-dehydrocarnitine, riboflavin, pantothenate, indolelactate, carnitine, pipecolate and uridine	Pyroglutamine			

GC-TOF-MS Gas chromatography-time-of-flight mass spectrometry
UHPLC-MS-MS Ultra-high performance liquid chromatography tandem mass spectrometry
GC-MS Gas chromatography mass spectrometry

amino acids (such as phenylalanyl-phenylalanine, threonine, glutamine, and serine) have been reported in diuretics-treated patients (Altmaier et al. 2014; Rotroff et al. 2015). Interestingly, this drug may impaired the glucose and lipid metabolism, resulted from the increased metabolite concentrations of ribonic acid, 1-hexadecanol, erythritol, glycero-gulo-heptose, dihydroabietic acid, 2-ketoisocaproic acid, aconitic acid, behenic acid, glucose 1-phosphate and glycine (Rotroff et al. 2015). Thiazide diuretic-induced hyperglycemia has been reported as one of the side-effects of this drug and associated with the increased risk of type 2 diabetes mellitus (Ellison and Loffing 2009). Thiazide diuretic-based treatments also induced the formation of tryptophan related metabolites, including C-glycosyltryptophan, pseudouridine and kynurenine (Altmaier et al. 2014; Rotroff et al. 2015). The role of tryptophan in hypertension is further supported by several *in vivo* and human studies, in which oral L-tryptophan administration successfully improve blood pressure, glucose metabolism and kidney function (Feltkamp et al. 1984; Wolf and Kuhn 1984; Fregly et al. 1989; Yonemura et al. 2004; Ardiansyah et al. 2011; Niewczas et al. 2014). Furthermore, an increased of urate and uric acid concentration are direct side-effect of thiazide diuretics, which may affect the risk of gout among patients with hypertension (McAdams DeMarco et al. 2012).

Angiotensin converting enzyme (ACE) inhibitors reduce blood pressure by blocking the conversion of angiotensin I to angiotensin II, a nature substance that induces vasoconstriction. Thus, ACE inhibitors help to dilate the blood vessels and consequently improve the blood circulation in heart (Sweitzer 2003). In hypertensive patients treated with ACE inhibitors, lower levels of aspartyl-phenylalanine and phenylalanylphenylalanine formed during ACE inhibition (Altmaier et al. 2014). Aspartyl-phenylalanine is a metabolite of aspartame that inhibits ACE activity in humans who consumed large amount of aspartame (Grobelny and Galardy 1985). On the other hand, the level of des-Arg9-bradykinin was increased after taking ACE inhibitors.

Bradykinin and its active metabolite des-Arg9-bradykinin are both the selective substrates for ACE (Skidgel and Erdös 1987; Cyr et al. 2001). Bradykinin potentiation is a metabolic process mediated by ACE inhibitors, via the inhibition of Bradykinin receptor B2 binding and prevents the degradation of des-Arg9-bradykinin (Tom et al. 2002). Therefore, the anti-hypertensive mechanisms of ACE inhibitors may act through the activation of bradykinin-releasing pathway, where the increase of bradykinin activity can dilates blood vessels and further lowering blood pressure (Sharma 2009).

Statins and fribates are both lipid-lowering drugs that can prevent the complications of hypertension. Several metabolic perturbations have been observed in hypertensive patients under these medications (Altmaier et al. 2014). Lipid levels such as lathosterol, glycochenodeoxycholate, 7-alpha-hydroxy-3-oxo-4-cholestenoate and 1-palmitoyl-glycero-phosphoinositol were significantly reduced in patients on statins, which further confirmed the direct action of this drug (Altmaier et al. 2014). For fibrates users, several intermediate metabolites of fenofibrate (2-hydroxyisobutyrate and 3-Dehydrocarnitine), amino acid derivative (indolelactate, carnitine and pipecolate) as well as vitamins and cofactors (riboflavin, pantothenate and uridine) were detected (Altmaier et al. 2014). Pyroglutamine level was decreased after fibrates treatment, but the opposite effect was observed among patients treated with beta-blockers (Altmaier et al. 2014). Pyroglutamine, a cyclic derivative of glutamine, has been reported in association with heart failure incident (Zheng et al. 2013a, b). Therefore, it is questionable whether the combination of beta-blockers and fibrates intake could balance the metabolic effects of these anti-hypertensive drugs.

12 Conclusions

Metabolomics has been applied in hypertension studies to gain new insights into pathophysiological processes underlying hypertension, discover metabolite markers for early risk prediction and monitor the efficacy and side effects of drugs treatment. A number of studies had highlighted perturbation in amino acids metabolism in hypertensive patients, notably increased concentration of alanine in blood and urine, as well as reduced concentrations of threonine and phenylalanine as risks for hypertension. In addition, the potential role of gut microflora warrants further investigation as microbial metabolites including lyxose, formate, hippurate and 4-hydroxyhippurate were found significantly changed in hypertensive patients. Taken altogether, future metabolomic, lipidomic and pharmacometabolomic studies in combination with other 'omics' technologies may act as a powerful platform to intensively study the molecular mechanisms of hypertension.

Acknowledgment The current work is funded by Ministry of Education, Malaysia under Fundamental Research Grant Scheme FRGS/1/2015/SKK08/UTAR/02/3.

References

Alonso A, Marsal S, Julià A (2015) Analytical methods in untargeted metabolomics: state of the art in 2015. Front Bioeng Biotechnol 3:23

Altmaier E, Fobo G, Heier M, Thorand B, Meisinger C, Romisch-Margl W et al (2014) Metabolomics approach reveals effects of antihypertensives and lipid-lowering drugs on the human metabolism. Eur J Epidemiol 29(5):325–336

Ardiansyah SH, Inagawa Y, Koseki T, Komai M (2011) Regulation of blood pressure and glucose metabolism induced by L-tryptophan in stroke-prone spontaneously hypertensive rats. Nutr Metabol 8(1):45–52

Bartel J, Krumsiek J, Theis FJ (2013) Statistical methods for the analysis of high-throughput metabolomics data. Comput Struct Biotechnol J 4(5):1–9

Beckonert O, Coen M, Keun HC, Wang Y, Ebbels TMD, Holmes E et al (2010) High-resolution magic-angle-spinning NMR spectroscopy for metabolic profiling of intact tissues. Nat Protoc 5(6):1019–1032

Bothwell JH, Griffin JL (2011) An introduction to biological nuclear magnetic resonance spectroscopy. Biol Rev Camb Philos Soc 86(2):493–510

Bruce SJ, Jonsson P, Antti H, Cloarec O, Trygg J, Marklund SL et al (2008) Evaluation of a protocol for metabolic profiling studies on human blood plasma by combined ultra-performance liquid chromatography/mass spectrometry: From extraction to data analysis. Anal Biochem 372(2):237–249

Cheng K-K, Akasaki Y, Lecommandeur E, Lindsay RT, Murfitt S, Walsh K et al (2014) Metabolomic analysis of akt1-mediated muscle hypertrophy in models of diet-induced obesity and age-related fat accumulation. J Proteome Res 14(1):342–352

Chobanian AV, Bakris GL, Black HR, Cushman WC, Green LA, Izzo JL et al (2003) Seventh report of the joint national committee on prevention, detection, evaluation, and treatment of high blood pressure. Hypertension 42(6):1206–1252

Cirillo M, Lombardi C, Laurenzi M, De Santo NG (2002) Relation of urinary urea to blood pressure: interaction with urinary sodium. J Hum Hypertens 16(3):205–212

Cyr M, Lepage Y, Blais C, Gervais N, Cugno M, Rouleau JL et al (2001) Bradykinin and des-Arg9-bradykinin metabolic pathways and kinetics of activation of human plasma. Am J Physiol Heart Circ Physiol 281 (1):H275–H283

de Jongh RT, Serné EH, Ijzerman RG, de Vries G, Stehouwer CDA (2004) Free fatty acid levels modulate microvascular function relevance for obesity-associated insulin resistance, hypertension, and microangiopathy. Diabetes 53(11):2873–2882

De Meyer T, Sinnaeve D, Van Gasse B, Tsiporkova E, Rietzschel ER, De Buyzere ML et al (2008) NMR-based characterization of metabolic alterations in hypertension using an adaptive, intelligent binning algorithm. Anal Chem 80(10):3783–3790

Deacon SP (1978) The effects of atenolol and propranolol upon lipolysis. Br J Clin Pharmacol 5(2):123–125

Duarte JD, Cooper-DeHoff RM (2010) Mechanisms for blood pressure lowering and metabolic effects of thiazide and thiazide-like diuretics. Expert Rev Cardiovasc 8(6):793–802

Dudley E, Yousef M, Wang Y, Griffiths WJ (2010) Targeted metabolomics and mass spectrometry. Adv Protein Chem Struct Biol 80:45–83

Dunn WB, Broadhurst DI, Atherton HJ, Goodacre R, Griffin JL (2011) Systems level studies of mammalian metabolomes: the roles of mass spectrometry and nuclear magnetic resonance spectroscopy. Chem Soc Rev 40(1):387–426

Ellison DH, Loffing J (2009) Thiazide effects and adverse effects: insights from molecular genetics. Hypertension 54(2):196–202

Fagot-Campagna A, Balkau B, Simon D, Warnet J-M, Claude J-R, Ducimetlèred P et al (1998) High free fatty acid concentration: an independent risk factor for hypertension in the Paris Prospective Study. Int J Epidemiol 27(5):808–813

Feltkamp H, Meurer KA, Godehardt E (1984) Tryptophan-induced lowering of blood pressure and changes of serotonin uptake by platelets in patients with essential hypertension. Klin Wochenschr 62 (23):1115–1119

Fregly MJ, Sumners C, Cade JR (1989) Effect of chronic dietary treatment with L-tryptophan on the maintenance of hypertension in spontaneously hypertensive rats. Can J Physiol Pharmacol 67(6):656–662

Frishman WH (1988) Beta-adrenergic blockers. Medic Clin North Am 72(1):37–81

Fuhrer T, Zamboni N (2015) High-throughput discovery metabolomics. Curr Opin Biotechnol 31:73–78

Gambardella S, Frontoni S, Pellegrinotti M, Testa G, Spallone V, Menzinger G (1993) Carbohydrate metabolism in hypertension: influence of treatment. J Cardiovasc Pharmacol 22:87–97

García-Puig J, Ruilope LM, Luque M, Fernández J, Ortega R, Dal-Ré R et al (2006) Glucose metabolism in patients with essential hypertension. Am J Medic 119(4):318–326

Graessler J, Schwudke D, Schwarz PEH, Herzog R, Shevchenko A, Bornstein SR (2009) Top-down lipidomics reveals ether lipid deficiency in blood plasma of hypertensive patients. PLoS ONE 4(7): e6261

Griffiths WJ, Koal T, Wang Y, Kohl M, Enot DP, Deigner HP (2010) Targeted metabolomics for biomarker discovery. Angew Chem Int Ed Engl 49(32):5426–5445

Grobelny D, Galardy RE (1985) A metabolite of aspartame inhibits angiotensin converting enzyme. Biochem Biophys Res Commun 128(2):960–964

Hannun YA, Obeid LM (2008) Principles of bioactive lipid signalling: lessons from sphingolipids. Nat Rev Mol Cell Biol 9(2):139–150

Hao Y, Wang Y, Xi L, Li G, Zhao F, Qi Y, et al (2016) A nested case-control study of association between metabolome and hypertension risk. BioMed Res Int 2016:7646979

Holmes E, Loo RL, Stamler J, Bictash M, Yap IKS, Chan Q et al (2008) Human metabolic phenotype diversity and its association with diet and blood pressure. Nature 453(7193):396–400

Hu C, Hoene M, Zhao X, Haring HU, Schleicher E, Lehmann R et al (2010) Lipidomics analysis reveals efficient storage of hepatic triacylglycerides enriched in unsaturated fatty acids after one bout of exercise in mice. PLoS ONE 5(10):e13318

Hu C, Kong H, Qu F, Li Y, Yu Z, Gao P et al (2011) Application of plasma lipidomics in studying the response of patients with essential hypertension to antihypertensive drug therapy. Mol Biosyst 7 (12):3271–3279

Jacobson TA, Zimmerman FH (2006) Fibrates in combination with statins in the management of dyslipidemia. J Clin Hypertens 8(1):35–41

Johnson CH, Ivanisevic J, Benton HP, Siuzdak G (2014) Bioinformatics: the next frontier of metabolomics. Anal Chem 87(1):147–156

Jung HR, Sylvänne T, Koistinen KM, Tarasov K, Kauhanen D, Ekroos K (2011) High throughput quantitative molecular lipidomics. Biochim Biophys Acta 1811(11):925–934

Kaddurah-Daouk R, Weinshilboum RM, Network PR (2014) Pharmacometabolomics: implications for clinical pharmacology and systems pharmacology. Clin Pharmacol Ther 95(2):154–167

Keun HC, Athersuch TJ (2011) Nuclear magnetic resonance (NMR)-based metabolomics. Methods Mol Biol 708:321–334

Kind T, Fiehn O (2010) Advances in structure elucidation of small molecules using mass spectrometry. Bioanal Rev 2(1–4):23–60

Kulkarni H, Meikle PJ, Mamtani M, Weir JM, Barlow CK, Jowett JB et al (2013) Plasma lipidomic profile signature of hypertension in Mexican American families: specific role of diacylglycerols. Hypertension 62(3):621–626

Lane AN (2012) Principles of NMR for Applications in Metabolomics. Handbook Metabol 127–197

Larive CK, Barding GA Jr, Dinges MM (2014) NMR spectroscopy for metabolomics and metabolic profiling. Anal Chem 87(1):133–146

Lenz EM, Wilson ID (2007) Analytical strategies in metabonomics. J Proteome Res 6(2):443–458

Liu Y, Chen T, Qiu Y, Cheng Y, Cao Y, Zhao A et al (2011) An ultrasonication-assisted extraction and derivatization protocol for GC/TOFMS-based metabolite profiling. Anal Bioanal Chem 400 (5):1405–1417

Ludwig C, Viant MR (2010) Two-dimensional J-resolved NMR spectroscopy: review of a key methodology in the metabolomics toolbox. Phytochem Anal 21 (1):22–32

Madsen R, Lundstedt T, Trygg J (2010) Chemometrics in metabolomics—a review in human disease diagnosis. Anal Chim Acta 659(1):23–33

Martin WF, Armstrong LE, Rodriguez NR (2005) Dietary protein intake and renal function. Nutr Metabol 2:25

McAdams DeMarco MA, Maynard JW, Baer AN, Gelber AC, Young JH, Alonso A et al (2012) Diuretic use, increased serum urate levels, and risk of incident gout in a population-based study of adults with hypertension: The Atherosclerosis Risk in Communities cohort study. Arthritis Rheum 64(1):121–129

Messerli FH, Williams B, Ritz E (2007) Essential hypertension. Lancet 370(9587):591–603

Millet L, Barbe P, Lafontan M, Berlan M, Galitzky J (1998) Catecholamine effects on lipolysis and blood flow in human abdominal and femoral adipose tissue. J Appl Physiol 85(1):181–188

Niewczas MA, Sirich TL, Mathew AV, Skupien J, Mohney RP, Warram JH et al (2014) Uremic solutes and risk of end-stage renal disease in type 2 diabetes: metabolomic study. Kidney Int 85(5):1214–1224

Nikolic SB, Sharman JE, Adams MJ, Edwards LM (2014) Metabolomics in hypertension. J Hypertens 32 (6):1159–1169

Patti GJ (2011) Separation strategies for untargeted metabolomics. J Sep Sci 34(24):3460–3469

Patti GJ, Yanes O, Siuzdak G (2012) Innovation: Metabolomics: the apogee of the omics trilogy. Nat Rev Mol Cell Biol 13(4):263–269

Pitt JJ (2009) Principles and applications of liquid chromatography-mass spectrometry in clinical biochemistry. Clin Biochem Rev 30(1):19–34

Poulter NR, Prabhakaran D, Caulfield M (2015) Hypertension. Lancet 386(9995):801–812

Psychogios N, Hau DD, Peng J, Guo AC, Mandal R, Bouatra S et al (2011) The human serum metabolome. PLoS ONE 6(2):e16957

Roberts LD, Souza AL, Gerszten RE, Clish CB (2012) Targeted metabolomics. Curr Protoc Mol Biol Chapter 30:Unit 30.2.1–24

Rotroff DM, Shahin MH, Gurley SB, Zhu H, Motsinger-Reif A, Meisner M et al (2015) Pharmacometabolomic Assessments of Atenolol and Hydrochlorothiazide Treatment Reveal Novel Drug Response Phenotypes. CPT Pharm Syst Pharmacol 4(11):669–679

Salek R, Cheng K-K, Griffin J (2011) The study of mammalian metabolism through NMR-based metabolomics. Methods Enzymol 500:337–351

Sapcariu SC, Kanashova T, Weindl D, Ghelfi J, Dittmar G, Hiller K (2014) Simultaneous extraction of proteins and metabolites from cells in culture. MethodsX 1:74–80

Sas KM, Karnovsky A, Michailidis G, Pennathur S (2015) Metabolomics and diabetes: analytical and computational approaches. Diabetes 64(3):718–732

Savica V, Bellinghieri G, Kopple JD (2010) The effect of nutrition on blood pressure. Annu Rev Nutr 30:365–401

Sechi LA, Catena C, Zingaro L, De Carli S, Bartoli E (1997) Hypertension and abnormalities of carbohydrate metabolism possible role of the sympathetic nervous system. Am J Hypertens 10(6):678–682

Sellick CA, Hansen R, Stephens GM, Goodacre R, Dickson AJ (2011) Metabolite extraction from suspension-cultured mammalian cells for global metabolite profiling. Nat Protoc 6(8):1241–1249

Sharma JN (2009) Hypertension and the bradykinin system. Curr Hypertens Rep 11(3):178–181

Shulaev V (2006) Metabolomics technology and bioinformatics. Brief Bioinform 7(2):128–139

Skidgel RA, Erdös EG (1987) The broad substrate specificity of human angiotensin I converting enzyme. Clin Exp Hypertens A 9(2–3):243–259

Spijkers LJA, van den Akker RFP, Janssen BJA, Debets JJ, De Mey JGR, Stroes ESG et al (2011) Hypertension is associated with marked alterations in sphingolipid biology: a potential role for ceramide. PLoS ONE 6(7):e21817

Sugimoto M, Kawakami M, Robert M, Soga T, Tomita M (2012) Bioinformatics tools for mass spectroscopy-based metabolomic data processing and analysis. Curr Bioinformatics 7(1):96–108

Sweitzer NK (2003) What is an angiotensin converting enzyme inhibitor? Circulation 108(3):e16–e18

Theodoridis G, Gika HG, Wilson ID (2011) Mass spectrometry-based holistic analytical approaches for metabolite profiling in systems biology studies. Mass Spectrom Rev 30(5):884–906

Thongboonkerd V (2005) Genomics, proteomics and integrative 'omics' in hypertension research. Curr Opin Nephrol Hypertens 14(2):133–139

Tom B, Dendorfer A, Rd V, Saxena PR, Jan Danser AH (2002) Bradykinin potentiation by ACE inhibitors: a matter of metabolism. Br J Pharmacol 137(2):276–284

van Deventer CA, Lindeque JZ, van Rensburg PJJ, Malan L, van der Westhuizen FH, Louw R (2013) Use of metabolomics to elucidate the metabolic perturbation associated with hypertension in a black South African male cohort: the SABPA study. J Am Soc Hypertens 9(2):104–114

Wang S, Ma A, Song S, Quan Q, Zhao X, Zheng X (2008) Fasting serum free fatty acid composition, waist/hip ratio and insulin activity in essential hypertensive patients. Hypertens Res 31(4):623–632

Wang L, Hou E, Wang L, Wang Y, Yang L, Zheng X et al (2015) Reconstruction and analysis of correlation networks based on GC–MS metabolomics data for young hypertensive men. Anal Chim Acta 854:95–105

Want EJ, Nordström A, Morita H, Siuzdak G (2007) From exogenous to endogenous: the inevitable imprint of mass spectrometry in metabolomics. J Proteome Res 6(2):459–468

Wei R, Li G, Seymour AB (2010) High-throughput and multiplexed LC/MS/MRM method for targeted metabolomics. Anal Chem 82(13):5527–5533

Wikoff WR, Frye RF, Zhu H, Gong Y, Boyle S, Churchill E et al (2013) Pharmacometabolomics reveals racial differences in response to atenolol treatment. PLoS ONE 8(3):e57639

Wolf WA, Kuhn DM (1984) Effects of L-tryptophan on blood pressure in normotensive and hypertensive rats. J Pharmacol Exp Ther 230(2):324–329

Wymann MP, Schneiter R (2008) Lipid signalling in disease. Nat Rev Mol Cell Biol 9(2):162–176

Xiao JF, Zhou B, Ressom HW (2012) Metabolite identification and quantitation in LC-MS/MS-based metabolomics. Trends Anal Chem 32:1–14

Yin P, Xu G (2014) Current state-of-the-art of nontargeted metabolomics based on liquid chromatography-mass spectrometry with special emphasis in clinical applications. J Chromatogr A 1374:1–13

Yin P, Lehmann R, Xu G (2015) Effects of pre-analytical processes on blood samples used in metabolomics studies. Anal Bioanal Chem 407(17):4879–4892

Yonemura K, Takahira R, Yonekawa O, Wada N, Hishida A (2004) The diagnostic value of serum concentrations of 2-(alpha-mannopyranosyl)-L-tryptophan for normal renal function. Kidney Int 65(4):1395–1399

Zheng Y, Yu B, Alexander D, Manolio TA, Aguilar D, Coresh J et al (2013a) Associations between metabolomic compounds and incident heart failure among African Americans: the ARIC Study. Am J Epidemiol 178:534–542

Zheng Y, Yu B, Alexander D, Mosley TH, Heiss G, Nettleton JA et al (2013b) Metabolomics and incident hypertension among blacks the atherosclerosis risk in communities study. Hypertension 62(2):398–403

Zhong L, Zhang JP, Nuermaimaiti AG, Yunusi KX (2014) Study on plasmatic metabolomics of Uygur patients with essential hypertension based on nuclear magnetic resonance technique. Eur Rev Med Pharmacol Sci 18(23):3673–3680

Zicha J, Kuneš J, Devynck MA (1999) Abnormalities of membrane function and lipid metabolism in hypertension: a review. Am J Hypertens 12(3):315–331

Adv Exp Med Biol - Advances in Internal Medicine (2017) 2: 615–631
DOI 10.1007/5584_2016

Index

A

Abdominal aortic aneurysms (AAAs), 424
Abdominal bruit, 210, 211
ABPM. *See* Ambulatory blood pressure measurement/
    monitoring (ABPM)
ACEI. *See* Angiotensin converting enzyme inhibitors
    (ACEI)
Acromegaly
    clinical features, 229
    diagnostic approach, 229
    management, 229–230
    pathophysiology, 228–229
Action in Diabetes and Vascular disease: preterAx and
    diamicroN-MR Controlled Evaluation
    (ADVANCE) study, 298
Acute dissection (AD), 429–430
Adenosine, 518
Adherence to treatment
    characteristics of patient and disease, 132
    characteristics of treatment, 132
    clinical expert consensus documents, 142–143
    cognitive losses, 132
    compliance
        assistance to scheduled appointments, 135
        Batalla test, 135
        compliers, 131
        definition, 131
        direct measuring methods, 133–134
        doctor-patient relationship, 136–137
        Haynes-Sackett/self-reported compliance test, 134
        health education to patients and professionals, 137
        health professional judgement, 135
        indirect measuring methods, 134
        MEMS, 135
        method based on improvement of treated
          disease, 135
        method based on medication collection, 135
        Morinsky-Green test, 134–135
        multiple interventions, 140, 141
        organizational interventions, 139
        pharmacists and nurses care, 138
        price of drugs, 139
        reminder systems, 137–138
        self-monitoring, 138–139
        social support and self-help groups, 139–140
        tablets count, 135
        treatment simplification, 138
    and concordance, 131
    definition, 131
    ESH/ESC guideline, 140–142
    functional illiteracy, 132
    interaction with professionals, 132
    JNC 8 guideline, 142
    lost in clinical follow-up, 132
    NICE guideline, 142
    noncompliance
        absolute breach, 131
        consequences, 130–131
        definition, 131
        drug holidays, 132
        medication abandonment, 132
        mixed non-compliers, 132
        partial non-compliance, 131
        persistence/secondary non adherence, 132
        predicted non-compliance, 132
        primary non adherence, 132
        time table non-compliance, 132
        white coat effect, 132
    patient-physician relationship, 132
    prevalence, 133
    psychopathology, 132
β1-Adrenergic receptor (ADRB1), 568
β2-Adrenergic receptor (ADRB2), 568
Adrenomedullin (AM)
    adrenomedullinergic system
        in cerebellum vermis, 544–546
        during hypertension(*see* (Cerebellar
          adrenomedullinergic system))
    in blood pressure control, 549–551
    blood pressure regulation, 542
    body fluid balance, 542
    in cardiovascular regulation, 553–555
    cerebellum as cardiovascular regulator, 551–553
    NAD(P)H oxidase stimulation, 542
    porcine precursor, 542
    preproadrenomedullin, 542
    receptors
        AM1 and AM2, 542, 543